THE ELBOW AND ITS DISORDERS

BERNARD F. MORREY, M.D.

Associate Professor of Surgery,
Mayo Medical School
Consultant in Orthopedic Surgery,
Mayo Clinic
Rochester, Minnesota

1985

W.B. SAUNDERS COMPANY
PHILADELPHIA □ LONDON □
TORONTO □ MEXICO CITY □
RIO DE JANEIRO □ SYDNEY □
TOKYO □

W. B. Saunders Company: West Washington Square
Philadelphia, PA 19105

1 St. Anne's Road
Eastbourne, East Sussex BN21 3UN, England

1 Goldthorne Avenue
Toronto, Ontario M8Z 5T9, Canada

Apartado 26370—Cedro 512
Mexico 4, D.F., Mexico

Rua Coronel Cabrita, 8
Sao Cristovao Caixa Postal 21176
Rio de Janeiro, Brazil

9 Waltham Street
Artarmon, N.S.W. 2064, Australia

Ichibancho, Central Bldg., 22-1 Ichibancho
Chiyoda-Ku, Tokyo 102, Japan

Library of Congress Cataloging in Publication Data
Main entry under title:

The elbow and its disorders.

    1. Elbow—Surgery.   2. Elbow—Diseases.
3. Elbow—Fractures.   I. Morrey, Bernard F.,
1943–   . [DNLM: 1. Elbow Joint.   2. Elbow Joint—
injuries.   3. Joint Diseases. WE 820 E383]

RD558.E43 1985   617'.574   84-13853

ISBN 0-7216-1097-8

The Elbow and Its Disorders   ISBN 0–7216–1097–8

Last digit is the print number: 9   8   7   6   5   4   3   2   1

To my parents—
For their encouragement and inspiration

To my wife, Carla, and children, Michael,
Matthew, Mark, and Maggie—
For their patience and understanding

To my teachers and colleagues—
For their instruction and generous participation

Contributors

Kai-Nan An, Ph.D.
Associate Professor of Bioengineering, Mayo Medical School; Consultant, Biomechanics Laboratory, Department of Orthopedic Surgery, Mayo Clinic, Rochester, Minnesota
Biomechanics of the Elbow; Functional Evaluation of the Elbow

Robert D. Beckenbaugh, M.D.
Associate Professor of Orthopedic Surgery, Mayo Medical School and Mayo Clinic; Orthopedic Surgeon, St. Marys Hospital and Rochester Methodist Hospital, Rochester, Minnesota
Arthrodesis

James B. Bennett, M.D.
Chief of Hand and Upper Extremity Section, Division of Orthopaedic Surgery, Baylor College of Medicine; Orthopedic Surgeon, Methodist Hospital, Ben Taub General Hospital, and Shrine Hospital, Houston, Texas
Ligamentous and Articular Injuries in the Athlete

Thomas H. Berquist, M.D.
Associate Professor of Diagnostic Radiology, Mayo Medical School; Radiologist, Saint Marys Hospital and Rochester Methodist Hospital, Rochester, Minnesota
Diagnostic Radiographic Techniques of the Elbow

Anthony J. Bianco, Jr., M.D.
Professor of Orthopedic Surgery, Mayo Medical School, and Chairman, Department of Orthopedic Surgery, Mayo Clinic; Orthopedic Surgeon, Saint Marys Hospital, Rochester Methodist Hospital, and Mayo Clinic, Rochester, Minnesota
Osteochondritis Dissecans

Richard S. Bryan, M.D., M.S. (Orthopedic Surgery)
Professor of Orthopedic Surgery, Mayo Medical School; Orthopedic Surgeon, Saint Marys Hospital, Rochester Methodist Hospital, and Mayo Clinic, Rochester, Minnesota
Fractures of the Distal Humerus; Total Joint Replacement

Ernest M. Burgess, M.D.
Clinical Professor of Orthopedic Surgery, University of Washington School of Medicine; Director, Amputation and Limb Viability Service, Veterans Administration Medical Center; Director, Prosthetics Research Center, Seattle, Washington
Amputation

Kenneth P. Butters, M.D.
Clinical Assistant Professor of Orthopedics, University of Oregon Health Science Center, Portland; Hand Surgeon, Sacred Heart Hospital, Eugene, Oregon
Septic Arthritis

Miguel E. Cabanela, M.D.
Associate Professor of Orthopedic Surgery, Mayo Medical School; Consultant, Orthopedic Surgery, Mayo Clinic, Rochester, Minnesota
Fractures of the Proximal Ulna and Olecranon

Edmund Y. S. Chao, Ph.D.
Professor of Bioengineering, Mayo Clinic; Consultant in Research, Department of Orthopedics, Mayo Clinic, Rochester, Minnesota
Functional Evaluation of the Elbow

William P. Cooney, III, M.D.
Associate Professor of Orthopedics, Mayo Medical School; Hand/Orthopedic Surgeon, St. Marys Hospital and Rochester Methodist Hospital, Rochester, Minnesota
Contractures and Burns

Ralph W. Coonrad M.D.
Associate Clinical Professor of Orthopedic Surgery, Duke University School of Medicine; Associate Clinical Professor of Orthopedic Surgery, Duke University Hospital and Medical Center; Medical Director and Chief Surgeon, Lenox Baker Childrens Hospital; Attending Orthopedic Surgeon, Durham General Hospital, Durham, North Carolina
Nonunion of the Olecranon and the Proximal Ulna

Mark B. Coventry, M.D.
Emeritus Professor of Orthopedic Surgery, Mayo Medical School; Emeritus Consultant, Orthopedic Surgery, Mayo Clinic, Rochester, Minnesota
Ectopic Ossification About the Elbow

David C. Dahlin, M.D.
Professor Emeritus of Pathology, Mayo Medical School; Consultant in Surgical Pathology, Mayo Clinic, Rochester, Minnesota
Neoplasms of the Elbow

James H. Dobyns, M.D.
Professor of Orthopedic Surgery, Mayo Medical School; Consultant in Orthopedic Surgery and Surgery of the Hand, Rochester Methodist Hospital and St. Marys Hospital, Rochester, Minnesota
Congenital Abnormalities of the Elbow

Morris A. Dodge, C.P.
Tacoma, Washington
Amputation

Gary S. Fanton, M.D.
Sports, Orthopedic and Rehabilitation Medicine Associates, Portola Valley, California
Nerve Injuries

Douglas E. Garland, M.D.
Associate Clinical Professor of Orthopedics, University of Southern California School of Medicine, Los Angeles; Chief, Head Trauma Service, Rancho Los Amigos Hospital, Downey, California
Spastic Dysfunction of the Elbow

Gerald S. Gilchrist, M.D.
Professor and Chairman, Department of Pediatrics, Mayo Medical School; Consultant in Pediatric Hematology and Oncology, and Director, Comprehensive Hemophilia Center, Mayo Clinic, Rochester, Minnesota
Hematologic Arthritis

Hymie Gordon, M.D., F.R.C.P.
Professor of Medical Genetics, Mayo Medical School; Chairman, Department of Medical Genetics, Mayo Clinic, Rochester, Minnesota
Embryology

Alan D. Hoffman, M.D.
Assistant Professor, Diagnostic Radiology, Mayo Medical School; Radiologist, Saint Mary's Hospital and Rochester Methodist Hospital, Rochester, Minnesota
Radiography of the Pediatric Elbow

M. Mark Hoffer, M.D.
Professor and Chief of Orthopedic Surgery, California College of Medicine, University of California, Irvine; Chief, Children's Orthopedics, Rancho Los Amigos Hospital, Downey, California
Spastic Dysfunction of the Elbow

Allan E. Inglis, M.D.
Professor of Clinical Surgery and Clinical Professor of Anatomy, Cornell University Medical College; Attending Orthopaedic Surgeon and Senior Scientist, Research Division, The Hospital for Special Surgery; Director, The Comprehensive Arthritis Program, The Hospital for Special Surgery, New York, New York
Rheumatoid Arthritis

Frank W. Jobe, M.D.
Associate Clinical Professor, Department of Orthopedics, University of Southern California School of Medicine, Los Angeles; Member, Southwestern Orthopedic Medical Group, Inglewood; Consultant, Centinela Hospital Medical Center, Inglewood, California
Nerve Injuries

Rudolph A. Klassen, M.D.
Assistant Professor of Orthopedic Surgery, Mayo Medical School; Consultant, Pediatric Orthopedics, Mayo Clinic, St. Marys Hospital and Methodist Hospital, Rochester, Minnesota
Supracondylar Fractures of the Elbow in Children

Merv Letts, M.D., F.R.C.S(C.)
Professor of Surgery, Faculty of Medicine, University of Manitoba; Head, Orthopaedics, Children's Hospital, Winnipeg, Canada
Dislocations of the Child's Elbow

Ronald L. Linscheid, M.D.
Professor of Orthopaedic Surgery, Mayo Medical School; Consultant in Orthopaedic Surgery and Surgery of the Hand, Mayo Clinic, Rochester, Minnesota
Elbow Dislocations; Nerve Entrapment Syndromes

James London, M.D.
Assistant Professor of Orthopedic Surgery, UCLA School of Medicine, Los Angeles; Staff Surgeon, San Pedro Peninsula Hospital, San Pedro, and

Harvor General Hospital, Harvor City, California
Custom Arthroplasty and Hemiarthroplasty of the Elbow

Bernard F. Morrey, M.D.
Associate Professor of Orthopedics, Mayo Medical School; Consultant in Orthopedics, Mayo Clinic; Orthopedic Surgeon, St. Marys Hospital, Rochester, Minnesota
Anatomy of the Elbow Joint; Biomechanics of the Elbow; The Physical Examination of the Elbow; Functional Evaluation of the Elbow; Arthroscopy of the Elbow; Surgical Exposures of the Elbow; Rehabilitation; Fractures of the Distal Humerus; Radial Head Fracture; Tendon Injury About the Elbow; Total Joint Replacement; Revision Joint Replacement; Septic Arthritis; Loose Bodies; Bursitis; The Elbow in Metabolic Disease.

Scott J. Mubarak, M.D.
Assistant Clinical Professor of Orthopedic Surgery, University of California, San Diego, School of Medicine; Pediatric Orthopedic Surgeon, Children's Hospital and Health Center, San Diego, California
Ischemia from Fractures and Injuries About the Elbow

Robert P. Nirschl, M.S., M.D.
Assistant Clinical Professor of Orthopedic Surgery, Georgetown University School of Medicine, Washington, D.C.; Attending Orthopedic Surgeon, Arlington Hospital, Arlington, Virginia
Muscle and Tendon Trauma: Tennis Elbow; Rehabilitation of the Athlete's Elbow

Eugene T. O'Brien, M.D.
Associate Clinical Professor of Orthopedic Surgery, University of Texas Health Science Center; Chief, Orthopedic Surgery, Methodist Hospital, San Antonio, Texas
Flaccid Dysfunction of the Elbow

Hamlet A. Peterson, M.D.
Professor of Orthopedic Surgery, Mayo Medical School; Consultant, Pediatric Orthopedics, Mayo Clinic, Rochester, Minnesota
Physeal Fractures

Douglas J. Pritchard, M.D.
Professor of Orthopedic Surgery, Mayo Medical School; Orthopedic Surgeon and Consultant, Mayo Clinic and Rochester Methodist Hospital, Rochester, Minnesota
Neoplasms of the Elbow

Franklin H. Sim, M.D.
Professor of Orthopedics, Mayo Medical School; Consultant, Mayo Clinic and Saint Marys Hospital, Rochester, Minnesota
Nonunion and Delayed Union of Distal Humeral Fractures

Morton Spinner, M.D.
Clinical Professor of Orthopedic Surgery, Albert Einstein College of Medicine, New York, New York
Nerve Entrapment Syndromes

J. Clarke Stevens, M.D., F.R.C.P.(C.)
Assistant Professor of Neurology, Mayo Medical School; Consultant, Department of Neurology, Mayo Clinic, Rochester, Minnesota
Neutrophic Arthritis

Marcus J. Steward, M.D.
Professor, Department of Orthopedic Surgery, University of Tennessee College of Medicine; Chief, Department of Orthopedics, Veterans Administration Medical Center, Memphis, Tennessee
Fascial Arthroplasty of the Elbow

Richard B. Tompkins, M.D.
Assistant Professor of Medicine, Mayo Medical School; Consultant, Internal Medicine and Rheumatology, Mayo Clinic, St. Marys Hospital, and Rochester Methodist Hospital, Rochester, Minnesota
Nonrheumatoid Inflammatory Arthritis

Hugh S. Tullos, M.D.
Head, Division of Orthopedic Surgery, Baylor College of Medicine; Chief, Orthopedic Service, Methodist Hospital and Ben Taub General Hospital, Houston, Texas
Ligamentous and Articular Injuries in the Athlete

Robert G. Volz, M.D., F.A.C.S.
Professor of Orthopedic Surgery, Arizona Health Science Center; Surgeon, University Hospital, Kino Hospital, and Veterans Administration Medical Center, Tucson, Arizona
The Physical Examination of the Elbow

Robert L. Waters, M.D.
Clinical Professor of Surgery, University of Southern California School of Medicine, Los Angeles; Chairman, Surgical Services, Rancho Los Amigos Hospital, Downey, California
Spastic Dysfunction of the Elbow

John H. Wedge, M.D., B.Sc., F.R.C.S.(C.)
Professor of Surgery (Orthopedics), University of Saskatchewan College of Medicine; Head of Orthopaedic Surgery, University Hospital, Saskatoon, Canada
Fractures of the Neck of the Radius in Children

Michael B. Wood, M.D.
Associate Professor of Orthopaedic Surgery, Mayo Medical School; Consultant, Department of Orthopaedic Surgery, Section of Hand Surgery, Mayo Clinic; Consultant, St. Marys Hospital and Rochester Methodist Hospital, Rochester, Minnesota
Replantation About the Elbow

Phillip E. Wright, II, M.D.
Clinical Associate Professor of Orthopaedic Surgery, School of Medicine, University of Tennessee; Active Staff, Campbell Clinic, Baptist Memorial Hospital, Regional Medical Center of Memphis, and University of Tennessee Hospital; Consultant Staff, Le Bonheur Children's Medical Center and Memphis Veterans Administration Medical Center, Memphis, Tennessee
Fascial Arthroplasty of the Elbow

Foreword

In creating the first definitive text on the elbow, Doctor Morrey and his contributors have passed a milestone in the understanding and treatment of this long-neglected joint. Many leading experts join in presenting, in depth, virtually every aspect of pathology and treatment. This book will be the basis of study for all serious students of the upper extremity and will become the classic reference on the subject.

The scope of *The Elbow and Its Disorders* is immense. It begins with a detailed consideration of the important current concepts regarding surgical anatomy and biomechanics, practical clinical appraisal, and the most advanced diagnostic aids, including diagnostic imaging and arthroscopy.

The initial chapter on embryology lays important groundwork for the eight-chapter section on pediatric disorders that follows. This is the most extensive consideration of conditions affecting the child's elbow ever to be published.

The large section on fractures and their complications is presented by nine authorities with salient references. It includes a chapter on replantation.

Five of the world's leading authorities on the elbow in sports join in creating a unique section on sports injuries. Eleven authorities discuss all aspects of the reconstructive procedures of the elbow, including various arthroplasties and replacements, arthrodesis, amputations, and the treatment of flaccid and spastic paralysis. In the final section, arthritic and systemic disorders, infections, neoplasms, and other lesions peculiar to the elbow are considered in detail, making this truly a complete work on the elbow.

Doctor Morrey is respected throughout the world for his astute leadership in the field of elbow surgery. His extensive clinical and research experience as well as that of the impressive group of contributors is reflected throughout the text. The detailed consideration given to each topic makes this a most valuable reference for all musculoskeletal surgeons as well as a hallmark in the advancement of elbow surgery.

CHARLES S. NEER, II, M.D.
Inaugural President
American Shoulder and Elbow Surgeons

Professor of Clinical Orthopaedic Surgery
Columbia University
New York, New York

Preface

While the elbow is not a frequent site of trauma and has no particular predilection for disease processes, injuries to this articulation are notoriously difficult to manage successfully. Unexpected loss of significant function after an apparently trivial insult has been a source of disappointment to the treating physicians and patients alike. Reconstructive procedures are limited in selection, difficult to execute, and prone to complications. The subcutaneous location and the intimate association with the major nerve account, in part, for the high complication rate associated with elbow afflictions and their management.

To date, relatively little attention has been given to problems of the elbow joint. There is a need for a comprehensive and detailed reference for the orthopedist. So that we might provide such a book, with the most authoritative information currently available, we sought to enlist the expertise of many knowledgeable associates who have generously contributed. We have attempted to synthesize and present the material in a format that is easy to read and understand and allows rapid access to any question at hand.

This undertaking was, therefore, stimulated by a desire to provide a single comprehensive source of reliable information to assist the practicing orthopedic surgeon in the management of problems at the elbow joint. We hope that this effort will result in greater confidence and satisfaction for all physicians who must deal with elbow conditions and better care and postoperative function for our patients.

B. F. MORREY, M.D.

Acknowledgment

We gratefully acknowledge Marlene Boyd, Connie Brown, and Sherry Koperski for their superb secretarial assistance and efforts in the preparation of this volume, and we wish to acknowledge the generous cooperation of the Mayo Medical Graphics and Photography Departments.

Some of the illustrations incorporated in this text consist of consultation material sent in by my colleagues. It would be impossible to acknowledge all of these sources independently but we acknowledge with grateful appreciation the use of their clinical cases.

Contents

Part II
CONDITIONS AFFECTING THE CHILD'S ELBOW

Part III
TRAUMA TO THE ADULT ELBOW

Part V
RECONSTRUCTIVE PROCEDURES OF THE ELBOW

Chapter 32
FASCIAL ARTHROPLASTY OF THE ELBOW 530
Phillip E. Wright, II, and Marcus J. Steward

Chapter 33
CUSTOM ARTHROPLASTY AND HEMIARTHROPLASTY
OF THE ELBOW 540
James London

Chapter 34
TOTAL JOINT REPLACEMENT 546
B. F. Morrey and R. S. Bryan

Chapter 35
REVISION JOINT REPLACEMENT 570
B. F. Morrey

Chapter 36
ARTHRODESIS... 582
Robert D. Beckenbaugh

Chapter 37
FLACCID DYSFUNCTION OF THE ELBOW 589
Eugene T. O'Brien

Chapter 38
SPASTIC DYSFUNCTION OF THE ELBOW 616
M. M. Hoffer, R. L. Waters, and D. E. Garland

Chapter 39
AMPUTATION 627
Ernest M. Burgess and Morris A. Dodge

Part VI
SEPTIC AND NONTRAUMATIC CONDITIONS OF THE ELBOW

Chapter 40
RHEUMATOID ARTHRITIS.. 638
Allan E. Inglis

Chapter 41
NONRHEUMATOID INFLAMMATORY ARTHRITIS 656
Richard B. Tompkins

Chapter 42
SEPTIC ARTHRITIS 664
K. P. Butters and B. F. Morrey

PART I

Fundamentals and General Considerations

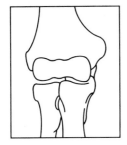

CHAPTER 1

Embryology

HYMIE GORDON

The upper limbs begin to develop on the twenty-sixth day after ovulation, when the developing human is about 3 mm long from crown to rump. The first signs of the upper limbs are buds that project from the sides of the body; they consist of cores of undifferentiated mesoderm covered by ectoderm. During the next 30 days, the buds elongate; nerves and blood vessels enter them; the mesenchyme differentiates into cartilage and muscle; condensation and segmentation lead to the demarcation of arm, forearm, wrist, hand, and phalanges; regression of tissue permits the separation of the fingers; and cavitation between the ends of the precursors of the tubular bones initiates the formation of the synovial joints, including the elbows.

In this chapter the events of those 30 days will be described with particular attention to the formation of the elbow. To begin with, the embryonic situation that exists just before the emergence of the limb buds will be described. Then a chronologic outline will be presented of the day-by-day development of the upper limbs. Next, a few special points will be made about the formation of a synovial joint. Finally, we will have a glimpse at some of the attempts that are being made to under-

stand the morphogenesis of the limb at the fundamental chemical and molecular levels.

THE PRELIMINARY STAGE

During the third week after ovulation, the cells of the paraxial mesoderm (at the sides of the neural tube) condense and segment into blocks, called somites. Within each somite, the mesodermal cells differentiate into a dorsolateral dermatome, an intermediate myotome, and a ventromedial sclerotome.

The dermatome is the precursor of the dermis. The myotome is the precursor of muscles. The sclerotome initially consists of young connective tissue cells (mesenchyme) that will differentiate into fibroblasts, chondroblasts, and osteoblasts (Fig. 1–1).

THE CHRONOLOGY OF THE DEVELOPMENT OF THE UPPER LIMBS

This account of the development of the upper limb is based on the observations of Bardeen and Lewis (1901),[2] Lewis (1902),[6] Windle (1944),[9] Gray and Gardner (1951),[5] Zwilling (1961),[10] Andersen (1962),[1] Gardner (1971),[4]

1

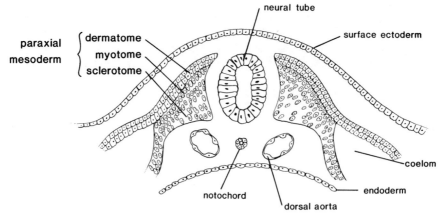

Figure 1–1. Diagrammatic cross-section of an embryo 15 to 21 days after ovulation, showing the antecedents of the constituents of the future limb buds.

and O'Rahilly and Gardner (1972 and 1975).[7, 8] The account is selectively biased to emphasize what is known about the development of the elbow.

The stages of development are given in days after ovulation and in the crown-rump length of the developing person. For each stage a brief description is given of the external appearance of the upper limb, followed by an account of the internal structures—nerves, blood vessels, muscles, bones, and joints.

Days 26–28; 3–6 mm

The upper limb buds appear as small lateral elevations opposite somites C3–8 and T1–2.

These elevations are pockets of ectoderm containing mesenchymal cells from the paraxial mesoderm. On the twenty-eighth day a few thin-walled blood vessels are present.

Days 28–32; 5–7 mm

The limb buds now are rounded protuberances that curve ventromedially and taper distally (Figs. 1–2 and 1–3A).

The ectoderm at the apex of the bud is thickened to form the apical ectodermal ridge. (Interactions between these cells and the underlying and nearby mesenchyme are important determinants of the morphogenesis of the hand.) A marginal blood vessel is forming beneath this ridge.

Spinal nerves C4–8 and T1 have appeared just proximal to the root of the bud.

Day 33; 7–9 mm

The distal end of the bud expands to form the hand plate.

The spinal nerves penetrate into the root of the bud. The mesenchyme along the central axis of the

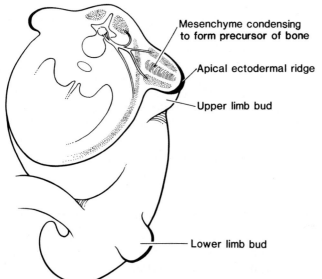

Mesenchyme condensing
to form precursor of bone

Apical ectodermal ridge

Upper limb bud

Lower limb bud

Figure 1–2. Diagram of cross-sectioned embryo at 32 days.

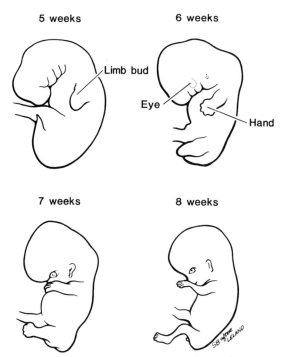

5 weeks 6 weeks

Limb bud

Eye

Hand

7 weeks 8 weeks

Figure 1–3. Embryonic development from 5 to 8 weeks (not drawn to scale), showing the external appearances of the upper limb. Note that by the eighth week, the position of the limb has changed so that the palms face downward and the elbows point caudally.

bud begins to condense—the first visible sign of the bones of the upper limb.

Days 34–40; 8–11 mm

Indications of carpus, metacarpus, and a distal digital flange can be seen on the hand plate.

Premuscle masses begin to form proximal to the bud. The pectoral premuscle mass can be distinguished.

The condensation of the central mesenchyme has advanced to a stage in which the humerus, radius, and ulna can be discerned. Chondrification begins in the humerus.

The brachial plexus has formed. In the proximal part of the bud, nerve fibers aggregate to form the peripheral nerve trunks; the dorsal fibers form the radial nerve; the ventral fibers form the median and ulnar nerves. These nerves reach as far as the level of the future elbow.

Days 41–43; 11–14 mm

Finger rays, which are indicative of longitudinal condensation of the mesenchyme, are visible on the dorsal surface of the hand plate (Fig. 1–3B).

Discrete muscle masses can now be discerned. The radius, ulna, and metacarpals begin to chondrify, and the radial, median, and ulnar nerves extend down to the hand plate.

Days 44–47; 13–17 mm

Finger rays are clearly visible and interdigital notches have appeared along the distal border of the hand plate. The elbow is now visible.

Most of the large muscles are identifiable, including the trapezius, pectoralis major and minor, deltoid, biceps, triceps, coracobrachialis, brachialis, and brachioradialis.

A mesenchymal clavicle is visible. Chondrification begins in the scapula, head of the humerus, carpal bones (except the pisiform), and proximal phalanges.

The joints are beginning to form. For instance, at the sites of some metacarpophalangeal joints, homogeneous interzones form between the carpal and metacarpal cartilages. At the same time, the mesenchyme around the interzones is condensing to initiate the formation of the ligaments and capsules of joints.

Days 48–50; 16–18 mm

The fingers are separated except for interdigital webs of skin. The upper limbs project forward, and their pre-axial borders are cranial; that is, the thumbs are uppermost and the right and left palms face each other.

Some of the components of the elbow joints are more clearly delineated. Homogeneous interzones have appeared between the ends of the bones. With increasing chondrification, the modeling of the distal ends of the bones has progressed to where the shapes of the olecranon and the humeral epicondyles can be recognized.

Similar developments are taking place elsewhere in the limb. A homogeneous interzone has appeared at the shoulder and at some of the intercarpal joints. Collateral and palmar ligaments are present at some of the metacarpophalangeal joints. Chondrification is occurring in the styloid processes of the radius and ulna. The middle phalanges are also beginning to chondrify.

Day 51; 18–22 mm

The interdigital webs are breaking down, beginning the separation of the fingers.

Modeling of the bones is continuing: the glenoid fossa and the acromion can now be seen. The distal phalanges are starting to chondrify.

Mesenchymal consensation and differentiation around the joints are progressing rapidly: the flexor retinaculum, the collateral ligaments of the wrist, and the carpal, metacarpal, and proximal interphalangeal ligaments are present. The annular ligament of the radius has appeared.

Days 52–53; 22–24 mm

The fingers have now separated. Active movements of the upper limb are now beginning and will promote the development of the joints.

All the muscles of the upper limb are now in place, and each muscle has an appropriate supply of nerves and blood vessels.

The humerus and, to a lesser extent, the radius are beginning to ossify.

Days 54–57; 23–31 mm

Growth, passive torsion, and active movements are turning the palms downward and pointing the elbows caudally.

The coronoid process of the ulna has chondrified; elsewhere the ulna is beginning to ossify. The head of the radius has assumed its concave form. The radial tuberosity is visible but not yet chondrified.

Cavitation now begins in the elbow, shoulder, and radioscaphoid joints. At the elbow, cavitation is first seen in the radiohumeral joint, then in the ulnohumeral and radioulnar joints. It begins in the center of the interzones and extends peripherally until all three cavities become confluent.

Blood vessels enter the loose mesenchyme adjacent to the interzones to form the primitive synovium of the elbow and other joints.

O'Rahilly and Gardner[8] have neatly summarized what has been accomplished by the end of the eighth week after ovulation: ". . . all the major skeletal, articular, muscular, neural, and vascular elements of the limbs are present in a form and arrangement closely resembling those of the adult. Most ligaments are discernible, cavitation is frequently beginning in the larger joints, some bursae may be present, and the periosteal ossification has begun in certain skeletal components." All this has happened during a period of 30 days in which the developing human has grown from 3 to 31 mm.

The primary development of the elbow itself takes place in even less time—just 1 week. On the fiftieth day, the cartilagenized olecranon and humeral epicondyles are visible, and a homogeneous interzone forms between the ends of the skeletal precursors. The annular ligament of the radius appears on the fifty-first day. Active movements of the elbow begin on the fifty-second day. By the fifty-sixth day, the position of the upper limbs has changed so that the elbows point caudally. On the fifty-seventh day, the joint cavity appears, with collateral ligaments and joint capsule in place and a blood supply to the primitive synovium.

THE DEVELOPMENT OF THE SYNOVIAL JOINT

Between the forty-eighth and fiftieth days, after chondrification of the humerus, radius, and ulna, the space between the ends of these three bones is occupied by a broad interzone of homogeneous mesenchyme, consisting of tightly packed cells with round or oval nuclei and scanty cytoplasm. This homogeneous interzone merges with the cartilaginous ends of the bones.

During the next 2 or 3 days the peripheral mesenchyme at the sides of the interzone condenses further to form the capsule and the ligaments, including the annular ligament of the radius. The cells lining the inside of the capsule and the ends of the bones become vascularized to form the primitive synovial membrane (Fig. 1–4). Blood vessels do not penetrate into the center of the interzone. With increasing movement of the joint, the synovium over the ends of the bones will disappear.

The cells in the center are now more loosely packed, and they stain metachromatically. This metachromasia becomes progressively more intense, indicating the accumulation of acid mucopolysaccharides (glycosaminoglycans)—specifically, chondroitin sulfate—in the cells and ground substance of the interzone.[1] This accumulation is at its peak on about the fifty-fifth day and is soon followed by cavitation (a non-necrotic loss of cells) in the center of the interzone. Cavitation usually appears first in the radiohumeral joint, then in the ulnohumeral and the radioulnar joints. As the cavities expand, they coalesce so that by about the fifty-seventh day only one joint cavity is present. It is lined by the primitive vascularized synovium and is supported by the capsule and ligaments.

MOLECULAR CONTROL OF CELL DIFFERENTIATION

Throughout this chapter the word *differentiate* has been used frequently—for instance ". . . the mesenchyme, which will differentiate into fibroblasts, chondroblasts, and osteoblasts." Ever since embryology has been studied at the microscopic level, this com-

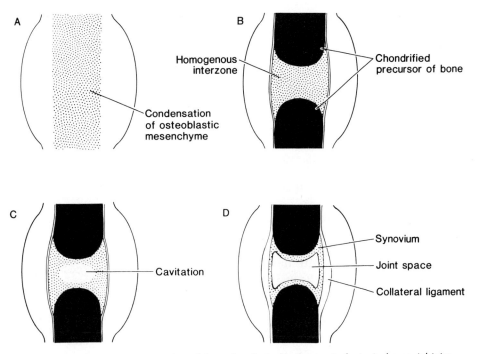

Figure 1–4. Schematic representation of the embryologic development of a typical synovial joint.

fortably nebulous word *differentiate* has been a popular item in the embryologists' jargon, permitting a rather carefree mental hop from a pluripotent cell to a specialized one. How does a mesenchymal cell become a chondroblast? "It differentiates." In recent years, embryologists have sought to explain what cellular differentiation really means by studying the process at the histochemical and the molecular levels. Some progress has been made, for instance, in understanding how the mesenchymal cells of the limb buds differentiate. One approach has been to investigate the chemical changes associated with differentiation.

In the experimental animal the chick the mesenchymal cells of the limb bud are pluripotent until day 4: they can differentiate into muscle or into cartilage cells. After day 4, a particular mesenchymal cell is committed to become either a muscle cell or a cartilage cell, but not both. This phenotypic commitment is determined by the relative positions of the mesenchymal cells in the limb bud and, hence, by their extracellular environment.

The more peripheral mesenchymal cells receive a richer nourishment from the primitive vascular system. One of the nutriments now under scrutiny is nicotinamide. When this "vitamin" enters a mesenchymal cell it is converted, with the participation of ATP, to nicotinamide adenine diphosphate (NAD). A rich supply of NAD will produce a high intracellular concentration of NAD; this will actively promote myogenesis while actively inhibiting chondrogenesis. Conversely, low intracellular levels of NAD will favor chondrogenesis and inhibit myogenesis.[3]

During the time when the mesenchymal cells are commiting themselves to their future form, a sharp increase occurs in the intracellular concentration of polyadenylic-diphosphoribose (polyADP-ribose). This unusual nucleic acid is derived from NAD. It binds covalently with the histone and nonhistone nucleoproteins. These are the proteins that are associated with the nuclear DNA and play important roles in controlling the genetic activity of DNA—the uncoiling of the double helix, the accessibility of exogenous inducers to DNA, the rate of transcription of the genetic code, and so on. In the case of histone, NAD binds preferentially with the basic amino acids, especially lysine and arginine, which are abundant at the carboxy- and amino-terminals of the histone molecules. Such polyADP-ribosylation of histone probably disrupts its interaction with DNA, thus promoting the transcription of messenger RNA.[3]

Perhaps the following sequence contributes to the early differentiation of the mesenchyme of the limb bud:

peripheral localization →
  richer supply of nicotinamide →
    more intracellular NAD →
      increased synthesis of polyADP-ribose →
        specific binding with nucleoprotein →
          derepression of specific sequences of DNA →
            transcription of specific messenger RNA →
              specific synthesis of muscle-cell components.

Much of this is speculation, but it illustrates the kinds of fundamental information that we need about the process of normal and abnormal morphogenesis. Then we will have a much better understanding of the normal and abnormal development of the parts of the body. Consequently, those of us who are interested in the elbow and its developmental disorders will be able to offer more valuable diagnostic opinions than "the head of the radius failed to form" or "the radius and ulna never separated." And, if our dreams come true, it may even be possible to prevent these disorders by rational periconceptional treatment.

References

1. Andersen, H.: Histochemical Studies of the Histiogenesis of the Human Elbow Joint. Acta Anat., **51**, 60–68, 1962.
2. Bardeen, C. R., and Lewis, W. H.: Development of the Limbs, Body-Wall and Back in Man. Am. J. Anat., **1**, 1–35, 1960.
3. Caplan, A. I.: The Molecular Basis for Limb Morphogenesis. *In* Littlefield, J. W., and de Groucy, J. (Eds.): Birth Defects. Proceedings of the Fifth International Conference. Amsterdam-Oxford, Excerpta Medica, 1978.
4. Gardner, E.: Osteogenesis in the Human Embryo and Fetus. *In* Bourne, G. H. (Ed.): The Biochemistry and Physiology of Bone, 2nd ed. pp. 77–118. New York, Academic Press, 1971.
5. Gray, D. J., and Gardner, E.: Prenatal Development of the Human Elbow Joint. Am. J. Anat., **88**, 429–470, 1951.
6. Lewis, W. H.: The Development of the Arm in Man. Am. J. Anat., **1**, 145–183, 1902.
7. O'Rahilly, R., and Gardner, E.: The Initial Appearance of Ossification in Staged Human Embryos. Am. J. Anat., **134**, 291–307, 1972.
8. O'Rahilly, R., and Gardner, E.: The Timing and Sequence of Events in the Development of the Limbs in the Human Embryo. Anat. Embryol., **148**, 1–23, 1975.
9. Windle, W. F.: Genesis of Somatic Motor Function in Mammalian Embryos: A Synthesizing Article. Physiol. Zoöl., **17**, 247–260, 1944.
10. Zwilling, E.: Limb Morphogenesis. Adv. Morphogens., **1**, 301–330, 1944.

CHAPTER 2

Anatomy of the Elbow Joint

B. F. MORREY

This chapter discusses the anatomy of the elbow region with special emphasis on the anatomic features of the joint. Detailed descriptions of the nerves, arteries, and muscles are available in standard anatomy textbooks. Specific pathologic anatomy is discussed in later chapters of this book dealing with the pertinent condition.

Topical Anatomy and General Survey

The skin overlying the elbow region is freely movable circumferentially about the brachial and forearm fascia. The contours of the biceps muscle and antecubital fossa are easily observed anteriorly (Fig. 2–1), and the triceps muscle and the tendon are readily palpable posteriorly. Laterally, the avascular interval between the brachioradialis and the triceps is an important palpable landmark for surgical exposures. In most individuals the tip of the olecranon and the medial and lateral epicondyles are readily palpated and are co-linear in extension, forming an inverted triangle when the elbow is flexed to 90 degrees (Fig. 2–2). Laterally, the tip of the olecranon, the lateral epicondyle, and the radial head also form an equilateral triangle and provide an important landmark for joint aspiration (see Chapter 4). The flexion crease of the elbow is on a line with the medial and lateral epicondyles and thus is actually 1 to 2 cm proximal to the joint line when the elbow is extended (Fig. 2–3). The inverted triangular depression on the anterior aspect of the extremity distal to the epicondyles is called the cubital (antecubital) fossa.

If the extremity is not obese, the superficial

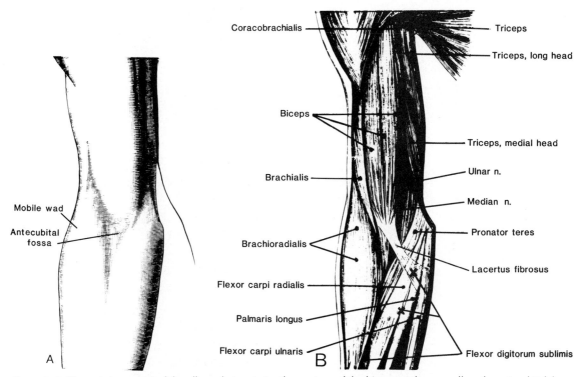

Figure 2–1. The anterior aspect of the elbow demonstrates the contour of the biceps tendon as well as the antecubital fossa (A). B, The underlying musculature.

7

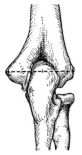
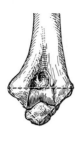

Figure 2–2. The palpable landmarks of the tip of the olecranon and the medial and lateral epicondyle form an inverted triangle posteriorly when the elbow is flexed 90 degrees but are colinear when the elbow is fully extended. (From Anson, B. J., and McVay, C. B.: Surgical Anatomy. Vol. 2, 5th ed. Philadelphia, W. B. Saunders Company, 1971.)

veins over the cubital fossa are easily observed. The cephalic and basilic veins are the most prominent superficial major contributions of the anterior venous system and communicate by way of the median cephalic and median basilic veins to form an M pattern over the cubital fossa (Fig. 2–4). These are the most commonly used veins for venipuncture.

The extensor forearm musculature origi-

nates from the lateral epicondyle and is termed the *mobile wad* by Henry.[37] The mobile wad forms the lateral margin of the antecubital fossa and the lateral contour of the forearm and comprises the brachioradialis and the extensor carpi radialis longus and brevis muscles. The muscles comprising the contour of the medial anterior forearm and forming the medial margin of the cubital fossa include the pronator teres, flexor carpi radialis, palmaris longus, and flexor carpi ulnaris. Henry has demonstrated that their relationship and location can be approximated by placing the opposing thumb and the index, long, and ring fingers over the anterior medial forearm as shown in Figure 2–5. The dorsum of the forearm is contoured by the extensor musculature, consisting of the anconeus, extensor carpi ulnaris, extensor digitorum quinti, and the extensor digitorum communis. The relationships of these muscles are depicted in Figure 2–6.

The cutaneous innervation of the upper extremity is somewhat variable. In general, the skin about the proximal elbow is provided innervation by the lower lateral cutaneous

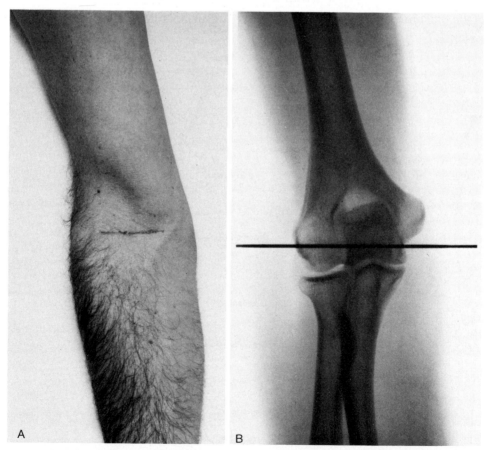

Figure 2–3. A line placed over the flexion crease *(A)* is actually situated about 1 cm above the elbow joint line *(B)*.

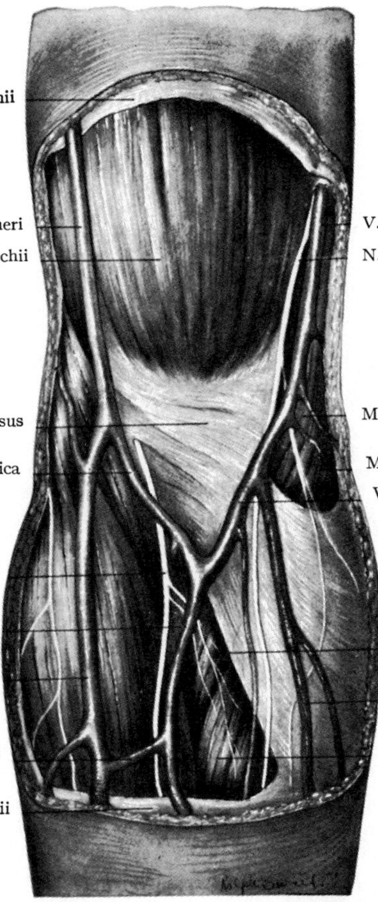

Figure 2–4. The superficial venous pattern of the anterior aspect of the elbow demonstrates a rather characteristic inverted M pattern formed by the median cephalic and median basilic veins. (From Anson, B. J., and McVay, C. B.: Surgical Anatomy. Vol. 2, 5th ed. Philadelphia, W. B. Saunders Company, 1971.)

(C5, C6) and medial cutaneous (radial nerve, C8, T1 and T2) nerves of the arm. The forearm skin is innervated by the medial (C8, T1), lateral (musculocutaneous, C5, C6), and posterior (radial nerve, C6–8) cutaneous nerves of the forearm (Fig. 2–7).

The lymphatic drainage of the elbow begins in the hand and traverses the forearm with the accompaniment of the superficial and deep veins. The brachial lymphatics originate from antecubital nodes and arise as two or three major conduits with the brachial vessels. The brachial lymphatics terminate in the central and lateral axillary nodes. One or two epitrochlear nodes are occasionally palpable just proximal to the medial epicondyle.

OSTEOLOGY

Humerus

The distal humerus consists of two condyles forming the articular surfaces of the trochlea and capitellum (Fig. 2–8).

Proximal to the trochlea the prominent medial epicondyle serves as a source of attach-

ment of the ulnar collateral ligament and the flexor pronator group of muscles. Laterally, the lateral epicondyle is located just above the capitellum and is much less prominent than the medial epicondyle. The lateral collateral ligament and the supinator-extensor muscle group originate from the flat, irregular surface of the lateral epicondyle. The posterior inferior aspect serves as a source of origin of the anconeus muscle.

Just above the articular surface of the capitellum the radial fossa serves to accommodate the margin of the radial head during flexion. Medial to the radial fossa, a large coronoid fossa is present anteriorly just above the trochlea. The coronoid inserts into this fossa during extremes of elbow flexion. Posteriorly, the olecranon fossa serves a similar purpose, receiving the tip of the olecranon during extension.

A thin membrane of bone separates the two fossae in about 90 percent of individuals, although there is some race and sex variation with this anatomic feature.[82] The coronoid and olecranon fossae are bordered on either side by the strong lateral supracondylar bony

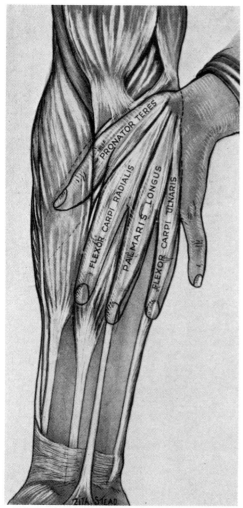

Figure 2–5. The orientation of the flexor or pronator muscles can be remembered by Henry's technique of placing the opposite hand over the medial aspect of the forearm as indicated. (From Henry, A. K.: Extensile Exposure. 2nd ed. Baltimore, The Williams & Wilkins Company, 1957.)

column and a smaller medial supracondylar bony column (Fig. 2–9). The difference in size of these two structures is important because the smaller medial column may be vulnerable to fracture during insertion of some designs of humeral components at the time of elbow prosthetic replacement surgery.[56] The posterior aspect of the lateral supracondylar column is flat, whereas the anterior surface is slightly curved. The prominent lateral supracondylar ridge separates the two surfaces into the so-called safe interval between the brachioradialis and extensor carpi radialis longus anteriorly and the triceps posteriorly. This serves as an important landmark for many lateral surgical approaches.

Proximal to the medial epicondyle, about 5 to 7 cm along the medial intramuscular sep-

tum, a supracondylar process is observed in 1 to 3 percent of individuals[45, 49, 76] (Fig. 2–10). A fibrous band termed the ligament of Strothers may originate from this process and attach to the medial epicondyle.[38] When present, this spur serves as an anomalous insertion of the coracobrachialis muscle and an origin of the pronator teres muscle.[33] Various pathologic processes have been associated with the supracondylar process, including fracture[45] and median[4] and ulnar nerve[38] entrapment (see Chapter 45).

Radius

The cross-sectional shape of the radius is almost cylindrical proximally, widening and becoming more elliptical distally. The proximal radius includes the radial head, which articulates with the capitellum and exhibits a

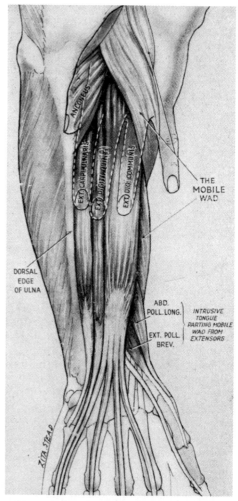

Figure 2–6. The relationship of the muscles forming the contour of the extensor aspect of the forearm is demonstrated by placing the opposite hand over the lateral aspect of the joint. (From Henry, A. K.: Extensile Exposure. 2nd ed. Baltimore, The Williams & Wilkins Company, 1966.)

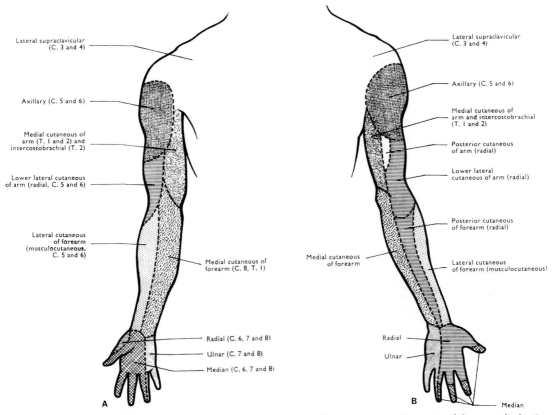

Figure 2–7. Typical distribution of the cutaneous nerves of the anterior *(A)* and posterior *(B)* aspects of the upper limb. (From Cunningham, D. J.: Textbook of Anatomy. 12th ed., G. J. Romanes, ed., New York, Oxford University Press, 1981.)

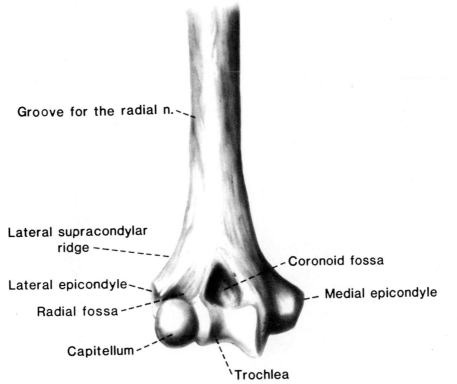

Figure 2–8. The bony landmarks of the anterior aspect of the distal humerus.

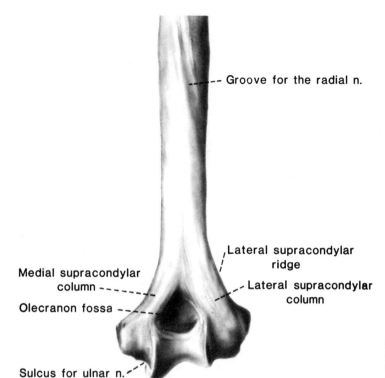

Groove for the radial n.

Lateral supracondylar ridge

Medial supracondylar column

Lateral supracondylar column

Olecranon fossa

Sulcus for ulnar n.

Figure 2–9. The prominent medial and lateral supracondylar bony columns as well as other landmarks of the posterior aspect of the distal humerus.

cylindrical shape with a depression in the midportion to accommodate the capitellum. The disc-shaped head is secured to the ulna by the annular ligament (Fig. 2–11). Distal to

the radial head the bone tapers to form the neck of the radius. The head and neck are frequently fractured, and this angular orientation of the articular part with respect to the shaft has been implicated in the mechanism of this fracture.[77] The radial tuberosity marks the distal aspect of the neck and has two distinct parts. The anterior surface is covered by bicipitoradial bursa protecting the tendon during full pronation (Fig. 2–35), but the biceps tendon does not originate here. The rough posterior aspect provides the source of attachment to the biceps tendon. This relationship and the dorsal position of the tu-

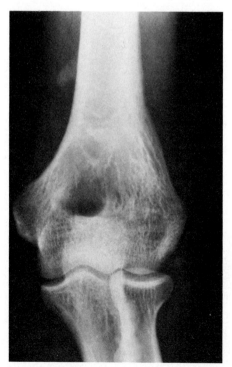

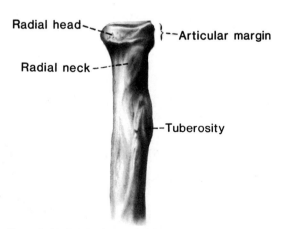

Radial head

Articular margin

Radial neck

Tuberosity

Figure 2–10. Typical supracondylar process located approximately 5 cm proximal to the medial epicondyle with its characteristic configuration.

Figure 2–11. Proximal aspect of the radius demonstrating the articular margin for articulation with the olecranon, the radial neck, and tuberosity.

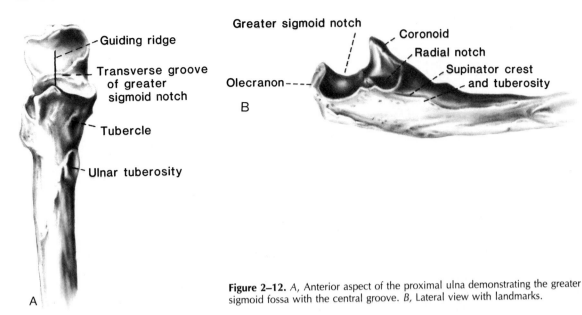

Figure 2–12. A, Anterior aspect of the proximal ulna demonstrating the greater sigmoid fossa with the central groove. B, Lateral view with landmarks.

berosity during full pronation allow exposure and repair of a ruptured biceps tendon through a posterior approach[14] (see Chapter 26). The orientation of the bicipital tuberosity has also been used as a means of determining axial alignment of the radius when it is fractured in its midportion.[25]

Ulna

The proximal ulna provides the major articulation of the elbow that is responsible for its inherent stability. With distal progression the bone quickly tapers to assume first a triangu-lar and then a cylindrical shape. The broad, thick, proximal aspect of the ulna consists of the greater sigmoid notch (incisura semilu-naris), which articulates with the trochlea of the humerus (Fig. 2–12). The anterior and distal aspect of the sigmoid notch is composed of the coronoid process with its artic-ular surface and a cortical surface that serves as the site of insertion of the brachialis muscle and of the oblique cord. The olecranon, com-prising the proximal aspect of the semilunar notch, provides the posterior articulation of the ulnohumeral joint. The external surface of the olecranon is the site of attachment for

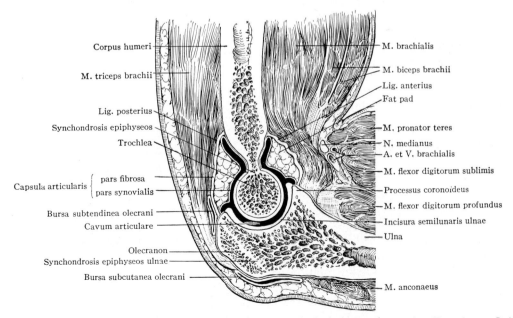

Figure 2–13. Sagittal section through the elbow region, demonstrating the high degree of congruity. (From Anson, B. J., and McVay C. B.: Surgical Anatomy. Vol. 2, 5th ed. Philadelphia, W. B. Saunders Company, 1971.)

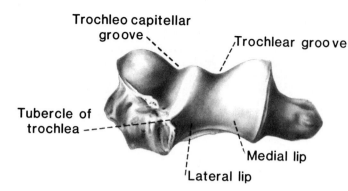

Trochleo capitellar groove
Trochlear groove
Tubercle of trochlea
Medial lip
Lateral lip

Figure 2–14. Axial view of the distal humerus shows the isometrical trochlea as well as the anterior position of the capitellum. The trochlear capitellar groove separates the trochlea from the capitellum.

the triceps tendon, the most proximal tip being separated from the tendon by the subtendinous bursa.

On the lateral aspect of the coronoid process, the lesser semilunar notch or the radial notch is oriented roughly perpendicular to the long axis of the bone. The circular margin of the radial head articulates with the radial notch and is stabilized by the annular ligament, which attaches to the anterior and posterior margins of the notch. A depression on the lateral surface of the proximal ulna extends distally from the proximal inferior border of the radial notch, the crest of which is the site of the ulnar origin of the supinator muscle. A tuberosity on the crest of this depression, the crista supinatoris, is the site of insertion of the accessory lateral collateral ligament, which serves as a tether for the annular ligament and a supplement to the radial collateral ligament.[58]

The medial aspect of the coronoid process serves as the site of attachment of the anterior portion of the medial collateral ligament. A tubercle serves as the ulnar origin of the flexor digitorum sublimis, below which is the ulnar origin and the flexor digitorum profundus. The ulnar portion of the pronator teres and the flexor policis longus also originate along the medial aspect of the coronoid process.

ELBOW JOINT STRUCTURE

Articulation

The elbow joint consists of two types of articulations and thus provides two types of motion. The ulnohumeral articulation resembles a hinge joint (ginglymus), allowing flexion and extension. The radiohumeral and proximal radioulnar joint allows axial rotation or a pivoting (trochoid) type of motion. Technically, therefore, the joint articulation is classified as a trochoginglymoid joint.[73]

Humerus

The trochlea is the hyperbaloid, pulleylike surface that articulates with the semilunar notch of the ulna (Fig. 2–13). A continuous surface of cartilage covers the anterior, distal, and posterior aspects, forming an arch of about 300[68] to 330 degrees.[42, 73] This generous articulation allows for a captive type of interface with the proximal ulna. The trochlea is not symmetrical because the medial lip is larger and projects more distally than does the lateral part (Fig. 2–14). The two surfaces are separated by a groove that courses in a helical manner from an anterolateral to a posteromedial direction.

The capitellum is almost spheroidal in

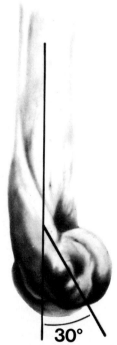

30°

Figure 2–15. Lateral view of the humerus shows the 30-degree anterior rotation of the articular condyles with respect to the long axis of the humerus.

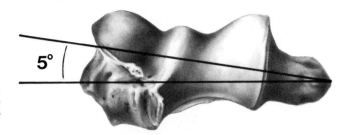

Figure 2–16. Axial view of the distal humerus demonstrates the 5- to 7-degree internal rotation of the articulation in reference to the line connecting the midportions of the epicondyles.

shape and is covered with hyaline cartilage, which is about 2 mm thick anteriorly. The posterior medial limit of the capitellum is marked by a prominent tubercle.[61] A groove separates the capitellum from the trochlea, and the rim of the radial head articulates with this groove throughout the arc of flexion and during pronation and supination.

Because the elbow is not a weight-bearing joint and is not frequently beset with severe degenerative arthritis, relatively little is known about the articular cartilage of this joint. In the dog, Simon et al.[69] have demonstrated that the cartilage is thickest in joints with the least congruity. In the human, the elbow is one of the most congruent joints of the body, so the articular surface should be relatively thin. Consistent with this observation, Morris[59] states that the cartilage of the distal humerus is thicker laterally over the capitellum, which is the less constrained portion of the joint. Several cadaver specimens were sectioned in our laboratory, and measurements revealed that the articular cartilage about the trochlea varies in width from 1 mm medially to 2 mm laterally. By comparison, the cartilage thickness of the tibial plafond and talus is about the same thickness. It should be noted that the precise definition of cartilage thickness is difficult to ascertain from cadaver specimens because use and water content cause variation in this measurement.[24]

The orientation of the articular surface of the distal humerus is not at a right angle to the long axis nor is it parallel to the epicondylar axis of the humerus. In the lateral plane the articulation is rotated anteriorly about 30 degrees with respect to the long axis of the humerus (Fig. 2–15). The center of the concentric arc formed by the trochlea and capitellum is on a line that is co-planar to the anterior distal cortex of the humerus.[55] London's data likewise reveal 3 to 8 degrees of internal rotation of the condyles with respect to a line joining the epicondyles when viewed in the axial plane of the humerus (Fig. 2–16).[49a] In the frontal plane, an average of approximately 6 degrees valgus tilt of the

condyles with respect to the long axis of the humerus[3] has been described (Fig. 2–17)[43, 47] (see Chapter 3).

Proximal Radius

Hyaline cartilage covers the depression of the radial head, which has an angular value of about 40 degrees,[73] as well as approximately 240 degrees of the outside circumference that articulates with the ulna (Fig. 2–18). The lesser sigmoid fossa forms an arc of approximately 60 to 80 degrees,[42, 73] leaving an excursion of about 180 degrees for pronation and supination. The anterolateral third of the circumference of the radial head is void of cartilage. This part of the radial head lacks subchondral bone and thus is not as strong as the part that supports the articular cartilage; this part has been demonstrated to be the portion

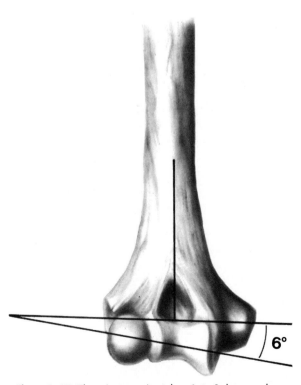

Figure 2–17. There is approximately a 6- to 8-degree valgus tilt of the distal humeral articulation with respect to the long axis of the humerus.

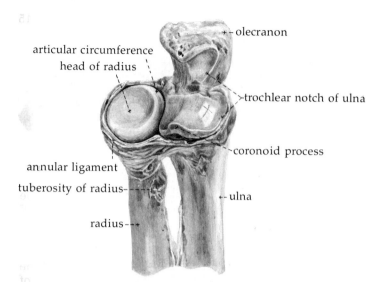

articular circumference
head of radius

annular ligament

tuberosity of radius

radius

olecranon

trochlear notch of ulna

coronoid process

ulna

Figure 2–18. Hyaline cartilage covers approximately 240 degrees of the outside circumference of the radial head, allowing its articulation with the proximal ulna at the radial notch of the ulna. (From Langman, J., and Woerdeman, M. W.: Atlas of Medical Anatomy. Philadelphia, W. B. Saunders Company, 1976.)

most often fractured.[77] The head and neck are not co-linear with the rest of the bone and form an angle of approximately 15 degrees with the shaft of the radius opposite the radial tuberosity[25] (Fig. 2–19).

Proximal Ulna

The sigmoid notch is not covered by a continuous surface of hyaline cartilage. In most individuals, a transverse portion composed of

fatty tissue divides the anterior articular cartilage that covers the coronoid and the posterior cartilage that covers the olecranon (Fig. 2–20). The semilunar notch is also divided longitudinally into medial and lateral por-

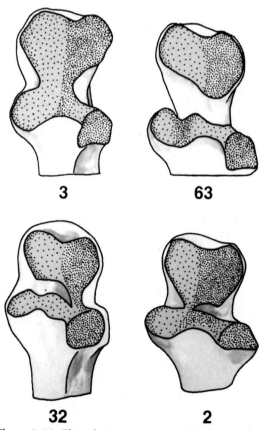

3   63

32   2

Figure 2–20. The relative percentage of hyaline cartilage distribution at the proximal ulna. (Redrawn from Tillmann, B.: A Contribution to the Function Morphology of Articular Surfaces. Translated by G. Konorza. Stuttgart, George Thieme, Publishers, P. S. G. Publishing Company, Mass., 1978.)

15°

Figure 2–19. The neck of the radius makes an angle of approximately 15 degrees with the long axis of the proximal radius.

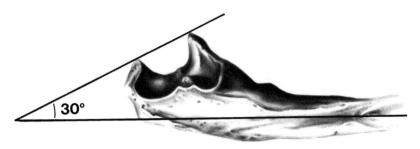

Figure 2–21. The greater sigmoid notch opens posteriorly with respect to the long axis of the ulna. This matches the 30-degree anterior rotation of the distal humerus, as shown in Figure 2–15.

tions by the "guiding ridge."[59] Hence, the proximal ulnar articulation consists of four articular parts, two anterior and two posterior.

In the lateral plane the sigmoid notch forms an arc of about 180 degrees (Fig. 2–21). Tillman has carefully studied the osseous trabecular pattern of the sigmoid notch. Predictably, the bone of the coronoid and olecranon is more dense than is that of the midportion of the sigmoid notch, which is consistent with its function of absorbing the force of articular contact.[79]

The opening of the sigmoid notch is oriented approximately 30 degrees posterior to the long axis of the bone (Fig. 2–21). In the frontal plane the shaft is angulated from about

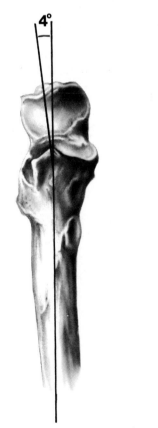

Figure 2–22. There is a slight (approximately 4 degrees) valgus angulation of the shaft of the ulna with respect to the greater sigmoid notch.

1 to 6 degrees[43, 47, 68] lateral to the articulation (Fig. 2–22). This angle contributes in part to the formation of the carrying angle, which is discussed in Chapter 3.

The lesser sigmoid notch consists of a depression with an arc of about 70 degrees and is situated just distal to the lateral aspect of the coronoid and articulates with the radial head. Because radial head rotation occurs at a right angle to flexion and extension, this surface is oriented almost perpendicular to the greater sigmoid notch.

Carrying Angle

The so-called carrying angle is the angle formed by the long axes of the humerus and the ulna with the elbow fully extended. This anatomic relationship is probably more of academic and cosmetic interest than of clinical importance. The valgus angle of the humeral articulation with the long axis of the humerus and the valgus angle of the proximal ulna account for the creation of the carrying angle. In the male the mean carrying angle is 11 to 14 degrees, and in the female it is 13 to 16 degrees,[3, 43] but Beals measured an angle of 17.8 degrees in adults with no difference between male and female.[10]

Joint Capsule

The anterior capsule inserts proximally above the coronoid and radial fossae (Fig. 2–23A). Distally, the capsule attaches to the anterior margin of the coronoid medially as well as to the annular ligament laterally. Posteriorly, the capsule attaches just above the olecranon fossa, distal along the supracondylar bony columns, and then down along the medial and lateral margins of the trochlea (Fig. 2–23B). Distally, attachment is along the medial and lateral articular margin of the sigmoid notch, and laterally it occurs along the lateral aspect of the sigmoid notch and blends with the annular ligament.

The anterior capsule is normally a thin transparent structure that allows visualization

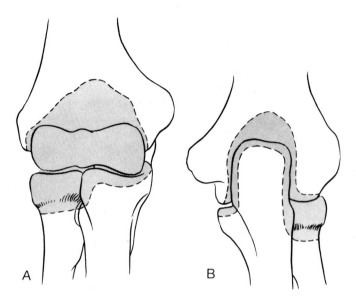

Figure 2–23. The insertion of the capsule of the elbow as viewed from the anterior aspect *(A)* as well as the posterior aspect *(B)*. (From Hollinshead, W. H.: The back and limbs. *In* Anatomy for Surgeons. Vol. 3. New York, Harper and Rowe, 1969, pp. 379–384.)

of the prominences of the articular condyles when the elbow is extended. This normal appearance suggests that it may not contribute to elbow stability.[61] Yet significant strength is provided by transverse and obliquely directed fibrous bands. These originate above the medial aspect of the trochlea and insert into the annular ligament.[58] A second prominent pattern originates above the capitellum and inserts along the lateral aspect of the coronoid[58] (Fig. 2–24). The anterior capsule is, of course, taut in extension but becomes lax in flexion, the greatest capacity occurring at about 60 degrees of flexion.[41] The joint capsule is innervated by branches from all major nerves crossing the joint, including the contribution

from the musculoskeletal nerve (Fig. 2–25). The variations and relative contributions have been carefully documented by Gardner.[28]

Synovial Membrane

The synovial membrane lines the joint capsule and is attached above the radial and coronoid fossae anteriorly to the medial and lateral margins of the articular surface and posteriorly to the superior margin of the olecranon fossa (Fig. 2–26A, B). Distally, it lines the annular ligament and is reflected over the radial neck, forming the sacciform recess (Fig. 2–24). A fold of synovial tissue has been described as projecting between the

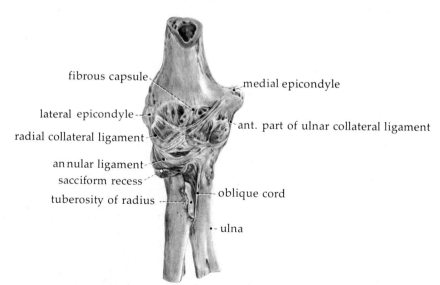

fibrous capsule

medial epicondyle

lateral epicondyle

ant. part of ulnar collateral ligament

radial collateral ligament

annular ligament

sacciform recess

tuberosity of radius

oblique cord

ulna

Figure 2–24. There is a cruciate orientation of the fibers of the anterior capsule that provides a good deal of its strength. (From Langman, J., and Woerdeman, M. W.: Atlas of Medical Anatomy. Philadelphia, W. B. Saunders Company, 1978.)

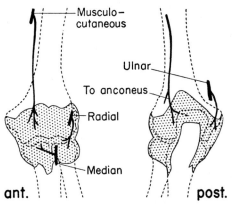

Figure 2–25. A typical distribution of the contributions of the musculocutaneous radial median and ulnar nerves to the joint capsule. (From Gardner, E.: The innervation of the elbow joint. Anat. Rec. 102:161–174, 1948.)

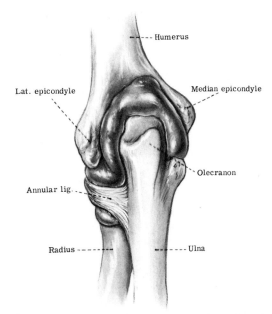

Figure 2–26. Distribution of the synovial membrane from the posterior aspect demonstrating the presence of the synovial recess under the annular ligament and about the proximal ulna. (From Beethman, W. P.: Physical Examination of the Joints. Philadelphia, W. B. Saunders Co., 1965.)

capitellum and the radial head, forming the "meniscus" of the radiohumeral joint. Between the synovium and the capsule a deposit of fatty tissue occupies the coronoid and olecranon fossae (Fig. 2–13). This anatomic feature is clinically significant as the so-called fat pad sign observed on lateral radiographic views in the presence of hemarthrosis or effusion (Chapter 6).

Ligaments

The ligaments of the elbow consist of specialized thickenings of the medial and lateral capsule that form medial and lateral collateral ligament complexes.

Medial Collateral Ligament Complex

The medial collateral ligament is traditionally described as consisting of three parts: anterior, posterior, and transverse segments (Fig. 2–27). The anterior bundle is the most discrete component, the posterior portion being

a thickening of the posterior capsule, and is well-defined only in about 90 degrees of flexion. The transverse ligament appears to contribute little or nothing to elbow stability because its fibers span the medial border of the semilunar notch from the coronoid to the olecranon. Although occasionally these fibers may be rather well demonstrated, frequently the so-called transverse ligament (ligament of Cooper) can hardly be defined.

The origin of the medial collateral ligament is at the undersurface of the medial apophysis during growth and from the entire inferior surface of the medial epicondyle in the adult (Fig. 2–28). On the lateral projection the origin of the anterior bundle of the medial collateral

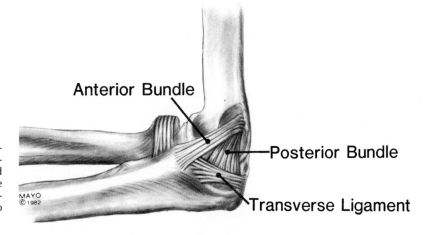

Figure 2–27. The classic orientation of the medial collateral ligament including the anterior and posterior bundles as well as the transverse ligament. This last structure contributes relatively little to elbow stability.

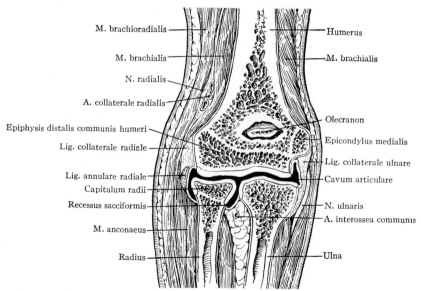

M. brachioradialis

M. brachialis

N. radialis

A. collaterale radialis

Epiphysis distalis communis humeri

Lig. collaterale radiale

Lig. annulare radiale

Capitulum radii

Recessus sacciformis

M. anconaeus

Radius

Humerus

M. brachialis

Olecranon

Epicondylus medialis

Lig. collaterale ulnare

Cavum articulare

N. ulnaris

A. interossea communis

Ulna

Figure 2–28. Sagittal view of the bones and joints of the elbow demonstrating the accurate origin of the mediocollateral ligament of the undersurface of the medial epicondyle. (From Anson, B. J., and McVay, C. B.: Surgical Anatomy. Vol. 2, 5th ed. Philadelphia, W. B. Saunders Company, 1971.)

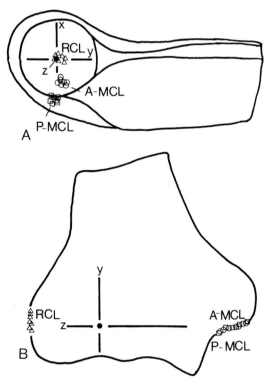

Figure 2–29. A, Lateral view of the distal aspect of the humerus demonstrating the locus of the medial and radial collateral ligaments referrable to the axis of rotation, Z. B, Frontal projection of the distal humerus showing the locus of the origin of the radial medial collateral ligaments. Note that of these various components only the radial collateral ligament lies in the axis of rotation Z, thereby explaining the length–tension relationship of these ligaments. (From Morrey, B. F., and An, K. N.: Functional Anatomy of the Elbow Ligaments. Biomechanical Assessment of the Ligaments of the Elbow. Clinical Orthopedics, in press, 1985)

ligament is just inferior to the axis of rotation, whereas the posterior component originates inferior and posterior to this axis (Fig. 2–29). The insertion of the anterior portion is along the medial aspect of the coronoid process. The posterior bundle inserts along the midportion of the medial margin of the semilunar notch. The mean length of the anterior component of the complex is about 27 mm compared with 24 mm for the posterior segment. The width of the anterior bundle is approximately 4 to 5 mm compared with 5 to 6 mm at the midportion of the fan-shaped posterior segment.[58]

The function of the ligamentous structures is discussed in detail below. The origin clearly is not along the axis of flexion as previously described;[61] thus some fibers of the anterior portion of the ligament are taut during extension[34, 67] and flexion,[58] whereas the posterior portion is taut during flexion. Clinically and experimentally, the anterior bundle is clearly the major portion of the medial ligament complex.

Lateral Ligament Complex

Unlike the rather consistent pattern of the medial collateral ligament complex, the lateral ligaments of the elbow joint are less discrete, and some individual variation is common. The radial collateral ligament is commonly described as originating from the lateral epicondyle and terminating diffusely in the annular ligament[5, 58, 42] as an ill-defined

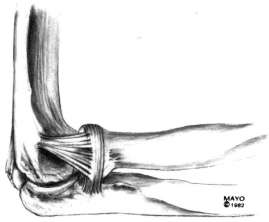

Figure 2–30. Typical perception of the lateral collateral ligament complex showing the relative thickening of the capsule that blends with the undersurface of the supinator muscle.

thickening of the capsule (Fig. 2–30). An anterior and posterior thickening has been frequently mentioned[31, 70] but is rarely demonstrable. Several investigators[29, 31, 41, 71] have described lateral ulnar attachment of components of the ligament complex in front of and behind the radial notch, but details are usually lacking. Because the lateral ligament is so variably described, we have studied the complex in our laboratory. Our investigation has suggested that several components comprise the lateral ligament complex: (1) the radial collateral ligament, (2) the lateral ulnar collateral ligament, (3) the accessory lateral collateral ligament, and (4) the annular ligament.

The Radial Collateral Ligament. This structure is not as well defined as its counterpart, the anterior bundle of the medial collateral ligament. It originates from the lateral epicondyle and terminates indistinguishably in the annular ligament (Fig. 2–31). Because its superficial aspect provides a source of origin for a portion of the supinator muscle, the dimensions of this particular segment are not readily measurable. In ten specimens the length averaged approximately 20 mm with a width of approximately 5 mm. This portion of the ligament is almost uniformly taut throughout the normal range of flexion and extension, indicating that the origin of the ligament is very near the axis of rotation, as was shown by our dissections (Fig. 2–29).

Lateral Ulnar Collateral Ligament. In five of the ten specimens, posterior fibers of the radial collateral ligament were noted to extend superficial to and across the annular ligament, terminating at a discrete attachment at the tubercle of the crista supinatoris of the ulna (Fig. 2–32). We have termed this portion the lateral ulnar collateral ligament, and its existence has been noted by others.[52]

Accessory Lateral Collateral Ligament. This definition has been applied to the ulnar insertion of discrete fibers on the tubercle of the supinator as described previously but without a demonstable contribution to the posterior portion of the radial collateral ligament. This pattern was noted in four of ten specimens. Proximally, the fibers tend to blend with the inferior margin of the annular ligament. This so-called accessory collateral ligament is taut only when varus stress is applied to the elbow and does not appear to be altered during elbow flexion and extension or pronation and supination. Its function is to further stabilize the annular ligament during varus stress. This description of the lateral collateral ligament

Figure 2–31. More detailed representation of the radial collateral ligament complex showing a portion termed the radial collateral ligament that extends from the humerus to the annular ligament. This is the portion that is most commonly meant when referring to the radial or lateral collateral ligament.

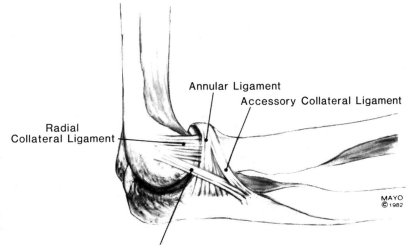

Annular Ligament

Accessory Collateral Ligament

Radial Collateral Ligament

Lateral Ulnar Collateral Ligament

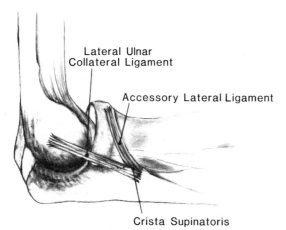

Figure 2–32. In about 50 percent of the specimens a lateral ulnar collateral ligament extends from the lateral epicondyle to the crista supinatoris.

complex is generally consistent with that of Gray and Martin.[52]

Annular Ligament. A strong band of tissue originating and inserting on the anterior and posterior margins of the lesser sigmoid notch comprises the annular ligament and maintains the radial head in contact with the ulna. The ligament is tapered distally to give the shape of a funnel and contributes about four-fifths of the fibro-osseous ring (Fig. 2–33). The structure may not be as simple as it appears. Martin has carefully studied the annular ligament in cadaver specimens and has described three layers: a deep, capsular structure; an intermediate layer forming the annular ligament proper; and a superficial portion that has been described above as the accessory lateral collateral ligament.[52] The upper margin of the ligament blends with the fibrous capsule and serves as a source of

origin of some of the oblique fibers that traverse the anterior capsule attaching to the humerus. A synovial reflection extends distal to the lower margin of the annular ligament, forming the sacciform recess. The radial head is not a pure circular disc;[72] thus, it has been observed that the anterior insertion becomes taut during supination and the posterior aspect becomes taut during extremes of pronation.[72]

A thin, fibrous layer covering the capsule between the inferior margin and the annular ligament and the ulna is referred to as the quadrate ligament[20, 59] or the ligament of Denucé.[72] Although usually described as a discrete entity, and accepted by the Nomina Anatomica Parisiensia (N.A.P.), Martin does not feel that the structure is of sufficient functional importance to warrant the designation of a ligament.[53] Spinner and Kaplan, on the other hand, have demonstrated a functional role for the structure, describing the anterior part as a stabilizer of the proximal radial ulnar joint during full supination.[72] The weaker posterior attachment stabilizes the joint in full pronation.

The oblique cord is a small and inconstant bundle of fibrous tissue formed by the fascia overlying the deep head of the supinator and extending from the lateral side of the tuberosity of the ulna to the radius just below the radial tuberosity (Fig. 2–24). Although the morphologic significance is debatable[53, 72] and the structure is not considered to be of great functional consequence,[31] it has been noted to become taut in full supination, and contracture of the oblique cord has been implicated in the etiology of idiopathic limitation of forearm supination.[12]

Bursae

Several consistent and other variably occurring bursae have been associated with the elbow joint. Lanz describes seven bursae including three associated with the triceps.[47] In general, these bursae may be described as superficial (subcutaneous) and deep. On the posterior aspect of the elbow, the superficial olecranon bursa between the olecranon process and the subcutaneous tissue is well known (Fig. 2–34). A very frequent deep intratendinous bursa is present in the substance of the triceps tendon as it inserts on the tip of the olecranon, and an occasional deep subtendinous bursa is likewise present between the tendon and the tip of the olecranon. A bursa has been described deep to the anconeus muscle in about 12 percent of subjects by

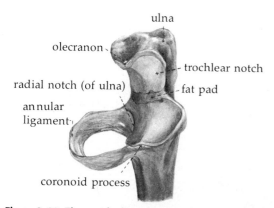

Figure 2–33. The annular ligament comprises approximately four-fifths of a complete circle and stabilizes the radial head in the radial notch of the ulna. (From Langman, J., and Woerdeman, M. W.: Atlas of Medical Anatomy. Philadelphia, W. B. Saunders Company, 1976.)

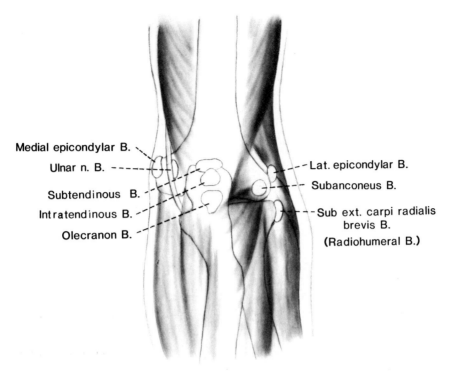

Figure 2–34. Posterior view of the elbow demonstrating the superficial and deep bursae that are present about this joint.

Henle.[36] On the medial and lateral aspects of the joint the subcutaneous medial epicondylar bursa is frequently present, and the lateral subcutaneous epicondylar bursa has been occasionally observed. The radiohumeral bursa lies deep to the common extensor tendon, below the extensor carpi radialis brevis and superficial to the radiohumeral joint capsule. This entity has been recognized and implicated by several authors[18, 62] in the etiology of lateral epicondylitis. The constant bicipito-radial bursa is known to all as the structure separating the biceps tendon from the tuberosity of the radius (Fig. 2–35). Less commonly

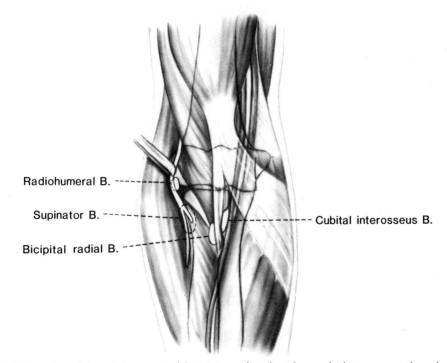

Figure 2–35. A deep view of the anterior aspect of the joint revealing the submuscular bursa present about the elbow joint.

appreciated is the deep cubital interosseous bursa lying between the lateral aspect of the biceps tendon and the ulna, brachialis, and supinator fascia. This bursa is present in about 20 percent of individuals,[71] and according to Spalteholz this structure is seen with increased frequency during later life. Finally, the uncommon occurrence of a bursa between the ulnar nerve and the medial epicondyle and margin of the triceps muscle has been mentioned by Hollinshead.[38] The clinical significance of the bursae about the elbow is described in Chapter 48.

VESSELS

Brachial Artery and Its Branches

The cross-sectional relationship of the vessels to the nerves, muscles, and bones is shown in Figure 2–36. The brachial artery descends in the arm, crossing in front of the intramus-cular septum to lie anterior to the medial aspect of the brachialis muscle. The median nerve crosses in front of and medial to the artery at this point, near the middle of the arm (Fig. 2–37). The artery continues distally at the medial margin of the biceps muscle and enters the antecubital space medial to the biceps tendon and lateral to the nerve (Fig. 2–38). At the level of the radial head, it gives off its terminal branches, the ulnar and radial arteries, which continue into the forearm.

The brachial artery is usually accompanied by medial and lateral brachial veins. Proximally, in addition to its numerous muscular and cutaneous branches, the large, deep brachial artery courses posteriorly and laterally to bifurcate into the medial and radial collateral arteries. The medial collateral artery continues posteriorly, supplying the medial head of the triceps and ultimately anastomosing with the interosseous recurrent artery at the posterior aspect of the elbow. The radial col-

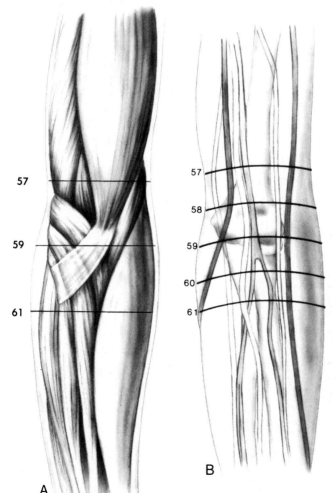

Figure 2–36. Cross-section relationships of the muscles *(A)* and the neurovascular bundles *(B).*

Illustration continued on opposite page

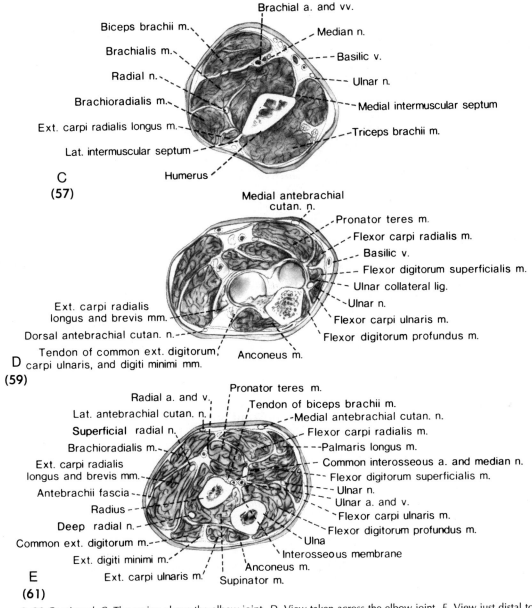

C
(57)

D
(59)

E
(61)

Figure 2–36 *Continued. C,* The region above the elbow joint. *D,* View taken across the elbow joint. *E,* View just distal to the articulation. (Redrawn from Eycleshymer, A. C., and Schoemaker, D. M.: A Cross-Section Anatomy. New York, D. Appleton and Company, 1930.)

lateral artery penetrates the lateral intermuscular septum and accompanies the radial nerve into the antecubital space, where it anastomoses with the radial recurrent artery at the level of the lateral epicondyle.

The other major branches of the brachial artery are the superior and inferior ulnar collateral arteries, which originate medial and distal to the profunda brachial artery. The superior ulnar collateral artery is given off just distal to the midportion of the brachium, penetrates the medial intermuscular septum, and accompanies the ulnar nerve to the medial epicondyle, where it terminates by anastomosing with the posterior ulnar recurrent

artery and variably with the inferior ulnar collateral artery (Fig. 2–39).

The inferior ulnar collateral artery arises from the medial aspect of the brachial artery about 4 cm proximal to the medial epicondyle. It continues distally for a short course, dividing into and anastomosing with branches of the anterior ulnar recurrent artery, and it supplies a portion of the pronator teres muscle. The vascular contribution of the brachial artery to the elbow joint is so variable that no two specimens studied by Polonskaja exhibited the same pattern. Hence, no discrete description of this circulation is available.

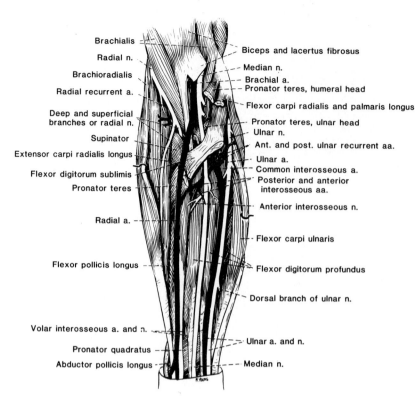

Figure 2–37. Anterior aspect of the elbow region demonstrating the intricate relationships between the muscles, nerves, and vessels. (From Hollinshead, W. H.: The back and limbs. *In* Anatomy for Surgeons. Vol. 3 New York, Harper and Rowe, 1969, pp. 379–384.)

Radial Artery

In most instances, the radial artery originates at the level of the radial head, emerges from the antecubital space between the brachioradialis and the pronator teres muscle, and continues down the forearm under the brachioradialis muscle. A more proximal origin occurs in up to 15 percent of individuals.[54] The radial recurrent artery originates laterally from the radial artery just distal to its origin.

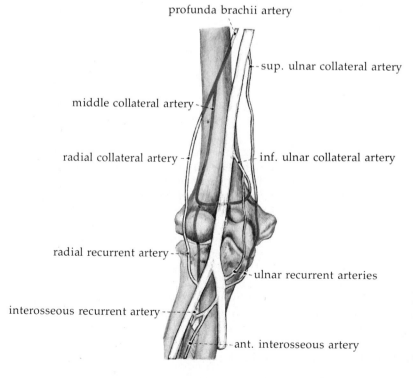

Figure 2–38. The anterior arterial vascular network about the elbow proximally and distally. (From Langman, J., and Woerdeman, M. W.: Atlas of Medical Anatomy. Philadelphia, W. B. Saunders Company, 1976.)

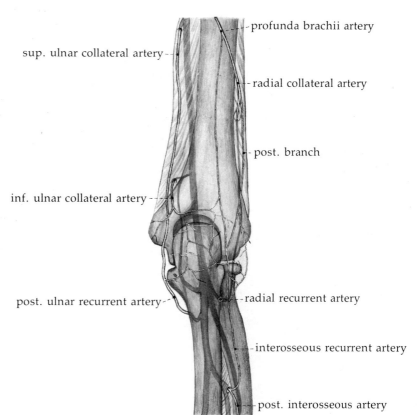

profunda brachii artery

sup. ulnar collateral artery

radial collateral artery

post. branch

inf. ulnar collateral artery

post. ulnar recurrent artery

radial recurrent artery

interosseous recurrent artery

post. interosseous artery

Figure 2–39. Posterior view of the elbow demonstrating the vascular anastomoses about the elbow region. (From Langman, J., and Woerdeman, M. W.: Atlas of Medical Anatomy. Philadelphia, W. B. Saunders Company, 1976.)

It ascends laterally on the supinator muscle to anastomose with the radial collateral artery at the level of the lateral epicondyle, to which it provides circulation. The radial recurrent artery is sometimes sacrificed with the anterior extensile exposure as described by Henry.

Ulnar Artery

The ulnar artery is the largest of the two terminal branches of the brachial artery. There is relatively little variation in its origin, which is usually at the level of the radial head. The artery traverses the pronator teres between its two heads and continues distally and medially behind the flexor digitorum superficialis muscle. It emerges medially to continue down the medial aspect of the forearm under the cover of the flexor carpi ulnaris. Two recurrent branches originate just distal to the origin of the ulnar artery. The anterior ulnar recurrent artery ascends deep to the humeral head of the pronator teres and deep to the medial aspect of the brachialis muscle to anastomose with the descending superior and inferior ulnar collateral arteries. The posterior ulnar recurrent artery originates with or just distal to the smaller anterior ulnar recurrent artery. The vessel then passes proximal and posterior between the superficial and deep flexors pos-

terior to the medial epicondyle. This artery continues proximally with the ulnar nerve under the flexor carpi ulnaris to anastomose with the superior ulnar collateral artery. Additional extensive communication with the inferior ulnar and middle collateral branches constitutes the rete articulare cubiti (Fig. 2–38).

The common interosseous artery is a large vessel originating 2½ cm distal to the origin of the ulnar artery. It passes posterior and distal between the flexor pollicis longus and the flexor digitorum profundus just distal to the oblique cord, dividing into anterior and posterior interosseous branches. The interosseous recurrent artery originates from the posterior interosseous branch. This artery runs proximally through the supinator muscle to anastomose with the vascular network of the olecranon (Fig. 2–39).

NERVES

Specific clinical and pertinent anatomic aspects of the nerves in the region of the elbow are discussed in subsequent chapters as appropriate. Although there are many anatomic variations,[39, 40, 48] a general survey of the common relative patterns and anatomy is given here (see Fig. 2–36).

Musculocutaneous Nerve

This nerve originates from C5–8 nerve roots and is a continuation of the lateral cord. The musculocutaneous nerve innervates the major elbow flexors, the biceps and brachialis, and continues through the brachial fascia lateral to the biceps tendon, terminating as the lateral antebrachial cutaneous nerve (Fig. 2–40). The motor branch enters the biceps approximately 15 cm distal to the acromion; it enters the brachialis approximately 20 cm below the tip of the acromion.[48]

Median Nerve

The median nerve arises from the C5–8 and T1 nerve roots. The nerve enters the anterior aspect of the brachium, crossing in front of the brachial artery as it passes across the intermuscular septum. It follows a straight course into the medial aspect of the antecubital fossa, medial to the biceps tendon and to the brachial artery. It then passes under the bicipital aponeurosis. The first motor branch is given to the pronator teres, through which it passes; this relationship is discussed in detail by Jamieson and Anson (Fig. 2–41).[2, 40] It enters the forearm and continues distally under the flexor digitorum superficialis within the fascial sheath of this muscle.

There are no branches of the median nerve in the arm (Fig. 2–42). In the cubital fossa a few small articular branches are given off before the motor branches to the pronator

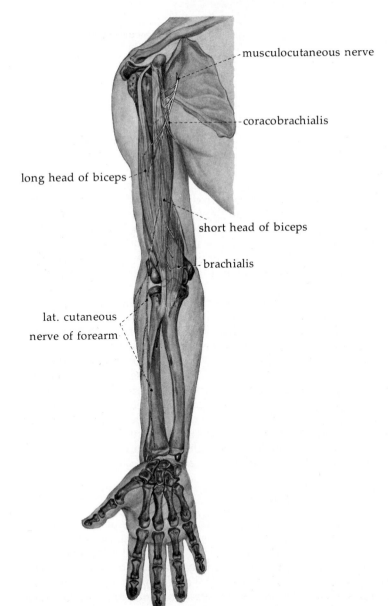

musculocutaneous nerve

coracobrachialis

long head of biceps

short head of biceps

brachialis

lat. cutaneous
nerve of forearm

Figure 2–40. The musculocutaneous nerve innervates the flexors of the elbow and continues distal to the joint as the lateral cutaneous nerve of the forearm. (From Langman, J., and Woerdeman, M. W.: Atlas of Medical Anatomy. Philadelphia, W. B. Saunders Company, 1976.)

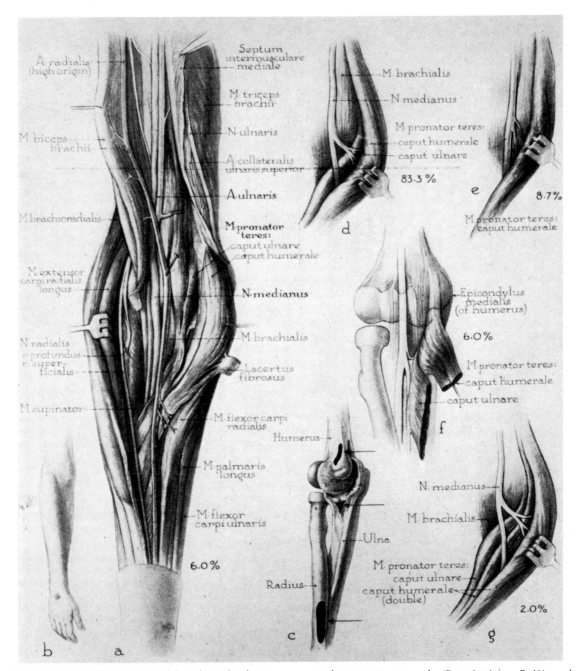

Figure 2–41. Relative frequency of the relationship between nerve and pronator teres muscle. (From Jamieson, R. W., and Anson, B. J.: Relation of the median nerve to the heads of origin of the pronator teres muscle: A study of 300 specimens. Quart. Bull., Northwestern University Medical School, 26:34–38, 1952.)

teres, the flexor carpi radialis, the palmaris longus, and the flexor digitorum superficialis. All of these arise medially, thus allowing safe medial retraction of the nerve during exposure of the anterior aspect of the elbow.

The anterior interosseous nerve arises from the median nerve near the inferior border of the pronator teres and travels along the anterior aspect of the interosseous membrane in the company of the anterior interosseous artery. This branch innervates the flexor pollicis longus and the lateral portion of the flexor digitorum profundus.

Radial Nerve

The radial nerve is a continuation of the posterior cord and originates from the C6, C7, and C8 nerve roots with variable contribu-

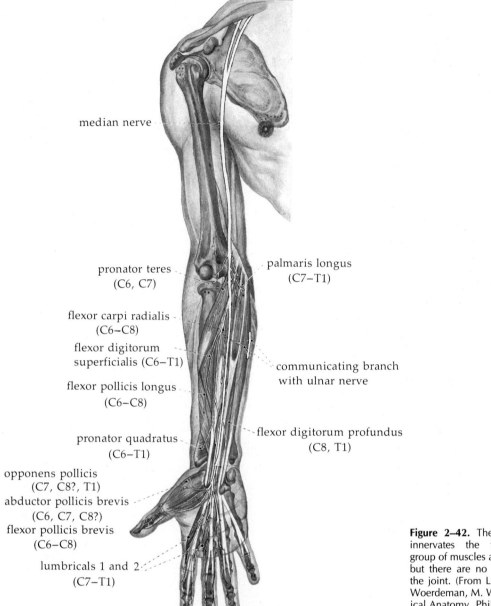

median nerve

pronator teres
(C6, C7)

palmaris longus
(C7–T1)

flexor carpi radialis
(C6–C8)

flexor digitorum
superficialis (C6–T1)

communicating branch
with ulnar nerve

flexor pollicis longus
(C6–C8)

pronator quadratus
(C6–T1)

flexor digitorum profundus
(C8, T1)

opponens pollicis
(C7, C8?, T1)
abductor pollicis brevis
(C6, C7, C8?)
flexor pollicis brevis
(C6–C8)

lumbricals 1 and 2
(C7–T1)

Figure 2–42. The median nerve
innervates the flexor pronator
group of muscles about the elbow,
but there are no branches above
the joint. (From Langman, J., and
Woerdeman, M. W.: Atlas of Medical Anatomy. Philadelphia, W. B.
Saunders Company, 1976.)

tions of the C5 and T1 roots. In the midportion
of the arm the nerve courses laterally to occupy the groove in the humerus that bears its
name. It then emerges in a spiral path inferiorly and laterally to penetrate the lateral intermuscular septum. Before entering the anterior aspect of the arm it gives off motor
branches to the medial and lateral head of the
triceps, accompanied by the deep branch of
the brachial artery. After penetrating the lateral intermuscular septum in the distal third
of the arm, it descends anterior to the lateral
epicondyle behind the brachioradialis and
brachialis. It innervates the brachioradialis

with a single branch to this muscle. In the
antecubital space the nerve divides into the
superficial and deep branches. The superficial
branch is a continuation of the radial nerve
and extends into the forearm to innervate the
mid-dorsal cutaneous aspect of the forearm
(Fig. 2–43).

The motor branches of the radial nerve are
given off to the triceps above the spiral
groove except for the branch to the medial
head of the triceps, which originates at the
entry to the spiral groove. This branch continues distally through the medial head to terminate as a muscular branch to the anconeus.

Hence, surgical approaches that reflect the anconeus[13, 44, 63] can be performed while preserving the innervation of the muscle.

In the antecubital space the recurrent radial nerve curves around the posterior lateral aspect of the radius, passing deep to the supinator muscle, which it innervates. During its course through the supinator muscle the nerve lies over a "bare area," which is distal to and opposite to the radial tuberosity.[22] The nerve is felt to be at risk at this site with fractures of the proximal radius. It emerges from the muscle as the posterior interosseous nerve, and the recurrent branch innervates the extensor digitorum minimi, the extensor carpi ulnaris, and occasionally, the anconeus. The posterior interosseous nerve is accompanied by the posterior interosseous artery and sends further muscle branches distally to supply the abductor pollicis longus, the extensor pollicis longus, the extensor pollicis brevis, and the extensor indicis on the dor-

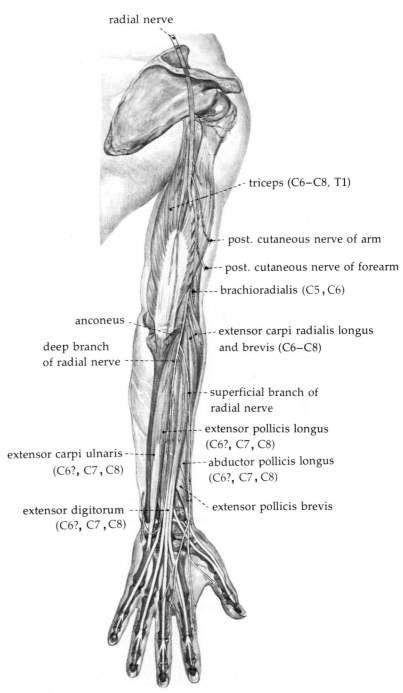

radial nerve

triceps (C6–C8, T1)

post. cutaneous nerve of arm

post. cutaneous nerve of forearm

brachioradialis (C5, C6)

anconeus

deep branch of radial nerve

extensor carpi radialis longus and brevis (C6–C8)

superficial branch of radial nerve

extensor pollicis longus (C6?, C7, C8)

extensor carpi ulnaris (C6?, C7, C8)

abductor pollicis longus (C6?, C7, C8)

extensor digitorum (C6?, C7, C8)

extensor pollicis brevis

Figure 2–43. The muscles innervated by the right radial nerve. (From Langman, J., and Woerdeman, M. W.: Atlas of Medical Anatomy. Philadelphia, W. B. Saunders Company, 1976.)

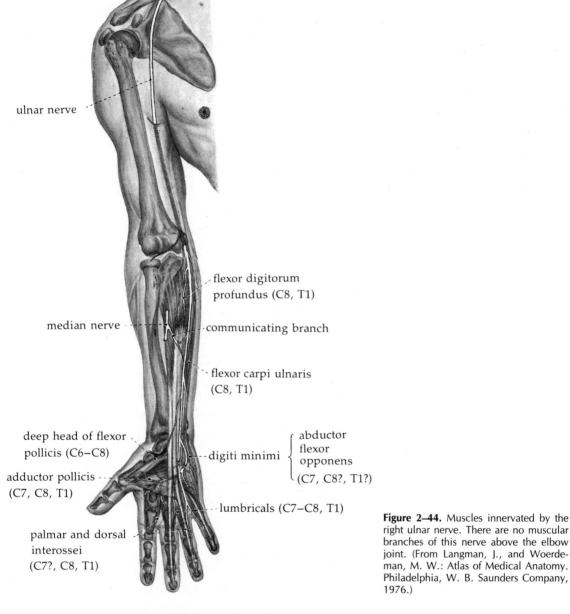

ulnar nerve

flexor digitorum
profundus (C8, T1)

median nerve

communicating branch

flexor carpi ulnaris
(C8, T1)

deep head of flexor
pollicis (C6–C8)

digiti minimi { abductor
flexor
opponens
(C7, C8?, T1?)

adductor pollicis
(C7, C8, T1)

lumbricals (C7–C8, T1)

palmar and dorsal
interossei
(C7?, C8, T1)

Figure 2–44. Muscles innervated by the right ulnar nerve. There are no muscular branches of this nerve above the elbow joint. (From Langman, J., and Woerdeman, M. W.: Atlas of Medical Anatomy. Philadelphia, W. B. Saunders Company, 1976.)

sum of the forearm. The nerve is subject to compression as it passes through the supinator muscle[17] or from synovial proliferation.[27] Compression and entrapment problems are described in detail in Chapter 45.

Ulnar Nerve

The ulnar nerve is derived from the medial cord of the brachial plexus from roots C8 and T1. In the midarm it passes posteriorly through the medial intermuscular septum and continues distally along the medial margin of the triceps in the company of the superior ulnar collateral branch of the brachial artery and the ulnar collateral branch of the radial

artery. There are no branches of this nerve in the brachium (Fig. 2–44). The ulnar nerve passes into the cubital tunnel under the medial epicondyle and rests against the posterior portion of the medial collateral ligament, where a groove in the ligament accommodates this structure. This relationship accounts for the well-recognized vulnerability of the nerve to compression and entrapment.[72] Similarly, elbow instability can compromise the integrity of the nerve.[51] A few small twigs are given to the elbow joint in this region and are the most obvious source of innervation of the capsule.[9] The first motor branch is a single nerve to the ulnar origin and another one to the epicondylar head of the flexor carpi ulnaris. Distally, the nerve sends a motor branch to the ulnar half of the flexor digitorum profundus. Two cutaneous nerves arise from the ulnar nerve in the distal half of the forearm and innervate the skin of the wrist and the hand.

MUSCLES

Relevant features of the origin, insertion, and function of the muscles of the elbow region are covered in other chapters dealing with surgical exposure, functional examination, and biomechanics. This information is also discussed in various chapters when dealing with specific pathology. The following description will serve as a simple overview of the origin, insertion, and function of the major musculature that crosses the elbow joint. The

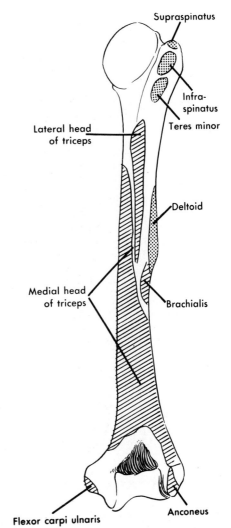

Figure 2–46. Posterior view of the humerus demonstrating the broad surface over which the origin of the triceps takes place.

origin and insertion of these muscle groups are illustrated in Figures 2–45 and 2–46, and the superficial musculature is shown in Figures 2–47 and 2–48.

Elbow Flexors

Biceps

The biceps covers the brachialis muscle in the distal arm and passes into the cubital fossa as the biceps tendon, which attaches to the posterior aspect of the radial tuberosity (Fig. 2–49). The constant bicipitoradial bursa separates the tendon from the anterior aspect of the tuberosity, and an interosseous cubital bursa has been described as separating the tendon from the ulna and the muscles covering the radius (Fig. 2–35). The bicipital aponeurosis, or lacertus fibrosus, is a broad, thin

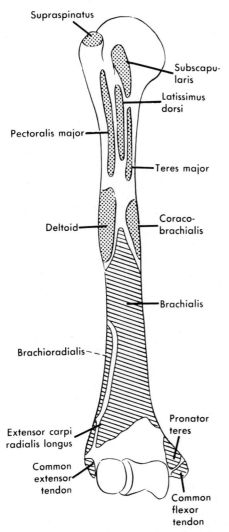

Figure 2–45. Anterior humeral origin and insertion of muscles that control the elbow joint.

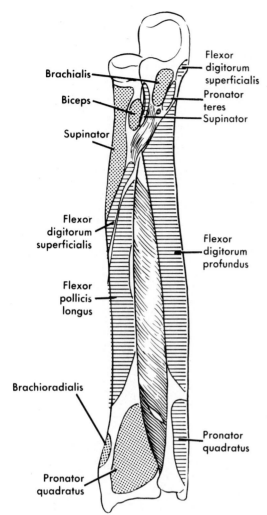

Figure 2–47. Anterior view of the radius and ulna demonstrating the insertion of the major motors of the elbow joint.

Brachialis

This muscle has the largest cross-sectional area of any of the elbow flexors but suffers from a poor mechanical advantage because it crosses so close to the axis of rotation. The origin consists of the entire anterior distal half of the humerus, and it extends medially and laterally to the respective intermuscular septa (Fig. 2–45). The muscle crosses the anterior capsule with some fibers inserting into the capsule that are said to help retract the capsule during elbow flexion. More than 95 percent of the cross-sectional area is muscle tissue at the elbow joint,[50] a relationship that accounts for the high incidence of trauma to this muscle and the development of myositis ossificans with elbow dislocation.[78] The insertion of the brachialis is along the base of the coronoid and into the tuberosity of the ulna.

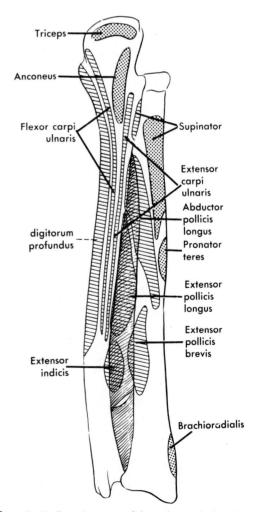

band of tissue that is a continuation of the anterior medial and distal muscle fasciae. It runs obliquely to cover the median nerve and brachial artery and inserts into the deep fasciae of the forearm and possibly into the ulna as well.[19] As the elbow is flexed to 90 degrees, the medial margin of the bicipital aponeurosis is readily palpable along the medial aspect of the cubital fossa.

The biceps is a major flexor of the elbow that has a large cross-sectional area but an intermediate mechanical advantage because it passes relatively close to the axis of rotation. In the pronated position the biceps is a strong supinator, but in this position it is probably unable to play a simultaneous major role as an elbow flexor.[7] The distal insertion occasionally undergoes spontaneous rupture,[57] and this condition is discussed in detail later (Chapter 26).

Figure 2–48. Posterior view of the radius and ulna demonstrating the insertion of the extensors of the elbow as well as the origin of the forearm musculature.

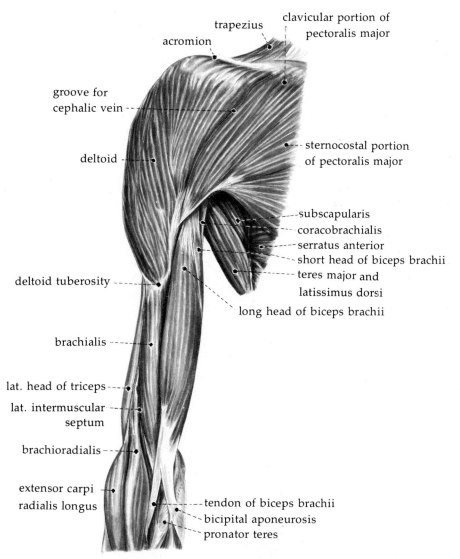

Figure 2–49. Anterior aspect of the arm and elbow region demonstrating the major flexors of the joint, the brachialis, and biceps muscles. (From Langman, J., and Woerdeman, M. W.: Atlas of Medical Anatomy. Philadelphia, W. B. Saunders Company, 1976.)

The muscle is innervated by the musculo-cutaneous nerve, and the lateral portion covers the radial nerve as it spirals around the distal humerus. The median nerve and brachial artery are superficial to the brachialis and lie behind the biceps in the distal humerus.

Brachioradialis

The brachioradialis has a lengthy origin along the lateral supracondylar bony column that extends proximally to the level of the junction of the mid and distal humerus (Fig. 2–45). The origin separates the lateral head of the triceps and the brachialis muscle. The lateral border of the cubital fossa is formed by this muscle, which crosses the elbow joint with the greatest mechanical advantage of any elbow flexor. It covers the proximal origin of the flexor carpi radialis longus (Fig. 2–50) and progresses distally to insert into the base of the radial styloid (Fig. 2–48). The muscle protects and is innervated by the radial nerve (C5, C6) as it emerges from the spiral groove. Its major function is elbow flexion. A possible role as a pronator and supinator has been debated,[38] but there are no conclusive data to resolve this issue. Rarely, the muscle may be ruptured.[35] The function of the muscle is further discussed in Chapter 3.

Extensor Carpi Radialis Longus

The extensor carpi radialis longus originates from the supracondylar bony column joint

just below the origin of the brachioradialis
(Fig. 2–50). The origin of this muscle is intermediate between the brachialis and the extensor carpi radialis brevis, being covered by the
former and in turn covering the latter. As it
continues into the midportion of the dorsum
of the forearm, it becomes largely tendinous
and inserts into the dorsal base of the second
metacarpal. Innervated by the radial nerve
(C6, C7), the motor branches arise just distal
to those of the brachioradialis muscle.

In addition to wrist extension, its orientation suggests that this muscle might function
as an elbow flexor. Its possible role as a
pronator and a supinator has likewise been
considered and is discussed in Chapter 3.

Clinically, the origin of this muscle and its
relationship with that of the extensor carpi
radialis brevis have been implicated in the
pathologic anatomy of tennis elbow by
Nirschl (Chapter 28).

Extensor Carpi Radialis Brevis

The extensor carpi radialis brevis originates
from the lateral inferior aspect of the lateral
epicondyle (Fig. 2–45). Its origin is the most
lateral of the extensor group and is covered
by the extensor carpi radialis longus. This
relationship is considered important by
Nirschl for the proper assessment of the pathologic anatomy of lateral epicondylitis, which
often involves the origin of this muscle at the
lateral epicondyle. The extensor digitorum
communis originates from the common extensor tendon and is just medial or ulnar to the
extensor carpi radialis brevis. In the proximal
forearm, the muscle fibers of the extensor
carpi radialis longus and the extensor digitorum are almost indistinguishable from those
of the extensor carpi radialis brevis (Fig.
2–50). The latter muscle shares the same extensor compartment as the longus as it crosses

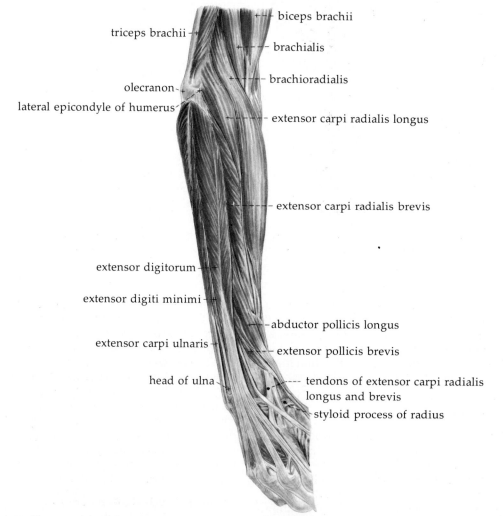

Figure 2–50. The musculature of the posterolateral aspect of the right forearm. (From Langman, J., and Woerdeman, M. W.:
Atlas of Medical Anatomy. Philadelphia, W. B. Saunders Company, 1976.)

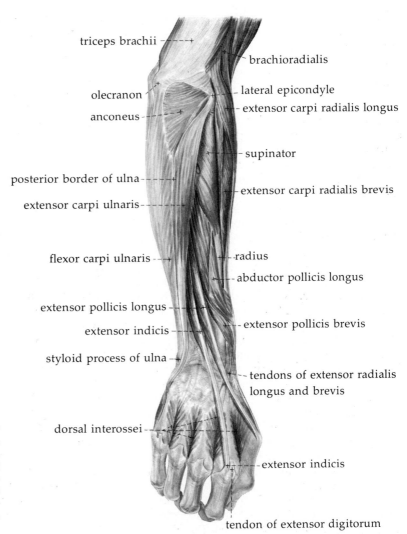

triceps brachii

brachioradialis

olecranon

lateral epicondyle

anconeus

extensor carpi radialis longus

supinator

posterior border of ulna

extensor carpi radialis brevis

extensor carpi ulnaris

flexor carpi ulnaris

radius

abductor pollicis longus

extensor pollicis longus

extensor pollicis brevis

extensor indicis

styloid process of ulna

tendons of extensor radialis
longus and brevis

dorsal interossei

extensor indicis

tendon of extensor digitorum

Figure 2–51. The extensor aspect of the forearm demonstrating the deep muscle layer after the extensor digitorum and extensor digiti minimi have been removed. (From Langman, J., and Woerdeman, M. W.: Atlas of Medical Anatomy. Philadelphia, W. B. Saunders Company, 1976.)

the wrist under the extensor retinaculum and inserts into the dorsal base of the third metacarpal. The function of the extensor carpi radialis brevis is pure wrist extension with little or no radial or ulnar deviation, although in selected functions radial deviation has been attributed to the muscle.[1] The extensor carpi radialis brevis is innervated by fibers of the sixth and seventh cervical nerves. The motor branch arises from the radial nerve in the region of its division into deep and superficial branches.

Extensor Digitorum Communis

Originating from the anterior distal aspect of the lateral epicondyle, the extensor digitorum communis accounts for most of the contour of the extensor surface of the forearm (Fig. 2–50). With a variable pattern of division, the three or four extensor tendons pass under the extensor retinaculum in a common compartment and contribute to the complex extensor

mechanism of the second through fifth fingers. The muscle extends and abducts the fingers. According to Wright, the muscle can assist in elbow flexion when the forearm is pronated. This observation is not, however, confirmed by our cross-sectional studies.[1] The innervation is from the deep branch of the radial nerve with contributions from the sixth through eighth cervical nerves.

Extensor Carpi Ulnaris

The extensor carpi ulnaris originates from two heads, one above and the other below the elbow joint. The humeral origin is the most medial of the common extensor group (Figs. 2–45 and 2–51). The ulnar attachment is along the aponeurosis of the anconeus and at the superior border of this muscle. The insertion is on the dorsal base of the fifth metacarpal after crossing the wrist in its own compartment under the extensor retinaculum. The extensor carpi ulnaris is a wrist extensor and ulnar deviator. Fibers of the sixth through eighth cervical nerve routes innervate the muscle from branches of the deep radial nerve.

Supinator

This flat muscle is characterized by the virtual absence of tendinous tissue and a complex origin and insertion. It originates from three sites above and below the elbow joint: (1) the lateral anterior aspect of the lateral epicondyle; (2) the lateral collateral ligament; and (3) the proximal anterior crest of the ulna along the crista supinatoris, which is just anterior to the depression for the insertion of the anconeus. The form of the muscle is approximately that of a rhomboid as it runs obliquely, distally, and radially to wrap around and insert diffusely on the proximal radius, beginning lateral and proximal to the radial tuberosity and continuing distal to the insertion of the pronator teres at the junction of the proximal and middle third of the radius (Fig. 2–51). It is important that the radial nerve passes through the supinator to gain access to the extensor surface of the forearm. This anatomic feature is clinically significant with regard to exposure of the lateral aspect of the elbow joint and the proximal radius and in certain entrapment syndromes.[72]

The muscle obviously supinates the forearm and is generally considered a weaker supinator than the biceps.[38] Our clinical data support this position (Chapter 3). Unlike the biceps, however, the effectiveness of the supinator is not altered by the position of elbow flexion. The innervation is derived from the muscular branch given off by the radial nerve just prior to and during its course through the muscle with nerve fibers derived primarily from the sixth cervical root.

Elbow Extensors

Triceps Brachii

The entire posterior musculature of the arm is composed of the triceps brachii (Fig. 2–43). Two of its three heads originate from the posterior aspect of the humerus (Fig. 2–46). The long head has a discrete origin from the infraglenoid tuberosity of the scapula. The lateral head originates in a linear fashion from the proximal lateral intramuscular septum on the posterior surface of the humerus. The medial head originates from the entire distal half of the posterior medial surface of the humerus bounded laterally by the radial

groove and medially by the intramuscular septum. Thus, each head originates distal to the other with progressively larger areas of origin. The long and lateral heads are superficial to the deep medial head, blending in the midline of the humerus to form a common muscle that then tapers into the triceps tendon and attaches to the tip of the olecranon with Sharpey's fibers. The tendon is usually separated from the olecranon by the subtendinous olecranon bursa. The distal 40 percent of the triceps mechanism consists of a layer of fascia that blends with the triceps distally. This is the structure reflected when the Campbell posterior approach to the elbow joint is used (see Chapter 8).

Innervated by the radial nerve, the long and lateral heads are supplied by branches that arise proximal to the entrance of the radial nerve into the groove. The medial head is innervated distal to the groove with a branch that enters proximally and passes through the entire medial head to terminate by innervating the anconeus, an anatomic feature of considerable importance when considering some approaches (e.g., Kocher, Bryan, Boyd, and Pankovitch) to the joint.

The function of the triceps is to extend the elbow. Lesions of the nerve in the midportion of the humerus do not usually prevent triceps function that is provided by the more proximally innervated lateral and long heads. The long head also serves to extend and adduct the humerus owing to its insertion across the glenohumeral joint.[38]

Anconeus

This muscle has little tendinous tissue because it originates from a rather broad site on the posterior aspect of the lateral epicondyle and inserts into the lateral dorsal surface of the proximal ulna (Fig. 2–51). It is innervated by the terminal branch of the nerve to the medial head of the triceps. Curiously, the function of this muscle has been the subject of considerable speculation. Travell[81] considered the anconeus an extensor of the elbow, but the function of abduction[23, 65] during pronation has likewise been attributed to this muscle. The most recent and possibly most accurate description of the anconeus function is that proposed by Basmajian and Griffin and by DaHora, who suggest that its primary role is that of a joint stabilizer. The muscle covers the lateral portion of the annular ligament and the radial head. For the surgeon, the major significance of this muscle is its position as a key landmark in various lateral and posterolateral exposures of the elbow joint.

Flexor Pronator Muscle Group

Pronator Teres

This is the most proximal of the flexor pronator group. There are usually two heads of origin; the largest arises from the anterior-superior aspect of the medial epicondyle and the second from the coronoid process of the ulna, which is absent in about 10 percent of individuals (Fig. 2–41).[40] The two origins of the pronator muscle provide an arch through which the median nerve typically passes to gain access to the forearm. This anatomic characteristic is a significant feature in the etiology of the median nerve entrapment syndrome and is discussed in detail in Chapter 45. The common muscle belly proceeds radially and distally under the brachioradialis, inserting at the junction of the proximal and middle portions of the radius by a discrete broad tendinous insertion into a tuberosity on the lateral aspect of the bone. Obviously a strong pronator of the forearm, it also is a weak flexor of the elbow joint.[1, 8] The muscle is usually innervated by two motor branches from the median nerve before the nerve leaves the cubital fossa.

Flexor Carpi Radialis

The flexor carpi radialis originates just inferior to the origin of the pronator teres and the common flexor tendon at the anterior-inferior aspect of the medial epicondyle (Fig. 2–45). It continues distally and radially to the wrist, where it can be readily palpated before it inserts into the base of the second and sometimes the third metacarpal. Proximally, the muscle belly partially covers the pronator teres and palmaris longus muscles and shares a common origin from the intermuscular septum, which it shares with these muscles. The innervation is from one or two twigs of the median nerve (C6, C7), and its chief function is as a wrist flexor. At the elbow no significant flexion moment is present,[1] but with the elbow flexed, it has been reported to assist with forearm pronation.[23]

Palmaris Longus

This muscle, when present, arises from the medial epicondyle and from the septa it shares with the flexor carpi radialis and flexor carpi ulnaris (Fig. 2–42). It becomes tendinous in the proximal portion of the forearm and inserts into and becomes continuous with the palmar aponeurosis. Morphologic variations of the muscle have been reported in about 10 percent of people, and it is absent in an additional 10 percent of extremities.[66] Its major function is wrist flexion and as a donor tendon for reconstructive surgery, and it is innervated by a branch of the median nerve.

Flexor Carpi Ulnaris

The flexor carpi ulnaris is the most posterior of the common flexor tendons originating from the medial epicondyle (Figs. 2–42 and 2–45). A second and larger source of origin is from the medial border of the coronoid and the proximal medial aspect of the ulna. The ulnar nerve enters and innervates (T7–8 and T1) the muscle between these two sites of origin with two or three motor branches given off just after the nerve has entered the muscle. These are the first motor branches of the ulnar nerve, and the function of the flexor carpi ulnaris is therefore useful in localizing the level of an ulnar nerve lesion. The muscle continues distally to insert into the pisiform, where the tendon is easily palpable because it serves as a wrist flexor and ulnar deviator. With an origin posterior to the axis of rotation, weak elbow extension may also be provided by the flexor carpi ulnaris.[1] It is significant that in the forearm the muscle covers the ulnar nerve and the accompanying artery, which lies superficial to the flexor digitorum profundus. By elevating the common flexor tendon and fascia, the ulnar nerve can be translated submuscularly as an effective means of treatment of the ulnar nerve entrapment syndrome (see Chapter 45).

Flexor Digitorum Superficialis

This muscle is deep to those originating from the common flexor tendon but superficial to the flexor digitorum profundus; thus, it is considered the intermediate muscle layer. This broad muscle has a complex origin (Fig. 2–52). Medially, it arises from the medial epicondyle by way of the common flexor tendon and possibly from the ulnar collateral ligament and the medial aspect of the coronoid.[38] The lateral head is smaller and thinner and arises from the proximal two thirds of the radius. The two origins converge to form the common muscle, which descends over the volar aspect of the forearm and divides into the four flexor tendons, which insert into the base of the middle phalanx of the second through fifth fingers. The unique origin of the muscle forms a fibrous margin under which

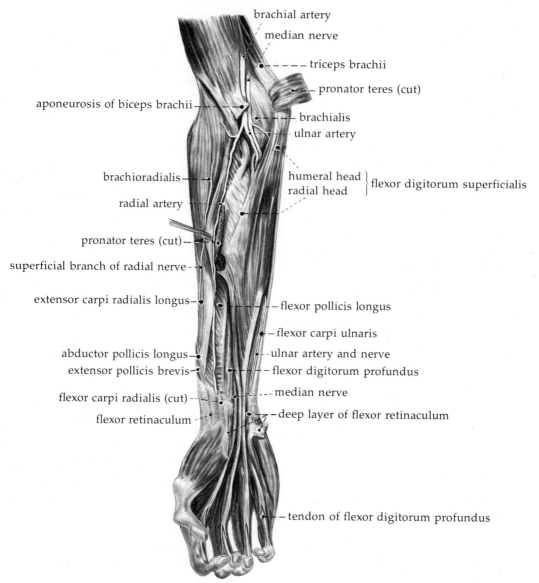

Figure 2–52. The flexor digitorum superficialis is demonstrated after the palmaris longus and flexor carpi radialis had been removed. The pronator teres has been transected and reflected. The important relationships of the nerves and arteries should be noted. (From Langman, J., and Woerdeman, M. W.: Atlas of Medical Anatomy. Philadelphia, W. B. Saunders Company, 1976.)

the median nerve and the ulnar artery emerge as they exit from the cubital fossa. These two structures occupy the interval between the superficial and deep flexor muscles in the forearm. The muscle is innervated by the median nerve (C7, C8, T1) with branches that originate before the median nerve enters the pronator teres. The action of the flexor digitorum superficialis is flexion of the proximal interphalangeal joints.

Flexor Digitorum Profundus

The flexor digitorum profundus originates from the proximal ulna distal to the elbow

joint and will be discussed only as appropriate for the given topic in subsequent chapters.

References

1. An, K. N., Hui, F. C., Morrey, B. F., Linscheid, R. L., and Chao, E. Y.: Muscles Across the Elbow Joint: A Biomechanical Analysis. J. Biomechan., **14(10)**:659–669, 1981.
2. Anson, B. J., and McVay, C. B.: Surgical Anatomy, 5th ed., vol. 2. Philadelphia, W. B. Saunders, 1971.
3. Atkinson, W. B., and Elftman, H.: The Carrying Angle of the Human Arm as a Secondary Sex Character. Anat. Rec., **91**:49, 1945.
4. Barnard, L. B., and McCoy, S. M.: The Supracondyloid Process of the Humerus. J. Bone Joint Surg., **28(4)**:845–850, 1946.

5. Basmajian, J. V.: The Unsung Virtues of Ligaments. Surg. Clin. North Am., **54(6)**:1259–1267, 1974.
6. Basmajian, J. V., and Griffin, W. R.: Function of Anconeus Muscle. J. Bone Joint Surg., **54A**:1712–1714, 1972.
7. Basmajian, J. V., and Latif, A.: Integrated Actions and Functions of the Two Flexors of the Elbow—A Detailed Myographic Analysis. J. Bone Joint Surg., **39A**:1106, 1957.
8. Basmajian, J. V., and Travell, A.: Electromyography of the Pronator Muscles in the Forearm. Anat. Rec., **139**:45, 1961.
9. Bateman, J. E.: Denervation of the Elbow Joint for the Relief of Pain—A Preliminary Report. J. Bone Joint Surg., **30B**:635, 1948.
10. Beals, R. K.: The Normal Carrying Angle of the Elbow. Clin. Orthop. Rel. Res., **119**:194–196, 1976.
11. Beetham, W. P.: Physical Examination of the Joints. Philadelphia, W. B. Saunders, 1965.
12. Bert, J. M., Linscheid, R. L., and McElfresh, E. C.: Rotatory Contracture of the Forearm. J. Bone Joint Surg., **62A**:1163–1168, 1980.
13. Boyd, H. B.: Surgical Exposure of the Ulna and Proximal Third of the Radius Through One Incision. Surg. Gynec. Obstet., **71**:86, 1940.
14. Boyd, H. D., and Anderson, L. D.: A Method for Reinsertion of the Biceps Tendon Brachii Tendon. J. Bone Joint Surg., **43A**:1141, 1961.
15. Bryan, R. S., and Morrey, B. F.: Extensive Posterior Exposure of the Elbow—A Triceps-Sparing Approach. Clin. Orthop., **166**:188–192, 1982.
16. Campbell, W. C.: Incision for Exposure of the Elbow Joint. Am. J. Surg., **15**:65, 1932.
17. Capener, N.: The Vulnerability of the Posterior Interosseous Nerve of the Forearm—A Case Report and Anatomic Study. J. Bone Joint Surg., **48B**:770, 1966.
18. Carp, L.: Tennis Elbow (Epicondylitis) Caused by Radiohumeral Bursitis. Arch. Surg., **24**:905–922, 1932.
19. Congdon, E. D., and Fish, H. S.: The Chief Insertion of the Biceps After Neurosis in the Ulna: A Study of Collagenous Bundle Patterns of Antebrachial Fascia and Bicepital Aponeurosis. Anat. Rec., **116**:395, 1953.
20. Cunningham, D. J.: Textbook of Anatomy, 12th ed. Edited by G. J. Romanes. New York, Oxford University Press, 1981.
21. DaHora, B.: Musculus Anconeus. Thesis, University of Recife, Recife, Brazil, 1959. Cited by Basmajian, J. V., and Griffin, W. R.: J. Bone Joint Surg., **54A**:1712–1714, 1972.
22. Davies, F., and Laird, M.: The Supinator Muscle and the Deep Radial (Posterior Interosseous Nerve). Anat. Rec., **101**:243, 1948.
23. Duchenne, G. B.: Physiology of Motion. Translated and edited by E. B. Kaplan. Philadelphia, J. B. Lippincott, 1949.
24. Ekholm, R., and Ingelmark, B. E.: Functional Thickness Variations of Human Articular Cartilage. Acta Societ. Medicor. Upsaliensis, **57**:39–59, 1952.
25. Evans, E. M.: Rotational Deformity in the Treatment of Fractures of Both Bones of the Forearm. J. Bone Joint Surg., **27**:373–379, 1945.
26. Eycleshymer, A. C., and Schoemaker, D. M.: A Cross-Section Anatomy. New York, D. Appleton, 1930.
27. Field, J. H.: Posterior Interosseous Nerve Palsy Secondary to Synovial Chondromatosis of the Elbow Joint. J. Hand Surg., **6(4)**:336–338, 1981.
28. Gardner, E.: The Innervation of the Elbow Joint. Anat. Rec., **102**:161–174, 1948.
29. Grant, J. C. B.: Atlas of Anatomy, 6th ed. Baltimore, Williams & Wilkins, 1972.
30. Grant, J. C. B.: Method of Anatomy, 6th ed. Edited by J. V. Basmajian. Baltimore, Williams & Wilkins, 1980.
31. Gray, H.: Anatomy, Descriptive and Applied, 35th ed. pp. 429–431. Edited by Warwick, R. and P. L. Williams. Philadelphia, W. B. Saunders, 1980.
32. Gruber, W.: Monographie Der Bursae Mucosae Cubitales. Mem. Acad. Sc. Petersburg, **VII(7)**:10, 1866.
33. Gruber, W.: Monographie Les Canalis Supracondylaideus Humeri. Mem. Acad. Sc. Petersburg. Cited by Morris, H.: Human Anatomy. Philadelphia, Blakiston, 2nd ed., p. 214, 1899; 3rd ed., 1953.
34. Guttierez, L. F.: A Contribution to the Study of the Limiting Factors of Elbow Fixation. Acta Anat., **56**:146–156, 1964.
35. Hamilton, A. T., and Raleigh, N. C.: Subcutaneous Rupture of the Brachioradialis Muscle. Surgery, **23**:806–807, 1948.
36. Henle, J.: Handbüch Der Systematischen Anatomie des Menschen Muskellehre. p. 224. Berlin, Braunschweig, 1866.
37. Henry, A. K.: Extensile Exposure, 2nd ed. Baltimore, Williams & Wilkins, 1957.
38. Hollinshead, W. H.: The Back and Limbs. In Anatomy for Surgeons, vol. 3, pp. 379–384. New York, Harper and Row, 1969.
39. Hollinshead, W. H., and Markee, J. E.: The Multiple Innervation of Limb Muscles in Man. J. Bone Joint Surg., **28**:721–731, 1946.
40. Jamieson, R. W., and Anson, B. J.: The Relation of the Median Nerve to the Heads of Origin of the Pronator Teres Muscle: A Study of 300 Specimens. Q. Bull Northwestern Univ. Med. School, **26**:34–38, 1952.
41. Johansson, O.: Capsular and Ligament Injuries of the Elbow Joint. Acta Chir. Scand. (Suppl.) 287, 1962.
42. Kapandji, I. A.: The Physiology of Joints. Vol. I: Upper Limb, 2nd ed. Baltimore, Williams & Wilkins, 1970.
43. Keats, T. E., Teeslink, R., Diamond, A. E., and Williams, J. H.: Normal Axial Relationships of the Major Joints. Radiology **87**:904–907, 1966.
44. Kocher, T.: Textbook of Operative Surgery, 3rd ed. Translated by H. J. Stiles and C. B. Paul. London, A. & C. Black, 1911.
45. Kolb, L. W., and Moore, R. D.: Fractures of the Supracondylar Process of the Humerus. J. Bone Joint Surg., **49A(3)**:532–534, 1967.
46. Langman, J., and Woerdeman, M. W.: Atlas of Medical Anatomy. Philadelphia, W. B. Saunders, 1976.
47. Lanz, T., and Wachsmuth, W.: Praktische Anatomie. ARM, Berlin, Springer, 1959.
48. Linell, E. A.: The Distribution of Nerves in the Upper Limb, With Reference to Variables and Their Clinical Significance. J. Anat. **55**:79, 1921.
49. Lipmann, K., and Rang, M.: Supracondylar Spur of the Humerus. J. Bone Joint Surg., **48B(4)**:765–769, 1966.
49a. London, J. T.: Kinematics of the Elbow. J. Bone Joint Surg. **63A**:529, 1981.
50. Loomis, L. K.: Reduction and After-Treatment of Posterior Dislocation of the Elbow: With Special Attention to the Brachialis Muscle and Myositis Ossificans. Am. J. Surg., **63**:56, 1944.
51. Malkawi, H.: Recurent Dislocation of the Elbow Accompanied by Ulnar Neuropathy: A Case Report and Review of the Literature. Clin. Orthop., **161**:170–174, 1981.
52. Martin, B. F.: The Annular Ligament of the Superior Radial Ulnar Joint. J. Anat., **52**:473–482, 1958(a).
53. Martin, B. F.: The Oblique Cord of the Forearm. J. Anat., **52**:609, 1958(b).

54. McCormick, L. J., Cauldwell, E. W., and Anson, B. J.: Brachial and Antebrachial Artery Patterns: A Study of 750 Extremities. Surg. Gynec. Obstet., **96**:43, 1953.

55. Morrey, B. F., and Chao, E. Y.: Passive Motion of the Elbow Joint. A Biomechanical Analysis. J. Bone Joint Surg., **58A**:501–508, 1976.

56. Morrey, B. F., Bryan, R. S., Dobyns, J. H., and Linscheid, R. L.: Total Elbow Arthroplasty—A Five-Year Experience at the Mayo Clinic. J. Bone Joint Surg., **63A**:1050–1063, 1981.

57. Morrey, B. F., An, K. N., and Aschew, L.: Rupture of the Insertion of the Biceps Tendon. A Biomechanical Study. Submitted to J. Bone Joint Surg.

58. Morrey, B. F., and An, K. N.: Functional Anatomy of the Elbow Ligaments. Submitted to Clin. Orthop.

59. Morris, H.: Human Anatomy, 11th ed. Edited by J. P. Schaeffer. Philadelphia, Blakiston, 1953.

60. Nirschl, R. P., and Pettsone, F. A.: Tennis Elbow. The Surgical Treatment of Lateral Epicondylitis. J. Bone Joint Surg., **61A**:832–839, 1979.

61. Ogilvie, W. H.: Discussion on Minor Injuries of the Elbow Joint. Proc. R. Soc. Med. 23:306–322, 1930.

62. Osgood, R. B.: Radiohumeral Bursitis, Epicondylitis, Epicondylalgia (Tennis Elbow). Arch Surg., 4:420–433, 1922.

63. Pankovich, A. M.: Anconeus Approach to the Elbow Joint and the Proximal Part of the Radius and Ulna. J. Bone Joint Surg., **59A**:124–126, 1977.

64. Polonskaja, R.: Zur Frage der Arterienanastomosen im Gobiete der Ellenbagenbeuge des Menschen. Anat. Anz., **74**:303, 1932.

65. Ray, R. D., Johnson, R. J., and Jamieson, R. M.: Rotation of the Forearm: An Experimental Study of Pronation and Supination. J. Bone Joint Surg., **33A**:993, 1951.

66. Reimann, A. F., Daseler, E. H., Anson, B. J., and Beaton, L. E.: The Palmaris Longus Muscle and Tendon: A Study of 1600 Extremities. Anat. Rec., **89**:495, 1944.

67. Schwab, G. H., Bennett, J. B., Woods, G. W. (as quoted by Lanz), and Tullos, H. S.: The Biomechanics of Elbow Stability: The Role of the Medial Collateral Ligament. Clin. Orthop. Rel. Res., **146**:42–52, 1980.

68. Shiba, R., Siu, D., and Sorbie, C.: Geometric Analysis of the Elbow Joint. Submitted to J. Bone Joint Surg.

69. Simon, W. H., Friedenberg, S., and Richardson, S.: Joint Congruence. J. Bone Joint Surg., **55A**:1614–1620, 1973.

70. Sobotta, J.: Human Anatomy: An Atlas and Textbook, vol. I. Philadelphia, W. B. Saunders, 1906.

71. Spalteholz, V.: Hand Atlas of Human Anatomy, 2nd ed. Edited and translated by L. F. Baker. Philadelphia, J. B. Lippincott, 1861.

72. Spinner, M., and Kaplan, E. B.: The Quadrate Ligament of the Elbow—Its Relationship to the Stability of the Proximal Radio-Ulnar Joint. Acta Orthop. Scand., **41**:632–647, 1970.

73. Steindler, A.: Kinesiology of the Human Body, 5th ed. Springfield, Ill., Charles C Thomas, 1977.

74. Stimson, H.: Traumatic Rupture of the Biceps Brachii. Am. J. Surg., **29**:472, 1935.

75. Strachan, J. H., and Ellis, B. W.: Vulnerability of the Posterior Interosseous Nerve During Radial Head Resection. J. Bone Joint Surg., **53B**:320–323, 1971.

76. Terry, R. J.: New Data on the Incidence of the Supracondylar Variation. Am. J. Phys. Anthropol., **9**:265, 1926.

77. Thomas, T. T.: A Contribution to the Mechanism of Fractures and Dislocations in the Elbow Region. Ann Surg., **89**:108–121, 1929.

78. Thompson, H. C., III, and Garcia, A.: Myositis Ossificans: Aftermath of Elbow Injuries. Clin. Orthop., **50**:129–134, 1967.

79. Tillman, B.: A Contribution to the Function Morphology of Articular Surfaces. Translated by G. Konorza. Stuttgart, Georg Thieme, P. S. G. Publishing, 1978.

80. Travell, A., and Basmajian, J. V.: Electromyography of the Supinators of the Forearm. Anat. Rec., **139**:557, 1961.

81. Travell, A. A.: Electromyographic Study of the Extensor Apparatus of the Forearm. Anat. Rec., **144**:373–376, 1962.

82. Trotter, M.: Septal Apertures in the Humerus of American Whites and Negros. Am. J. Phys. Anthropol., **19**:213, 1934.

83. Van Gorder, G. W.: Surgical Approach in Supracondylar "T" Fractures of the Humerus Requiring Open Reduction. J. Bone Joint Surg., **22**:278, 1940.

84. Wright, W. B.: Muscle Function. New York, Hoeber, 1928; Hafner, 1962.

CHAPTER 3

Biomechanics of the Elbow

K. N. AN and B. F. MORREY

Normal use of the hand depends largely on a well-functioning elbow joint. The elbow is a complex joint that acts as a component link of the lever arm system that positions the hand, as a fulcrum of the forearm lever, and as a load-carrying joint. Mobility and stability of the elbow joint are necessary for daily, recreational, and professional activities. Loss of joint congruity or destruction of both elbow joints, as in rheumatoid arthritis, will jeopardize the patient's independent existence. The importance of a more thorough appreciation of biomechanics is reflected in clinical practice. Total joint replacement has been an important development in the care of rheumatoid and post-traumatic arthritis. Unfortunately, little basic research directed at fully understanding the resultant or distributive forces at the elbow joint was conducted prior to clinical usage of total elbow prostheses. Predictably, therefore, a large percentage of failures from loosening or dislocation has occurred. Similarly, dislocations of the less constrained prostheses resulted from a lack of in-depth knowledge of the soft tissue constraints of the elbow. A complete understanding of the biomechanics of the elbow joint will be valuable in providing basic guidelines and a rationale for complex surgical procedures and rehabilitation programs.

This chapter will first review elbow kinematics and then discuss the load transmitted through the joint during static and dynamic functions. Finally, the mechanism of elbow joint stability will be analyzed.

KINEMATICS

The bony components of the elbow joint include the trochlea and capitellum on the medial and lateral aspects of the bifurcated distal humerus, and distally, the upper end of the ulna and the head of the radius. The joint is composed of three articulations: the radiohumeral (between the capitellum and the radial head); the ulnohumeral (between the trochlea and the trochlear notch of the ulna); and the radioulnar (between the radial

head and the radial notch of the ulna). The elbow is generally described as a trochoginglymoid joint. That is, it possesses two degrees of freedom in motion: flexion-extension and supination-pronation. However, with the complex geometry of the articulations, description of elbow joint motion in terms of three-dimensional rotational components has also been attempted.

Flexion-Extension

Because of the congruity at the ulnohumeral articulation and surrounding soft tissue constraint, the elbow joint, especially the ulnohumeral joint, is generally considered to be a hinge joint. However, the axis of motion in flexion and extension has been the subject of many investigations and is still controversial. Fischer (1909), using Reuleaux's technique to determine the location of the axis of elbow flexion, found a so-called locus of the instant center of rotation that he considered to be an area 2 to 3 mm in diameter at the center of the trochlea (Fig. 3–1). This observation was later verified in a three-dimensional study of passive motion of the elbow joint by using the biplanar x-ray technique.[40] Using Reuleaux's method, Ewald concluded that the elbow joint has a constantly changing center of rotation during flexion-extension that occurs along the so-called pathway of the instant center.[19] Our studies, however, indicate that Reuleaux's method is not adequate to study elbow joint motion.

The concept of an instantaneous axis, or instantaneous screw displacement axis, has also been used to define elbow joint flexion-extension motion. The transverse axis, about which the ulna rotates during flexion-extension, runs through the center of the trochlea. Based on direct experimental study as well as analytic investigation, Youm et al. concluded that the axis does not change during flexion-extension.[54] A three-dimensional study of passive motion at the elbow revealed that the elbow is not a true hinge joint.[29, 40] However, the pathway of the axis, as meas-

43

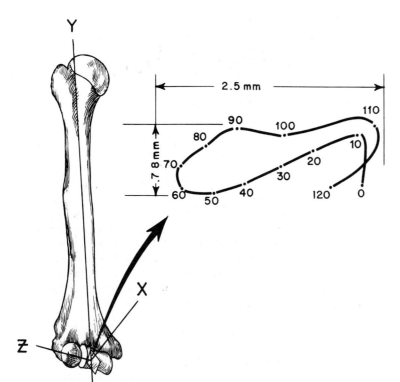

Figure 3–1. Configuration and dimensions of the locus of the instant center of rotation of the elbow. (From Morrey, B. F., and Chao, E. Y. S.: Passive motion of the elbow joint. J. Bone Joint Surg. 58A:501–508, 1976.)

ured from the intersection of the instantaneous axis with the sagittal plane, follows an irregular pattern. The instantaneous axis deviates within 17 degrees in the intact specimen and within about 29 degrees after excision of the radial head. A similar type of helical motion of the flexion axis was previously suggested[28, 38] and was attributed to the obliquity of the trochlear groove along which the ulna moves.[30]

Nevertheless, from a practical point of view, the deviation of the center of joint rotation, or instantaneous axis of rotation, for flexion-extension is certainly minimal and possibly appears irregular due to limitations of experimental design. Thus, the ulnohumeral joint could well be assumed to move as a uniaxial articulation except at the extremes of flexion and extension. The axis of rotation passes through the center of the arcs formed by the trochlear sulcus and capitellum (Fig. 3–2; see also Chapter 6).[36] As seen from below, the axis of rotation is internally rotated 3 to 8 degrees relative to the plane of the epicondyles. As seen from the front, a line perpendicular to the axis of rotation forms a proximally and laterally opening angle of 4 to 8 degrees with the long axis of the humerus.[33] Viewed from the side, the axis lies anterior to the midline of the humerus[46] and lies on a line that is co-linear with the anterior cortex of the distal humerus[40] (Chapter 2).

Forearm Rotation

The radiohumeral joint, which forms the lateral half of the elbow joint, has a common transverse axis with the elbow joint that coincides wih the ulnohumeral axis during flexion-extension. In addition, the radius also rotates around the ulna, allowing for forearm rotation, or supination-pronation. In general, the longitudinal axis of the forearm is considered to pass through the convex head of the radius in the proximal radioulnar joint and

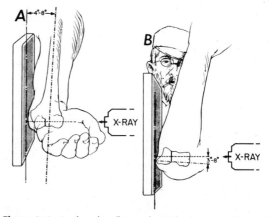

Figure 3–2. As the ulna flexes about the humerus, the path it follows is dictated by the deep sulcus in the trochlea. The axis of rotation for elbow flexion is not coincidental with the line through the epicondyles. (From London, J. T.: Kinematics of the elbow. J. Bone Joint Surg. 63-A:529–535, 1981.)

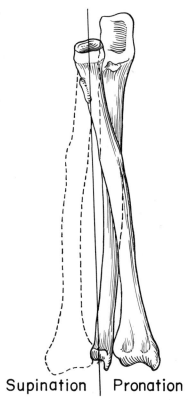

Supination | Pronation

Figure 3–3. The longitudinal axis of pronation-supination runs proximally from the distal end of the ulna to the center of the radial head.

through the convex articular surface of the ulna at the distal radioulnar joint.[48] The axis, therefore, is oblique to the longitudial axes of both the radius and the ulna (Fig. 3–3).

In the past, ulnar rotation was described as being coupled with forearm rotation. At the terminal range of elbow joint flexion and extension, a certain amount of axial rotation was attributed to the proximal ulnohumeral joint.[52] But this observation could not be reproduced in a recent study by Youm et al.[54]

By using a metal rod introduced transversely into the ulna, extension, lateral rotation, and then flexion of the ulna were described with rotation from pronation to supination. The axial rotationl movements of the ulna were also observed by others.[7, 13, 18, 26, 40, 45, 54]

Ray et al. also suggested that varus-valgus movement of the ulna occurs depending on the rotational axis of the forearm.[45] That is, if the forearm rotates on an axis extending from the head of the radius to the index finger, then this ulnar motion would occur. However, if motion occurred about an axis extending through the ring finger—that is, along the more normal axis—such movement of the ulna would be reduced considerably.

If flexion and forearm rotation are carried out simultaneously, the combined axis of both motions of the radius is given by the hypotenuse of a right-angle triangle, the acute angle representing the deflection of the rotatory motion from the transverse flexion-extension axis (Fig. 3–4).[48]

Carrying Angle

The carrying angle, which is defined as the angle formed by the long axis of the humerus and the long axis of the ulna, is measured in the frontal plane with the elbow joint in the extended position and averages 10 to 15 degrees in men and about 5 degrees more in women.[11, 32, 48]

However, when the term *carrying angle* is generalized to account for the angular relationship of the long axis of the ulna and humerus as the elbow is flexed, conflicting observations result. Dempster described a change in the carrying angle during elbow flexion that followed an oscillatory pattern.[16] Morrey and Chao reported that the carrying angle changed linearly with respect to the degree of flexion and extension, being greatest

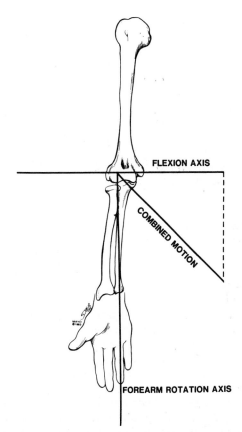

FLEXION AXIS

COMBINED MOTION

FOREARM ROTATION AXIS

Figure 3–4. The axis of simultaneous flexion and forearm rotation is oriented obliquely to these two axes (Steindler).

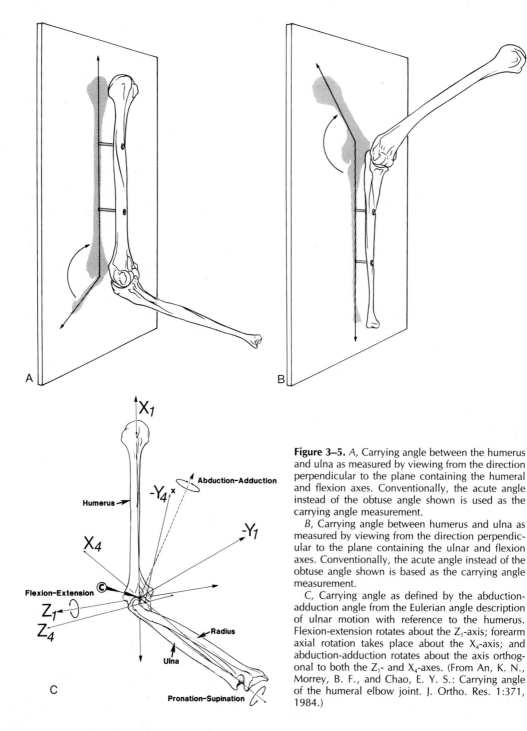

Figure 3–5. *A,* Carrying angle between the humerus and ulna as measured by viewing from the direction perpendicular to the plane containing the humeral and flexion axes. Conventionally, the acute angle instead of the obtuse angle shown is used as the carrying angle measurement.

B, Carrying angle between humerus and ulna as measured by viewing from the direction perpendicular to the plane containing the ulnar and flexion axes. Conventionally, the acute angle instead of the obtuse angle shown is based as the carrying angle measurement.

C, Carrying angle as defined by the abduction-adduction angle from the Eulerian angle description of ulnar motion with reference to the humerus. Flexion-extension rotates about the Z_1-axis; forearm axial rotation takes place about the X_4-axis; and abduction-adduction rotates about the axis orthogonal to both the Z_1- and X_4-axes. (From An, K. N., Morrey, B. F., and Chao, E. Y. S.: Carrying angle of the humeral elbow joint. J. Ortho. Res. 1:371, 1984.)

at full extension and diminishing during flexion.[40] Both patterns have been recorded from three-dimensional experiments.[1, 54] These variations of the carrying angle during joint flexion as explained by Kapandji were due to the obliquity, or helices, of the trochlear groove.[30] More recently, these findings have been challenged with the hypothesis that the carrying angle of the elbow joint remains constant as the elbow flexes.[36] The confusion arises because three different definitions have been adopted for the measurement of carrying angle changes.[6]

Definition 1. The carrying angle is defined as the acute angle formed by the long axis of the humerus and the projection of the long axis of the ulna onto the plane containing the humerus (Fig. 3–5A).

Definition 2. The carrying angle is defined as the acute angle formed by the long axis of the ulna and the projection of the long axis of the humerus onto the plane of the ulna (Fig. 3–5B).

Definition 3. For the finite three-dimensional angular displacement of the ulna about the humerus, the three Eulerian angles are defined as flexion-extension, abduction-adduction, and ulnar axial rotation (Fig. 3–5C). The carrying angle is analytically defined as the abduction-adduction angle of the ulna with respect to the humerus when using Eulerian angles to describe arm motion.

From an anatomic point of view, it is not difficult to conclude that the existence of the carrying angle is due to the existence of obliquities, or cubital angles, between the proximal humeral shaft, trochlea, and distal ulnar shaft, respectively. By assuming that the ulnohumeral joint is a pure hinge joint and that the axis of rotation coincides with the axis of the trochlea, the change in the carrying angle during flexion can be defined as a function of anatomic variations of the obliquity of the articulations according to simple trigonometric calculations.[6] If the first or second definition is accepted, the carrying angle changes minimally during flexion. The analytic calculation of the Eulerian angle shows progressive decrease with elbow flexion.

Limitation of the Range of Motion

In the normal situation, elbow motion ranges from 0 degrees in the extended or slightly hyperextended position up to about 150 degrees in flexion and from about 75 degrees in pronation to 85 degrees in supination (see Chapter 2). The cartilage of the trochlea forms an arc of about 320 degrees, whereas the sigmoid notch creates an arch of about 180 degrees. The arc of the radial depression is about 40 degrees,[48] which articulates with the capitulum, presenting an angle of 180 degrees. In general, these ranges of motion are thought to be limited by the geometry of the joint surfaces, surrounding bone, capsules, ligaments, and muscles. However, there is disagreement about the extent to which these various structures limit the range of motion.

Kapandji pointed out the significance of the 30-degree anterior angulation of the trochlea with the 30-degree posterior orientation of the greater sigmoid notch in promoting flexion and extension of the elbow joint (see Chapter 2).[30] He suggests that the factors limiting joint extension are the impact of the olecranon process on the olecranon fossa, the tension of the anterior ligament and capsule, and the

flexor muscles. The anterior muscle bulk of the arm and forearm along with contraction of the triceps prevents active flexion beyond 145 degrees. However, the factors limiting passive flexion include the impact of the head of the radius against the radial fossa, of the coronoid process against the coronoid fossa and, also, tension from the capsule and triceps.

For pronation and supination, Braune and Flügel found that passive resistance of the stretched antagonist muscle restricts the excursion range more than that of the checking ligamentous structures.[12] Spinner and Kaplan, however, have shown that the quadrate ligament does provide some static constraint to forearm rotation.[47] Impingement of tissue restrains pronation, especially by the flexor pollicis longus, which is forced against the deep finger flexors. The entire range of active excursion in an intact arm is about 150 degrees, whereas when the muscles are removed from a cadaver specimen, the range increases to 185 to 190 degrees. When the ligaments are cut, the range increases up to 205 to 210 degrees.

Contact Area of the Elbow Joint

The contact area on the articular surface during elbow joint motion has been investigated by Goodfellow and Bullough.[24] They found that on the proximal radial head, the central depression articulates with the dome of the capitulum and that the medial triangular facet was always in contact with the ulna. The upper rim of the radial head made no contact at all. At the ulnohumeral joint, the articular surfaces were always in contact during some phases of movement. At a particular angle, there were two narrow bands of contact across the trochlear surface in young specimens, but a more diffuse contact area was present in older specimens. More recently, Walker[53] reproduced this experiment by using engineer's blue and confirmed the findings of Goodfellow and Bullough. A double narrow band was reproduced on the trochlea. The contact area on the ulna occurred anteriorly and posteriorly and tended to move together and slightly inward from each side from 0 to 90 degrees of flexion (Fig. 3–6). Goel studied the elbow joint contact areas by using wax as a casting material.[23] The shape and size of the contact areas changed in different elbow positions. In full extension, the contact was observed to be on the lower medial aspect of the ulna, whereas in other postures, the pres-

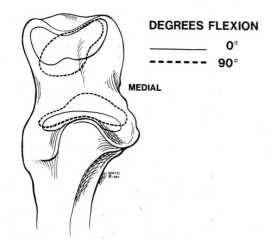

DEGREES FLEXION

—————— 0°

- - - - - - 90°

MEDIAL

Figure 3–6. Contact in the sigmoid fossa moves toward the center of the fossa during elbow flexion. (Redrawn from Walker, P. S.: Human Joints and Their Artificial Replacements. Springfield, IL., Charles C Thomas, 1977.)

sure areas described a strip extending from posterolateral to anteromedial. The radiocapitellar joint also revealed contact during flexion under no externally applied load.

FORCE ACROSS THE ELBOW JOINT

Study of the force across the elbow joint is not an easy task. The analysis can be performed at various degrees of sophistication. It can be either two-dimensional or three-dimensional, static or dynamic, and with or without hand activities. The clinical implications of these forces is obvious, but the magnitudes are not common knowledge. Consequently, in this section, the factors that affect the force passing through the elbow joint will first be analyzed in detail based on two-dimensional considerations. Then, more realistic data based on three-dimensional analysis will be presented.

Two-Dimensional Elbow Force Analysis

In sagittal plane motion, the elbow joint is assumed to be a hinge joint. Forces and moments created at the joint, due to the loads applied at the hand, are balanced by the (1) muscles, (2) tendons, (3) ligaments, and (4) contact forces on the articular surfaces. The amount of tension in the muscles and the magnitude and direction of the joint forces are determined by the external loading conditions as well as by the responses of muscles, i.e., force distribution among these muscles.

To calculate these forces, a free-body anal-

ysis of the forearm and hand isolated at the elbow joint is required. From this analysis, a set of equilibrium equations is obtained:

$$\Sigma\, M_i\, f_{xi} + R_x + P_x = 0$$
$$\Sigma\, M_i\, f_{yi} + R_y + P_y = 0 \qquad [1]$$
$$\Sigma\, M_i\, r_i + P\, r_p = 0$$

in which M_i = magnitude of the tension in i^{th} muscle;

f_{xi}, f_{yi} = components in x and y direction for the unit vector along the line of action of muscle;

R_x, R_y = x and y components of the joint contact force;

P, P_x, P_y = magnitude of the applied forces on the forearm and its associated components; and

r_i, r_p = moment arms of the muscle force and the applied force to the elbow joint center, respectively.

The lines of action of muscles crossing the joint have been reported.[2, 5, 44] In the sagittal plane, based on the magnitude of moment arms, the major elbow muscles consist of biceps (BIC), brachialis (BRA), brachioradialis (BRD), extensor carpi radialis longus (ECRL), triceps (TRI), and anconeus (ANC) (Table 3–1). The other forearm muscles for the hand and wrist provide various, but limited, contributions to elbow flexion-extension. Unfortunately, the contributions of these forearm muscles are not consistently reported in the literature.

Assuming friction and ligament forces are negligible, the resultant joint constraint force vector should be perpendicular to the arc of the articular surface and pass through the center of curvature of this arc. Thus, the problem of elbow force analysis may be reduced to one of solving the unknown variables R_x, R_y, and M_i in the equations of [1]. However, in reality, even for a simple task, multiple muscles are involved, making the force calculation an indeterminate problem. Methods for resolving these indeterminate problems are thus required.

Single Muscle Analysis

The simplest case is to consider only a single muscle involved in resisting an external force. This type of consideration has been used widely in the literature for two-dimensional force analysis of the musculoskeletal system. Based on the parameters shown in Figure 3–7, the magnitude of the muscle force, M, and the magnitude and orientation of joint reac-

Table 3–1. **Physiological Cross-Sectional Area (PCSA), Unit Force Vector (F_x, F_y), and Moment Arms (r) of Elbow Muscles in Sagittal Plane**

| Muscle | PCSA[a] | Elbow Joint Flexion Angle (degrees) | | | | | | | | | | | |
| | | (0°) | | | (30°) | | | (90°) | | | (120°) | | |
		r[b]	F_x	F_y	r	F_x	F_y	r	F_x	F_y	r	F_x	F_y
BIC	4.6	20.7	.86	.50	20.7	.86	.50	45.5	.17	.99	40.0	.35	.93
BRA	7.0	15.2	.82	.57	15.2	.82	.57	33.5	.36	.92	33.8	.12	.97
BRD	1.5	30.8	.99	−.11	30.8	.99	.04	75.0	.92	.39	79.9	.89	.41
FCR	2.0	2.0	1.0	.04	2.0	1.0	.04	5.0	1.0	.04	5.9	1.0	.04
ECRL	2.4	8.6	.99	.16	8.6	.99	.16	29.3	.97	.25	32.0	.97	.26
FCU	1.6	0.0	1.0	.04	0.0	.99	.04	0.0	1.0	.04	0.0	1.0	.04
TRI	18.8	−23.0	1.0	.09	−26.0	.81	.59	−20.0	.05	1.0	−17.0	.05	1.0
ECRB	1.5	−1.0	.99	.17	−1.0	.99	.17	−2.0	.96	.28	−2.5	.96	.28
ECU	1.7	−2.0	.99	.16	−9.0	.99	.16	−9.0	.98	.19	−8.0	.98	.19
EDC	3.8	0.0	.99	.17	0.0	.99	.17	−2.0	.98	.22	−2.0	.99	.23
FDS	3.0	−4.0	1.0	.04	−3.0	1.0	.05	−3.5	1.0	.04	−3.5	1.0	.04

[a]PCSA = cm²
[b]r = mm

Table 3–2. **Muscle and Joint Forces with Single Muscle**[a]

| Muscle | Elbow Position (flexion angles, degrees) | | | | | | | | | | | |
| | (0°) | | | (30°) | | | (90°) | | | (120°) | | |
	M/P	R/P	φ	M/P	R/P	φ	M/P	R/P	φ	M/P	R/P	φ
BIC	15.5	15.5	27.0	15.5	15.0	27.0	7.0	6.1	78.7	8.0	7.1	66.4
BRA	21.1	20.5	32.0	21.1	20.5	32.0	9.6	8.6	66.3	9.5	8.5	82.6
BRD	10.4	10.4	−3.2	10.4	10.4	−3.2	4.3	4.0	9.6	4.0	3.7	10.5
TRI	13.9	14.5	39.3	13.9	12.9	39.7	16.0	17.0	87.3	18.8	19.8	87.2

[a]r_p = 320 mm; D = 15 mm; ψ = 90° for flexion; ψ = 270° for extension. (See Fig. 3–7 for definitions.)
M = muscle force; P = applied force; R = resultant joint force
φ = angle between R and long ulnar axis

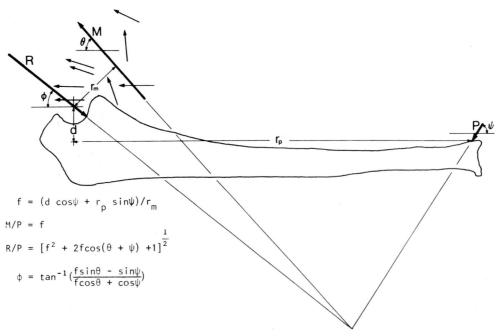

$$f = (d\ cos\psi + r_p\ sin\psi)/r_m$$

$$M/P = f$$

$$R/P = [f^2 + 2fcos(\theta + \psi) + 1]^{\frac{1}{2}}$$

$$\phi = tan^{-1}\left(\frac{f sin\theta - sin\psi}{f cos\theta + cos\psi}\right)$$

Figure 3–7. Free-body diagram of isolated forearm. External force, P, applied at r_p from the joint center with an angle of ψ to the ulnar axis. Combined muscle force, M, has moment arm r_m and is oriented θ with the ulnar axis. The resultant joint force, R, is oriented with the ulnar axis by an angle, ϕ. All forces applied to the ulna are under equilibrium conditions.

tion force, R and ϕ, can be obtained by solving equation [1] with i = 1.

$$f = \frac{M}{P} = [\ Cos\psi\ \frac{d}{r_F} + Sin\psi\ \frac{r_P}{r_F}]$$

$$\frac{R}{P} = \sqrt{f^2 + 2fCos(\theta + \psi) + 1} \qquad [2]$$

$$\phi = tan^{-1}\ \frac{f\ Sin\theta - Sin\psi}{f\ Cos\theta + Cos\psi}$$

An intimate relationship between the joint force and the muscle forces in balancing the externally applied force on the forearm (Table 3–2) thus exists. The magnitude of muscle force required to balance the external force reflects the changes of the muscle's moment arm, or mechanical advantage, with changes of the joint configuration.

Effect of Muscle Moment Arm. The effect of a changing muscle moment arm on the resultant joint force is demonstrated graphically in Figure 3–8. If the loading configuration does not change, both the muscle force and the joint reaction force decrease as the muscle moment arm increases. The orientation of the resultant force also changes from the middle portion of the trochlear notch toward the border of the articular cartilage.

Effect of Orientation on Muscle Line of Action. Under the same loading conditions, the

effect of changing the orientation of the muscle line of action under a constant moment arm is demonstrated (Fig. 3–9). The applied force is assumed again to be perpendicular to the forearm. Both magnitudes of muscle and joint reaction forces change slightly with the change of the muscle's line of action. How-

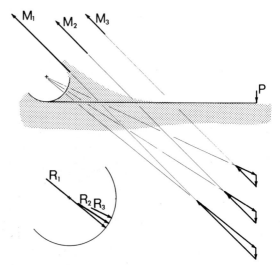

Figure 3–8. Effect on the muscle and joint forces by changing the moment arm of the muscle force. For a given externally applied force, the longer moment arm decreases the muscle and joint forces. Also, the resultant joint force and orientation (R_1, R_2, R_3) are affected by the magnitude of the muscle moment arm.

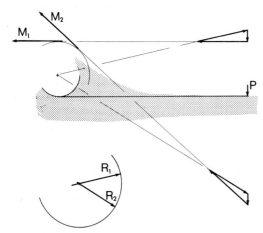

Figure 3–9. Effect of changing the orientation of the muscle line of action on the muscle and joint force under a given load. The magnitudes of both muscle and joint forces are not changed but their orientations are.

ever, the orientation of the resultant joint force is quite sensitive to changes of the muscle force line. The orientation of the resultant joint force, therefore, moves from the central portion of the trochlea toward the rim as the direction of muscle pull relative to the forearm changes from vertical to parallel. This is especially true for the resultant joint force in the trochlear notch brought about by the contraction of the upper arm muscles whose direction relative to the forearm axis changes with the elbow joint flexion angle. On the other hand, the directions of forearm muscles with respect to the trochlear notch are relatively constant, so the direction of the resul-

tant joint forces are thus reasonably constant. When considering the direction of resultant joint forces applied on the trochlea, the effects of upper arm and forearm muscles are just reversed.

Effect of the Moment Arm of External Force. With the orientations and moment arms of the muscles kept constant, the magnitude of the muscle force and joint force created to resist the externally applied force decreases proportionally with the decrease of the moment arm of the external force. This is obviously true, simply because the resultant segmental moment created at the elbow joint due to externally applied load decreases when the moment arm decreases. It should be noticed that the direction of resultant joint force also changes slightly. From the above results, it is also easy to realize that the magnitude of the muscle force and joint force increases proportionally with increases of the magnitude of external force. Therefore, in general, the results are usually expressed in terms of ratio to the external load.

Effect of the Direction of the Externally Applied Force. When the force applied at the wrist changes direction from vertical to horizontal, the effective moment arm of this applied force changes. The resultant segmental moment about the elbow joint center due to this force changes as well (Fig. 3–10). Furthermore, when the resultant segmental moments change from flexion to extension, the required muscles will also change from flexors to extensors.

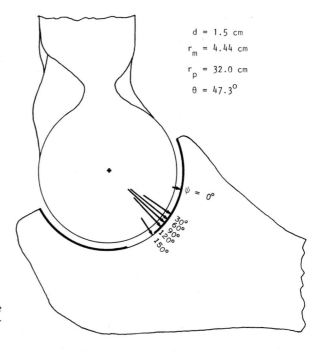

$d = 1.5$ cm

$r_m = 4.44$ cm

$r_p = 32.0$ cm

$\theta = 47.3°$

$\psi = 0°$

Figure 3–10. Effect of changes in the orientation of the applied force (ψ) on the joint force, where 90° is perpendicular to the long axis of the forearm (see Fig. 3–7).

In summary, the parametric analysis demonstrates that the magnitude and orientation of the resultant joint forces in the trochlear notch depend very much on whether the upper arm or the forearm muscle is used, the location and orientation of the external load applied on the forearm, and also the joint flexion angle that alters the moment arm and orientation of the muscle line of action.

Multiple Muscle Analysis

In reality, when external loads are applied on the forearm, multiple muscles are involved, and this makes the analytic determination of muscle and joint forces difficult. Because the magnitude and orientation of the resultant joint force are two unknown variables, if more than one muscle force is involved, then the number of unknown variables exceeds the number of available equations. This makes the problem indeterminate, and a nonunique solution will result.

Several methods have been employed to resolve the indeterminate problem. Electromyographic data (EMG) and the physiological cross-sectional area may be used to provide an additional equation. The most commonly adopted techniques are analytical reduction and optimization methods.

In the reduction method, the redundant unknown variables are systematically eliminated, making the remaining system uniquely solvable. In a two-dimensional analysis, this method is more or less the same as that which considers only a single muscle, as described in the previous section. This method can usually provide the ranges of magnitude and orientation of the resultant joint forces for a given task. However, the technique may give physiologically unreasonable solutions, such as using a single forearm muscle to resist the forearm load. Additional judgment and screening are thus required.

When using the optimization method, a unique solution to an indeterminate problem is obtained by minimizing a preselected objective function or cost function. Although the solution to the problem is still nonunique, each solution is generally associated with some physiologic phenomenon or condition on which the objective function is constructed and selected. This technique has been described in more detail elsewhere.[5a]

The most commonly used objective functions for resolving the indeterminate force analysis problem include linear and nonlinear weighted combinations of the unknown variables. A specific analytical technique used to optimize the linear objective function for solution is called linear programming.

Major Elbow Muscles. We are now in a position to consider several muscles in the solution: these include the biceps (BIC), triceps (TRI), brachialis (BRA), and brachioradialis (BRD).

For the loading case of force applied at the wrist in the sagittal plane, with the elbow in 90 degrees of flexion, the solutions of two types of optimization procedures are shown in Table 3–3. The magnitude and direction of the resultant joint force at four elbow flexion positions, when the external force is applied perpendicular to the forearm, are also shown (Fig. 3–11). It is observed that results vary according to the optimization criterion selected, the loading conditions, and the joint positions. For example, when the forearm muscles carry the dominant forces, the resultant joint force on the proximal ulna will be consistently toward the rim of the coronary process throughout the elbow flexion range. On the other hand, for a given task, if the upper arm muscles carry the dominant forces, then the resultant joint force will have more variation along the articular surface with changes of joint flexion. This is because the

Table 3–3. **Muscle and Joint Forces in Resisting Flexion Moment by Three Major Flexors**[a]

	Optimization Methods for Solutions (elbow joint angle = 90°)									
		$Obj^a = \Sigma$ *(Muscle stress[b])²*					$Obj^a = \sigma$; *Muscle stress $\leq \sigma$*			
ψ^c	BIC[d]	BRA[d]	BRD[d]	R^e	ϕ^e	BIC	BRA	BRD	R	ϕ
0°	.13	.22	.02	1.17	17.0	.12	.19	.04	1.17	15.6
30°	1.49	2.55	.26	4.14	56.5	1.43	2.18	.47	3.89	53.3
60°	2.46	4.19	.43	6.30	63.3	2.35	3.58	.77	5.86	60.3
90°	2.76	4.71	.49	6.83	67.4	2.65	4.03	.86	6.31	64.6
120°	2.33	3.97	.41	5.56	72.1	2.23	3.39	.73	5.10	69.6
150°	1.27	2.17	.22	2.88	83.2	1.22	1.85	.40	2.60	81.7

[a]Obj = objective function used in optimization method.
[b]Muscle stress = muscle force/PSCA.
[c]ψ = angle between the applied force and the long ulnar axis (see Fig. 3–7 for definition).
[d]BIC, BRA, BRD = muscle forces, as expressed in the unit of externally applied force, of associated muscles.
[e]R = resultant joint force; ϕ = angle between R and long ulnar axis.

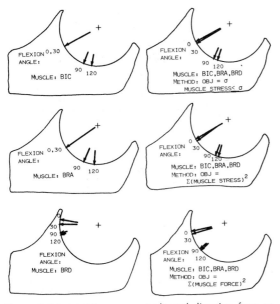

Figure 3–11. Joint force magnitude and direction from an applied load at the wrist at various elbow flexion angles. Family of solutions by using different muscle combinations and solution techniques.

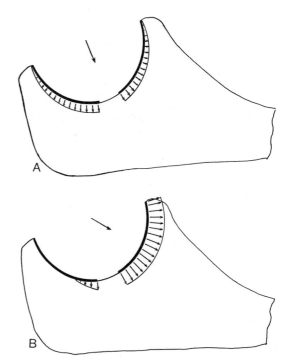

Figure 3–12. The contact pressure depends on the direction and magnitude of the resultant compressive force.

A, When the resultant force is oriented toward the center of the trochlear notch, a more uniform distribution of pressure is observed.

B, When the line of action of the resultant joint force is directed to the rim of the trochlear notch, the weight-bearing surface becomes smaller, and maximum compressive stress increases.

line of action of the upper arm muscle undergoes a tremendous change in direction with respect to the ulnar axis during flexion, as discussed earlier.

The maximum elbow flexion strength occurs at 90 degrees (see Chapter 5). From the measured lifting strength data, the maximal muscle force per unit of cross-sectional area can be calculated to be in the range of 10 to 14 kg/cm². About one third or one half of the maximum lifting force can be generated with the elbow in the extended or 30-degree flexed position. At these positions, a force three times the body weight can be encountered in the elbow joint during strenuous lifting (Table 3–4).

Contact Stress on the Joint Articular Surface

With the magnitude, direction, and point of application of the resultant joint force available, the stress on the articular cartilage can

now be determined. Because the joint is not a simple geometric shape,[44] the problem of contact of two rigid bodies must be solved.[31] If the line of action of the resultant force is at the middle of the articular surface, the stress is almost equally distributed throughout the entire articular surface (Fig. 3–12A). On the other hand, as the resultant force is directed toward the margin of the articulation anteriorly or posteriorly, the weight-bearing surface becomes smaller, the maximum compressive stress becomes elevated, and the stress distribution over the joint surface becomes more uneven (Fig. 3–12B). It should be

Table 3–4. **Muscle and Joint Forces Under Maximum Flexion Forces**

Elbow Flexion Angle (degree)	Maximum Flexion[a] Strength at Wrist (Newtown)	Muscle Force			Resultant Joint Force
		BIC	BRA	BRD	
		(× body weight)			
0°	90–150	0.79–1.19	1.2–1.81	0.29–0.39	2.15–3.2
30°	110–190	1.00–1.48	1.5–2.26	0.32–0.49	2.70–4.1
90°	220–383	0.90–1.33	1.3–2.02	0.29–0.43	2.10–3.1
120°	178–307	0.72–1.08	1.1–1.66	0.24–0.31	1.70–2.6

[a]Based on average body weight of 670 Newtons.

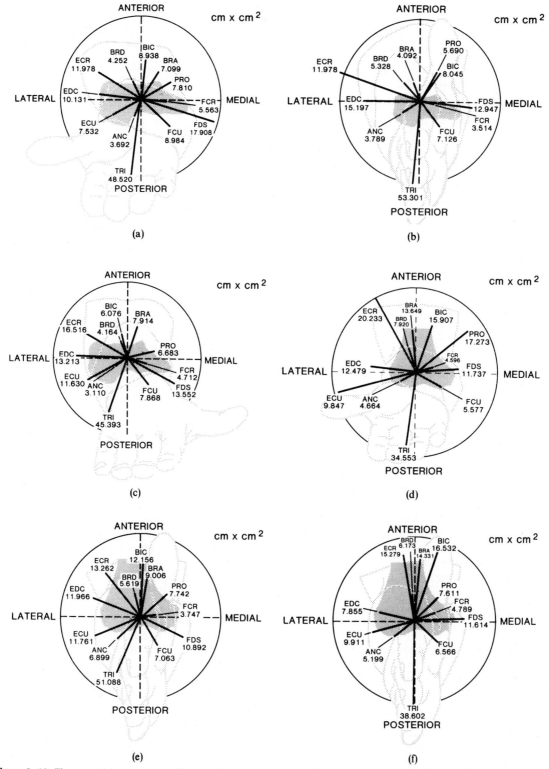

Figure 3–13. The potential moment contribution of each muscle at the elbow joint was estimated by multiplying the moment arm (cm) of the muscle by its physiological cross-section area (cm²). These diagrams show the contributions to flexion-extension and varus-valgus rotation about the joint center at six elbow and forearm configurations. *A,* Extended/supinated; *B,* Extended/neutral; *C,* Extended/pronated; *D,* Semiflexed/supinated; *E,* Semiflexed/neutral; *F,* Flexed/neutral. (From An, K. N., et al.: Muscles across the elbow joint: A biomechanical analysis. J. Biomechanics 14:659, 1981.)

further noticed that the position of maximum stress does not necessarily correspond with the point of intersection of the resultant joint force through the articular surface.

Three-Dimensional Analysis

For more practical applications, a three-dimensional analysis of the forces occurring in the elbow joint is required. In formulating the three-dimensional analysis, four additional force and moment equations in the frontal plane as well as the transverse plane are required. In addition, sometimes the moment equilibrium equation to ensure balance of the forearm pronation-supination rotation is required.

Contribution of Muscle Force

In determining the muscle forces crossing the elbow joint three-dimensionally, an indeterminate problem is encountered again, and either the reduction or optimization method is required for solution. In this section, an alternative concept for solution under the special case is considered. During strenuous actions, the maximum tension that could possibly be provided by each individual muscle is usually considered to be proportional to the physiologic cross-sectional area. This has been carefully measured for muscles crossing the elbow.[5] The potential moment contribution of each muscle at the elbow joint can thus be estimated by multiplying its moment arm by its physiologic cross-sectional area. The moment contributions for all of the muscles crossing the elbow joint have been calculated (Fig. 3–13). Of note, the potential moment in varus appears to be balanced by the valgus moment under all of the functional configurations. When flexed, the flexion potential moment seems to be balanced by the extension moment. However, the extension moment exceeds the flexion moment when the elbow is extended.

In constructing these moment potential diagrams, it is assumed that all muscles are simultaneously and maximally contracted to their optimal lengths. To apply these data for more general conditions, consideration should be given and adjustment made for length-tension and force-velocity relationships. In addition, when activities involve submaximal contraction, a proper scaling system based on experimental measurements such as electromyograms is required.[3, 15, 20, 22, 39]

Electromyographic Activities of Elbow Muscles

Electromyographic analysis is used to provide scaling systems for the muscle force calculations during submaximal contraction and to show the phasic distribution of muscular activities for a given task.

Flexors. Surface electrodes along the belly of the biceps were first used to record electrical activity during dynamic flexion and extension, with and without load.[50] This early study showed that there was a decrease in biceps activity in the pronation compared with the supination position and that the biceps acted in extension to "brake" the forearm.

Subsequent studies have presented inconsistent data, but in almost all investigations the biceps demonstrates no[9] or decreased activity when flexion occurs in pronation.[22, 37, 49] As expected, little influence is reflected in the brachialis muscle with forearm rotation.[22, 49] The brachioradialis demonstrates electrical activity with flexion, especially when the forearm is rotated to the neutral position[10, 17] or in pronation.[22, 34, 49]

These data are summarized for the 90-degree flexion position because this is the position of maximum strength[9, 34] and of greatest electrical activity of the elbow flexors (Fig. 3–14).[22]

Extensors. Electromyographic investigations of the elbow extensor muscles were first completed by Travill in 1962. The medial head of the triceps and anconeus muscles were found to be active during extension; the lateral and long head of the triceps acted as auxillaries. The anconeus was also active during resisted pronation and supination. In fact, the anconeus has been demonstrated to be active during flexion and abduction-adduction resisted motions.[22, 43] Thus, the anconeus may be considered a stabilizer of the elbow joint because it is active with almost all motions.

Currier, in 1972, studied the same muscles at 60 degrees, 90 degrees, and 120 degrees of elbow flexion. The greatest electrical activity occurred at the 90- and 120-degree positions, consistent with the position of greatest strength.[8] Others found that there was no difference between position and muscular electrical activity.[35]

Conclusion. Electromyographic data of the elbow muscles have thus provided the following information: (1) the biceps is generally less active in full pronation of the forearm,

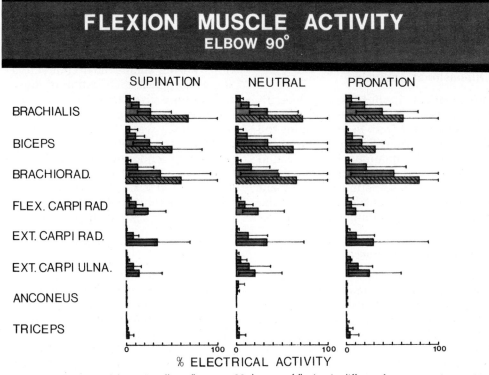

Figure 3–14. Electrical activity of the major elbow flexors at 90 degrees of flexion in different forearm rotation positions (From Funk, D.: An EMG analysis of muscles controlling elbow motion. M. S. Thesis, Mayo Clinic, 1984.)

probably due to its secondary role as a supinator; (2) the brachialis is active in most ranges of function and is felt to be the "workhorse" of flexion; (3) there is an increase in electrical activity of the triceps with increased elbow flexion, probably secondary to an increased stretch reflex; (4) the anconeus shows activity in all positions and hence is considered a dynamic joint stabilizer; and (5) generally speaking, the different heads of the triceps and biceps are active in the same manner through most motion.

Distributive Forces on the Articular Surfaces

Joint compressive forces on various facets of the elbow joint have been reported in the literature.[3, 42] During activities involving resistance of flexion and extension moments at various elbow joint positions, the components of force along the medial-lateral direction, causing varus-valgus stress, are small compared with those acting in the sagittal plane directed anteriorly or posteriorly. The resul-

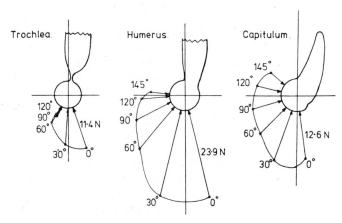

Figure 3–15. Orientation and magnitude of forces at the humeral articular surface during flexion, per unit of force at the hand. (From Amis, A. A., Dowson, D., and Wright, V.: Elbow joint force predictions for some strenuous isometric actions. J. Biomechanics 13:765, 1980.)

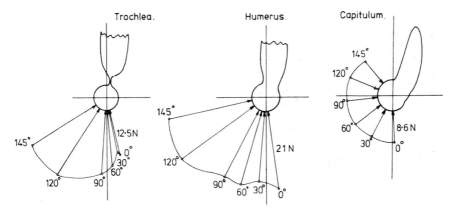

Figure 3–16. Orientation and magnitude of forces at the humeral articulating surface during extension, per unit of force at the hand. (From Amis, A. A., Dowson, D., and Wright, V.: Elbow joint force predictions for some strenuous isometric actions. J. Biomechanics 13:765, 1980.)

tant joint forces on the trochlea and capitulum have been described in the sagittal plane for flexion (Fig. 3–15) and extension (Fig. 3–16) isometric loads. Because of the poor mechanical advantage when the elbow is in extension, the largest isometric flexion forces occur in this position (Fig. 3–16).[3, 27] Isometric extension produces a posterior-superior compressive stress across the distal humerus (Fig. 3–16). When the elbow is extended and axially loaded, the distribution of stress across the joint has been calculated to be approxi-

mately 40 percent across the ulnohumeral joint and 60 percent across the radiohumeral articulation (Fig. 3–17).[25, 53]

When the elbow is flexed, inward rotation of the forearm against resistance imposes large torques to the joint. The magnitudes have been calculated as approaching twice body weight tension in the medial collateral ligament and three times body weight at the radiohumeral joint.[4]

Considerably less knowledge is available regarding the distributed forces at the elbow during use. Nicol has demonstrated significant forces with daily activities occurring at the radiohumeral, ulnohumeral, and collateral ligaments.[42] An example of such force patterns is shown in Figure 3–18.

Applied Force

40% **60%**

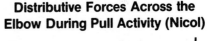

Figure 3–17. Static compression of the extended elbow places more force on the radiohumeral than on the ulnohumeral joint.

Distributive Forces Across the Elbow During Pull Activity (Nicol)

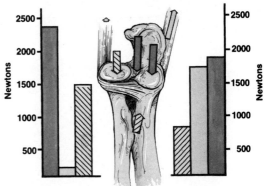

Figure 3–18. Distribution of articular and soft tissue forces across the elbow for a selected activity. (Data from Nichol, A. C., Berme, N., and Paul, J. P.: A biomechanical analysis of elbow joint function. *In* Joint Replacement in the Upper Limb. London, Institute of Mechanical Engineers, 1977.)

ELBOW STABILITY

The elbow is one of the most congruous joints of the musculoskeletal system and as such is one of the most stable. This feature is the result of an almost equal contribution from the soft tissue constraints and the articular surfaces.[41]

The static soft tissue stabilizers include the collateral ligament complexes and the anterior capsule. The anatomy of the lateral col-

lateral ligament has been discussed earlier (see Chapter 2). It originates from the lateral condyle at a point through which the axis of rotation passes. Conversely, the medial collateral ligament has two discrete components, neither of which originates at a site that lies on the axis of rotation. Because elbow joint motion occurs about a near perfect hinge axis though the center of the capitellum and trochlea, different parts of the medial collateral ligament complex will be taut at different

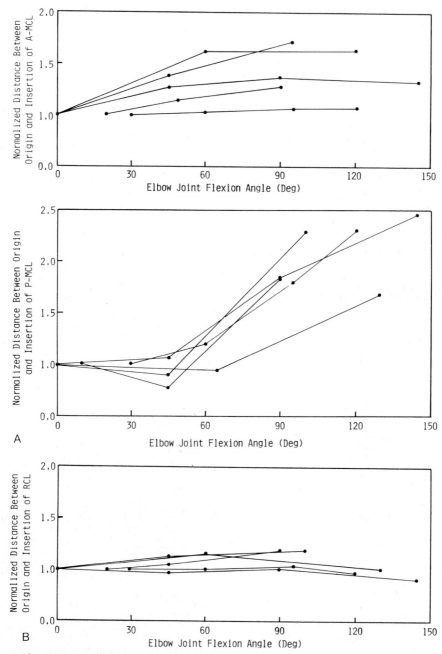

Figure 3–19. A, The anterior medial collateral ligament remains more taut during elbow flexion than does the posterior segment of the ligament. B, The radial collateral ligament originates at the axis of rotation for elbow flexion, hence has little length variation during flexion and extension.

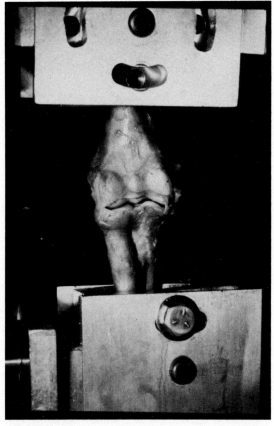

Figure 3–20. An elbow specimen mounted in the material testing fixtures. The anterior capsule has been excised.

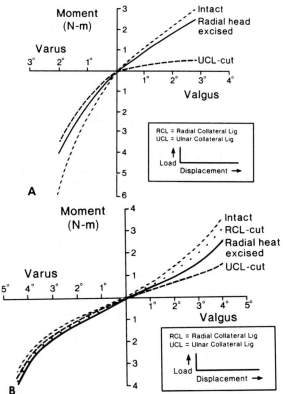

Figure 3–21. Force displacement curves demonstrate relative contribution of elements to elbow stability in extension (A) and flexion (B). (From B. F., and An, K. N.: Articular and Ligamentous contributions to the stablity of the elbow joint. Am. J. Sports Med. 11:315, 1983.)

positions of elbow flexion (Fig. 3–19A). The lateral collateral ligament lying on the axis of rotation, however, will assume a rather uniform tension regardless of elbow position (Fig. 3–19B).

The constraining influence of each ligamentous and articular component has been studied by using the materials testing machine and imparting a given and controlled displacement to the elbow (Fig. 3–20).[41] The

relative contribution of each stabilizing structure can be demonstrated by sequentially eliminating each element and observing the load recorded by the load cell for the constant displacement imparted, usually 2 to 5 degrees (Fig. 3–21). For the extended and 90-degree flexed positions, distraction and varus-valgus stability have been studied. A simplified summary of the observations is shown in Table 3–5. In extension, the anterior capsule pro-

Table 3–5. **Percentage Contribution of Restraining Force During Displacement (Rotational or Distractional)**

Position	Stabilizing Element	Distraction	Varus	Valgus
Extension	MCL[a]	12	—	31
	LCL[b]	10	14	—
	Capsule	78	32	38
	Articulation	—	54	31
Flexion	MCL[a]	80	—	54
	LCL[b]	10	9	—
	Capsule	10	13	10
	Articulation	—	78	36

[a]MCL = Medial collateral ligament complex
[b]LCL = Lateral collateral ligament complex

vides about 70 percent of the soft tissue restraint to distraction, whereas the medial collateral ligament assumes this function at 90 degrees of flexion. Varus stress is limited in extension equally by the joint articulation (55 percent) and the soft tissue, lateral collateral ligament, and capsule. In flexion, the articulation provides 75 percent of the varus stability. Valgus stress in extension is equally divided between the medial collateral ligament, the capsule, and the joint surfaces. With flexion, the capsular contribution is assumed by the medial collateral ligament, which is the primary stabilizer (54 percent) to valgus stress at this position. Further, for all practical purposes, the anterior portion of the medial collateral ligament provides virtually all of this structure's function.

The contribution of the articular geometry was further evaluated by serial removal of portions of the proximal ulna, as shown in Figure 3–22. Valgus stress, both in extension and at 90 degrees of flexion, was primarily (75 to 85 percent) resisted by the proximal half of the sigmoid notch, whereas varus stress was resisted primarily by the distal half, or coronoid portion, of the articulation, both in extension (67 percent) and in flexion (60 percent).

Internal and external rotation of the ulna is limited primarily by the distal coronoid portion of the joint. In flexion, the entire constraint arises from the distal 50 percent and the associated soft tissue attachments. In general, direct loads across the ulnohumeral joint are absorbed in a measure proportional to the amount of proximal ulna present (Fig. 3–23).

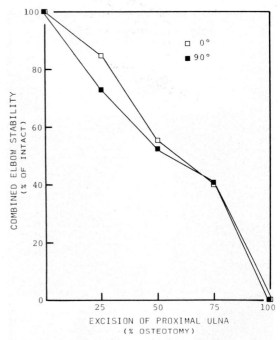

Figure 3–23. A linear decrease of combined stability is observed with removal of the olecranon. Note a similar effect for both the extended and 90-degree flexed positions.

References

1. Amis, A. A., Dowson, D., Unsworth, A., Miller, J. H., and Wright, V.: An Examination of the Elbow Articulation with Particular Reference to Variation of the Carrying Angle. Engrg. Med., **6**:76–80, 1977.
2. Amis, A. A., Dowson, D., and Wright V.: Muscle Strengths and Musculoskeletal Geometry of the Upper Limb. Engrg. Med., **8**:41–48, 1979.
3. Amis, A. A., Dowson, D., and Wright, V.: Elbow Joint Force Predictions for Some Strenuous Isometric Actions. J. Biomechan., **13**:765–775, 1980.
4. Amis, A. A., Miller, J. H., Dawson, D., and Wright, V.: Biomechanical Aspects of the Elbow: Joint Forces Related to Prosthesis Design. Engrg. Med., **10**:65, 1981.
5. An, K. N., Hui, F. C., Morrey, B. F., Linscheid, R. L., and Chao, E. Y.: Muscles Across the Elbow Joint: A Biomechanical Analysis. J. Biomechan., **14**:659–669, 1981.
5a. An, K. N., Kwak, B. M., Chao, E. Y., and Morrey, B. F.: Determination of Muscle and Joint Forces Across Human Elbow Joint. In Advances in Bioengineering, ASME, pp. 70–71, 1983.
6. An, K. N., Morrey, B. F., and Chao, E. Y.: Carrying Angle of Human Elbow Joint. (In press, J. Orthop. Res., 1984.)
7. Anderson, R.: Rotation of the Forearm. Lancet, **2**:1333–1334, 1901.
8. Askew, L. J., An, K. N., Morrey, B. F., and Chao, E. Y.: Functional Evaluation of the Elbow: Normal Motion Requirements and Strength Determinations. In Transactions of the 27th Annual Meeting, Orthopaedic Research Society, **6**:183, 1981.
9. Basmajian, J. V., and Latif, S.: Integrated Actions and Functions of the Chief Flexors of the Elbow. J. Bone Joint Surg., **39A**:1106–1118, 1957.
10. Basmajian, J. V., and Travill, A. A.: Electromyogra-

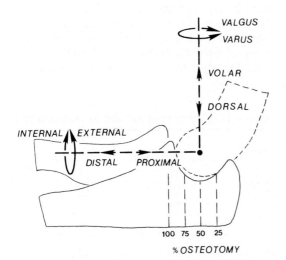

Figure 3–22. Removal of successive portions of the proximal ulna was studied for effect on various modes of joint stability.

phy of the Pronator Muscles in the Forearm. Anat. Rec., **139**:45–49, 1961.

11. Beals, R. K.: The Normal Carrying Angle of the Elbow. Clin. Orthop., **119**:194, 1976.

12. Braune, W., and Flügel, A.: Über Pronation und Supination des menschlichen Vorderarms und der Hand. Arch. Anat. Physiol. Anat., Abt. 1882.

13. Capner, N.: The Hand in Surgery. J. Bone Joint Surg., **38B**:128–151, 1956.

14. Currier, D. P.: Maximal Isometric Tension of the Elbow Extensors at Varied Positions. Part 2. Assessment of Extensor Components at Quantitative Electromyography. Phys. Therap., **52**:1265–1276, 1972.

15. Dempster, W. T., and Finerty, J. C.: Relative Activity of Wrist Moving Muscles in Static Support of the Wrist Joint: An Electromyographic Study. Am. J. Physiol., **150**:596–606, 1947.

16. Dempster, W. T.: Space Requirements of the Seated Operator. Geometrical, Kinematic and Mechanical Aspects of the Body with Special Reference to the Limb. Wright Air Development Center, Project No. 7214, Wright-Patterson AFB, Ohio, 1955.

17. De Sousa, O. M., De Moraes, J. L., and De Moraes Vieira, F. L.: Electromyographic Study of the Brachioradialis Muscle. Anat. Rec., **139**:125–131, 1961.

18. Dwight, T.: The Movements of the Ulna in Rotation of the Forearm. J. Anat. Physiol., **19**:186–189, 1884.

19. Ewald, F. C.: Total Elbow Replacement. Orthop. Clin. N. Am., **6**:685–696, 1975.

20. Fidelus, K.: The Significance of the Stabilizing Function in the Process of Controlling the Muscle Groups of Upper Extremities. In Medicine and Sport, Vol. 8, Biomechanics III, pp. 129–133. Basel, Karger, 1973.

21. Fischer, G., cited by Fick, R.: Handbüch der Anatomie und Mechanik du Gelenke, unter Berücksichtigung der Bewegenden Muskeln, Vol. 2, p. 299. Jena, G. Fischer, 1911.

22. Funk, D.: An EMG Analysis of Muscles Controlling Elbow Motion. M. S. Thesis, Minneapolis, Mayo Clinic, 1984.

23. Goel, V. K., Singh, D., and Bijlani, V.: Contact Areas in Human Elbow Joints. J. Biomechan. Engrg., **104**:169–175, 1982.

24. Goodfellow, J. W., and Bullough, P. G.: The Pattern of Aging of the Articular Cartilage of the Elbow Joint. J. Bone Joint Surg., **49B**:175, 1967.

25. Halls, A. A., and Travill, R.: Transmission of Pressures across the Elbow Joint. Anat. Rec., **150**:243, 1964.

26. Heiberg, J.: The Movement of the Ulna in Rotation of the Forearm. J. Anat. Physiol., **19**:237–240, 1884.

27. Hui, F. C., Chao, E. Y., and An, K. N.: Muscle and Joint Forces at the Elbow During Isometric Lifting (abstract). Orthop. Trans., **2**:169, 1978.

28. Hultkrantz, J. W.: Das Ellbogengelenk und seine Mechanik, Jena, G. Fischer 1897.

29. Ishizuki, M.: Functional Anatomy of the Elbow Joint and Three-Dimensional Quantitative Motion Analysis of the Elbow Joint. J. Jap. Orthop. Assn., **53**:989–996, 1979.

30. Kapandji, I. A.: The Physiology of the Joints: The Elbow: Flexion and Extension, Vol. 1, 2nd ed. Baltimore, The Williams & Wilkins Company, 1970.

31. Kawai, T., and Takenchi, N.: A Discrete Method of Limit Analysis with Simplified Elements. In International Conference on Computing in Civil Engineering. New York, ASCE, 1981.

32. Keats, T. E., Tuslink, R., Diamond, A. E., and Williams, J. H.: Normal Axial Relationships of the Major Joints. Radiology, **87**:904, 1966.

33. Lanz, T., and Wachsmuth, W.: Praktische Anatomie. Berlin, Springer-Verlag, 1959.

34. Larson, R. F.: Forearm Positioning on Maximal Elbow-Flexor Force. Phys. Therap., **49**:748–756, 1969.

35. Le Bozec, S., Maton, B., and Cnockaert, J. C.: The Synergy of Elbow Extensor Muscles During Static Work in Man. Europ. J. Appl. Physiol., **43**:57–68, 1980.

36. London, J. T.: Kinematics of the Elbow. J. Bone Joint Surg., **63A**:529–535, 1981.

37. Maton, B., and Bouisset, S.: The Distribution of Activity Among the Muscles of a Single Group During Isometric Contraction. Europ. J. Appl. Physiol., **37**:101–109, 1977.

38. Meissner, G.: Lokomotion des Ellbogengelenkes. Ber. Üb.d. Fortschr. d. Anat. u. Physiol., Vol. 7, 1856.

39. Messier, R. H., Duffy, J., Litchman, H. M., Pasley, P. R., Soechting, J., and Stewart, P. A.: The Electromyogram as a Measure of Tension in the Human Biceps and Triceps Muscles. Int. J. Mech. Sci., **13**:585–598, 1971.

40. Morrey, B. F., and Chao, E. Y. S.: Passive Motion of the Elbow Joint. J. Bone Joint Surg., **58A**:501–508, 1976.

41. Morrey, B. F., and An, K. N.: Articular and Ligamentous Contributions to the Stability of the Elbow Joint. Am. J. Sports Med., **11**:315, 1983.

42. Nicol, A. C., Berme, N., and Paul, J. P.: A Biomechanical Analysis of Elbow Joint Function. In Joint Replacement in the Upper Limb, p. 45. London, Institute of Mechanical Engineers, 1977.

43. Pauly, J. E., Rushing, J. L., and Schieving, L. E.: An Electromyographic Study of Some Muscles Crossing the Elbow Joint. Anat. Rec., **159**:47–54, 1967.

44. Pauwels, F.: Biomechanics of Locomotor Apparatus. Translated by P. Maquet and R. Furlong. New York, Springer-Verlag, 1980.

45. Ray, R. D., Johnson, R. J., and Jamieson, R. W.: Rotation of the Forearm, an Experimental Study of Pronation Supination. J. Bone Joint Surg., **33A**:993–996, 1951.

46. Schlein, A. P.: Semiconstrained Total Elbow Arthroplasty. Clin. Orthop., **121**:222–229, 1976.

47. Spinner, M., and Kaplan, E. B.: The Quadrate Ligament of the Elbow, Its Relationship to the Stability of the Proximal Radioulnar Joint. Acta Orthop. Scand., **41**:632, 1970.

48. Steindler, A.: Kinesiology of the Human Body under Normal and Pathological Conditions, pp. 493–494. Springfield, Il., Charles C Thomas, 1955.

49. Stevens, A., Stijns, H., Reybrouck, T., Bonte, G., Michels, A., Rosselle, N., Roelandts, P., Krauss, E., and Verheyen, G.: A Polyelectromyographical Study of the Arm Muscles at Gradual Isometric Loading. Electromyogr. Clin. Neurophysiol., **13**:465–476, 1973.

50. Sullivan, W. E., Mortensen, O. A., Miles, M., and Greene, L. S.: Electromyographic Studies of m. biceps brachii During Normal Voluntary Movement at the Elbow. Anat. Rec., **107**:243–251, 1950.

51. Travill, A. A.: Electromyographic Study of the Extensor Apparatus of the Forearm. Anat. Rec., **144**:373–376, 1962.

52. Von Meyer, H., cited in Steindler, A.: Kinesiology of the Human Body under Normal and Pathological Conditions, pp. 490–507. Springfield, Il., Charles C Thomas, 1955.

53. Walker, P. S.: Human Joints and Their Artificial Replacements, pp. 182–183. Springfield, Il., Charles C Thomas, 1977.

54. Youm, Y., Dryer, R. F., Thambyrajah, K., Flatt, A. E., and Sprague, B. L.: Biomechanical Analysis of Forearm Pronation-Supination and Elbow Flexion-Extension. J. Biomechan., **12**:245–255, 1979.

CHAPTER 4

The Physical Examination of the Elbow

R. G. VOLZ and B. F. MORREY

GENERAL CONSIDERATIONS

Routine systematic elbow examination has been discussed elsewhere.[5, 9, 11, 15] This chapter will relate the physical findings with the pathologic condition.

The examination of a patient presenting with complaints of the elbow region begins with the taking of a precise history. Primary attention should be focused upon this aspect of the assessment because patients are often unable to identify accurately the singular nature of their problem. Not infrequently, the patient who has lived with chronic pain, such as that accompanying rheumatoid arthritis, has learned certain accommodative activities that have assisted in lessening or eliminating pain from a conscious level. Such patients may complain only of a sudden inability to lift objects against gravity, of an unexplainable dropping of objects, or of a decrease in muscle power of the upper extremity. Under such circumstances, the examining physician should be suspicious that the resulting compromise in function is due to reflex inhibition caused by pain. In other patients the underlying primary disability may be loss of a functional range of motion. Such patients may merely complain of an inability to perform certain activities of daily living such as combing their hair or placing the hand in a certain position in space. Because the elbow is one of three important joints of the upper extremity that permit the hand to be placed in an infinite variety of positions, the examiner must be aware of the interplay of shoulder and wrist function as they complement the usefulness of the elbow.

Functionally, the elbow is the most important joint of the upper extremity because it provides the intermediate linkage that allows the hand to be brought to the torso, head, or mouth. An inability to perform such necessary daily activities should focus attention upon the elbow as the source of the problem, although disabilities of the shoulder and wrist can cause similar complaints. However, a considerable limitation of elevation and abduction function can exist at the shoulder complex without producing an appreciable compromise in most activities of daily living. This is true because only a relatively small amount of shoulder flexion and rotation is necessary to place the hand about the head or posteriorly about the waist or hip, and scapulothoracic motion can compensate for glenohumeral dysfunction.

The patient's history may also suggest elbow dysfunction if there is a loss of forearm rotation such as might exist with an inability to accept change in the supinated hand. But the maintenance of normal forearm rotation reflects more than normal elbow function. Full supination and pronation can be achieved only when both the proximal and the distal radioulnar joints are normal in their relationship, the relative length of the radius and ulna is anatomic, and the interosseous membrane is unaltered. Thus a loss of forearm rotation may suggest not only a problem with the elbow but also a mechanical problem at the distal radioulnar joint, residual deformity secondary to fracture, skeletal growth abnormality of the radius or ulna, or even an idiopathic condition.[6]

The patterns of pain related to problems in or about the elbow can be somewhat variable. Conditions involving the lateral compartment of the elbow—that is, the radiocapitellar articulation—generally provoke a pattern of pain that extends over the lateral area of the elbow and forearm. The symptom is frequently of a "deep" nature and is perceived in the area of the proximal common extensor muscle mass that is supplied by the deep branch of the radial nerve. When a more diffuse pathologic condition involves the elbow joint, such as the destructive changes associated with rheumatoid arthritis, symptoms are generally more periarticular in distribution. An ulnar neuropathy arising at the elbow will usually be described as paresthetic in nature and extends from the ulnar notch distally into the sensory distribution of the hand and fingers. Less commonly, a nonspecific ache, poorly localized to the medial aspect of the elbow, can represent ulnar nerve pathology. Symptoms arising from cervical radiculopathy can be distinguished by a more proximal point of origin and specific distribution into the hand. A history is commonly elicited from the patient of provocation of pain by changes in the posture of the cervical spine, attempts at elevation of the upper extremity above the horizon, or lifting activities.

PHYSICAL EXAMINATION

Inspection

The trained examiner can gain considerable information from visual inspection of the elbow joint. Since much of the joint is subcutaneous, any appreciable alteration in the skeletal anatomy is often detectable. Gross soft tissue swelling or muscle atrophy is also visible.

Axial Alignment

An alteration in the carrying angle of the elbow when compared with the opposite side suggests prior trauma or a skeletal growth disturbance. To determine the carrying angle, the forearm and hand should be supinated and the elbow extended; the angle formed by

the humerus and forearm is then determined (Fig. 4–1A). As a general rule, women have a carrying angle that is 2 to 3 degrees greater than that of men. Although there is considerable variation with race, age, sex, and thin or heavy individuals, an average of 10 degrees for men and 13 degrees for women has been calculated as the mean carrying angle from several reports.[3, 4, 13, 14]

Although angular deformities, such as cubitus varus or valgus, are easily identifiable (Fig. 4–1B) and suggest prior trauma or a disturbance in distal epiphyseal growth, rotational deformities following supracondylar or other fractures of the humeral shaft may be difficult to perceive. Bowing of the forearm, usually in an ulnar direction, from malunion of the radius or ulna is a relatively common deformity.

Lateral Aspect

Fullness about the infracondylar recess located just inferior to the lateral condyle of the humerus suggests either an increase in synovial fluid, synovial tissue proliferation, or radial head pathology such as fracture, subluxation, or dislocation (Fig. 4–2).

Thin, taut, adherent skin over the lateral epicondyle may be indicative of excessive cortisone injections in this area for refractory lateral epicondylitis.

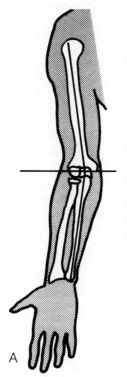

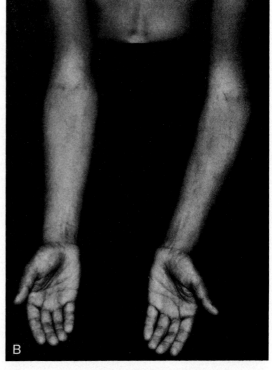

Figure 4–1. *A,* The carrying angle is a clinical measurement of the angle formed by the forearm and the humerus with the elbow extended. *B,* The normal 10 to 15 degrees carrying angle can be altered by injury about the elbow, causing a varus carrying angle or the so-called gunstock deformity.

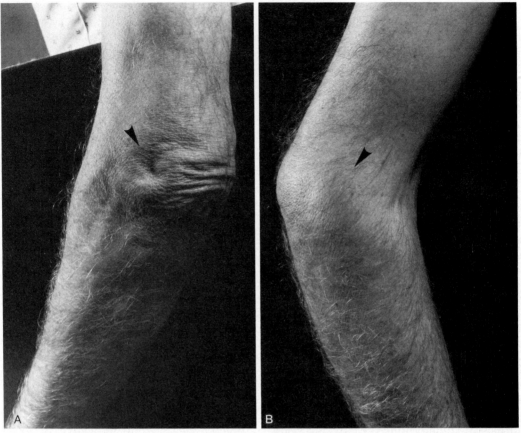

Figure 4–2. A normal depression in the contour of the skin in the intracondylar recess (arrow) *(A)* becomes obliterated in the presence of synovitis or effusion *(B)*.

Posterior Aspect

A prominent olecranon tip or posterior displacement of the forearm suggests destructive loss of bone of the ulnohumeral interface with posterior subluxation or migration of the forearm upon the arm (Fig. 4–3). Rupture of the triceps tendon at its insertion should be suspected if this finding is accompanied by loss of active extension. Unquestionably, a loss of extension at the elbow is a sensitive indicator of intra-articular pathology because elbow extension is the first motion lost and the last to be regained with intra-articular injury or disease.

The prominent subcutaneous olecranon bursa is readily observed posteriorly when it is inflamed or distended (Fig. 4–4). Rheumatoid nodules are frequently found on the subcutaneous border of the ulna (see Chapter 48).

Medial Aspect

Few landmarks are observable from the medial aspect of the joint. The prominent medial epicondyle is evident unless the patient is

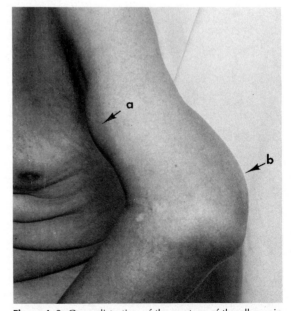

Figure 4–3. Gross distortion of the contour of the elbow, in this instance, due to posterior displacement of the forearm *(b)* from a Charcot joint. The humerus is anterior *(a)*. (From Polley, H. F., and Hunder, G. G.: Rheumatologic Interviewing and Physical Examination of the Joints, 2nd ed. Philadelphia, W. B. Saunders Company, 1978.)

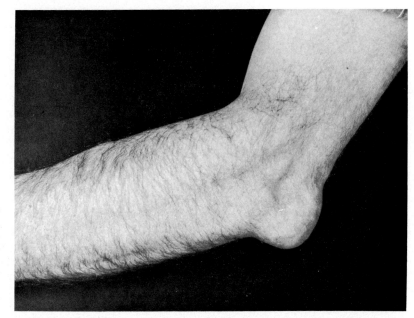

Figure 4–4. An inflamed or enlarged olecranon bursa is one of the more dramatic diagnoses made by observation in the region of the elbow. (From Polley, H. F., and Hunder, G. G.: Rheumatologic Interviewing and Physical Examination of the Joints, 2nd ed. Philadelphia, W. B. Saunders Company, 1978.)

obese. Rarely, the ulnar nerve may be observed and may displace anteriorly during flexion in certain individuals with recurrent subluxation of the ulnar nerve.[8]

Associated Joints

No examination of the elbow or forearm is complete without an evaluation of the wrist, especially the distal radioulnar joint. For normal forearm rotation, there must be a normal anatomic relationship between the proximal and distal radioulnar joint. Frequently, a loss of forearm rotation will result from inflammatory changes involving either the elbow or the wrist or both. A disruption of the normal relationship of the distal radioulnar joint will be characterized by a dorsally displaced prominence of the distal ulna. Dorsal displacement of the distal ulna is exaggerated by pronation and is lessened by supination. Because pronation is the common resting position of the hand, dorsal subluxation of the ulna at the wrist is often readily identifiable by inspection.

PALPATION

Bony Landmarks

Careful palpation of the elbow and periarticular soft tissue should proceed in a systematic manner. Palpation of the tips of the medial and lateral epicondyles and the tip of the olecranon should, when viewed from the posterior, form an equilateral triangle (Fig. 4–5). Fracture, malunion, unreduced dislocation, or

growth disturbances involving the distal end of the humerus can be assessed clinically in this fashion.

Lateral Aspect

The avascular interval in the lateral supracondylar region is readily palpable and is a valuable landmark during lateral surgical exposures (Fig. 4–6; see also Chapter 8). Examination of the radial head is easily performed provided a joint effusion is not present. Digital pressure over the peripheral artic-

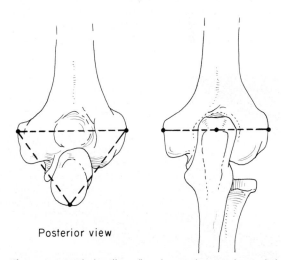

Posterior view

Figure 4–5. With the elbow flexed to 90 degrees, the medial and lateral epicondyles and tip of the olecranon form an eqilateral triangle when viewed from posterior. When the elbow is extended, this relationship is changed to a straight line connecting these three bony landmarks.

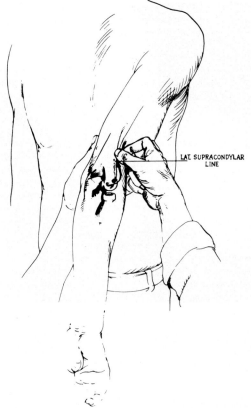

LAT. SUPRACONDYLAR LINE

Figure 4–6. The lateral supracondylar interval is an avascular area that can be readily palpated and serves as an important landmark in many surgical exposures to the elbow. (From Hoppenfeld, S.: Physical Examination of the Spine and Extremities. New York, Appleton-Century-Crofts, 1976.)

ular surface of the radial head, when combined with pronation and supination of the forearm in varying degrees of elbow flexion, will offer valuable information about this bony structure. If painful, this examination should be done gently. Radial head fracture

may be thus suspected even when the roentgenogram is negative. An effusion of the elbow is most easily identified by palpation over the lateral border of the radial head or about the posterior recess located just between the radial head and the lateral border of the olecranon (Fig. 4–7). Ballottement may produce increased pressure over the medial aspect of the joint at the ulnar border of the olecranon. As with other joints, significant effusions will limit extremes of motion, especially extension.

Medial Aspect

Because of the scant amount of synovial tissue present on the medial side of the olecranon, greater difficulty is encountered in palpable assessment of the soft tissues in this area. Palpation of the ulnar notch is easily performed (Fig. 4–8) and may be helpful in identifying ulnar nerve entrapment at this level or synovial proliferation such as that observed in patients with rheumatoid arthritis.

Posterior Aspect

Although the triceps mechanism covers the tip of the olecranon, its muscle fibers are not directly attached at its most proximal prominence. Thus, with deep pressure the tip of the olecranon may be palpated, provided the elbow is not held in full extension, because in this position the olecranon tip is terminally impacted against the trochlear notch. If malunion or deformity involves the olecranon, this may serve to limit normal extension of the elbow. With elbow flexion, the olecranon fossa may be identified in a thin person by careful palpation (Fig. 4–9). A tense effusion

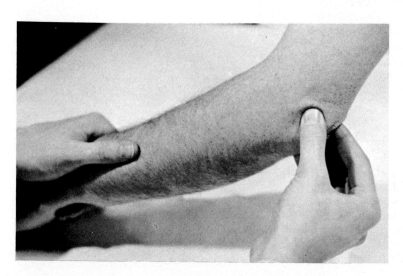

Figure 4–7. The radial head may be readily palpated. The contour and integrity of the structure may be further appreciated by pronating and supinating the forearm during this examination. (From Polley, H. F., and Hunder, G. G.: Rheumatological Interviewing and Physical Examination of the Joints, 2nd ed. Philadelphia, W. B. Saunders Company, 1978.)

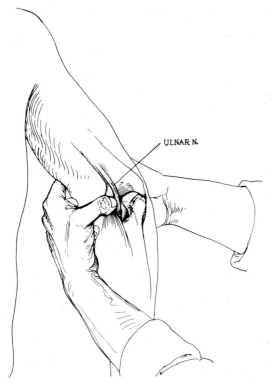

Figure 4–8. Palpation of the cubital tunnel just anterior to the medial aspect of the olecranon allows assessment of the ulnar nerve as it passes the posterior aspect of the elbow. (From Hoppenfeld, S.: Physical Examination of the Spine and Extremities. New York, Appleton-Century-Crofts, 1976.)

is likewise detectable from this aspect as well. The subcutaneous border of the olecranon and proximal ulna are also readily appreciated by palpation along the posterior aspect of the distal elbow region.

Anterior Aspect

The cubital fossa is bound laterally by the mobile wad of muscles that includes the brachioradialis and the extensor carpi radialis longus and brevis. The brachioradialis is a significant elbow flexor and becomes tense with elbow flexion against resistance. The medial aspect of the cubital fossa contains the biceps tendon, which is readily palpable, particularly with flexion against resistance. The lacertus fibrosus may be palpated just medial to the tendon, and the pulsation of the brachial artery is easily located lying deep to the lacterus fibrosus.

MOTION

Perhaps no portion of the physical examination is more important than the assessment of the range of motion of the elbow. This motion occurs about two axes: flexion and extension, and forearm rotation (pronation and supination). A change in the carrying angle from valgus to varus can be noted in most people as the forearm is supinated and as it is moved from a position of extension into full flexion.[16, 22] Emphasis is again placed on the importance of the loss of full extension, because this is the first plane of motion usually altered and the last to be regained with intrinsic problems of the elbow joint.

Normally, the arc of flexion and extension, although variable, ranges from about 0 to 140 degrees plus or minus 10 degrees[1, 7, 20] (Fig. 4–10). This range far exceeds what is normally required for activities of daily living.[17] Pronation and supination may vary to a greater

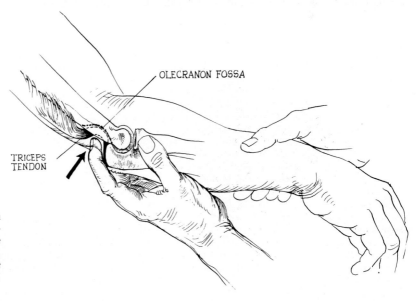

Figure 4–9. The olecranon fossa may be palpated in some individuals with the elbow flexed and the triceps relaxed. (From Hoppenfeld, S.: Physical Examination of the Spine and Extremities. New York, Appleton-Century-Crofts, 1976.)

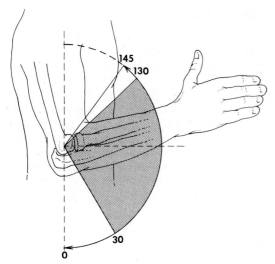

Figure 4–10. The normal flexion and extension of the elbow is from zero to approximately 145 degrees. The functional arc of flexion and extension about which most daily activities are achieved is 30 to 130 degrees.

extent than the arc of flexion and extension. Acceptable norms of motion are pronation, 70 degrees and supination, 85 degrees (Fig. 4–11). In assessing the range of motion, the examiner should record both active and passive values while being certain to immobilize the humerus in a vertical position when evaluating the arc of forearm rotation. Patients often tend to accommodate for a loss of forearm rotation by enlisting abduction or adduction shoulder motion. Any significant difference between active and passive ranges of motion tends to suggest that pain is the inhibiting factor.

Assessment of crepitation should first be performed by a passive range of motion fol-

lowed by active assistance on the patient's part. Active contraction of the skeletal muscles will often accentuate or provoke crepitance that is otherwise barely discernible on passive motion of the joint.

The patient may sometimes have difficulty in identifying a mechanical explanation for an inability to perform a certain task such as combing his hair or reaching the ipsilateral side of the face. In such a case, the patient should be asked to perform these motions before the examiner, who can then make a careful assessment of any compromised motion at the shoulder, elbow, or wrist. Often the disability will arise from a combination of factors not previously considered, but it should be stressed that a full range of motion at the elbow is not essential for performance of the activities of daily living. The essential arc of elbow flexion and extension required for daily activities ranges from about 30 to 130 degrees[17] (Fig. 4–10). Because the loss of extension up to a certain degree only shortens the lever arm of the upper extremity, flexion contractures of less than 45 degrees may have little practical significance, although patients will sometimes be concerned about the cosmetic appearance.

Because the primary functions of the shoulder and elbow are to assist the hand in its placement within space, the practical significance of a loss of motion at both the shoulder and the elbow must be carefully evaluated against the individual's need. Thus, patients with rheumatoid arthritis are not necessarily handicapped by their inability to elevate the arm above the horizon, a function of shoulder motion, but they are handicapped when they do not possess sufficient shoulder or elbow motion to bring the hand to the head, torso,

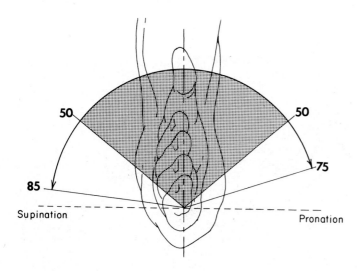

Supination   Pronation

Figure 4–11. Normal pronation and supination is about 75 to 85 degrees respectively. The functional arc of forearm rotation consists of approximately 50 degrees of pronation and 50 degrees of supination.

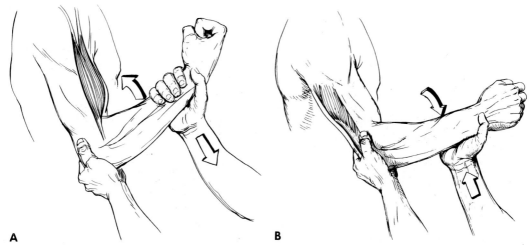

Figure 4–12. Flexion strength is best assessed with the elbow flexed to 90 degrees and the forearm in neutral rotation. Flexion resistance is assessed while the examiner attempts to extend the elbow *(A)*. To test extension strength, the examiner applies resistance to the patient's ability to extend the elbow with the joint in approximately 90 degrees of flexion and the forearm in neutral (or pronated) position *(B)*. (From Hoppenfeld, S.: Orthopedic Neurology. Philadelphia, J. B. Lippincott Company, 1977.)

or mouth. This practical analysis of disability versus need should be considered in the course of the assessment (see Chapter 5).

Similar observations may be made concerning the arc of forearm rotation. The useful arc is between 50 degrees pronation and 50 degrees supination[17] (Fig. 4–11). For most individuals pronation is the primary arc of motion on the dominant side for eating and writing, and loss of pronation is compensated by shoulder abduction to accomplish these tasks. On the other hand, a loss of supination of the nondominant side may significantly hinder personal hygiene needs, the taking of change in the palm, and the opening of door handles. These tasks are poorly compensated by shoulder or wrist motions.

STRENGTH

Strength assessment is an additional aspect of the physical examination of the elbow. Only gross estimates of strength are attainable in the clinical setting. Flexion and extension strength testing (Fig. 4–12) is conducted against resistance with the forearm in neutral rotation and the elbow at 90 degrees of flexion. Extension strength is normally 70 percent that of flexion strength[2] and is best measured with the elbow at 90 degrees of flexion with the forearm in neutral rotation.[10, 18, 19, 21] Pronation (Fig. 4–13A), supination (Fig. 4–13B), and grip strength are also best studied with the elbow at 90 degrees of flexion and the forearm in neutral rotation. Supination

strength is normally about 15 percent greater than pronation strength.[2] The dominant extremity is about 5 to 10 percent stronger than the nondominant side, and females are 50 percent as strong as males[2] (see Chapter 5).

The patient's ability to lift a given weight with the elbow flexed against gravity offers additional confirmation concerning the extent of the patient's disability, especially as it relates to arthritic involvement. Many patients will exhibit a surprising inability to lift objects of any appreciable weight, even a cup of coffee or a plate. This, of course, is due to the marked magnification of any weight held in the hand because of the lever arm length of the forearm. Biomechanical studies have shown that a 1 kg weight held in the hand with the elbow flexed at 90° may generate a 10 kg joint reactive force of the elbow.

Reflexes

The fifth, sixth, and seventh cervical nerve roots may be tested by their function about the elbow. The C5 root is tested by the biceps reflex, C6 by the brachioradialis reflex, and C7 by the triceps reflex (Fig. 4–14).

INSTABILITY

In the absence of articular cartilage loss, the mechanical integrity of the radial and ulnar collateral ligaments is difficult to assess because of the intrinsic stability offered by the closely approximated surfaces of the olecra-

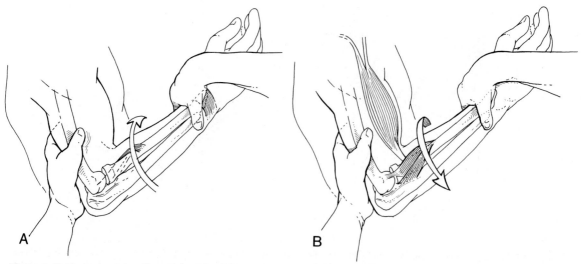

Figure 4–13. Pronation strength is evaluated with the patient comfortable and the elbow at 90 degrees of flexion. Pronation strength is usually measured by grasping the wrist or, less commonly, the hand with the forearm in neutral or in supination rotation (A). To test supination strength, the forearm is in neutral or pronation (B).

non and trochlea and the buttressing effect of the radial head against the capitellum. However, when articular cartilage has been destroyed, as it is in rheumatoid arthritis, or removed, as with radial head excision, collateral ligament stability can be determined by the application of varus and valgus stresses. Whereas the fibers of the anterior bundle of the medial collateral ligament offer stability through nearly the entire arc of flexion and extension, the posterior portion contributes stability only through an arc of approximately 60 to 135 degrees of flexion and extension (see Chapter 3). The radial collateral ligament resists varus stress throughout the arc of el-

bow flexion with varying contributions of the anterior capsule and articular surface in extension (see Chapter 3). To properly assess collateral ligament integrity, the elbow should be flexed to about 15 degrees. This relaxes the anterior capsule and removes the olecranon from the fossa. Varus stress is best applied with the humeus in full internal rotation (Fig. 4–15A). Valgus instability is best measured with the arm in full external rotation (Fig. 4–15B). Anterior and posterior instability, if present, is usually very obvious. Laxity in the anterior plane may also be due to cartilage loss from rheumatoid arthritis and is best determined with the elbow at 90 degrees of flexion and exerting an anterior-posterior force on the forearm.

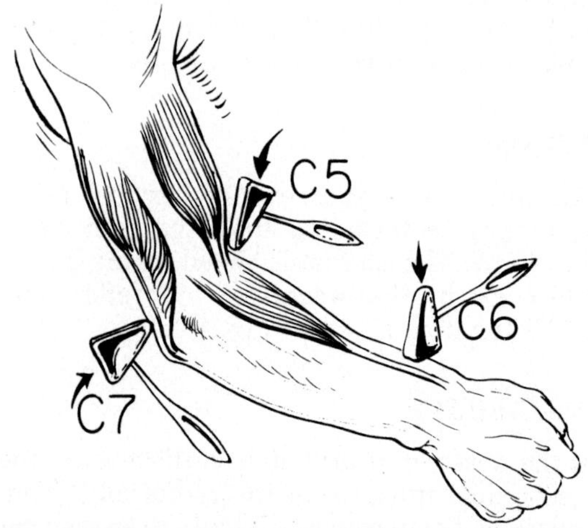

LOCALIZATION OF PATHOLOGY

Distinction between intra-articular and peri-articular pathology may be difficult at times. The dilemma may be resolved by the intra-articular injection of 2 to 3 ml of a 1 percent lidocaine hydrochloride (Xylocaine) solution. Joint aspiration or injection is best performed by positioning the elbow at 90 degrees of flexion with the forearm comfortably supported on a desk or table or across the chest. Entrance to the joint space is most easily gained by insertion of the needle between the radial head and the radial border of the adjacent ulna (Fig. 4–16). Aspiration is particularly easy if a joint effusion is present. The patient's expression of pain relief, if obtained following such a diagnostic injection, can

Figure 4–14. The biceps, brachioradialis, and triceps reflexes allow evaluation of the C5, C6, and C7 nerve roots, respectively. (From Hoppenfeld, S.: Orthopedic Neurology, Philadelphia, J. B. Lippincott Company, 1977.)

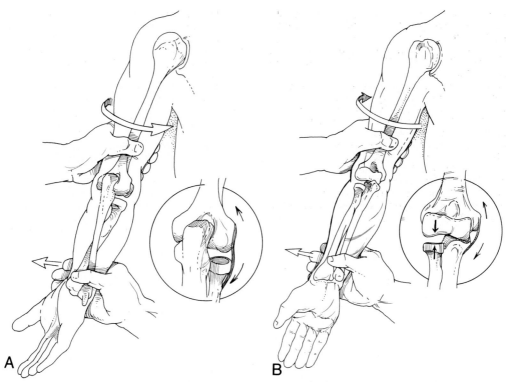

Figure 4–15. *A,* Varus in stability of the elbow is measured with the humerus in full internal rotation and a varus stress applied to the slightly flexed joint. *B,* Valgus instability is evaluated with the humerus in full external rotation while a valgus stress is applied to the slightly flexed joint.

generally be taken as strong evidence of an intrarticular source of disability.

Similarly, the patient's ability to lift increased amounts of weight and perform more functions, for instance, following arthroplasty of the elbow, is consistent with lessening of pain and an increase in functional capabili-

ties, and resembles the effect observed in the lower extremity following total joint replacement.

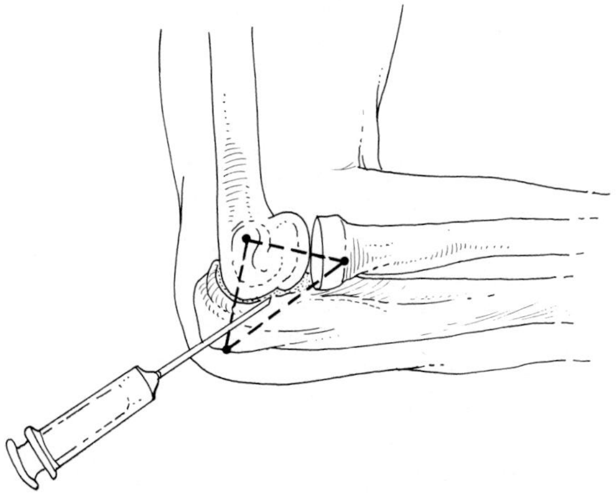

Figure 4–16. Elbow joint aspiration or injection is readily performed by inserting the needle in the midportion of the triangular space formed by the lateral epicondyle, radial head, and tip of the olecranon. This area is coincident with the infracondylar recess, which becomes distended if an effusion is present (see Fig. 4–2).

References

1. American Academy of Orthopedic Surgeons: Joint Motion: Method of Measuring and Recording. Chicago, American Academy of Orthopedic Surgeons, 1965.
2. Askew, L. J., An, K. N., Morrey, B. F., and Chao, E. Y.: Functional Evaluation of the Elbow: Normal Motion Requirements and Strength Determination. Orthop. Trans. **5**:304, 1981.
3. Atkinson, W. B., and Elftman, H.: The Carrying Angle of the Human Arm as a Secondary Symptom Character. Anat. Rec. **91**:49, 1945.
4. Beals, R. K.: The Normal Carrying Angle of the Elbow. Clin. Orthop. **119**:194, 1976.
5. Beetham, W. P., Jr., Polley, H. F., Slocumb, C. H., and Weaver, W. F.: Physical Examination of the Joints. Philadelphia, W. B. Saunders Co., 1965.
6. Bert, J. M., Linscheid, R. L., and McElfresh, E. C.: Rotatory Contracture of the Forearm. J. Bone Joint Surg. **62A**:1163, 1980.
7. Boone, D. C., and Azen, S. P.: Normal Range of Motion of Joints in Male Subjects. J. Bone Joint Surg. **61A**:756, 1979.
8. Childress, H. M.: Recurrent Ulnar Nerve Dislocation at the Elbow. Clin. Orthop. **108**:168, 1975.
9. Daniels, L., Williams, M., and Worthingham, C.: Muscle Testing: Techniques of Manual Examination, 2nd ed. Philadelphia, W. B. Saunders Co., 1946.

10. Elkins, E. C., Ursula, M. L., and Khalil, G. W.: Objective Recording of the Strength of Normal Muscles. Arch. Phys. Med. **33**:639, 1951.

11. Hoppenfeld, S.: Physical Examination of the Spine and Extremities. New York, Appleton-Century-Crofts, 1976.

12. Johansson, O.: Capsular and Ligament Injuries of the Elbow Joint. Acta Chir. Scand. Suppl. **287**, 1962.

13. Keats, T. E., Teeslink, R., Diamond, A. E., and Williams, J. H.: Normal Axial Relationships of the Major Joints. Radiology **87**:904, 1966.

14. Lanz, T., and Wachsmuth, W.: Praktische Anatomie. Berlin, ARM, Springer-Verlag, 1959.

15. McRae, R.: Clinical Orthopedic Examination. London, Churchill Livingstone, 1976.

16. Morrey, B. F., and Chao, E. Y.: Passive Motion of the Elbow Joint: A Biomechanical Study. J. Bone Joint Surg. **61A**:63, 1979.

17. Morrey, B. F., Askew, L. J., An, K. N., and Chao, E. Y.: A Biomechanical Study of Normal Functional Elbow Motion. J. Bone Joint Surg. **63A**(6):872, 1981.

18. Provins, K. A., and Salter, N.: Maximum Torque Exerted About the Elbow Joint. J. Appl. Physiol. **7**:393, 1955.

19. Rasch, P. J.: Effect of Position of Forearm on Strength of Elbow Flexion. Res. Q. **27**:333, 1955.

20. Wagner, C.: Determination of the Rotary Flexibility of the Elbow Joint. Europ. J. Appl. Physiol. **37**:47, 1977.

21. Williams, M., and Stutzman, L.: Strength Variation Through the Range of Motion. Phys. Ther. Rev. **39**:145, 1959.

22. Youm, Y., Dryer, R. F., Thambyrajahk, K., Flatt, A. E., and Sprague, B. L.: Biomechanical Analysis of Forearm Pronation-Supination and Elbow Flexion-Extension. J. Biomechan. **12**:245, 1979.

CHAPTER 5

Functional Evaluation of the Elbow*

B. F. MORREY, K. N. AN and E. Y. S. CHAO

Functional compromise of the upper extremity is relatively common. Involvement of the upper limb accounts for about 10 percent of all compensation paid in the United States for disabling work-related injuries.[30, 44] In addition, dysfunction of the upper extremity cost about 5.5 million lost work days in 1977.[43] It is, therefore, appropriate that physicians should become better acquainted with some of the elements that compromise normal elbow function and the significance of each.

The elbow is essential for and its function may be summarized in three activities: (1) to allow the hand to be positioned in space; (2) to provide the power to perform lifting activities; and (3) to stabilize the upper extremity linkage for power and fine work activities. Hence, assessment of the joint should include these three components: measurement of useful motion; an estimate of static, dynamic, and endurance strength; and finally, evaluation of joint stability.

ELBOW MOTION

Normal Motion

Normal flexion and extension and pronation and supination of the elbow are estimated clinically with the hand-held goniometer. Such measurement devices were described centuries ago.[49] Forearm rotation is measured with the elbow at 90 degrees of flexion, often with the subject holding a linear object to make the measurement more objective.[53] The reliability of these measurements is based on

the type of device, the technique of examination, and the anatomic features of the joint and skill of the examiner.[24] In spite of obvious limitations, investigators have concluded that the standard hand-held goniometric examination by a skilled observer allows measurement of elbow flexion-extension and pronation-supination with an error of less than about 5 percent.[24, 64]

Normal passive elbow flexion has been reported to range between 0 and 140 to 150 degrees.[1, 8, 28, 53] Greater variation of normal forearm rotation has been described but averages about 75 degrees pronation and 85 degrees supination.[1, 8, 28, 59] What is of particular importance, however, is the amount of motion used for daily activity. These data can be determined only by measuring the active and simultaneous motion of elbow flexion, pronation, and supination. The hand-held goniometer is inadequate for this purpose and has led to the design of an instrument that allows such measurements.

Measurement Techniques—The Electrogoniometer

To measure three-dimensional joint motion in daily activities, any one of several rather sophisticated experimental techniques can be used.[11, 64] For the elbow joint, a method was selected based on the following criteria: (1) convenience of use, (2) capability of accurate measurement of most daily activities, (3) avoidance of a tedious data reduction process, and (4) capability of simultaneous measurement of active elbow flexion and forearm rotation. The triaxial electrogoniometer satisfies these criteria[3, 12, 42] and can be easily adapted to the subject for examination of a wide spectrum of daily activities (Fig. 5–1).

*We acknowledge the effort of L. J. Askew, R.P.T., who has conducted many of the motion and strength measurements referred to in this chapter.

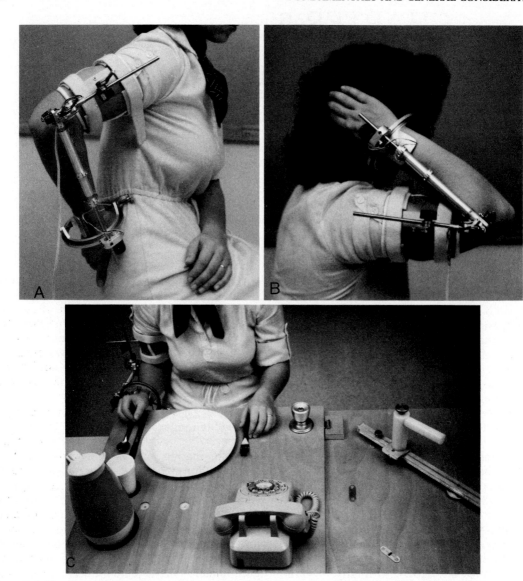

Figure 5–1. The elbow electrogoniometer may be used to measure activities of daily living. Elbow flexion and forearm rotation to reach the sacrum *(A)* or the back of the head *(B)* may be recorded. The subject is sitting at the activities table *(C)*. (From Morrey, B. F., et al.: A biomechanical study of normal functional elbow motion. J. Bone Joint Surg. 63A:872, 1981.)

In addition to flexion and rotation a change in carrying angle can also be recorded by this device.

The axes of rotation for the components of motion are defined in Figure 5–2 and are replicated by the electrogoniometer as demonstrated in Figure 5–3. The three electropotentiometers record the rotational angles along each axis in terms of electrical voltage. A four-channel strip chart recorder is used to provide motion sequencing data directly for each activity (Fig. 5–4), and a minicomputer allows conversion to the magnitude and pattern of each rotation.

Experimental measurements obtained with the electrogoniometer closely duplicate actual motions that occur in a joint model. Repeated testing of individual subjects at different times demonstrates the high reproducibility and reliability of this instrument.[38] Application of the device to the patient requires less than 10 minutes but is subject to error unless it is done by an experienced examiner. The entire sequence of such a functional evaluation takes about 20 minutes, and the data are analyzed and reported within 1 hour after the evaluation. The electrogoniometer has proved to be a valuable tool for research purposes and is presently being used for special clinical evaluations as well.

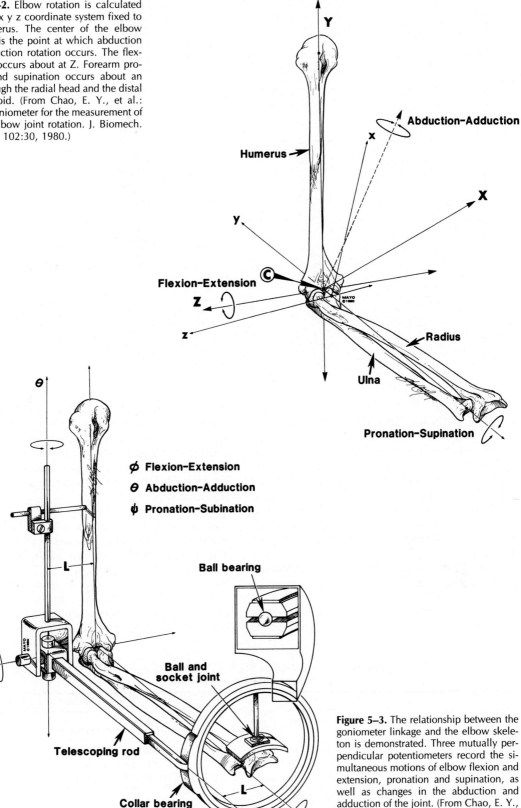

Figure 5–2. Elbow rotation is calculated using an x y z coordinate system fixed to the humerus. The center of the elbow joint (C) is the point at which abduction and adduction rotation occurs. The flexion axis occurs about at Z. Forearm pronation and supination occurs about an axis through the radial head and the distal ulna styloid. (From Chao, E. Y., et al.: Electrogoniometer for the measurement of human elbow joint rotation. J. Biomech. Engineer. 102:30, 1980.)

Humerus

Abduction-Adduction

x

X

y

Flexion-Extension

Z

z

C

Radius

Ulna

Pronation-Supination

ϕ Flexion-Extension
θ Abduction-Adduction
ψ Pronation-Subination

θ

L

ϕ

Ball bearing

Ball and socket joint

Telescoping rod

L

Collar bearing

ψ

Figure 5–3. The relationship between the goniometer linkage and the elbow skeleton is demonstrated. Three mutually perpendicular potentiometers record the simultaneous motions of elbow flexion and extension, pronation and supination, as well as changes in the abduction and adduction of the joint. (From Chao, E. Y., et al.: Electrogoniometer for the measurement of human elbow joint rotation. J. Biomech. Engineer. 102:301, 1980.)

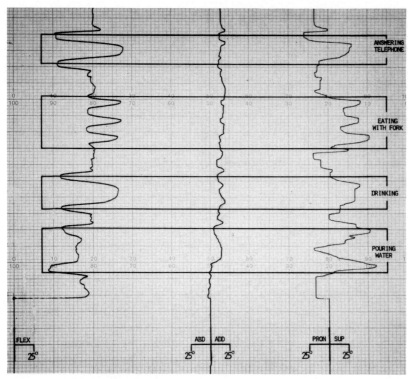

Figure 5–4. Typical electrogoniometric tracings of routine daily activities, for example, answering a phone, eating, drinking, and using table utensils. (From Morrey, B. F., et al.: A biomechanical study of normal functional elbow motion. J. Bone Joint Surg. 63A:872, 1981.)

Functional Motion

For most activities, the full potential of elbow motion is not needed or used. Loss of terminal flexion is more disabling than the same degree of loss of terminal extension. Ogilvie[47] has stated that the elbow was "designed" for use between 10 and 110 degrees of flexion. Carstam[10] placed the greatest clinical relevance in an arc of motion of 30 to 120 degrees, with 60 to 120 degrees being the most important portion.

Using the electrogoniometer described above, fifteen activities of daily living were accomplished using an arc of elbow flexion of 15 to 140 degrees.[42] The same activities required forearm motion of about 55 degrees

of pronation and 55 degrees of supination (Tables 5–1 and 5–2). In general, most activities can be performed using an arc of 100 degrees of flexion between 30 and 130 degrees (Fig. 5–5) and 100 degrees of forearm rotation equally divided between pronation and supination (Fig. 5–6).

The motion requirements of the elbow joint needed for daily activities are really a measurement of the reaching ability of the hand. The extent to which this function is impaired by loss of elbow flexion or extension can also be estimated analytically. In the sagittal plane, assuming normal shoulder motion, a surface of reach potential can be defined on the basis of a varying degree of elbow motion with an

Table 5–1. **Positions of the Elbow During Routine Activities of Personal Care and Hygiene**
(Mean and Standard Deviation)

Position	Elbow Flexion (degrees)	Forearm Rotation (degrees)	
		Supination	*Pronation*
Hand to:			
Head (vertex)	118.6 ± 6.1	46.6 ± 16.0	—
Head (occiput)	144.0 ± 7.0	2.0 ± 23	—
Shirt (waist)	100.4 ± 13.2	11.9 ± 23.8	—
Shirt (chest)	120.0 ± 8.2	29.4 ± 19.2	—
Shirt (neck)	134.7 ± 5.2	40.9 ± 16.3	—
Sacrum	69.7 ± 12.4	55.8 ± 20.1	—
Shoe	16.0 ± 6.3	—	19.0 ± 17.2

From Morrey, B. F., Askew, L. J., An, K. N., and Chao, E. Y.: A biomechanical study of normal elbow motion. J. Bone Joint Surg., 63A:872, 1981.

Table 5–2. **Amount of Elbow Motion Required to Carry Out Selected Daily Activities**

| Activity | Mean Flexion (degrees) | | | Mean Rotation (degrees) | | |
	Minimum	Maximum	Arc	Pronation	Supination[a]	Arc
Pour from a pitcher	35.6	58.3	22.7	42.9	21.9	64.8
Put glass to mouth	44.8	130.0	85.2	10.1	13.4	23.5
Cut with a knife	89.2	106.7	17.5	41.9	− 26.9	15.0
Put fork to mouth	85.1	128.3	43.2	10.4	51.8	62.2
Use a telephone	42.8	135.6	92.8	40.9	22.6	63.5
Read a newspaper	77.9	104.3	26.4	48.8	− 7.3	41.5
Rise from a chair	20.3	94.5	74.2	33.8	− 9.5	24.3
Open a door	24.0	57.4	33.4	35.4	23.4	58.8

[a]A negative value indicates pronation.

From Morrey, B. F., Askew, L. J., An, K. N., and Chao, E. Y.: A biomechanical study of normal elbow motion. J. Bone, Joint Surg. **63A**:872, 1981.

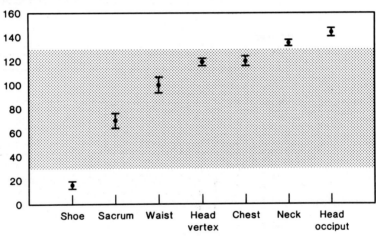

A   Activity requiring positioning of elbow

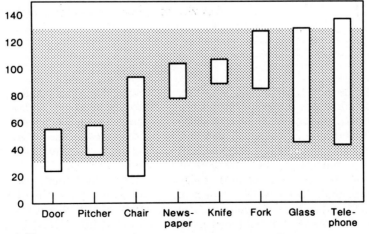

B   Activity requiring arc of elbow motion

Figure 5–5. Normal elbow flexion positions for activities of hygiene (A) and those requiring arcs of motion (B) are demonstrated. Most functions can be performed between 30 and 130 degrees of elbow flexion. (From Morrey, B. F., et al.: A biomechanical study of normal functional elbow motion. J. Bone Joint Surg. 63A:872, 1981.)

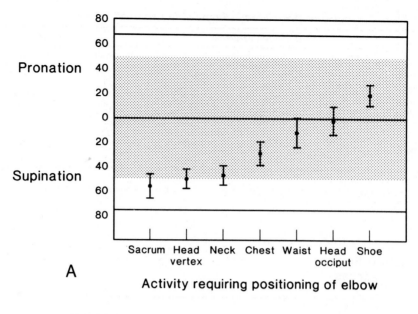

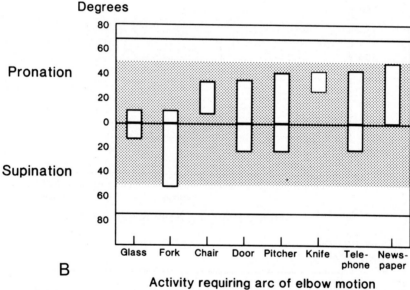

Figure 5–6. Routine daily activities requiring pronation and supination *(A)* or arcs of motion *(B)* are performed between 50 degrees pronation and 50 degrees supination. (From Morrey, B. F., et al.: A biomechanical study of normal functional elbow motion. J. Bone Joint Surg. 63A:872, 1981.)

anatomic range of from 0 to 150 degrees (Fig. 5–7). If an individual has limited motion from 30 to 130 degrees, the potential area reached by the hand is reduced by about 20 percent. Thus, the range of elbow flexion between 30 to 130 degrees defined by the goniometer study as the amount needed for most daily activities corresponds to about 80 percent of the normal reach capacity of the forearm and hand in a selected plane of shoulder motion. Figure 5–8 demonstrates the inter-relationship between the area of reach and different amounts of flexion and extension loss for an

assumed normal range of elbow flexion from 0 to 150 degrees. A modest limitation of full elbow extension is well tolerated clinically and corresponds to the analytical solution that demonstrates only minimal decrease of the reach area.

These data, then, provide some insight into the inter-relationship between the reach capacity of the elbow and the motion required for activities of daily living. Such data can be quite useful in occupational medicine and in studies of the work environment. Disability might be predicated not only on the percent-

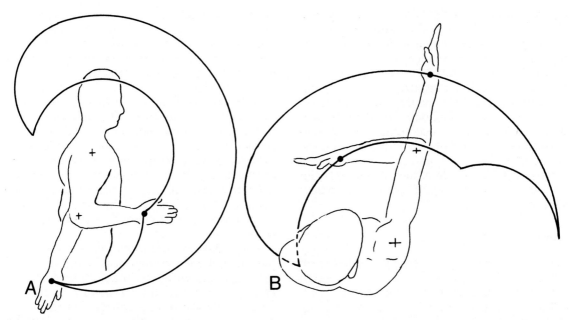

Figure 5–7. The reaching area of the hand in the sagittal (A) and transverse planes (B) with simultaneous movement of the elbow and shoulder. If the elbow is held at approximately 90 degrees of flexion, marked reduction of reach potential occurs.

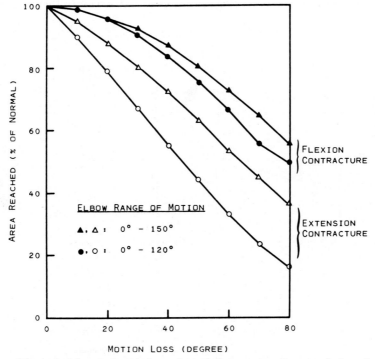

Figure 5–8. Reduction of the potential area of reach due to loss of elbow motion. For normal elbow flexion of 150 degrees, a 20-degree loss of extension results in a 20 percent loss of area. An 80-degree flexion contracture loses 60 percent of the normally attained area of reach.

age of motion loss but also on the specific part of the arc that is limited and the effect of this impairment on daily activities as reflected by limitation of the reach area.

Additional investigation is necessary to determine the motions required in various occupations as well as to analyze in more detail the coordination of flexion-extension and pronation-supination in accomplishing special tasks. The more complex function of compensation by the shoulder and wrist must also be considered. Nonetheless, the present data can be used to assess the significance of lost elbow motion.

STRENGTH

The usual assessment of strength is based on gross clinical measurements that are often rather subjective, more qualitative than quantitative, not well controlled, and not readily reproducible. To understand the value and limitations of clinical strength assessment, it will be helpful to review briefly the types of muscle contraction, the major factors affecting strength, different measurement techniques, and the results of previous studies.

Background

Types of Muscle Contraction. Because great emphasis is currently being placed on muscle

physiology, testing, and rehabilitation, a brief review of the subject is appropriate here. There are several types of muscle contraction, and they are classified according to changes in length, force, and velocity of contraction[23, 40, 60] (Fig. 5–9). If there is no change of muscle length during a contraction, it is called an isometric contraction. Although contractile components do shorten, in clinical usage an isometric contraction is one in which the external length of the muscle remains unchanged, i.e., the joint position is unchanged. Isometric contraction is sometimes called static contraction and is the type of muscle contraction most frequently assessed clinically.

When the external force exceeds the internal force of a shortened muscle and the muscle lengthens while maintaining tension, the contraction is called an *eccentric* or lengthening contraction. In eccentric contraction, a muscle can usually sustain a greater tension than it can develop in isometric contraction at a given equivalent static condition. In contrast, if the muscle shortens while maintaining tension, a *concentric* contraction occurs. For elbow flexion, eccentric force exceeds isometric force by about 20 percent; and isometric force exceeds concentric force by about 20 percent[58] (Fig. 5–10).

If the muscle produces a constant internal force that exceeds the external force of the

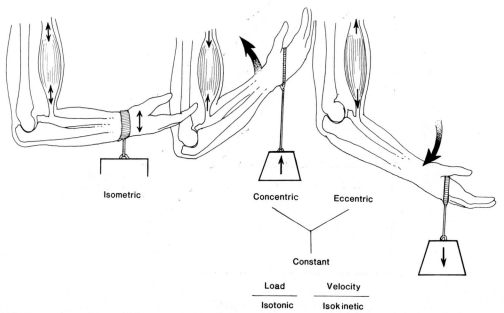

Figure 5–9. Types of muscle contractions classified according to change in muscle length. An isometric contraction results in no change of muscle length with a constant load and velocity. The concentric contraction is defined as a shortening of the muscle, whereas the eccentric contraction occurs with lengthening of the muscle. These latter two contractions may be subclassified according to whether a constant load (isotonic) or a constant velocity (isokinetic) condition is met.

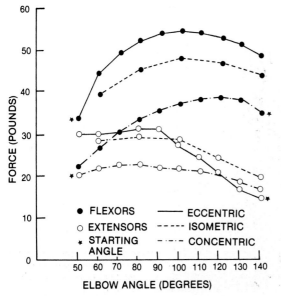

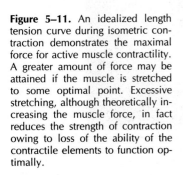

Figure 5–10. Comparison of isometric, concentric, and eccentric flexion and extension contraction strength for different positions of elbow flexion. Note that approximately 20 percent greater strength may be generated with an eccentric than with an isometric contraction; the isometric contraction, on the other hand, is approximately 20 percent greater than the concentric type of contraction. (Modified from Singh, M.: Isotonic and isometric forces of forearm flexors and extensors. J. Appl. Physiol., 21:1436, 1966.)

resistance, the muscle shortens and the contraction is further characterized as *isotonic.* Energy utilization in this case is larger than that required to produce tension, which will balance the load, and the extra energy is used to shorten the muscle.

If the speed of rotation of an exercising limb is predetermined and held constant, changes occur in the amount of tension de-

veloped in the muscles causing the motion. This is called an *isokinetic* contraction and may be of the concentric or eccentric type.

Components of each of these types of contraction occur during routine daily activity and are described in detail in Chapter 9.

Factors Affecting Maximum Muscle Tension

Muscle Length at Contraction. The maximum muscle tension that can be developed under static conditions is directly related to the length of the muscle at contraction, which is dependent on the position of the joint. The relationship of muscle tension to muscle length is recognized by most clinicians and is presented graphically in the form of a length-tension curve of an isolated muscle (Fig. 5–11). The exact nature of the relationship varies from muscle to muscle, depending on its specific function.

Speed of Contraction

A rapidly contracting muscle generates less force than one contracting more slowly. In isotonic contraction, the maximum shortening velocity decreases as the load is increased. In an isometric contraction, the velocity is zero because the resistance exceeds the ability of the muscle to move the joint. In sports, rates of motion exceeding 300 degrees per second are common.

Technique of Strength Measurement

When evaluating strength, either the *torque* created about the joint or the *force* generated

Figure 5–11. An idealized length tension curve during isometric contraction demonstrates the maximal force for active muscle contractility. A greater amount of force may be attained if the muscle is stretched to some optimal point. Excessive stretching, although theoretically increasing the muscle force, in fact reduces the strength of contraction owing to loss of the ability of the contractile elements to function optimally.

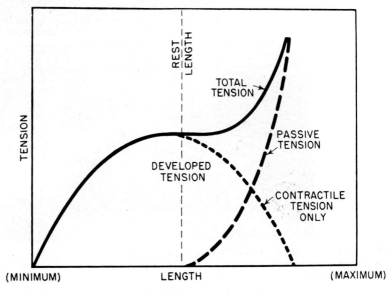

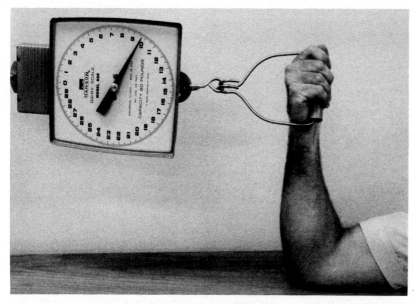

Figure 5–12. A simple spring tensiometer, which is used in the clinical setting to estimate elbow flexion strength.

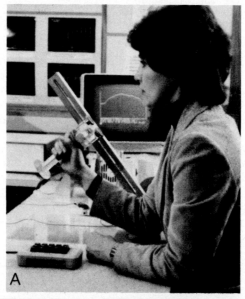

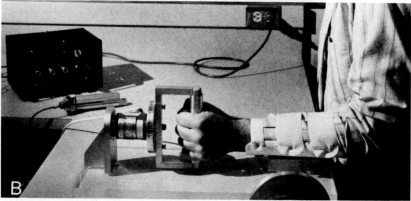

Figure 5–13. *A,* A torque cell may be used to calculate elbow flexion and extension strength. Notice that the device allows adjustment for an adequate fit of the individual being tested. *B,* A similar device may be employed to measure supination and pronation strength.

in the hand and forearm in resisting joint rotation is measured. Either static or dynamic measuring devices may be used.

The most common state measured clinically is static or isometric flexion-extension strength using a simple tensiometer, or spring device[13, 34] (Fig. 5–12). More sophisticated devices such as a strain gauge tensiometer[20] in conjunction with a cable and pulley arrangement, or a strain gauge–instrumented bar dynamometer[17, 51] have also been used. For more accurate investigative studies, the application of a torque cell has been adapted to measure elbow joint torque[3, 41] (Fig. 5–13A). For static axial forearm rotation, supination or pronation torque can be transmitted to a transducer with a metal bar gripped by the hand (Fig. 5–13B).

For dynamic isotonic elbow strength measurement, the maximum weight that can be moved through the range of movement is determined.[9] Dynamometers have been designed for this purpose that use a strain gauge load cell and various sized pulleys.[19, 58]

Isokinetic strength is a more specific measurement of dynamic elbow flexion and extension function. In an isokinetic muscular movement, the speed of rotation of the limb is held constant despite changes in the amount of tension developed. This isokinetic movement can be measured by means of an accommodating resistance dynamometer. Because of the accommodating load cell, the velocity of an exercising limb cannot be increased.[40, 48] As more force is exerted against the lever arm of the dynamometer, more resistance is encountered by the limb, and rotation occurs only at the predetermined constant speed. These devices accurately measure peak torque, the joint angle position at peak torque, the range of motion, and endurance.[6] Currently, several devices are commercially available for isokinetic elbow strength assessment. This technique is becoming increasingly useful for the measurement of elbow

strength and endurance and for more accurate study of the role of fatigue in arriving at disability estimates.[57]

ELBOW STRENGTH

Static Function

Flexion-Extension Strength of the Elbow. Many reports address the question of flexion strength of the elbow joint.[3, 20, 37, 63] Absolute strength measurements are not exactly comparable owing to variations in study technique and even greater differences between individual subjects, yet the general trends are relatively consistent.

On the average, the maximum isometric torque created at the elbow joint is about 7 kg-m for males and 3.5 kg-m for females[3] (Table 5–3). Overall, males are about 50 percent stronger than females and the dominant extremity is 5 to 10 percent stronger than the nondominant side.[3] Muscle power is greatest during flexion at joint positions between 90 and 110 degrees.[20] At elbow angles of 45 and 135 degrees, only about 75 percent of the maximum elbow flexion strength is generated.[27, 29] Maximum flexion strength is generated in forearm supination; forearm pronation is associated with the weakest flexion strength. Most of the torque occurs from the biceps, brachialis, and brachioradialis function.[22] A composite diagram summarizing the findings of several investigators depicts elbow flexion strength at various elbow joint angles (Fig. 5–14).

Forearm rotation position has been shown to alter elbow flexion strength to various degrees. The average difference in isometric flexion force among the three forearm positions at various flexion angles is about 5 percent for females and 10 percent for males.[20] We have noticed variations of up to 50 percent between pronation and supination flexion strength in some clinical settings being

Table 5–3. **Normal Isometric Elbow Strength**[a]

	Flexion (Kg-cm)		Extension (Kg-cm)		Pronation (Kg-cm)		Supination (Kg-cm)		Grip (Kg)	
	Dom	Non	Dom	Non	Dom	Non	Dom	Non	Dom	Non
Males	725	708	421	406	73	68	91	80	53	51
N = 50	±154	±156	±109	±106	±17	±17	±23	±21	±12	±11
Females	336	323	210	194	36	33	44	41	30	27
N = 54	±80	±77	±61	±49	±8	±10	±12	±10	±10	±9

[a]Ages: Males, $\overline{age}$ = 41 ± 12
    Females, $\overline{age}$ = 45 ± 16
    N = 104

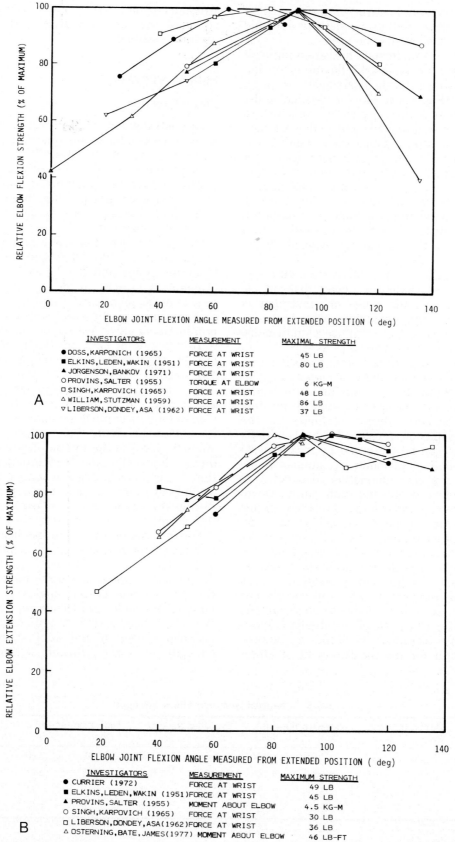

Figure 5–14. A composite of several studies demonstrating maximum elbow flexion *(A)* and extension *(B)* strength as a function of the elbow joint angle.

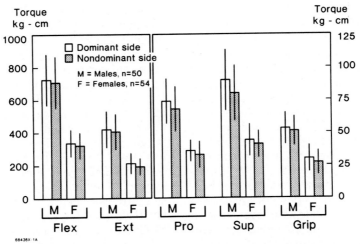

Figure 5–15. Mayo Clinic Biomechanics Laboratory study of normal elbow strength. Notice that males are approximately twice as strong as females and that a 5 to 10 percent difference is noted between the dominant and nondominant extremities.

evaluated in the biomechanics laboratory. Strengths at the neutral forearm position were slightly greater than those at the supinated and pronated positions.[20, 27, 51, 54, 60] Electromyographic studies suggest that inhibition of the biceps muscle due to pronation of the forearm is a likely explanation for less flexion strength at the pronated position.[27]

For elbow extension, the average maximum torque strength is about 4 kg-m for males and 2 kg-m for females[3] (Fig. 5–15). Observations for 14 female and 10 male subjects showed a gradual increase in strength as the elbow is extended. Although peak extension strength has been recorded at 60[62] to 140 degrees,[14] most reports show that the 90-degree position generates the greatest isometric extension force.[16, 22, 35, 51] In general, the dominant extremity is about 5 to 10 percent stronger than the nondominant side, and males are about twice as strong as females in most positions (Fig. 5–15). The isometric force of the flexors is about 40 percent greater than the isometric force of the extensors.[3, 29]

Supination and Pronation Strength

Strength measurements of forearm supination and pronation have been studied only occasionally. A linear relationship exists between strength and forearm rotation. The greatest supination strength is generated from the pronated position; the converse relationship is also true. In the majority of shoulder-elbow positions, the average torque of supination exceeded that of pronation by about 15 to 20 degrees for males and females. This was particularly marked when the elbow was extended. The available data from our laboratory indicate that, on the average, pronation and supination strengths for males are 80 kg-cm and 90 kg-cm, respectively, and for females, 35 kg-cm and 55 kg-cm, respectively. The dominant and nondominant strength difference in these two types of function averaged about 10 percent (Fig. 5–15).

Less studied but also worthy of note is the influence of body position during testing.[13] For example, elbow extension strength obtained from the prone position is significantly greater than that in the supine position.[37]

Dynamic Function. In practice, a patient may sometimes demonstrate normal isometric strength at a given position but be unable to perform some functions properly because of inadequate dynamics or fatigue. Fatigue is an important consideration in altered function because the conduct of routine activities requires repetitive actions that may exceed one million cycles per year.[18] Therefore, it is important to assess functional strength under dynamic conditions. Because of limited facilities and the uncertainty of interpretation, this is rarely done in the routine clinical setting.

The relative value of different strength testing modalities is a debated issue. For example, there have been conflicting reports that no difference exists between isometric and isotonic strength measurements,[54] marked differences exist between the two measurements,[7] or the results are too variable to draw any conclusions[50, 52] The dilemma has been clarified somewhat by Carlson, who found a consistent relationship between isometric and isotonic testing strengths. Isometric test results were about 13 percent higher than the results of isotonic tests. It was concluded that if the purpose of the test is to distinguish *relative* strength compared to some standard, isometric test results are valid. If the purpose is to determine the *absolute amount* of strength, isometric data are of a poor reflection of isotonic test results. This conclusion is of practical significance because of the ease of making clinical isometric measurements and applying such data to disability statements.

The rate and strength of muscle contractions have also been analyzed.[2, 4, 27, 45, 61] Interestingly, with the forearm pronated, the flexion force curve is 10 to 15 percent lower than the force wave obtained with the forearm supinated. Although this is consistent with the isotonic and electromyographic (EMG) data,[22] it contradicts the prediction of Fick,[21] in which the performance of the elbow flexors was predicted to be better with the forearm pronated than supinated, based on the assumption that innervation of all elbow flexors is independent of the degree of forearm position.

The relationship between strength and speed of movement has also been studied. Most of the earlier investigations[39, 50, 52, 61] consistently supported the hypothesis that maximum strength and the rate of movement were independent of each other.[45] This hypothesis was challenged by a study showing a statistically significant relationship between static strength and speed of movement.[34, 45] The relationship between isokinetic torques and maximum isometric force measurement is a frequent topic of study. To date, reports have been contradictory, and this question is still unsettled.[5]

Additional Variables of Strength Assessment

Besides the factors discussed above such as type of contraction, measurement apparatus, joint and forearm position, and body position, all of which will affect the result, the investigator should be aware of other factors when performing muscle strength assessment. These include motivation, the learning effect of repetitive tests, the actual psychologic benefit derived from repetitive testing, and the influence of the time of day of the test. Each of these variables has been investigated.

The subject's motivation to give his best effort is a variable that is well recognized but difficult to control, quantitate, or eliminate.[15, 31, 58] The rate of strength buildup during repetitive exertion has been suggested as

a possible objective criterion for judging whether or not a subject is exerting his full muscular strength in a routine test.[31]

Kroll[32, 33] has identified some so-called nonpertinent variables of strength testing that will influence the reliability of the test-retest studies: effect of trial and effect of day. The trial effect is the decrease of strength with serial testing on the same day, apparently due to fatigue. The day effect is the improved performance that results from repeated testing over several days. This increase in mean strength, whether attributable to actual strength gain per se or to a learning effect, has been noted by several investigators.[25, 33, 65] McGarvey et al.[38] have even shown that a normal variation of about 5 percent in some strength functions occurs during the day, but this is not considered significant in the routine clinical setting.

STABILITY

By virtue of the inherent stability afforded by the joint articulation, clinical instability of the elbow is an uncommon problem. A recent report has called attention to the isolated ligamentous lesion.[46] Ligamentous injury, however, usually occurs in association with radial head fracture[26, 56] or elbow dislocation. The tendency toward adequate spontaneous healing of the elbow ligament is demonstrated by the fact that only 1 to 2 percent of elbow dislocations result in recurrent instability.[36] In this setting, both the lateral and the medial collateral ligamentous complexes may be involved. The most common clinical presentations of an unstable joint occur in patients with rheumatoid arthritis or following severe trauma, soft tissue arthroplasty, or radial head resection with associated medial collateral ligamentous injury after certain forms of sepsis or due to congenital laxity of the joints.

Demonstration of instability is difficult. With the elbow extended, the olecranon is seated in the olecranon fossa, the anterior capsule is taut, and the articulation stabilizes the joint independent of ligamentous competency. Varus-valgus stability is therefore examined with the joint flexed about 20 degrees to relax the capsule and remove the tip of the olecranon from its fossa, but flexion causes a rotation of the humerus with varus or valgus stress. Full internal rotation of the shoulder stabilizes the brachium and allows a more accurate assessment of varus laxity. Similarly, full external rotation of the humerus provides a more reliable estimate of valgus instability

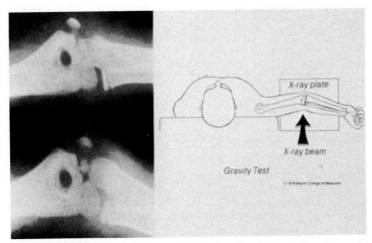

Figure 5–16. Demonstration of the radiographic technique of placing a valgus stress on the elbow. The patient lies supine on the x-ray table with the brachium in full external rotation. (From Schwab, G. H., et al.: Biomechanics of elbow instability: The role of the medial collateral ligament Clin. Orthop. 146:46, 1980.)

(see Chapter 4). Anterior-posterior stability is assessed with the elbow in 90 degrees of flexion. No well-defined standard currently exists to grade clinically detected instability.

Roentgenographic confirmation of elbow instability has been discussed in Chapter 30. To control the effect of humeral rotation, full external rotation is obtained by positioning the patient supine with the arm held over the edge of the table. Gravity allows valgus stress to open the joint medially (Fig. 5–16). A similar technique is used to visualize varus instability, but the patient is positioned prone on the table. In each instance, complete muscle relaxation is essential for a proper study. We have arbitrarily defined less than 5 mm or a 5-degree opening as mild, less than 10 mm or 10 degrees as moderate, and greater than 10 mm or 10 degrees widening of the joint as severe instability.

PATIENT EVALUATION

An objective and reproducible means of evaluating elbow function is obviously desirable. A trade-off exists between a complex but too detailed assessment protocol and one that is oversimplified. A complete and comprehensive assessment that might be available in a research facility is not practical clinically. For a clinician, a useful rating system should be both complete and amenable to an office practice. A single parameter or index composed of all pertinent variables should accurately reflect the gradation of objective function as discussed above. To be of further value, the rating system should include the presence of pain and specific daily functions as reflections of all these variables as they apply to discrete activity.

The ability to measure motion accurately with the hand goniometer is accessible to all. Accurate objective strength measurement is difficult to perform and interpret, and the results vary depending on the facilities available. Hence, the traditional muscle strength grading system developed during the polio era is an acceptable (Table 5–4) alternative, although it does suffer from placing too much emphasis on weakness and not enough on slight decreases from normal strength. Stability of the elbow has not been subjected to any specific grading system, so its importance is not completely known.

Given the limitations of available facilities and the lack of real knowledge of the relative importance of these variables, the following simplified rating system (Fig. 5–17) has proved helpful in our practice and may provide a useful guide for the clinician.

Table 5–4. **Clinical Muscle Grading Systems**

Grade	Definition	Per-cent	Explanation
0	Absent	0	No function
1	Trace	10	Slight contraction, no motion
2	Poor	25	Complete motion gravity eliminated
3	Fair	50	Complete motion against gravity
4	Good	75	Complete motion against gravity and some resistance
5	Normal	100	Apparently normal strength

Elbow Evaluation

Name: _____ UH#: _____ Elbow: _____ R/L

Procedure: _____ Date: _____ Dominant: _____ R/L

Date of Exam (month/day/year)

Pain (maximum points)

5 = none (30); 4 = slight—with continuous activity, no medication (25); 3 = moderate—with occasional activity, some medication (15); 2 = moderately severe—much pain, frequent medication (10); 1 = severe—constant pain, markedly limited activity (5); 0 = complete disability (0)

Motion degrees (37 points maximum)

Extension   Flexion
(8 pts max)   (17 pts max)

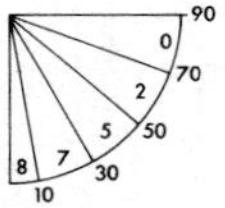

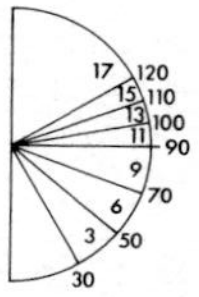

Pronation/Supination

(pt) = 0.1 per degree—6 maximum

	Extension	° ( )
	Flexion	° ( )
	Pronation	° ( )
	Supination	° ( )

Strength (15 points maximum)

5 = normal; 4 = good; 3 = fair; 2 = poor; 1 = trace; 0 = paralysis; NA = not available

	Flex.	Ext.	Pro.	Sup.
Normal	5	(5)	(4)	(3)	(3)
Good	4	(4)	(3)	(2)	(2)
Fair	3	(3)	(2)	(1)	(1)
Poor	2	(2)	(1)	(0)	(0)
Trace	1	(1)	(0)	(0)	(0)
None	0	(0)	(0)	(0)	(0)

	Extension	( )
	Flexion	( )
	Pronation	( )
	Supination	( )

Instability (6 points maximum)

	Ant./Post.	Med./Lat.
None	3	3
Mild <5 mm, <5°	2	2
Moderate <10 mm, <10°	1	1
Severe >10 mm, >10°	0	0

| | Ant./Post. | _____ |
| | Med./Lat. | _____ |

Function (12 points maximum)

4 = normal (1); 3 = mild compromise (0.75); 2 = difficulty (0.5); 1 = with aid (0.25); 0 = unable (0); NA = not applicable

(Index—multiply × 0.25)

1. Use back pocket ( )
2. Rise from chair ( )
3. Perineal care ( )
4. Wash opposite axilla ( )
5. Eat with utensil ( )
6. Comb hair ( )
7. Carry 10–15 pounds with arm at side ( )
8. Dress ( )
9. Pulling ( )
10. Throwing ( )
11. Do usual work ( )
    Specify work:
12. Do usual sport ( )
    Specify sport:

Patient Response

3 = much better; 2 = better; 1 = same; 0 = worse; NA = not available/not applicable _____

Completed By: Name of Examiner

Index

Key: 95–100 = excellent; 80–95 = good; 50–80 = fair; <50 = poor ( ) ( ) ( ) ( )

Figure 5–17. A clinically useful elbow evaluation sheet provides objective data retrieval and grading (A) as well as information about function (B). The use of such a rating index in the clinical setting provides an objective means of comparing different treatment options.

References

1. American Academy of Orthopaedic Surgeons: Joint Motion: Method of Measuring and Recording. Chicago, American Academy of Orthopaedic Surgeons, 1965.
2. Abbott, B. D., Bigland, B., and Ritchie, J. M.: The Physiological Cost of Negative Work. J. Physiol. (London) **117**:380, 1952.
3. Askew, L. J., An, K. N., Morrey, B. F., and Chao, E. Y.: Functional Evaluation of the Elbow. Normal Motion Requirements and Strength Determinations. Orthop. Trans. 5:304, 1981.
4. Asmussen, E., Hansen, O., and Lammert, O.: The Relation Between Isometric and Dynamic Muscle Strength in Man. Danish Nat. Assoc. Infant Paral. **20**, 1965.
5. Astrand, P. O., and Rodahl, K.: Textbook of Work Physiology. New York, McGraw-Hill Book Co., 1970.
6. Barnes, W. S.: The Relationship Between Maximum Isokinetic Strength and Isometric Endurance. Res. Q. Exerc. Sport **51**:714, 1980.
7. Berger, R. A.: Comparison of Static and Dynamic Strength Increases. Res. Q. **33**:329, 1962.
8. Boone, D. C., and Azen, S. P.: Normal Range of Motion of Joints in Male Subjects. J. Bone Joint Surg. **61A**:756, 1979.
9. Carlson, B. R., and Kroll, W.: The Use of Analysis of Variance in Estimating Reliability of Isometric Elbow Flexion Strength. Res. Q. **41**:129, 1970.
10. Carstam, N.: Operative Treatment of Fractures of the Head and Neck of the Radius. Acta Orthop. Scand. **19**:502, 1950.
11. Chao, E. Y.: Experimental Methods for Biomechanical Measurements of Joint Kinematics. CRC Handbook of Engineering in Medicine and Biology, Section B: Instruments and Measurements. West Palm Beach, CRC Press, 1978.
12. Chao, E. Y., An, K. N., Askew, L. J., and Morrey, B. F.: Electrogoniometer for the Measurement of Human Elbow Joint Rotation. J. Biomechan. Engin., **102**:301, 1980.
13. Clarke, H. H., and Bailey, T. L.: Strength Curves for Fourteen Joint Movements. J. Assoc. Phys. Ment. Rehab. 4:12, 1950.
14. Clarke, H. H., Elkins, E. C., Martin, G. M., et al.: Relationship Between Body Position and the Application of Muscle Power to Movements of the Joint. Arch. Phys. Med. **31**:81, 1950.
15. Cooper, D. F., et al.: Perception of Effort in Isometric and Dynamic Muscular Contraction. Europ. J. Appl. Physiol. **41**:173, 1979.
16. Currier, D. P.: Maximal Isometric Tension of the Elbow Extensor at Various Positions, Part I. Assessment by Cable Tensiometer. Phys. Ther. **52**:1043, 1972.
17. Darcus, H. D.: The Maximum Torques Developed in Pronation and Supination of the Right Hand. J. Anat. **85**:55, 1951.
18. Davis, P. R.: Some Significant Aspect of Normal Upper Limb Functions. Conference on Joint Replacement of the Upper Extremity. London, Institute of Mechanical Engineers, 1977.
19. Doss, W. S., and Karpovich, P. V.: A Comparison of Concentric, Eccentric, and Isometric Strength of the Elbow Flexion. J. Appl. Physiol. **20**:351, 1965.
20. Elkins, E. C., Leden, U. M., and Wakim, K. G.: Objective Recording of the Strength of Normal Muscles. Arch. Phys. Med. **32**:639, 1951.
21. Fick, K.: Handbüch der Anatomie und Mechanic der Gelenke, Vol. 3. Jena, 1911, p. 3201.
22. Funk, D.: EMG Investigation of Muscular Contrac-

tions About the Human Elbow. MS Thesis, Mayo Graduate School of Medicine, 1984.
23. Gowitzke, B. A., and Miller, M.: Understanding the Scientific Basis of Movement. 2nd ed. Baltimore, The Williams & Wilkins Co., 1980.
24. Hellebrandt, F. A., Duvall, E. N., and Moore, M. L.: The Measurement of Joint Motion: Part III. Reliability of Goniometry. Phys. Ther. Rev. **29**:302, 1949.
25. Hood, L. B., and Forward, E. M. M.: Strength Variations in Two Determinations of Maximal Isometric Contractions. J. Am. Phys. Ther. Assoc. **45**:1046, 1965.
26. Johansson, O.: Caspular and Ligament Injuries of the Elbow Joint. Acta Orthop. Scand. Suppl. **287**, 1962.
27. Jorgensen, K., and Bankov, S.: Maximum Strength of Elbow Flexors with Pronated and Supinated Forearm. Med. Sport Biomechan. II, **6**:174, 1971.
28. Kapandji, I. A.: The Physiology of the Joints. Vol. I: Upper Limb. 2nd ed. Baltimore, The Williams & Wilkins Co., 1970.
29. Karpovich, P. V., and Singh, M.: Isotonic and Isometric Forces of Forearm Flexors and Extensors. J. Appl. Physiol. **21**:1435, 1966.
30. Kelsey, J. L., Pastides, H., Kreiger, N., Harris, C., and Chernow, R. A.: Upper Extremity Disorders. A Study of Their Frequency and Cost in the United States. St. Louis, C. V. Mosby Co., 1980.
31. Kroemer, K. H. E., and Marras, W. S.: Towards an Objective Assessment of the "Maximal Voluntary Contraction" Component in Routine Muscle Strength Measurements. Europ. J. Appl. Physiol. **45**:1, 1980.
32. Kroll, W.: Reliability of a Selected Measure of Human Strength. Res. **33**:410, 1962.
33. Kroll, W.: Reliability Variations of Strength in Test-Retest Situations. Res. Q. **34**:50, 1963.
34. Larson, C. L., and Nelson, R. C.: An Analysis of Strength, Speed and Acceleration of Elbow Flexion. Arch. Phys. Med. Rehab. **50**:274, 1969.
35. Liberson, W. T., Dondey, M., and Asa, M. M.: Brief Repeated Isometric Maximal Exercises. Am. J. Phys. Med. **41**:3, 1962.
36. Linschied, R. L., and Wheeler, D. K.: Elbow Dislocations. J.A.M.A. **194**:1171, 1965.
37. Little, A. D., and Lehmkuhl, D.: Elbow Extension Force: Measured in Three Test Positions. J. Am. Phys. Ther. Assoc. **46**:7, 1966.
38. McGarvey, S., Morrey, B. F., Askew, L. J., and An, K. N.: Reliability of Isometric Strength Testing: Temporal Factors and Strength Variation. Clin. Orthop. Rel Res. **185**:301, 1984.
39. Masley, J. W., Hairabedian, A., and Donaldson, D. N.: Training in Relation to Strength, Speed and Coordination. Res. Q. **24**:308, 1953.
40. Moffroid, M., et al.: Rehabilitation. Monograph 40: Guidelines for Clinical Use of Isokinetic Exercise. New York, Institute of Rehabilitation Medicine, New York University Medical Center, 1969.
41. Morrey, B. F., Chao, E. Y., and Hui, F. C.: Biomechanical Study of the Elbow Following Excision of the Radial Head. J. Bone Joint Surg. **61A**:63, 1979.
42. Morrey, B. F., Askew, L. J., An, K. N., and Chao, E. Y.: A Biomechanical Study of Normal Elbow Motion. J. Bone Joint Surg. **63A**:872, 1981.
43. National Center for Health Statistics, 1977. Cited by Kelsey et al. (op. cit.).
44. National Safety Council, 1976. Cited by Kelsey et al. (op. cit.).
45. Nelson, R. C., and Fahrney, R. A.: Relationship Between Strength and Speed of Elbow Flexion. Res. Q. **36**:455, 1963.
46. Norwood, L. A., et al.: Acute Medial Elbow Ligament Ruptures. Am. J. Sports Med. **9**:16, 1981.

47. Ogilvie, W. H.: Discussion on Minor Injuries of the Elbow Joint. Proc. Roy. Soc. Med. **23**:306, 1930.
48. Osternig, L. R., Bates, B. T., and James, S. L.: Isokinetic and Isometric Torque Force Relationships. Arch. Phys. Med. Rehabil. **58**:254, 1977.
49. Pearn, J.: Two Early Dynamometers: An Historical Account of the Earliest Measurements to Study Muscular Strength. J. Neurol. Sci. **34**:127, 1978.
50. Pierson, W. R., and Rasch, P. J.: Strength and Speed. Perceptual Motor Skills **14**:144, 1962.
51. Provins, K. A., and Salter, N.: Maximum Torque Exerted About the Elbow Joint. J. Appl. Physiol. **7**:393, 1955.
52. Rasch, P. J.: Effect of Position of Forearm on Strength of Elbow Flexion. Res. Q. **27**:333, 1956.
53. Russe, O.: An Atlas of Examination, Standard Measurements and Diagnosis in Orthopedics and Traumatology. Vienna, Hans Huber, 1972.
54. Salter, N.: The Effect on Muscle Strength of Maximum Isometric and Isotonic Contractions at Different Repetition Rates. J. Physiol. (London), **130**:109, 1955.
55. Schenck, J. M., and Forward, E. M.: Quantitative Strength Changes with Test Repetitions. J. Am. Phys. Ther. Assoc. **45**:562, 1965.
56. Schwab, G. H., et al.: Biomechanics of Elbow Instability: The Role of the Medial Collateral Ligament. Clin. Orthop. **146**:42, 1980.
57. Simmons, J. W., Rath, D., and Merta, R.: Calculation of Disability Using the Cybex II System. Orthopedics, **5**:181, 1982.
58. Singh, M., and Karpovich, P. V.: Isotonic and Isometric Forces of Forearm Flexors and Extensors. J. Appl. Physiol. **21**:1435, 1966.
59. Wagner, C.: Determination of the Rotatory Flexibility of the Elbow Joint. Europ. J. Appl. Physiol. **37**:47, 1977.
60. Wells, K.: Kinesiology, 2nd ed. Philadelphia, W. B. Saunders Co., 1955.
61. Wilkie, D. R.: The Relation Between Force and Velocity in Human Muscle. J. Physiol. (London), **110**:249, 1950.
62. Williams, M., and Stutzman, L.: Strength Variation Through the Range of Joint Motion. Phys. Ther. Rev. **39**:145, 1959.
63. Williams, M., Toberlin, J. A., and Robertson, K. J.: Muscle Force Curves of School Children. Phys. Ther. **45**:539, 1965.
64. Wilmer, H. A., and Elkins, E. C.: An Optical Goniometer for Observing Range of Motion of Joints. Arch. Phys. Med. **28**:695, 1947.
65. Worshal, D.: The Reliability of Isometric Strength Gain in Therapeutic Assessment. Am. Correct. Ther. J. **33**:188, 1979.

CHAPTER 6

Diagnostic Radiographic Techniques of the Elbow

T. H. BERQUIST

Although the imaging techniques available to clinicians and radiologists continue to expand (Table 6–1), evaluation of the elbow still relies heavily upon routine radiographic techniques. So many advances have occurred in tomography that complex motion tomography is more commonly utilized than conventional linear motion tomography. Computed tomography has assisted in the evaluation of numerous bone and soft tissue disorders.[12, 19, 29] In addition, arthrography can also be an important tool in the diagnosis of intra-articular disorders of the elbow.

A new modality, nuclear magnetic resonance imaging (MRI), is presently being evaluated. This technique uses magnetic gradients and radiofrequency pulses that produce images that are similar to those of computed tomography. Nuclear magnetic resonance has already demonstrated its clinical usefulness in the field of neuroradiology. This modality promises to be useful in evaluating musculoskeletal diseases as well.[6, 3, 31]

Within the scope of this chapter the indications for these diagnostic options as well as

their usefulness in given clinical situations will be discussed. Sufficient background information to aid in determining the best modality for a given situation will also be presented.

ROUTINE RADIOGRAPHY

An understanding of the process by which routine radiographs are obtained is essential. Factors such as the type of equipment, patient positioning, and radiation dose must be kept in mind when determining the necessary views in a given clinical setting.[2, 5] In obtaining views of the elbow we routinely use a 48-inch target-film distance with 50 to 60 kvp, 600 ma, and an exposure time of 0.0125 seconds. Kodak XL–1 film with Kodak X-omat regular cassettes measuring 10 × 12 inches are routinely employed.

A minimum of two projections is necessary for evaluation of the elbow.[2, 5] Anteroposterior (AP) and lateral views of the elbow are taken at 90-degree angles and fulfill these criteria. In trauma patients we routinely obtain oblique views as well.

Anteroposterior

The AP view (beam enters the patient anteriorly and the film is posterior) is obtained by placing the patient adjacent to the radiographic table in a sitting position (the supine position may be used if the patient is injured). The patient should be positioned with the extended elbow at the same level as the cassette so that the extremity is in contact with the full length of the cassette.[2, 5] The hand is supinated, and the beam is centered perpendicular to the elbow (Fig. 6–1A). The AP view demonstrates the medial and lateral epicondyles and the radiocapitellar articular surface (Fig. 6–1B). Assessment of the trochlear articular surface and at least a portion of the olecranon fossa is also possible. The normal carrying angle (5 to 20 degrees, average 15 degrees) can be measured on the AP view.[4, 41]

Table 6–1. **Radiographic Techniques in Evaluation of the Elbow**

Routine radiography
  Skeletal techniques
  Stress views
  Soft tissue techniques (low KV)
  Xeroradiography
  Magnification

Tomography
  Linear
  Complex motion
  Transaxial

Arthrography
  Single contrast ⎫ with or without tomography
  Double contrast ⎭
  Subtraction

Angiography
  Computed tomography
  Scintigraphic imaging
  Ultrasound
  Nuclear magnetic resonance imaging

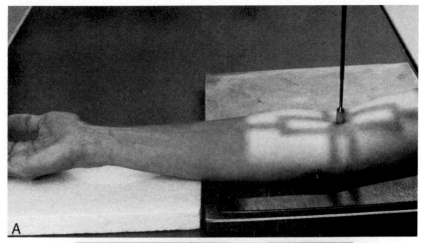

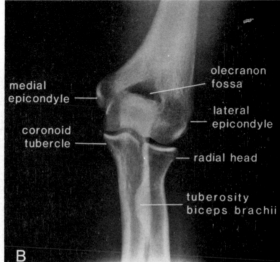

Figure 6–1. A, Patient positioned for the AP view of the elbow. The arm is level with the cassette with the hand palm up. The central beam (line) is perpendicular to the elbow. B, Radiograph of the elbow in the AP projection with anatomic labels.

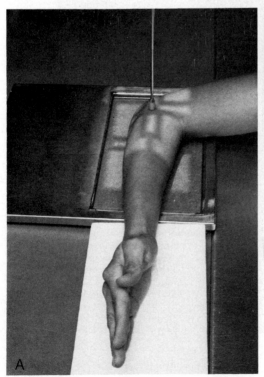

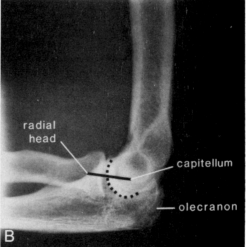

Figure 6–2. A, Patient positioned for the lateral view with the elbow flexed 90 degrees and the beam (pointer) perpendicular to the joint. The shoulder is at the same level as the cassette. This position is required to obtain a true lateral view. B, The projected image.

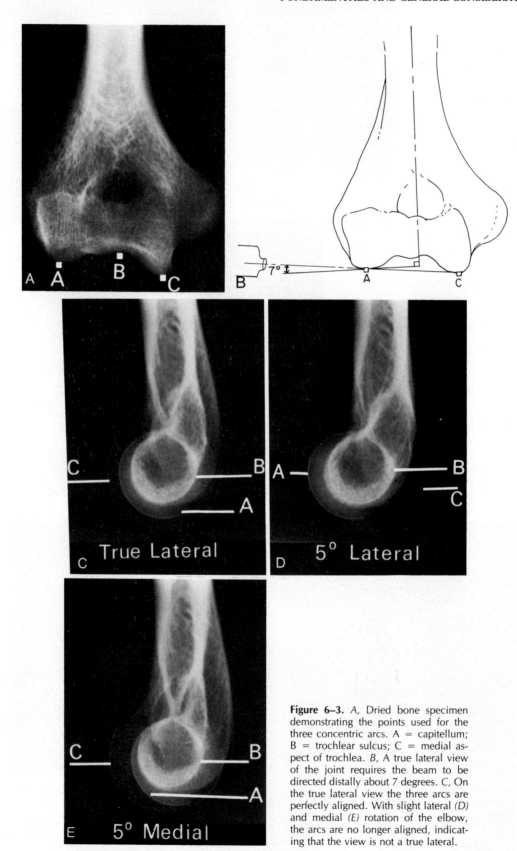

Figure 6–3. *A,* Dried bone specimen demonstrating the points used for the three concentric arcs. A = capitellum; B = trochlear sulcus; C = medial aspect of trochlea. *B,* A true lateral view of the joint requires the beam to be directed distally about 7 degrees. *C,* On the true lateral view the three arcs are perfectly aligned. With slight lateral *(D)* and medial *(E)* rotation of the elbow, the arcs are no longer aligned, indicating that the view is not a true lateral.

Lateral View

The lateral view is obtained by flexing the elbow 90 degrees and placing it directly on the cassette. The hand is positioned with the thumb up so that the forearm is in the neutral position; the beam is perpendicular to the humerus (Fig. 6–2A).[2, 5] This view provides good detail of the distal humerus, elbow joint, and proximal forearm. The coronoid of the ulna, which cannot be readily seen on the AP view, and the olecranon are well visualized on the lateral view (Fig. 6–2B). Since the articular surface makes a valgus angle of about 7 degrees to the long axis of the humerus (Chapter 2), a lateral view of the arm does not provide a lateral view of the joint. If the x-ray beam is parallel to the articular surface, three concentric arcs can be identified (Fig. 6–3A–E).[27] The smaller arc is the trochlear sulcus, the intermediate arc represents the capitellum, and the largest arc is the medial aspect of the trochlea. If the arcs are interrupted, a true lateral view has not been obtained. Unfortunately, in patients with acute injury, true AP and lateral views are often difficult to obtain. Patients are frequently unable to extend or flex the elbow fully. In these situations the tube must be angled and the cassette positioned to simulate these views as closely as possible.

Oblique Views

Oblique views are obtained by initially positioning the arm as if one were taking the AP

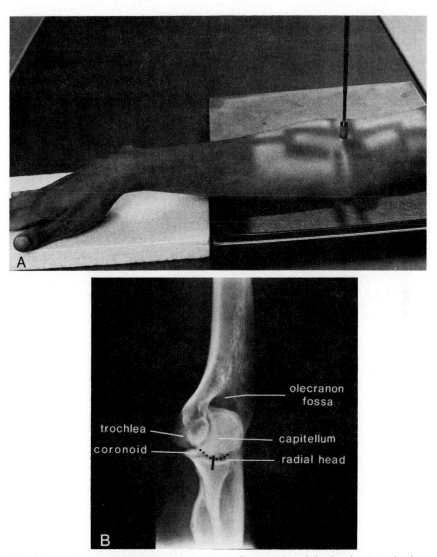

Figure 6–4. Medial oblique view. A, The patient's arm is internally rotated and the hand pronated. The central beam is perpendicular to the elbow. B, Radiograph of the medial oblique view. The radial head is obscured by the ulna. Note the constant relationship of the radial head and the capitellum.

view. For the medial oblique projection (Fig. 6–4A and B), the arm is positioned with the forearm and arm internally rotated approximately 45 degrees (Fig. 6–4A).[2] This view allows improved visualization of the trochlea, olecranon, and coronoid (Fig. 6–4B). The radial head is obscured by the proximal ulna. The lateral oblique view is taken with the forearm, hand, and arm rotated externally (Fig. 6–5A).[2] This projection provides excellent visualization of the radiocapitellar joint, medial epicondyle, radioulnar joint, and coronoid tubercle (Fig. 6–5B).

Radial Head View

Radial head fractures are a common clinical problem and are often difficult to visualize radiographically. The radial head view may define the fracture more clearly.[21, 22, 40, 41] This projection (Fig. 6–6A–C) is easily accomplished by positioning the patient as one would for the routine lateral view. The tube is angled 45 degrees toward the shoulder joint (Fig. 6–6A).[21, 22] This view projects the radial head away from the ulna, allowing subtle changes to be more easily identified (Fig. 6–6C), and it may also allow better visualization of the fat pads.

Axial Views

Occasionally, suspected pathology of the olecranon or epicondyles prompts further evaluation with axial views. Figures 6–7A and B demonstrate the axial projection used to eval-

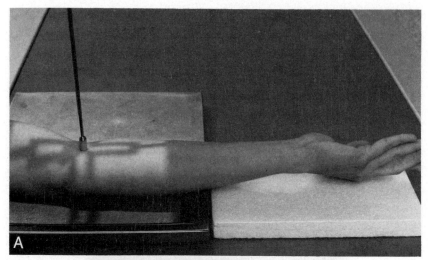

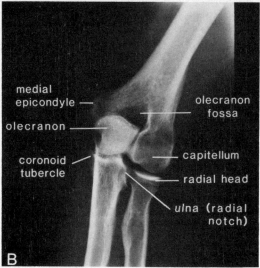

Figure 6–5. Lateral oblique view. *A,* The patient is positioned with the arm externally rotated, the forearm supinated, and the central beam perpendicular to the elbow. *B,* Radiograph of the lateral oblique view. Note the visualization of the radial head and capitellum, medial epicondyle, and radioulnar joint.

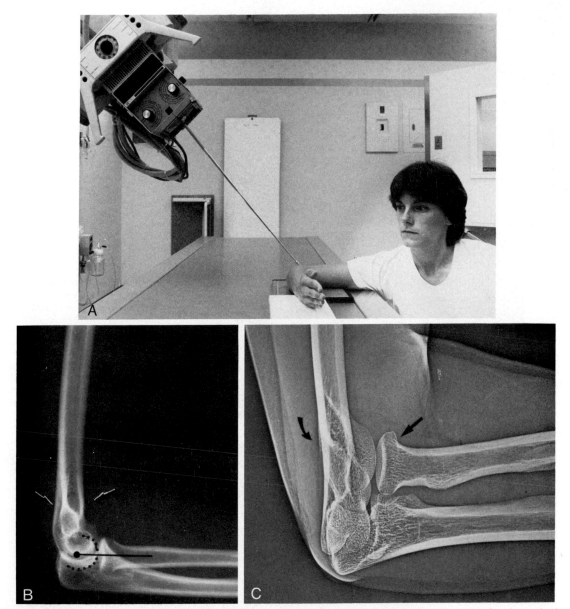

Figure 6–6. Radial head view. *A*, The patient is positioned as if a routine lateral view (see Fig. 2A) were to be obtained. The tube is angled 45 degrees toward the humeral head rather than perpendicular to the joint. *B*, Routine lateral view with normal radiocapitellar relationship (radial head = line, capitellum = broken circle). The anterior and posterior fat pads (arrow) are the only abnormal findings. *C*, Radial head view with xerographic technique demonstrates an impacted radial head fracture (arrow). The fat pads are also more clearly seen (arrow).

uate the epicondyles, olecranon fossa, and ulnar sulcus. The patient's elbow is flexed approximately 110 degrees with the forearm on the cassette and the beam directed perpendicular to the cassette.[2] This view is also helpful in detecting subtle calcification in patients with tendonitis. The olecranon process may be better seen on the reverse axial projection (Fig. 6–8A and B).[2]

Other views of the elbow may also be used,[2, 5] but those discussed above are usually sufficient.

Radiographic Assessment of Routine Radiographs

Assessment of the above views should be complete and systematic. Certain findings should be checked consistently and, if necessary, further views or techniques employed.

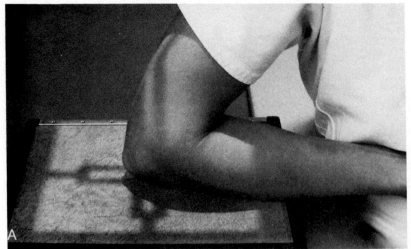

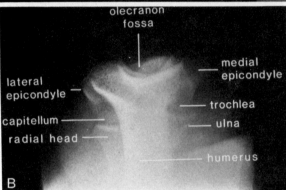

olecranon
fossa

lateral
epicondyle

capitellum

radial head

medial
epicondyle

trochlea

ulna

humerus

B

Figure 6–7. *A,* Patient positioned for the axial view of the distal humerus. The elbow is flexed approximately 110 degrees with the forearm and elbow on the cassette. The central beam is perpendicular to the cassette and centered on the olecranon fossa. *B,* The radiograph provides excellent visualization of the epicondyles, ulnar sulcus, and radiocapitellar and ulnotrochlear articulations.

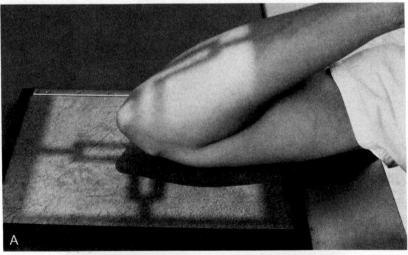

A

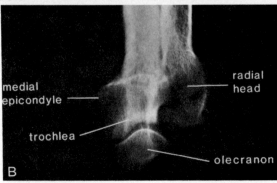

medial
epicondyle

trochlea

radial
head

olecranon

B

Figure 6–8. *A,* The patient's arm is placed on the cassette with the elbow completely flexed. The central beam is perpendicular to the cassette. *B,* The radiograph demonstrates the olecranon, trochlea, and medial epicondyle. Contrast this view with that of Fig. 6–7*B.*

The relationship of the radial head to the capitellum should be constant regardless of the view obtained (Fig. 6–9A–C).[34] The radius is normally bowed at the level of the tubercle. Therefore, the line should be drawn in the midpoint of the radial head, not extended to include this portion of the radial shaft.

Careful evaluation of the fat pads and supinator fat stripe is essential. These structures are best seen on the lateral and radial head views. The anterior and posterior fat pads are intracapsular but extrasynovial.[8, 26, 34, 40, 41] The anterior fat pad is normally visible on the lateral view. The posterior fat pad is obscured

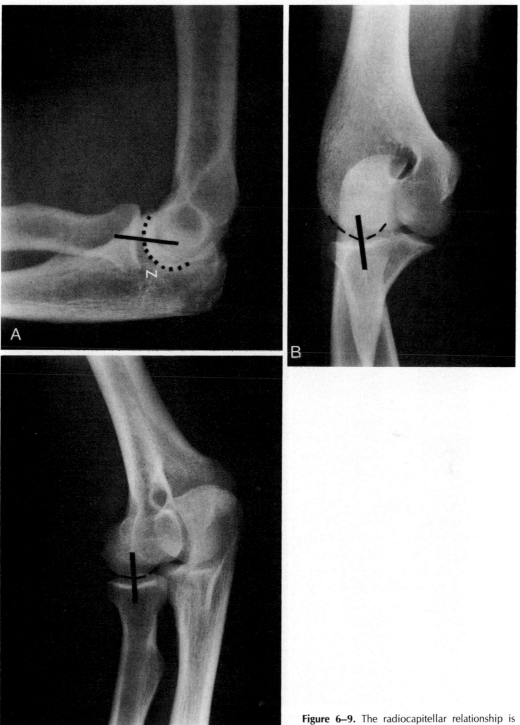

Figure 6–9. The radiocapitellar relationship is constant regardless of the view. *A,* Lateral view. *B,* Medial oblique view. *C,* Lateral oblique view.

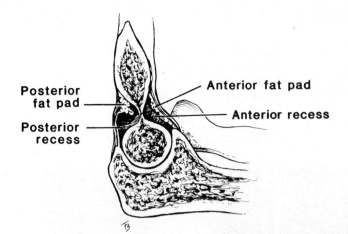

Posterior fat pad

Posterior recess

Anterior fat pad

Anterior recess

Figure 6–10. Lateral illustration of the elbow demonstrating the anterior and posterior fat pads. These structures are intracapsular but extrasynovial.

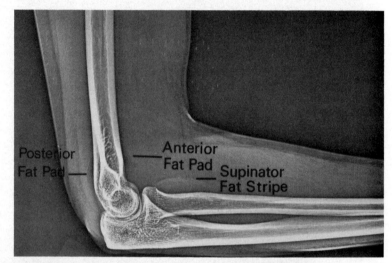

Posterior Fat Pad

Anterior Fat Pad

Supinator Fat Stripe

Figure 6–11. Xerogram of the elbow demonstrating the fat pads and supinator fat stripe due to subtle radial head fracture.

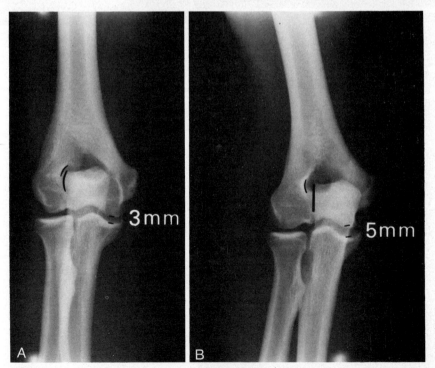

3 mm

5 mm

A

B

Figure 6–12. AP views of the elbow in neural *(A)* and valgus *(B)* stress. Note that the joint space has increased from 3 to 5 mm, indicating the presence of a ligamentous injury. The valgus angle is also subtly changed. The ulna has changed its relationship to the olecranon fossa (curved lines).

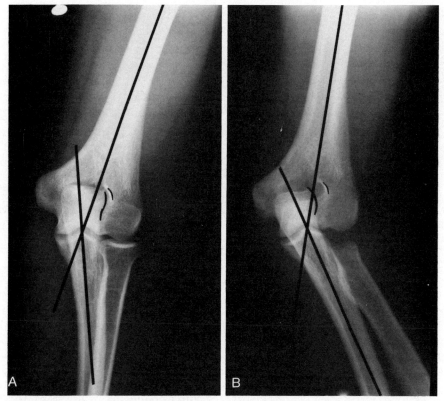

Figure 6–13. A, Stress views of the normal elbow. B, Opposite elbow (previous radial head resection). Note the increased valgus angle on the operated side and the change of position of the ulna in the olecranon fossa.

owing to its position in the olecranon fossa (Fig. 6–10). Displacement of the fat pads, particularly the posterior fat pad, is indicative of an intra-articular fluid collection due to inflammation or hemarthrosis due to trauma.[1, 5–7, 33, 34, 41, 44] Norell[34] reported that 90 per cent of children with displaced posterior fat pads had elbow fractures. This finding is somewhat less specific in adults, but if present in patients following trauma a fracture is likely. Cross-table lateral views may be more specific. A lipohemarthrosis, which is more specific for an intra-articular fracture, may be evident.[1, 40, 49]

The supinator fat stripe lies anterior to the radial head and neck on the surface of the supinator muscle. Fractures of the elbow will frequently displace or obliterate this structure, providing a clue to the underlying injury (Fig. 6–11). Rogers and MacEwan[41] reported changes in the fat stripe in 100 percent of fractures of the radial head and neck and 82 per cent of other elbow fractures.

The anterior humeral line helps to detect

Figure 6–14. Demonstration of fulcrum level (tomographic plane), tube angle, and film motion. The shaded area is the level of the tomogram. The remaining structures will be blurred. (From McCullough, E. C., and Coulam, C. M.: Physical and dosimetric aspects of diagnostic geometrical and computer-assisted tomography. Radiol. Clin. N. Am. 14:3–13, 1976.)

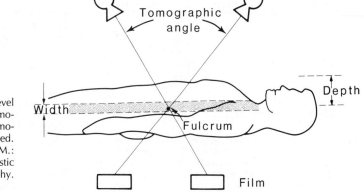

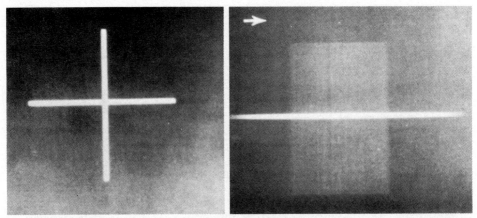

Figure 6–15. Imaging of crosswire: (1) With linear tomography. The path of the tube (arrow in 2) blurs the wire perpendicular to the tube travel but not the wire parallel to the tube motion. This should be kept in mind when imaging patients with metal implants. (From McCullough, E. C., and Coulam, C. M.: Physical and dosimetric aspects of diagnostic geometrical and computer-assisted tomography. Radiol. Clin. N. Am. 14:3–13, 1976.)

subtle supracondylar fractures in children but is not as frequently used for adults.[40] This line, drawn along the anterior humeral cortex, should pass through the middle third of the capitellum.

Stress Views

In patients with suspected ligament disruption or instability, varus and valgus stress views are desirable and may be diagnostic. Ideally, these examinations should be performed with fluoroscopic guidance. This allows proper positioning of the elbows. Also, visualization of subtle changes in the articular distance may be evident while stress is being applied. Spot films should be obtained in the neutral position and during valgus and varus stress. Accuracy may be hindered by guarding

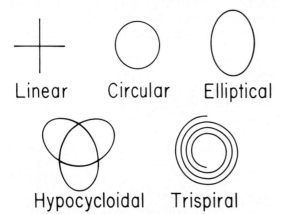

Figure 6–16. Illustration of the types of tomographic motion. (From McCullouogh, E. C., and Coulam, C. M.: Physical and dosimetric aspects of diagnostic geometrical and computer-assisted tomography. Radiol. Clin. N. Am. 14:3–13, 1976.)

and swelling following acute injury. In this situation anesthetic injection should be performed prior to the examination. In the normal elbow the joint should not open when stress is applied. We have arbitrarily chosen an increase in the joint space of greater than 1 mm as being abnormal (Figs. 6–12A and B). The relationship of the tip of the olecranon in the fossa is also helpful in interpreting radiographic instability. The normal elbow carrying angle may also increase significantly if ligament instability is present (Figs. 6–13A and B).

TOMOGRAPHY

Tomography is frequently required for evaluation of areas of interest that are not clearly depicted on routine radiographs. Tomography provides a method of studying a specific plane by blurring the anatomic structures not located in this region. The degree of blurring is dependent upon the distance the tube travels, the distance of the object from the focal point, the orientation of the tube (type of motion), and the distance from the body part to the film (Fig. 6–14).[13, 28] With linear tomography, objects parallel to the tube motion are not blurred significantly even if they are outside of the focal plane (Fig. 6–15).

The type of motion (linear or complex—see Fig. 6–16) is important in orthopedic practice, especially when metal fixation devices are present in the area to be studied. Complex motion may cause a splaying effect of the metal, reducing the adjacent bone detail (Fig. 6–17A). Linear motion parallel to the metal

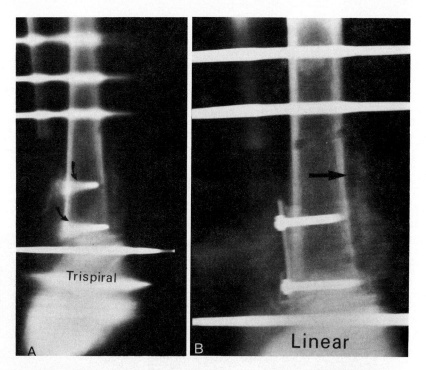

Figure 6–17. External fixation and bone grafting of the tibia. *A,* The trispiral tomogram causes more metal blurring with some loss of adjacent bone detail. *B,* The metal effect is less with linear tomography parallel to the metal (arrow = tube direction).

Trispiral

Linear

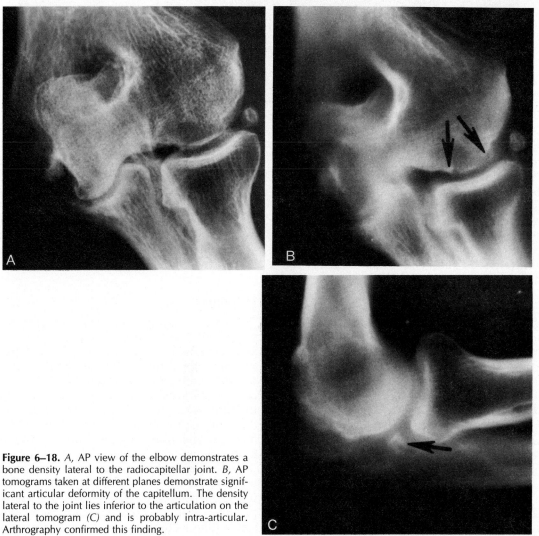

Figure 6–18. *A,* AP view of the elbow demonstrates a bone density lateral to the radiocapitellar joint. *B,* AP tomograms taken at different planes demonstrate significant articular deformity of the capitellum. The density lateral to the joint lies inferior to the articulation on the lateral tomogram *(C)* and is probably intra-articular. Arthrography confirmed this finding.

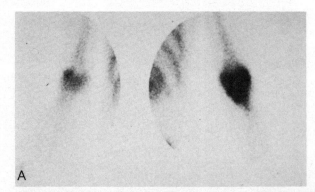

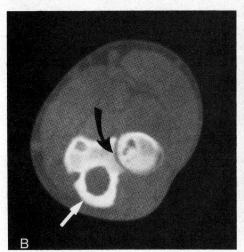
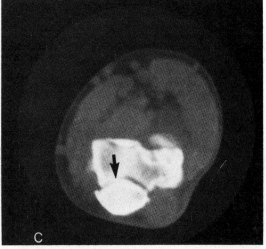

Figure 6–19. *A,* Isotope scan of the elbow in a patient with chronic elbow pain. There is diffusely increased uptake in the elbow region. *B* and *C,* CT scans demonstrate degenerative changes with a degenerative cyst (white arrow) and degenerative changes in the radioulnar (curved black arrow in *B*) and ulnartrochlear articulations (straight arrow in *C*).

results in less metal blurring and better bone detail (Fig. 6–17*B*).

Tomography should be performed in more than one plane in most situations. In the elbow, AP and lateral tomograms are commonly performed. If no metal is present, thin-section (less than 5 mm), trispiral tomography provides the best detail. Tomography is useful in the study of subtle trabecular and articular changes. Detection of calcified or ossified loose bodies (Fig. 6–18) is also possible.

Computed tomography (CT) is useful in the evaluation of bone and soft tissue tumors.[19, 29] Occasionally, CT may be useful in defining articular relationships and excluding a suspected neoplasm (Fig. 6–19).

ARTHROGRAPHY

Elbow arthrography provides valuable information about the capsule size, the synovial lining, and articular surfaces of the joints. The most common indication for this procedure is the detection of possible loose bodies and the demonstration of capsular leaks.[17] Loose bodies may be osteocartilaginous owing to

osteochondromatosis or osteochondral fragments due to acute trauma, or they may be due to osteochondritis dissecans. The articular surface and synovium in the various arthridities may also be evaluated. Less commonly, arthrograms are performed to evaluate capsule size and disruption of the ligaments or capsule in patients with chronic elbow instability.[17, 30, 45]

Technique

To obtain maximum information, arthrography should be performed by an experienced physician with a thorough understanding of the patient's clinical situation. Review of the routine radiographs is essential. These films often provide clues that dictate subtle changes in film technique following the injection of the contrast material. The choice of contrast material and indications for tomography are highly dependent on the clinical setting.

The radiographic equipment used is important in obtaining an arthrogram of high quality. We prefer an overhead tube because this provides better geometry and more work space than a conventional fluoroscopic unit.

Table 6–2. **Elbow Arthrography: Indications and Techniques**

Indication	Procedure
Loose bodies	Double contrast with or
Osteochondromatosis	without tomography
Osteochondritis dissecans	
Fracture fragments from acute trauma	
Ligament and capsule tears	Single contrast
Synovitis	Double contrast with
	tomograpy
Synovial cysts	Single contrast
Articular cartilage	Double contrast with
abnormalities	tomography
Capsule size	Single contrast
Needle position prior to	Single contrast
aspiration	
Postoperative	
Total joint replacement	Subtraction technique for
	TEA's
Other	Double contrast with
	tomography

Contrast agents include air, positive contrast material, or a combination of the two. Several contrast media are available. We commonly use Hypaque-M 60 (Winthrop). Renografin-60 and Reno-M-60 (Squibb) are also commonly used. Because of the increased osmolality and rapid absorption, the contrast medium becomes rapidly diluted, resulting in loss of detail if filming is delayed. A change in the appearance of the contrast medium may develop as early as 5 to 10 minutes following injection. This phenomenon can be prevented by combining 0.3 ml of 1:1000 epinephrine with the contrast agent. This step is especially helpful if tomography is to be performed.[17, 23, 46]

Multiple techniques have been described for performing elbow arthrograms.[16, 17, 20, 25, 36, 39, 46] As previously mentioned, the technique chosen is largely determined by the patient's clinical symptoms (Table 6–2). In most cases, we use a double-contrast technique with 1 ml of contrast agent and 10 to 12 cc of room air because it provides better detail of the articular surface and the synovium. Air alone may be used in patients with an allergy to the contrast material. In this situation, tomography or even computed tomography is helpful in obtaining an adequate examination. Single-contrast injections of 5 to 6 ml are useful in evaluating capsule tears and synovial cysts (Table 6–2). Subtle changes can be obscured if single-contrast technique is used routinely.[25, 26, 36] We often use trispiral tomography to increase the articular and capsular detail. Linear tomography may be used if complex motion equipment is not available.[16]

The patient is positioned either sitting adjacent to the radiographic table or lying prone on the table (Fig. 6–20). In either position the elbow is flexed 90 degrees with the lateral aspect toward the examiner. Determination of the best position depends on the equipment available and the patient's condition. Prior to the injection of contrast agent, fluoroscopic evaluation of range of motion, and evidence of possible ligament stability or loose bodies should be accomplished.

The elbow is then prepared using sterile technique. One of two injection sites may be used. In most cases, a lateral approach into the radiocapitellar joint is chosen. In patients with previous radial head resection or suspected lateral ligament injury, a posterior ap-

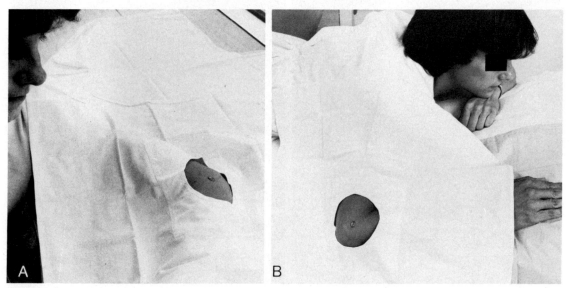

Figure 6–20. Patient positioned for lateral elbow arthrography, sitting (A) and prone (B) with the elbow flexed and the metal marker over the radiocapitellar joint.

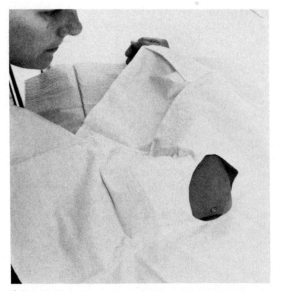

Figure 6–21. Patient positioned for a posterior injection. The elbow is flexed with the marker above the olecranon.

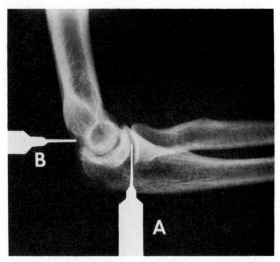

Figure 6–22. Illustration of the position of the needle tip for the posterior (B) and lateral (A) injections.

proach is more suitable. With the posterior approach, the elbow is again flexed 90 degrees, and the medial and lateral epicondyles and olecranon are palpated. The needle is placed an equal distance between these points (Fig. 6–21) and is positioned fluoroscopically (Fig. 6–22). If properly positioned, the contrast medium will flow away from the needle

tip as it is injected. If not properly positioned, the contrast collects at the needle tip and significant resistance is encountered.

Following the injection the needle is removed and the elbow is studied fluoroscopically. This step is essential in evaluating stability of the joint and loose bodies. Routine films include AP, lateral, and both oblique views. Medial and lateral cross-table lateral views provide additional information with double-contrast technique.

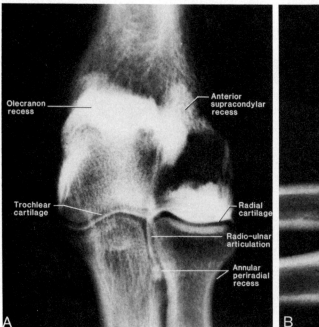

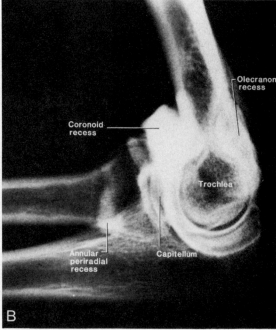

Figure 6–23. Routine projections for single contrast arthrogram with normal anatomy labeled. A, AP view. B, Lateral view.
Illustration continued on opposite page

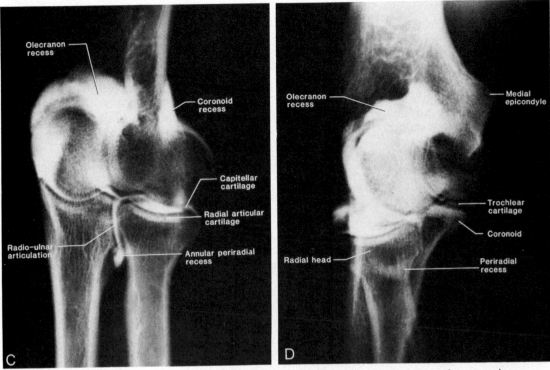

Figure 6–23 *Continued. C* and *D,* Oblique views. Normal double contrast arthrograms with tomography.

Normal Findings

In the normal arthrogram (Fig. 6–23A–D), the radiocapitellar, ulnartrochlear, and radioulnar joints can be identified. The anterior (coronoid), posterior (olecranon), and annular recesses are also visualized. Double-contrast tomograms (Fig. 6–24A and B) in the AP and lateral positions demonstrate the synovium and articular surfaces to better advantage.

The normal joint capacity is 10 to 12 ml. This may increase to 18 to 22 ml in patients with chronic instability, or it may be decreased in patients with capsulitis or flexion contracture.[25]

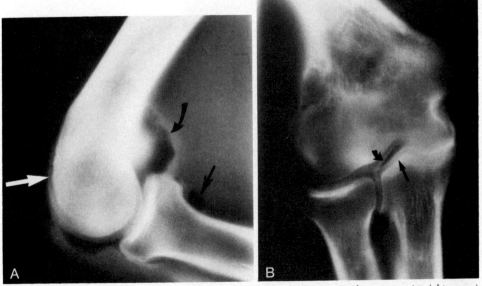

Figure 6–24. *A,* Lateral view demonstrates the synovial lining of the annular or sacciform recess (straight arrow), anterior (curved arrow), and posterior (white arrow) recesses. *B,* AP view demonstrates the articular cartilage to better advantage (arrows).

Abnormal Findings

Though tomograms may occasionally be helpful in demonstrating loose bodies, arthrography is more definitive. The density must be calcified if tomography is to be useful (Fig. 6–25). Loose bodies may be either attached to the synovium or actually free within the joint. If they are free they can be seen fluoroscopically or demonstrated on film by contrast that completely surrounds the structure (Fig. 6–26). Differentiation of a loose body in the olecranon fossa from the normal os supratrochlear dorsale is possible because of the nature of the trabecular pattern and the cortical thickness.[35] Most symptomatic densities in the olecranon fossa have prominent trabeculae and sclerotic cortical margins. The normal ossicle has sparse trabeculae and a thin cortical rim (Fig. 6–27A and B).

Occasionally, arthrography is performed to exclude capsular tears following trauma or surgical procedures. In this situation a single-contrast technique is usually adequate (Table 6–2). Extravasation of contrast material indicates a tear (Fig. 6–28A–D). Care must be taken not to mistake extravasation at the needle site for a rent of the capsule. Therefore, the needle should not be placed near the area of suspected injury. If a lateral tear is suspected, a posterior approach should be used.

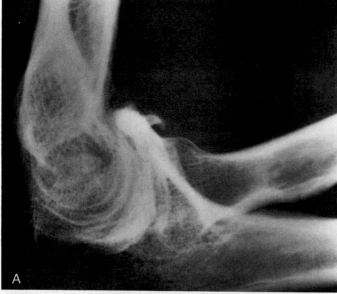

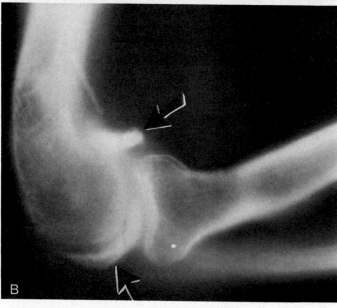

Figure 6–25. A, Lateral view of the elbow demonstrates increased density in the radiocapitellar joint with spurring near the coronoid. B, Lateral tomogram reveals that these findings are due to osteochondral fragments (arrows).

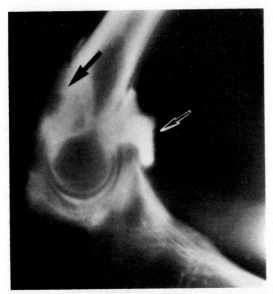

Figure 6–26. Single contrast arthrogram. The contrast medium completely surrounds the lucent loose body in the olecranon fossa. The capsule is flattened anteriorly (small arrow) owing to capsulitis. The joint capacity was only 6 cc.

Complications

Complications due to elbow arthrography are rare. Freiberger[17] reports an incidence of infection of approximately 1 in 25,000 cases.

Effusions may occur whether contrast material or air is utilized; they usually occur within 12 hours and may result in pain and joint stiffness.[23, 32] The joint fluid may have a turbid appearance owing to the high eosinophil count.[24, 32] Pain and effusion are reported less frequently following use of the double-contrast technique,[23] possibly due to the smaller amounts of contrast used.

The patient should be questioned about possible allergy to the contrast medium. Although rare (0.1 percent),[17] this complication must be kept in mind. Urticaria is the most common reaction experienced, and often no treatment is necessary. In more severe cases, antihistamines may be required. Most allergic reactions occur in the first 30 minutes after the injection. Premedication with an antihistamine may be used in patients with suspected allergy. These patients can be observed for 1 or 2 hours following the procedure.

XERORADIOGRAPHY

The image provided by xeroradiography results from an electrostatic process rather than the chemical process that produces the conventional radiographic film. This technique provides greater detail between objects of different densities such as bone and soft tis-

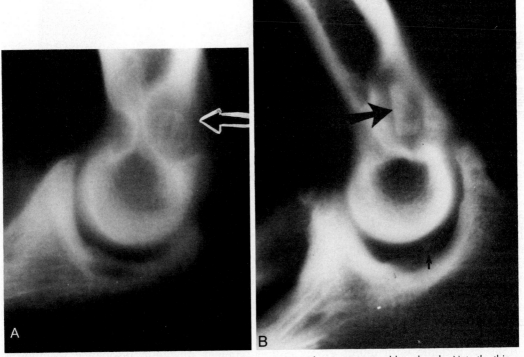

Figure 6–27. Lateral tomograms of the elbow. *A,* Asymptomatic patient with an os supratrochlear dorsale. Note the thin cortex and lack of trabeculae (arrow). *B,* Symptomatic patient with a density in the same region with thick cortex (large arrow) representing a loose body. There is a second smaller density in the joint space inferiorly (small arrow).

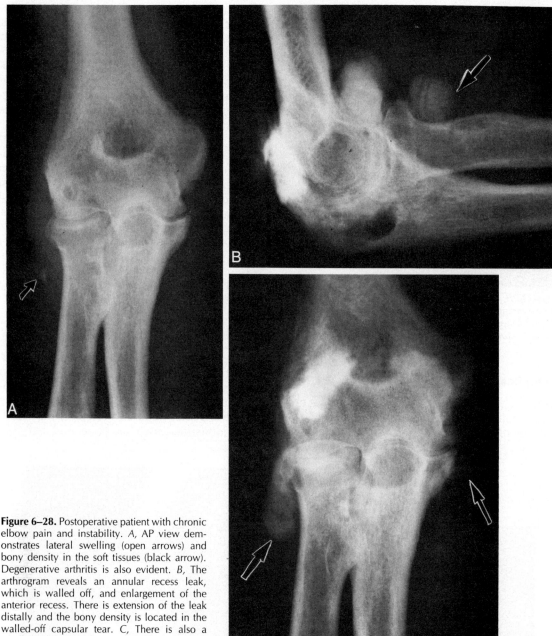

Figure 6–28. Postoperative patient with chronic elbow pain and instability. *A,* AP view demonstrates lateral swelling (open arrows) and bony density in the soft tissues (black arrow). Degenerative arthritis is also evident. *B,* The arthrogram reveals an annular recess leak, which is walled off, and enlargement of the anterior recess. There is extension of the leak distally and the bony density is located in the walled-off capsular tear. *C,* There is also a small capsular disruption medially on the AP arthrogram.

sue,[11, 15, 47, 48] a phenomenon referred to as edge enhancement.

For many years this modality was used primarily for mammography, but it has also proved to be useful for the study of soft tissues in the extremities and for evaluation of subtle skeletal changes in arthritis and metabolic bone disease.[11, 48] Subtle fractures may also be more easily detected (Fig. 6–6C). Fine calcifications in patients with tennis elbow and nonopaque foreign bodies may also be visible with xerographic technique (Fig. 6–29).

The major disadvantage of xeroradiography is the increased radiation doses,[48] which approach 7 to 10 times the dose required for routine radiography. Improvements in screen-film combinations have greatly reduced the use of xerograms.

MAGNETIC RESONANCE IMAGING

Nuclear magnetic resonance imaging (MRI) has been used for chemical analysis for some time. Recent advances in imaging technique

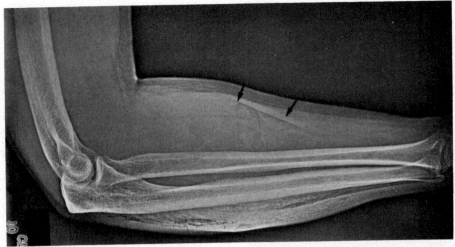

Figure 6–29. Xerogram of the forearm in a patient with a nonopaque foreign body. Large wood sliver (arrows) in the soft tissues that was not evident on the routine radiographs. Note the subcutaneous emphysema over the posterior portion of the forearm.

have demonstrated the potential usefulness of this technique in the clinical setting. Nuclear magnetic resonance images are obtained by placing the patient in a magnetic field and applying magnetic gradients and radiofrequency pulses that differentiate the tissue characteristics of the patient.[37] The tissue is differentiated by its proton density (hydrogen is used primarily owing to its abundance and strong signal), and the relaxation time of the sample. It is beyond the scope of this chapter

to discuss in detail the complex physical principles involved in magnetic resonance imaging. However, it can be said that the two relaxation times of the nuclei, T2 spin-spin relaxation and T1 spin-lattice relaxation, assist in differentiating tissues.

Early work in orthopedic practice has demonstrated that most patients are suitable candidates for this mode of imaging. Orthopedic appliances are not as a rule ferromagnetic, and therefore they are not affected by the

Figure 6–30. Metal artifact with computed tomography and MRI. *A,* Metal plates on the lower extremities with CT scan causes a significant "star burst" artifact. *B,* The same metal on the MRI with a free induction decay sequence results in less artifact (arrows). *C,* When a spin-echo sequence is used the artifact is almost nonexistent.

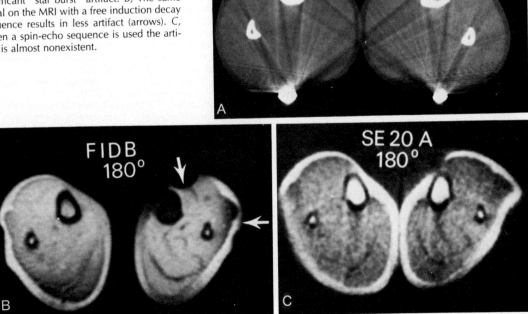

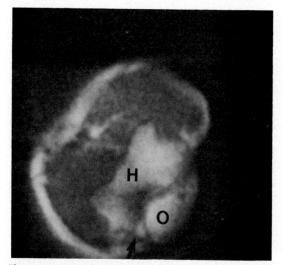

Figure 6–31. Axial scan of the elbow with MRI. Note the high intensity signal of the medullary cavity of the humerus (H) and the olecranon (O). The subcutaneous fat and ulnar nerve (arrow) are also of high intensity due to the increased proton density and short relaxation time. The muscle is of intermediate density. Cortical bone gives little signal.

magnet. Depending on the amount of metal present and its location, some artifact may be obtained (Fig. 6–30A–C). In certain situations this is less prohibitive than metal in CT scans. Cast material does not interfere with the quality of the image as it does in conventional radiographs. At this time it is believed that patients with ferromagnetic devices (e.g., aneurysm clips) and pacemakers should not be studied by MRI.

Early clinical investigations have shown that the anatomy of the soft tissues and tendons is clearly seen with MRI. Bone and soft tissue tumors, disc disease, avascular necrosis, infection, and fracture healing may all prove to be better studied with MRI than with conventional techniques (Fig. 6–31).[6, 9, 31] This technique uses no radiation, and to date it involves no known biologic hazards.[6, 42] However, more complete assessment of MRI is required before its precise usefulness as a clinical imaging modality will be evident.

References

1. Arger, P. H., et al.: Lipohemarthrosis. Am. J. Roentgenol. **121**:97, 1974.
2. Ballinger, P. W.: Merrill's Atlas of Radiographic Positions and Radiologic Procedures. St. Louis, C. V. Mosby Co., 1982.
3. Bassett, L. W., et al.: Post-traumatic Osteochondral "Loose Body" of the Olecranon Fossa. Radiology **141**:635, 1981.
4. Beals, R. K.: The Normal Carrying Angle of the Elbow: A Radiographic Study of 422 Patients. Clin. Orthop. **119**:194, 1976.
5. Bernau, A., and Berquist, T. H.: Positioning Techniques in Orthopedic Radiology. Orthopedic Positioning in Diagnostic Radiology. Baltimore, Urban and Schwartzenberg, 1983.
6. Berquist, T. H.: Magnetic Resonance Imaging: Preliminary Experience in Orthopedic Radiology. Magnetic Resonance Imaging, **2**:41, 1984.
7. Bledsoe, R. C., and Izenstark, J. L.: Displacement of Fat Pads in Disease and Injury of the Elbow. A New Radiographic Sign. Radiology **73**:717, 1959.
8. Bohrer, S. P.: The Fat Pad Sign Following Elbow Trauma. Clin. Radiol. **21**:90, 1970.
9. Brady, T. J., et al.: NMR Imaging of Forearms in Healthy Volunteers and Patients with Giant Cell Tumor of Bone. Radiology **144**:549, 1982.
10. Brown, R., et al.: Osteochondritis of the Capitellum. J. Sports Med. **2**:27, 1974.
11. Campbell, C. J., Roach, J., and Grisiola, A.: Comparative Study of Xeroradiography and Routine Roentgenography in Recording Roentgen Images of Bone Specimens. J. Bone Joint Surg. **39A**:577, 1957.
12. Carlson, D. H.: CT evaluation of Intra-Articular Fractures. South. Med. J. **73**:820, 1980.
13. Christianson, E. E., Curry, T. S., and Nunnally, J.: An Introduction to the Physics of Diagnostic Radiology. Philadelphia, Lea & Febiger, 1972.
14. Corbett, R. H.: Displaced Fat Pads in Trauma to the Elbow. Injury **9**:297, 1978.
15. Crowe, J. K.: Pulmonary Application of Xeroradiography and Xero-Tomography. Ph.D. Thesis, University of Minnesota, December, 1976.
16. Eto, R. T., Anderson, P. W., and Harley, J. D.: Elbow Arthrography with the Application of Tomography. Radiology **115**:283, 1975.
17. Freiberger, R. H., and Kaye, J. J.: Arthrography. New York, Appleton-Century-Crofts, 1979.
18. Fullerton, G. D.: Basic Concepts for Nuclear Magnetic Resonance Imaging. Magnetic Resonance Imaging **1**:39, 1982.
19. Genant, H. K., et al.: CT of the Musculoskeletal System. J. Bone Joint Surg. **62A**:1088, 1980.
20. Godefray, G., et al.: Arthrography of the Elbow: Anatomical and Radiological Considerations and Technical Considerations. Radiology **62**:441, 1981.
21. Greenspan, A., and Norman, A.: The Radial Head, Capitellar View. Useful Technique in Elbow Trauma. Am. J. Roentgenol. **138**:1186, 1982.
22. Greenspan, A., and Norman, A.: The Radial Head, Capitellar View. Another Example of its Usefulness. Am. J. Roentgenol. **139**:193, 1982.
23. Hall, F. H.: Morbidity from Shoulder Arthrography. Am. J. Roentgenol. **136**:59, 1981.
24. Hasselbacker, P.: Synovial Fluid Eosinophilia Following Arthrography. J. Rheumatol. **5**:173, 1978.
25. Hudson, T. M.: Elbow Arthrography. Radiol. Clin. North. Am. **19**:227, 1981.
26. Kohn, A. M.: Soft Tissue Alterations in Elbow Trauma. Am. J. Roentgenol. **82**:867, 1959.
27. London, J. T.: Kinematics of the Elbow. J. Bone Joint Surg. **63A**:329, 1981.
28. McCullough, C., and Coulam, C. M.: Physical and Dosimetric Aspects of Diagnostic Geometrical and Computer Assisted Tomography. Radiol. Clin. North Am. **14**:3, 1976.
29. McLeod, R. A., et al.: Computed Tomography of the Skeletal System. Semin. Roentgenol. **13**:235, 1978.
30. Mink, J. H., Eckardt, J. J., and Grant, T. T.: Arthrography in Recurrent Dislocation of the Elbow. Am. J. Roentgenol. **136**:1242, 1981.

31. Moon, K. L., et al.: Musculoskeletal Applications of NMR. Radiology **147**:161, 1983.
32. Murry, R. C.: Transitory Eosinophilia Localized to the Knee Joint. J. Bone Joint Surg. **32**:74, 1950.
33. Murry, W. A., and Siegel, M. J.: Elbow Fat Pads With New Signs and Extended Differential Diagnosis. Radiology **124**:659, 1977.
34. Norell, H. G.: Roentgenologic Visualization of the Extracapsular Fat. Its Importance in the Diagnosis of Traumatic Injuries to the Elbow. Acta Radiol. **42**:205, 1954.
35. Obermann, W. R., and Loose, H. W. C.: The Os Supratrochlear Dorsale: A Normal Variant That May Cause Symptoms. Am. J. Roentgenol. **141**:123, 1983.
36. Pavlov, H., Ghelman, B., and Warren, R. F.: Double Contrast Arthrography of the Elbow. Radiology **130**:87, 1979.
37. Pykett, I. L., Newhouse, J. H., et al.: Principles of Nuclear Magnetic Resonance Imaging. Radiology. **143**:157, 1982.
38. Resnick, D., et al.: Diagnosis of Bone and Joint Diseases. Philadelphia, W. B. Saunders Co., 1981.
39. Roback, D. L.: Elbow Arthrography: Brief Technical Considerations. Clin. Radiol. **30**:311, 1979.
40. Rogers, L. F.: Radiology of Skeletal Trauma. New York, Churchill Livingstone, 1982.
41. Rogers, S. L., and MacEwan, D. W.: Changes Due to Trauma in the Fat Plane Overlying the Supinator Muscle: A Radiographic Sign. Radiology **92**:954, 1969.
42. Saunders, R. D.: Biological Effects of NMR Clinical Imaging. Appl. Radiol. Sept.-Oct., 43–45, 1982.
43. Schwartz, J. L., and Crooks, L. E.: NMR Imaging Produces No Observable Mutations or Cytotoxicity in Mammalian Cells. Am. J. Roentgenol. **139**:583, 1982.
44. Smith, D. N., and Lee, J. R.: The Radiological Diagnosis of Post-Traumatic Effusion of the Elbow Joint and Its Clinical Significance: The Displaced Fat Pad Sign. Injury **10**:115, 1978.
45. Weisman, J., and Reimate, A.: Contrast Arthrography in Diagnosis of Soft Tissue Injuries of the Elbow Joint. RoFo **136**:313, 1982.
46. Weston, W. J., and Dalinka, M. K.: Arthrography. New York, Springer-Verlag, 1980.
47. Wolfe, J. N.: Xeroradiography: Image Content and Comparison with Film Roentgenograms. Am. J. Roentgenol. **117**:690, 1973.
48. Wolfe, J. N.: Xeroradiography of Bones, Joints, and Soft Tissues. Radiology **93**:583, 1969.
49. Yousefzadeh, D. K., and Jackson, J. H.: Lipohemarthrosis of the Elbow Joint. Radiology **128**:643, 1978.

CHAPTER 7

Arthroscopy of the Elbow

B. F. MORREY

The technique of elbow arthroscopy is somewhat challenging because the high degree of joint congruence provides limited tolerances with which to work. The indications, diagnostic information, and treatment options are all limited, thus further restricting this procedure as a means of diagnosis or treatment of routine elbow pathology. Nonetheless, in some instances, elbow arthroscopy can be of value. We feel that both a sound knowledge of elbow anatomy as well as experience with knee arthroscopy are prerequi-

sites to this procedure. Little has been written about elbow arthroscopy to date.[2, 3, 5]

INDICATIONS

Diagnostic Arthroscopy

In general, elbow arthroscopy is indicated in patients in whom intra-articular pathology is not readily definable by other noninvasive means. Some investigators[5] feel that the risk of elbow arthroscopy may be greater than any

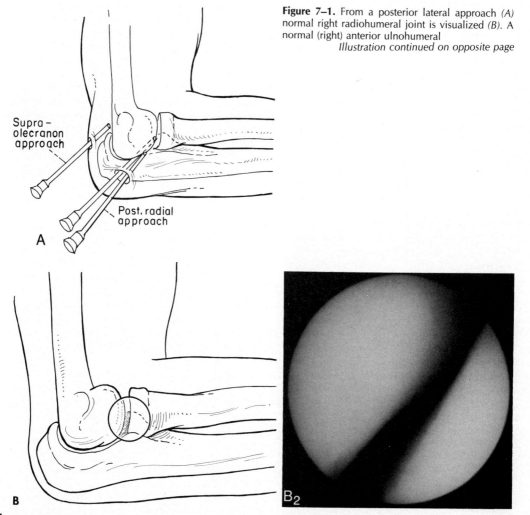

Figure 7–1. From a posterior lateral approach *(A)* normal right radiohumeral joint is visualized *(B)*. A normal (right) anterior ulnohumeral

Illustration continued on opposite page

Supra-olecranon approach

Post. radial approach

A

B

B₂

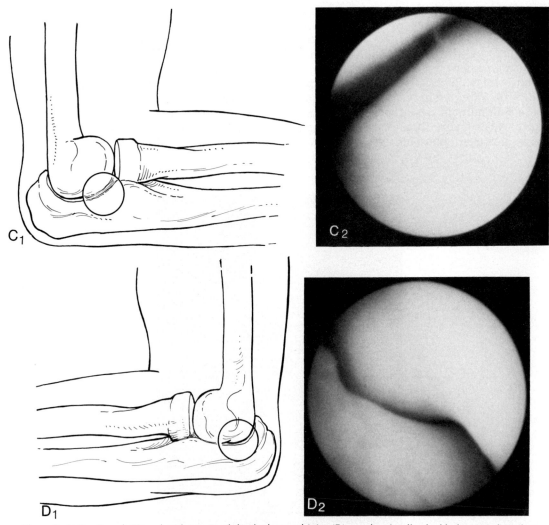

Figure 7–1. *Continued. (C)* and midposterior *(left)* ulnohumeral joint *(D)* may be visualized with the same insertion.

potential benefit. Yet because virtually all of the joint can be visualized by arthroscopy it provides considerable diagnostic potential (Fig. 7–1).

Degenerative Arthritis. Changes of the radiohumeral or ulnohumeral joint may be symptomatic but cannot be demonstrated by routine radiographs. In such cases arthroscopy may be capable of defining the nature and extent of the process (Fig. 7–2).

Post-traumatic Fibrosis and Arthritis. Type I fractures of the radial head may be present with inexplicable pain, loss of motion, or a grating sensation. In this setting, elbow arthroscopy has been helpful in the diagnosis of intra-articular adhesions and incongruity of the articular surface (Fig. 7–3).

Synovitis. Synovitis as a result of trauma or underlying disease may be diagnosed with arthroscopy much more readily than by physical examination (Fig. 7–2B).

Loose Bodies. Radiolucent cartilaginous loose bodies due to trauma or spontaneous formation are more reliably diagnosed by arthroscopy than by arthrograms (Fig. 7–4).

Other Uses. The potential for further delineation of the pathology present in epicondylitis, bursitis, and tendinitis has been suggested as a further application of arthroscopy,[2] but at this time, such applications must be considered to be purely speculative.

Operative Arthroscopy

The spectrum of useful arthroscopic operative procedures in the elbow is limited.

Loose Bodies. The removal of loose bodies is the procedure most amenable to operative arthroscopy of the elbow joint. When a loose body is present in the olecranon fossa, access is attained by inserting the scope from the posterior lateral route (Fig. 7–4). Occasionally, a fragment will be too large to be grasped by the loose body forceps. Even in this setting, localization is facilitated by arthroscopy, which permits a limited incision to remove the loose fragment.

Synovectomy. Subtotal synovectomy is possible in the elbow. This requires a triangulation technique with insertion of the scope or surgical instrument from a medial portal, which, however, may increase the risk of injury to the ulnar or median nerve. Before this procedure is undertaken, the risk-benefit ratio must be seriously considered. Using the high-speed bur in a patient with soft arthritic bone, arthroscopic removal of the radial head and synovectomy may be technically possible in a patient with rheumatoid arthritis, but we have not had experience with this.

Joint Débridement or Lavage. Arthroscopic lysis or excision of fibrous bands, joint lavage,

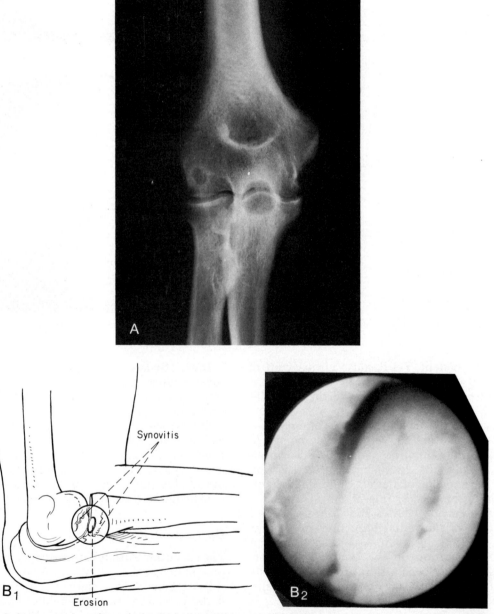

Figure 7–2. Anteroposterior radiograph showing extensive degenerated cysts, but the radiohumeral joint looks normal (A). A posterior lateral portal demonstrates an erosion in the radial head and synovitis B.

Illustration continued on opposite page

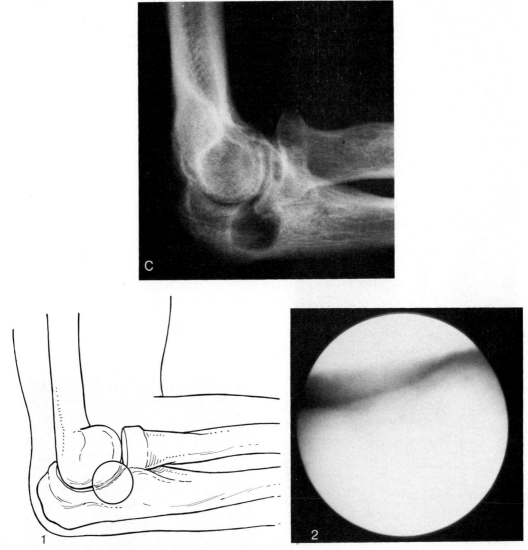

Figure 7–2. *Continued.* The lateral radiograph suggests cartilage disruption of the olecranon *(C)*, which is demonstrated to be in continuity by arthroscopy *(D).*

and joint debridément may be accomplished with variable success (Fig. 7–3C). Inability to effectively separate the joint limits exposure and hence may limit the surgeon's ability to perform adequate débridement.

Soft Tissue Release. Some surgeons have performed anterior capsular incision under arthroscopic control, with limited success to date.*

TECHNIQUE

For arthroscopy of the elbow, the patient is placed in the supine position with the shoul-

der over the side of the operating table and the arm suspended (Fig. 7–5). The upper extremity is prepared in the usual manner from the midhumerus to the wrist and is draped free to allow manipulation. Regional or local anesthesia may be employed, but we prefer a general anesthetic. The examiner sits, and the arm is brought over the chest (Fig. 7–6). The small (2.7 mm) arthroscopic system is used, and a syringe introduced through a separate insertion site allows constant irrigation and distention of the joint.

Several potential insertion sites provide access to the joint (Fig. 7–7). We prefer the anterior or posterior lateral insertions for most diagnostic studies. The radial head, tip of the olecranon, and lateral epicondyle are pal-

---

*Andrews, J.: Personal communication, 1983; Johnson, L.L.: Personal communication, 1983.

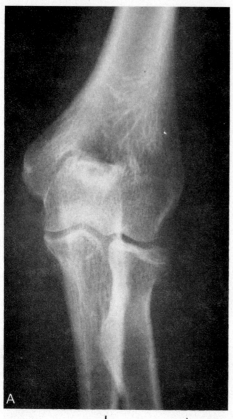

Figure 7–3. A 30-year-old female with a healed type I fracture of the radial head (A). However, the patient had persistent discomfort with a clicking sensation. Arthroscopic assessment revealed grade 3 changes of the radial head (B), which was treated by débridement (C). The patient was considerably relieved of her symptoms 3 months after the procedure.

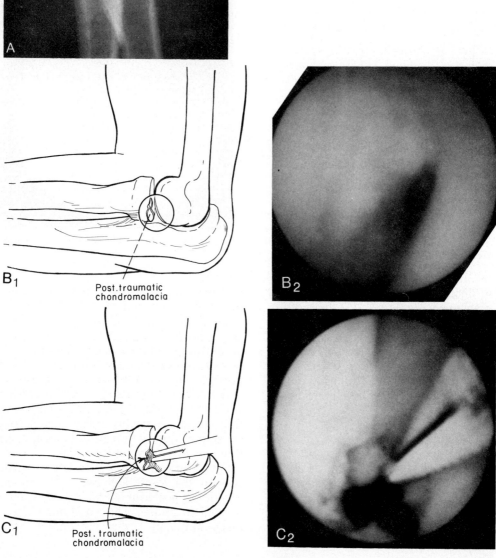

Post.traumatic
chondromalacia

Post. traumatic
chondromalacia

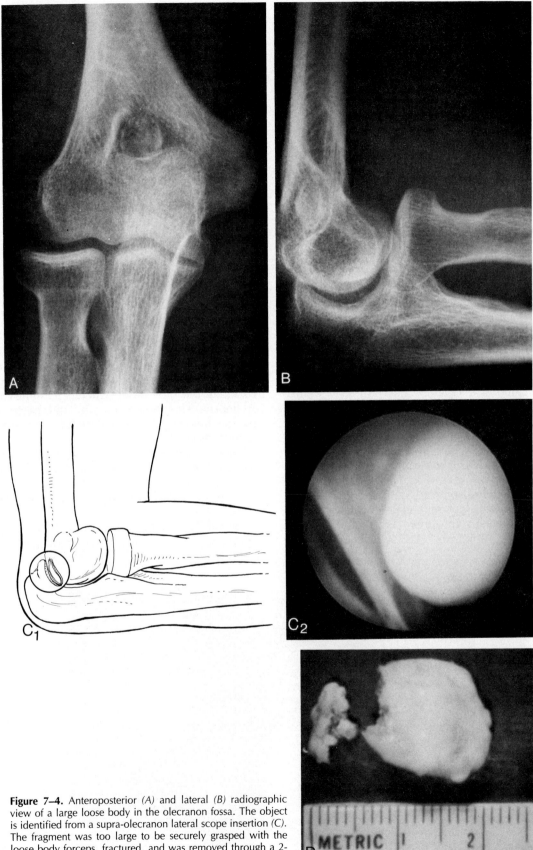

Figure 7–4. Anteroposterior (A) and lateral (B) radiographic view of a large loose body in the olecranon fossa. The object is identified from a supra-olecranon lateral scope insertion (C). The fragment was too large to be securely grasped with the loose body forceps, fractured, and was removed through a 2-cm incision (D).

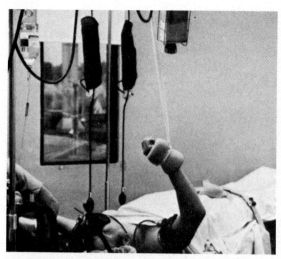

Figure 7–5. The patient is positioned with the shoulder over the side of the table, and the extremity is prepared from the wrist to the midhumerus and draped free. (From Johnson, L. L.: Diagnostic and Surgical Arthroscopy: The Knee and Other Joints, 2nd ed. St. Louis, C.V. Mosby Company, 1981.)

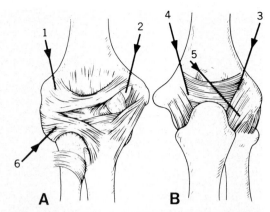

Figure 7–7. Several anterior (A) and posterior (B) portals of entry are possible for elbow arthroscopy. We avoid the medial sites of insertion for fear of injury to the ulnar nerve. (From Watanabe, N., Takeda, S., and Ikeuchi, H.: Atlas of Arthroscopy, 3rd ed. Tokyo, Igaku-Shoin, 1979.)

pated. Rotation of the forearm confirms the location of the radial head, and the joint is distended with an 18-gauge needle through the same or a separate insertion site. Manipulation of the radial head by pronation and supination and by flexion and extension of the joint is helpful to attain and remain oriented as well as to help visualize certain parts of the joint. Varus and valgus stress is difficult to impart and is of little value. Axial distraction is used to some advantage, but in general the elbow is not amenable to manipulative techniques to improve visualization. Thus, multiple puncture sites are needed (Table 7–1).

Posterior Insertions

The olecranon fossa may be entered posteriorly either from the medial (site 4) or the lateral (site 3) entry point. We prefer the lateral approach because this avoids possible injury to the ulnar nerve. If arthritis is present, visualization may be obstructed by synovitis or debris. The transolecranon and posterior approaches are particularly useful for removal of loose bodies.

Lateral Approach. The posterior lateral insertion (site 5) allows visualization of the radiohumeral articulation as well as most of the lateral ulnohumeral articulations (Fig. 7–1).

Medial Approach. Some surgeons have recommended the ulnar or medial approach[2] because they feel that it provides better visu-

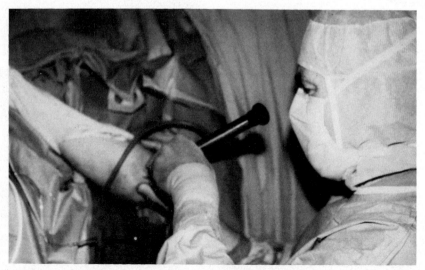

Figure 7–6. The arthroscopist sits during arthroscopy from the lateral approach, and the arm is brought across the chest.

Table 7–1. **Possible Insertion Sites for Elbow Arthroscopy**

Sites	Comments
Supracondylar anterior radial approach	Offers relatively little benefit
Supracondylar anterior ulnar approach	Preferred by some for ulnohumeral and radiohumeral inspection
Supraolecranon radial approach	Loose body removal and fossa inspection
Supraolecranon ulnar approach	Dangerous, should be avoided
Posterior radial approach	Author's preferred approach
Anterior radial approach	Limited visualization, primarily of soft tissue

alization of the radial head or better access for débridement or capsular release.* We have no experience with medial insertion of the scope and have avoided anterior insertion for fear of damage to the median nerve and posterior medial insertion for fear of injury to the ulnar nerve.

Multiple Insertion Sites

Débridement or loose body removal requires the use of a second insertion site. For osseous loose bodies, localization by routine radiography helps the surgeon plan the insertion site of the scope. Classic triangulation techniques are used for loose body removal. The location of the object is first performed with arthroscopy. The proper orientation and angle needed to effect removal is estimated by using a spinal needle percutaneously placed through the skin. Finally, the skin is incised and the loose body grasped and removed.

COMPLICATIONS

No complications of elbow arthroscopy have been published, but undoubtedly they must occur. The personal experience of well known arthroscopists who have performed elbow arthroscopy fails to contribute any complications of this procedure.† The close tolerances and high degree of congruence of the elbow joint place the articular cartilage at some risk of injury even with simple diagnostic procedures. Use of the medial approach has the potential to injure the ulnar nerve either directly or indirectly from pressure in the cubital tunnel owing to extravasation of fluid from the joint. For this reason, we feel that medial insertion of the scope should be

reserved for those who are both well versed in arthroscopy and thoroughly familiar with the anatomy of this joint.

RESULTS

No critical report of the effectiveness of diagnostic or therapeutic elbow arthroscopy has yet appeared. Our experience indicates that the major benefit has been the diagnosis of an arthritic process that exceeds the degree suggested by routine radiographs (Figs. 7–2 and 7–3). The most successful surgical procedure has been the removal of loose bodies. The beneficial effect of lavage, observed regularly with knee arthroscopy, has, in our experience, not been duplicated after this procedure at the elbow.

CONCLUSION

Although elbow arthroscopy is technically possible, one must constantly address the question of the real value of this procedure. A critical analysis not just of the technique but also of the ways in which treatment has been altered as a result of arthroscopy is indicated. A similar study of shoulder arthroscopy has been performed by Cofield, and it is only through such studies that the true value of this technique will be accurately defined.

References

1. Cofield, R. H.: Arthroscopy of the Shoulder. Mayo Clinic Proceedings. **58**:501, 1983.
2. Johnson, L. L.: Diagnostic and Surgical Arthroscopy: The Knee and Other Joints, 2nd ed. St. Louis, The C. V. Mosby Co., 1981.
3. McGinty, J. B.: Arthroscopic Removal of Loose Bodies. Orthop. Clin. North Am. **13**:313, 1982.
4. Watanabe, N., Takeda, S., and Ikeuchi, H.: Atlas of Arthroscopy, 3rd ed. Tokyo, Igaku-Shoin, 1979.
5. Zarins, B.: Arthroscopic Surgery in a Sports Medicine Practice. Orthop. Clin. North Am. **13**:415, 1982.

*Andrews, J.: Personal communication, 1983.

†Andrews, J.: Personal communication, 1983; Johnson, L.L.: Personal communcation, 1983.

CHAPTER 8

Surgical Exposures of the Elbow

B. F. MORREY

Few joints require familiarity with as many surgical exposures as does the elbow. The intricate anatomy and range of pathologic processes it may undergo account for the numerous techniques that have been described to provide appropriate surgical access to the elbow region. Depending on the pathology and the surgical goal, the joint and the surrounding region may be approached from the lateral, posterior, medial, or anterior direction. Only the anterior medial aspect of the joint is considered inaccessible to direct exposure because of the vulnerability of the median nerve and the brachial artery.

In general, a carefully planned and limited exposure from the medial and lateral aspects allows the removal of loose bodies and the treatment of certain localized fractures without risk of injury to any vital structure. Because a variety of extensile posterior exposures are used for most complex fractures and joint reconstructive procedures, this might be considered the universal approach to the joint. The extensile anterior approach of Henry is an uncommon but valuable technique for certain contractures, biceps tendon pathology, and similar lesions.

Several authors have presented variants of the more commonly used approaches to the elbow joint.[8, 13, 14, 27] It is not the purpose of this chapter to discuss all of the approaches to the joint but rather to provide a comprehensive collection and critique of those exposures that may prove helpful to the practicing orthopedic surgeon.

GENERAL PRINCIPLES

As others have noted in the past,[7, 8, 28] rigorous adherence to the principles of good surgical technique is of no greater importance in any other anatomic part than it is in the elbow region. Selection of the most appropriate surgical approach to the elbow region depends on the specific goal of the surgical procedure as well as the pathology involved. As with any orthopedic procedure, the choice of surgical approach should be based on the following criteria:

1. Potential to be extended to meet any unforeseen circumstances that should arise.
2. Capability of providing adequate visualization to define and correct the specific pathology completely.
3. Safety: avoidance of vital structures or visualization of these structures to avoid injury during the procedure.
4. Preservation of the normal anatomy as much as possible during the exposure, the procedure, and at closure.
5. Dissection along natural tissue planes rather than across muscle, tendon, or ligamentous structures.
6. Provision of careful hemostasis and adequate drainage after extensile exposures.
7. Satisfactory soft tissue closure that ensures rapid and predictable rehabilitation.

Knowledge of and adherence to these guidelines is of great importance for a predictable and uncomplicated surgical result. A thorough understanding of the anatomy of the elbow region is important in selecting the exposure that best satisfies these considerations. The cross-sectional anatomy of this region is depected in Figure 8–1.

Figure 8–1. A–G, Cross-sectional anatomy shows the important neurovascular and muscular relationships that must be understood for a complication-free exposure of the elbow. (Modified from Eycleshymer, A.C., and Schoemaker, D.M.: A Cross Section Anatomy. New York, Appleton and Company, 1930. *In* Darrach, W.: Surgical approaches for surgery of the extremities. Am. J. Surg. 67:93, 1945.

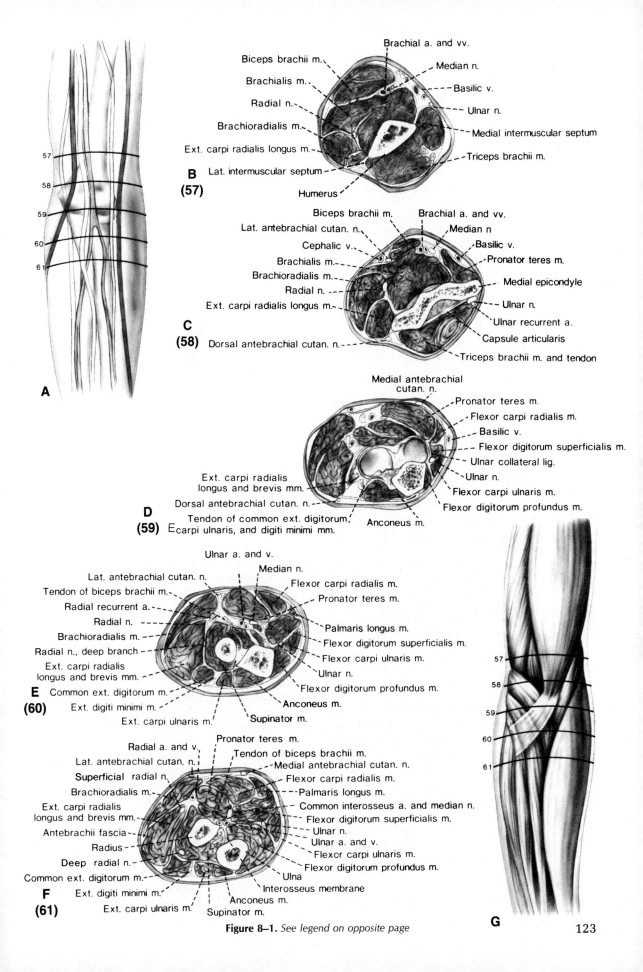

B
(57)

Biceps brachii m.
Brachialis m.
Radial n.
Brachioradialis m.
Ext. carpi radialis longus m.
Lat. intermuscular septum

Brachial a. and vv.
Median n.
Basilic v.
Ulnar n.
Medial intermuscular septum
Triceps brachii m.
Humerus

C
(58)

Biceps brachii m.
Lat. antebrachial cutan. n.
Cephalic v.
Brachialis m.
Brachioradialis m.
Radial n.
Ext. carpi radialis longus m.
Dorsal antebrachial cutan. n.

Brachial a. and vv.
Median n
Basilic v.
Pronator teres m.
Medial epicondyle
Ulnar n.
Ulnar recurrent a.
Capsule articularis
Triceps brachii m. and tendon

D
(59) **E**

Medial antebrachial cutan. n.
Pronator teres m.
Flexor carpi radialis m.
Basilic v.
Flexor digitorum superficialis m.
Ulnar collateral lig.
Ulnar n.
Flexor carpi ulnaris m.
Flexor digitorum profundus m.

Ext. carpi radialis longus and brevis mm.
Dorsal antebrachial cutan. n.
Tendon of common ext. digitorum, carpi ulnaris, and digiti minimi mm.
Anconeus m.

E
(60)

Ulnar a. and v.
Median n.
Lat. antebrachial cutan. n.
Tendon of biceps brachii m.
Radial recurrent a.
Radial n.
Brachioradialis m.
Radial n., deep branch
Ext. carpi radialis longus and brevis mm.
Common ext. digitorum m.
Ext. digiti minimi m.
Ext. carpi ulnaris m.

Flexor carpi radialis m.
Pronator teres m.
Palmaris longus m.
Flexor digitorum superficialis m.
Flexor carpi ulnaris m.
Ulnar n.
Flexor digitorum profundus m.
Anconeus m.
Supinator m.

F
(61)

Radial a. and v.
Lat. antebrachial cutan. n.
Superficial radial n.
Brachioradialis m.
Ext. carpi radialis longus and brevis mm.
Antebrachii fascia
Radius
Deep radial n.
Common ext. digitorum m.
Ext. digiti minimi m.
Ext. carpi ulnaris m.

Pronator teres m.
Tendon of biceps brachii m.
Medial antebrachial cutan. n.
Flexor carpi radialis m.
Palmaris longus m.
Common interosseus a. and median n.
Flexor digitorum superficialis m.
Ulnar n.
Ulnar a. and v.
Flexor carpi ulnaris m.
Flexor digitorum profundus m.
Ulna
Interosseus membrane
Supinator m.
Anconeus m.

A

G

Figure 8–1. *See legend on opposite page*

123

LATERAL APPROACHES

The lateral exposure is probably the most commonly used approach to the elbow joint and offers the greatest variation. It is used for radial head excision, removal of loose bodies, and repair of lateral condylar and Monteggia fractures. Access to the radiohumeral articulation has been described by several authors.[6, 16, 19, 21, 30] The techniques differ according to the muscle interval entered or the means of reflecting the muscle mass from the proximal ulna. An ever-present awareness of the possibility of injury to the recurrent branch of the radial nerve is assumed with any of the lateral exposures to the joint or to the proximal radius.

No attempt is made here to present every technique that has been described for exposure of the lateral aspect of the elbow joint, but the more common and useful approaches will be discussed.

APPROACH. Lateral (Kaplan, 1941)[19]—between the extensor digitorum communis and the extensor carpi radialis longus.

Indication. Removal of the radial head.

Comment. Kaplan has described an approach through the interval between the extensor digitorum communis and the extensor carpi radialis longus and brevis muscles. Because of the proximity of the radial nerve, pronation of the forearm during exposure has been recommended to assist in carrying the radial nerve out of the surgical field. The effect of this maneuver has been quantified by Strachan and Ellis, who found that approximately 1 cm of medial-lateral radial nerve translation can occur with forearm pronation (Fig. 8–2).[35] However, even with this maneuver, the radial nerve is precariously close to the surgical field, and thus this approach is used less commonly than that described by Kocher.

Description of Technique. The patient is placed in a prone position. The incision begins directly over and about 5 cm proximal to the lateral epicondyle and is continued for about 6 cm distally to the radiohumeral joint (Fig. 8–3). With the forearm supinated, the dissection is carried down to bone between the brachioradialis and the common extensor muscles laterally and the extensor digitorum communis medially. This interval is then retracted, exposing the supinator muscle in the depths of the wound. The muscle is released from its humeral and ulnar attachments and retracted medially as necessary to provide

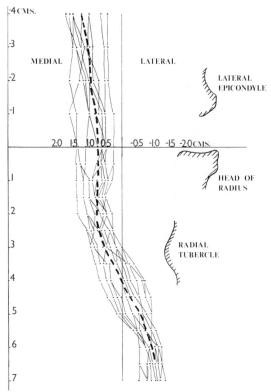

Figure 8–2. Approximately 1 cm of medial-to-lateral translation of the posterior interosseous nerve occurs as the forearm is rotated from supination to pronation. (From Strachan, J. H., and Ellis, B. W.: Vulnerability of the posterior interosseous nerve during radial head resection. J. Bone Joint Surg. 53B:320, 1971.)

exposure of the annular ligament. The radial head and neck are exposed by incising the annular ligament. The effect of forearm pronation and supination is contrasted in Figures 8–2A and B.

APPROACH. Lateral (Kocher, 1911)[21]—between the extensor carpi ulnaris and anconeus.

Indications. Excision of the radial head, removal of loose bodies; it may be converted to an extensile posterolateral exposure if needed.

Comment. The most common approach to the radial head is through this safer, more posterior interval, as described by Kocher. In contrast to the direct lateral approach of Kaplan, this exposure enters the joint through the interval of the anconeus and extensor carpi ulnaris, thus providing a source of protection to the deep radial nerve. In addition to providing a limited exposure for radial head excision and loose body removal, the particular value of this technique is that it may be

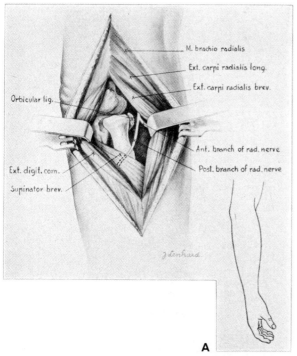
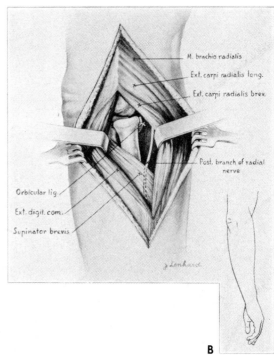

Figure 8–3. The Kaplan approach. A 10- to 11-cm incision is centered over the radial humeral joint extending proximally along the posterior aspect of the brachialis and distally down the forearm over the extensor carpi radialis longus and brevis muscles. The interval between the common extensor tendon and the extensor carpi radialis longus and brevis is identified and developed to expose the supinator muscle as it covers the proximal radius. The ulnar and humeral origins of the supinator are released and retracted to expose the annular ligament, which is incised to expose the joint *(A)*. With full pronation of the forearm the posterior interosseous nerve is translated to approximately 1 cm, further protecting the nerve from insult at the time of surgery *(B)*. (From Kaplan, E. B.: Surgical approaches to the proximal end of the radius and its use in fractures of the head and neck of the radius. J. Bone Joint Surg. 23:86, 1941.)

converted to an extensile posterolateral approach to the entire distal humerus (see below).

Description of Technique. The distal Kocher exposure begins with a skin incision just proximal to the lateral epicondyle of the humerus in the avascular interval. It is extended distally and posteriorly approximately 6 cm in an oblique manner over the fascia of the anconeus and extensor carpi ulnaris muscles (Fig. 8–4). This interval is developed, and the dissection is carried down to the joint capsule. The nerve is a safe distance from the dissection and is protected by the extensor carpi ulnaris and extensor digitorum communis muscle mass. The origin of the anconeus is released subperiosteally from the humerus and retracted posteriorly to permit adequate exposure of the capsule. A longitudinal incision is made across the capsule to expose the radiocapitellar joint.

APPROACH. Transepicondylar lateral approach (Campbell, 1971).[11]

Indications. Fracture of the lateral condyle.

Comment. Excellent exposure of the radiohumeral articulation may be realized by performing an osteotomy of the lateral epicondyle. The clinical applications of this exposure are probably limited, however, because other techniques provide similarly adequate visualization of the joint without requiring the osteotomy and union of the common extensor origin.

Description of Technique. The incision is begun approximately 5 cm proximal to the lateral epicondyle of the humerus and extends distally over the avascular interval and across the epicondyle, ending about 3 to 4 cm distal to the joint along the posterolateral surface of the forearm (Fig. 8–5). The lateral border of the humerus is exposed by subperiosteal dissection of the triceps posteriorly and the origin of the extensor carpi radialis longus and the brachioradialis anteriorly. The radial nerve is avoided because it lies in close proximity to the proximal angle of the wound. With a small osteotome, the lateral epicon-

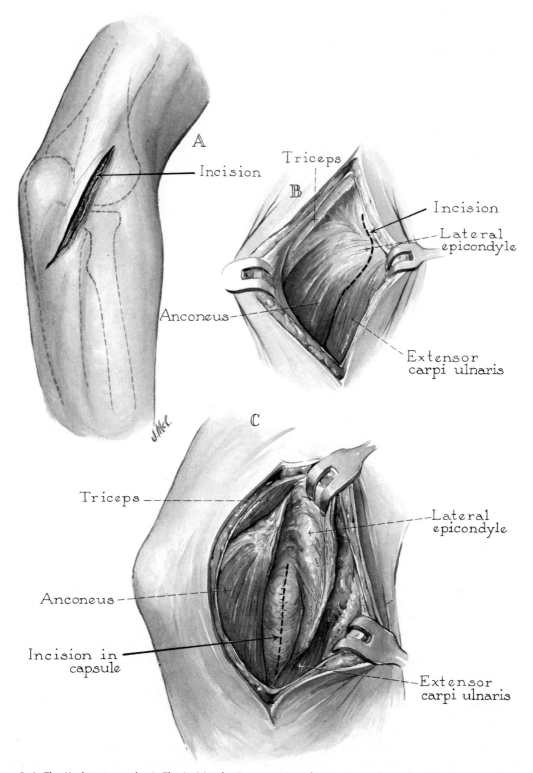

Figure 8–4. The Koeber approach. *A*, The incision begins approximately 2 to 3 cm above the lateral epicondyle over the supracondylar bony ridge and extends distally and posteriorly for approximately 4 cm. *B*, The interval between the anconeus and the extensor carpi ulnaris is identified. *C*, Development of this interval reveals the capsule.

Illustration continued on opposite page

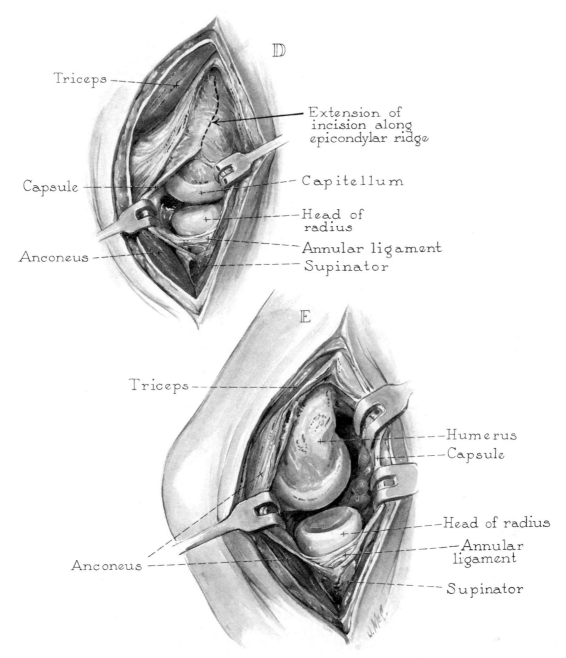

Figure 8–4. *Continued.* The joint capsule may be entered proximal to the annular ligament *(D)*, and a more extensive exposure may be obtained by extending the capsular incision proximally *(E)*, thereby providing adequate exposure of the radiohumeral articulation. (From Banks, S. W., and Laufman, H.: An Atlas of Surgical Exposures of the Extremities. Philadelphia, W. B. Saunders Co., 1953).

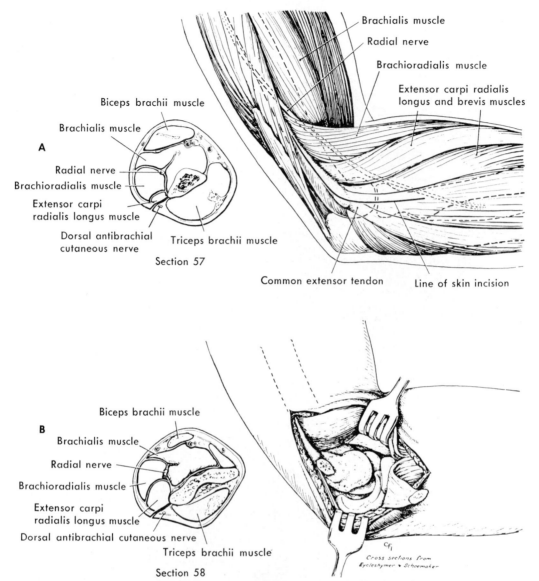

Figure 8–5. Lateral Campbell approach. *A,* Cross section through the distal humerus (left) and the skin incision with its relationship to the underlying muscles (right). *B,* A cross section of the humerus just above the joint shows the interval being developed (left). To expose the lateral epicondyle, the epicondyle has been osteotomized and the muscle reflected distally, exposing the joint (right). (From Crenshaw, A. H.: Surgical Approaches. *In* Edmonson, A. S., and Crenshaw, A. H. (eds.): Campbell's Operative Orthopaedics, 6th ed. St. Louis, The C. V. Mosby Co., 1980; cross sections modified from Eycleshymer, A. C., and Schoemaker, D. M.: A Cross-Section Anatomy. New York, D. Appleton & Co., 1930.)

dyle, with a common origin of the extensor muscle mass and the radial collateral ligament, is removed and the complex is retracted distally, exposing the radiohumeral joint. The deep branch of the radial nerve is protected as it enters the supinator muscle. The brachioradialis and the extensor carpi radialis longus muscles are elevated as they originate on the anterior aspect of the distal humerus, and the capsule is incised to expose the lateral aspect of the elbow joint.

Comment. Not only can this technique be used for fracture of the proximal ulna com-

plicated by radial head dislocation, but it can also be extended to allow a safe exposure of the proximal one-fourth of the radius as well.[11] Care must be taken to repair the annular ligament, however, because this provides varus stability to the elbow as well as stability for the radial head (see Chapter 2).

POSTEROLATERAL EXPOSURES

When exposure of the olecranon as well as the radiohumeral joint is required, several variations of a posterolateral approach may be used. Depending on the desired exposure of the proximal ulna or the distal humerus, these approaches can be extended, thus providing a significant element of versatility.[34]

APPROACH. Posterolateral exposure of the radial head and proximal ulna (Boyd, 1940).[6]
Indication. Monteggia fracture.
Comment. This approach has been modified to function as an extensile exposure of the elbow joint.[30]
Description of Technique. Begin the incision just posterior to the lateral epicondyle and lateral to the triceps tendon and continue it distally to the lateral tip of the olecranon and then down the subcutaneous border of the ulna to the junction of its proximal and middle thirds or as necessary to expose the fracture (Fig. 8–6). The anconeus and extensor carpi ulnaris are stripped subperiosteally from the ulna beginning on the lateral subcutaneous crest of the bone and reflecting the muscles volarward. The supinator is released subperiosteally from its ulnar insertion, and the entire muscle mass is reflected anteriorly. Thus, the lateral surface of the ulna and the proximal portion of the radius are adequately exposed. The substance of the reflected supinator protects the deep branch of the radial nerve. If greater exposure of the radius is desired, the recurrent interosseous artery (not the dorsal interosseous artery) is divided in the proximal portion of the wound, and the muscle mass is further reflected volarward to expose the interosseous membrane. The deep branch of the radial nerve remains protected.

APPROACH. Posterior lateral exposure of the elbow region (Pankovich, 1977).[30]
Indication. An extensile exposure is used by the author for radial head fractures, Monteggia fractures, lateral ligament reconstruction, and any severe injury to the lateral joint.
Comment. No adverse neurovascular effects to the anconeus muscle have been appreciated by Pankovich with this approach, but the need to preserve the proximal triceps-anconeus relationship must be recognized.
Description of Technique. The patient is placed in a semilateral position with a sandbag under the scapula; the extremity is placed over the chest. The incision begins 2 cm proximal to the olecranon, extends over the lateral border of the triceps tendon, and curves distally around the olecranon, ending 4 to 5 cm down the posterior ridge of the ulna, depending on the length of the anconeus muscle (Fig. 8–7). The well-defined fascia over the extensor muscles is released from

the ulna along the dorsal margin of the anconeus muscle. The interval between the anconeus and the extensor carpi ulnaris is entered, and the entire ulnar insertion of the anconeus is reflected proximally by subperiosteal dissection. The relationship between the triceps and the anconeus is identified, and the medial portion is released to provide adequate exposure of the radiohumeral joint. Because the neurovascular supply to the anconeus muscle passes through the triceps, the entire anconeus can be reflected in a distal to proximal direction. The posterolateral capsule of the elbow joint is readily observed as well as the origin of the deep portion of the supinator, the radial collateral ligament complex, and the proximal ulna. The joint capsule may be excised, thus exposing the radiohumeral aspect of the elbow joint. At the end of the procedure, the anconeus muscle should be returned to its normal position and secured with several resorbable sutures. No attempt is made to close the fascia, and the wound is closed in layers as desired.

For more extensive visualization of the elbow joint, the origin of the radial collateral ligament and the common extensor origin are detached from the humerus, thus allowing posterior dislocation of the joint. The anterior compartment of the elbow joint and the coronoid process are thus exposed. Reattachment of the capsule-ligament complex is accomplished by passing nonabsorbable sutures through drill holes in the lateral epicondyle and tying them with the elbow in extension. Postoperatively, the elbow may be mobilized in a few days without risk of recurrent dislocation.

This approach may also be extended distally in the manner described by Boyd if further exposure of the ulna is required.

APPROACH. Posterolateral (Gordon, 1967).[16]
Indication. Monteggia fractures.
Comment. To preserve the soft tissue attachment of the anconeus to fracture fragments of the proximal ulna, Gordon has combined features from both the Boyd and Kocher exposures. The soft tissue attachments to the fracture fragments are preserved by exposing the fracture from the ulno-anconeus interval as well as from the anconeus–extensor carpi ulnaris interval. Although we have not used this exposure we would be concerned that it would be somewhat limited by the attempt to preserve these muscular attachments. In addition, the value of this technique appears to be somewhat theoretical because nonunion is uncommon and avascular necrosis has not

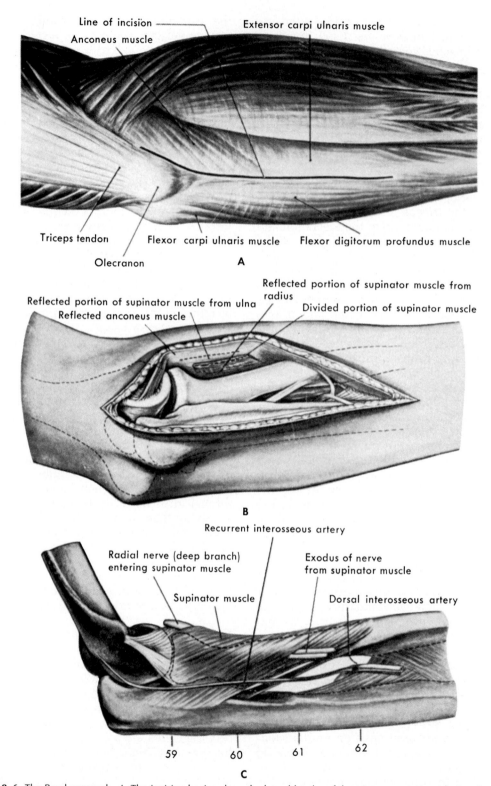

Figure 8–6. The Boyd approach. *A*, The incision begins along the lateral border of the triceps approximately 2 to 3 cm above the epicondyle and extends distally over the lateral subcutaneous border of the ulna for approximately 6 to 8 cm past the tip of the olecranon. The ulnar insertion of the anconeus and the origin of the supinator muscles are elevated subperiosteally. More distally, the subperiosteal reflection includes the abductor pollicus longus and extensor carpi ulnaris as well as the extensor pollicus longus muscle. The origin of the supinator at the crista supinatorus of the ulna is released, and the entire muscle flap is retracted radially, exposing the radiohumeral joint *(B)*. The posterior interosseous nerve is protected in the substance of the supinator, which must be gently retracted. *C*, To extend the incision more distally the dorsal interosseous artery must be ligated. *Illustration continued on opposite page*

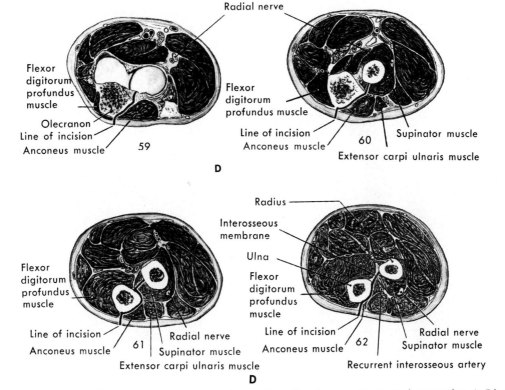

Figure 8–6. *Continued. D,* Cross-section relationship is shown. (From Crenshaw, A. H.: Surgical Approaches. *In* Edmonson, A. S., and Crenshaw, A. H. (eds.): Campbell's Operative Orthopaedics, 6th ed. St. Louis, The C. V. Mosby Co., 1980. *A* and *B* modified from Boyd, H. B.: Surg. Gynecol. Obstet. *71*:86, 1940; *D* modified from Eycleshymer, A. C., and Schoemaker, D. M.: A Cross-Section Anatomy. New York, D. Appleton & Co., 1930.)

been a recognized clinical problem if the fracture of the olecranon is adequately fixed. Thus, although this approach may have theoretical advantages in some instances, from a practical standpoint its use is probably rather limited.

Description of Technique. The skin incision is similar to that described for the Boyd approach. The ulna is exposed subperiosteally and the fracture is fixed, but the anconeus is not detached from the fracture. The interval between the anconeus and the extensor carpi ulnaris is then entered, and the radial head is reduced, excised, or repaired as indicated.

POSTERIOR EXPOSURES

A posterior exposure of the elbow joint may be used with a variety of surgical indications. The dissection may be readily extended and thus may be considered the universal approach to the joint, because distal humeral and proximal ulnar fractures, joint reconstruction, tumors, infections, and synovial processes are amenable to treatment with a posterior exposure. Several skin incisions and techniques have been described. Although MacAusland used a transverse incision, most posterior skin incisions are longitudinal. The S incision of Ollier is not as commonly used today as the straighter incision recommended by Langenbeck. Probably the most important aspect of any incision is that it should not cross the tip of the olecranon. Smith also attributed better healing to a medial incision as apposed to a lateral incision. The method of joint exposure is primarily either soft tissue release of the triceps or osteotomy of the triceps insertion on the olecranon.

TRICEPS PROCEDURES

Transverse section of the triceps mechanism at its musculotendinous junction has been described but does not afford adequate repair for optimal rehabilitation.[38] Releasing the triceps at its attachment to the olecranon[23] is not advisable owing to the difficulty of adequate repair and possible disruption during rehabilitation.[9] A midline splitting incision was described as early as 1918 by James Thompson from Galveston, Texas, to expose the distal humerus for fractures, but it did not include release from the ulna to provide exposure of the joint itself.[37] Splitting the triceps in line with the muscle fibers and at its

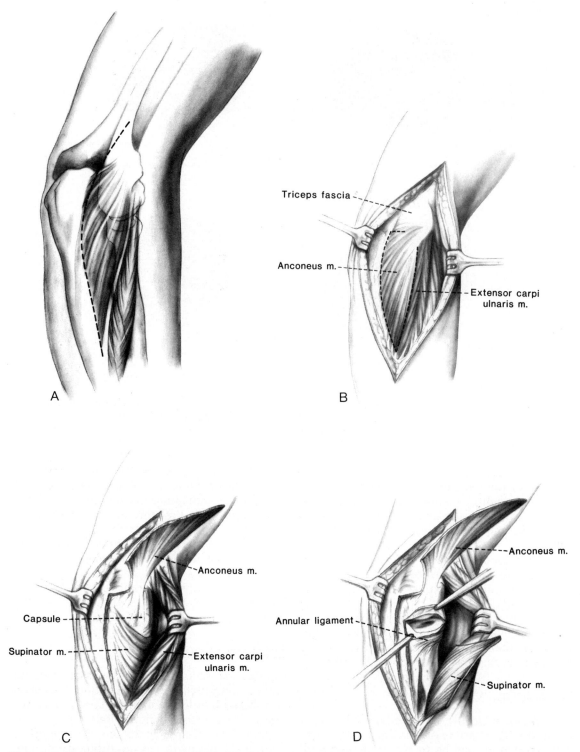

Figure 8–7. The Pankovich approach. *A,* The incision begins 2 cm proximal to the tip of the olecranon and extends over the lateral border of the triceps tendon, curving distally around the olecranon and ending 4 to 5 cm along the posterior ridge of the ulna. *B,* The interval between the anconeus and the extensor carpi ulnaris is identified along with the ulnar insertion of the muscle. The insertion of this muscle is then reflected subperiosteally and proximally to the posterior common fascial attachment with the triceps, which is divided, leaving the pedicle containing the motor branch to the muscle intact. *C,* The entire muscle is then retracted proximally exposing the supinator muscle. *D,* The supinator is released from its ulnar and humeral attachments and retracted, exposing the capsule, which may be entered transversely or horizontally. The approach may be extended distally according to the description of Boyd.

insertion to expose the humerus and the elbow joint was described by Langenback and Willis Campbell. If contracture was present Campbell first separated the tendon from the muscle as an inverted V and then released the muscle fibers longitudinally. This technique, recommended later by Van Gorder for distal humerus fractures, allows lengthening of the musculotendinous unit, which may be necessary to fully mobilize the ankylosed joint. Alonso-Llames has described a triceps-sparing approach from both the medial and lateral aspects, giving Ollier credit for an earlier description.

APPROACH. Posterior triceps splitting (Campbell, 1932).[10]

Indications. Elbow arthroplasty, unreduced elbow dislocation, distal humeral fracture, posterior exposure of the joint for ankylosis, sepsis, synovectomy.

Comment. Care must be exercised to maintain the medial portion of the triceps expansion over the forearm fascia in continuity with the flexor carpi ulnaris. Laterally, the anconeus and triceps form a more stable composite structure that has less chance of disruption.

Description of Technique. The skin incision begins in the midline over the triceps approximately 10 cm above the joint line, curves gently laterally or medially at the tip of the olecranon, and continues distally over the lateral aspect of the subcutaneous border of the proximal ulna for a distance of approximately 5 to 6 cm. If the incision is curved medially at the olecranon the scar may have less tendency to contract.[31]

The triceps is exposed along with the proximal 4 cm of the ulna. A midline incision is made through the triceps, fascia, and tendon and is continued distally across the insertion of the triceps tendon at the tip of the olecranon and down the subcutaneous crest of the ulna (Fig. 8–8). The triceps tendon and muscle are split longitudinally, exposing the distal humerus. The anconeus is then reflected subperiosteally laterally while the flexor carpi ulnaris is similarly retracted medially. The insertion of the triceps is carefully released from the olecranon, leaving the extensor mechanism in continuity with the forearm fascia and muscles medially and laterally. The ulnar nerve is visualized and protected in the cubital tunnel. Closure of the triceps fascia

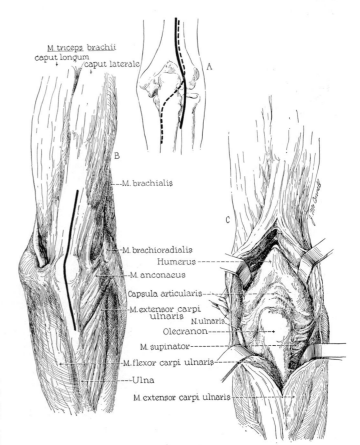

Figure 8–8. The Campbell posterior approach. The original description calls for a curved incision, but we prefer a straight one just lateral to the tip of the olecranon and the subcutaneous border of the ulna. (From Anson, B. J., and Maddock, W. G.: Callander's Surgical Anatomy, 4th ed. Philadelphia, W. B. Saunders Co., 1958.)

only is required proximally, but the insertion may be supplemented with a suture passed through the tip of the olecranon. The incision is then closed in layers.

APPROACH. Triceps reflection (Campbell, 1932; Van Gorder, 1940).[10, 39]

Indications. Same as for the midline splitting approach just described with elbow contracture and unreduced elbow dislocations.

Comment. This variation of the technique described above may be considered when more than 50 degrees of elbow flexion improvement is anticipated after the surgical procedure, because this technique allows lengthening of the triceps mechanism.

Description of Technique. The skin incision is begun 10 cm proximal to the medial epicondyle, lateral to the midline, and extends over the lateral aspect of the proximal ulna, ending 3 cm distal to the joint (Fig. 8–9). The triceps fascia and aponeurosis are exposed along with the tendinous insertion into the ulna. The tendon is reflected from the muscle in a proximal to distal direction, freeing the underlying muscle fibers while preserving the tendinous attachment to the olecranon. The triceps muscle is then split in the midline, and the distal humerus is exposed subperios-

teally. The periosteum and triceps are elevated for a distance of approximately 5 cm proximal to the olecranon fossa, exposing the posterior aspect of the elbow joint (Fig. 8–9). If greater exposure is desired, the subperiosteal dissection is extended to the level of the joint, exposing the condyles both medially and laterally. The ulnar nerve should be identified and protected to avoid excessive traction or damage to the nerve during the surgical procedure. The radial head can be visualized by excising the lateral capsule. If the radial collateral ligament is released, it should be carefully repaired. After the procedure, if an elbow contracture has been corrected, the joint should be maximally flexed. The tendon will slide distally from its initial position, and the proximal muscle and tendon are reapproximated at the lengthened relationship. The distal part of the triceps is then securely sutured to the fascia of the triceps expansion, and the remainder of the wound is closed in layers.

Reflection of the Triceps in Continuity

The triceps mechanism may be preserved in continuity and simply reflected to one side or the other. Two surgical approaches have been

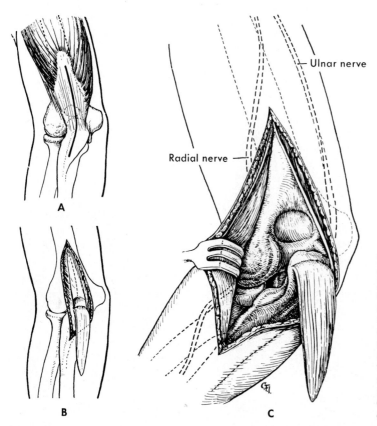

Figure 8–9. The Campbell (Van Gorder) approach. A, The straight incision is placed just lateral to the midline approximately 10 cm proximal and 3 cm distal to the joint. B, The triceps aponeurosis is identified and reflected distally. C, The remaining fibers of the triceps are then split in the midline and reflected from the humerus, and the anconeus is reflected subperiosteally from the ulna to expose the joint. (From Crenshaw, A. H.: Surgical Approaches. In Edmonson, A. S., and Crenshaw, A. H. (eds.): Campbell's Operative Anthopaedics, 6th ed. St. Louis, The C. V. Mosby Co., 1980.)

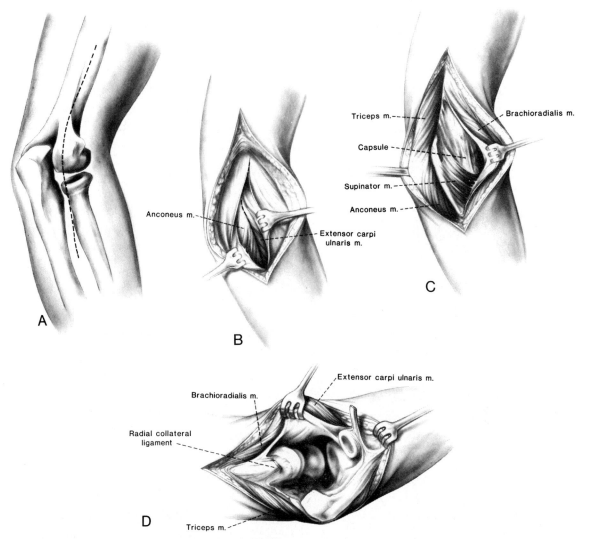

Figure 8–10. *A,* The incision 8 cm proximal to the joint just posterior to supracondylar bony ridge and extending distally over the anconeus for approximately 6 cm. *B,* The interval between the anconeus and the extensor carpi ulnaris is identified and entered. *C,* The anconeus is reflected subperiosteally from the proximal ulna along with its fascial attachment to the triceps, which is likewise reflected medially exposing the supinator muscle. The insertion of the triceps on the tip of the olecranon is released by sharp dissection, and the supinator muscle is released from the proximal portion of the ulna and the humerus as necessary to expose the capsule, which is entered with a longitudinal incision. *D,* The release of the radiocollateral ligament at its humeral origin allows the joint to sublux, exposing the entire distal humerus.

described that preserve the triceps muscle and tendon in continuity with the distal musculature and forearm fascia and expose the entire joint. These exposures allow rapid rehabilitation without concern for the possibility of triceps disruption. A third approach was described by Alonso-Llames[3], exposing the distal posterior humerus for intercondylar fractures.

APPROACH. Posterolateral, extensile triceps-sparing (Kocher, 1911).[21]
Indications. Joint arthroplasty, ankylosis, complex fractures of the distal humerus, synovectomy, radial head excision, and infection.

Description of Technique. The limited or distal exposure has been described above. For more extensile exposures the skin incision begins 8 cm proximal to the joint just posterior to the supracondylar bony ridge and continues distally over the anconeus approximately 6 cm distal to the tip of the olecranon (Fig. 8–10). Proximally, the triceps is identified and freed from the brachioradialis and extensor carpi radialis longus along the intramuscular septum to the level of the joint capsule. The interval between the extensor carpi radialis longus and anconeus is then identified proximally, and that between the extensor carpi ulnaris and anconeus is iden-

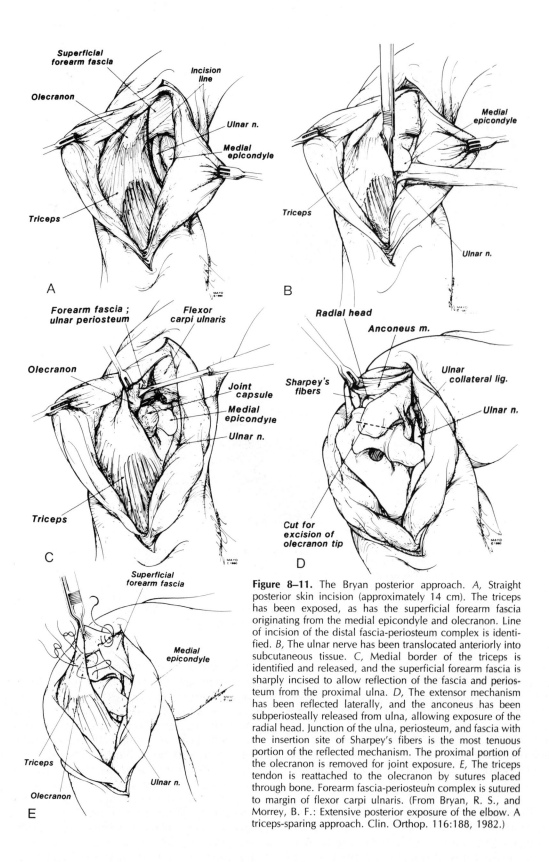

Figure 8–11. The Bryan posterior approach. *A,* Straight posterior skin incision (approximately 14 cm). The triceps has been exposed, as has the superficial forearm fascia originating from the medial epicondyle and olecranon. Line of incision of the distal fascia-periosteum complex is identified. *B,* The ulnar nerve has been translocated anteriorly into subcutaneous tissue. *C,* Medial border of the triceps is identified and released, and the superficial forearm fascia is sharply incised to allow reflection of the fascia and periosteum from the proximal ulna. *D,* The extensor mechanism has been reflected laterally, and the anconeus has been subperiosteally released from ulna, allowing exposure of the radial head. Junction of the ulna, periosteum, and fascia with the insertion site of Sharpey's fibers is the most tenuous portion of the reflected mechanism. The proximal portion of the olecranon is removed for joint exposure. *E,* The triceps tendon is reattached to the olecranon by sutures placed through bone. Forearm fascia-periosteum complex is sutured to margin of flexor carpi ulnaris. (From Bryan, R. S., and Morrey, B. F.: Extensive posterior exposure of the elbow. A triceps-sparing approach. Clin. Orthop. 116:188, 1982.)

tified distally, and these are developed to expose the capsule of the radiohumeral joint (Figs. 8–4 and 8–10B). The anconeus is reflected subperiosteally from the proximal ulna. Sharp dissection frees the bony attachment of the triceps expansion to the anconeus at the lateral epicondyle. The insertion of the triceps tendon to the tip of the olecranon is then sharply released, and the entire musculofascial composite is reflected medially. The joint may be dislocated with varus stress, providing generous exposure after the subperiosteal release of the radiocollateral ligament from the humerus (Fig. 8–10D). Routine closure in layers is performed, but the radiocollateral ligament should be reattached to the bone through holes placed in the lateral epicondyle.

APPROACH. Posteromedial, extensile triceps-sparing exposure (Bryan and Morrey, 1982).[9]

Indications. Joint arthroplasty, elbow dislocation, supracondylar T and Y fractures, synovial disease, infection, ulnar nerve or medial collateral ligament pathology.

Comment. This exposure is selected when exposure of the ulnar collateral ligament or ulnar nerve is desired as well as extensive joint exposure.

Description of Technique. The patient is placed in the lateral decubitus or supine position with a sandbag under the scapula. A sterile pneumatic tourniquet is applied high on the arm, which is brought across the chest (Fig. 8–11). A straight posterior incision is made medial to the midline, approximately 9 cm proximal and 8 cm distal to the tip of the olecranon. The ulnar nerve is identified proximally in the epineural fat at the margin of the medial head of the triceps and, depending on the procedure, is either protected or carefully dissected free of the cubital tunnel to its first motor branch. For joint arthroplasty, the nerve is routinely transferred anteriorly into the subcutaneous tissue.

The medial aspect of the triceps is elevated from the humerus along the intramuscular septum to the level of the posterior capsule. The superficial fascia of the forearm is then incised distally, for about 6 cm, to the periosteum of the medial aspect of the proximal ulna. The periosteum and fascia complex is carefully reflected laterally. The medial part of the complex is the weakest portion of the reflected tissue, so care must be exerted to maintain continuity of the triceps mechanism at this point. After the triceps has been released from the olecranon, the remaining por-

tion of the triceps mechanism is reflected. If exposure of the radial head is desired, the anconeus is removed subperiosteally from the proximal ulna, thus widely exposing the entire joint.

The tip of the olecranon may be removed for clear visualization of the trochlea. If the ligaments have been released from the humerus to obtain a more extensive view of the joint surface, these must be carefully repaired at the completion of the procedure. The triceps is returned to its anatomic position and sutured directly to the bone of the proximal end of the ulna. The periosteum is then sutured to the superficial forearm fascia as far as the margin of the flexor carpi ulnaris. The tourniquet is deflated, hemostasis is secured, and the wound is drained and closed in layers.

Posterior Transosseous Exposures

Posterior access to the elbow may be accomplished by detaching the triceps by an oblique osteotomy of the proximal ulna,[26] by an osteotomy through the midportion of the greater sigmoid notch,[24] or by a V-shaped osteotomy of the proximal ulna.[2] Because this last osteotomy involves cortical bone, requires unnecessary distal exposure, and provides no better access to the joint itself, it has little to recommend it at this time, and only the first two techniques will be described.

APPROACH Oblique osteotomy of the olecranon (Muller, 1970).[26]

Indications. T or Y condylar fracture.

Description of Technique. A 14-cm incision is made just lateral to the midline, extending past the tip of the olecranon. The insertion of the triceps tendon to the proximal ulna is carefully identified, and a 3.2-mm hole is drilled through the tip of the olecranon, centered down the medullary canal and on the insertion of the triceps tendon (Fig. 8–12). The triceps attachment is then carefully isolated and osteotomized in an oblique fashion with an oscillating saw. The muscle with its attachment to the osteotomized segment is reflected proximally. At the completion of the procedure the osteotomized fragment is reattached with a lag screw, and the wound is closed in layers.

APPROACH. Transolecranon osteotomy (MacAusland, 1915).[24]

Indication. Ankylosed joints; T or Y condylar fracture.

Comment. The intra-articular osteotomy first described by MacAusland was originally

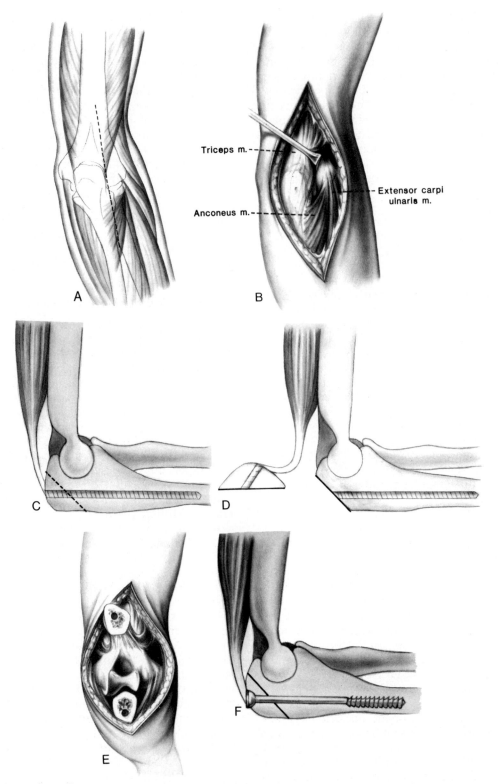

Figure 8–12. The Muller posterior approach. *A,* A straight longitudinal incision is made over the lateral aspect of the elbow extending approximately 6 cm proximal and 8 cm distal from the tip of the olecranon. *B,* The lateral margin of the triceps is identified and reflected medially in order to expose the distal humerus. *C,* The proximal ulna is predrilled for reattachment later. *D,* An oblique extra-articular osteotomy including the attachment of the triceps is made across the proximal ulna. *E,* The triceps with its attachment to bone is then reflected proximally, and as the elbow is flexed, the entire distal humerus and elbow joint may be exposed. *F,* After the procedure the triceps is reattached with a malleolar or cancellous-type screw, which provides good compression across the osteotomy site. (From Muller, M. E., et al.: Manual of Internal Fixation: Technique Recommended by the AO-Group. New York, Springer-Verlag, 1970.)

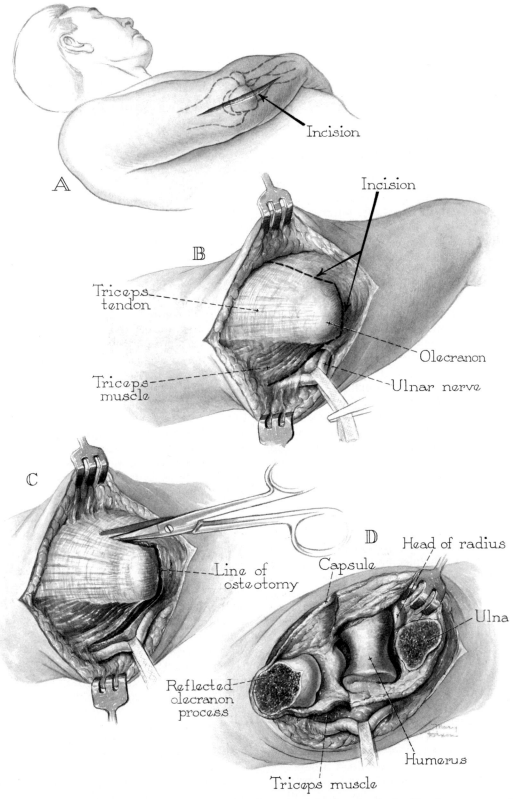

Figure 8–13. MacAusland posterior approach. *A,* A straight incision is made just lateral to the tip of the olecranon approximately 7 cm proximal and 7 cm distal to the tip of the olecranon. *B,* The proximal ulna is predrilled with a 3.2-mm drill, and the margins of the triceps are identified. *C,* The triceps is released medially and laterally, protecting the ulnar nerve, and the ulna is osteotomized in the midportion of the sigmoid fossa with the proximal portion containing the triceps tendon retracted proximally *(D),* exposing the elbow joint. (From Banks, S. W., and Laufman, H.: An Atlas of Surgical Exposures of the Extremities. Philadelphia, W. B. Saunders Co., 1953.)

recommended for ankylosed joints. It has been adopted by some[18] for radial head excision and synovectomy and used or modified by others[12] for T and Y condylar fractures. However, in rheumatoid arthritics this portion of the bone may be quite thin, and therefore, this is not a suitable exposure for total elbow arthroplasty. Rehabilitation must be adjusted according to the progress of healing of the osteotomy.

Description of Technique. Originally, a transverse incision across the elbow was described. Currently, a straight incision is recommended; it is made posteriorly just lateral to the midline and measures approximately 14 cm centered on the olecranon (Fig. 8–13). The ulnar nerve is isolated and dissected from the cubital tunnel and protected. A 3.2-mm drill hole crosses the proposed osteotomy site for anatomic replacement at the completion of the procedure. The joint is exposed at the midportion of the greater sigmoid notch and is then osteotomized with an oscillating saw; care is taken to avoid damage to the trochlea. Because in most individuals the midportion of the olecranon is free of articular cartilage, osteotomy can be made through this area with impunity (see Chapter 2). The capsular attachments, including the posterior portion of the ulnar collateral ligament, are released. The triceps tendon, along with the osteotomized portion of the olecranon, may then be retracted proximally, and by flexing the elbow the joint can be exposed. Occasionally, the radial or medial collateral ligament may be released for better exposure, but if this is done it must be reattached to the bone to avoid instability. At the completion of the procedure, the tip of the olecranon is secured with a single cancellous screw. The elbow is usually immobilized for 2 to 3 weeks, after which time a gentle, active rehabilitation program may be instituted if clinically indicated.

MEDIAL APPROACHES

There are relatively few indications for exposure of the elbow joint from a medial approach. A transverse exposure through the posterior aspect of the capsule of the ulnotrochlear articulation allows limited access to the joint for removal of loose bodies. The transcondylar approach described independently by Molesworth and Campbell does provide excellent exposure of the joint, but it involves dissection of the ulnar nerve as well as healing of the osteotomized epicondyle, both of which increase the complexity and thus limit the utility of this approach. It is of

value, however, to be familiar with the technique if one is confronted with medial joint pathology with associated ulnar nerve symptoms. In 1969, Taylor and Scham described a medial approach to the proximal ulna that was useful for fractures in this region.

APPROACH. Limited approach to the medial capsule (Banks, 1953).[5]

Indications. Removal of loose bodies.

Comment. This incision traverses only the weak posterior portion of the ulnar collateral ligament, which is not essential for elbow stability. The anterior bundle, the major stabilizing element of the ulnar collateral ligament complex, is not violated.

Description of Technique. A longitudinal 6-cm incision is centered over the posterior aspect of the elbow joint approximately midway between the medial epicondyle and the olecranon process of the ulna (Fig. 8–14). The deep fascia is incised, and the flap is undermined medially as far as the medial epicondyle and as far as the margin of the olecranon. The ulnar nerve is identified and retracted anteriorly but is not necessarily translocated. If necessary, the overlying fascia is excised so that the nerve can be further visualized during the remainder of the procedure (Fig. 8–14B). The dissection is continued proximally to separate the fibers of the adjacent portion of the triceps muscle and tendon. The proximal fibers of the flexor carpi ulnaris muscle in the distal wound are retracted away from the ulna. The joint cavity is exposed by opening the posterior capsule. Closure is routine but should include a secure closure of the posterior capsule to restore the posterior ulnar collateral ligament (Fig. 8–14C).

APPROACH. Transepicondylar approach (Molesworth, 1930; Campbell, 1932).[10, 25]

Indications. Medial epicondylar fractures, loose bodies, medial pathology with symptoms requiring ulnar nerve exploration.

Comment. This procedure was described independently by Molesworth in England and Willis Campbell in Memphis. Because this procedure requires osteotomy of the medial epicondyle, which involves more concern about reattachment and healing compared with other exposures, the indications for its use today are limited.

Description of Technique. With the elbow flexed at 90 degrees, a medial incision is made from 5 cm above to approximately 5 cm below the elbow over the medial epicondyle (Fig. 8–15). The ulnar nerve is identified, released, and retracted from the medial epicondyle,

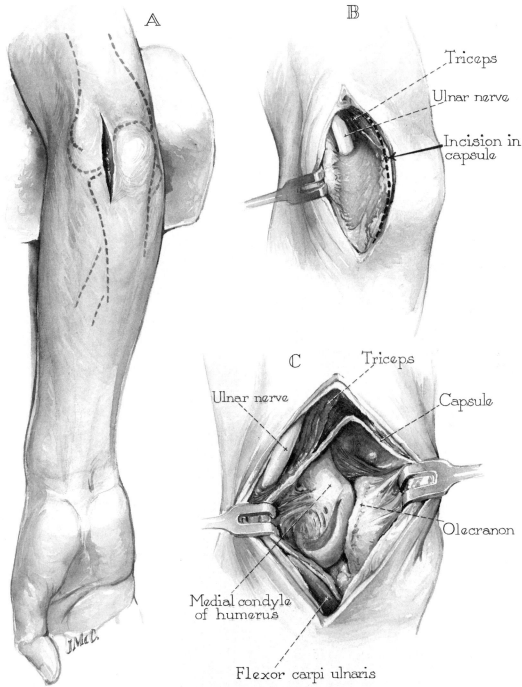

Figure 8–14. Medial approach. *A,* A 6-cm incision is made just medial to the olecranon. The ulnar nerve is then identified and the capsule is released from the medial aspect of the sigmoid fossa *(B). C,* The ulnar nerve along with the capsule is retracted anteriorly, providing limited exposure to the posterior ulnohumeral joint. (From Banks, S. W., and Laufman, H.: An Atlas of Surgical Exposures of the Extremities. Philadelphia, W. B. Saunders Co., 1953.)

which is freed from soft tissue. It is helpful to make a longitudinal incision in the capsule just anterior to the ulnar collateral ligament and to place a periosteal elevator under the ligament as a landmark prior to performing the osteotomy. In this way, healing of the osteotomy restores the integrity of the ulnar collateral ligament. With a small osteotome the epicondyle is freed and turned downward with its muscular attachments. Blunt dissection allows distal retraction of the flexor muscles, and careful technique avoids injury to the innervation of the muscle mass. The medial aspect of the coronoid process is exposed

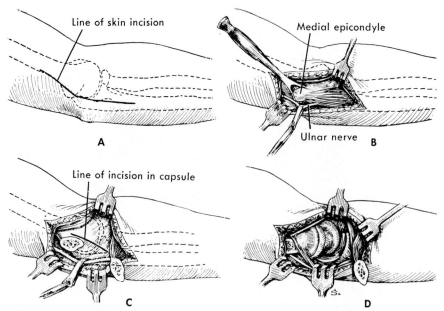

Figure 8–15. Molesworth medial approach. *A,* A 10-cm incision is centered on the medial epicondyle. *B,* The medial epicondyle is then identified, and the ulnar nerve is released and protected. *C,* The epicondyle is osteotomized, and the capsule is excised anterior to the epicondyle. *D,* By reflecting the medial epicondyle and its muscle attachments distally, the joint may be exposed with a valgus stress imparted to the forearm. (From Crenshaw, A. H.: Surgical approaches. *In* Edmonson, A. S., and Crenshaw, A. H. (eds.): Campbell's Operative Orthopaedics, 6th ed. St. Louis, The C. V. Mosby Co., 1980.)

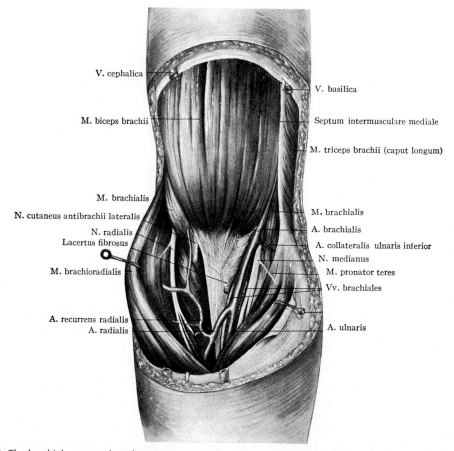

Figure 8–16. The brachial artery and median nerve occupy the anterior medial aspect of the elbow joint, thus excluding the possibility of an anterior medial approach to the joint. (From Anson, B. J., and Maddock, W. G.: Callander's Surgical Anatomy, 4th ed. Philadelphia, W. B. Saunders Co., 1958.)

as well as the anterior and posterior capsules which may be reflected from the humerus as required for additional exposure. Valgus stress hinges the joint on the lateral ligament and the remaining portions of the capsule and provides generous exposure of virtually the entire elbow joint. Care must be taken to protect the median nerve as it passes over the anterior aspect of the joint. The epicondyle is returned to its anatomic position and secured with a small screw or with sutures placed through the bone. This step is important because the quality of the repair will influence the integrity of the ulnar collateral ligament, which is so essential to the stability of the elbow joint.

ANTERIOR EXPOSURE OF THE ELBOW REGION

Because of the vulnerability of the brachial artery and median nerve, the anterior medial approach to the elbow is not recommended (Fig. 8–16). The extensile exposure described by Henry as modified from Fiolle and Delmas is the best known and the most useful anterior exposure of the joint. Minor modifications of the Henry approach have been described,[20, 32] and a limited anterolateral exposure has been described by Darrach.[14]

APPROACH. Extensile anterior exposure of the elbow region (Henry, 1957).[17]

Indications. Anteriorly displaced fracture fragments, excision of tumors in this region, reattachment of the biceps tendon to the radial tuberosity, exploration of entrapment syndromes, and anterior capsule release for contracture.

Description of Technique (Modified Henry). The skin incision begins about 5 cm proximal and lateral to the flexor crease of the elbow joint and extends distally along the anterior margin of the brachioradialis muscle (Fig. 8–17). Below the elbow joint, the incision turns medially to avoid crossing the flexor crease at a right angle, thus discouraging hypertrophic scar formation. The incision continues transversely to the biceps tendon and then turns distally over the medial volar aspect of the forearm, ending approximately 6 or 7 cm distal to the flexion crease. The interval between the brachioradialis laterally and the biceps and brachialis medially is identified and entered. The fascia is released distally between the brachioradialis and the pronator teres.

The interval is then entered proximally, and a gentle, blunt dissection demonstrates the radial nerve coursing on the inner surface of the brachioradialis muscle. Care is taken to avoid injury to the superficial sensory branch of the radial nerve. Because the radial nerve gives off its branches laterally it can be safely retracted with the brachioradialis muscle. At the level of the elbow joint, as the brachioradialis is retracted laterally and the pronator gently retracted medially, the radial artery can be observed where it emerges from the medial aspect of the biceps tendon giving off its muscular and recurrent branches in a medial-to-lateral direction. The muscular branch is ligated, but the recurrent radial artery should be sacrificed only if the pathology warrants the more extensive exposure that can be realized with this maneuver.

The dorsal interosseous nerve enters the supinator and continues along the dorsum of the forearm distally. The dissection continues distally, exposing the supinator muscle, which covers the proximal aspect of the radius and the anterolateral aspect of the capsule. Muscular attachments to the anterior aspect of the radius and those distal to the supinator include the discrete tendinous insertion of the pronator teres as well as the origins of the flexor digitorum sublimis and the flexor pollicis longus. The brachialis muscle is identified, elevated, and retracted medially to expose the proximal capsule.

If more distal exposure is needed, the forearm is fully supinated, demonstrating the insertion of the supinator muscle on the proximal radius. This is incised, and the supinator is retracted laterally in a subperiosteal manner. The supinator serves as protection to the deep interosseous branch of the radial nerve, but excessive retraction of the muscle should be avoided. The proximal aspect of the radius as well as the capitellum is thereby exposed. Additional visualization may be obtained both proximally and distally because the radial nerve has been identified and can be avoided proximally. The posterior interosseous nerve is protected distally by the supinator muscle, and the radial artery is visualized and protected medially if a more extensile exposure is required.

NOTE: The recurrent and muscular branches of the radial artery and vein should be ligated prior to their release to avoid hematoma formation, which could cause ischemic contracture of the forearm (see Chapter 17). Retraction of the brachioradialis and the extensor carpi radialis longus and brevis muscles is facilitated if the elbow is flexed at 90 degrees. This allows an easier exposure of

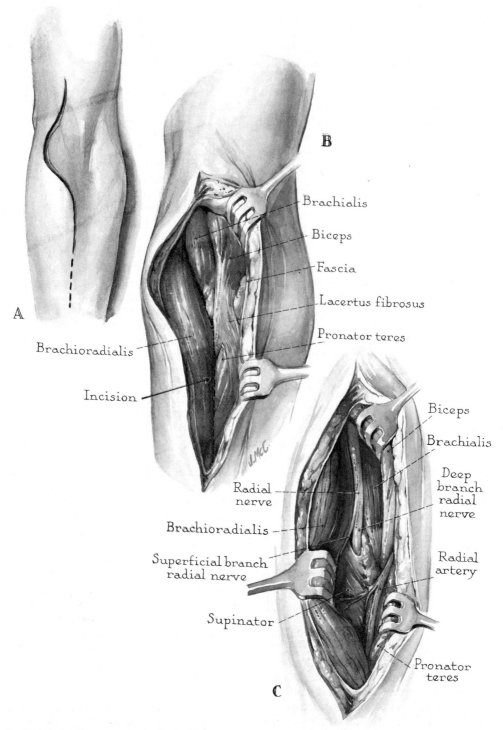

Figure 8–17. Anterior Henry approach. *A,* An incision is made approximately 5 cm proximal to the elbow crease on the lateral margin of the biceps tendon. It extends transversely across the joint line and curves distally over the medial aspect of the forearm. *B,* The interval between the brachioradialis and brachialis proximally and the biceps tendon and pronator teres in the distal portion of the wound is identified. The radial nerve is protected and retracted along with the brachialis muscle. *C,* The radial recurrent branches of the radial artery as well as its muscular branches are identified and sacrificed if more extensive exposure is required. The biceps tendon along with the brachialis muscle is retracted medially.

Illustration continued on opposite page

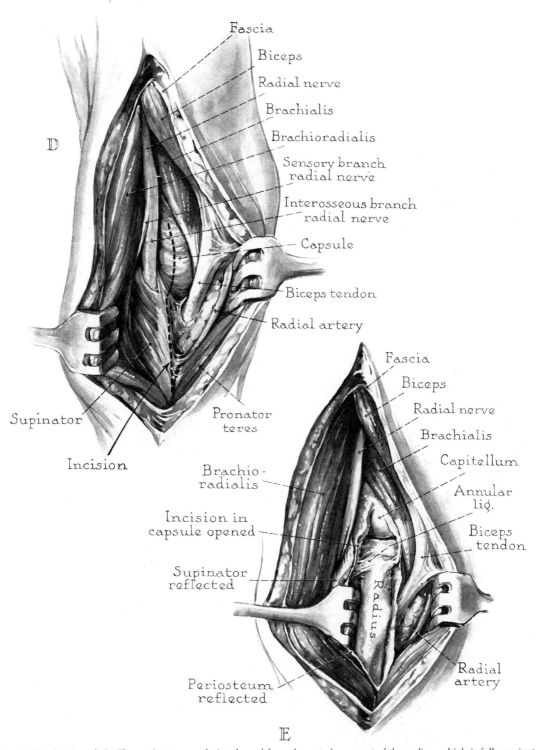

Figure 8–17. *Continued. D,* The supinator muscle is released from the anterior aspect of the radius, which is fully supinated. *E,* This interval may now be developed to expose the entire anterior aspect of the elbow joint including the capitellum, the proximal radius, and the radial tuberosity. (From Banks, S. W., and Laufman, H.: An Atlas of Surgical Exposures of the Extremities. Philadelphia, W. B. Saunders Co., 1953.)

the supinator muscle. When the supinator muscle is stripped subperiosteally from the radius, the bursa between the biceps tendon and the radius is usually identified and should be entered, facilitating the subperiosteal exposure of the muscle. The proximal radius is further exposed by subperiosteal dissection as the forearm is being pronated and supinated.

References

1. Abbott, L. C., Larsen, L. J., Jones, E. W., Lucas, D. B., Saunders, J. B., and Dec, M.: Surgical Approaches to the Joints. In Cole, W. H.: Operative Technique in Specialty Surgery. Vol. 2. New York, Appleton-Century-Crofts, 1949, p. 539.
2. Albee, F. H.: Arthroplasty of the Elbow. J. Bone Joint Surg. 15:979, 1933.
3. Alonso-Llames, M.: Bilaterotricipital Approach to the Elbow. Acta Orthop. Scand. 42:479, 1972.
4. Anson, B. J., and Maddock, W. G.: Callander's Surgical Anatomy, 4th ed. Philadelphia, W. B. Saunders Co., 1958.
5. Banks, S. W., and Laufman, H.: An Atlas of Surgical Exposures of the Extremities. Philadelphia, W. B. Saunders Co., 1953.
6. Boyd, H. B.: Surgical Exposure of the Ulna and Proximal Third of the Radius Through One Incision. Surg. Gynecol. Obstet. 71:86, 1940.
7. Boyd, H. B.: Surgical Approaches to the Elbow Joint. In American Academy of Orthopaedic Surgeons: Instructional Course Lectures, Vol. 4. Ann Arbor, J. W. Edwards, 1947, p. 147.
8. Bost, F. C., Schottstaedt, E. R., Larsen, L., and Abbott, L.: Surgical Approaches to the Elbow Joint. In American Academy of Orthopaedic Surgeons: Instructional Course Lectures, Vol. 10. Ann Arbor, J. W. Edwards, 1953, p. 180.
9. Bryan, R. S., and Morrey, B. F.: Extensive Posterior Exposure of the Elbow: A Triceps-Sparing Approach. Clin. Orthop. 166:188, 1982.
10. Campbell, W. C.: Incision for Exposure of the Elbow Joint. Am. J. Surg. 15:65, 1932.
11. Campbell, W. C., Edmonson, A. S., and Crehnshaw, A. H. (eds.): Campbell's Operative Orthopedics. In Surgical Approaches, 6th ed., Vol. I. St. Louis, The C. V. Mosby Co., 1971, p. 119.
12. Casselbaum, W. H.: Operative Treatment of T and Y Fractures of the Lower End of the Humerus. Am. J. Surg. 83:265, 1952.
13. Consentino, R.: Atlas of Anatomy and Surgical Approaches in Orthopaedic Surgery. Springfield, Il., Charles C Thomas, 1960.
14. Darrach, W.: Surgical Approaches for Surgery of the Extremities. Am. J. Surg. 67:93, 1945.
15. Eycleshymer, A. C., and Schoemaker, D. M.: A Cross-Section Anatomy. New York, D. Appleton and Co., 1930.
16. Gordon, M. L.: Monteggia Fracture. A Combined Surgical Approach Employing a Single Lateral Incision. Clin. Orthop. 50:87, 1967.
17. Henry, A. K.: Extensile Exposure, 2nd ed. Baltimore, The Williams & Wilkins Co., 1957.
18. Inglis, A. E., Ranawat, C. S., and Straub, L. R.: Synovectomy and Debridement of the Elbow in Rheumatoid Arthritis. J. Bone Joint Surg. 53A:652, 1971.
19. Kaplan, E. B.: Surgical Approaches to the Proximal End of the Radius and Its Use in Fractures of the Head and Neck of the Radius. J. Bone Joint Surg. 23:86, 1941.
20. Kelly, R. P., and Griffin, T. W.: Open Reduction of T-Condylar Fractures of the Humerus Through an Anterior Approach. J. Trauma 9:901, 1969.
21. Kocher, T.: Text-Book of Operative Surgery, 3rd ed. H. J. Stiles and C. B. Paul, Transls. London, A. and C. Black, 1911.
22. Langenbeck (1864): Cited by Alonso-Llames, M.: Bilaterotricipital Approach to the Elbow. Acta Orthop. Scand. 43:479, 1972.
23. Lexer (1919): Cited by Alonso-Llames, M.: Bilaterotricipital Approach to the Elbow. Acta Orthop. Scand. 43:479, 1972.
24. MacAusland, W. R.: Ankylosis of the Elbow: With Report of Four Cases Treated by Arthroplasty. J.A.M.A. 64:312, 1915.
25. Molesworth, W. H. L.: Operation for Complete Exposure of the Elbow Joint. Br. J. Surg.. 18:303, 1930.
26. Muller, M. E., Allgower, M., and Willenegger, H.: Manual of Internal Fixation: Technique Recommended by the AO-Group. New York, Springer-Verlag, 1970.
27. Nicola, T.: Atlas of Surgical Approaches to Bones and Joints. New York, The Macmillian Co., 1945.
28. Ogilvie, W. H.: Discussion of Minor Injuries of the Elbow Joint. Proc. Roy. Soc. Med. 23:306, 1929.
29. Ollier (1888): Cited by Alonso-Llames, M.: Bilaterotricipital Approach to the Elbow. Acta Orthop. Scand. 43:479, 1972.
30. Pankovich, A. M.: Anconeus Approach to the Elbow Joint and the Proximal Part of the Radius and Ulna. J. Bone Joint Surg. 59A:124, 1977.
31. Smith, F. M.: Surgery of the Elbow, 2nd ed. Philadelphia, W. B. Saunders Co., 1972.
32. Sorrell, E., and Longuet, Y. J.: La Voie Transbrachiale Antérieure Dans La Chirurgie des Fractures Supracondyliennes de l'Humérus Chez l'Enfant. Rev. Orthop. 32:117, 1946.
33. Speed, J. S.: An Operation for Unreduced Posterior Dislocation of the Elbow. South Med J. 18:193, 1925.
34. Speed, J. S., and Boyd, H. B.: Treatment of Fractures of Ulna With Dislocation of Head of Radius (Monteggia Fracture). J.A.M.A. 115:1699, 1940.
35. Strachan, J. H., and Ellis, B. W.: Vulnerability of the Posterior Interosseous Nerve During Radial Head Reaction. J. Bone Joint Surg. 53B:320, 1971.
36. Taylor, T. K. F., and Scham, S. M.: A Posteromedial Approach to the Proximal End of the Ulna for the Internal Fixation of Olecranon Fractures. J. Trauma 9:594, 1969.
37. Thompson, J. E.: Anatomical Methods of Approach in Operations on the Long Bones of the Extremities. Ann. Surg. 68:309, 1918.
38. Van Gorder, G. W.: Surgical Approach in Old Posterior Dislocation of the Elbow. J. Bone Surg. 14:127, 1932.
39. Van Gorder, G. W.: Surgical Approach in Supracondylar "T" Fractures of the Humerus Requiring Open Reduction. J. Bone Joint Surg. 22:278, 1940.

CHAPTER 9

Rehabilitation

R. P. NIRSCHL and B. F. MORREY

The elbow has received relatively little attention in regard to rehabilitation. The concepts discussed in this chapter are mainly the result of our experience over the last decade. Although the specific applications may vary, the principles have been expanded to encompass the broad scope of elbow pathology. It is our intention to present an organized and systematic basis for the rehabilitative process. The details of rehabilitation for the athlete are discussed in detail in Chapter 31.

ANATOMIC CONSIDERATIONS

The anatomy of the elbow regions has been discussed in Chapter 2. Some aspects that influence the rehabilitation plan or philosophy should be emphasized. The unique three bone, four joint articulation has a high degree of congruence and accounts for much of the difficulty experienced in obtaining normal function after injury or surgery.

Articulations

Ulnohumeral Joint. The high degree of congruence of the ulnohumeral joint originates in part from the presence of the posterior articular facets of the olecranon. The need to accommodate the olecranon in extension makes the elbow vulnerable to a mechanical block in the olecranon fossa. This effect on the capacity of the elbow to attain full extension is an important consideration in rehabilitation.

Radiohumeral Joint. This articulation is involved in flexion-extension movement as well as in forearm rotation. Any mechanical distortion of the lateral compartment will directly affect flexion and may occasionally be a severely compromising factor in the rehabilitative process.

Proximal and Distal Radioulnar Joints. The elbow is unique in that it provides pronation and supination motions. The two articulations that allow this function are intimately related, and the distal joint can affect the return of normal elbow function.

Ligaments

The anterior capsule of the elbow joint is usually a relatively thin, pliable structure. The capsule is, however, very sensitive to injury, and major alterations in its anatomy are a common clinical factor compromising normal elbow flexion and extension (Fig. 9–1). The medial ligamentous structures originate primarily from the medial epicondyle to insert at the proximal ulna and are the prime stabilizer of the elbow. The medial ligament is subject to rupture, contracture, and occasionally calcification, the effects of which can severely compromise normal motion. Post-traumatic thickening of the lateral ligamentous structures can cause impingement and snapping with flexion or rotation. The annular ligament may also give rise to pain or restrictive motion when the radial head is deformed or misshapen.

Musculotendinous Factors

With the exception of the pronator teres, the muscles of common flexor origin comprising the flexor carpi radialis and ulnaris and the palmaris longus traverse both the elbow and

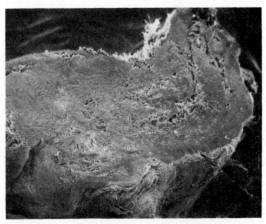

Figure 9–1. The normal anterior capsule of the elbow is thin and translucent. When injured, this structure becomes thickened to 3 to 4 mm, which accounts for the typical flexion contracture seen after elbow injury. This scanning electron micrograph is magnified ×30.

the wrist joints. Major alterations of these muscle-tendon units can severely compromise elbow function, which may be aggravated by wrist dysfunction or pathology.

Muscles originating from the lateral epicondyle area, the common origin of the extensor tendons, the extensor carpi radialis brevis and longus, and the brachioradialis may all affect normal elbow excursion and strength. These muscle-tendon units, except the brachioradialis, again cross both the elbow and the wrist joints. In addition, the extensor brevis originates just anterior and distal to the lateral epicondyle. During elbow flexion and extension this muscle origin glides over the outer lateral capsule and over the bony aspects of the lateral condyle. Alterations in the shape of the lateral condyle or scar tissue at the undersurface of the extensor brevis can alter normal elbow extension.

The anterior anatomy of the elbow is unique because the brachialis muscle inserts into the capsule and crosses the anterior aspect as a muscle, not as tendinous tissue. Hemorrhage into the brachialis at this level, therefore, has a high potential for significant scar formation and joint contracture or even ectopic bone formation (e.g., myositis ossificans).

Neurovascular Considerations

In a chronic flexion contracture, rehabilitative attempts to attain full extension may cause mechanical compression of either the brachial artery, the median nerve, or both. Because the ulnar nerve has little tolerance as it passes through the cubital tunnel, it is vulnerable to compression or inflammation during rehabilitative efforts.

SPECIFIC REHABILITATIVE CONSIDERATIONS

As with other joints, rehabilitation of the elbow will vary according to the specific pathology involved: overuse, single event trauma, surgical trauma, systemic inflammatory process, and the like. The stages of rehabilitation include control of the inflammatory response, allowance of healing, and restoration of function (Table 9–1). It does

Table 9–1. **Stages of Rehabilitation**

Control inflammation
Allow and encourage healing
Restore function
Strength
Flexibility (motion)
Endurance

Table 9–2. **Mnemonic Used to Remember the Elements Used to Control Inflammation**

P—Protection
R—Rest
I—Ice
C—Compression
E—Elevation

little good to know the appropriate concepts but to apply them with poor timing or improper implementation. A more detailed discussion of these elements is appropriate.

Relief of Inflammation

It should be kept in mind that rehabilitation essentially starts at the time of injury. If the inflammatory phase of healing can be minimized, more complete and rapid rehabilitation will be attained. The time-tested scheme represented by the mnemonic PRICE (Table 9–2) is highly appropriate in the early stages of healing of any tissue, whether bone, articular, ligamentous, or muscular.

Protection. Protection does not necessarily imply immobilization or lack of use of the injured parts. The technique of protection with various types of immobilization devices is discussed below.

Rest. Rest implies restriction of the functional use or abusive aggravation of the injured area, not total inactivity. Although not always possible, every effort should be made to encourage activity of the uninjured adjacent joints.

Ice. Ice is a time-honored modality used to minimize edema and hemorrhage and to control inflammatory exudation.[7] It is used on a regular basis in the early phase of inflammation and intermittently after exercise in the later stages of rehabilitation.

Compression. Compression is useful in the early stages of injury or after surgery. Both static and intermittent air-compression devices may be used.

Elevation. The elbow is relatively easy to elevate, at least to a moderate extent, above the level of the heart. Prolonged periods of elevation may be difficult if the shoulder is also involved with disease as in rheumatoid arthritis.

Drugs. The inflammatory process can also be controlled by pharmacologic methods. Aspirin is ill-advised, however, in very acute stages of trauma if there is a potential for further local hemorrhage. In some instances, high voltage galvanic stimulation has also proved helpful in controlling the inflammatory process by initiating involuntary muscle contractions that relieve edema and provide muscle re-education. If immobilization is necessary, a device may be designed that allows the application of this additional modality. We rarely use plaster immobilization for elbow soft tissue problems.

Allowance and Promotion of Healing

The healing process involves an inflammatory phase, but relief of pain by medication, such as cortisone injections or oral administration, must not be misinterpreted as assisting the healing process. If a patient is allowed to return to full activity without an appropriate period of rehabilitation, the underlying problem will merely recur or become worse once the effects of the anti-inflammatory agent have ceased. It is therefore extremely important to distinguish the aspects of a rehabilitative program that provide pain relief from those that assist the true healing process.

The following rehabilitative elements are, in our opinion, capable of and used for promotion of healing:

1. Early exercise of non-injured areas.
2. Early protected exercises for injured areas.
3. High voltage galvanic stimulation.
4. Continuous passive motion.

Early Exercise of Noninjured Areas. Basic research at the cellular level is incomplete, but there is little question about the positive beneficial effects of this modality.[1, 2, 11] Observed clinical events include apparent enhancement of local circulation, maintenance of strength and tissue compliance, and reduction of edema or fluid extravasation.[3, 9] The exercise programs, of course, must be designed in such a manner that the injured part is not violated.

Early Protective Exercise for Injured Areas. Observations of bone and cartilage healing have demonstrated the effectiveness of protective exercise for promoting this process.[11] The same principles apply to soft tissue injury. To prevent further injury, the program must have an appropriate timing sequence and must be supervised closely to achieve the rehabilitative objectives. Semirigid immobilization is appropriate at this stage. Motion is allowed to occur in a safe, prescribed arc that can be attained actively or passively without excessive pain or stress to the healing tissue. Extremes of position that may injure bone ligament or muscle should be avoided. Protection, therefore, during the healing and rehabilitative phases can and should be modi-

fied according to the specific need of the individual. If the injury has caused instability due to fracture or ligament damage, rigid immobilization is appropriate. In most instances, however, because the joint is so congruent, early motion is often allowed with a ligament injury if proper protective splinting is provided.

Electrical Stimulation. Electrical (galvanic) stimulation is known to play a role in the enhancement of bone healing and may possibly have a role in soft tissue healing as well. The benefits of high voltage galvanic stimulation may be summarized as follows:

1. The short time sequence of skin penetration eliminates the heat build-up, pain, and potential burning that have been noted with low voltage stimulation.

2. The process has the capacity to enhance involuntary muscle contracture.

3. It enhances local blood flow.

4. It has an analgesic effect.

5. It dissipates edema and hemorrhage, possibly partly owing to stimulating muscle contracture.

Continuous Passive Motion. Continuous passive motion is prescribed in the safe arc that will not injure tissue (Fig. 9–2). Decreased wound edema, lessened joint effusion, and increased range of motion have been observed in both postsurgical[3] and post-traumatic[6] joints. Our experience with the results of continuous passive motion at the elbow is similar to these reports. However, this modality should be strictly avoided in patients with poor tissue or circulatory impairment; rest rather than motion is prescribed for such patients.

Restore Function

Once the inflammatory process is under control and an appropriate stage of healing has been attained, restoration of function to the injured area can be undertaken. There are significant differences in the goals and potential recovery of function in post-traumatic, rheumatoid, and athletic patients. For example, a difference of severalfold in the demand and hence in the oxygen consumption of skeletal muscle has been documented in sedentary and in highly trained individuals.[12] In many athletic patients with soft tissue injury, an overuse syndrome is present. Thus, full flexibility arcs of motion are generally best introduced after there has been some reasonable progress in the program to increase strength, and endurance should be sought near the end of the process. This strategy may

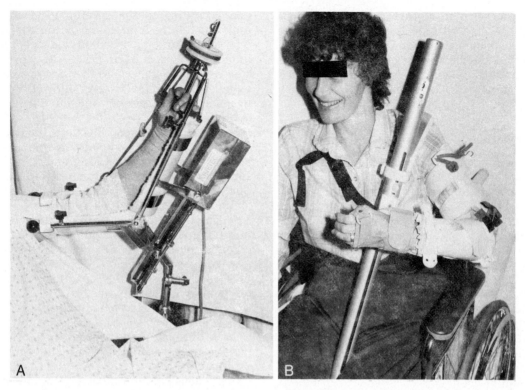

Figure 9–2. Continuous passive motion machines are becoming available for use in treating the elbow. Both flexion-extension and pronation-supination features are incorporated in these devices. These may be used both for the hospitalized patient (A) as well as for an individual for whom local ambulation is desirable or permitted (B).

be entirely different from the goals and rehabilitation sequence sought in persons suffering from a generalized arthritic process or in those who have sustained an injury that has damaged multiple tissues around the joint. The general guidelines of the rehabilitation program are described below, and the program for the athlete is detailed in Chapter 31.

Motion

Because of the tight congruity of the elbow joint, the closely applied and vulnerable soft tissues, and the proximity of the muscles that move the elbow, stiffness is extremely difficult to overcome. Immobilization adversely influences the orientation and mechanical properties of periarticular soft tissue.[1] Joint stiffness is felt to be due not only to scarred static structures (Fig. 9–1) but also in part to the actin-myosin in cross bridges[8] that cause muscle stiffness, and thus this aspect must be addressed. Further, excessive passive stretch of the joint is to be assiduously avoided. The generally accepted principle of resting damaged tissue by prolonged immobilization[5] was challenged by Willems[15] after the "great war" in 1919. The scientific basis of the benefits of early motion is emerging as the harmful influence of increased synthesis of collagen cross-linking during immobilization is becoming

more clear.[2] Passive joint motion not only provides nourishment to the articular cartilage[11] but also has the beneficial effect of clearing hematoma formation from the joint.[9] Therefore, early active motion must be initiated as soon as the inflammatory process has been controlled and to the extent that the healing phase will allow. The initial arc of motion should be limited to one that does not aggravate inflammation or retard healing. As applied to the elbow, the availability of continuous passive motion devices is limited (Fig. 9–2). Our early experience suggests that the beneficial effects of these devices that have been observed in the knee[3] are also obtained in the elbow, but precise prescriptions for duration and rate of use and the like are not yet available. In joints that are unstable, the use of a hinge brace may be employed.

If joint stiffness has occurred or if stiffness is anticipated, dynamic bracing may also be used. A slow continuous force that stretches the damaged contracted tissue must be distinguished from the sudden, quick maneuver (manipulation) that tears tissue and may evoke a response that results in further contracture. The value of progressive stretching of the contracted tissues in the subacute phase of healing implies the presence of immature and mature scar formation. This was recognized by Steindler[14] and popularized by Green,[4] who recommended the use of a turnbuckle type of splint in this setting. For several years, we have used a dynamic brace (Fig. 9–3) in the early healing phase (1 to 2 weeks), continuing into the rehabilitation program. With this device, adjustments to encourage flexion or extension or both may be made. We recommended that the splint be worn with the dynamic stretch applied in the direction of the motion that is most desired during the night with the opposite stretch during the day.

In spite of the above measures, loss of joint motion remains one of the most difficult problems in the elbow joint and offers considerable potential for further research and improvement.

Strength

A description of the types of muscle contraction is presented in Chapter 5 and the specifics of strength training are described in Chap-

ter 31. In the less motivated patient or in one suffering from a generalized arthritic process, limited benefits should be anticipated. In such an individual, isometric exercises to improve flexion and extension, pronation, supination, and grip strengths are readily performed at home. The isometric contraction is held for 3 seconds and is followed by 3 seconds of relaxation. It is usually recommended that the elbow be held at 90 degrees for flexion and extension exercises and that the forearm be placed in the neutral position for pronation and supination exercises. A series of 15 to 20 efforts performed two to three times a day is the usual recommendation. Complete relaxation is needed during the exercise period, and total muscle relaxation between contractures is important.[10]

Probably the most common method of rehabilitation of elbow flexion and extension strength is the use of weights. The elbow is ideally suited to exert flexion and extension motions against the resistance of a hand-held

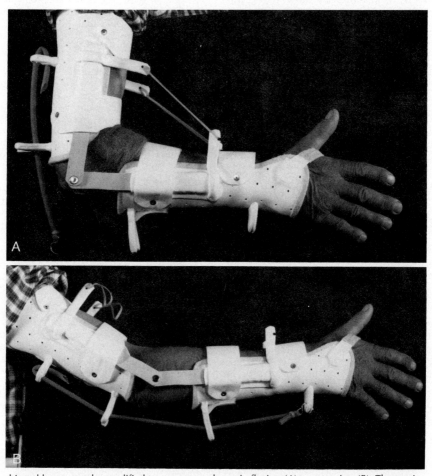

Figure 9–3. The hinged brace may be modified to encourage dynamic flexion (A) or extension (B). The tension of the dynamic component is provided by a rubber band or a round rubber tube that may be adjusted by the patient. The splint is used at night in the direction of the motion that is most required. Use of this device may begin in the early healing phase of treatment but should be monitored to prevent inflammation.

weight. Such exercises result in concentric contracture of the muscles, and because the weight (force) is constant, the effect is further classified as an isotonic exercise.*

Although such exercises may be extremely difficult or impossible to perform in a patient with rheumatoid arthritis, isotonic or "isoflex" concentric contracture is an important feature in the rehabilitation program of the patient with a post-traumatic injury to the elbow region. A series of 15 to 20 efforts performed two to three times a day is the usual program, starting with approximately 1 kg of weight. The exercise is performed in the sitting position for flexion with the elbow initially fully extended and then flexed through an arc of 130 to 140 degrees in 1 to 3 seconds. It should be noted that the more rapid rates of movement result in less force across the joint. Extension exercises are conducted with the patient either lying supine with the elbow flexed and the arm elevated at a right angle to the torso or standing with the arm raised overhead. In this way, the effect of gravity is negated and the extensor musculature may be adequately exercised. Starting with a weight of approximately 1 kg, additional weight is added in 1-kg increments to attain the goal of maximum force that has been determined according to the patient's needs and goals and the status of the joint. For more specific details about strength testing see Chapter 5. When used in a patient with a limited arc of motion, strength exercises should not be delayed until a full range of motion is obtained but should be begun simultaneously with flexibility exercises.

Additional Factors

Personal motivation and pending litigation are also important and cannot be ignored when attempting to return the elbow to normal function. Although it may seem trite to mention these factors, awareness of such "nonmedical" aspects of the patient has existed for many years.[13] Realistic expectations must also be clearly set forth prior to initiating the rehabilitation effort. The person with severe rheumatoid arthritis and adjacent joint involvement is markedly improved with a total elbow replacement offering 100 degrees of painless motion. In this patient, occupa-

tional therapy may be the most effective means not only of restoring motion but also of encouraging the use of other joints on a regular basis. For the competitive athlete, on the other hand, anything short of normal function with the potential of obtaining above-average strength and endurance is inadequate. Implicit in this discussion, therefore, is the recommendation that the physician devote adequate time to clearly explaining the goals of the treatment offered and carefully supervising the rehabilitation process.

References

1. Akeson, W. H., Amiel, D., and Woo, S. L. Y.: Immobility Effects on Synovial Joints. The Pathomechanics of Joint Contracture. Biorheology 17:95, 1980.
2. Amiel, D., Akeson, W. H., Harwood, F. L., and Frank, C. B.: Stress Deprivation Effect on Metabolic Turnover of the Medial Collateral Ligament Collagen—A Comparison Between 9 and 12 Week Immobilization. Clin. Orthop. 172:265, 1983.
3. Coutts, R. D., Toth, C., and Kaita, J.: The Role of Continuous Passive Motion in the Rehabilitation of the Total Knee Patient. In Hungerford, D. (ed.): Total Knee Arthroplasty—A Comprehensive Approach. Baltimore, The Williams & Williams Co., 1983. (In press.)
4. Green, D. P., and McCoy, H.: Turnbuckle Orthotic Correction of Elbow-Flexion Contractures. J. Bone Joint Surg. 61A:1092, 1979.
5. Keith, A.: Menders of the Maimed Tendon. London Oxford University Press, 1919.
6. Korcok, M.: Motion, Not Immobility, Advocated for Healing Synovial Joints. J.A.M.A. 246:2005, 1981.
7. Lehman, J.: Therapeutic Heat and Cold, pp. 404–407, 563–566. Baltimore, The Williams & Wilkins Co., 1982.
8. Margar, D. L.: Separation of Active and Passive Components of Short-Range Stiffness of Muscle. Am. J. Physiol. 232:45, 1977.
9. O'Driscoll, S. W., Kumar, A., and Salter, R. B.: The Effect of Continuous Passive Motion on the Clearance of a Hemarthrosis From a Synovial Joint: An Experimental Investigation in the Rabbit (Abstract). Proc. Orth. Res. Soc. 8:32, 1983.
10. Sainbury, P., and Gebson, T. G.: Symptoms in Anxiety and Tension and the Accompanying Physiological Changes in the Muscular System. J. Neurol. Neurosurg. Pyschiatr. 17:216, 1954.
11. Salter, R. B., Simmonds, D. F., Malcolm, B. W., Rumble, E. J., MacMichael, D., and Clements, N.: The Effects of Continuous Passive Motion on Healing of Full Thickness Defects in Articular Cartilage. J. Bone Joint Surg. 62A:1232, 1980.
12. Saltin, B.: Fiber Types and Metabolic Potential of Skeletal Muscles in Sedentary Men and Endurance Runners. Ann. N.Y. Grad. Sci. 301:3, 1977.
13. Smith, F. M.: Surgery of the Elbow, 2nd ed. Philadelphia, W. B. Saunders Co., 1972.
14. Steindler, A.: The Traumatic Deformities and Disabilities of the Upper Extremity. Springfield, Ill., Charles C Thomas, 1946.
15. Willems, C.: Treatment of Purulent Arthritis by Wide Arthrotomy Followed by Immediate Active Mobilization. Surg. Gynec. Obstet. 28:546, 1919.

---

*Although the mechanical advantage of the muscles changes with joint position, the resistance decreases with successive flexion motions. By using an elastic tension cord, a progressive increase in tension occurs with increasing elbow flexion, thus accommodating the improved mechanical advantage of the muscles.

PART II

Conditions Affecting the Child's Elbow

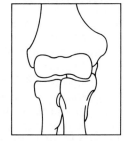

CHAPTER 10

Radiography of the Pediatric Elbow

ALAN D. HOFFMAN

IMAGING METHODS

The ability to obtain adequate and appropriate radiographs of the elbow depends on a number of variables. Often the pattern and timing of the appearance of the numerous secondary ossifications centers at the elbow is a source of confusion to those who deal infrequently with children. To obtain diagnostic radiographs consistently requires well-maintained, modern equipment and technologists who pay careful attention to the details of radiographic technique. Radiology technicians are generally empathetic with the anxiety that a child (and an accompanying parent or guardian) may feel when confronted with the need to enter a radiology exposure room with its ominous appearing, bulky machinery. It is always helpful to reassure the patient gently that the examination is easy and will not cause any discomfort.

The radiographic views used for examining a child's elbow do not differ in the routine case from those obtained for adults. The initial examination consists of anteroposterior and lateral views. The anteroposterior view is obtained with the forearm supine and the elbow in as full extension as possible. If

significantly less than full extension is possible, this should be noted on the film. Alternatively, two anteroposterior views can be obtained—one of the humerus and the other of the forearm. The lateral film is obtained with the elbow in 90 degrees of flexion and the forearm in a neutral position halfway between pronation and supination. Particularly for evaluation of the humeral "fat pads," it is essential that the humerus be held in as true a lateral position as possible.

In certain situations, especially in an elbow that has undergone trauma when a fracture is not seen on the initial radiographs, oblique views may be obtained. They are particularly helpful in the delineation of fractures of the radial head or coronoid process of the ulna that may otherwise remain undetected.

In certain instances fluoroscopic examinations of the elbow may yield valuable information by virtue of the examiner's ability to obtain just the precise degree of obliquity necessary to show an abnormality. Either spot films or conventional radiographic films may then be obtained.

Tomography using either a simple linear method or complex motion systems can be utilized in the evaluation of growth plates that may have closed prematurely following trauma. Computed tomography has been increasingly used in the evaluation of problems in the extremities. Delineation of the extent of a tumor may be uniquely shown with the cross-sectional imaging capabilities of this method. Another newer imaging modality, magnetic resonance imaging (MRI), will undoubtedly be able to add useful diagnostic information about pathologic processes of the elbow. This technique, which does not rely on ionizing radiation, can obtain direct image slices in any projection.

Other currently available modalities in the armamentarium of the diagnostic radiologist are also used in the evaluation of disorders involving the elbow. Ultrasonography, radionuclide bone scanning, and angiography may occasionally be indicated. Elbow arthrography, although infrequently used in pediatric patients, also may be performed. These specialized radiographic techniques are discussed in detail in Chapter 6.

The only portion of the skeleton in which routine use of the comparison view of the contralateral side exceeds that for the elbow is the hip. However, depending on the experience of those interpreting radiographs of the pediatric elbow, it is probably necessary to obtain comparison views in only selected cases.[5, 6]

NORMAL DEVELOPMENT

The maturation sequence at the elbow is more variable than that at the hand and wrist, which is the most valuable area for determination of skeletal maturation. Nonetheless, an appreciation of the normal sequence and timing of the appearance of ossification centers and maturation patterns is important for an understanding of the radiographic appearances of the elbow in children (Fig. 10–1). Several mnemonics have been suggested to help remember the time of appearance of the ossification of these centers. We find that the cross (Fig. 10–1B) connecting ossification centers is particularly helpful in remembering at least the order of ossification of these centers. An atlas, *Radiology of the Elbow*,[2] shows standards for elbow maturation in children.

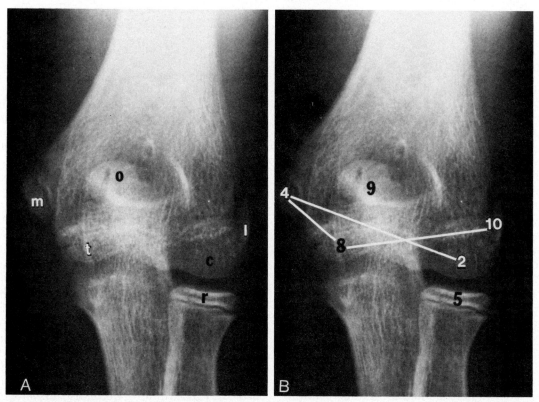

Figure 10–1. *A,* Normal left elbow showing the secondary centers: capitellum (c); medial epicondyle (m); radial head (r); trochlea (t); olecranon (o); and lateral epicondyle (1). *B,* The approximate age at time of appearance of these centers is indicated in years. The cross connecting the secondary centers of the distal humerus serves as a reminder of the order of ossification of these centers (Modified from Brodeur, A. E., et al.: The basic tenets for appropriate evaluation of the elbow in pediatrics. Curr. Probl. Diag. Radiol. 12(5):1, September/October, 1983.)

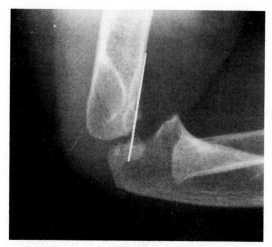

Figure 10–2. Two-year-old girl, lateral elbow radiograph. The posterior portion of the physis of the capitellum is broader than the anterior portion. A line along the anterior shaft of the distal humeral shaft, the anterior humeral line (AHL), normally intersects the anterior third of the ossific nucleus of the capitellum.

The description that follows is a brief discussion of some of the major points in the development of secondary centers at the elbow.

Capitellum. The capitellum is the first of the six elbow ossification centers to appear. It is the most variable in its pattern of ossification and time of appearance. Generally, it is visualized radiographically in children between 1 and 2 years old. As with most of the ossification centers, the capitellum initially ossifies as a sphere and then flattens with further development into its normal mature shape. On the lateral projection the posterior portion of the physis is broader than the anterior portion until about 8 years (Fig. 10–2). The capitellum frequently fuses with the trochlea or with the lateral epicondyle before it unites with the humeral shaft (Fig. 10–3).

The orientation of the capitellum with the humeral shaft can be a source of confusion. On a true lateral projection the anterior humeral line (AHL) will allow proper interpretation of this relationship (Fig. 10–2). Brodeur[1] uses the humeral shaft line (HSL) parallel to the long axis of the shaft rather than the AHL, which is drawn along the anterior humeral surface.

The radiocapitellar line is a line drawn through the long axis of the proximal radial shaft that should, in the absence of dislocation, pass through the middle of the capitellum ossification center. This is generally true in anteroposterior, lateral, or any oblique projection. In early development, however, the radial metaphysis is wedged so that on the anteroposterior projection a normal radial shaft line may appear to extend lateral to the capitellum. However, on the lateral projection the normal radiocapitellar line can be appreciated (Fig. 10–4). In older patients, although it may appear that the radiocapitellar line is normal in one projection in a patient with a radial head dislocation, it will invariably be abnormal in the projection taken at right angles, generally the lateral projection.

Medial Epicondyle. The medial epicondyle is the second elbow ossification center to appear in the normal sequence, usually at about 4 years. Lying posteromedially, it is often best appreciated on the lateral projection (Fig. 10–5). It may arise from more than one ossific nucleus. Although it is the second humeral ossification center to appear, its development is slow and it is usually the last center to unite with the humeral shaft in the normal child, sometimes as late as 15 or 16 years. This center may fuse with the trochlea before uniting with the humeral shaft. Injuries involving the nonunited medial epicondyle are relatively common and are among the most difficult to evaluate. Consequently, to avoid errors Rogers suggests making a habit of identifying the presence and position of the medial epicondyle ossification center in each case.[7] A classic example of the importance of appreciating the sequence of humeral

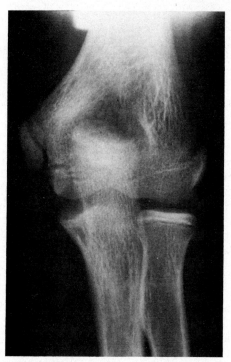

Figure 10–3. Thirteen-year-old girl in whom the capitellum has joined with the lateral epicondyle and trochlea prior to fusion with the humeral shaft. Note the normal sclerotic radial epiphysis that is wider than the radial neck.

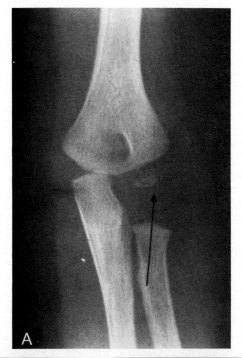

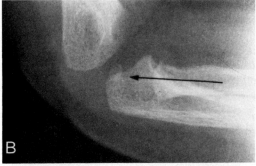

Figure 10–4. A, Normal seven-month-old girl with apparent abnormal radiocapitellar line on the anteroposterior radiograph because of wedging of the metaphysis. B, The relationship between the radial shaft and capitellum is normal on the lateral radiograph.

ossification center appearance is avulsion and displacement of the medial epicondyle ossification center. This frequently results in the displacement of the medial epicondyle into the normal position of the trochlear ossification center. In a child between 4 and 8 years of age—the time of appearance of the medial epicondyle and trochlear ossification centers—a radiograph suggesting a trochlear ossification center, without visualization of a medial epicondyle center, should suggest that in fact fracture and dislocation of the medial epicondyle has occurred.

Radial Head Epiphysis. The initial ossification of this epiphysis is fairly predictable and usually occurs in the fifth year (Fig. 10–1B). Although usually beginning as a sphere, it often matures as one or more flat sclerotic

centers. This pattern may be mistakenly interpreted as a fracture. With maturation, the physis on the anterorposterior radiograph is wider laterally than medially and this appearance, combined with the medial angulation of the radius at the junction of its shaft and neck, may suggest dislocation on anteroposterior views, Lateral projection of the elbow will not confirm the suggestion of dislocation. With further maturation of ossification of the proximal radial ossification center, the normal relationship of the radius and capitellum can be seen on anteroposterior radiographs. Notches or clefts of the metaphysis of the proximal radius are often seen as normal variations of ossification during maturation.[3, 4]

The elbow joint is attached to the proximal radius by the annular ligament. Since fractures of the radial neck are extracapsular, they will not be associated with hemarthrosis and abnormalities of the humeral fat pads. Radial head fractures, which are more common in children, are intracapsular and can be expected to show displacement of the distal humeral fat pads.

Trochlear Epiphysis. The next ossification center of the elbow to appear is that of the trochlea. Unlike the centers that appear earlier, the trochlea generally begins from several centers (Fig. 10–6). Later it often has an irregular outline, and this appearance should not be confused with such abnormal processes as trauma or avascular necrosis (Fig. 10–9). These ossification centers typically appear between 8 and 10 years of age.

Olecranon. The normal development of the epiphysis and physis of the olecranon is frequently mistaken for a fracture. There are subtle features that should be understood to prevent such errors. The appearance time of the olecranon ossification center is between 8 and 10 years, with fusion to the ulnar shaft occurring at 14 to 14½ years. Prior to the appearance of the olecranon epiphysis, metaphyseal sclerosis of the proximal olecranon and deepening of the olecranon fossa frequently occur. Often there are two or more nuclei, and the anterior center is almost always smaller than the posterior one (Fig. 10–7).

The olecranon physis has prominent sclerotic margins just prior to closure. Fusion proceeds posteriorly from the joint side or anterior surface (Fig. 10–8). During its development the physeal line remains relatively perpendicular to the ulnar shaft. As a result of differential growth, often with maturation, the olecranon growth plate, which initially is proximal to the elbow joint comes to lie at a

Figure 10–5. *A,* Ten-year-old boy with a normal poster-omedially lying ossification center for the medial epicondyle (arrows) seen posterior to the humeral shaft on the lateral projection. *B,* Another 10-year-old boy who sustained trauma resulting in avulsion of the medial epicondyle, which is displaced anteriorly (arrows) on the lateral projection, and displaced medially *C,* and rotated on the anteroposterior projection.

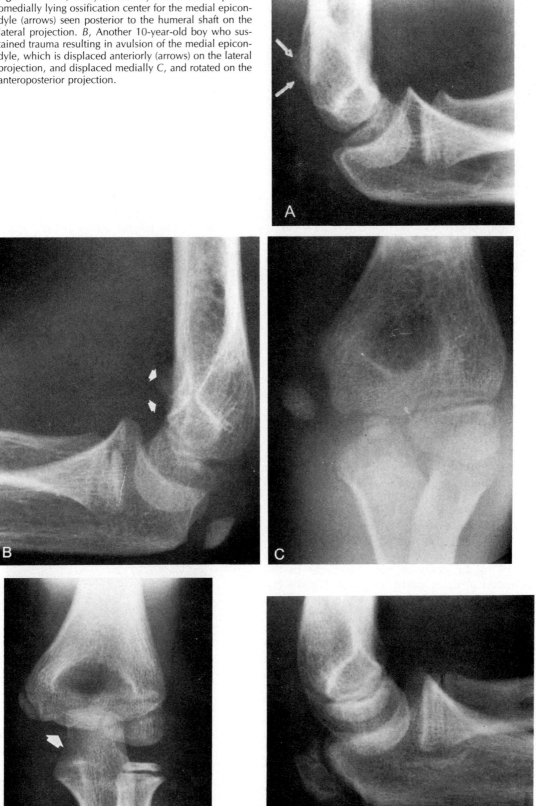

Figure 10–6. Multiple ossification nuclei of developing trochlea (arrows) in a 9-year-old boy.

Figure 10–7. Thirteen-year-old boy with double ossification center of the olecranon. The anterior nucleus is smaller.

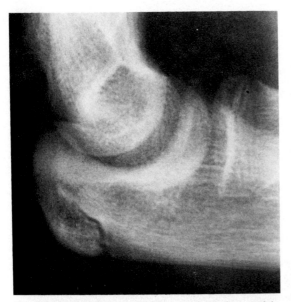

Figure 10–8. Fourteen-year-old boy in whom closure of the olecranon growth plate has begun anteriorly. Note the sclerotic margin of that portion of the growth plate that remains unfused.

mid–elbow joint level by the time of fusion. This "wandering physeal line of the olecranon" does not occur in all individuals.[2]

Although the majority of olecranon fractures are intracapsular and are associated with alterations of fat pads, some are not. The tip of the olecranon is not within the capsule in some individuals. The only other common site of fracture related to the elbow that lies outside the joint capsule is the radial neck (see Chapter 14).

Lateral Epicondyle. The ossification center of the lateral epicondyle is the last of the elbow centers to appear. It is usually first seen at 10 or 11 years of age and fuses to the humeral shaft at about 14 years. Unlike the other ossification centers of the elbow, the lateral epicondyle appears first as a thin sliver rather than as a round or spherical ossific nucleus (Fig. 10–9). Ossification commences in the lateral portion of the cartilaginous mold so that the physis appears particularly wide. As maturation proceeds, this center generally fuses to the capitellum before closure of the growth plate occurs.

Because of the relatively short time between the appearance and fusion of this center, it is not always certain in individual cases whether ossification is delayed or fusion to the humerus has already occurred. To avoid confusion about this point, it must be realized that prior to ossification the humerus has a

sharp, straight, sloping metaphyseal line that changes to a sloping, curving margin at the capitellum. The fused lateral epicondyle, on the other hand, has a smooth, curved margin that is continuous with the capitellum (Fig. 10–10).

NORMAL VARIANTS

In addition to the confusing appearances caused by the normally developing elbow, there are a few variations from normal or unusual appearances that should be noted.

The normal radial tuberosity, which is the site of insertion of the biceps brachii, lies medially at the junction of the medial shaft and neck. On lateral views it may appear as an undermineralized focus and may be misinterpreted as a destructive lesion of the bone (Fig. 10–11). On the anteroposterior view of the elbow, the thin humeral olecranon fossa occasionally appears to be entirely lucent, the so-called perforated olecranon fossa (Fig. 10–12). In some instances there is a bridge of bone crossing or a separate ossicle within a perforated olecranon fossa.

A rare anatomic anomaly is a bony projection from the anterior medial distal humerus known as the supracondylar process (Fig. 10–13), which is discussed in Chapters 2 and 18.

An appreciation of these variations of the patterns of development of the secondary centers of ossification of this joint is essential for

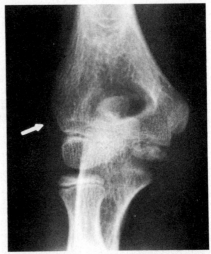

Figure 10–9. Nine-year-old boy with beginning ossification of the lateral epicondyle (arrow) from a thin sliver widely separated from the metaphysis. Note the irregular outline of the developing ossification center of the trochlea.

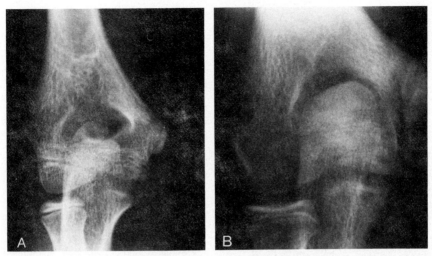

Figure 10–10. *A,* Nine-year-old boy in whom ossification of the lateral epicondyle is about to begin. The metaphysis has a sharp, straight, sloping margin. *B,* The fusing lateral epicondyle in this 4-year-old boy, in contrast, has a smoother, rounded margin.

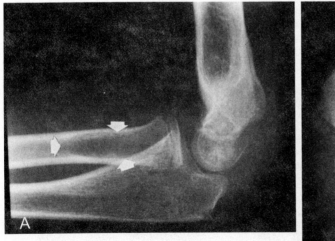

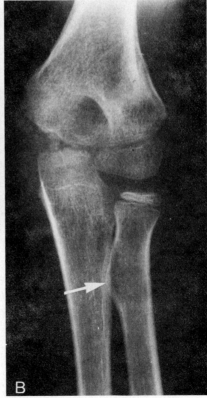

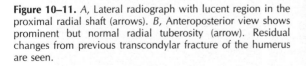

Figure 10–11. *A,* Lateral radiograph with lucent region in the proximal radial shaft (arrows). *B,* Anteroposterior view shows prominent but normal radial tuberosity (arrow). Residual changes from previous transcondylar fracture of the humerus are seen.

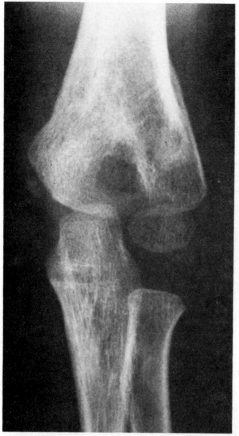

Figure 10–12. Six-year-old boy with perforated olecranon fossa. There has been a previous supracondylar fracture.

proper radiographic diagnosis of abnormalities in the pediatric elbow.

References

1. Brodeur, A. E., Silberstein, M. J., Graviss, E. R., and Luisiri, A.: The Basic Tenets for Appropriate Evaluation of the Elbow in Pediatrics. Curr. Probl. Diag. Radiol. **12(5)**:1, Sept./Oct., 1983.
2. Brodeur, A. E., Silberstein, M. J., and Graviss, E. R.: Radiology of the Pediatric Elbow. Boston, G. K. Hall, 1981.
3. Keats, T. E.: An Atlas of Normal Roentgen Variants That May Simulate Disease, 2nd ed., pp. 241–268. Chicago, Year Book Medical Publishers, 1979.
4. Kohler, A., and Zimmer, E. A.: Borderlands of the Normal and Early Pathologic in Skeletal Roentgenology, 3rd ed. New York, Grune & Stratton, 1968.
5. McCauley, R. G. K., Schwartz, A. M., Leonidas, J. C., Darling, D. B., Bankoff, M. S., and Swan, C. S., II: Comparison Views in Extremity Injury in Children: An Efficacy Study. Radiology **131**:95, 1979.
6. Merten, D. F.: Comparison Radiographs in Extremity Injuries of Childhood: Current Application in Radiological Practice. Radiology **126**:209, 1978.
7. Rodgers, L. F.: Radiology of Skeletal Trauma. pp. 435–501. New York, Churchill Livingstone, 1982.
8. Silberstein, M. J., Brodeur, A. E., Graviss, E. R., and Luisiri, A.: Some Vagaries of the Olecranon. J. Bone Joint Surg. **63A(5)**:722, 1981.
9. Silberstein, M. J., Brodeur, A. E., Graviss, E. R., and Luisiri, A.: Some Vagaries of the Medial Epicondyle. J. Bone Joint Surg. **63A(4)**:524, 1981.
10. Silberstein, M. J., Brodeur, A. E., and Graviss, E. R.: Some Vagaries of the Capitellum. J. Bone Joint Surg. **61A(2)**:244, 1979.
11. Silberstein, M. J., Brodeur, A. E., and Graviss, E. R.: Some Vagaries of the Radial Head and Neck. J. Bone Joint Surg. **64A(8)**:1153, 1982.

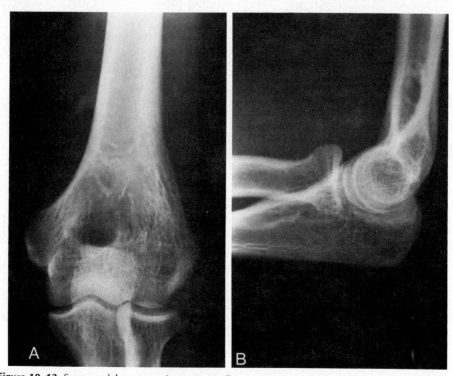

Figure 10–13. Supracondylar process in a mature elbow. *A,* Anteroposterior and *B,* lateral radiographs.

CHAPTER 11

Congenital Abnormalities of the Elbow

J. H. DOBYNS

The elbow seems to be not only positioned between the shoulder and hand but also lost between the shoulder and hand when congenital anomalies of the upper limb are being discussed. Such problems in the elbow region are seldom mentioned, much less emphasized. The best known problem in the elbow area, congenital synostosis, is plagued by nihilism and controversy about treatment methods. With this background, it can be readily believed that the future holds the promise of more information about the management of congenital elbow problems than the past has yet produced. Elbow function and configuration are affected by conditions both proximal and distal to the elbow. Nevertheless, in this chapter discussion will center on that portion of the upper limb lying between the shaft-metaphyseal junction of the humerus proximally and the bicipital tuberosity distally.

CAUSES OF CONGENITAL ANOMALIES

The causes of congenital elbow anomalies follow the same patterns of genetic or chromosomal damage or direct damage to the embryo that are seen in other congenital anomalies. The most common problem, that of radial head subluxation or dislocation, may be induced by a relatively trivial injury or merely by a short ulna from any cause, so statistics for this problem are unreliable. Because so much of the elbow area is cartilaginous at birth, it is difficult to rule out trauma as a possible agent in some dislocations and deformities. In addition, pyogenic sepsis and other infections, tumors (congenital or infantile), and diseases (e.g., hemophilia) occasionally involve the elbow. Conditions that quite commonly involve the elbow are constitutional diseases of bone, metabolic abnormalities, and syndromes featuring limb formation and differentiation failures[26, 29, 53, 56] (Table 11–1).[35] Some of the syndromes can be

grouped under such broad categories as osteochondrodysplasia,[3, 23, 24, 25, 56] dysostoses,[13] primary growth disturbances, primary metabolic abnormalities, and so on.

CLASSIFICATION

I use a simple tissue defect classification based on the most obvious and most inhibiting tissue defect known to be present, though often accompanied by some degree of defect in other tissues. The classification consists of three major categories: (1) bone and joint anomalies, (2) soft tissue anomalies, and (3) anomalies of all tissues. Bone and joint abnormalities at the elbow may include major absences, but more commonly the skeletal structures are present but malformed. The common bone and joint problems are synostosis (Fig. 11–1), ankylosis (Figs. 11–2 to 11–4), and instability (Fig. 11–5). Soft tissue anomalies include malformations with contractures, control deficiencies, isolated tissue anomalies (Fig. 11–6), and congenital tumors (Fig. 11–7). Complete absence or disorganization of the whole limb including elbow structures occurs as in phocomelia (Fig. 11–8), but usually recognizable though dysplastic structures are present (Fig. 11–9). Similar involvement but more isolated to the elbow area occurs in the pterygium syndromes.

DIAGNOSIS

Bone and Joint Anomalies

Synostosis. Synostoses may occur between all or any two of the three bones present at the elbow. The most common synostosis is that between the radius and the ulna proximally in the forearm near the elbow (Fig. 11–10), but these two bones may also be synostosed at any point in their paired course in the forearm. In addition, radiohumeral synostosis, ulnohumeral synostosis, or synostosis

Text continued on page 169

Table 11-1. Elbow Deformities in Congenital Syndromes

Syndrome	Syndrome Characteristics[a]	Catalog Numbers[b]	Inheritance[c]	Number of Patients[d]
1. Achondroplasia	O-1	10080	ASD	> 100
2. Mesolmelic dwarfism	O-1	15623, 24970	ASD, ASR	> 100
3. Nievergelt's	O-1	16340	ASD	< 50
4. Werner's	O-1	27770	ASR	> 100
5. Ellis-Van Creveld's	O-1	22550	ASR	< 50
6. Acrodysostosis	O-1	10180	ASD	< 50
7. Acromesomelic dwarfism	O-1	20125	ASR	< 50
8. Ulna, fibula hypoplasia	O-1	19140	ASD	< 25
9. Type 1 acrocephalopolysyndactyly	O-1	10110, 20100, 10112, 20102, 16420, 10120, 10130, 10140, 10160	ASD	> 100
10. Multiple cartilaginous exostoses	O-2	13370	ASD, ASR	> 100
11. Metaphyseal chondrodysplasia	O-3	26040, 25401, 20090, 25022, 25023, 25025, 15640, 25030, 15650, 24270, 15640, 15650, 21505, 25022, 25023, 25025, 25030, 25040, 25041	ASD	< 100
12. Cranial dysostosis	D-1	12350, 12290, 21835, 30411	ASD	< 100
13. Familial radioulnar synostosis	D-3	17930	ASD	< 100
14. Pterygium	D-3	26500, 31215, 19100, 11950, 19360, 17820	ASD, ASR	> 50
15. Radial aplasia	D-3	21860	ASD, S	> 100
16. Idiopathic osteolysis		26580, 26570, 27795, 25960, 16630	ASD, S	< 50
17. Mucopolysaccharidoses	PMA	25270, 23000, 22380, 25280, 30990, 25290, 25292, 25293, 25294, 25300, 25301, 25320, 25322, 25323	ASR	> 100
18. Mucolipidoses	PMA	25240, 25250, 25260, 25265	ASR	> 100
19. Lipidoses	PMA	21280, 30150, 24680, 23050, 23060, 23065, 21208, 25010, 25720	ASR	< 50
20. VATER complex		19235, 10748	ASD	< 50
21. Craniocarpotarsal dystrophy		19370, 27772	ASD	> 50
22. Craniosynostosis		12310, 27235, 20100, 10120, 10160, 10140, 20155, 31410, 21850, 21853, 21855, 21860, 25922, 12315	ASD	> 100
23. De Lange dwarfism		12247	ASD	> 100
24. Diastrophic dysplasia		22260	ASR	< 50
25. Nail-patella	D-2	16120	ASD	< 50
26. Otopalatodigital		31130	X	< 100
27. Rubenstein-Taybi's		26860	ASR	> 100
28. Silver-Russell's		27005	ASR	> 50

No.	Condition	Catalog numbers[b]	Inheritance[c]	Approx. no.[d]
29.	Klinefelter's	27330	ASR	> 50
30.	Thalidomide embryopathy	27360	T, ASR	> 100
31.	Holt-Oram's	14290	ASD	> 50
32.	Acrofacial dyostosis (Nager)	15440	S, ASD	> 50
33.	LADD	14973	ASD, S	< 50
34.	Fanconi's anemia	22765, 22766	ASR	> 100
35.	TAR	27400	ASR	> 100
36.	Auriculo-osteodysplasia	10900	ASD	< 25
37.	Ehlers-Danlos	13000, 13001, 13002, 13005, 22535, 30520, 22540, 13006, 22541, 13008, 30415, 22531, 14790	ASD, ASR	> 100
38.	Phocomelia	26900	ASR	< 50
39.	Larsen's	15025, 24560	ASD, ASR	> 50
40.	Oculomelic complexes	16420, 25790, 25792, 16430, 25795, 16431	ASD, ASR	
41.	Otopalatodigital	31130	X	< 50
42.	Amelia of arm	10440	S, ASD	< 25
43.	Peromelia of humerus	10030, 10330	ASD	< 25
44.	Humeroradial synostosis	14305, 23640	ASD, ASR	> 50
45.	Femoral-fibula-ulna complex	22820	ASR	> 100
46.	Focal dermal hypoplasia (Goltz)	30560	X	> 50
47.	Split hand	18360	ASD	> 100
48.	Ulnar mammary	19145	ASD	< 25
49.	Ulnar deficiency	13575, 19140, 20070, 24960, 10790, 31436, 27170, 20060, 20061	ASD, ASR	> 100

[a]O–1, Defects of growth of tubular bones
O–2, Disorganized development of cartilage and fibrous skeletal elements
O–3, Abnormalities of diaphyseal cortical density or metaphyseal modeling
D–1, Dysostosis with cranial and facial involvement
D–2, Dysostosis with predominant axial involvement
D–3, Dysostosis with predominant extremity involvement
PMA, Primary metabolic abnormalities
PGD, Primary growth disturbances
[b]Catalog numbers are those used in McKusick, V. A.: Mendelian Inheritance in Man. 6th ed. Baltimore, The Johns Hopkins University Press, 1983.
[c]ASD, Autosomal dominant
ASR, Autosomal recessive
S, Sporadic
X, Linked to sex chromosome
T, Teratogenic
[d]Approximate number so far reported.

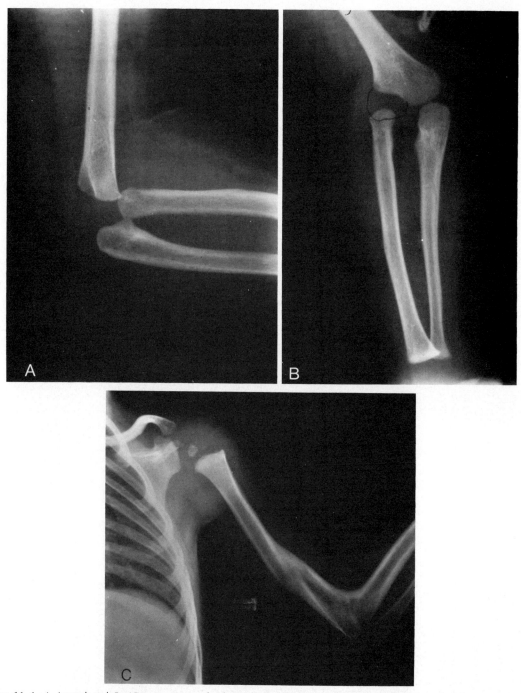

Figure 11–1. *A,* Lateral and *B,* AP x-ray views of a hypoplastic distal humerus and an apparent radial head subluxation certainly reveal a deformity but probably not a subluxation. Clinically, there was no evidence of a dislocated radial head. *C,* The opposite elbow showed a radiohumeral synostosis and also a recent fracture just proximal to the synostosis. This case demonstrates the difficulties of differentiation between subluxation, dislocation, and synostosis about the elbow.

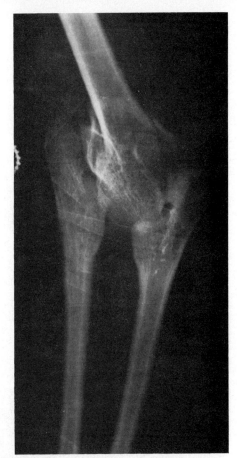

Figure 11–2. This AP view of an elbow in ulnar dimelia shows no radiohumeral joint but two ulnohumeral joints. The appearance is unusual as expected, but no dislocation is noted. Both elbow and forearm motion are limited more than 50 percent.

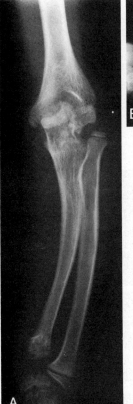

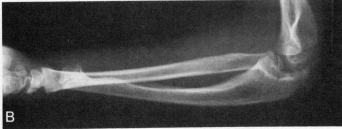

Figure 11–3. *A,* Elbow and forearm function are, to date, nearly normal in this teenage boy in whom the AP x-ray view shows ulnar hypoplasia and bowing, distortion of the distal ulnar physis-metaphysis, and subluxation of the radial head. *B,* The lateral x-ray view shows a similar epiphysis-physis-metaphysis distortion of the proximal ulna with associated joint surface irregularity and shaft bowing. No diagnosis has been confirmed, but this is probably an osteochondrodysplasia.

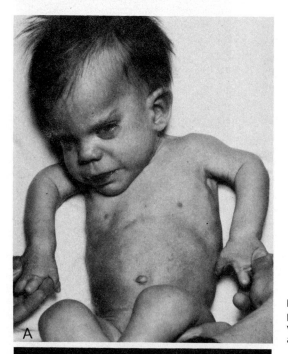

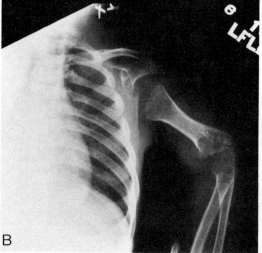

Figure 11–4. *A,* This 18-month-old infant with chondrodysplasia punctata has contractures of many joints including the elbows, where broad metaphyses and irregular, calcified epiphyses *(B)* are seen.

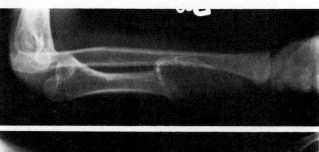

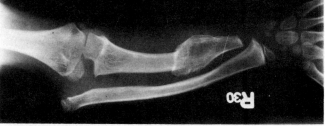

Figure 11–5. This case further demonstrates the overlap between congenital and developmental abnormalities of the elbow. Gradual radial head subluxation due to unequal length of forearm bones is well known in multiple exostosis. These AP and lateral x-rays demonstrate a severe dislocation of the radial head that was present at birth and was associated with a severe osteochondroma deformity of the distal ulna with inhibition of ulnar growth.

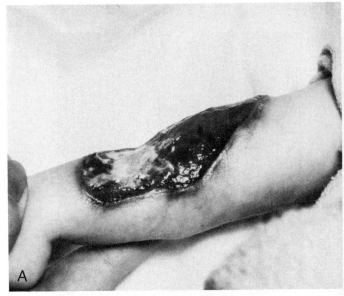

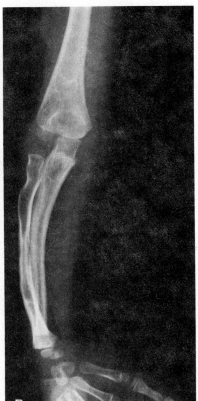

Figure 11–6. *A,* Congenital aplasia of skin and soft tissues at the elbow and proximal forearm results in *(B)* secondary bone changes in the forearm and elbow.

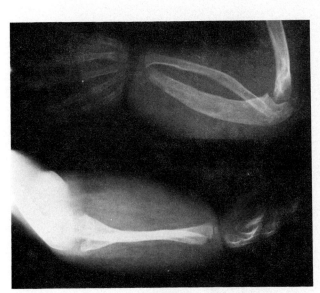

Fig. 11–7

Fig. 11–8

Figure 11–7. The AP and lateral x-rays of the elbow and forearm in a patient with juvenile fibromatosis reveal marked enlargement of the ulna, posterolateral subluxation of the radial head, moderate enlargement of the distal humerus, and surface irregularities at all aspects of the joint.

Figure 11–8. This x-ray of the upper limb of a patient with phocomelia shows a fairly well developed shoulder and arm, a very hypoplastic hand, and fusion of all elbow elements with the short ulna protruding at right angles to the radius and forearm.

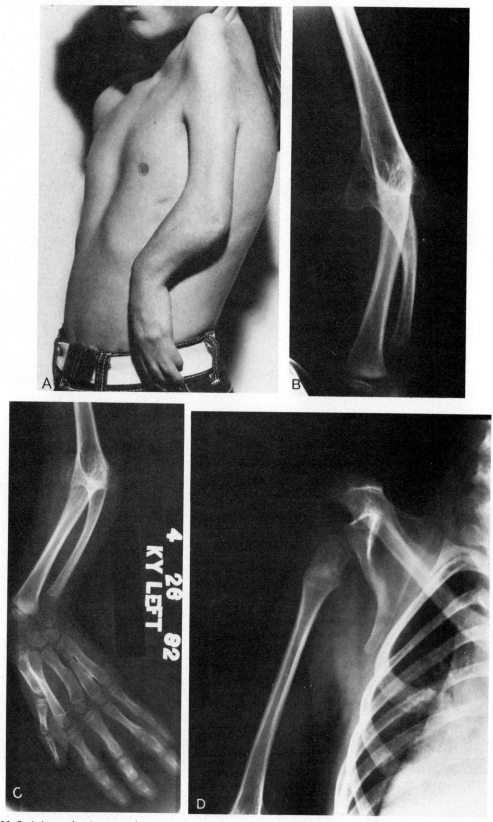

Figure 11–9. *A,* In another instance of generalized hypoplasia of the upper limb all segments from the shoulder girdle through the hand are equally and severely affected. *B,* Synostosis of all components of the elbow is present (C), correlated with a hypoplastic and asymmetric forearm plus a hypoplastic hand. *D,* Hypoplasia of the arm, shoulder and shoulder girdle is also obvious on this radiograph.

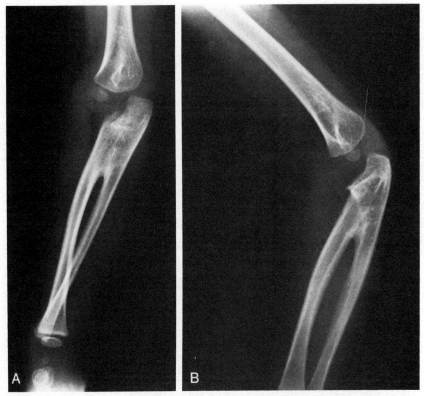

Figure 11–10. A, X-ray view of a typical proximal, radioulnar, congenital synostosis. B, The lateral view of the same synostosis is seen but demonstrates no radial head posterior subluxation, though this is commonly seen.

between the radius, humerus, and ulna may be present. Posterior dislocation of the radial head is a common accompaniment of many of these syndromes. Incomplete synostosis may occur, but often this is a radiologic appearance rather than an actual occurrence because complete synostosis is usually present by maturity, both clinically and radiographically.[21, 26, 33, 53]

Ankylosis. Partial ankylosis of the elbow or the proximal radioulnar joint is often overlooked because limited elbow-forearm motion is common in infancy[22] and unremarkable in childhood. Causes include failure of complete synostosis as just mentioned, intrinsic abnormalities of the joint or surface formation mechanism, or abnormalities of the surrounding soft tissues. The joint must be formed correctly, must have adequate surface material and ligamentous support, and must move soon after its formation or it will become ankylosed. There are instances when all or part of the elbow appears to be dislocated but proves to be only malformed and limited in motion (Fig. 11–11).

Instability. Instability of the elbow area seldom resembles the post-traumatic condition except in those situations in which there is controversy about whether the cause is post-traumatic or congenital. Ulnohumeral dislocation is infrequent except in severe multitissue hypoplasia such as phocomelia, severe ulnar hypoplasia, and severe pterygium syndrome. Ligament laxity sufficient to produce instability in the presence of normal skeletal and articular structures could occur in theory but has not been reported.

By far the most common problem of instability at the elbow is that of radial head subluxation or dislocation.[1, 2, 8, 15, 17, 20, 30, 31, 32, 39, 42, 43, 48, 49] Not only is this the most frequent congenital elbow abnormality, it is also the most controversial in regard to the precise definition of its pathogenesis. Our perception differs in emphasis from that presented in Chapter 16. When subluxation is an isolated phenomenon there is considerable doubt about whether it is congenital or merely an infantile posttraumatic event.[10, 15, 28, 30, 34] The pulled elbow of infancy is a well-known clinical problem that is associated with trivial trauma and laxity or minor tears of the annular ligament.[39, 44, 45, 51] Children have been seen at birth or shortly thereafter with similar

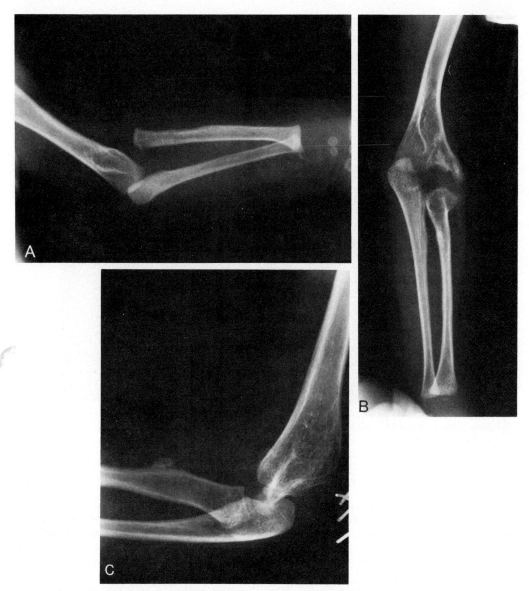

Figure 11–11. *A,* AP x-ray view of an *apparent* radiohumeral dislocation similar to that shown in Figure 11–2 is seen preoperatively. *B,* A postoperative AP x-ray view 4 years later shows repositioning of what was determined to be a displaced radiohumeral joint but not a dislocation of the radial head. *C,* A lateral postoperative view of the same elbow. Repositioning was obtained when the radius was shortened by removing a segment of the radial shaft. This segment of excised radius was then used to block the repositioned lateral condyle in its new position. This surgical procedure improved the x-ray position of the elbow but did not change function, which demonstrated both pre- and postoperatively mild loss of extension-flexion and moderate loss of supination-pronation.

problems.[10, 39, 46] Furthermore, such subluxations in the infant, if not treated by closed reduction or other means, may result in deformities similar to those described as indicative of congenital dislocation of the radial head. However, the degree of deformity in the few cases of known infantile dislocation that have been untreated but followed suggest that the resulting deformity is somewhat milder than that seen in definite congenital hypoplasia at the elbow (Fig. 11–12). When traumatic dislocation is unreduced in the older child, the development of the radial head and the capitellum remains fairly normal, displaying only minimally those radiographic features said to be characteristic of congenital radial head dislocation—i.e., (1) dislocated or subluxed radial head, (2) underdeveloped radial head, (3) flat or dome-shaped radial head, (4) a more slender radius than normal, (5) a longer radius than normal, (6) underdeveloped capitellum humeri, and (7) lack of anterior angulation of the distal humerus.[15, 41, 55]

The criteria used in the past to support a diagnosis of congenital dislocation of the radial head have been summarized as follows: (1) hypoplastic or absent capitellum, (2) dome-shaped radial head, (3) short ulna or long radius, (4) bilateral involvement, (5) concurrence of other congenital anomalies, (6) familial occurrence, (7) no history of trauma, and (8) dislocation seen at birth. Not one of these criteria is absolutely reliable. There may be only one absolute criterion of congenital elbow dislocation—dislocation with severe hypoplasia of all osseous elements of the elbow. Absence of the capitellum is probably an example of congenital aplasia, but hypo-

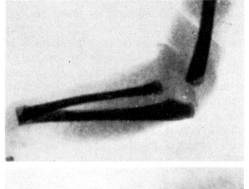

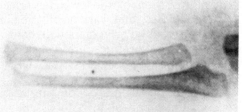

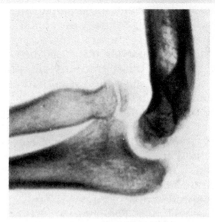

Figure 11–12. Anterior dislocation of the radial head is demonstrated at initial diagnosis (age 2 weeks), at age 4 months, and at age 11 years. In addition to the dislocation there is a reversal of the ulnar curve and some convexity of the radial head.

plasia of the capitellum may occur after dislocation from any cause, as may a deformity of the radial head. The short ulna–long radius configuration, regardless of etiology, usually results in radial head subluxation. Such subluxation is therefore more of a secondary phenomenon than a primary congenital abnormality.[32] Subluxation of the radial head due to trivial trauma is quite common, particularly in infants.[39, 45] Such subluxation does not occur because the radial head is smaller than the neck; in fact, most studies have indicated that it is larger by 30 to 60 percent.[44] However, when the forearm is in pronation it is quite easy to produce a transverse tear in the thin distal attachment of the annular ligament to the periosteum of the radial neck. Once this transverse tear is present, the anterior portion of the radial head can escape from beneath the anterior part of the annular ligament, which then displaces over the radial head. Because the infantile radial head has an oval shape and an articular surface that is not completely perpendicular, there is less discrepancy between the diameter of the metaphysis and the epiphysis when the forearm is in pronation, permitting the annular ligament to displace occasionally even without tearing.[39] There have now been several recorded instances of traumatic subluxation of the radial head in early infancy,[10, 39, 46] and another is recorded in this chapter. When recognized, the condition is treated by either closed or open reduction methods as required. It is therefore very difficult to sustain a diagnosis of congenital dislocation unless there is a considerable amount of hypoplasia in the elbow area generally.

When radial head dislocation is familial or occurs with other musculoskeletal anomalies, particularly anomalies in the same upper limb, the evidence is more convincing that the radial head dislocation is congenital. However, even in such a case, the instability of the radial head is often associated with a discrepancy in length of the paired forearm bones. It is well known that inadequate length of the ulna from any cause will result in increased compressive stresses along the radius, leading gradually to a subluxation and perhaps to a dislocation of the radial head.[28, 31, 49]

Soft Tissue Anomalies

Soft tissues anomalies or absences may interfere with elbow function as much as bone or joint deformities. These anomalies have been subdivided into malformations with contractures, control deficiencies, isolated tissue anomalies, and congenital soft tissue tumors.

Contractures. The classic malformation with contracture is pterygium cubitale, in which almost every soft tissue is abnormal and a severe flexion contracture exists.[18, 26] The condition has also been called cutaneous webs and webbed elbow; it is but one manifestation of a congenital syndrome that may affect the neck, axilla, elbow, knee, or digits. This pterygium syndrome is known as the Bonnevie-Ullrich syndrome. A survey of 240 cases of cutaneous webs reported in the literature included 29 in the region of the elbow.[18] The web may be unilateral or bilateral, symmetrical or asymmetrical. The condition has been reported to result from both an autosomal dominant and a recessive gene. Associated abnormalities involving almost every body system have been reported.[26, 53]

Control Deficiencies. Arthrogryposis and its related syndromes are included in this group but are discussed in another chapter (Chapter 37). Both flaccid and spastic palsies will affect elbow control and range of motion. Simple absences or deficiencies of tissue will also affect elbow control. Hypoplasia of the part includes deficient growth not only of osseous structures but also of the related soft tissue control elements and cover structures.[9, 37, 52]

Isolated Tissue Anomalies. The skin may be deficient or missing with absence, hypoplasia, or scarring of the underlying tissues. Nerve, vascular, and lymphatic anomalies in the region of the elbow are common. A more common problem, said by Spinner[40] to be present in as many as 70 percent of arms, is the arcade of Struthers, which is a fascial and sometimes muscular connection from the medial head of the triceps to the medial intermuscular septum that passes over the ulnar nerve. The anconeus epitrochlearis is occasionally present as an anomalous muscle and may cover the ulnar nerve in the cubital tunnel area, contributing to the possibility of entrapment. Other anomalous muscles that may cause nerve entrapment problems are (1) Gantzer's muscle, an anomalous head of the flexor pollicis longus or flexor profundus that usually originates from the medial epicondyle or the coronoid process of the ulna and occasionally is a factor in anterior interosseous nerve compression; (2) a solitary head of the supinator and other anomalies of this muscle; (3) accessory muscles of the anterolateral aspect of the elbow including the accessory brachialis or accessory brachioradialis; (4) variations in the head, origin, or insertion of the pronator teres; (5) variations of a similar nature in the flexor carpi radialis, the flexor carpi ulnaris, and the palmaris longus;[54] (6) an aberrant medial head of the triceps, which may snap over the medial epicondyle and irritate the ulnar nerve.[12]

Congenital Soft Tissue Tumors. Tumors of the soft tissue are rare but include a wide variety of abnormalities ranging from overgrowth to neoplasms and from multitissue hamartomas to single tissue entities. Probably most common in the infant is one of the fibromatoses; next in frequency is one of the vascular tumors. If the elbow area is involved, there is usually some limitation of motion.

Combined Bone and Soft Tissue Anomalies

Soft tissue anomalies may co-exist with mild osseous anomalies such as those related to the supracondyloid process.[9, 52, 54] The supracondyloid process is an anomalous bony prominence extending from the anteromedial aspect of the distal third of the humerus. Struthers[52] in 1848 described the ligament associated with this process, and since then various anomalies have been reported in connection with it. These include a more proximal branching of the ulnar artery off the brachial artery above the bony spur, a more proximal insertion of the pronator teres on the bony process, and various relationships of the neurovascular structures with bone and ligament. The symptoms are usually neuralgic—that is, pain, tingling, numbness, and so on—but they may be vascular.

Many of the congenital anomalies already discussed are manifest in both osseous and soft tissues but appear predominantly in one or the other. In this category the abnormalities of skin and soft tissue are roughly equal, as with the mild changes just described in association with the supracondyloid process. More severe changes are seen with severe pterygium cubitale and severe forms of ulnar hypoplasia and phocomelia. In pterygium cubitale, or congenital webbed elbow, a skin web extends from the upper arm across the volar elbow to the forearm. Flexion is usually possible, but extension, pronation, and supination are all severely limited. The muscles and neurovascular structures are incompletely developed. The bones are hypoplastic and deformed, and the elbow joint is often dislocated or severely hypoplastic. Fibrous strands represent missing muscles or tendons. Muscle hypoplasia is present posteriorly as well as anteriorly.

Severe ulnar hypoplasia is marked by radial head dislocation, diminishing segments (ranging from small to nonexistent) of the proximal ulna, variable but seldom normal motion and stability, and muscle and neurovascular abnormalities. Proximal to the elbow conditions are more normal, but distally more abnormalities are apparent; the ulnar forearm and hand structures are particularly dysplastic. Phocomelia may present with similar findings, or the elbow may be even more dysplastic or absent altogether (hand, wrist, or forearm may be attached directly to the shoulder or trunk).

TREATMENT OF BONE AND JOINT DYSPLASIAS

Treatment of Synostosis

The treatment of synostosis at the elbow level, whether radiohumeral[38] or ulnohumeral, is dictated by the position of the forearm-wrist-hand unit. Usually only one forearm bone is well represented and this is often bowed or deformed in some manner as well as short. In addition, there may be a rotational deformity. The forearm-wrist-hand unit may point directly posterior when the upper limb is in its usual dependent position beside the torso. It has been suggested that these rotational deformities can be corrected by derotation of the humeral shaft, perhaps even in the proximal humeral metaphysis. This is undoubtedly true, but there are usually multiplane deformities that must be corrected, and it is generally preferable to correct them at the site of maximum deformity—i.e., the humeral-forearm junction—perhaps extending the correction distally in the forearm (Fig. 11–13). In fact, the author's favorite method involves a posterior approach and a multiple-segment corrective osteotomy, making one or more of the segments trapezoidal in shape and rotating it 180 degrees, if necessary, to realign the unit as desired. If only one limb is involved, this desired position is usually at maximum length with the forearm, wrist, and hand in the midposition. Derotation should be accomplished in the direction that causes the least torsion of the neurovascular structures, commonly from an internally rotated position through a clockwise rotation to a forearm midposition. Hyperextension, if present, is corrected simply to neutral or slight flexion, and the osteotomy segments are adjusted to make the best contact in the desired position; a segment may be excised if this is needed for contouring. If both limbs are involved, enough elbow flexion angle should be

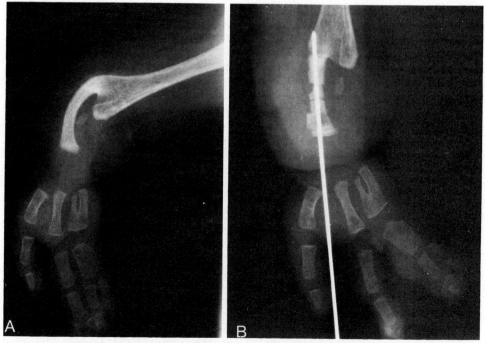

Figure 11–13. A, Typical radiohumeral synostosis with marked curving of the radial segment. B, A "shish kabob" corrective osteotomy was carried out with temporary internal fixation. Excellent correction resulted and there were no complications. The elbow synostosis resulted in a posterior pointing forearm, wrist, and hand.

included on one side to allow one of the limbs to reach the face and head.

Proximal forearm synostosis may occur with elbow synostosis, in which case the elbow is derotated as described previously. If, however, it occurs in the presence of a functioning elbow joint, derotation of the forearm alone may be required. Although many authors have attempted and a few have claimed success for passive and even active mobilization of the forearm,[5, 11, 14, 21, 27, 36] there is still no body of literature that substantiates these results in a significant number of patients who have been followed for an adequate period of time. When attempted, these procedures usually involve excision of the proximal radius including the synostotic mass, division of the entire length of the interosseous membrane, interposition of some material between the contact areas of the radius and the ulna, and tendon transfers such as rerouting the extensor carpi radialis longus to the volar wrist for supination and the flexor carpi radialis to the dorsal wrist for pronation. A similar procedure involving the interposition of a metallic swivel has been described by Kelikian and Doumanian,[27] but few long-term results have been described in the literature.

A more reliable procedure is that of derotation osteotomy.[21] This procedure is best outlined by Green and Mital,[19, 36] who perform the rotational osteotomy through the synostosis itself. The synostosis is approached through a dorsal incision and transversely osteotomized. A radioulnar (in the coronal plane) K-wire or Steinmann pin is then placed distal to the osteotomy site and is left protruding externally on both sides. A longitudinal (in the sagittal plane) pin is then placed from the olecranon across the osteotomy site, and corrective rotation is carried out as desired. In most instances, 70 to 90 degrees of rotation from pronation toward supination is required. If circulatory deficits appear during or after this derotation, less rotation is accepted, although an additional amount may be carried out 10 to 15 days later. The radioulnar pin may be fixed by either a plaster cast or an external fixation apparatus. Internal fixation should not be used because it may require alteration of forearm rotation to diminish circulatory difficulties. Goldner et al.[16] claim that these circulatory problems may be minimized by the use of derotation in the distal forearm (radius only in younger patients, radius and ulna in older patients). Their results have yet to appear in the literature except in abstract form, but the rationale seems reasonable and the technique appropriate. They recommend cross-pin fixation in children and plate fixation in adolescents or adults.

Treatment of Ankylosis

Ankylosis that does not involve synostosis, subluxation, or dislocation of the elbow may occur. Paralyses, muscle disease, and other soft tissue abnormalities commonly restrict motion; treatment of these is discussed elsewhere (see Chapters 37 and 38). Abnormalities of joint shape and joint cartilage occur but are usually treated only by physical therapy. Rotation ankylosis due to soft tissue abnormalities occurs but has minimal effect on the elbow; its treatment requires release not only of the proximal radioulnar area but also in the forearm and wrist.[4]

Treatment of Instability

Treatment of a dislocation of the radial head that is present at birth or shortly thereafter depends on the degree of hypoplasia present in the elbow area. If in doubt about the configuration of the various components of the elbow joint, an arthrogram should be performed;[39] this may show that there is no dislocation at all but merely a deformed elbow joint with the radiocapitellar joint displaced from the usual position. However, if a definite subluxation or dislocation of the radial head does exist and if a capitellum is present, reduction may be carried out as soon as the patient's general health and other priorities permit (Fig. 11–14). Most dislocations of the radial head are more unstable in pronation. If supination will reduce the dislocation completely, this should be done, followed by a period of support in that position. If reduction is not complete or is not maintained, open reduction may be carried out. Either a lateral, posterolateral, or posterior approach is satisfactory. The annular ligament, which is usually damaged or deficient and is often interposed between the radial head and the capitellum, should be repaired or reconstructed (reconstruction may be done by using a strip of triceps tendon left attached distally, looped around the radial neck, and then sutured to the adjacent ulna).[6, 14, 30, 36, 39, 46] Quadrate ligament hypoplasia may be a factor,[50] but reconstruction of this ligament has not been reported. The most stable configuration of the radial head against the capitellum should be obtained and temporarily fixed with a Kirschner-wire drilled from a posterior

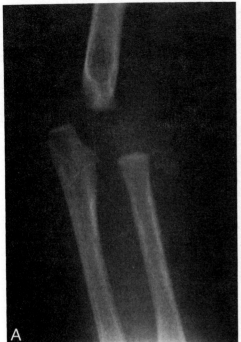

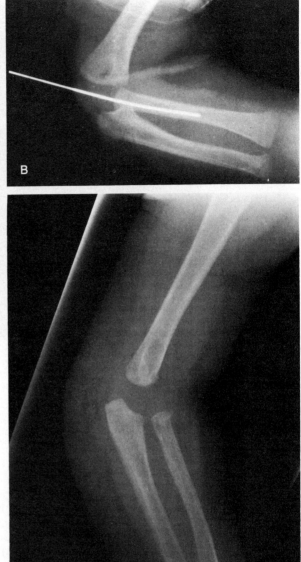

Figure 11–14. *A,* This x-ray view of an infant's elbow is difficult to interpret as abnormal, although the axial line of the radial shaft seems to be directed slightly more anteriorly than usual. Clinically, there was no question that this radial head clicked and moved into two different positions, one of which seemed more normal than the other. *B,* This abnormality was confirmed at surgery when the annular ligament was found to be interposed in the radiohumeral joint but would still permit reasonably normal alignment in one position (more then 90 degrees flexion). The ligament was removed from the joint, the joint was reduced, and the ligament was reconstructed in its normal position. Fixation was obtained by a transcondylar, transradial head K-wire (many current practitioners prefer a K-wire fixing the ulna to the radius rather than crossing the radiocapitellar joint). *C,* At 2 months after the operation the reduced position is maintained.

direction through the capitellum into the radial head with the radial head maintained in reduction and the elbow flexed at about 90 degrees. Although it is well recognized that fracture of the pin may occur, even in a cast, we have used this method routinely without encountering this complication. In some instances stability may not be satisfactory without shortening of the radial shaft, which is often best carried out at the midshaft of the radius.[14] This too can be fixed temporarily with a wire (Fig. 11–15).

The alternative to attempted reduction of congenital or infantile radial head dislocation is to accept the imposed disability (some limitation of forearm rotation ranging from a few degrees to more than 90 degrees, occasional limitation of elbow motion, and infrequent pain) and proceed with radial head excision, if needed, at maturity.[14, 15, 17, 26, 32, 49]

TREATMENT OF SOFT TISSUE DYSPLASIAS

Treatment of most soft tissue problems at the elbow level is discussed in other chapters. Arthrogryposis, as well as other flaccid palsies, is covered in Chapter 37. Spastic neurogenic problems are discussed in Chapter 38 and nerve entrapment around the elbow in Chapter 45. Successful treatment for other soft

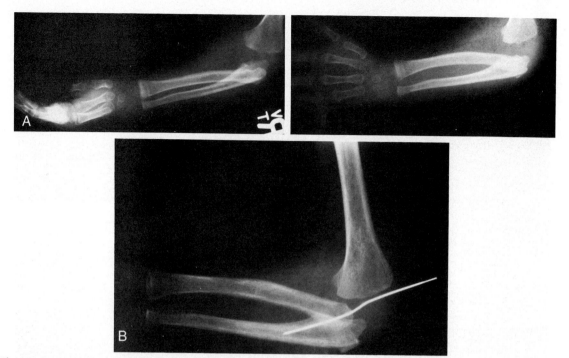

Figure 11–15. *A,* AP and lateral x-ray views of a radial head dislocation in a limb with other congenital anomalies. This completely fulfills the requirements usually listed for congenital dislocation; nevertheless, the dislocation may simply be developmental, related to the unequal length of the two forearm bones. Hypoplasia of the capitellum may be a factor, but hypoplasia of the ulna may be the principal factor. These x-rays are almost identical to the initial preoperative x-rays but represent recurrent dislocation after an initial procedure. Repositioning of the head and tightening of the capsule were the only procedures done at the first operation, but redislocation occurred. *B,* Postoperative lateral x-rays after open reduction of the dislocated radial head and internal fixation. A second operation was carried out a year later, at which time the radius was shortened and the annular ligaments were reconstructed; repeat reduction of the radial head was also performed.

tissue dysplasias at the elbow is rare. Aplasia cutis congenita has occurred in the elbow area. In the author's experience, it was associated with scarring and hypoplasia of the regional forearm muscles plus reactive deformity of the underlying bones. Resurfacing with a skin and subcutaneous flap was eventually necessary, followed by tendon transfers, which in this instance were required to provide extensor function of the wrist and hand. Muscle anomalies may result in either mechanical problems (snapping or catching)[12] or neurovascular entrapment as discussed in Chapter 45.

TREATMENT FOR COMBINED BONE AND SOFT TISSUE DYSPLASIAS

Pterygium cubitale remains an unsolved challenge. Attempts at treatment have included Z-plasty, skin grafts, and release of other tight structures. Improvement has been limited, and risks are high.[18, 26] Because there is no substantial report in the literature describing a reliable and useful method of treatment, for

the time being no recommendations for surgical treatment are offered. To my knowledge, techniques of bone shortening to permit a greater safe excursion of the neurovascular structures or techniques of vascular and nerve grafting have not yet been attempted. The hands in pterygium cubitale are often deficient also, but because limited excursion of the elbow is available in flexion, they are at least usually able to reach the upper trunk, face and head.

In severe forms of ulnar dysplasia the elbow often displays adequate range and stability. Occasionally the displaced radial head is sufficiently limiting or symptom-provoking that treatment is offered. Although excision of the radial head and a sufficient portion of the shaft to resolve the mechanical block might suffice, the desire to stabilize and lengthen the forearm plus the fear of recurrent encroachment by the radial shaft usually lead to a recommendation for a one-bone forearm procedure (Fig. 11–16).[7] This is carried out as follows:

1. Use a long lateral incision that covers

the distal half of the arm, elbow, and proximal half of the forearm.

2. Mobilize the anterior flap, identify and protect the radial nerve, and identify and mobilize the anteriorly and radially dislocated radius.

3. Mobilize the posterior flap, identify the short ulnar fragment, and uncover the interosseous space.

4. With both bones visualized through both anterior and posterior intervals (obviously the procedure can be done through an anterior approach only or through a proximal anterior and a distal posterior approach, but I have found that access and safety are preferable this way), the maximum forearm length that the soft tissue will accept is judged by manual displacement.

5. The radius is then osteotomized at the length just determined, and the proximal fragment is removed.

6. The distal fragment is aligned with the short ulnar fragment, and contact is maintained by an intramedullary pin drilled through the olecranon, along the ulnar medullary cavity, across the osteotomy site, and along the radial intramedullar space until it penetrates the radial cortex at some point. (The forearm position—usually the midportion—should be set before this distal penetration occurs.)

7. The usual support dressings (long arm splint-dressing combination initially, perhaps changed to a long arm cast later for the older child) are used until healing occurs (4 to 6 weeks). The supports are then discontinued, and the pin is removed.

In phocomelia the elbow is seldom the site of the infrequent surgical attention given to this condition, but there may be an occasional indication for a one-bone forearm procedure or for simultaneous lengthening and stabilization at an unstable elbow segment.[47]

Obviously, many of the surgical procedures used for congenital anomalies in the elbow area are not yet developed or are unproved.

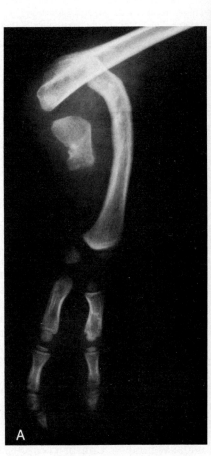 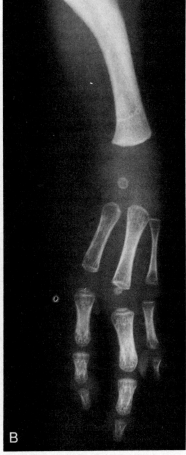

Figure 11–16. *A*, A lateral view of an elbow in ulnar agenesis shows an apparent dislocation proximally and anteriorly of the radial head. Clinical findings suggested that this was a true dislocation. *B*, There is occasional need for excision of the dislocated radial head and combination of the proximal ulna and distal radius to form a one-bone forearm as seen here. This changes both the appearance and the function of the elbow as well as the forearm (the range of motion of the elbow is usually improved; the forearm position becomes fixed).

Table 11–2. **Summary of Indications and Contraindications**

Congenital Bone or Joint Dysplasias

Humeroradial synostosis: Corrective osteotomy

Indications:	1. Nonfunctional position of hand
	2. Cosmetic deficiency of hand position
Contraindication:	Acceptable cosmetic and functional hand position

Proximal radioulnar synostosis: Corrective osteotomy

Indications and contraindications are the same as those listed for humeroradial synostosis. In both instances correction may need to be staged if circulatory deficits are noted.

Dislocation of radial head: Open reduction

Indications:	1. Near-normal appearance of bone and joint structures
	2. Failure of closed reduction
	3. Short-term (less than 1 year) presence of dislocation
Contraindications:	1. Dysplastic bone or joint structures, particularly when dislocation is actually a malformation
	2. Successful closed reduction
	3. Long-term dislocation (more than 1 year)

Dislocation of radial head: Excision

Indications:	1. Pain due to the dislocation
	2. Limitation of motion due to the dislocation
	3. Neural or vascular impingement from the dislocated head
Contraindications:	1. Presence of continued physis growth
	2. Likelihood of increasing elbow or forearm instability
	3. Likelihood of progressive forearm shortening

Congenital Soft Tissue Dysplasias

Procedures for arthrogryposis, spastic and flaccid palsies, anomalous structures, nerve entrapments, and tumors are covered in other chapters. Procedures are occasionally required for other problems, but there is no standard procedure.

Congenital Combined Bone, Joint, and Soft Tissue Dysplasias

Severe ulnar hemimelia: One-bone forearm procedure

Indications:	1. Limitation of elbow motion (30 percent or more)
	2. Discomfort, instability during useful function is a noticeable and annoying deformity
Contraindications:	1. Comfortable, functional arc of elbow range of motion
	2. Patient requires forearm motion

For those few procedures that can be considered standard at this time a short summary of indications, contraindications, and results is offered (Tables 11–2 and 11–3).

COMPLICATIONS

Unwarranted Treatment Due to Misdiagnosis. This problem, present in any medical management situation, is a particular hazard with congenital anomalies. In the infant, testing of the neurovascular supply, dynamic and static control elements, and structural and support elements is difficult and uncertain. Interpretation of x-rays when so much of the skeletal tissue is still cartilaginous is deceptive. Nevertheless, the best review possible is needed if surgery is contemplated. This may require examination under sedation or special radiographic techniques such as arthrography or CT scans or combinations of these, image intensifier motion and stress studies, and others.

Infection. This is a serious problem after any surgical procedure, and the usual wound management preventive measures are employed. The ability to apply a splint-dressing that will maintain the desired position and stay in place is very important in infants. Also important is a high index of suspicion; dressing removal and wound inspection are carried out if there is any doubt about infection.

Vascular Compromise. Vascular damage due to direct insults, compartment pressure increase, or indirect damage from stretch or torsion does occur. The stretch-torsion injury is a particular risk in the corrective osteotomies used to treat synostosis. For this reason circulation should be checked during the osteotomy procedure. For osteotomies in the proximal forearm or elbow, fixation that can be moved or adjusted to decrease vascular stress is necessary. The circulatory pattern is almost always abnormal; if an extensive alteration is anticipated, preliminary angiography may be helpful.

Nerve Damage. Nerve injury due to dissection or compression at anatomic entrapment points during postoperative reaction, stretch, or torque stress may also occur. Torque stress can usually be controlled by monitoring the effect of the stress on the vascular supply. The other possibilities are best controlled by adequate exposure and careful dissection.

Physis Damage. Partial or total destruction of the physis may result from bone cutting, pin or other fixation, or damage to the local physis circulation. Care should be taken to avoid it, particularly because most such limbs are hypoplastic and short already. A pin passing near the center and at right angles to the plate of the physis may do no serious damage, but other modes of fixation and other positions should be avoided.

Joint Damage. Incongruous, malformed, and abnormally surfaced joints are common with congenital problems, and the investing soft tissue, motor units, and even skin may also limit normal joint function. Careful preservation of the available joint structures is therefore important, and this includes avoiding pin breakage in the elbow joint. Many surgeons, for instance, fix the ulna and radius rather than the humerus and radius to minimize the chances of intra-articular pin breakage after radial head reduction. Recurring elbow or forearm stiffness after operations for congenital elbow area anomalies is the most depressingly common complication of all. Suppression of scar formation and early continuous passive motion should help, and both treatments should be available soon.

Table 11–3. **Results of Surgery**

Congenital Bone and Joint Dysplasias

Elbow synostosis: Corrective osteotomy
  Goal of functional or cosmetic repositioning of the functional unit, the hand, is nearly always achieved, although full correction may require two stages of the same operation or two operations.

Proximal forearm synostosis: Corrective osteotomy[16, 19, 36]
  Same as for elbow synostosis.

Elbow synostosis: Mobilization for range of motion
  Experience inadequate for comment.

Proximal forearm synostosis: Mobilization for range of motion[2, 5, 6, 14, 27, 30, 34, 36]
  There is much experience, but most of it has achieved poor results or reasonable results not confirmed by others.

Radial head dislocation: Excision[14, 15, 17, 26, 32, 49]
  Results are good if excision is deferred until bone growth ceases, although range of motion does not always improve.

Radial head dislocation: Open reduction and reconstruction of ligament[6, 14, 30, 36, 39, 46]
  The body of experience here is small, with more hearsay than documented reports. Furthermore, the more dysplastic the radiographic and clinical (operative) appearance of the elbow structures, the less likely the result is to be satisfactory. This may mean that instances in which a successful result is obtained are post-traumatic dislocations or subluxations and not truly congenital dislocations.

Elbow dislocation: Open reduction
  Experience with surgical treatment is too limited to comment.

Elbow malformation: Reconstruction
  Same as that described for elbow dislocation

Congenital Soft Tissue Dysplasias

Elbow contracture: Release
  Experience with these problems due to congenital causes (most are post-traumatic) is too variable for meaningful comment. The mild contractures are seldom treated, and the severe ones involve bone and joint as well as soft tissues. Some are due to tissue absence (aplasia cutis) or abnormal tissue (fibromatosis, hemangiomatosis), and primary treatment is directed at the tissue absence, excess, or abnormality. Results, reported individually, are highly variable.

Elbow Control Problems

All surgical results for this condition are reported in other chapters.

Elbow Muscle Anomalies and Nerve Entrapments

Surgical results are reported in other chapters.

Congenital Bone, Joint, and Soft Tissue Dysplasias

Elbow contracture: Release
  This is an even more difficult surgical procedure than that needed when soft tissues only are involved, and attempts to date have given poor results.

Elbow instability correlated with short ulna and dislocated radius: One-bone forearm procedure
  Results are excellent, but only a small percentage of patients with this problem need treatment.

Elbow instability correlated with dislocation or extreme hypoplasia of all joint structures: Stabilization
  Experience here is minimal and is associated almost entirely with phocomelia. No meaningful comment about results can be made.

Summary

Congenital elbow dysplasia is a more common problem than is generally realized. If mild, elbow function is minimally affected; if severe, problems of the entire limb or the wrist and hand often take precedence. In the few instances when the elbow abnormality is isolated and relatively severe, surgical assistance is available but is less than satisfying. The most provoking problem is that of radial head subluxation-dislocation, in which the abnormality may be partly truly congenital, traumatic, and developmental (resulting from congenital, traumatic, infectious, tumor, or other cause). Progress in management of these problems is long overdue.

References

1. Abbott, F. C.: Congenital Dislocation of Radius. Lancet 1:800, 1892.
2. Almquist, E. E., Gordon, L. H., and Blue, A. L.: Congenital Dislocation of the Head of the Radius. J. Bone Joint Surg. 51A:1118, 1969.
3. Bailey, J. A.: Elbow and Other Upper Limb Deformities in Achondroplasia. Clin. Orthop. 80:75, 1971.
4. Bert, J. M., McElfresh, E. C., and Linscheid, R. L.: Rotary Contracture of the Forearm. J. Bone Joint Surg. 62A:1163, 1980.
5. Brady, L. P., and Jewett, E. L.: A New Treatment of Radio-ulnar Synostosis. South. Med. J. 53:507, 1960.
6. Brennan, J. J., Krause, M. E. H., and Harvey, D. M.: Annular Ligament Construction for Congenital Anterior Dislocation of Both Radial Heads. Clin. Orthop. 29:205, 1963.
7. Broudy, A. S., and Smith, R. J.: Deformities of the Hand and Wrist with Ulnar Deficiency. J. Hand Surg. 4:304, 1979.
8. Caravias, D. E.: Some Observations on Congenital Dislocations of the Head of the Radius. J. Bone Joint Surg. 39B:86, 1957.
9. Crotti, F. M., et al.: Supracondyloid Process and Anomalous Insertion of Pronator Teres as Sources of Median Nerve Neuralgia. J. Neurolog. Sci. 25:41, 1981.
10. Danielsson, L. G., and Theander, G.: Traumatic Dislocation of the Radial Head at Birth. Acta Radiolog. 22:379, 1981.
11. Dawson, H. G. W.: A Congenital Deformity of the Forearm and Its Operative Treatment. Br. Med. J. 2:833, 1912.
12. Dreyfuss, U., and Kessler, I.: Snapping Elbow Due to Dislocation of the Medial Head of the Triceps. J. Bone Joint Surg. 60B:56, 1978.
13. Falvo, K. A., and Freidenberg, Z. B.: Osteo-Onychodysplasia. Clin. Orthop. 81:130, 1971.
14. Ferguson, A. B., Jr.: Orthopedic Surgery in Infancy and Childhood. 2nd ed. Baltimore , The Williams & Wilkins Co., 1963.
15. Fox, K. W., and Griffen, L. L.: Congenital Dislocation of the Radial Head. Clin. Orthop. 18:234, 1960.
16. Goldner, J. L., and Lipton, M. A.: Congenital Radioulnar Synostosis: Diagnosis and Treatment Based on Anatomic and Functional Assessment. Orthop. Transac. 6:466, 1982.
17. Good, C. J., and Wicks, M. H.: Developmental Posterior Dislocation of the Radial Head. J. Bone Joint Surg. 65B:64, 1983.
18. Green , D. C.: Operative Hand Surgery. New York, Churchill-Livingstone, 1982, pp. 267–277; 308–312.
19. Green, W. T., and Mital, M. A.: Congenital Radioulnar Synostosis: Surgical Treatment. J. Bone Joint Surg. 61A:738, 1979.
20. Gunn, D. R., and Pillay, V. K.: Congenital Posterior Dislocation of the Head of the Radius. Clin. Orthop. 34:108, 1964.
21. Hansen, O. H., and Anderson, N. O.: Congenital Radio-ulnar Synostosis: Report of 37 cases. Acta Orthop. Scand. 41:225, 1970.
22. Hoffer, M. M.: Joint Motion Limitation in Newborns. Clin. Orthop. 148:94, 1980.
23. Hollister, D. W., and Lachman, R. S.: Diastrophic Dwarfism. Clin. Orthop. 114:61, 1976.
24. Kaitila, I. I., Leistei, J. T., and Rimoin, D. L.: Mesomelic Skeletal Dysplasias. Clin. Orthop. 114:94, 1976.
25. Kaufmann, H. J.: Classification of the Skeletal Dysplasias and of the Radiologic Approach to Their Differentiation. Clin. Orthop. 114:12, 1976.
26. Kelikian, H.: Congenital Deformities of the Hand and Forearm. Philadelphia, W. B. Saunders Co., 1974, pp. 310–407, 714–752, 902–975.
27. Kelikian, H., and Doumanian, A.: Swivel for Proximal Radio-ulnar Synostosis. J. Bone Joint Surg. 39A:945, 1957.
28. Kelly, D. W.: Congenital Dislocation of the Radial Head Spectrum and Natural History. J. Pediatr. Orthop. 1(3):245, 1981.
29. Lenz, W.: Genetics and Limb Deficiencies. Clin. Orthop. 148:9, 1980.
30. Lloyd-Roberts, G. C., and Bucknill, T. M.: Anterior Dislocation of the Radial Head in Children: Aetiology, Natural History and Management. J. Bone Joint Surg. 59B:402, 1977.
31. Mann, R. A., Johnston, J. O., and Ford, J.: Developmental Posterior Dislocation of the Radial Head: Ten Cases Resulting from Ulnar Hypoplasia. Presented at the 38th Annual Meeting of the Western Orthopedic Association, Honolulu, Hawaii, October 5–12, 1974.
32. Mardam-Bey, T., and Ger, E.: Congenital Radial Head Dislocation. J. Hand Surg. 4:316, 1979.
33. McCredie, J.: Congenital Fusion of Bones: Radiology, Embryology, and Pathogenesis. Clin. Radiol. 26:47, 1975.
34. McFarland, B.: Congenital Dislocation of the Head of the Radius. Br. J. Surg. 24:41, 1936.
35. McKusick, V. A.: Mendelian Inheritance in Man. 6th ed. Baltimore, The Johns Hopkins Press, 1983.
36. Mitral, M. A.: Congenital Radioulnar Synostosis and Congenital Dislocation of the Radial Head. Orthop. Clin. North Am. 7:375, 1976.
37. Murakami, Y., and Komiyama, Y.: Hypoplasia of the Trochlea and the Medial Epicondyle of the Humerus Associated with Ulnar Neuropathy. J. Bone Joint Surg. 60B:225, 1978.
38. Murphy, H. S., and Hansen, C. G.: Congenital Humeroradial Synostosis. J. Bone Joint Surg. 27:712, 1945.
39. Ogden, J. A.: Skeletal Injury in the Child. Philadelphia, Lea & Febiger, Pennsylvania, 1982, pp. 319–321.
40. Omer, G. E., and Spinner, M. (eds.): Management of Peripheral Nerve Problems. Philadelphia, W. B. Saunders Co., 1980.
41. Pfeiffer, R.: Die angeborene Verrenkung des Speichenkopfchens als Teilerscheinung anderer kongenitaler Ellenbogengelenkmissbildungen. Mensch. Vererb. Konstitutionslehre 21:530, 1938.

42. Phillips, S.: Congenital Dislocation of Radii. Brit. Med. J. 1:773, 1883.
43. Powers, C. A.: Congenital Dislocations of the Radius. J.A.M.A. 41:165, 1903.
44. Ryan, J. R.: The Relationship of the Radial Head to Radial Neck Diameters in Fetuses and Adults with Reference to Radial Head Subluxation in Children. J. Bone Joint Surg. 51A:781, 1969.
45. Salter, R., and Zaltz, C.: Anatomic Investigations of the Mechanism of Injury and Pathologic Anatomy of "Pulled Elbow" in Children. Clin. Orthop. 77:134, 1971.
46. Schubert, J. J.: Dislocation of the Radial Head in the Newborn Infant. J. Bone Joint Surg. 47A:1019, 1965.
47. Smith, R. J., and Lipke, R. W.: Treatment of Congenital Deformities of the Hand and Forearm, Part II. N. Engl. J. Med. 300:402, 1979.
48. Smith, R. W.: Congenital Luxations of the Radius. Dublin Q. J. Med. Sci. 13:208, 1852.
49. Southmayd, W., and Ehrlich, M. G.: Idiopathic Sub-luxation of the Radial Head. Clin. Orthop. 121:271, 1976.
50. Spinner, M., and Kaplan, E. B.: Quadrate Ligament of the Elbow, Relation to the Stability of the Proximal Radioulnar Joint. Orthop. Scand. 41:623, 1970.
51. Stone, C. A.: Subluxation of the Head of the Radius: Report of a Case and Anatomical Experiments. J.A.M.A. 1:28, 1916.
52. Struthers, J.: A Peculiarity of the Humerus and Humeral Artery. Monthly J. Med. Sci. 28:264, 1848.
53. Temtamy, S. A., and McKusick, V. A.: Carpal/tarsal Synostosis. Birth Defects 14:502, 1978.
54. Tubiana, R.: The Hand. Philadelphia, W. B. Saunders Col, 1981.
55. Windfeld, P.: On Congenital and Acquired Luxation of the Capitellum Radii with Discussion of Some Associated Problems. Acta Orthop. Scand. 16:126, 1946.
56. Wynne-Davies, R.: Heritable Disorders in Orthopaedic Practice. Oxford, Blackwell Scientific Publications, 1973.

CHAPTER 12

Supracondylar Fractures of the Elbow in Children

RUDOLPH A. KLASSEN

Supracondylar, dicondylar, transcondylar, and intercondylar fractures of the humerus represent 50 to 60 percent of all fractures about the elbow in children. Holmberg[49] and Lipscomb[59a] reported that 60 to 70 percent of these fractures occurred in boys aged 4 to 10, and the left elbow is involved almost twice as frequently as the right.[19, 26, 28, 49, 59a, 61, 63, 64, 83b] Current authors show an equal sex ratio.[45, 48, 66, 67, 70, 81, 83, 94] Left-sided fractures probably occur more often because the left arm is more frequently used in the motion of protection and guarding when falling. Ninety-eight percent of these fractures occur when falling with the arm extended and the wrist in dorsiflexion at the moment of impact. In about 65 percent of fractures the distal fragment is displaced medially and posteriorly, and in the rest it is displaced laterally or directly posteriorly; the fracture line is usually angled posteriorly (Fig. 12–1). Fractures occurring with the elbow in the flexed position at the moment of impact result in either an anteriorly displaced distal fragment (Fig. 12–2) or, if there is a direct blow to the elbow, an intercondylar fracture (Fig. 12–3).[61, 64, 70, 72]

HISTORICAL REVIEW

Orthopedists have shown a great interest in the management of supracondylar fractures during the past century, producing a voluminous literature on the subject. Bardenheuer in 1889 introduced skin traction with the elbow in a right-angled position.[42] Roberts in 1892 noted that of 103 surgeons 86 percent preferred to treat supracondylar fractures with closed reduction and splinting with the elbow in a flexed position at right angles. The rest advocated keeping the elbow in extension to control angular and rotational deformities.[32, 78a] Smith in 1893 performed a series of experimental supracondylar fractures in ca-

davers and noted that extension-type fractures were best reduced with the elbow in acute flexion and pronation.[84] Poland in 1898 suggested that many persistent deformities following supracondylar fractures were secondary to injuries of the physis and subsequent altered growth.[73] Ingebrigtsen introduced overhead traction in 1908.[42, 45] Hey Groves in 1916 and Attenborough in 1953 noted that absolute anatomic reduction of the fracture fragments was not necessary to achieve an "excellent" functional result.[7, 41a] The fragments could be left translocated medially or laterally as long as they were not tilted. The distal fragment could be left in a moderately retroverted or anteverted position as long as the overall alignment was maintained. Remodeling of the fracture would result in excellent function in the young child.[7]

Bauman in 1929 disputed Poland's observation and indicated that the deformities were due to malunion, not physeal injury.[11] Key in 1924 described management of supracondylar fractures by using percutaneous fixation with Kirschner-type pins.[15] Bohler in 1930, like Smith in 1893, advised reduction with placement of the forearm in pronation.[15b] Bergenfeldt in 1932 used both medial and lateral condylar pinning techniques, noting that although these pins could cause epiphyseal injury there was no significant deformity in his patients from this cause. He also demonstrated that persistent deformity was due to malunion, not to growth disturbance.[15] Collie in 1933 reported excellent results in the management of these fractures with the use of overhead traction and an olecranon pin.[15] In 1929 Dunlop demonstrated that straight lateral traction resulted in a high degree of success with minimal neurovascular or malunion complications.[28, 26] MacLemman in 1947, recounting his experience since 1911, strongly advised open reduction and internal

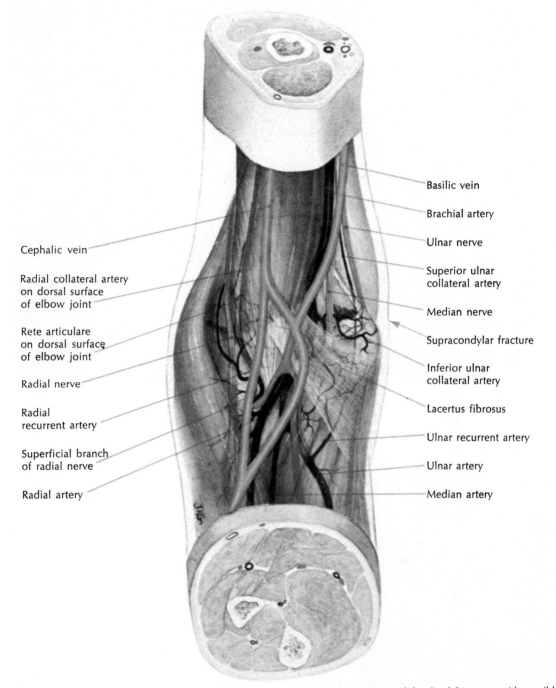

Cephalic vein

Radial collateral artery
on dorsal surface
of elbow joint

Rete articulare
on dorsal surface
of elbow joint

Radial nerve

Radial
recurrent artery

Superficial branch
of radial nerve

Radial artery

Basilic vein

Brachial artery

Ulnar nerve

Superior ulnar
collateral artery

Median nerve

Supracondylar fracture

Inferior ulnar
collateral artery

Lacertus fibrosus

Ulnar recurrent artery

Ulnar artery

Median artery

Figure 12–1. Most supracondylar fractures result in posterior and medial displacement of the distal fragment, with possible injury of the brachial artery and median nerve by the distal end of the proximal fragment, as well as stretching of the radial and ulnar nerves. (From Micheli, L. J., et al.: Supracondylar fractures in the humerus of children. Am. Fam. Phys. 19(3):111, 1979.)

fixation of displaced supracondylar fractures.[63] Current methods of management employ the principles set forth by these authors because little has been added in the last fifty years in the management and understanding of this problem.

ANATOMY

The basic anatomy of the elbow joint, radiographic techniques, pediatric roentgenographic anatomy and elbow dislocations are all addressed in other chapters (see Chapters

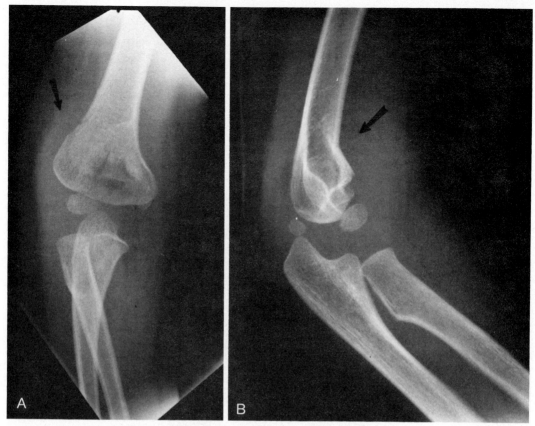

Figure 12–2. *A,* Flexion type of supracondylar fracture with anterior and medial angulation. *B,* Lateral view. Note also that what appears to be an avulsion of the medial epicondyle is really due to the rotation of the distal humerus and obliquity of the film.

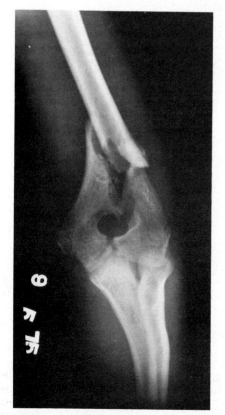

Figure 12–3. Intercondylar fracture in a 14-year-old boy due to a direct fall on the elbow.

Figure 12–4. An experimentally produced fracture shows the medial periosteal hinge and offers a glimpse of the posterior hinge. After reduction, the soft tissues hold the fragments in place. The better the reduction, the greater the security. (From Rang, M.: Children's Fractures, 2nd ed. Philadelphia, J. B. Lippincott Company, 1983.)

Figure 12–5. *A,* Transverse and sagittal sections of distal humerus. The shaft diameter is wide above the supracondylar foramen. *B,* However, if a cut is made through the supracondylar foramen, the "bicolumnar" nature of this region becomes evident, as seen in *C* looking proximally, and in *D* looking distally. (From Ogden, J.: Skeletal Injury in the Child. Philadelphia, Lea & Febiger, 1983.)

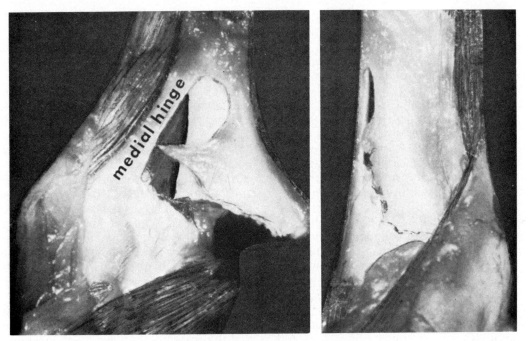

Figure 12–4. *See legend on opposite page*

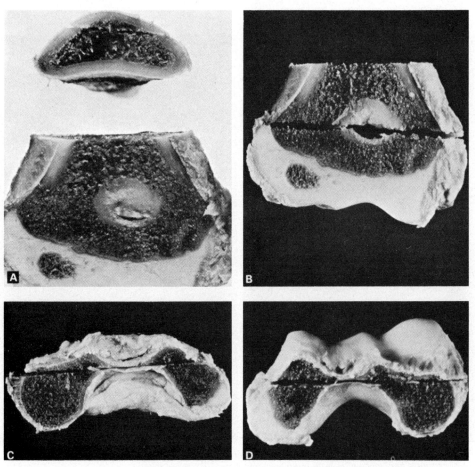

Figure 12–5. *See legend on opposite page*

2, 6, 10, and 16). Graham's anatomic observations are of interest, however, because they assist in management of these fractures. He noted that the stability of the elbow is achieved by bony and soft tissue structures.[39, 40, 70, 77] Soft tissue stability on the lateral aspect of the elbow is provided by an expansion of the triceps, anconeus, brachioradialis, and extensor carpi radialis longus. Extension of the triceps mechanism provides posterior posterior stability as well. The thickened periosteum of a young child, both medially and laterally, is an important additional stabilizer of the fracture fragment and provides a medial or lateral hinge that is used as a tether during attempted reduction (Fig. 12–4). The distal humeral fragment is also locked into the ulna through the olecranon and the trochlea. The distinctive shape of the humeral metaphysis with the medial and lateral condyles and columns (Fig. 12–5) and the narrow midpoint of the olecranon fossa (which Rang likens to a fishtail configuration) adds to the instability of the fracture, particularly when there is distal rotation and tilting of the fragments.[70, 71] In most instances the fragment line is oblique in the sagittal as well

as the anteroposterior plane, which adds to the anatomic instability (Fig. 12–6).

Angular deformities, varus or valgus, are the most common complications in the management of these fractures. Therefore, the normal variations in pediatric anatomy should be understood. The carrying angle of the elbow joint in children is not constant.[2, 85] Smith noted that of 150 children aged 3 to 11 the carrying angle in boys averaged 5.4 degrees and ranged from 0 to 11 degrees, whereas in girls it averaged 6 degrees and ranged from 0 to 12 degrees. Nine percent had no carrying angle, and 48 percent had a carrying angle of less than 5 degrees (Figs. 12–7 and 12–8).[85] Aebi noted that in clinical measurements of 100 patients the carrying angle in males averaged 6.5 degrees, ranging from 0 to 14 degrees; in females it averaged 13 degrees with a range of 4 to 20 degrees.[2] He also observed that the measurements were not constant and changed as the child matured. After fracture the radiographic evaluation of the carrying angle resulted in a 50 percent error in correlating diagnosis and prognosis using standard anteroposterior films. Aebi therefore used a clinical method of assessing the carrying an-

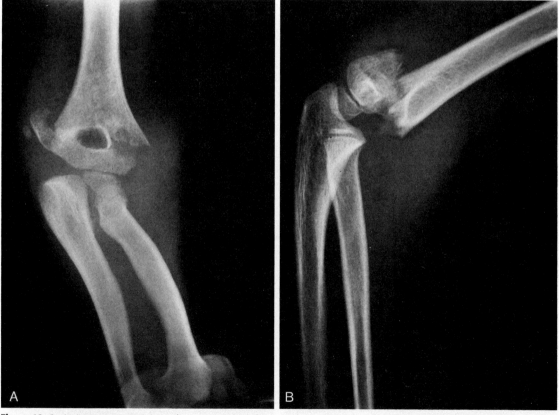

Figure 12–6. *A,* Anteroposterior view of a supracondylar fracture. Note the medial obliquity; *B,* Note the posterior obliquity; this is the most common displacement seen in these fractures.

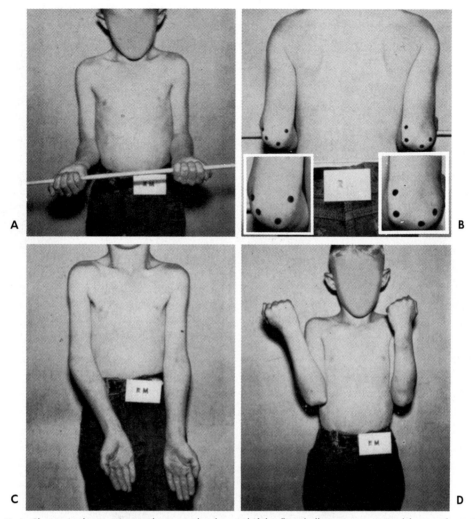

Figure 12–7. *A,* Change in the carrying angle cannot be detected if the flexed elbows are examined from in front. *B,* Change in the carrying angle is quite apparent, however, if the flexed elbows are examined posteriorly. On the right, the bone prominences (marked with black dots) can be seen to have tilted medially. *C,* With the arms extended, a 25-degree varus deformity of the right arm can be seen in a 9-year-old boy 2 years after a supracondylar fracture of the right arm. There is no limitation of motion. Note that the normal carrying angle of the left arm is 0 degrees. *D,* When the varus elbow is acutely flexed, the hand points laterally away from the shoulder joint. This view also demonstrates the medial tilt of the bone prominences. (From Smith, L.: Deformity following supracondylar fractures. J. Bone Joint Surg. 42A:236, 1960.)

gle deformity by measuring the angles subtended by lines drawn from the midpoint of the wrist to the midpoint of the antecubital space and the midpoint of the humeral head to the antecubital space. The elbows were fully extended, and the humerus was externally rotated with the forearm supinated.[2] Gray, quoted by Smith, used the visual method of observation and compared the results with those from the opposite elbow.[85] Bauman described a radiographic method of evaluation, observing that a line drawn along the axis of the humerus and a line drawn along the physeal line of the capitellum sub-

tended at angle of 70 to 75 degrees (see Fig. 12–9). The angles of both the normal and injured elbows must be measured and compared.

CLASSIFICATION AND ROENTGENOGRAPHIC EVALUATION

Fractures of the distal humerus are classified according to their level of fracture. Supracondylar and transcondylar fractures are identical fractures in terms of etiology and treatment

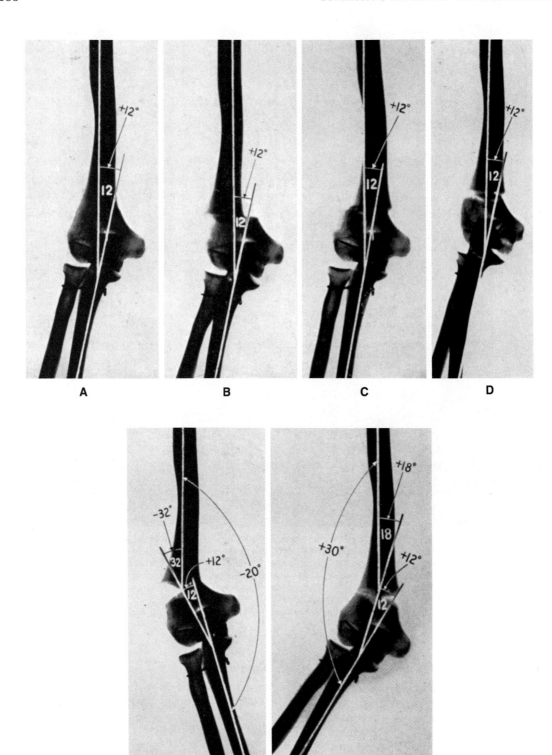

Figure 12–8. Effect on the carrying angle of various displacements of the fragments. *A,* The carrying angle of this elbow is 12 degrees of valgus. *B,* The distal fragment is displaced medially, and the carrying angle did not change from its 12 degrees. *C,* The carrying angle does not change with lateral displacement of the distal fragment. *D,* The distal fragment is rotated internally 15 degrees, and the carrying angle does not change. *E,* The distal fragment is tilted medially 32 degrees, and the carrying angle changes to 20 degrees of varus. *F,* The distal fragment is tilted laterally 18 degrees, and the carrying angle increases to 30 degrees of valgus. (From Smith, L.: Deformity following supracondylar fractures. J. Bone Joint Surg. 42A:238, 1960.)

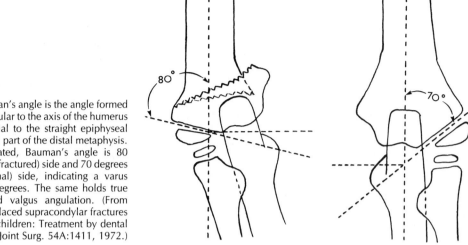

Figure 12–9. Bauman's angle is the angle formed by a line perpendicular to the axis of the humerus and a line tangential to the straight epiphyseal border of the lateral part of the distal metaphysis. In the case illustrated, Bauman's angle is 80 degrees on the left (fractured) side and 70 degrees on the right (normal) side, indicating a varus angulation of 10 degrees. The same holds true for lateral tilt and valgus angulation. (From Dodge, H. S.: Displaced supracondylar fractures of the humerus in children: Treatment by dental extraction. J. Bone Joint Surg. 54A:1411, 1972.)

but occur at slightly different levels above or through the olecranon fossa. Epiphyseal injuries are rare (see Chapter 13).[15, 66, 73] Intercondylar fractures are also uncommon in children, usually occurring in the more mature adolescent and adult.[68]

Numerous classifications of these fractures have been devised. Most consider (1) the mechanism of injury, (2) the degree of displacement, (3) the degree of angulation and displacement, and (4) displacement and its relationship to prognosis. These fractures are best classified, defined, and evaluated radiographically.[79] Fractures in a young child with incomplete ossification of the elbow are often the most difficult to define, and comparative views of the uninjured elbow are often imperative for proper assessment of the injury. The anterior or posterior fat pad sign may be positive. That is, elevation of the soft tissue structures from the bone in the supracondylar area is frequently a clue that the fracture has occurred in this area even if bony deformity is not initially evident. Bauman's angle in the anteroposterior projection (Fig. 12–9) and the anterior humeral line in the lateral projection (Fig. 12–10) should be drawn and the relationship to the metaphysis and capitellum noted. Normally, the anterior humeral line will transect the capitellum through its middle third, denoting normal anteversion.[11]

Bergenfeldt relates that Kocher preferred a classification of fractures according to the mechanism of injury and the radiographic findings, and defined them simply as flexion- and extension-type fractures.[15] Holmberg expanded on this classification and divided the fractures into four categories: (1) none or minimally displaced, tilted, or rotated, (2)

moderate displacement, (3) moderate displacement with rotational deformity, and (4) marked displacement.[49]

Rogers and El-Ahwany's classifications are perhaps most useful in achieving an understanding of these fractures and relating the changes seen to the management and prognosis. Each of these classifications emphasizes some factor that is useful in defining and managing supracondylar fractures. Rogers divided Holmberg's type I fractures as follows: (1) incomplete fractures due to plastic

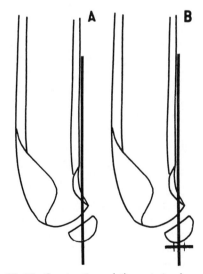

Figure 12–10. Construction of the anterior humeral line (AHL). *A,* A line is drawn down the anterior humeral cortex. *B,* A second line is drawn perpendicular to the AHL from the anterior to the posterior extent of the capitellum. This line is divided into thirds. In normal cases the AHL passes through the middle third of the capitellum. (From Rogers, L. F., et al.: Plastic bowing, torus and greenstick supracondylar fractures of the humerus: Radiographic clues to obscure fractures of the elbow in children. Radiology 128:146, 1978.)

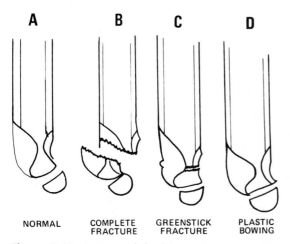

A **B** **C** **D**

NORMAL   COMPLETE   GREENSTICK   PLASTIC
          FRACTURE   FRACTURE   BOWING

Figure 12–11. *A,* A normal distal humerus as seen on the lateral view with 40 degrees anteversion of the capitellum. *B,* Complete fracture with separation and posterior displacement of the distal fragment. *C,* Combination of greenstick fracture (anterior cortex) and a torus fracture (posterior cortex). *D,* In plastic bowing fractures there is a change in the normal anteversion of the distal humerus. No fracture can be identified. (From Rogers, L. F., et al.: Plastic bowing, torus and greenstick supracondylar fractures of the humerus: Radiographic clues to obscure fractures of the elbow in children. Radiology 128:146, 1978.)

onstrates the tilting of the distal fragment, whereas the lateral view shows rotation best. These are the views that are most helpful following reduction of the fracture (Fig. 12–12). Using this radiographic technique, five types of fractures are defined: (1) A fracture that passes transversely through the olecranon fossa with minimal displacement. (2) A fracture in which the fracture line begins above the capitellum and extends through the olecranon fossa and then descends medially. (3) A short oblique fracture in which the fracture line passes obliquely from lateral to medial. Displacement is usually medial, rotation is common, temporary neurovascular compromise is present in 20 percent of these cases, and malunion and cubitus varus are common. (4) A common fracture that passes obliquely from medial to lateral. Displacement is usually lateral, and external rotation of the medial fragment is common. Eighty percent of these patients had neurovascular compromise requiring treatment. Malunion for cubitus valgus may occur. (5) A transcondylar fracture distal to the olecranon fossa. It is often angled anteriorly, the lesion being more common after age 6 (Fig. 12–13).

bowing, (2) torus or impacted fractures, and (3) greenstick fractures (Fig. 12–11).[79] Accurate radiographic analysis must be made to prevent malunion in these fractures. Hendrickson classified these fractures according to the appearance of the lateral roentgenogram as follows: (1) no displacement, (2) apical angulation of less than 20 degrees dorsally and anterior displacement of less than the breadth of the bone, (3) angle of greater than 20 degrees dorsally or anterior displacement of the breadth of the bone, and (4) angle of greater than 20 degrees.[48]

El-Ahwany's classification is perhaps the most useful in the management of these fractures. He correlates the radiographic findings with methods of management, complications, and prognosis.[31] Three standardized roentgenograms are taken, preferably under anesthesia for very painful and displaced fractures. An anteroposterior view is obtained with the elbow as straight as possible and the forearm supinated in line with the humeral bicipital groove anteriorly. An axial view is taken with the elbow flexed and the x-ray film placed posteriorly to the elbow; the x-ray beam is directed at a right angle to the supinated forearm. The lateral view is taken with the elbow flexed to a right angle and the forearm in neutral position. The axial view best dem-

TREATMENT

The goal of all treatment is the anatomic restoration of the humerus and resolution of any complications with subsequent healing of the fracture with normal alignment and function. Several general principles must be considered. The fracture should be promptly assessed clinically, and the neurovascular status and radiographic features should be noted before treatment is undertaken. Treatment of the compromised neurovascular structures is the first priority (see Chapter 17).[1, 8, 16, 18, 71, 76, 80, 86, 96] Marked displacement of the fracture fragment frequently results in laceration of the deep soft tissue structures including the lacertus fibrosus and brachialis muscles, so that the sharp end of the proximal fractured metaphysis may be tenting the skin as well as the neurovascular structures (Fig. 12– 14).[16–20, 25, 33, 41, 43, 51, 58b, 69, 70] The limb should be splinted in a position that presents the least risk to the neurovascular structures. This is usually a position of some flexion because extension of the elbow may cause further stretching of the neurovascular structures, whereas excessive flexion may cause buckling or pinching (Fig. 12–16).[70] Functional alignment of these fractures is satisfactory in the young child who has at least 2

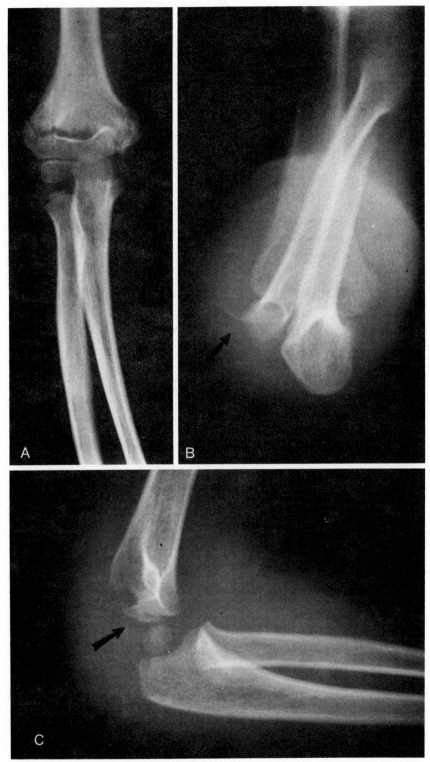

Figure 12–12. *A,* Anteroposterior roentgenogram of the elbow provides excellent visualization of the fracture, but this view is difficult to take with a severely displaced fracture. If attempted after reduction, it will often result in loss of reduction. *B,* Axial view permits excellent visualization of the alignment of the distal humerus with the elbow flexed. This view is preferred after a closed reduction. *C,* The lateral view demonstrates rotation, anterior posterior inclination, and displacement well.

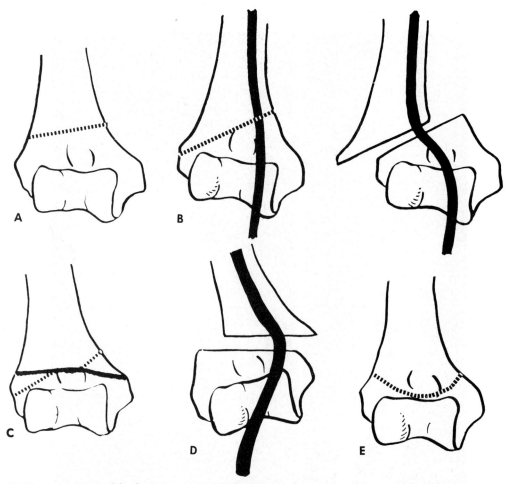

Figure 12–13. *A,* A supracondylar fracture, type 1. A high transverse fracture. *B,* A supracondylar fracture, type 2. A short oblique fracture. *C,* A supracondylar fracture, type 3. Pro-varus, steep oblique fracture; it is unstable, and liable to produce cubitus varus. *D,* A supracondylar fracture, type 4. Pro-varus, steep oblique fracture, liable to immediate neurovascular complications. It is an unstable fracture. *E,* A low transverse fracture—the so-called transcondylar fracture. Forward displacement is common. (From El-Ahwany, M. D.: Supracondylar fractures of the humerus in children with a note on the surgical correction of late cubitus varus. Injury 6(1):46, 1973.

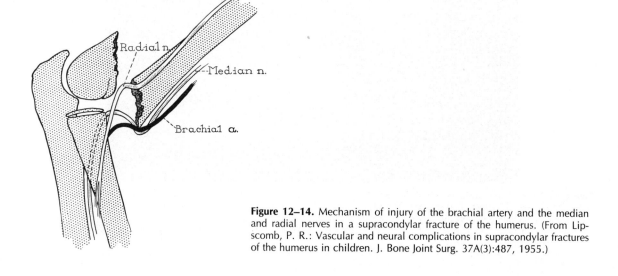

Figure 12–14. Mechanism of injury of the brachial artery and the median and radial nerves in a supracondylar fracture of the humerus. (From Lipscomb, P. R.: Vascular and neural complications in supracondylar fractures of the humerus in children. J. Bone Joint Surg. 37A(3):487, 1955.)

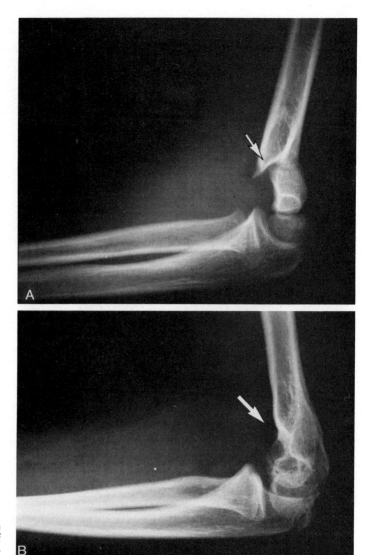

Figure 12–15. A, Supracondylar fracture with posterior angulation. B, Treated wtih flexion of the elbow and casting, the injury shows excellent early alignment and remodeling.

years of growth left, because normal remodeling of the fracture will result in reconstitution of the bone (Fig. 12–15).[7] Anteroposterior, lateral, and axial roentgenograms including the entire forearm should be taken at the initial assessment to be sure no other injuries are present and to allow an appropriate choice of treatment. More detailed radiographs can be taken under anesthesia if the initial roentgenograms are unsatisfactory for full evaluation of the deformity. This is true even with apparently minor injuries such as a minimally displaced or torus fracture, which may be difficult to recognize in the young patient. These may not be innocuous injuries, however, and may result in malunion (Fig. 12–17).[70, 77, 79] The fat pad sign is usually positive, and comparative roentgenograms are often necessary for proper assessment of these lesions.

Following the initial assessment, treatment is chosen according to the type of fracture. In my opinion, the choices include the following: (1) splinting for minimally displaced or angulated fractures (I use a simple collar and cuff [see Fig. 12–18]), (2) closed reduction for moderately displaced fractures with minimal to moderate swelling, (3) traction for fractures that are severely displaced and swollen (I prefer to use skeletal rather than cutaneous traction), (4) closed reduction and percutaneous pinning for fractures that can be readily reduced but are unstable, and (5) open reduction with pinning and splinting for open fractures and fractures with significant neurovascular compromise.[68, 79]

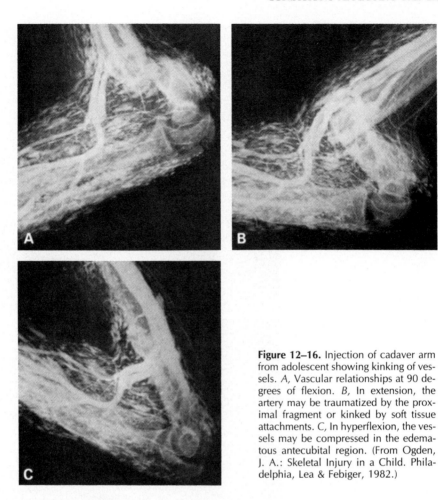

Figure 12–16. Injection of cadaver arm from adolescent showing kinking of vessels. *A,* Vascular relationships at 90 degrees of flexion. *B,* In extension, the artery may be traumatized by the proximal fragment or kinked by soft tissue attachments. *C,* In hyperflexion, the vessels may be compressed in the edematous antecubital region. (From Ogden, J. A.: Skeletal Injury in a Child. Philadelphia, Lea & Febiger, 1982.)

Figure 12–17. *A,* Schematic view of greenstick fracture causing a medial trabecular-cortical compression leading to cubitus varus. This must be corrected with manipulation. *B,* Acute cubitus varus in a 5-year-old. This was not corrected. *C,* Mild cubitus varus 2 years later. (From Ogden, J. A.: Skeletal Injury in a Child. Philadelphia, Lea & Febiger, 1982.)

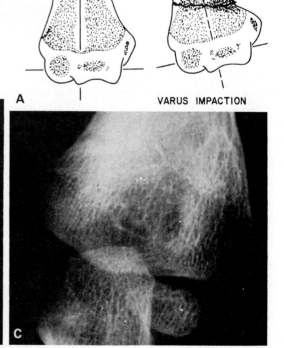

VARUS IMPACTION

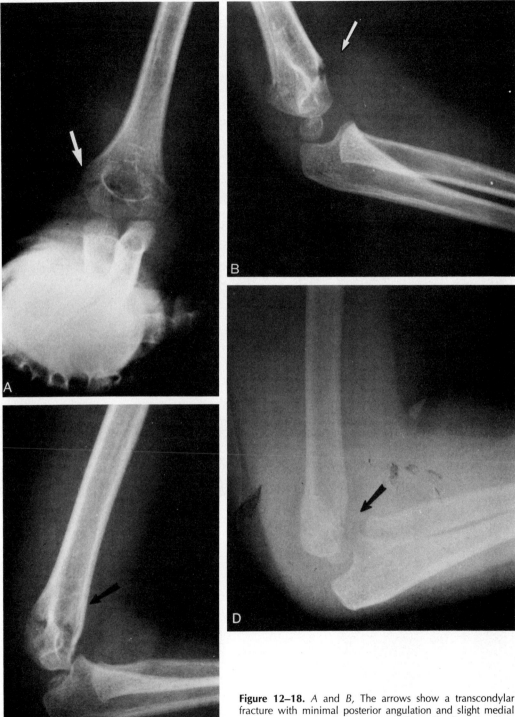

Figure 12–18. *A* and *B*, The arrows show a transcondylar fracture with minimal posterior angulation and slight medial tilting. *C*, Treated in flexion with a collar and cuff. *D*, Excellent remodeling.

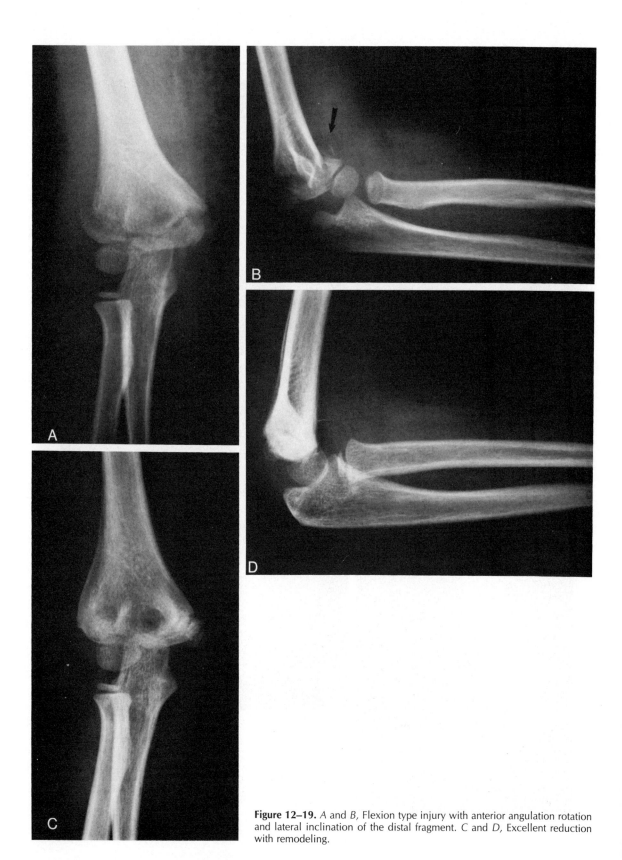

Figure 12–19. *A* and *B*, Flexion type injury with anterior angulation rotation and lateral inclination of the distal fragment. *C* and *D*, Excellent reduction with remodeling.

Closed Reduction

Most supracondylar fractures can be treated by closed reduction (Fig. 12–19).[1, 3, 10] Accurate assessment of the clinical status and the roentgenograms is important. Minimally displaced fractures are treated by flexion of the elbow to about 120 degrees followed by application of a collar and cuff or a posterior splint. Failure to maintain the elbow in this degree of flexion will result in loss of reduction.[67, 68a] Regional or preferably general anesthesia is necessary for reduction of most displaced fractures. Although these fractures may vary in complexity, if the guidelines noted in the classification of these fractures are followed, the reduction process can be simplified.[31] In 80 to 85 percent of these fractures the distal fragment is displaced posteriorly and medially, and the remainder are displaced laterally or posteriorly. Reduction is usually achieved by traction on the forearm with the elbow in the partially flexed position.[30, 67] Hyperextension should be avoided because it may result in compromise of a neurovascular structure (Fig. 12–16).[70] Countertraction is applied to the upper arm, and medial or lateral displacement and posteriorly overriding are overcome by manual manipulation of the distal fragment. The elbow is then flexed while the posteriorly displaced fragment is manipulated anteriorly. The medial or lateral thickened periosteal sleeve acts as a hinge and aids in achieving a reduction if it is not torn (Fig. 12–4). Fractures with medially displaced fragments are therefore usually treated with the forearm placed in pronation because this helps to close the fracture gap and fix the fragments. Similarly, the arm in placed in supination if the displacement is lateral.[6, 9, 24, 70, 77] Some fractures are quite stable in the neutral position, and these maneuvers are not necessary. The elbow is then placed in a splint or cast and held at about 120 degrees of flexion (Fig. 12–20). Excessive edema may prevent this degree of flexion and will render the fracture unstable. If the fracture is unstable after reduction, the cause must be promptly determined (Fig. 12–21). Repeated manipulation should be avoided because it usually results in further instability owing to comminution of the fracture fragments or tearing of the soft tissues and subsequent increased edema. Failure to achieve reduction is usually due to inadequate reduction or soft tissue interposition. Reduction can be readily assessed with the use of an image intensifier, which we prefer to use, or serial roentgenograms.[68a] Comminuted fractures (Fig. 12–3), which usually occur in the older child, or fractures through the olecranon fossa, in which the central segment of the metaphysis is very thin and the medial and lateral condylar pillows are narrow, may make maintenance of the reduction very difficult (Fig. 12–5).[77] Soft tissue interposition, particularly neurovascular structures, may also prevent reduction (Fig. 12–22).[33, 89, 90, 92, 96] The soft tissues may be so massively swollen and the hematoma so large that manipulation, reduction, and maintenance of the fractures are not possible. Skeletal traction, percutaneous pinning or open reduction and pin fixation (Fig. 12–23), or a combination of these, is then the treatment of choice.

Traction

Traction may be used routinely in the management of any displaced supracondylar fracture.[13, 26, 28, 29, 53, 54, 62, 64, 81, 85, 89, 94] It has been considered the standard of care with which all other forms of treatment should be compared.[13, 26, 24, 29, 48] Traction is a safe means of achieving and maintaining a reduction in most instances. The severely displaced fragment, particularly if neurovascular compromise is present, is best managed if it is first reduced under anesthesia, noting the neurovascular status, and then placed in skeletal traction. Neurovascular compromise must be resolved prior to replacement of traction because traction itself may cause or aggravate this complication if the fragments are locked or if soft tissue structures are interposed in the fracture site.[58, 74, 89, 90] Dislocation of the elbow joint has also been reported as a complication with this form of treatment.[47] We prefer to use skeletal traction when there is marked swelling at the fracture site, particularly in the young or multiply injured child when other injuries might take priority in management. Reduction of the fracture should be achieved within the first 24 hours of treatment. Traction must be applied, however, until the fracture has stabilized, which usually takes 7 to 10 days. Stability implies that the fracture has developed sufficient early callus formation to prevent it from displacing with the application of a splint or cast and that satisfactory alignment is maintained. This is a clinical as well as a radiographic assessment.

Two forms of traction have been traditionally used: cutaneous or Dunlop's traction and skeletal traction. Dunlop's traction is applied

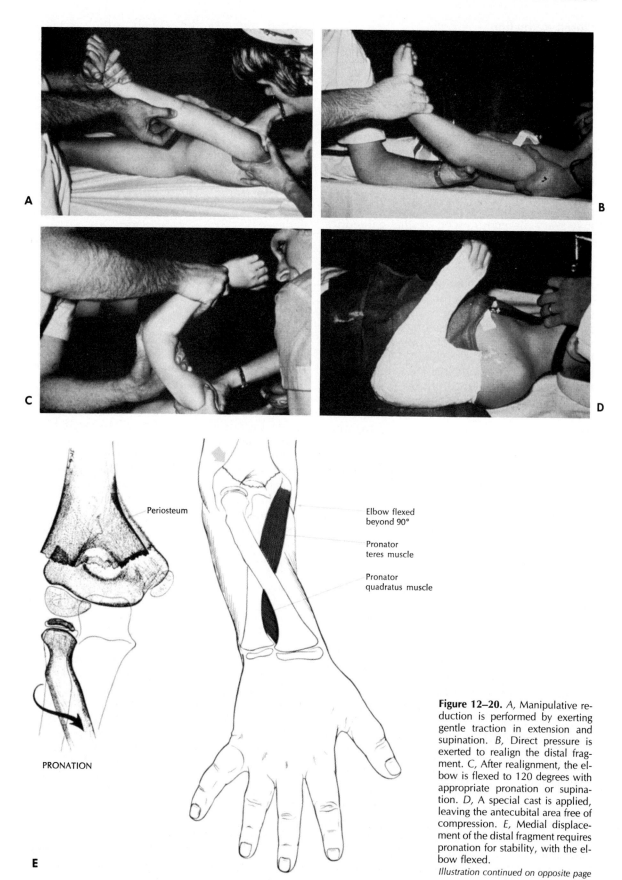

Figure 12–20. *A,* Manipulative reduction is performed by exerting gentle traction in extension and supination. *B,* Direct pressure is exerted to realign the distal fragment. *C,* After realignment, the elbow is flexed to 120 degrees with appropriate pronation or supination. *D,* A special cast is applied, leaving the antecubital area free of compression. *E,* Medial displacement of the distal fragment requires pronation for stability, with the elbow flexed.

Illustration continued on opposite page

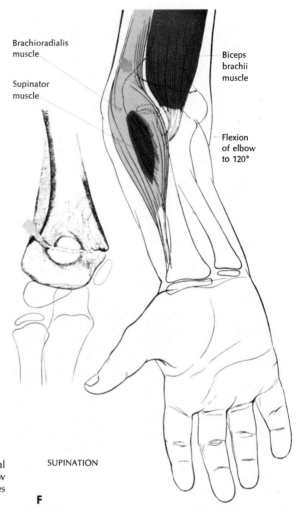

Brachioradialis
muscle

Supinator
muscle

Biceps
brachii
muscle

Flexion
of elbow
to 120°

SUPINATION

F

Figure 12–20 *Continued. F,* Lateral displacement of the distal fragment requires supination for stability, with the elbow flexed. (From Micheli, L. J., et al.: Supracondylar fractures of the humerus in children. AFP 19(3):100, 1979.)

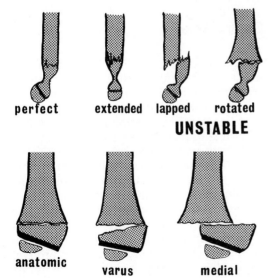

perfect   extended   lapped   rotated

UNSTABLE

anatomic   varus   medial

Figure 12–21. Possible appearances in the anteroposterior and lateral radiographs. In the anteroposterior film, observe Bauman's angle; the thick, black line should be at 70 to 80 degrees of the humeral shaft. (From Rang, M.: Children's Fractures, 2nd ed. Philadelphia, J. B. Lippincott Company, 1983.)

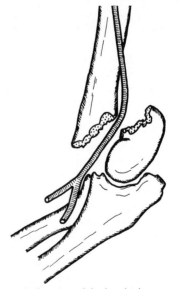

Figure 12–22. Dislocation of the brachial artery with supracondylar fracture of the humerus. (From Staples, O. S.: Dislocation of the brachial artery: A complication of supracondylar fracture of the humerus in children. J. Bone Joint Surg. 47A(8):1525, 1965.)

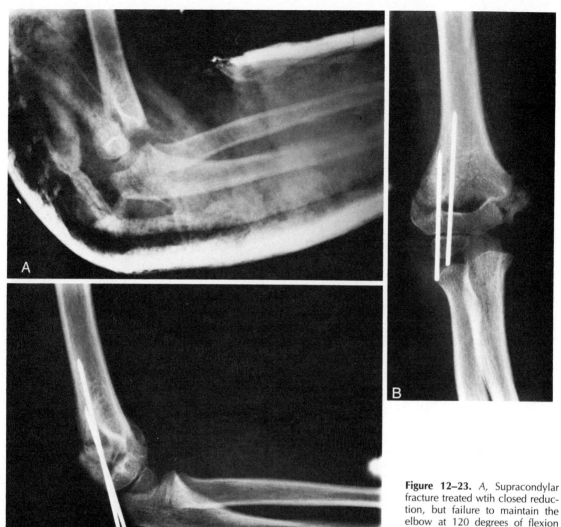

Figure 12–23. A, Supracondylar fracture treated wtih closed reduction, but failure to maintain the elbow at 120 degrees of flexion and pronation has resulted in loss of the reduction. B and C, Definitive treatment with pin fixation.

in a lateral direction with the patient in a supine position (Fig. 12–24). Pronation and supination of the forearm and varus or valgus tilt of the distal fragment have been difficult to control and correct with this method of traction. The forearm tends to rotate into supination, resulting in a loss of stability that is ordinarily achieved when the forearm is maintained in the pronated position in most common fractures.[3, 6, 9, 10, 12, 13, 29, 41, 45, 54] This position also places the distal fracture fragment in some extension, but this deformity is usually corrected either when the arm is splinted in flexion or when remodeling of the fracture occurs. Because of these disadvantages, we prefer to use skeletal traction with the arm maintained in an overhead position.[21, 53, 68a] Under general or regional anesthesia a Kirschner wire may be inserted through the proximal ulna at the palpable tip

of the olecranon (see Fig. 12–26A). An olecranon screw, which is inserted at the same level, is simpler to insert and avoids risk to the ulnar nerve. Predrilling of the ulna and the use of image intensification (see Fig. 12–28C) are helpful in inserting this device.

If there is gross displacement, it is corrected at this time, and the arm is then suspended from an overhead frame with the sling under the forearm to control its position. Three to five pounds of traction are usually sufficient to reduce and stabilize the fracture. Excess weight results in elevating the shoulder and twisting the thorax, causing the child to shift his position, thereby losing control of the fracture fragment. Suspension of the forearm in this position permits rapid reduction of edema and good control of elbow flexion. Rotational deformity can be controlled by placing the arm in either a cephalad or caudad

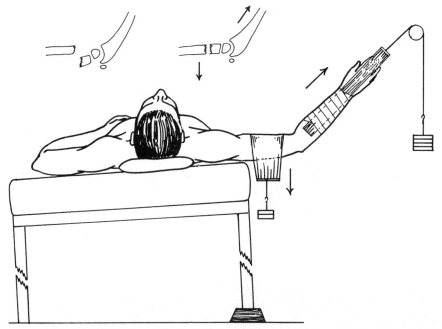

Figure 12–24. Supracondylar fracture of the humerus being treated in Dunlop's traction. (From Smith, F. M.: Children's elbow injuries: Fractures and dislocations. Clin. Orthop. Rel. Res. 50:14, 1967.)

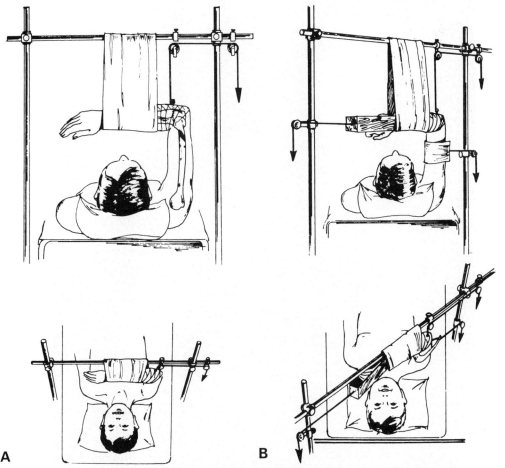

A

B

Figure 12–25. A, Position of patient in bed relative to overhead traction. B, Angulation of the traction controls reduction. (From Ogden, J. A.: Skeletal Injury in a Child. Philadelphia, Lea & Febiger, 1982.)

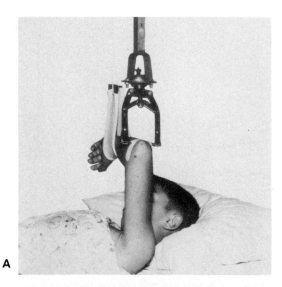

Figure 12–26. *A,* Traction arrangement. *B,* Supracondylar fracture with a Kirschner wire through the olecranon; the bone prominences are aligned in conformity with the appearance of the other elbow. *C,* For demonstration purposes, the distal fragment has been tilted into valgus deformity. *D,* The distal fragment has been tilted into varus deformity. *E,* Roentgenogram of the elbow as it appeared in *A.* Lead dots were placed on the ink markings, and a wire was taped over the axis of the humerus. The lateral displacement of the distal fragment will have no effect on the carrying angle or function. (From Smith, L.: Deformity following supracondylar fractures. J. Bone Joint Surg. 42A(2):244, 1960.)

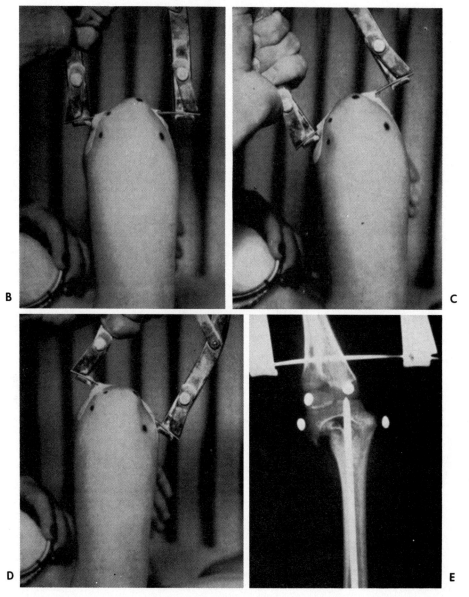

position. If necessary, a lateral sling around the upper arm may also provide lateral traction to correct anterior displacement of the proximal fragment (Fig. 12–25).[70] Smith uses a traction bail attached to a Kirschner wire to provide more precise control of the tilt of the fracture, thereby correcting the varus and valgus positions (Fig. 12–26).[85] He has documented the most successful use of traction with this method, noting absence of all complications. Serial roentgenograms must be taken and may require some ingenuity on the part of the technician and direction on the part of the physician to obtain adequate films. The lateral projection is usually obtained without difficulty, but the axial view requires some means of overcoming the obstruction of the overhead frame.

Percutaneous Pin Fixation

Percutaneous pinning is used to maintain the reduction of an unstable fracture.[5, 16, 22, 34, 36, 38, 44, 56, 68, 68a, 70, 77, 91] Our indications for pinning

are as follows: (1) gross swelling that may prohibit sufficient flexion of the elbow to allow locking of the fragments (see Fig. 12–23); (2) torn soft tissues and a comminuted fracture, making it difficult to maintain a reduction; (3) failure of traction to achieve reduction of the fragments (closed reduction and pinning are used after swelling has subsided); (4) multiple injuries, particularly multiple fractures and ipsilateral trauma. It is apparent from this list that there is some overlap in the indications for the use of traction versus pinning and fixation in maintaining a reduction; clinical judgment and skill are the deciding factors. Pinning is an exacting techniquue, particularly in the small child, in whom the osseous structures are ill-defined, but it is readily mastered with some experience. The advantages of percutaneous pinning are that (1) the elbow need not be maintained in an acutely flexed position following reduction and fixation of the fracture, (2) loss of position is infrequent, (3) alignment can be readily assessed clinically and radio-

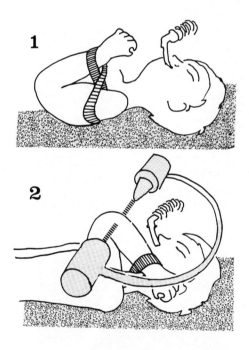

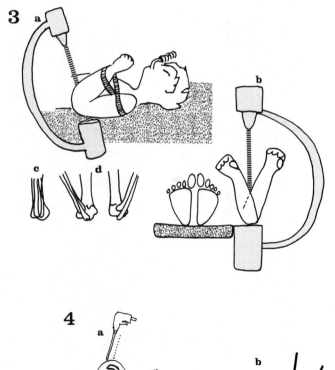

Figure 12–27. The steps in percutaneous pinning. (1) Hold reduction with a figure-of-8 bandage; use several turns. (2) Check reduction with the image intensifier. Twist the C arm, not the child's arm. (3) Check anteroposterior appearance; use two oblique views to yield images (d) which are easier to interpret than the usual superimposed view (c). (4) Use a power driver to insert the pins. Owing to anterior angulation of the distal humerus, start the pins just posterior to the intercondylar line. (From Rang, M.: Children's Fractures, 2nd ed. Philadelphia, J. B. Lippincott Company, 1983.)

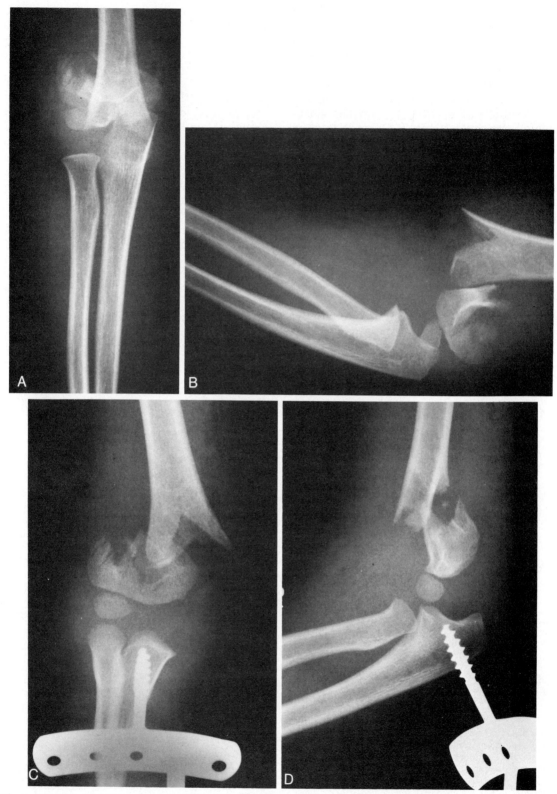

Figure 12–28 *A* and *B,* Severe fracture with rotation, posterior and lateral displacement, and neurovascular compromise. *C,* Traction screw has been inserted too proximally and can enter the joint. The lateral and posterior displacement should be reduced before application of traction. *D,* Traction was not satisfactory, and percutaneous pinning was required. Note that the screw track indicates that the screw entered the joint and could contaminate the joint.

Illustration continued on opposite page

graphically and (4) hospitalization is minimized.

Procedure

The patient is placed in the supine position and anesthetized.[77] Some surgeons prefer the prone position, but I feel that this only adds another anesthetic risk. The fracture is reduced as described under Closed Reduction (above) and verified by the image intensifier. Smith has noted that the bony landmarks of the olecranon and the medial and lateral condyles form an equilateral triangle when the fracture is reduced, aiding in making a clinical assessment of the reduction.[85] Assessment is difficult, however, if significant swelling occurs. Because cartilaginous structures are present in the young child, radiographic analysis is also difficult, so two straight needles may be inserted as markers to identify the medial and lateral condyles following the attempted reduction. Once the fracture is reduced under radiographic control, the elbow is supported, keeping the humerus parallel to the floor. A small Kirschner wire is then inserted with a power drill from the lateral condyle across the fracture site to engage the opposite cortex if possible (Fig. 12–27). Occasionally, the fracture is angled transversely or medially, and because the pin cannot be angled in this manner it is extended up the

medullary canal. Following placement of the pin, reduction of the fracture is then checked in both planes, rotating the C-arm rather than the humerus.

I prefer to place the first pin in the most lateral position near the epicondyle. The second pin is then placed parallel and medial to the first one. The pins must not cross at the fracture line because this will allow rotation at this site (Fig. 12–28). If the pins cross they should do so in the metaphysis proximal to the fracture line. If the pins are placed too obliquely and do not engage the opposite cortex, they may well ride up along the inner surface of the medullary canal, resulting in displacement of the fragment by levering the fragment into either a varus or valgus position. Pins that penetrate the opposite cortex are subject to migration and may result in penetration of neurovascular structures medially. Lateral pin placement is preferable to medial placement because it avoids the posibility of injuring the ulnar nerve (Fig. 12–29). Medial and lateral placement of the pins is preferred by numerous authors and is an alternate method.

Following pinning, the elbow may be maintained in 90 degrees of flexion or less, depending on the swelling and neurovascular status of the elbow. A splint or cast similar to those used in closed reduction may be ap-

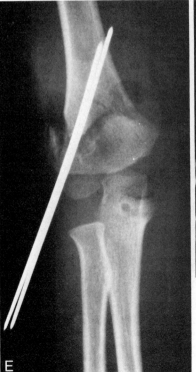

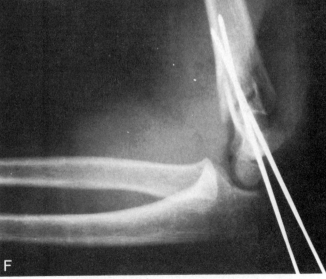

Figure 12–28 *Continued. E* and *F*, The problem was resolved by removal of the screw, reduction, and pinning.

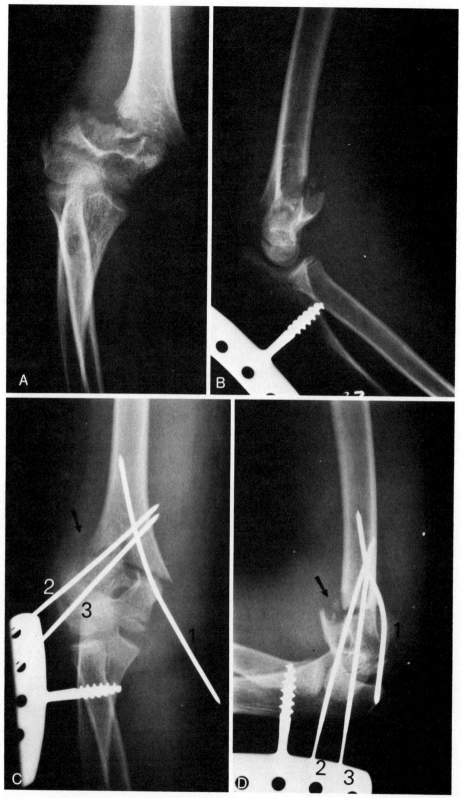

Figure 12–29. *A,* Extension type fracture with rotation, posterior angulation, and lateral displacement. *B,* Traction screw should be inserted at the level of the coronoid process. The insertion shown is too distal. *C,* Percutaneous pin number one has missed the distal fragment, is intramedullar, and has ridden up along the cortex, causing it to lever the distal fragment into a tilted and laterally displaced position. Pins two and three penetrate the medial cortex and are liable to migrate. *D,* Pin one is not engaging the distal fragment, and pins two and three have fixed the distal fragment in a position of rotation and extension.

Illustration continued on opposite page

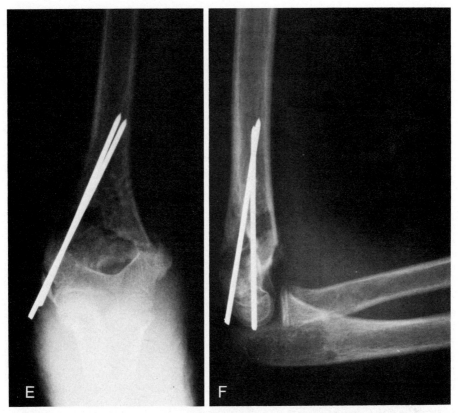

Figure 12–29 *Continued. E* and *F,* Remanipulation and proper pin fixation have resolved the problem.

plied. I prefer to use a cast with an antecubital opening as well as an opening over the wrist so that the radial pulse may be noted. The forearm is maintained in a neutral position with the fingers free to allow observation of their function (see Fig. 12–20D). The patient is hospitalized if any problems are anticipated. The arm should be immobilized with a sling in a manner that will prevent rotation of the shoulder whenever a reduction has been required. This precaution is frequently overlooked, resulting in loss of correction, particularly in patients treated with closed reduction without fixation. I prefer to cut the pins so that the tips are located subcutaneously, thus reducing the possibility of irritation and infection; the pins can readily be removed under local anesthesia.

Intracondylar fractures of the distal humerus, which usually occur in adolescents and adults, can sometimes be managed by closed reduction and pinning.[68] If the fragments are large, they can be manipulated and held in position by a transfixing pin or an external clamp, and the rest of the pins can then be placed across the fracture site. If the fragments are very unstable they may be partially reduced and the fragment manipulated into

place and cross-pinned. Occasionally, only the condylar fragments and the transverse element of supracondylar fractures are pinned. A cast is then applied as described previously. This technique avoids the use of open reduction, extensive dissection, and use of plates and screws that require removal (Fig. 12–30). Percutaneous pins are usually removed 3 weeks after injury under local anesthesia.

The child is permitted to use a sling for comfort for another week to 10 days but is encouraged to mobilize the elbow at his own leisure without assistance from others.[77] The elbow is usually quite functional at 6 weeks following injury, but a full range of motion may not return for 3 to 12 months. Evaluation of malalignment or epiphyseal injury and function should be done at regular intervals. Usually, epiphyseal injury is noted only when the fracture line has entered the physis or the pins have been infected or have been left in for an excessively long period of time.[15] There are, however, exceptions (Fig. 12–31).[66, 68, 69] Bergenfeldt noted that no clinical deformities secondary to growth alteration occurred following pinning of these fractures. However, on x-ray evaluation he found that three in-

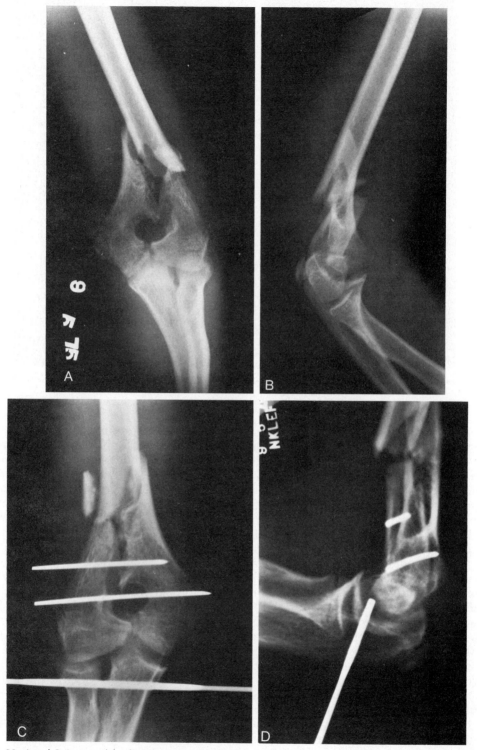

Figure 12–30. *A* and *B,* Intercondylar fracture with mild displacement. *C* and *D,* Percutaneous pinning of the condyles with insertion of an ulnar pin to maintain alignment while pinning.

Illustration continued on opposite page

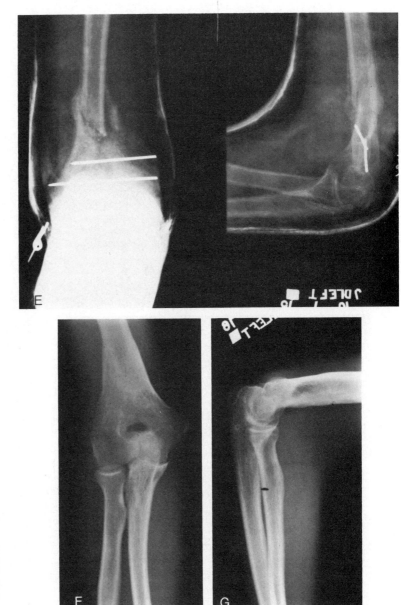

Figure 12–30 *Continued. E,* The transverse metaphyseal fracture component was treated in a cast. *F* and *G,* Satisfactory alignment and remodeling. This is preferable to plating in the adolescent.

stances of partial epiphyseal arrest occurred in patients in whom the pins had been left in for an extended period of time.[15]

Open Reduction

Indications for open reduction of supracondylar fractures are as follows: (1) open fracture requiring debridement; (2) severely displaced or compound fractures with neurovascular compromise; (3) persistent neurovascular compromise following attempted reduction; and (4) unreducible fractures due to soft tissue interposition.[8, 12, 13, 18, 20, 24, 33, 36, 42, 43, 46, 50, 52, 55, 74, 76, 80, 82, 86, 88–90, 92, 95, 96] Severely displaced and

open fractures usually lacerate the anterior muscles and ligaments, leaving the neurovascular structures at risk, tented over the fracture fragment. Excessive stretching or entrapment of these structures, particularly in the fracture site or more distally at the fibrous arch in the proximal third of the forearm, can result in loss of function of the anterior interosseous nerve (see Chapter 45). Surgical approaches to this area have been directed toward reducing the fracture, and evaluating and repairing, if necessary, the neurovascular bundle. Sorrel recommended the anteromedial approach along the internal bicipital groove as the approach of choice[85a] (see Chap-

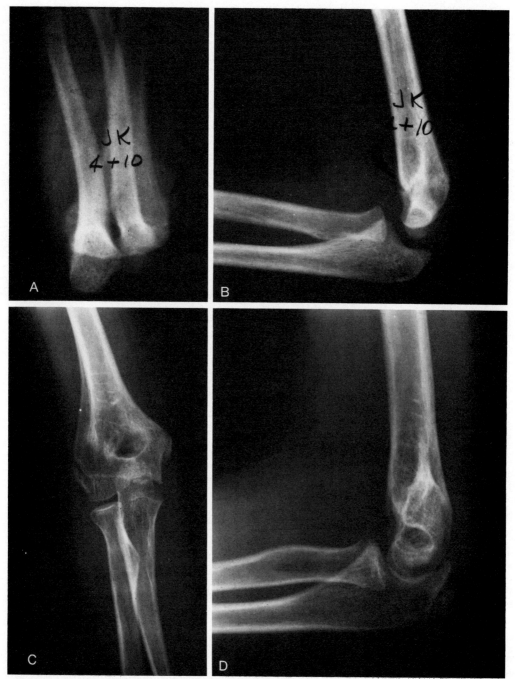

Figure 12–31. Supracondylar fracture in a child 4 years and 10 months of age. There is minimal displacement and no comminution on the axial (A) and lateral (B) views. C, Six years after injury note the sequelae of a symptomatic severe epiphyseal injury. D, Patient has limited motion and deformity of the radial head.

Illustration continued on opposite page

ter 8). He noted the ease of accessibility to the fracture site and neurovascular structures with this approach. Postoperatively, there was excellent return of function with minimal deformity. Carcassonne et al. favored a similar approach followed by percutaneous pinning of the medial and lateral condyles.[20] They achieved excellent clinical results in 97 percent of 40 cases with minimal loss of function, but 25 percent of patients did have a cubitus varus deformity and 10 percent had loss of some flexion or extension (Fig. 12–32). They felt that these complications were due to technical errors, such as failure to recognize

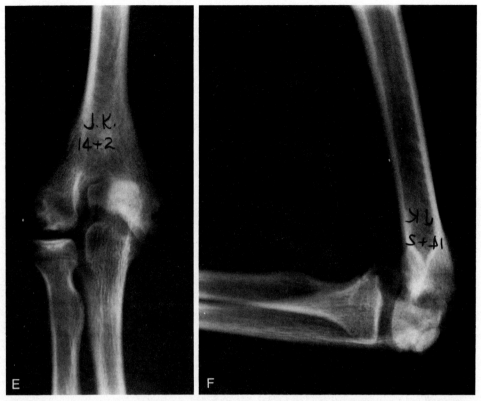

Figure 12–31 *Continued. E,* Ten years after injury she has a disabled elbow with degenerative changes of the capitellum as well as of the trochlea. *F,* Note the degenerative changes of the radial head. (Courtesy of L. Johnson, M.D., Minneapolis Shriners Hospital.)

Figure 12–32. Incision to expose brachial vessels and median nerve. This exposure results in the least complications. (From Staples, O. S.: Dislocation of the brachial artery: A complication of supracondylar fracture of the humerus in children. J. Bone Joint Surg. 47A(8):1526, 1965.)

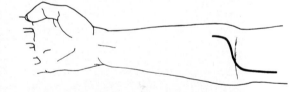

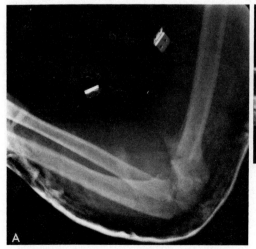

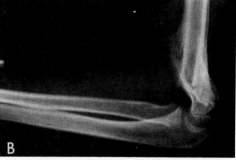

Figure 12–33. *A,* Supracondylar fracture with massive myositis ossificans and a rigid elbow. The patient also had an associated head injury. *B,* Spontaneous resorption and remodeling with restoration of excellent function lacking only 20 degrees of motion, 7 months after injury. (From Weiland, A. J., Meier, S., Tolo, V. T., Berg, H. L. and Mueller, J., Surgical treatment of displaced supracondylar fractures of the humerus in children, J. Bone Joint Surg. 60A(5):660, 1978.)

the deformity, which could be overcome. Medial, lateral, and posterior surgical approaches have also been used; however, the incidence of malunion and loss of function is greater with these approaches. Shifrin et al. suggested that all severely displaced supracondylar fractures should be treated with open reduction and pin fixation. They used a medial approach that produced uniformly good results and minimal complications, but offered no documentation of their results.[82] Routine open reduction of fractures does not appear to im-

prove the overall results. When indicated, the anteromedial surgical approach appears to give the best results and is the approach that we employ.

COMPLICATIONS

Complications in the management of supracondylar fractures may be due to the fracture itself (Fig. 12–31), its treatment, or a combination of both (Fig. 12–29). Simple or minimally displaced fractures are associated with

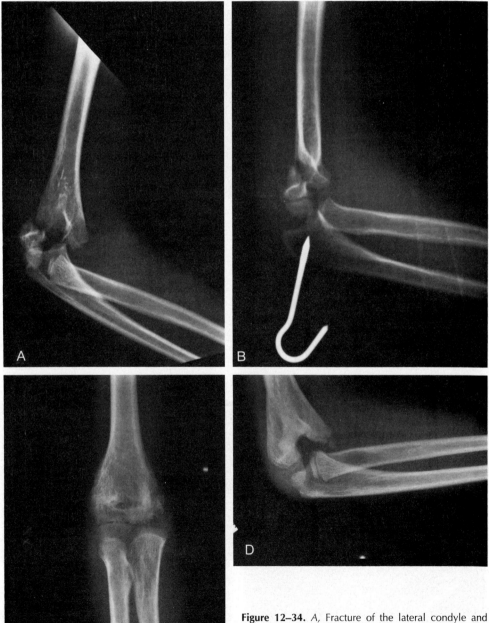

Figure 12–34. A, Fracture of the lateral condyle and dislocation misdiagnosed as a supracondylar fracture. B, Treated as a supracondylar fracture in traction. C and D, Note the marked malunion and limitation of motion.

few complications except failure to recognize a valgus or varus impaction injury (Fig. 12–17). Loss of anteversion such as occurs in a plane of flexion and extension is usually overcome with remodeling, and normal function returns (Fig. 12–19). Epiphyseal injuries may occur if the fracture line goes through the physis, resulting in alteration of growth or avascular necrosis of the segment of the physis, but these complications are rare (see Fig. 12–31 and Chapter 13). Failure to recognize and diagnose the type of fracture (for instance, a condylar fracture being mistaken for a supracondylar fracture) will result in malunion (Fig. 12–34).[35] A transcondylar or epiphyseal injury in a very young child may be diagnosed as a dislocation.

So-called myositis ossificans occurs infrequently. Siris noted only seven cases among 330 patients, and only three instances were noted in 450 supracondylar fractures in our institution.[17, 21b, 83a] The incidence is increased with concurrent central nervous system injury.[21a] The initial swelling may be quite marked and is out of proportion to the apparent injury, and the region may have the appearance of rampant cellulitis. The swelling gradually subsides, leaving a large indurated area. Ossification occurs initially, gradually disappearing with the return of function of the elbow, but some persistent loss of motion may be expected (Fig. 12–33). Complete os-

sification of the brachialis muscle may occur with complete ankylosis of the joint, and repeated manipulation of the elbow may also result in ankylosis.* The ossification may be excised when it is mature, usually after 1 year when the borders of the ossification are clearly defined and unchanging. Neurovascular injuries represent a major complication (see Chapter 17). Lipscomb reported an incidence of 4 percent of vascular injuries at our institution.[59a] Staples and Elstrom reported dislocation of the brachial artery and vein and median nerve at the fracture site, resulting in an irreducible fracture.[33, 89] Thrombosis[18] and rupture[86] of the brachial artery have been reported, and Wray documented progressive vascular compromise.[96] All of these lesions will result in ischemic muscle contracture (see Chapter 17). Management of vascular complications needs prompt recognition and appropriate intervention including reduction of the fracture and exploration of the structures if function does not return promptly.

Entrapment of median, ulnar, and radial nerves has been described with this fracture. Siris noted that the radial and ulnar nerves were almost equally involved, and involvement of the median nerve occurred less frequently.[83a] Symeonides et al. noted entrap-

---

*Personal communication, B.J.S. Grogono, 1984.

Table 12–1. **Complications of Treatment**

Treatment	Author(s)	No. of Fractures	Length of Follow-up	Patients with Varus Deformity (Per cent)	Patients with Decreased Range of Motion (Per cent)
Overhead skeletal traction	Smith (1960)	10	6 mos.	10	40
	Smith (1967)	62	—	0	0
Dunlop's traction	Dodge (1972)	48	6 mos.–6 yrs.	27	23
	Mitchell and Adams (1961)	16	10 yrs.	18	19
Closed red., immed. immobilization	Madsen (1955)	30	3–8 yrs.	20	7
	Mitchell and Adams (1961)	42	10 yrs.	60	94
Closed red., percutaneous pinning	Fowles and Kassab (1974)	80	2 yrs.	36	23
Open red., internal fixation	Gruber and Hudson (1964)	23	1–5 yrs.	0	27
	Sandegard (1943)	79	1–15 yrs.	53	91
	Alonso-Llames (1972)	31	4 mos.–2 yrs.	10	90
	Ramsey and Griz (1973)	15	3 mos.–4 yrs.	20	0
	Holmberg (1945)	54	—	32	24
	Present study	52	5–15 yrs.	25	10

From Weiland, A. J., et al.: Surgical treatment of displaced supracondylar fractures of the humerus in children. J. Bone Joint Surg. 60A(5):660, 1978.

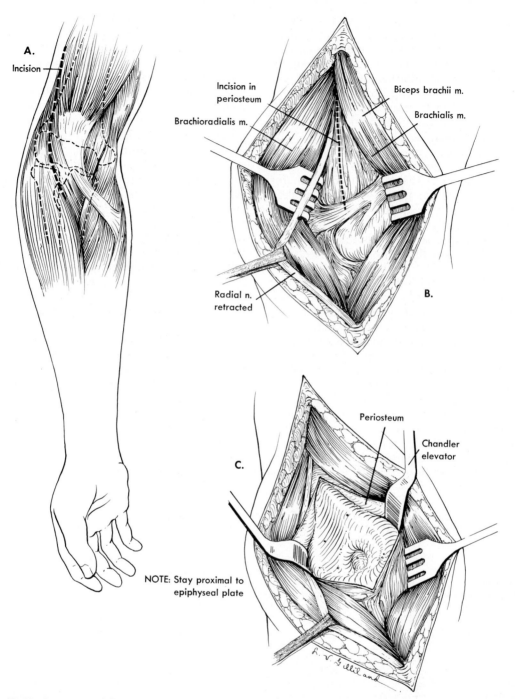

Figure 12–35. Osteotomy of distal humerus for correction of cubitus varus. *A,* A longitudinal incision is made over the anterolateral aspect of the distal third of the arm, wtih the anterior margin of the brachioradialis muscle serving as an anatomic landmark. It begins 1 cm proximal and anterior to the lateral epicondyle of the humerus and extends proximally for a distance of approximately 7 cm.

B, The subcutaneous tissue and fascia are divided in line with the skin incision. The skin flaps are mobilized and retracted. The anterior margin of the brachioradialis muscle laterally and the lateral margin of the biceps muscle medially are identified, and the radial nerve is located by blunt dissection in the loose areolar tissue between these two muscles. A moist hernia tape is passed around the radial nerve for gentle handling and traction.

The biceps muscle is retracted medially, exposing the lateral half of the brachialis muscle beneath it. By blunt dissection wtih a periosteal elevator, the lateral one third to one half of the muscle fibers of the brachialis are raised, exposing the periosteum on the front of the lower end of the humerus. The periosteum is incised longitudinally as shown in the illustration, its distal end stopping 1 cm proximal to the capsule of the elbow joint.

C, The periosteum is reflected with a periosteal elevator, and the lower end of the shaft of the humerus is exposed. It is essential not to disturb the growth of the epiphyseal plates and to keep out of the elbow joint.

Illustration continued on opposite page

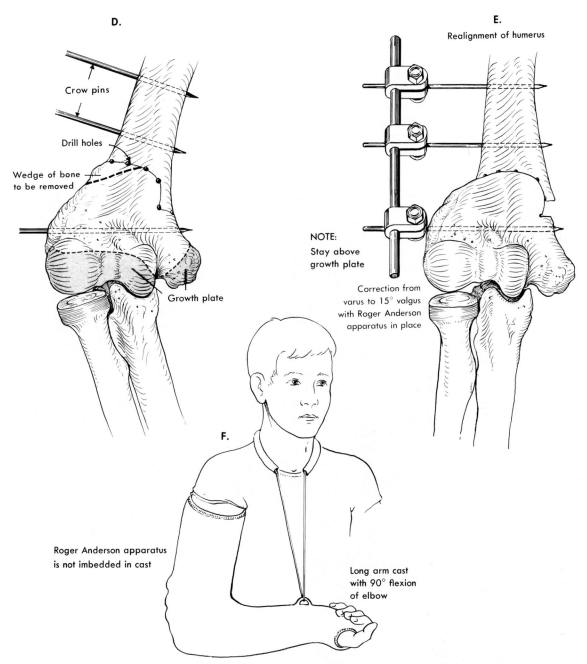

Figure 12–35 *Continued. D,* With a starter and drill, the line of a dome-shaped osteotomy is outlined with drill holes through both anterior and posterior cortices. The medial arch of the dome should be deeper and 1 to 1.5 cm longer than the lateral arch, which is almost transverse.

Next, through stab wounds separate from the skin incision, two 1/8-inch Crow pins are drilled transversely across the distal portion of the proximal fragment. The pins should be perpendicular to the shaft of the humerus, 3 cm apart, and should engage the medial cortex of the humerus. It is essential to drill the pins across the humerus under direct vision and lift the radial nerve anteriorly to protect it from injury. Then a third Crow pin is placed into the distal fragment at a predetermined angle so that when the varus deformity is corrected, the distal pin should be parallel to the proximal pins.

The distal pin should not cross the osteotomy line, and it should engage the medial cortex of the distal fragment. A Roger Anderson apparatus is applied to the Crow pins, and the bolts are loosely fitted. With sharp thin osteotomes, the osteotomy is completed, great care being taken not to split the medial cortex of the dome of the proximal fragment.

E, The bone fragments are manipulated and the angular and rotational deformities are corrected. If necessary, a wedge of bone may be removed from the lateral side of the distal fragment with a rongeur. The osteotomy fragments are anchored together by fixing the Roger Anderson apparatus firmly. Roentgenograms are taken with the elbow in extension to check the correction of the deformity and the position of the Crow pins. The periosteum and the wound are closed in the usual manner.

F, Abundant sheath wadding and petrolatum gauze are placed over the Roger Anderson apparatus, and a long arm cast is applied with the elbow in 90 degrees of flexion. (From Tachdjian, M.: Pediatric Orthopedics, Vol. 2. Philadelphia, W. B. Saunders Company, 1972.)

ment of the radial nerve in callus and bone about the fracture site.[92] Post described a similar entrapment of the median nerve with complete loss of function requiring partial resection of the nerve and reconstruction.[74] Compression of the anterior interosseous nerve has occurred from stretching of the neurovascular bundle and compression by the fibrous tunnel of the upper arm against the nerve.[87] Neurovascular complications may also be a result of treatment in which manip-

ulation has resulted in the above noted injuries.

Complications of Treatment

The primary complication of treatment is malunion, which occurs in 10 to 35 percent of patients in most series. Table 12–1 documents the findings of several representative series. Cubitus varus is the most common and persistent deformity. Increased or decreased anteversion of the distal humerus occurs fre-

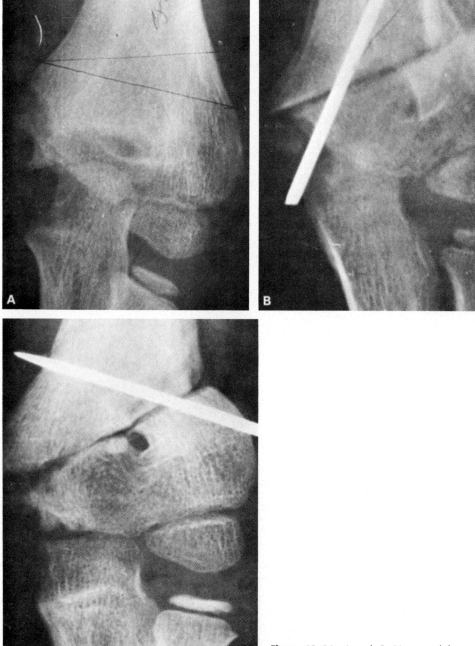

Figure 12–36. A and B, Varus and hyperextension following supracondylar fracture. C, Closing wedge osteotomy with pin fixation.

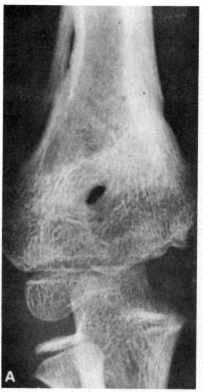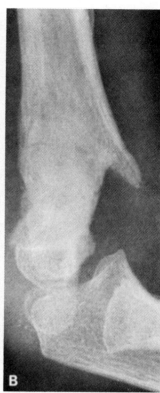

Figure 12–37. *A,* The corrective osteotomy is properly outlined preoperatively. *B,* However, the final osteotomy was too close to the medial epicondyle, and the fixation pin should be in bone, not epiphysis. (From Ogden, J. A.: Skeletal Injury in a Child. Philadephia, Lea & Febiger, 1982.)

quently with initial loss of flexion or extension but rarely presents a long-term problem because remodeling takes place. Malunion is usually noticed soon after treatment in contrast to growth disturbances, which appear as progressive deformities. Growth disturbances that may occur are secondary to the stimulation of growth of one of the condyles by the reaction of fracture healing or are due to direct injury to the physis that results in premature arrest of growth in the affected area (Fig. 12–31). Malunion occurs because of failure to recognize the deformity at the time of treatment. Once again, accurate radiographic evaluation is mandatory but is often difficult to achieve because it is necessary to take the anteroposterior view of the distal humerus with the elbow in a flexed position after the application of a cast. Smith has already demonstrated that precise traction techniques controlling pronation or supination as necessary will prevent or minimize deformity.[6, 9, 12, 13, 24, 27] Closed reduction with percutaneous pinning and open reduction and pin fixation can reduce the severity but will not necessarily decrease the incidence of these deformities.[20, 24, 25, 27, 57, 95]

Treatment of Complications

Treatment of malunion depends on the severity of the deformity. Cubitus valgus is usually mild and does not present a cosmetic disability. Cubitus varus, on the other hand, has a much more displeasing cosmetic appearance (Fig. 12–7). Because function is rarely affected, the major indications for treatment is improvement of the cosmetic defect.[31, 37, 42, 57, 59, 70, 93] Surgical management is usually achieved by performing a lateral closing wedge osteotomy and simultaneously correcting any rotational deformity that may be present. Accurate preoperative radiographs of both elbows should be taken with the elbow fully extended and the forearm supinated so that the deformity may be accurately defined and compared with the normal extremity. Preoperatively, a paper cut-out model of the intended osteotomy may be very helpful in judging the degree of wedge excision necessary. Several techniques have been described, and the same surgical approach is used in all methods (Fig. 12–35). Following surgical exposure of the distal humerus, Tachdjian suggests a rather complex closing wedge osteotomy following by fixation of the fragments with an external fixation device (Fig. 12–36).[93] Ogden has suggested a simple closing wedge osteotomy with fixation by K-wires (Fig. 12–37).[70] Bayer reported fewer complications using this technique compared with others.[11a] Both of these techniques result in correction of the general alignment, but a very prominent

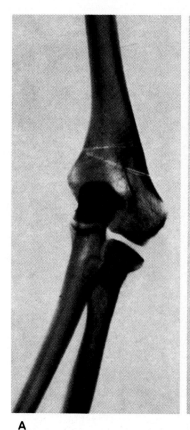
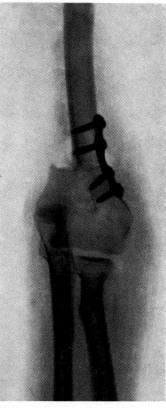

A   **B**

Figure 12–38. *A*, Cubitus varus in a girl aged 18 years following supracondylar fracture at the age of 3 years. *B*, The same elbow radiographed on the operating table immediately after correction of varus and rotation deformity and fixation by a bent metal plate. The lateral condyle is less prominent with translocation of the metaphyses and has a better cosmetic result. (From Langenskiold, A., and Kivilaakso, R.: Varus and valgus deformity on the elbow following supracondylar fractures. Acta Orthop. Scand. 38:316, 1967.)

medial condyle persists. Langenskiolde uses a technique that provides a better cosmetic result by performing a closing wedge osteotomy followed by translocation of the metaphysis medially and fixation with a small customized plate and screws (Fig. 12–38).[59] This gives the best cosmetic result and is our technique of choice. Plate removal does, however, require a second operation.

El-Ahwany has suggested a posterior surgical approach in which he places the patient in a prone position. A posteromedial incision exposes the triceps, which is transected into an inverted V; a closing wedge osteotomy is performed without any internal fixation.[31] The correction is held with a cast. This technique appears to be subject to the complication of loss of alignment.

Bayer and Rang have pointed out that complication of these osteotomies, such as loss of correction, pin problems, stiffness, neuropraxia, and unsightly scars, are not uncommon, occurring in 24 percent of Bayer's series, who had 12 unsatisfactory and 33 satisfactory results, and in 14 of 25 procedures in Rang's series. Therefore, corrective osteotomy should be used only when the deformity is moderately severe (Table 12–2).[11a, 77]

SUMMARY

Several large series of almost 50 cases such as those of Siris and D'Ambrosia have shown that good functional cosmetic results are obtained in at least 80 to 85 percent of patients treated by various modalities.[24, 83a] Attention to detail is the key to satisfactory management of these fractures, and perfection can be achieved, as demonstrated by Smith's series of 100 patients, in which no neurovascular or structural deformities occurred using his meticulous technique.[85] Gruber, utilizing an open reduction and fixation technique, had

Table 12–2. **Complications in 25 Patients**

General	
Poor scar	3
Stiffness	2
No internal fixation	
Displaced	3/7
Neuropraxia	1/7
Internal fixation	
Displaced	2/18
Pin problems*	3/18
	14/25

From Rang, M.: Children's Fractures, 2nd ed. Philadelphia, J. B. Lippincott, 1983.

similar results.[42] In Flynn's series, using closed reduction and percutaneous pinning, there was a 4 percent incidence of cubitus varus deformity.[34] Traction techniques usually require hospitalization of a week to 10 days, which had made this technique less attractive to many patients because of high medical costs. However, it still appears to be the safest way to manage a displaced supracondylar fracture of the elbow. Percutaneous pinning of these fractures in the hands of experienced surgeons offers a reasonable alternative to this form of treatment.

References

1. Abulfotooh, M.: Reduction of Displaced Supracondylar Fracture of the Humerus in Children by Manipulation in Flexion. Acta Orthop Scand. **49**:39, 1978.
2. Aebi, H.: Der Ellbogenwinkel, seine Beziehungen zu Geschlecht Körperbau und Hüfthreite. Acta Anat **3**:228, 1947.
3. Alcott, W. H., Boyd, W. B., and Miller, P. R.: Displaced Supracondylar Fractures of the Humerus in Children: Long-Term Follow-Up of 69 Patients. Am. Osteopath. Assoc. **76**:910, 1977.
4. Ambrosia, R. D.: Supracondylar Fractures of the Humerus: Prevention of Cubitus Varus. J. Bone Joint Surg. **54A**:60, 1972.
5. Arino, V. L., Lluch, E. E., Ramirex, A. M., Ferrer, J., Rodriguez, L., and Baixauli, F.: Percutaneous Fixation of Supracondylar Fractures of the Humerus in Children. J. Bone Joint Surg. **59A**(7):914, 1977.
6. Arnold, J. A., Nasca, R. J., and Nelson, C. L.: Supracondylar Fractures of the Humerus. The Role of Dynamic Factors in Prevention of Deformity. J. Bone Joint Surg. **59A**(5):589, 1977.
7. Attenborough, C. G.: Remodelling of the Humerus After Supracondylar Fractures in Childhood. J. Bone Joint Surg. **35B**(3):386, 1953.
8. Baily, G. G., Jr.: Nerve Injuries in Supracondylar Fractures of the Humerus in Children. N. Engl. J. Med. **221**(7):260, 1939.
9. Bakalim, G., and Wilppula, E.: Supracondylar Humerus Fractures in Children. Causes of Changes in the Carrying Angle of the Elbow. Acta Orthop Scand. **43**:366, 1972.
10. Bason, W.: Supracondylar and Transcondylar Fractures in Children. Clin Orthop, **1**:43, 1953.
11. Bauman, E.: Beitrage zur Kenntnis der Frakturen am Ellbogengelenk. Beur. Klin. Chir. **146**:1, 1929.
11a. Bayer, M. E., Oppenheim, W. L., Cledar, T., and Smith, C. F.: Supracondylar Osteotomy of the Humerus for Cubitus Varus Deformity in Children. A.A.O.S. Annual Meeting, Atlanta, February, 1984.
12. Bender, J.: Cubitus Varus After Supracondylar Fractures of the Humerus in Children: Can This Deformity be Prevented? Reconstr. Surg. Traumatol. **17**:100, 1979.
13. Bender, J., and Busch, C. A.: Results of Treatment of Supracondylar Fractures of the Humerus in Children With Special Reference to the Cause and Prevention of Cubitus Varus. Arch. Chir. Neerland. **30**:29, 1978.
14. Bensahel, H., and Desgrippes, Y.: Les Luxations Residuelles de la Tete Radial dans les Fractures de Monteggia. Ann. Chir. Infant. Paris **14**(3):229, 1973.
15. Bergenfeldt, E.: Über Schaden an der Epiphysenfuge bei operativer Behandlung von Frakturen am unteren Humerusende. Acta Chir Scand. **71**:103, 1932.

15a. Bohler, L.: Technik der Knochenbruchbehandlung. Vienna, Mandrich, 1930.
16. Bongers, K. J., and Ponsen, R. J. G.: Use of Kirschner Wires for Percutaneous Stabilization of Supracondylar Fractures of the Humerus in Children. Arch. Chir. Neerland. **31**(4):203, 1979.
17. Bristow, W. R.: Myositis Ossificans and Volkmann's Paralysis. Notes on Two Cases Illustrating the Rarer Complication of Supracondylar Fracture of the Humerus. Br. J. Surg. **10**:475, 1923.
18. Broudy, A. S., Jupiter, J., and May, J. W., Jr.: Management of Supracondylar Fracture With Brachial Artery Thrombosis in a Child: Case Report and Literature Review. J Trauma **19**(7):540, 1907.
19. Buhl, O., and Hellberg, S.: Displaced Supracondylar Fractures of the Humerus in Children. Acta Orthop Scand. **53**:67, 1982.
20. Carcassone, M., Bergoin, M., and Hornung, H.: Results of Operative Treatment of Severe Supracondylar Fractures of the Elbow in Children. J Pediatr Surg. **7**:676, 1972.
21. Carli, C.: Wire Traction for Supracondylar Fracture of the Elbow in Children. Chir Organi Mov. **18**:311, 1933.
21a. Carlson, W., and Klassen, R. A.: Myositis Ossificans in the Upper Extremity in Children. (In press, 1984.)
22. Coventry, M. B., and Henderson, C. C.: Supracondylar Fractures of the Humerus: A Critical Analysis of 49 Cases in Children. Meeting of the Wyoming State Medical Society, Laramie, Wyoming, June 13 to 15, 1955.
23. Cuendet, M. C.: Supracondylar Fractures of the Humerus in Children. Am. Fam. Phys. **12**(3), 1973.
24. D'Ambrosia, R. D.: Supracondylar Fractures of Humerus—Prevention of Cubitus Varus. J. Bone Joint Surg. **54A**:60, 1972.
25. Danielsson, L., and Pettersson, H.: Open Reduction and Pin Fixation of Severely Displaced Supracondylar Fractures of the Humerus in Children. Acta Orthop Scand. **51**:249, 1980.
26. Dodge, H. S.: Displaced Supracondylar Fractures of the Humerus in Children—Treatment by Dunlop's Traction. J. Bone Joint Surg. **54A**:1408, 1972.
27. Dowd, G. S. E., and Hopcroft, P. W.: Varus Deformity in Supracondylar Fractures of the Humerus in Children. Injury **10**:297, 1979.
28. Dunlop, J.: Transcondylar Fractures of the Humerus in Childhood. J. Bone Joint Surg. **21**(1):59, 1939.
29. Edman, P., and Lohr, G.: Supracondylar Fractures of the Humerus Treated With Olecranon Traction. Acta Chir Scand. **126**:505, 1963.
30. Eid, A. M.: Reduction of Displaced Supracondylar Fractures of the Humerus in Children by Manipulation in Flexion. Acta Orthop Scand. **49**:39, 1978.
31. El-Ahwany, M. D.: Supracondylar Fractures of the Humerus in Children With a Note on the Surgical Correction of Late Cubitus Varus. Injury **16**(1):45, 1973–1975.
32. El-Sharkawi, A., and Fattah, H.: Treatment of Displaced Supracondylar Fractures of the Humerus in Children in Full Extension and Supination. J. Bone Joint Surg. **47B**:273, 1965.
33. Elstrom, J. A., Pankovich, A. M., and Kassab, M. T.: Irreducible Supracondylar Fractures of the Humerus in Children. A Report of Two Cases. J. Bone Joint Surg. **57A**(5):680, 1975.
34. Flynn, J. C., Matthews, J. G., and Benoit, R. L.: Blind Pinning of Displaced Supracondylar Fractures of the Humerus in Children. Sixteen Years' Experience With Long-Term Follow-Up. J. Bone Joint Surg. **56A**(2):263, 1974.
35. Flynn, J. C., Richards, J. F., Jr., and Saltzman, R. I.:

Nonunion of Minimally Displaced Fractures of the Lateral Condyle of the Humerus in Children. A Scientific Exhibit Presented at the Forty-First Annual meeting, American Academy of Orthopedic Surgeons, Dallas, Texas, January, 1974.

36. Fowles, J. V., and Kassab, M. T.: Displaced Supracondylar Fractures of the Elbow in Children. J. Bone Joint Surg. **56B**:490, 1974.

37. French, P. R.: Varus Deformity of the Elbow Following Supracondylar Fractures of the Humerus in Children. Lancet **1**:439, 1959.

38. Gjerloff, C., and Sojbjerg, J. O.: Percutaneous Pinning of Supracondylar Fractures of the Humerus. Acta Orthop Scand **49**:597, 1978.

39. Graham, H. A.: Supracondylar Fractures of the Elbow of Children. Part I. Clin. Orthop. **58**:85, 1967.

40. Graham, H. A.: Supracondylar Fractures of the Elbow of Children. Part II. Clin. Orthop. **54**:93, 1967.

41. Griffin, P. P.: Supracondylar Fractures of the Humerus. Treatment and Complication. Symposium on Childhood Trauma. Pediatr. Clin. North Am. **22**(2):477, 1975.

41a. Groves, E. W. H.: Direct skeletal traction in the treatment of fractures. Br. J. Surg. **16**:149, 1929.

42. Gruder, M. A., and Hudson, O. E.: Supracondylar Fractures of the Humerus in Childhood: End Results in Study of Open Reduction. J. Bone Joint Surg. **46A**:1245, 1964.

43. Griffiths, D. L.: The Management of Acute Circulatory Failure in an Injured Limb. J. Bone Joint Surg. **30B**(2):280, 1948.

44. Haddad, R. J., Jr., Saer, K. J., and Riordan, D. C.: Percutaneous Pinning of Displaced Supracondylar Fractures of the Elbow in Children. Clin. Orthop. **71**:112, 1970.

45. Hagen, R.: Skin Traction Treatment of Supracondylar Fractures of the Humerus in Children. Acta Orthop. Scand. **35**:138, 1964.

46. Hart, G. M., Wilson, D. W., and Arden, G. P.: The Operative Management of the Difficult Supracondylar Fractures of the Humerus in the Child. Injury **9**(1):30, 1977.

47. Heilbronner, D. M., Manoli, A., II, and Little, R. E.: Elbow Dislocation During Overhead Skeletal Traction Therapy: A Case Report. Clin. Orthop. **154**:185, 1981.

48. Henrikson, B.: Supracondylar Fractures of the Humerus in Children. Acta. Chir. Scand. Suppl. **369**:1–73, 1966.

49. Holmberg, L.: Fractures in the Distal End of the Humerus in Children. Acta Orthop. Scand. (Suppl.), **92**:103, 1945.

50. Holms, J. C., Skolnick, M. D., and Hall, J. E.: Untreated Median Nerve Entrapment in Bone after Fracture of the Distal and of the Humerus: Postmortem Findings After Forty-Seven Years. Report of a Case. J. Bone Joint Surg. **61A**(2):309, 1979.

51. Hordegen, K. M.: Neurologische Komplikationen bei kindlichen suprakondylaren Humerusfrakturen. Arch. Orthop. Unfallchir. **68**:294, 1970.

52. Hovelius, L., and Tuvesson, T.: Anterior Interosseous Nerve Paralysis as a Complication of Supracondylar Fractures of the Humerus in Children. A Report of Two Cases. Orthop. Traumatol. Surg. **96**:59, 1980.

53. Hoyer, A.: Treatment of Supracondylar Fractures of the Humerus by Skeletal Traction in an Abduction Splint. J. Bone Joint Surg. **34A**:623, 1952.

54. Jefferiss, C. D.: "Straight Lateral Traction " in Selected Supracondylar Fractures of the Humerus in Children. Injury **8**:213, 1977.

55. Jones, E. T., and Louis, D. S.: Median Nerve Injuries Associated with Supracondylar Fractures of the Humerus in Children. Clin. Orthop. **150**:181, 1980.

56. Jones, K. G.: Percutaneous Pin Fixation of Fractures of the Lower End of the Humerus. Clin. Orthop. **50**:53, 1967.

57. Kagan, N., and Herold, H. Z.: Correction of Axial Deviations After Supracondylar Fractures of the Humerus in Children. Int. Surg. **58**:735, 1973.

58a. Kamal, A. S., and Austin, R. T.: Dislocation of the Median Nerve and Brachial Artery in Supracondylar Fractures of the Humerus. Injury **12**:161, 1980.

58b. Kekomaki, M., Luoma, R., Rehalaenen, H., and Vilkki, P.: Operative Reduction and Fixation of a Difficult Supracondylar Extension Fracture of the Humerus. J. Pediatr. Orthop. **4**:13, 1984.

59. Langenskiold, A., and Kivilaakso, R.: Varus and Valgus Deformity of the Elbow Following Supracondylar Fractures of the Humerus. Acta Orthop. Scand. **38**:313, 1967.

59a. Lipscomb, P.: Vascular and Neural Complications in Supracondylar Fractures of the Humerus in Children. J. Bone Joint Surg. **37A**:487, 1955.

60. Lugnegard, H., Walheim, G., and Wennberg, A.: Operative Treatment of Ulnar Nerve Neuropathy in the Elbow Region. Acta Orthop. Scand. **48**:168, 1977.

61. Lund-Kristensen, J., and Vibild, O.: Supracondylar Fractures of the Humerus in Children. Acta Orthop. Scand. **47**:375, 1976.

62. Mann, T. S.: Prognosis in Supracondylar Fractures. J. Bone Joint Surg. **45B**:516, 1963.

63. MacLemman, A.: Common Fractures About the Elbow in Children. Surg. Gynec. Obstet. **64**:447, 1947.

64. Maylahn, D. J., and Fahey, J. J.: Fractures of the Elbow in Children. Review of Three Hundred Consecutive Cases. J.A.M.A. **166**:220, 1958.

65. McCarty, S. M., and Ogden, J. A.: Radiology of Postnatal Skeletal Development. V. Distal Humerus. Skeletal Radiol. **7**:239, 1982.

66. Micheli, L. J., Santore, R., and Stanitski, C. L.: Epiphyseal Fractures of the Elbow in Children. Am. Fam. Phys. **22**(5):107, 1980.

67. Micheli, L. J., Skolnick, D., and Hall, J. E.: Supracondylar Fractures in the Humerus in Children. Am. Fam. Phys. **19**(3):100, 1979.

68. Miller, O. E.: Blind Nailing of the Fracture of the Lower End of the Humerus Which Involves the Joint. J. Bone Joint Surg. **21**:933, 1939.

68a. Millis, M. B., Hall, J. E., Singer, I.: Supracondylar Fracture in Children Further experience with a Study in Orthopedic Decision Making AAOS Annual Meeting, Atlanta, Feb. 1984.

69. Mizuno, K., Hirohata, K., and Kashiwagi, D.: Fractures—Separation of the Distal Humerus Epiphysis in Young Children. J. Bone Joint Surg. **61A**, (4):570, 1979.

70. Ogden, J.: Skeletal Injury in the Child. Philadelphia, Lea & Febiger, 1982, p. 240.

71. Ottolenghi, C. E.: Prophylactic due Syndrome de Volkmann dans des Humerus Supracondyliennes du Coude chez l'Enfant. Rev. Chir. Orthop. **57**:517, 1971.

72. Palmer, E. E., Niemann, K. M. W., Vesely, D., and Armstrong, J. H.: Supracondylar Fractures of the Humerus in Children. J. Bone Joint Surg. **60A**(5):653, 1978.

73. Poland, J.: Traumatic Separation of Epiphysis. London, Smith, Elder and Co., 1898.

74. Post, M., and Haskell, S. S.: Reconstruction of the Median Nerve Following Entrapment in Supracondylar Fractures of the Humerus. J. Trauma **14**:252, 1974.

75. Preitto, C. A.: Supracondylar Fractures of the Humerus. J. Bone Joint Surg. **61A**(3):425, 1979.

76. Ramsey, R. H., and Griz, J.: Immediate Open Reduction and Internal Fixation of Severely Displaced Supracondylar Fractures of the Humerus in Children. Clin. Orthop **90**:130, 1973.

77. Rang, M.: Children's Fractures, 2nd ed. Philadelphia, J. B. Lippincott, 1983.

78. Reinaerts, H. H. M., and Cheriex, E. C.: Assessment of Dislocation in the Supracondylar Fractures of the Humerus, Treated by Overhead Traction. Reconstr. Surg. Traumatol. **17**:92, 1979.

79. Rogers, L. F., Malave, S., Jr., White, H., and Tachdjian, M. O.: Plastic Bowing, Torus and Greenstick Supracondylar Fractures of the Humerus: Radiographic Clues to Obscure Fractures of the Elbow in Children. Radiology **128**:145, 1978.

80. Rowell, P. J. W.: Arterial Occlusion in Juvenile Humerus Supracondylar Fracture. Injury **6**(3):254, 1976.

81. Schickendanz, H., Schramm, H., Herrmann, K., and Jager, S.: Fractures and Dislocations in the Elbow in Childhood. Am. Fam. Phys. **13**(2), 1973.

82. Shifrin, P. G., Gehring, H. W., and Igelsias, L J.: Open Reduction and Internal Fixation of Displaced Supracondylar Fractures of the Humerus in Children. Orthop. Clin. North Am. **7**(3):573, 1976.

83. Smith, F. M.: Children's Elbow Injuries. Fractures and Dislocations. Clin. Orthop. **50**:7, 1967.

83a. Siris, J. E.: Supracondylar Fractures of the Humerus Analyzed 330 Cases. Surg. Gynec. Obstet. **68**:201, 1939.

84. Smith, H. C.: Position in the Treatment of Elbow Joint Fractures: An Experimental Study. Boston Med. Surgeons J. **131**:386, 1894.

85. Smith, L.: Deformity Following Supracondylar Fractures. J. Bone Joint Surg. **42A**:235, 1960.

85a. Sorrel, E., Longuet, V.: La voi transbrachial anterieure dans la chirurgie des fractures supra condy-

liennes de l'humerus chez L'enfant. Rev. Chir. Orthop. **32**:3, 1946.

86. Spear, H. C., and Janes, J. M.: Rupture of the Brachial Artery Accompanying Dislocation of the Elbow or Supracondylar Fracture. J. Bone Joint Surg. **33A**:889, 1951.

87. Spinner, M., and Schreiber, S.: Anterior Interosseous Nerve Paralysis—A Complication of Supracondylar Fractures of the Humerus in Children. J. Bone Joint Surg. **51A**:1584, 1969.

88. Stanitski, C. L., and Micheli, L. J.: Simultaneous Ipsilateral Fractures of the Arm and Forearm in Children. Clin. Orthop. **153**:218, 1980.

89. Staples, O. S.: Complication of Traction Treatment of Supracondylar Fractures of the Humerus in Children. J. Bone Joint Surg. **41A**:369, 1959.

90. Staples, O. S.: Dislocation of the Brachial Artery. A Complication of Supracondylar Fractures of the Humerus in Childhood. J. Bone Joint Surg. **47A**:1525, 1965.

91. Swenson, A. L.: The Treatment of Supracondylar Fractures of the Humerus by Kirschner-Wire Fixation. J. Bone Joint Surg. **30A**:993, 1948.

92. Symeonides, P. P., Paschaloglou, C., and Pagalides, T.: Radial Nerve Enclosed in the Callus of a Supracondylar Fracture. J. Bone Joint Surg. **57B**:523, 1975.

93. Tachdjian, M.: Pediatric Orthopedics, Vol. 2. Philadelphia, W. B. Saunders Co., 1972.

94. Vahvanen, V., and Aalto, K.: Supracondylar Fractures of the Humerus in Children. A Long-Term Follow-Up Study of 107 Cases. Acta Orthop. Scand. **49**:225, 1978.

95. Weiland, A. J., Meyer, S., Tolo, V. T., Berg, H. L., and Mueller, J.: Surgical Treatment of Displaced Supracondylar Fractures of the Humerus in Children. J. Bone Joint Surg. **60A**(5):657, 1978.

96. Wray, J.: Management of Supracondylar Fractures With Vascular Insufficiency. Arch. Surg. **90**:279, 1965.

CHAPTER 13

Physeal Fractures

HAMLET A. PETERSON

The incidence of injury involving the epiphyseal growth plates (physes) of the elbow is unknown. Some information has been gathered about the relative frequency of physeal injuries.[36] Approximately 19 percent of all growth plate injuries occur at the elbow: 14.8 percent in the distal humerus, 3.6 percent in the proximal radius, and 0.7 percent in the proximal ulna (Table 13–1.) These data, however, may not be completely accurate. For example, when considering the distal humerus, three authors stated that injuries of the medial epicondyle were included. Because the remaining authors made no such statement, there is a question about whether they included this structure or not. In addition, the relative frequency of injuries to various physes of the elbow varies greatly in different series (Table 13–1). For example, the percentage of injuries occurring in the distal humerus varied from 6.7 per cent to 59 percent. This wide discrepancy may be explained by the difficulty in distinguishing between supracondylar fractures, which are much more common, and fractures that actually involve the physis.

A similar situation exists for the proximal radius, where it may be difficult to distinguish between a fracture through the proximal portion of the metaphyseal neck of the radius and one that actually enters the physis. For example, in the last four studies of physeal injuries (Table 13–1), Lipschultz, Peterson and Peterson,[36] and Ogden[28] found only six cases of injury to the proximal radial physis out of 1153 injuries (0.52 percent), whereas Neer found 124 cases out of 2368 (5.2 percent). The relative frequency in Neer's study is therefore 10 times greater than that in the combined group. One would question whether some fractures through the neck of the radius were included in Neer's series. Because this series comprises over half of the total recorded physeal injuries in the literature, such a change in his data would significantly alter the total percentage of proximal radial physeal injuries (3.6 percent).

Physeal injuries of the proximal ulna are rare in all series.

Injuries of the distal humeral physes have several peculiarities when they are compared with injuries to other physes.[36] For example, the distal physis of every long bone is injured more frequently than the proximal end. This is true of all long bones except the humerus in some series. The age range for injuries is also different for fractures of the distal humerus compared with all other physes. The age distribution for all physeal injuries is a bell-shaped curve with the peak at age 12 and 13 years except for the distal humerus, which has a bimodal age distribution with the peak occurring in one group from 2 to 8 years and a second peak occurring at 11 to 15 years. The typical age range for injury to all physes is from 6 to 16 years, with a maximal incidence for girls at age 12 to 13 years and for boys at age 13 to 14 years. In the distal humerus, however, the age range is from 1 to 15; the age of maximal incidence for girls is 4 to 5 years and for boys, 5 to 8 years. The male-female ratio for all physeal injuries varies from 1:1 to 5:1, except for the distal humerus, which has a male predominance of 9:1.

The earlier peak incidence of distal humeral physeal injuries may be related to the difficulty in differentiating supracondylar (actually transcondylar) fractures from physeal injuries. Humeral supracondylar fractures are also frequent at this early age (age 4 to 8 years) (see Chapter 12). Because it may be difficult to determine whether a fracture line in the metaphysis extends into either the medial or the lateral cartilaginous epiphysis, many fractures recorded as physeal injuries may in fact be completely proximal to the physis. Any attempt to explain these discrepancies of distal humeral injuries compared with injuries to other physes requires a review of elbow epiphyseal development.

ANATOMY

Most long bones have one epiphyseal growth center and one physis at each end. Most joints are made up of the articulating epiphyses of two bones and two epiphyses (for example,

Table 13–1. **Relative Frequency of Physeal Injuries**

Site	1915 Bowen	1924 Smith	1933 Bergen-feldt	1934 Eliason & Ferguson	1935 Compere	1937 Bisgard & Martenson	1937 Lipschultz	1960 Neer	1972 Peterson & Peterson	1981[28] Ogden	Total	Per-cent
1. Distal Radius	21	12	137	48	6	9	234	1,096	98	114	1,775	43.3
2. Distal Humerus	2	10	70[a]	36[a]	11	29	43[a]	332	20	56	609	14.8
3. Distal Tibia	4	4	44	4	9	4	59	238	59	60	485	11.8
4. Distal Fibula	1		16	2	5	1	4	302	21	15	367	8.9
5. Distal Ulna		2	24	9	2	2	15	136	12	11	213	5.2
6. Proximal Humerus		3	5	2	1	1	18	72	22	27	151	3.7
7. Proximal Radius	4		8	1	2	1		124	1	5	146	3.6
8. Phalanges (fingers)									39	41	80	1.9
9. Distal Femur	2		1	3	4	2	3	28	18	17	78	1.9
10. Proximal Tibia			1					17	6	20	44	1.1
11. Phalanges (toes)									11	21	32	0.8
12. Proximal Ulna			2	1				21		3	27	0.7
13. Metacarpal	4	2							10	8	24	0.6
14. Pelvis										23	23	0.6
15. Proximal Femur (head)				2	2				7	9	20	0.5
16. Lesser Trochanter		2	2	2			4			4	12	0.3
17. Metatarsals									6	3	9	0.2
18. Proximal Fibula								2		2	4	0.1
19. Proximal Clavicle										3	3	0.1
20. Distal Clavicle										1	1	0.1
Total	38	33	310	110	42	49	380	2,368	330	443	4,103	100.0

[a]Includes injuries of the epicondyles.

(Adapted from Peterson, C. A., and Peterson, H. A.: Analysis of the incidence of injuries to the epiphyseal growth plate. J. Trauma 12:275–281, 1972. © 1972, The Williams & Wilkins Co., Baltimore.)

the knee). The articulating surfaces of the elbow, however, involve three bones. These three bones have six separate epiphyseal ossification centers, four of which participate in articulation.

Initially, the distal humeral epiphysis is one large mass of cartilage (Fig. 13–1). The epiphyseal growth plate is transverse at birth, which contributes to a predisposition to total separation of the epiphysis if significant trauma occurs (Fig. 13–2). During maturation separate ossification centers develop for the capitellum, the medial epicondyle, the trochlea, and the lateral epicondyle. In early youth the growth plate gradually extends obliquely downward and medially from a point just above the lateral epicondyle to below the medial epicondyle. This obliquity of the epiphyseal line may account in part for the frequent lateral displacement of the epiphysis and the difficulty of maintaining accurate reduction.

By age 4 years the growth plate becomes more irregular, and metaphyseal bone begins to project between the medial epicondyle and the capitellum. Both of these factors aid stability, and total separation of the epiphyses becomes more difficult.

The three lateral centers (lateral epicondyle, capitellum, and trochlea) unite in approximately the thirteenth year (earlier in females) to form the distal humeral epiphysis and articulating surfaces. This epiphysis later fuses with the shaft in the sixteenth year. Once fused, growth ceases and growth alteration following injury is no longer possible. The medial epicondylar epiphysis is extra-articular. It remains open and unites to the shaft as late as the nineteenth year. Some authors feel that osseous injury of the medial epicondyle that occurs after closure of the distal humeral physis is not a physeal injury. Thus, separation of the medial epicondyle that occurs in the later teens, which is not infrequent, may have been overlooked in the statistic analysis.

Anatomic peculiarities of the distal humerus may therefore explain the differences in age distribution of these injuries. These anatomic differences at various ages also account for the different types of physeal injuries that are seen at each age. There has been no documentation in the literature relating the type of distal humeral physeal injury to age or sex.

Many classifications of physeal injuries have been proposed. The classification of Salter and Harris[38] is the most frequently used and will, therefore, be used in the remainder of this chapter. There have been no case reports of physeal compression injury (Salter and Harris type V) recorded in the literature in the elbow or in the upper extremity, despite the fact that 73.8 percent of all physeal injuries occur in the upper extremity (Table 13–1). Recent speculation suggests that compression

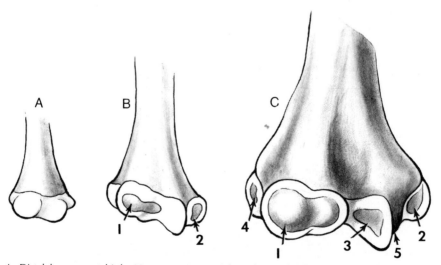

Figure 13–1. *A,* Distal humerus at birth. Note transverse epiphyseal growth plate and single cartilaginous epiphysis; no ossification centers are present. *B,* Distal humerus at age 5 years. Note obliquity of epiphyseal growth plate to longitudinal axis of humerus and single epiphysis; ossification centers [capitellum (1) and medial epicondyle (2)] have appeared. *C,* Distal humerus at age 12 years. Note irregular epiphyseal growth plate and projection of bone (5), which separates medial epicondyle (2) from the major distal epiphysis, which contains three ossification centers [capitellum (1), trochlea (3), and lateral epicondyle (4)]. (From Peterson C. A., and Peterson, H. A.: Analysis of the incidence of injuries to the epiphyseal growth plate. J. Trauma 12:275–281, 1972.)

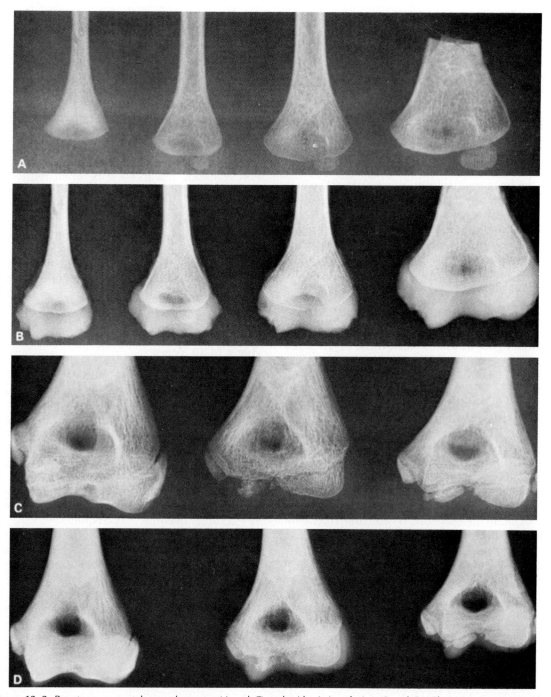

Figure 13–2. Roentgenograms taken under water (A and C) and with air interfacing (B and D). The water immersion films duplicate the clinical situation of radiolucent cartilage. A and B are specimens from children aged newborn, 15 months, 24 months, and 36 months, respectively (left to right). C and D are from children aged 14, 11, and 10 years, respectively (left to right). (From Ogden, J. A.: Skeletal Injury in the Child. Philadelphia, Lea & Febiger, 1982.)

injury (type V) of any physis is unlikely and may not exist.[35] It will therefore be omitted from discussion in the remainder of this chapter.

Anteroposterior and lateral roentgenograms of the injured elbow are essential for evalua-tion. Views of the opposite elbow in the same position provide a valuable basis for compar-ison in assessing injury. Intra-articular he-matoma may displace the posterior fat pad of the distal humerus (the "fat pad sign"), which may be the only demonstrable change in an undisplaced or spontaneously reduced fracture.[1, 25] Several recent excellent texts and atlases review the radiographic anatomy of the elbow at different ages in both sexes, variations in development, and treatment of fractures.[1, 8, 29, 47, 50, 51]

DISTAL HUMERUS

Age Birth to 3 Years

The epiphysis of the distal end of the humerus is one large cartilaginous mass during the first 3 years of life (Fig. 13–3). Its interface with the metaphysis is smooth and transverse. The ossification center of the capitellum appears as early as 6 months and always before age 2.[40] This ossification center initially remains oval and does not affect the contour of the adjacent metaphysis.

Most injuries in the newborn[12, 39] and infants,[3, 7, 13, 15, 19, 23] therefore, are transverse shear-type injuries along the line of the epiphyseal growth plate. Thus, these injuries are typically Salter and Harris types I and II (Fig. 13–3). The entire epiphysis may be displaced anteriorly,[8, 20] posteriorly, medially,[15, 19, 37] or laterally depending on the mechanism of the injury, but displacement is usually postero-medial.[7, 15] Rotatory malalignment may accompany displacement or occur alone. Injuries of types III and IV are theoretically possible but extremely rare (Fig. 13–4). Because the epiphysis is primarily cartilaginous in very young children, the type of injury may be difficult to diagnose by routine roentgenograms. Injury with mild displacement may go undetected in "battered" children who are brought for medical attention late. Epiphyseal injury is frequently misdiagnosed as a fracture of the lateral humeral condyle or an elbow dislocation.[3, 7, 19, 23, 30, 33, 37, 46] Arthrography in these young children may aid in establishing the correct diagnosis.[3, 13, 26, 42] Because the entire epiphyseal growth plate usually remains with the epiphysis, damage to the growth plate is uncommon, and the potential for resumption of normal growth is very good.

Treatment consists of aligning the epiphysis with the metaphysis. Precise anatomic reduction is desirable but not necessary. This can usually be obtained by closed manipulation or traction.[3, 19, 23, 37, 46] Immobilization with the elbow in 90 degrees of flexion and forearm pronation for 3 weeks is usually adequate.[7, 23] Percutaneous pin fixation or open reduction is rarely indicated. Three cases have been reported in which the authors performed late open reduction and internal fixation because of severe malalignment or interposition of soft tissue.[30, 45] The prognosis in these cases is favorable; minor malalignment usually corrects itself with normal growth and development, and physeal growth arrest is uncommon.

Age 4 to 10 Years

By age 4 the epiphyseal growth plate begins to become irregular (Figs. 13–1B and 13–5A). The plate becomes more oblique downward and medial from a point just above the lateral epicondyle to below the medial epicondyle. A projection of metaphyseal bone begins to separate the medial epicondyle from the trochlea, adding additional stability to the epiphyseal growth plate. Therefore, shear-type injuries, such as Salter and Harris types I and II fractures, become less frequent.[19]

On transverse section the physis remains irregularly oval, while that of the metaphysis becomes elongated transversely and thin in the sagittal plane. The strength of the physis is, at this age, therefore greater than that of the bone of the metaphysis. Thus, most injuries in this age group are supracondylar fractures. The decreased area of fracture contact

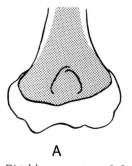 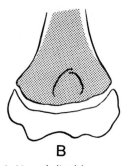 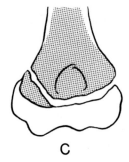

| A | B | C |

Figure 13–3. Distal humerus at age 0–3 years. *A,* Normal distal humerus. *B,* Salter and Harris type I injury. *C,* Salter and Harris type II injury. The radiographic appearance of the piece of metaphyseal bone attached to the epiphysis *(C)* may range in thickness from a thin, faintly visible line of ossification to a thick line including most of the condyle and is sometimes referred to as the Thurstan Holland sign.[16]

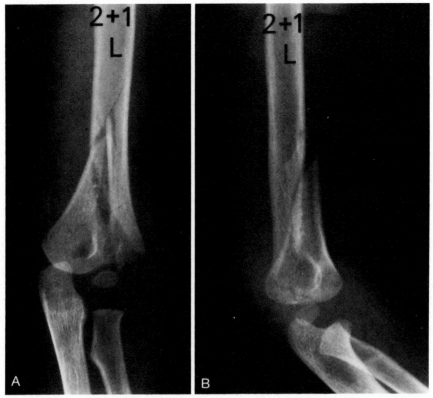

Figure 13–4. *A,* Anteroposterior and *B,* lateral roentgenograms of a girl 2 years and 1 month old whose elbow was run over by an automobile wheel. Joint effusion suggests intra-articular extension of the fracture lateral to the ossification center of the capitellum (Salter and Harris type IV injury). This case illustrates the difficulty of determining the precise nature and type of injury of fractures about the elbow.

in supracondylar fractures makes possible rotation and subsequent tilting of the distal fragment (cubitus varus). Because the area of fracture contact is much greater through the physis, rotation, tilt, and subsequent cubitus varus are less likely.[7]

Injuries involving the physis, when they do occur, are usually longitudinal Salter and Harris type IV of either the lateral or the medial condyle (Fig. 13–5*B, C*). Fractures of the lateral condyle are relatively common, comprising approximately 10 to 15 percent of all fractures in the region of the elbow. They occur in children between the ages of 2 and

14 years but are most common between 5 and 10 years. The mechanism of injury is usually a valgus stress with the elbow in extension.

The portion of metaphyseal bone attached to the capitellar and lateral epicondylar epiphysis may be large or small. The most important consideration is that this fracture is both intra-articular and transphyseal. The intra-articular portion of the fracture may traverse the ossification center of the capitellum, but the fracture line is usually entirely through cartilage and therefore is not visible on roentgenograms.

Because this fracture involves both the ar-

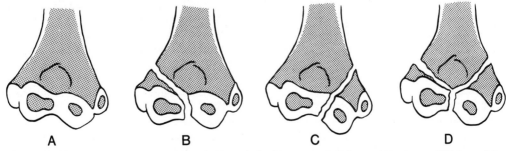

Figure 13–5. Distal humerus at age 4 to 10 years. *A,* Normal distal humerus. *B,* Salter and Harris type IV injury of the lateral condyle, *C,* medial condyle and *D,* both medial and lateral condyles.

ticular surface and the physis, anatomic reduction is necessary and must be held until the fracture has united. This usually requires internal fixation. If the fracture is undisplaced and stable, external immobilization by a long arm cast for 4 weeks will suffice. If there is displacement or evidence that there has been displacement (for example, instability or significant swelling), reduction and internal fixation will prevent redisplacement. If the fracture can be reduced closed, pins inserted percutaneously may be utilized for fixation to prevent redisplacement.[18] In most instances, however, open reduction and accurate replacement by direct vision will be necessary. The reduction must be held by firm internal fixation, preferably metal rather than suture.[11, 14, 17] Smooth pins as small in diameter as possible seem appropriate. Insertion from metaphysis to metaphysis and epiphysis to epiphysis is preferred. However, because the trochlear cartilage is not visible on roentgenograms, the pins may necessarily pass from epiphysis to metaphysis, crossing the physis obliquely. These pins should be removed within 3 weeks to prevent premature partial growth arrest. Threaded pins predispose to premature partial physeal arrest and should not be used across a physis. There is no place for the use of traction.[14]

Premature physeal closure has been noted in approximately 20 percent of lateral humeral injuries. The premature fusion may be of two types. In the first type the capitellar epiphysis fuses to the metaphysis and leads to a disturbance of growth commonly referred to as a fishtail deformity. In the second type the capitellar and trochlear epiphyses fuse together and to the metaphysis. Radial shift of the ulna can follow either type and result in cubitus valgus. The valgus deformity may cause impaired motion but is rarely severe enough to cause unsightly deformity.[4, 8, 49]

Untreated cases are frequently complicated by malunion and nonunion, and these cause deformity, loss of motion, traumatic arthritis, and tardy ulnar neuropathy. There is no agreement on the management of these complications.[14]

Overgrowth of the capitellum is an interesting phenomenon that may occasionally occur following even successful management of a lateral condylar fracture.[49] Although this may produce measurable cubitus varus, functional or cosmetic impairment is rare, and treatment is seldom necessary. Overgrowth of the capitellum is more frequent following supracondylar fractures (perhaps because

these are more common) than following fractures of the lateral condyle.

Fractures of the medial condyle are less frequent (Fig. 13–5C).[2, 10, 17, 21] Only 25 cases had been reported up to July, 1975.[9] The fracture is rare before the age of 8 years, and most occur between the ages of 8 and 10 when the medial half of the trochlea is not ossified. The displaced fragment therefore consists of a large piece of bone from the medial side of the lower humeral metaphysis, including the cartilaginous trochlea and the ossified medial epicondyle. Therefore, the unossified portion of the trochlea is not seen on the roentgenogram. If the fracture occurs before ossification of the trochlea, it may be mistaken for a fracture of the medial epicondyle. If the diagnosis is not made and the injury is treated nonoperatively as a fracture-separation of the medial epicondyle, a poor functional result can be anticipated.[6, 10]

Fractures of the medial condyle may result from a fall on the apex of the flexed elbow or from an avulsion valgus stress injury on an extended elbow.[9, 21, 23]

In addition to the factors of articular congruity and growth plate alignment, this fracture is important because of its proximity to the ulnar nerve. Anatomic reduction is therefore mandatory to avoid tardy ulnar palsy as well as nonunion or malunion. These fractures usually require open reduction and rigid internal fixation. Only if the fracture is undisplaced and there is no evidence that it was displaced may this fracture be treated by cast immobilization alone.

Fractures may involve both condyles with a split through the center of the articular surfaces (Fig. 13–5D). This is analogous to the adult T fracture and is an unstable situation that requires open reduction and internal fixation.[51]

Age 11 to Maturity

At this age the growth plate has again become more transverse but also more irregular (Fig. 13–1C). The medial epicondyle and the trochlea are completely separated by a projection of metaphyseal bone (Fig. 13–6A). The medial epicondyle does not articulate with the ulna or contribute to the longitudinal length of the humerus. All four ossification centers are now visible roentgenographically. Trochlear ossification is frequently irregular and fragmented, simulating fracture (Fig. 13–2C, D). The trochlea, capitellum, and lateral epicondyle usually fuse together before uniting with

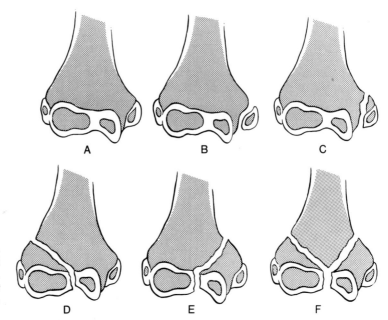

Figure 13–6. Distal humerus at age 11 years to maturity. *A*, Normal distal humerus. *B*, Medial epicondyle, Salter and Harris type I and *C*, type II injury. *D*, Salter and Harris type IV injury of the lateral condyle, *E*, medial condyle, and *F*, both medial and lateral condyles.

the humerus.[40] Transverse shear-type epiphyseal injuries of the Salter-Harris types I and II are now virtually impossible (except for the medial epicondyle).

Injuries involving the physis at this age are nearly always of type IV. Lateral and medial condyle fractures both occur in this age group (Fig. 13–6*D*, *E*). Medial condyle fractures are more common than they are at younger ages but are still less common than lateral condyle fractures. Both require open anatomic reduction and internal fixation. The T-type fracture is more frequent than at younger ages and also requires open reduction and internal fixation (Fig. 13–6*F*).[51]

The triplane fracture is rarely found anywhere other than the distal tibia. It has been reported in the distal humerus,[34] and because it involves both articular and physeal cartilage should be treated by anatomic reduction.

Premature closure of the physis is very frequent at this age with any type of injury. The premature closure, however, is nearly always complete, and angular deformity, which would result from partial physeal closure, is uncommon. Because the distal humerus contributes only 10 percent of the longitudinal length of the entire arm, growth arrest at this age rarely causes any noticeable arm length discrepancy.

MEDIAL EPICONDYLE

The ossification center of the medial epicondyle appears roentgenographically, on the average, at the age of about 4 years. Multicentric ossification centers have been demonstrated

and give a fragmented appearance. Awareness of this normal variant may obviate misdiagnosis. The medial epicondyle matures slowly and is the last of the six epiphyses of the elbow to unite with the humeral shaft.[43]

The medial epicondyle is located slightly posterior rather than strictly medial and therefore may cause confusion in roentgenographic interpretation.[43] Oblique roentgenograms of both elbows are sometimes necessary to determine whether the epicondyle on the injured side is in an abnormal position.

Fractures of the medial epicondyle usually occur between 9 and 15 years of age[4] and constitute approximately 10 percent of all injuries of the elbow region. The injury is unusual in younger children. The mechanism of injury is usually a valgus stress of the joint, which produces traction on the medial epicondyle through the flexor muscles. The injury is usually of Salter-Harris type I or II (Fig. 13–6*B*, *C*), although types III and IV have been noted as well. The epicondyle is always displaced inferiorly due to pull of flexor pronator origin, or it may be dislocated into and entrapped in the elbow joint owing to the opening of the joint by valgus stress. The entrapped epicondyle must be removed from the joint. The injury is frequent with posterolateral dislocation of the elbow; about half of the cases are associated with partial or complete dislocation of the elbow.

If the medial epicondyle is displaced less than 2 mm the elbow should be immobilized for 3 weeks in a long arm cast with the elbow in moderate flexion and the forearm in pronation. Comparison roentgenograms of the normal opposite elbow may be helpful in determining the degree of displacement. If the medial epicondyle is displaced more than 2 mm or rotated, or if the elbow joint is unstable on application of valgus stress, open reduction and internal fixation are indicated. The gravity stress test is a useful diagnostic test for acute medial instability.[52]

The medial epicondyle can frequently be reduced anatomically by closed means but cannot be held reduced. Percutaneous pinning is hazardous because of the proximity of the ulnar nerve. Therefore, open reduction and internal fixation with two smooth Kirschner wires is the safest method of treatment. It is usually not necessary to mobilize the ulnar nerve, although in severe injuries this maneuver may be helpful in gaining exposure. The wires should be removed after 3 weeks and active motion begun. After injury the physis of the epicondyle usually closes, but because the physis does not contribute to longitudinal length[4, 21] and because the epiphysis does not articulate with the ulna, growth arrest problems are rare or nonexistent. This is particularly true because

most of these children are near maturity, and the other physes about the elbow have already closed.

Any hypesthesia, paresthesia, or paralysis in the ulnar nerve distribution is an adequate reason for exploration, inspection of the nerve, and replacement of the fragment. If the ulnar nerve is found to be constricted or contused, it may be transposed anterior to the medial condyle.[46] This is rarely necessary.[5, 21]

Displaced fractures of the medial epicondyle, if left untreated, frequently progress to malunion or nonunion (Fig. 13–7). Tardy ulnar palsy is a common late problem, despite relatively good elbow motion and freedom from symptoms for several years. Severe chronic medial instability, although rare, may occur after fibrous union of a displaced fracture.[52] Treatment options include osteosynthesis of the fragment to the condyle or excision of the fragment. Because of the proximity of the ulnar collateral ligament, elbow stability should be examined after fracture healing.

LATERAL EPICONDYLE

The ossification center of the lateral epicondyle appears about the age of 10 years and fuses with the lateral condyle at 14 years of age. Its ossification characteristics are prone to misinterpretation as an avulsion or chip fracture because (1) it ossifies as a smooth, thin, curved sliver of bone; (2) it is well separated from the humerus; and (3) the distal part of the epiphysis usually fuses with the capitellum before the proximal part unites with the adjacent humeral shaft. As the epiphysis matures, its outline usually becomes smooth and well defined, but it may be quite irregular.[41]

Isolated injury of the lateral epicondyle is rare.[20] The lateral epicondylar ossification center is often irregular and may be confused with fracture. Injury may accompany elbow dislocation (Fig. 13–8). In most cases, there is relatively little displacement of the fragment. Immobilization of the elbow for 3 to 4 weeks usually is sufficient. Open reduction and internal fixation are usually unnecessary because these injuries tend to occur only in children approaching the age of skeletal maturity. The risk of associated growth arrest is minimal.

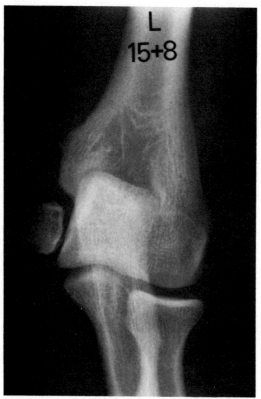

Figure 13–7. Fifteen-year eight-month old boy with tardy ulnar palsy secondary to nonunion of the medial epicondyle. Note hypertrophy of the epicondyle but lack of growth of the proximal portion of the condyle.

PROXIMAL RADIUS

The epiphysis of the radial head begins to ossify at about the age of 5 years. Although it

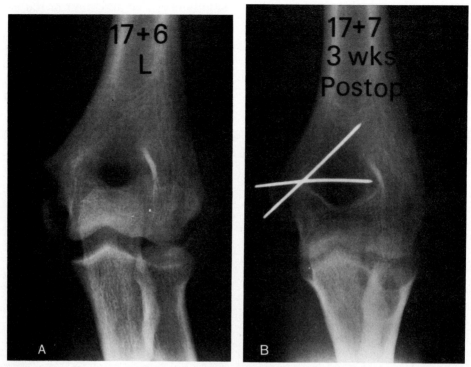

Figure 13–8. Seventeen-year six-month old girl who sustained a traumatic posterior elbow dislocation from a gymnastics injury. Note distal displacement of both the medial and lateral epicondyles *(A)*. The lateral epicondyle became entrapped in the joint following closed reduction of the elbow dislocation. Intra-articular entrapment of the lateral epicondyle is rare. Incisions medially and laterally were used to reduce the epicondyles. The lateral condyle was replaced and held by suture through drill holes in the lateral condyle. The medial epicondyle was reduced and pinned with two Kirschner wires. Three weeks later *(B)* the wires were removed. Elbow motion was regained rapidly, and the patient returned to competitive gymnastics 6 months later.

may appear first as a sphere, ossification soon advances into one or occasionally two ovoid, flat, or wedge-shaped nuclei, which may be interpreted as avulsion fractures of the metaphysis (Fig. 13–9A). Notches and clefts in the proximal radial metaphysis may closely resemble post-traumatic appearances.[42]

Radial neck fractures have been discussed in detail elsewhere (see Chapter 14) but will be reviewed here with emphasis on the phy-

seal nature of the injury. Although fractures of the neck of the proximal radius (Fig. 13–9F) are common in children, fractures involving the epiphyseal growth plate are not. They account for only 3.6 percent of all physeal injuries (Table 13–1), but even this figure may be inaccurately high, as mentioned earlier. The normal carrying angle of the elbow makes valgus injury more likely with a fall on the outstretched arm. The mechanism of injury

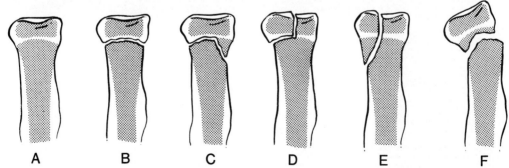

Figure 13–9. Proximal radius. *A,* Normal proximal radius. *B,* Salter and Harris type I, *C,* type II, *D,* type III, and *E,* type IV injury. Fracture of the proximal radial neck *(F)* is the most common injury to the proximal radius but does not involve the physis.

of a fall on the outstretched hand drives the capitellum against the outer side of the head of the radius, tilting it and displacing it outward. The fracture may be, therefore, either a Salter-Harris type I, II, III, or IV (Fig. 13–9B–E). A second mechanism is associated with posterior dislocation of the elbow with simultaneous compression of the capitellum on the head of the radius.[27]

The joint capsule is attached to the radius along the annular ligament. Because the radial neck lies outside the joint capsule, fracture of the neck does not ordinarily cause joint effusion or fat pad displacement. Fracture of the

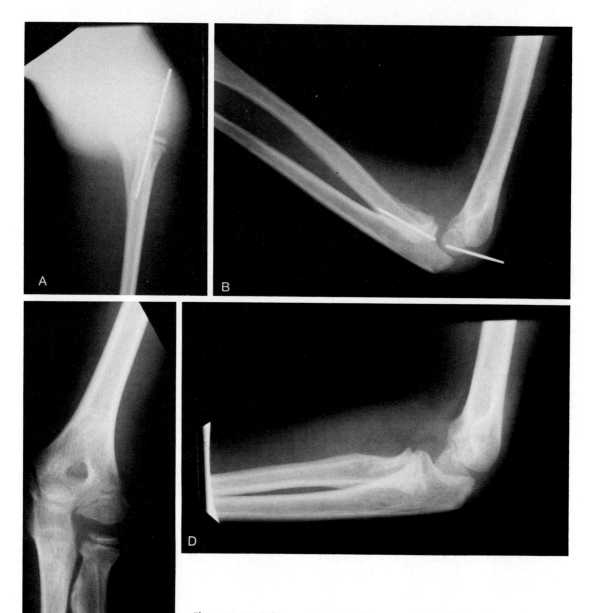

Figure 13–10. Eight-year six-month old boy sustained a displaced type II fracture of the proximal left radius during a fall. *A,* Open reduction wtih insertion of a longitudinal, smooth Kirschner wire through a capitellum, joint, and radial head and into radial diaphysis. A long arm cast was applied with elbow in 90-degree flexion, the forearm in neutral rotation. *B,* Five weeks later the cast was removed, and the roentgenogram revealed that the Kirschner wire was broken. Arthrotomy and varus stress were required to remove the distal portion of the wire. *C* and *D,* Anteroposterior and lateral roentgenograms 1 year after injury, at age 9 years 6 months. The patient was normally active and asymptomatic. There was full forearm rotation, but he lacked 10 degrees full elbow flexion and 5 degrees full extension. Normal physeal growth and elbow carrying angle.

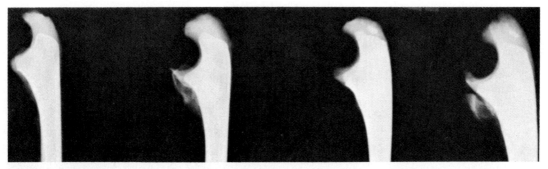

Figure 13–11. Serial roentgenographic development of the proximal ulna at 4, 6, 8, and 9 years (left to right, successively). Note that an extensive cartilaginous olecranon is present in all four specimens, and that it continues along the articular surface to the coronoid process. All of this cartilage, from the coronoid process to the olecranon processes, comprises the composite proximal chondroepiphysis. The specimen from the 9-year-old child, although morphologically larger, had a smaller ossification center than the specimen from the 8-year-old, demonstrating variation in this region, much like the rest of the elbow epiphyses. (From Ogden, J. A.: Skeletal Injury in the Child. Philadelphia, Lea & Febiger, 1982.)

radial head, however, usually produces elbow effusion and a positive fat pad sign.[42]

If a type I or type II injury is minimally displaced or can be manually reduced, immobilization for 3 to 4 weeks will suffice. Occasionally the entire head will be displaced through the joint capsule, and closed reduction is not possible. In this instance open reduction is necessary. Often, after surgical reduction, the fracture is stable, and no internal fixation is necessary.[32] Immobilization with the elbow in 90 degrees of flexion and the forearm in neutral rotation is satisfactory.

If the surgical reduction is unstable, internal fixation with two crossed Kirschner wires or one longitudinal wire through the capitellum ossification center extending across the radiocapitellar joint into the intramedullary cavity of the radial diaphysis can be considered.[24, 32] Each method of internal fixation should be supplemented with a long arm cast. The wires should be removed in 3 weeks, and gentle protected motion begun. If a single longitudinal wire is used it should be stout enough to avoid breakage at the joint level (Fig. 13–10). If this occurs, removal of the piece of wire embedded in the radius can be difficult, and it may be less damaging to leave the wire permanently in the radius.

Type III and IV injuries require precise anatomic reduction to restore articular congruity. Open reduction and internal fixation with tiny transverse or oblique Kirschner wires is necessary to prevent displacement of the fragments during healing. Premature closure of the physis nearly always occurs,[27] but because the proximal radius accounts for only 20 percent of the growth of the radius and because type III and IV injuries usually occur

in older children, problems from growth arrest are uncommon. Functional impairment, however, particularly limited forearm rotation, is common after type III and IV injuries.

With type I and II injuries the radial head should not be excised, even if all periosteal attachments are severed. Replacement of the head has not resulted in a high incidence of avascular necrosis. Only if the epiphyseal head is comminuted (type III or IV injuries) beyond repair may the fragments be excised. In this rare case, radial head Silastic replacement may be considered in an attempt to prevent variance of the distal radioulnar length.

Some radial head epiphyseal injuries develop growth disturbances with eccentric enlargement of the radial head. Abnormal cam motion may occur with forearm rotation. If the patient reaches adulthood with joint pain or limited motion, the radial head may be excised with little risk of development of wrist deformity.[46]

PROXIMAL ULNA

The epiphysis of the proximal ulna is unusual in that it is the only traction epiphysis of a long bone that contributes both a significant part of the longitudinal length of the bone and a major portion of its articulating surface.[31] The average time of appearance of the ossification center of the olecranon is age 9 years (Fig. 13–11), and it usually fuses at the age of 14½ years. Ossification of the olecranon begins in two or more centers that commonly fuse with each other before fusing with the parent bone (Fig. 13–12). They may be widely separated from the metaphysis in the

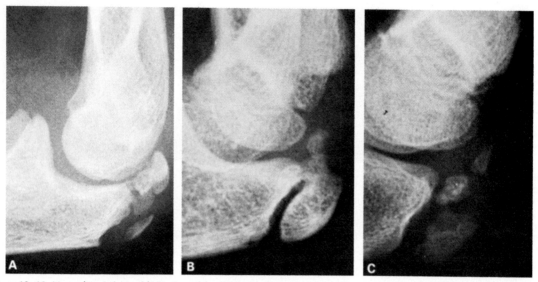

Figure 13–12. Normal variations of formation of the olecranon secondary ossification center. These could easily be interpreted as a fracture during the evaluation of acute trauma. *A,* Large ossification center with superior irregularity. *B,* Large superior segments with smaller distal portion. *C,* Multifocal early ossification. (From Ogden, J. A.: Skeletal Injury in the Child. Philadelphia, Lea & Febiger, 1982.)

early stages. The physis of the olecranon may be irregular, simulating a fracture.[44]

Injury to its growth plate, however, is infrequent and accounts for only 0.7 percent of all physeal injuries (Table 13–1). The major portion of the articulating surface of the olecranon is composed of the metaphyseal segment of the bone. The entire coronoid portion of the articulation is metaphyseal bone, and only the proximal small part of the olecranon portion is epiphyseal. As maturity progresses, the proportion of articular surface supplied by the olecranon epiphysis diminishes (Fig. 13–13). This is the so-called wandering physeal line of the olecranon.

Most injuries of the proximal ulna involve only metaphyseal bone, distal to the physis (Fig. 13–14D).[46] If the physis is involved the injury is nearly always a Salter-Harris type I or II (Fig. 13–14A, B, C). In type II injuries,

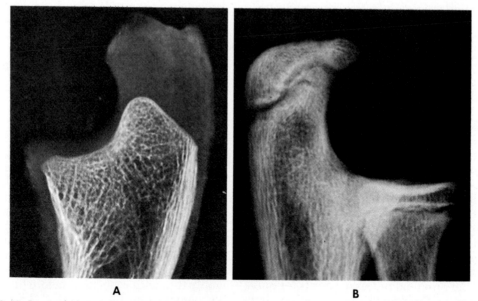

A   B

Figure 13–13. Proximal ulna. *A,* Five-year-old child. Note the large portion of articular surface supplied by the cartilaginous epiphysis. *B,* 14-year-old child. Note the irregular physis and that only a small portion of the articular surface is supplied by the epiphysis. (From Ogden, J. A.: Skeletal Injury in the Child. Philadelphia, Lea & Febiger, 1982.)

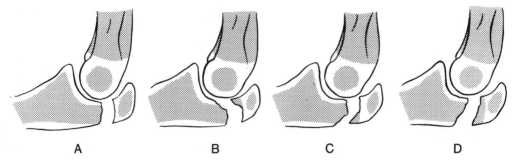

Figure 13–14. Proximal ulna. Salter and Harris type I *(A)* and II *(B and C)* injuries. Fracture of the proximal ulnar metaphysis *(D)* is the most common proximal ulnar fracture in children but does not involve the physis.

the fracture line in the metaphysis may be oblique (as shown) or may enter the ulnar shaft more longitudinally. Because the fragment contains articular surface, these fractures require anatomic reduction and maintenance of reduction until the fracture has united. This can frequently be accomplished by closed means, immobilizing the elbow in extension. If displacement is more than 2 to 3 mm, however, open reduction and internal fixation should be done. Fixation may be accomplished by longitudinal Kirschner wire, a wire loop, or both. A longitudinal screw should not be used if significant growth remains. Growth arrest problems are uncommon. Excision of the fragment, which is often performed in adults, should be avoided, particularly in young children.

GROWTH ARREST

The distal humeral physes and the proximal radius and ulnar physes contribute only 20 percent of the longitudinal growth of the humerus and forearm respectively. Because the amount of growth in these bones is minimal during and following an injury, the growth arrest lines that usually occur after any significant physeal injury are indistinct at best. Rarely can these be used as a measure of growth or an indicator of a growth arrest problem to the same extent that they are in other long bones.

Cubitus varus or cubitus valgus secondary to injury of the distal humeral physis that results in premature partial closure of the physis is possible but not nearly as common as angular deformity following malunion of a supracondylar fracture. Supracondylar osteotomy to correct malalignment due to premature partial physeal closure is therefore infrequently necessary. Although physeal bars may develop between the metaphysis and the epiphysis of the capitellum or tro-

chlea, they are not commonly reported. Bar excision for premature partial physeal closure has been performed at the Mayo Clinic in more than 50 cases during the period 1968 to 1980. None involved the elbow.[22]

A frequent concern is damage to the physeal cells between the metaphysis and the trochlea in young children. However, because the trochlear ossification center is not radiographically visible at this early age, this damage cannot be diagnosed by routine roentgenograms, tomograms, arthrograms, CT scan, or scintigraphy. Because repeated osteotomies for partial closure are rarely necessary, it is best to observe these cases for months or years before making the diagnosis of premature partial physeal arrest.

Injuries about the elbow in older children frequently result in complete closure of the physis or physes of the injured bone or even of all the physes of the elbow. Because these children are usually nearing maturity and because the distal humeral physes and the proximal radial and ulnar physes each contribute only 10 percent of the longitudinal growth of the entire arm, the resulting arm length discrepancy is usually minimal. This discrepancy causes no functional impairment, and clothes-fitting problems usually consist of coat sleeve alterations at most. Even if complete closure of all the physes about the elbow occurred in a young child, arrest of the physes of the contralateral normal elbow or surgical lengthening of the involved humerus or forearm would rarely, if ever, be indicated.

References

1. Brodeur, A. E., Silberstein, M. J., and Graviss, E. R.: Radiology of the Pediatric Elbow. Boston, G. K. Hall Medical Publishers, 1981.
2. Chacha, P. B.: Fracture of the Medial Condyle of the Humerus with Rotational Displacement. Report of Two Cases. J. Bone Joint Surg. **52A**:1453, 1970.
3. Chand, K.: Epiphyseal Separation of Distal Humeral

Epiphysis in an Infant. A Case Report and Review of the Literature. J. Trauma **14**:521, 1974.

4. Chessare, J. W., Rogers, L. F., White, H., and Tachdjian, M. O.: Injuries of the Medial Epicondylar Ossification Center of the Humerus. Am. J. Roentgenol. **129**:49, 1977.

5. Collins, R., and Lavine, S. A.: Fractures of the Medial Epicondyle of the Humerus with Ulnar Nerve Paralysis. Clin. Proc. Child. Hosp. D. C. **20**:274, 1964.

6. Cothay, D. M.: Injury of the Lower Medial Epiphysis of the Humerus Before Development of the Ossification Centre. Report of a Case. J. Bone Joint Surg. **49B**:766, 1967.

7. DeLee, J. C., Wilkins, K. E., Rogers, L. F., and Rockwood, C. A.: Fracture-Separation of the Distal Humeral Epiphysis. J. Bone Joint Surg. **62A**:46, 1980.

8. DePalma, A. F.: The Management of Fractures and Dislocations: An Atlas. Philadelphia, W. B. Saunders Co., 1970.

9. El Ghawabi, M. E.: Fracture of the Medial Condyle of the Humerus. J. Bone Joint Surg. **57A**:677, 1975.

10. Fahey, J. J., and O'Brien, E. T.: Fracture-Separation of the Medial Humeral Condyle in a Child Confused With Fracture of the Medial Epicondyle. J. Bone Joint Surg. **53A**:1102, 1971.

11. Flynn, J. C., and Richards, J. F.: Non-union of Minimally Displaced Fractures of the Lateral Condyle of the Humerus in Children. J. Bone Joint Surg. **53A**:1096, 1971.

12. Haliburton, R. A., Barber, J. R., and Fraser, R. L.: Pseudodislocation, An Unusual Birth Injury. Canad. J. Surg. **10**:455, 1967.

13. Hansen, P. E., Barnes, D. A., and Tullos, H. S.: Arthrographic Diagnosis of an Injury Pattern in the Distal Humerus of an Infant. J. Pediatr. Orthop. **2**:569, 1982.

14. Hardacre, J. A., Nahigian, S. H., Froimson, A. I., and Brown, J. E.: Fractures of the Lateral Condyle of the Humerus in Children. J. Bone Joint Surg., **53A**:1083, 1971.

15. Holda, M. E., Manoli, A., and LaMont, R. L.: Epiphyseal Separation of the Distal End of the Humerus with Medial Displacement. J. Bone Joint Surg. **62A**:52, 1980.

16. Holland, C. T.: A Radiographic Note of Injuries to the Distal Epiphyses of the Radius and Ulna. Proc. R. Soc. Med. **22**:695, 1929.

17. Ingersol, R. E.: Fractures of the Humeral Condyles in Children. Clin. Orthop. **41**:32, 1965.

18. Jones, K. G.: Percutaneous Pin Fixation of Fractures of the Lower End of the Humerus. Clin. Orthop. **50**:53, 1967.

19. Kaplan, S. S., and Reckling, F. W.: Fracture Separation of the Lower Humeral Epiphysis with Medial Displacement. J. Bone Joint Surg. **53A**:1105, 1971.

20. Keon-Cohen, B. T.: Fractures of the Elbow. J. Bone Joint Surg. **48A**:1623, 1966.

21. Kilfoyle, R. M.: Fractures of the Medial Condyle and Epicondyle of the Elbow in Children. Clin. Orthop. **41**:43, 1963.

22. Klassen, R. A., and Peterson, H. A.: Excision of Physeal Bars (Abstract). Orthop. Transac. **6**:65, 1982.

23. Marmor, L., and Bechtol, C. O.: Fracture Separation of the Lower Humeral Epiphysis. Report of a Case. J. Bone Joint Surg. **42A**:333, 1960.

24. McBride, E. E., and Monnet, J. C.: Epiphyseal Fractures of the Head of the Radius in Children. Clin. Orthop. **16**:264, 1960.

25. Micheli, L. J., Santori, R., and Stanitski, C. L.: Epiphyseal Fractures of the Elbow in Children. Am. Fam. Physician **22**:107, 1980.

26. Mizuno, K., Hirohata, K., and Kashiwagi, D.: Fracture-Separation of the Distal Humeral Epiphysis in Young Children. J. Bone Joint Surg. **61A**:570, 1979.

27. O'Brien, P. I.: Fractures Involving the Proximal Radial Epiphysis. Clin. Orthop. **41**:51, 1965.

28. Ogden, J. A.: Injury to the Growth Mechanisms of the Immature Skeleton. Skeletal Radiol. **6**:237, 1981.

29. Ogden, J. A.: Skeletal Injury in the Child. Philadelphia, Lea & Febiger, 1982.

30. Omer, G. E., Jr., and Simmons, J. W.: Fractures of the Distal Humeral Growth Plate. South. Med. J. **61**:651, 1968.

31. Parsons, F. G.: Observations on Traction Epiphyses. J. Anat. Physiol. **38**:248, 1903–1904.

32. Payne, J. F., and Earle, J. L.: Fracture Dislocation of the Proximal Radial Epiphysis. Minn. Med. **52**:479, 1969.

33. Perio, A., Mut, T., Aracil, J., and Martos, F.: Fracture-Separation of the Lower Humeral Epiphysis in Young Children. Acta Orthop. Scand. **52**:295, 1981.

34. Peterson, H. A.: Triplane Fracture of the Distal Humeral Epiphysis. J. Pediatr. Orthop. **3**:81, 1983.

35. Peterson, H. A., and Burkhart, S. S.: Compression Injury of the Epiphyseal Growth Plate: Fact or Fiction? J. Pediatr. Orthop. **1**:377, 1981.

36. Peterson, C. A., and Peterson, H. A.: Analysis of the Incidence of Injuries to the Epiphyseal Growth Plate. J. Trauma **12**:275, 1972.

37. Rogers, L. F., and Rockwood, C. A.: Separation of the Entire Distal Humeral Epiphysis. Radiology **106**:393, 1973.

38. Salter, R. B., and Harris, W. R.: Injuries Involving the Epiphyseal Plate. J. Bone Joint Surg. **45A**:587, 1963.

39. Siffert, R. S.: Displacement of the Distal Humeral Epiphysis in the Newborn Infant. J. Bone Joint Surg. **45A**:165, 1963.

40. Silberstein, M. J., Brodeur, A. E., and Graviss, E. R.: Some Vagaries of the Capitellum. J. Bone Joint Surg. **61A**:244, 1979.

41. Silberstein, M. J., Brodeur, A. E., and Graviss, E. R.: Some Vagaries of the Lateral Epicondyle. J. Bone Joint Surg. **64A**:444, 1982.

42. Silberstein, M. J., Brodeur, A. E., and Graviss, E. R.: Some Vagaries of the Radial Head and Neck. J. Bone Joint Surg. **64A**:1153, 1982.

43. Silberstein, M. J., Brodeur, A. E., Graviss, E. R., and Luisiri, A.: Some Vagaries of the Medial Epicondyle. J. Bone Joint Surg. **63A**:524, 1981.

44. Silberstein, M. J., Brodeur, A. E., Graviss, E. R., and Luisiri, A.: Some Vagaries of the Olecranon. J. Bone Joint Surg. **63A**:722, 1981.

45. Sutherland, D. H., and Wrobel, L.: Displacement of the Entire Distal Humeral Epiphysis. In Proceedings of the Western Orthopedic Association. J. Bone Joint Surg **56A**:206, 1974.

46. Smith, F. M.: Children's Elbow Injuries: Fractures and Dislocations. Clin. Orthop. **50**:7, 1967.

47. Smith, F. M.: Surgery of the Elbow, 2nd ed. Philadelphia, W. B. Saunders Co., 1972.

48. Wadsworth, T. G.: Premature Epiphyseal Fusion After Injury of the Capitellum. J. Bone Joint Surg. **46B**:46, 1964.

49. Wadsworth, T. G.: Injuries of the Capitellar (Lateral Humeral Condylar) Epiphysis. Clin. Orthop. **85**:127, 1972.

50. Wadsworth, T. G.: The Elbow. New York, Churchill Livingstone, 1982.

51. Weber, B. G., Brunner, C., and Freuler, F.: Treatment of Fractures in Children and Adolescents. New York, Springer-Verlag, 1981.

52. Woods, G. W., and Tullos, H. S.: Elbow Instability and Medial Epicondylar Fractures. Am. J. Sports **5**:23, 1977.

CHAPTER 14

Fractures of the Neck of the Radius in Children

JOHN H. WEDGE

Fractures of the neck and head of the radius in children are relatively rare, constituting 4 to 7 percent of elbow fractures and dislocations.[1, 4, 10, 13, 15] A review of the early literature reveals considerable controversy on the significance, treatment, and late results of this injury.[8, 14, 15]

Sex frequency varies from series to series, but overall there seems to be a slight female preponderance. The age range is from 4 to 14 years with the mean between 10 and 12 years. Thirty to 50 percent of patients have associated injuries to the elbow region (Figs. 14–1 to 14–3).[6, 9, 20, 23]

The prognosis following this fracture seems to depend more on the severity of the injury, the associated injuries about the elbow, and the type of treatment than on the accuracy of the reduction.[6, 10, 14, 16] Although emphasis has been placed on the angulation of the radial head, it is actually the displacement of the fracture that is the more important component of the deformity.

The classic discussion on this subject is that of Jeffery.[6] His observations in 1950 clarified the nature of the fracture, the mechanism of injury, the radiologic assessment, the method of reduction, and the prognosis. Complete remodeling of a fracture was demonstrated with perfect function after a residual angulation of 50 degrees.

Closed reduction seems to produce better results than open reduction even taking into account that more severe injuries are more likely to come to operation.[14, 16] However, the functional result following this fracture, regardless of the type of treatment, is generally good.[23]

MECHANISM OF THE FRACTURE

A fall on the outstretched arm produces a valgus thrust on the elbow that fractures the radial neck and often avulses structures on the medial side of the joint. The radial head tilts laterally because the forearm is usually supinated, but the exact direction of the tilt depends on the rotational position of the forearm at impact. This is the most common mechanism, but a direct blow to an elbow that has posteriorly dislocated momentarily reduces spontaneously, leaving the separated radial epiphysis tilted 90 degrees posteriorly beneath the capitellum of the humerus (Figs. 14–4, 14–10).[6, 7] Alternatively, axial compression on the elbow during a posterior dislocation can result in anterior displacement of the radial head as the proximal radius, while moving posteriorly, is obstructed by the capitellum. Less frequent injuries include anterior dislocation of the head of the radius with an associated fracture of the radial neck; a shear fracture through the neck of the radius with medial displacement of the shaft, which may become locked medial to the coronoid process of the ulna.[11]

Associated injuries thus include fracture of the olecranon, avulsion of the medial epicondyle of the humerus, dislocation of the elbow, and avulsion of the medial collateral ligament from the distal humerus.[6] As many as 50 percent of these fractures have one of these injuries, which are not only important in themselves but also have implications in regard to prognosis and treatment (Figs. 14–1 to 14–3).[10, 23]

CLASSIFICATION

The fracture may be classified according to the degree of angulation of the radial head,[15, 17] the mechanism of injury,[6] the type of epiphyseal plate disruption,[17, 18] the amount of fracture displacement, or combinations of these.[14]

O'Brien[15] divided these fractures into three groups according to the degree of angulation:

Type I: 0 to 30 degrees
Type II: 30 to 60 degrees
Type III: > 60 degrees

He also described an impaction fracture of the articular surface of the head. This fracture

237

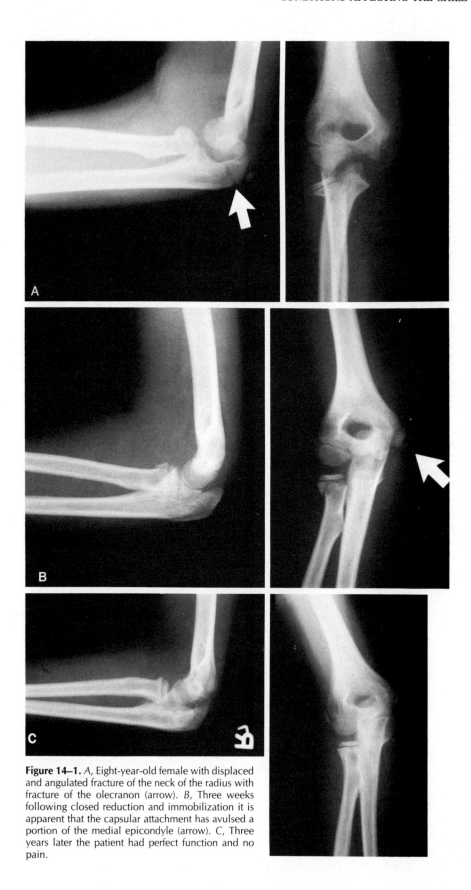

Figure 14–1. *A,* Eight-year-old female with displaced and angulated fracture of the neck of the radius with fracture of the olecranon (arrow). *B,* Three weeks following closed reduction and immobilization it is apparent that the capsular attachment has avulsed a portion of the medial epicondyle (arrow). *C,* Three years later the patient had perfect function and no pain.

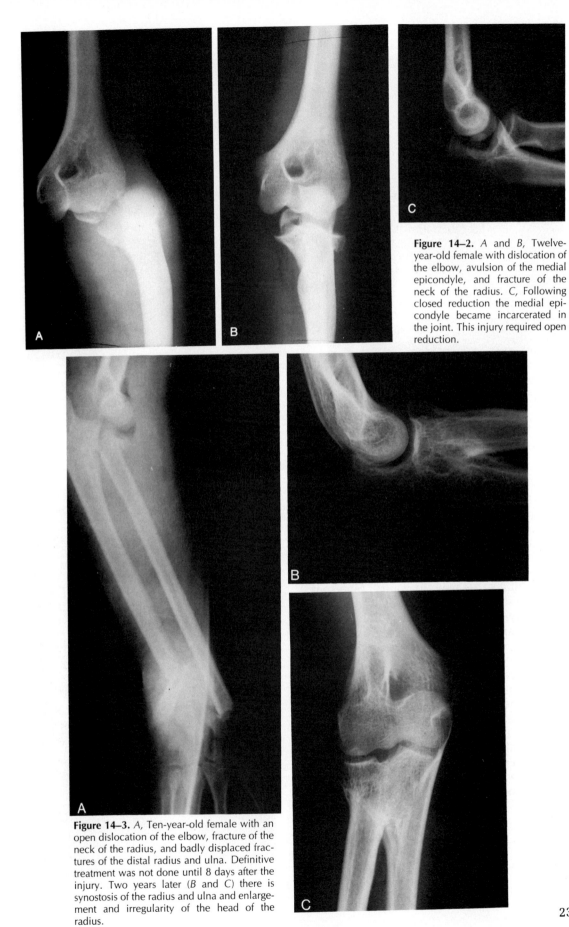

Figure 14–2. *A* and *B*, Twelve-year-old female with dislocation of the elbow, avulsion of the medial epicondyle, and fracture of the neck of the radius. *C*, Following closed reduction the medial epicondyle became incarcerated in the joint. This injury required open reduction.

Figure 14–3. *A*, Ten-year-old female with an open dislocation of the elbow, fracture of the neck of the radius, and badly displaced fractures of the distal radius and ulna. Definitive treatment was not done until 8 days after the injury. Two years later (*B* and *C*) there is synostosis of the radius and ulna and enlargement and irregularity of the head of the radius.

239

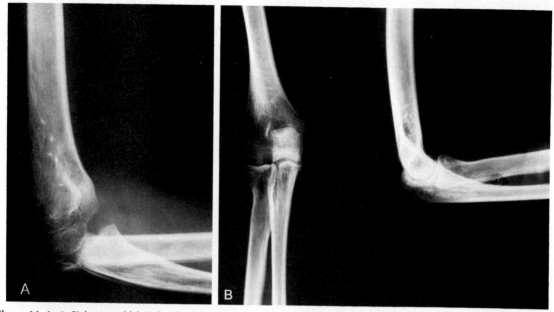

Figure 14–4. *A,* Eight-year-old female who fell 6 weeks before this radiograph was made. Note that the radial head is tilted 90 degrees posteriorly and is not articulating with the joint surface of the capitellum. The presumed mechanism of this fracture pattern is a direct blow to a posteriorly dislocated elbow, resulting in reduction of the joint but leaving the radial head displaced. *B,* The same patient 22 years after open reduction. Note the enlargement and irregularity of the radial head. She had a full range of motion and no pain. This is the only exception in our experience to the rule that stiffness usually follows late open reduction.

is more likely to be associated with lesser degrees of angulation.

It is important to recognize that the neck of the radius normally subtends an angle of 165 to 170 degrees with the shaft (see Chapter 2). The radius is not a straight bone even in its proximal third.[10, 21] Thus, a measured angulation of 50 degrees may, in reality, represent only 35 to 40 degrees of true angulation. As with many pediatric injuries, comparison with the uninjured elbow is often helpful or even essential for accurate assessment of this feature.

The injury may also be classified according to the type of epiphyseal plate injury. Although some authors believe that the fracture may occur entirely through the metaphysis of the neck of the radius,[8, 22] this is unusual both in the literature[14] and in our experience.[23]

The pattern of proximal radial physeal injuries as traditionally classified by Salter and Harris includes the following types:

Type I: rare and usually associated with dislocation of the radial head or elbow

Type II: the commonest pattern of fracture through the neck of the radius

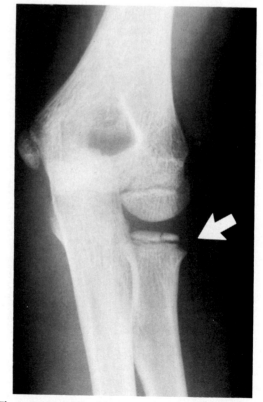

Figure 14–5. A Salter-Harris type III fracture of the proximal radius in an 8-year-old girl.

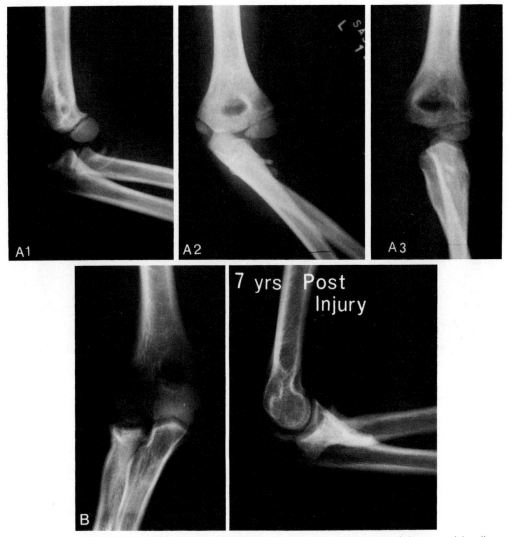

Figure 14–6. *A,* Eight-year-old boy with a type IV fracture of the radial head accompanying a dislocation of the elbow. *B,* The free fragment was excised, along with the radial head (*left*). Seven years later (*right*) he had very little forearm rotation, limited extension, irregularity of the articular surface, and valgus deformity.

Type III: rare (Fig. 14–5)

Type IV: second in frequency (five in our series)[23] and associated with a poorer prognosis due to marked displacement, irregularity of the radial head, and radioulnar synostosis (Figs. 14–6, 14–7)

Type V: seen in association with type II injuries. The crushing of the plate cannot be detected initially but is manifest by premature fusion of the physeal plate.

I prefer the classificaton of Newman[14] because it describes the deformity to be corrected and suggests the severity of the injury, thus indicating the prognosis.

Group 1:   lateral angulation

Group 2:   posterior displacement and angulation

Group 3:   anterior angulation and dislocation

Group 4:   lateral displacement

Group 5:   radial head fracture dislocation

TREATMENT

Assessment of Injury

The entire extremity should be thoroughly examined for open wounds, other injuries, and neurovascular impairment. A fall on the outstretched hand can result in injury at multiple levels. As in the adult, injury about the

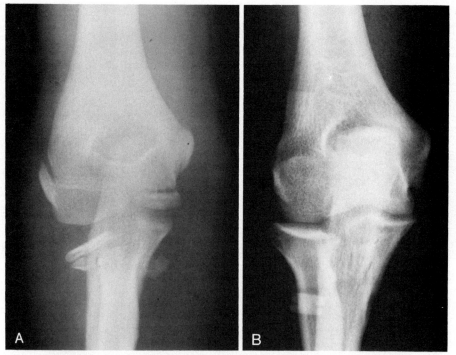

Figure 14–7. *A,* Thirteen-year-old boy with a comminuted fracture of the head of the radius. Note the free fragment, which consisted of epiphysis, growth plate, and metaphysis on the medial aspect of the ulna. The radial neck fracture was reduced open and the fragment excised. *B,* Four years later he had full flexion, extension, and pronation but no supination. Note the defect on the medial aspect of the head of the radius. He had only occasional pain in the elbow.

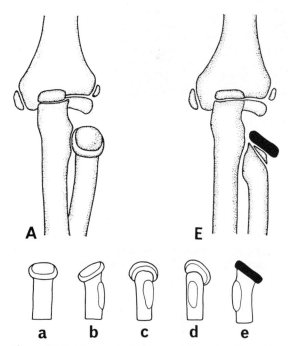

Figure 14–8. Diagrammatic representation of radiographic appearance of the head of the radius in varying degrees of rotation, where A equals a and E equals e. When the film is taken at right angles to the plane of maximum angulation, the radial head is rectangular in shape as in Ee (shaded epiphysis).

wrist must be specifically excluded, and fracture of the scaphoid has been reported (Fig. 14–3).[6]

Anteroposterior and lateral radiographs of both the elbow and the entire forearm should be examined for concomitant injuries, particularly about the elbow. An estimate of the degree of angulation of the radial head and the amount of displacement should also be made.

The degree of angulation can be accurately determined only by an anteroposterior radiograph with the forearm in the position of rotation at the moment of impact. Jeffery[6] demonstrated that this is best achieved by taking radiographs in varying degrees of forearm rotation so that the radial head will cast shadows of different shapes. When the radial head forms as near a perfect rectangle as possible, the real degree of angulation can be determined. Oval shapes indicate that the radiographs have not been taken at a right angle to the plane of maximal angulation (Fig. 14–8). Comparison views of the uninjured forearm in the same degree of rotation are helpful in assessing the degree of angulation. Also, in the child there are normal variations in the radiographic appearance of the proximal radius that must be considered when assessing injury.[19] Again, it is a basic principle of treating elbow fractures in children to compare radiographs with films of the opposite uninjured side.

Indications for Reduction

It is generally agreed that a fracture with an angulation of more than 60 degrees or with more than 3 mm of displacement may produce problems if it is not corrected.[1, 4, 14, 15, 23] It is also agreed, with the exception of some of the older literature, that fractures of less than 30 degrees angulation can safely be accepted.[6, 16, 21] There is also some support for the position that fractures of up to 45 degrees angulation do not require open reducton.[1, 14, 15, 20, 23] Treatment is controversial when angulation is between 45 and 60 degrees. There is support both for and against open reduction of these fractures.[4, 12, 16, 17, 20, 23] Those advocating open reduction believe that significant loss of forearm rotation will ensue without it. Those expressing a preference for closed reduction or acceptance of deformity believe that the complications of open reduction do not justify the risks considering the minimal disability present in those fractures left with 50 to 55 degrees of angulation.

In our experience angulation of less than 60 degrees may be accepted without late pain or significant loss of function. It is displace-ment rather than angulation that leads to loss of forearm rotation. Angulation results in a defect at the joint surface and therefore does not obstruct rotation. The lack of complete contact between articular surfaces is theoretically harmful, but enough remodeling usually occurs so that the lack of congruence appears to resolve. Displacement, on the other hand, results in radial neck deformity and abutment on the edges of the radial notch (Fig. 14–9). This produces a cam effect during rotation, which we have confirmed in cadaver studies. The radial neck was divided by a saw and fixed with Kirschner wires without angulation but with varying degrees of displacement. The effect on forearm rotation was observed. Displacement greater than 3 mm resulted in loss of forearm rotation because of abutment against the ulna.

Closed or open reduction more than 5 to 7 days after injury leads to loss of forearm rotation and radioulnar synostosis.[12, 14, 20, 23] Because of this, a fracture more than a week old represents a relative contraindication to reduction. It is better to accept deformity.

Principles of Treatment

Review of the literature indicates that, regardless of the severity of the injury, closed treatment gives better results than open treatment. Those fractures that require internal fixation also tend to have poorer results than those

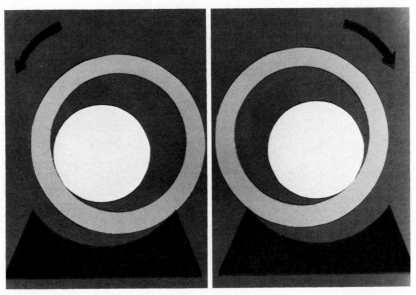

Figure 14–9. Diagram illustrating the effect of union with displacement of the fracture. The white circle represents the shaft of the radius just distal to the fracture. The gray circle represents the head of the radius. The black area represents the radial notch on the ulna. Rotation of the radius after union with persistent displacement results in abutment on the margin of the radial notch of the ulna. The degree of limitation of pronation and supination is proportional to the degree of displacement.

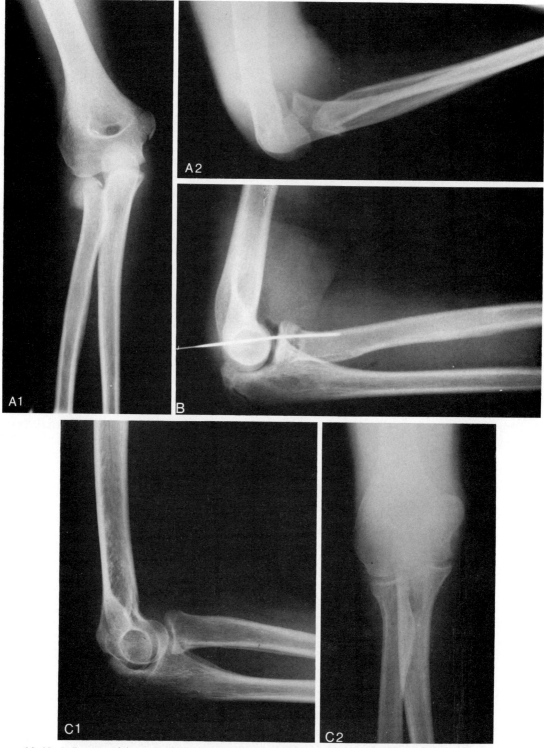

Figure 14–10. *A*, Fracture of the neck of the radius in a 13-year-old girl with dislocation of the elbow and marked posterior angulation. *B*, This was treated by open reduction and internal fixation with a wire passed through the capitellum into the radius. The high rate of complications with this method of fixation makes it an undesirable method of treatment. *C*, Three years later there is deformity of the head of the radius, subluxation, and marked restriction of forearm rotation.

treated by open reduction without internal fixation. Thus, as little internal fixation as possible should be utilized.[1, 23] Transcapitellar fixation, with a Kirschner wire passed through the capitellum of the humerus and across the joint into the head and medullary canal of the radius, leads to significant complications. These include possible infection of the joint and breakage of the wire in the joint leading to damage of the articular surface and making removal very difficult (Fig. 14–10).[5, 14] Immobilization of the elbow for more than 3 to 4 weeks leads to stiffness, even in children.

Thus, the following principles should be considered when treating this type of fracture:

1. Closed treatment generally gives better results than open reduction.

2. If open reduction is necessary use as little internal fixation as possible.

3. Treat promptly.

4. Do not use transcapitellar wires.

5. Do not immobilize the fracture for more than 3 weeks.

RESULTS

When assessing the published results of fractures of the neck of the radius it is apparent that pain, if present following this injury, is seldom disabling.[5, 13, 20, 23] Unsatisfactory results are consistently based on the degree of restriction of forearm motion.[4, 6, 14, ,17] It may be that permanent stiffness develops not only because of a mechanical block to rotation but also possibly because of reflex inhibition to avoid a painful arc of motion. Even when irregularity of the joint surface results in stiffness, there is usually surprisingly little pain. On the other hand, a "successful" open reduction with a perfect anatomic result may also be associated with significant loss of forearm rotation. Our series of patients followed for up to 22 years confirms this impression because pain was not a prominent feature and was not the reason for poor results.[23]

Loss of 20 degrees of supination or up to 40 degrees of pronation is not disabling, particularly when it occurs at a young age. "Fair" and "poor" results occur when there is greater than 40 degrees loss of forearm rotation. Unlike the situation in the adult, loss of elbow flexion and extension is less frequent and not as disabling as loss of rotation. When it does occur it is usually extension that is lost and seldom more than 30 to 35 degrees.

Avascular necrosis of the radial head, radioulnar synostosis,[2, 12, 14, 23] and removal of the radial head lead to poor results.[2, 14, 23] The incidence of radioulnar synostosis and avascular necrosis of a sufficient portion of the head of the radius is difficult to determine because of the small series of fractures of the neck of the radius in children. The problem is further complicated by the fact that these complications are associated with widely displaced fractures, those treated over-enthusiastically, those treated late, and those accompanying dislocations of the elbow. These injuries in turn make up a smaller part of the total number of fractures. It is enough to say that almost every series mentions these complications. In our experience avascular necrosis and synostosis complicate 5 to 10 percent of fractures, and are frequently seen together, usually after open reduction and fixation.

The unanticipated good result following acceptance of considerable deformity is related to remodeling of the deformity.[3, 5, 6, 12] This is somewhat surprising because the plane of the fracture is at right angles to the plane of motion of both the elbow and the radioulnar joints. This would seem to be an exception to the rule that remodeling in the child can be expected only if the fracture deformity is in the same plane of motion as the nearby joint. This remodeling may explain why younger children do better following fracture of the neck of the radius than older children.

Premature fusion of the proximal radial epiphysis is frequent but does not appear to influence the final result.[14, 15] It does not lead to significant shortening of the radius nor valgus deformity at the elbow.[6, 14] This is because most of the growth occurs at the distal end, and the fracture causes a stimulation of the growth rate initially.

Thus, the result largely depends on the degree of restriction of motion. In our experience composite loss of pronation, supination, flexion, and extension of greater than 90 degrees leads to functional disability and a poor result. Results are directly related to the severity of the injury, concomitant injuries about the elbow, and the extent of treatment necessary to reduce the fracture.

COMPLICATIONS

Complications Related to the Injury

Radioulnar Synostosis. This dreaded complication (Figs. 14–3, 14–11)[2, 12, 14, 15, 16, 23] is seen in widely displaced fractures and is usually associated with dislocation of the elbow.

Premature Fusion of the Epiphyseal Plate. This is frequent but of little consequence.[3, 5, 6, 12, 17]

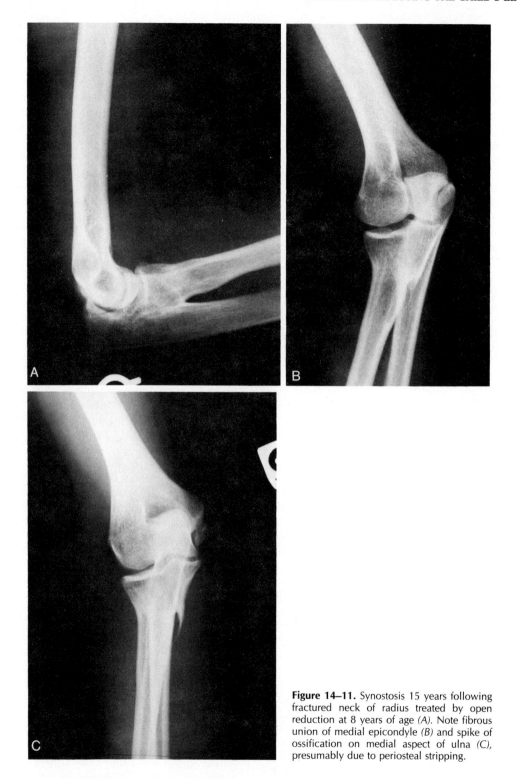

Figure 14–11. Synostosis 15 years following fractured neck of radius treated by open reduction at 8 years of age *(A)*. Note fibrous union of medial epicondyle *(B)* and spike of ossification on medial aspect of ulna *(C)*, presumably due to periosteal stripping.

Avascular Necrosis. This is most frequently seen (Fig. 14–12)[8, 12, 14, 20, 23] following open reduction but can occur with widely displaced fractures treated by closed reduction and is due to loss of soft tissue attachments. Although this complication probably occurs to a certain extent in many of these serious injuries, the eventual effect is determined by the degree of loss of blood supply.

Enlargement of the Head of the Neck of the Radius and Increase in Diameter of the Neck of the Radius. This is often seen and is accompanied by a compensatory enlargement of the capitellum of the humerus.[14, 15, 17] Due to stimulation of growth because of increased vascularity during the healing phase, the event is of little significance.

Ectopic Calcification. This is again frequent but is usually limited and has little effect on the outcome (Fig. 14–13).[14, 16, 17, 21, 23]

Vascular and Peripheral Nerve Injury. These complications are not frequent following this injury. When vascular injury occurs, it is usually related to accompanying dislocation of the elbow. Nerve damage occurs, but permanent paralysis is unusual.

Impaction Injury to the Articular Surface of the Radial Head. This is difficult to diagnose because it occurs in fractures resulting in less angulation, and the joint injury is not directly visualized.[15] When present it may lead to elbow stiffness and premature physeal closure due to crushing of the growth plate.

Complications Related to Treatment

Avascular Necrosis. This complication occurs (Fig. 14–12)[8, 10, 12, 14, 23] not only in widely

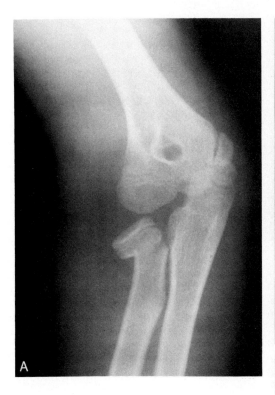

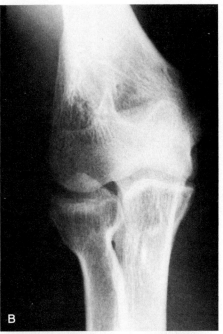

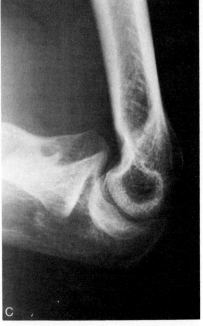

Figure 14–12. *A,* Fracture of neck of radius treated by open reduction and transcapitellar wiring in a 14-year-old boy. *B* and *C,* Treatment was complicated by avascular necrosis. These films were taken 7 years later. Patient has pain on activity and marked restriction of forearm rotation.

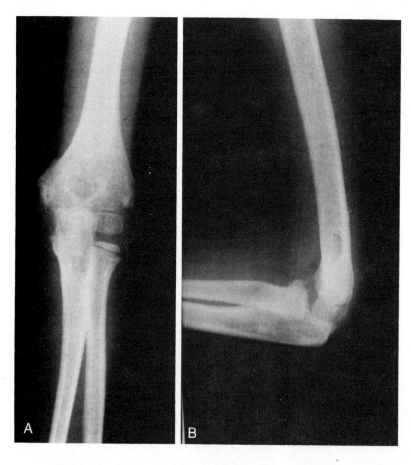

Figure 14–13. *A,* Two years following open reduction of a fracture of the neck of the radius in a 7-year-old boy. Note the ectopic calcification about the distal humerus. Despite this he had an almost full range of elbow and forearm motion *(B).*

displaced fractures but also in injuries with a lesser degree of displacement treated by open reduction. It can be avoided by carefully preserving the soft tissue attachments. It is seldom seen with closed treatment.

Radioulnar Synostosis. This may also result from less severe injuries that have undergone the trauma of open reduction and late closed reduction (Figs. 14–3, 14–11)[2, 6] If there is an unrecognized complete dislocation of the radial head or a dislocation of the elbow, reduction should probably be attempted up to 3 months following injury (Fig. 14–4). In this setting the parents must be warned that significant stiffness will result.

Infection. Postoperative infection (Fig. 14–14)[23] is always a concern with open procedures and can result in dissolution of the articular surface and ankylosis.

Nonunion. This is rare but when it occurs, it does so almost always following open re-

duction (Fig. 14–15). A poor result is universal.[3, 17, 23] There may be, however, surprisingly little pain, and excision should be delayed until skeletal maturity. Bone grafting should never be attempted because radioulnar synostosis regularly ensues.

A rare cause of nonunion may be complete reversal of the head of the radius when the fracture surface faces the capitellum of the humerus and the articular surface faces the distal fragment.[16] The radial head should be returned to its proper orientation even if it has lost all its soft tissue attachments. It should not be excised.

Damage to the Articular Surface. This may result from breakage of wires inserted across the joint to fix the fracture. This technique is also associated with stiffness and should be avoided.

Loss of Motion. Excessive stiffness results from closed or open reduction performed

Figure 14–14. *A,* A displaced fracture of the neck of the radius with 90 degrees of posterior angulation in an 11-year-old boy treated by open reduction and no internal fixation. He developed a staphylococcal wound infection. *B,* Because of necrosis of the head of the radius and marked pain, the radial head was excised 1 year later. *C,* Eight years following excision the patient had pain in the elbow and wrist. He also had marked restriction of elbow and forearm motion. Note the marked heterotopic bone formation at the site of excision of the head of the radius.

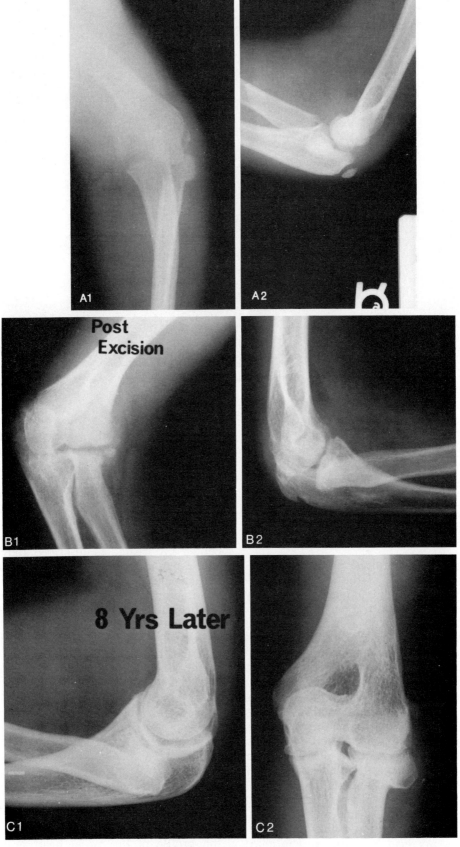

Figure 14–14. *See legend on opposite page*

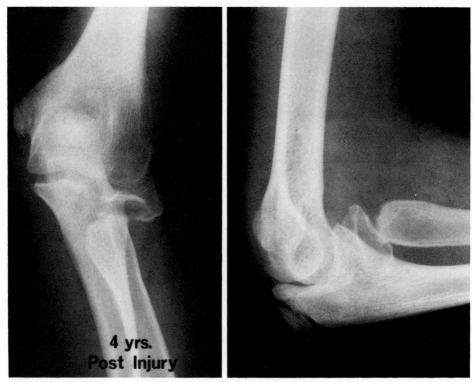

Figure 14–15. Nonunion of the neck of the radius 4 years following open reduction and fixation with a transcapitellar wire in a 12-year-old boy.

more than 1 week after injury. Immobilization of the elbow more than 4 weeks after injury should be discouraged because it is almost invariably associated with restricted forearm rotation.

AUTHOR'S PREFERRED METHOD OF TREATMENT

Selection of the technique of treatment depends on the nature of the injury. The sequence and method of treatment preferred by the author is based on a personal zeal for treating these injuries in a closed manner if at all possible. This position is substantiated by the improved clinical results that have been documented to follow closed reduction.

1. Angulation of less than 45 degrees and displacement of less than 3 mm. An above elbow cast with the elbow flexed 90 degrees and the forearm in neutral rotation for 3 weeks is appropriate. Radiographs should be done after 3 to 4 days to check the position. After immobilization is discontinued resumption of normal activity may be permitted. Physiotherapy is not necessary, and attempts at increasing the range of elbow motion by lifting heavy objects should be discouraged because this may lead to stiffness. The child

should be seen in 3 weeks and again in 3 months, by which time a full range of motion should have returned.

2. Angulation between 45 and 60 degrees with displacement of less than 3 mm. Gentle closed reduction by the method described below should be attempted. However, if this is unsuccessful the deformity should be accepted and treated as described above.

3. Angulation greater than 60 degrees and displacement of more than 3 mm. Every possible attempt should be made to reduce the fracture closed. It is, however, equally important to be gentle in all attempts.

Under appropriate anesthesia, usually general anesthesia in a child, rotate the forearm while palpating for the maximal prominence of the head of the radius at different degrees of flexion. Have an assistant apply a varus stress to the elbow to open the joint laterally and increase the prominence of the radial head. Apply firm pressure to the radial head in a medial and cranial direction. Confirm the reduction by radiographs, recognizing that several views may be necessary.

If the elbow region is too swollen, take radiographs in varying degrees of forearm rotation, beginning with full supination, until the profile of the radial head is as nearly rectangular as possible (Fig. 14–8). Then perform the above manipulation. A "C-arm" fluoroscope greatly facilitates reduction.

If this maneuver fails to achieve reduction, tightly wrap an Esmarch bandage around the elbow and repeat the radiographs. Occasionally this results in reduction.

If reduction is still not adequate, the arm is prepared and draped, but before making an incison an attempt to achieve a percutaneous reduction may be made. Under fluoroscopic control a sharp Steinmann pin is introduced through the skin, and the radial head is pushed into proper position. If reduction is achieved, apply a long arm cast with the elbow flexed 90 degrees and the forearm in a natural position. Take radiographs to confirm the maintenance of reduction.

If open reduction is necessary, make a 5-cm incision commencing on the lateral aspect of the capitellum and angling posteriorly over the radial head. This is the central portion of the Kocher posterolateral incision at the interval between the extensor carpi ulnaris and the anconeus muscles (see Chapter 8). Do not make the incision distal to the bicipital tuberosity of the radius to avoid damage to the posterior interosseous nerve. Enter the elbow joint anterior to the anconeus muscle. Do not interfere with the orbicular ligament even if torn, or stiffness may result. Lever the radial head into its proper position. It is usually sufficiently stable to make internal fixation unnecessary (Figs. 14–16, 14–17). If it is unstable, the child's bone is often sufficiently soft to allow use of a heavy absorbable suture on a stout cutting needle to suture it in place, introducing the needle at the articular margin of the radial head and passing it across the fracture into the neck of the radius and through the cortex. If this does not seem feasible, introduce one or two fine, smooth Kirschner wires at the articular margin of the radial head across the fracture and just through the cortex of the neck of the radius. They should be cut off just deep to the skin to facilitate removal in 3 weeks.

The radial head must never be excised in

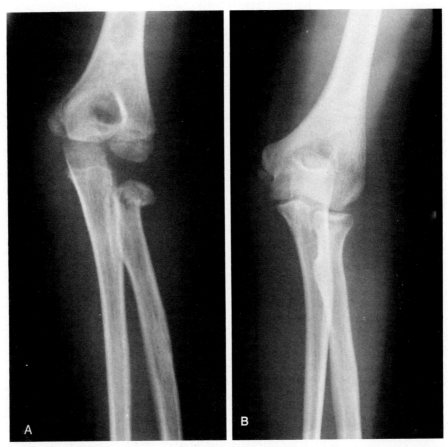

Figure 14–16. A, Displaced but not markedly angulated fracture of the neck of the radius in a 7-year-old girl. Closed reduction was unsuccessful, so open reduction without internal fixation was done. B, A satifisfactory result was obtained.

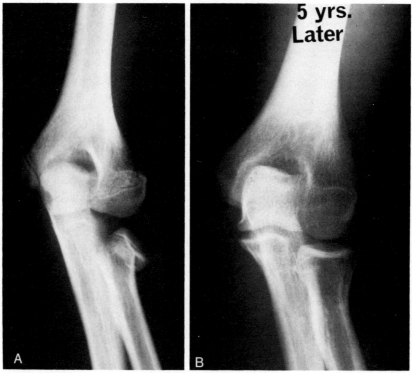

Figure 14–17. *A,* Fracture of the neck of the radius in a 13-year-old boy that was treated by open reduction without internal fixation. *B,* Five years following injury he had a full range of motion and no pain.

the growing child. Excision results in pain, increased carrying angle, radioulnar synostosis, or distal radioulnar dysfunction (Figs. 14–6, 14–14).[1, 2, 9] If stable reduction cannot be achieved, accept a less than optimal reduction and excise the radial head at skeletal maturity. However, more often than not, it will not be necessary to do a delayed resection.

The rare Salter type IV injury produces a dilemma. The displaced fragment is often too small to be fixed. In this case it may be excised. The result may not be very good, but the loss of motion after this fracture may be due to other factors because the injury is usually produced by considerable violence (Figs. 14–6, 14–7).

Immobilization following open reduction is as described for closed treatment and should be continued for no more than 3 to 4 weeks. If Kirschner wires have been used they should be removed at this time. Rehabilitation and follow-up are exactly as described for closed treatment.

SUMMARY

Fractures of the neck of the radius are rare but serious injuries, particularly if they are associated with marked angulation and displacement or with concomitant injuries to the elbow region. Every possible attempt should be made to treat this injury closed. Even though more serious fractures are treated by open reduction, the reported and personal experience suggest that surgical intervention has an adverse effect on the outcome.

When open reduction is necessary, dissection and internal fixation should be kept to a minimum. Treatment after 1 week following injury leads to stiffness, as does external immobilization for more than 4 weeks.

References

1. Blount, W. P.: Fractures in Children. Baltimore, The Williams & Wilkins Co., 1955, pp. 56–57.
2. Bohrer, J. V.: Fractures of the Head and Neck of the Radius. Ann. Surg. 97:204, 1933.
3. Conn, J., and Wade, P. A.: Injuries of the Elbow. A Ten Year Review. J. Trauma 1:248, 1961.
4. Dougall, A. J.: Severe Fracture of the Neck of the Radius in Children. R. Coll. Surg. Edinburgh J. 14:220, 1969.
5. Henriksen, B.: Isolated Fractures of the Proximal End of the Radius in Children. Epidemiology, Treatment and Prognosis. Acta Orthop. Scand. 40:246, 1969.
6. Jeffery, C. C.: Fractures of the Radius in Children. J. Bone Joint Surg. 32B:314, 1950.
7. Jeffery, C. C.: Fractures of the Neck of the Radius in Children. Mechanism of Causation. J. Bone Joint Surg. 54B:717, 1972.

8. Jones, E. R. L., and Esch, M.: Displaced Fractures of the Neck of the Radius in Children. J. Bone Joint Surg. **53B**:429, 1971.
9. Lewis, R. W., and Thibodeau, A. A.: Deformity of the Wrist Following Resection of the Radial Head. Surg. Gynec. Obstet. **64**:1079, 1937.
10. Lindham, S., and Hugosson, C.: The Significance of Associated Lesions Including Dislocation in Fractures of the Neck of the Radius in Children. Acta Orthop. Scand. **50**:79, 1979.
11. Manoli, A.: Medial Displacement of the Shaft of the Radius with a Fracture of the Radial Neck. Report of a Case. J. Bone Joint Surg. **61A**:788, 1979.
12. McBride, E. D., and Monnet, J. C.: Epiphyseal Fractures of the Head of the Radius in Children. Clin. Orthop. **16**:264, 1960.
13. Murray, R. C.: Fractures of the Head and Neck of the Radius. Br. J. Surg. **9**:114, 1977.
14. Newman, J. H.: Displaced Radial Neck Fractures in Children. Injury **9**:114, 1977.
15. O'Brien, P. I.: Injuries Involving the Proximal Radial Epiphysis. Clin. Orthop. **41**:51, 1965.
16. Rang, M.: Children's Fractures. Toronto, J. B. Lippincott Co., 1974, pp. 112–118.
17. Reidy, J. A., and Van Gorder, G. W.: Treatment of Displacement of the Proximal Radial Epiphysis. J. Bone Joint Surg. **45A**:1355, 1963.
18. Salter, R. B., and Harris, W. R.: Injuries Involving the Epiphyseal Plate. J. Bone Joint Surg. **45A**:587, 1963.
19. Silberstein, M. J., Brodeur, A. E., and Graviss, E. R.: Some Vagaries of the Radial Neck and Head. J. Bone Joint Surg. **64A**:1153, 1982.
20. Tibone, J. E., and Stoltz, M.: Fractures of the Radial Head and Neck in Children. J. Bone Joint Surg. **63A**:100, 1981.
21. Vahvanen, V., and Gripenberg, L.: Fracture of the Radial Neck in Children. A Long-Term Follow-Up Study of 43 Cases. Acta Orthop. Scand. **49**:32, 1978.
22. Weber, B. G., Brunner, C. H., and Freuler, F.: Treatment of Fractures in Children and Adolescents. Berlin, Springer-Verlag, 1980, pp. 172–178.
23. Wedge, J. H., and Robertson, D. E.: Displaced Fractures of the Neck of the Radius in Children. J. Bone Joint Surg. **64B**:256, 1982.

CHAPTER 15

Osteochondritis Dissecans

A. J. BIANCO

Chronic elbow pain in the older child or young adolescent is not an everyday diagnostic problem, but neither is it rare or unusual. The patient is usually male, and the right elbow is most often involved. The pain is dull and aching and is aggravated by activity, particularly throwing a ball or some other violent repetitive motion. The elbow may be swollen, and motion, particularly extension, is limited. Rest often relieves the pain, sometimes completely. In the child (ages 7 to 12) the most frequent cause of this chronic elbow pain is osteochondrosis of the capitellum. In the teenager (aged 13 to 16), in whom growth is beginning to end, the most common cause of chronic recurrent elbow pain and limited motion is osteochondritis dissecans of the capitellum.

Occasionally the patient may be female instead of male, or the left or nondominant elbow may be involved instead of the right. The pain may even be bilateral. These situations are unusual, however, compared with the more common situation of the young immature male with a chronically sore and swollen right elbow.

The difference between osteochondrosis of the capitellum and osteochondritis dissecans of the capitellum is one of age and degree of involvement of the capitellar secondary ossification center. The radiologic appearance and prognosis in these two entities are also different.

OSTEOCHONDROSIS—DEFINITIONS

Osteochondrosis is defined as a "disease of the growth or ossification centers in children that begins as a degeneration or necrosis followed by regeneration or recalcification." Osteochondrosis of the capitellum is also called Panner's disease or osteochondrosis deformans capitelli humeri (in Dorland's Medical Dictionary).

Clinical Characteristics

This condition is characterized by dull aching pain in the elbow, usually aggravated by motion or use, particularly throwing or other violent motions. It usually occurs in boys and always during the period of active ossification of the capitellar epiphysis (ages 7 to 12 with a peak at 9 years). In addition to pain, limited extension of the elbow is common, and local swelling and tenderness over the lateral side of the elbow is not unusual.[6]

Osteochondroses of the capitellum is a focal or localized lesion of the subchondral bone of the capitellum and its overlying articular cartilage.[3] The area of involvement is usually anterior and central in the area of the capitellum that is in maximum contact with the articular surface of the head of the radius.

Roentgenographic Characteristics

The capitellar ossification center appears to be fragmented owing to irregular patches of relative sclerosis alternating with areas of rarefaction (Fig. 15–1A, B). The outline of the epiphysis may be slightly irregular and smaller than the opposite normal capitellar epiphysis. The entire epiphysis may be involved. As growth progresses, the capitellar epiphysis eventually assumes a normal appearance in size, contour, and internal architecture. Pain and tenderness also subside in time. This, then, is obviously a self-limited condition not requiring any treatment except rest.

Osteochondrosis of the capitellum has been frequently compared with Perthe's disease of the capital femoral epiphysis in both the age of occurrence and the similarity of the roentgenographic findings.[7] However, deformity and collapse of the articular surface of the capitellum as a late sequelum is not as common in osteochondrosis as the late deformity of the femoral articular surface that results from total involvement of the capital epiphysis in severe Perthe's disease.

OSTEOCHONDRITIS—DEFINITIONS

Osteochondritis is defined as an "inflammation of both bone and cartilage." Osteochondritis dissecans is described as "osteochon-

254

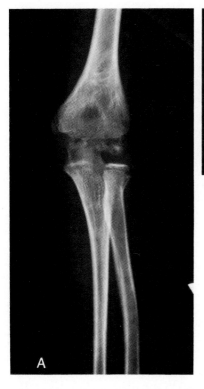
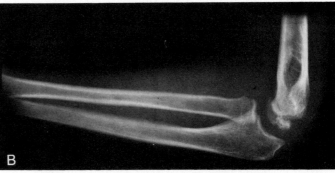

Figure 15–1. *A,* AP view of the right elbow of a 9-year-old boy showing involvement of the entire capitellum in alternating irregular areas of sclerosis and patchy rarefaction. *B,* Lateral view: osteochondrosis.

dritis resulting in the splitting of pieces of cartilage into the joint" (in Dorland's Medical Dictionary). *Osteochondritis dissecans of the capitellum* is similar to osteochondritis dissecans in other joints such as the knee in that it involves localized areas of subchondral bone and the adjacent articular cartilage. Because it occurs in an age group (early adolescence) in which the capitellum has almost completely ossified, although the physis is still actively functioning, it should not be confused with osteochondrosis of the capitellum (Panner's disease), nor is it due to an "inflammation" in spite of the definition for osteochondritis quoted above.[10] *Osteochondrosis dissecans* has been suggested as a more appropriate term.

From a practical standpoint the localized area of osteochondritis, consisting of articular cartilage and underlying bone, either remains in situ and eventually heals or separates from the capitellum and becomes a loose body in the joint.

Clinical Characteristics

Pain in the elbow is the most common complaint. It is usually dull and poorly localized and it is aggravated by use, particulary by athletic endeavors that involve throwing. Use aggravates the condition and rest relieves it.

A second complaint is that of limitation of motion of the elbow, particularly extension. Limitation of flexion of the elbow and pronation and supination of the forearm also occur but are less common.

Local tenderness over the lateral aspect of the elbow and crepitus with motion are also frequent complaints but are not as common as the dull pain that occurs with use and limited extension. Later in the course of the disease, locking of the elbow joint with severe pain may be a prominent complaint; this usually represents separation of fragments.

Roentgenographic Characteristics

Early in the disease radiographic changes are most commonly confined to the capitellum.[9] Rarefaction, irregular ossification, and a rarefied crater adjacent to the articular surface are frequent findings (Fig. 15–2). The crater of rarefaction in the capitellum usually has a sclerotic rim of subchondral bone adjacent to the articular surface.

If the central fragment separates, one or more ossific loose bodies may be seen in the joint, and the articular surface of the capitellum may appear to be irregular or flattened, particularly on the lateral view. In most instances the anteroposterior view will show rarefaction of the capitellum and in some cases irregular sclerosis of the subchondral bone. The lateral view will most likely show

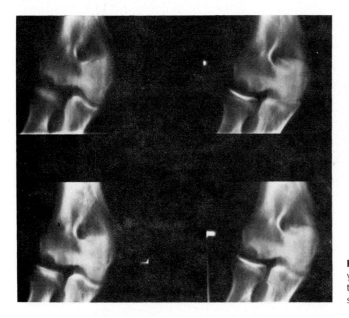

Figure 15–2. Tomograms of the right elbow of a 16-year-old boy with osteochondritis dissecans. Note the rarefied crater adjacent to the capitellar articular surface (type I lesion).

flattening and irregularity of the capitellar articular surface and the presence of loose fragments in the joint (Fig. 15–3).

Anteroposterior and lateral tomograms using a contrast medium may be the most accurate method of both establishing the diagnosis and determining if an area of articular surface and subchondral bone is in the process of dissecting from the capitellum.

Arthroscopy of the joint may also be valuable in determining whether the lesion is intact or partially separated. However, if the lesion is obviously loose in the joint the diagnosis can usually be made by routine radiographs or tomograms. Arthroscopy is also valuable in removing an obviously loose body if its size permits removal through the scope. The condition of the articular surfaces of the capitellum and radius can also be visualized by this method (see Chapter 7).

Several other radiographic changes are worth noting; however, most of these occur relatively late in the disease. Occasionally the radial head appears to be larger than the normal radial head of the opposite elbow on comparison views.

In a few instances, premature skeletal maturity (shown by early growth plate closure) is evident in the affected elbow compared with the normal unaffected side.

Late in the course of disease, degenerative changes characterized by irregularity and incongruity of both the capitellar and radial head articular surfaces are evident; these changes are the most important late sequelae of this condition.

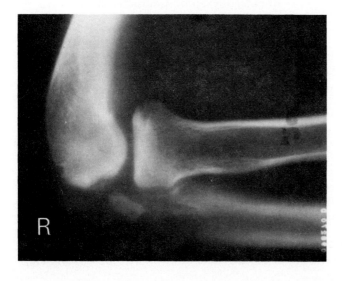

Figure 15–3. Lateral tomogram of the right elbow of a 16-year-old boy with osteochondritis dissecans. Note the irregular capitellar articular surface and a loose body in the elbow joint (type III lesion).

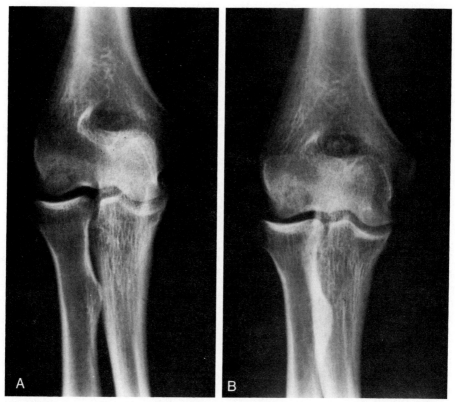

Figure 15–4. *A*, AP view, type I lesion in a 14-year-old boy with osteochondritis dissecans. *B*, AP view 1½ years later. The zone of rarefaction surrounding the lesion is becoming less distinct, and the patient is asymptomatic.

If sequestration does not occur, the central sclerotic fragment gradually becomes less distinct and opaque in time, the surrounding area of rarefaction gradually ossifies, and the lesion heals without significant sequelae. This radiographic evidence of healing may take several years, lasting even into adult life, long after pain, swelling, and limitation of motion have dissappeared (Fig. 15–4*A*, *B*).

ETIOLOGY

Most of the speculation about the cause of osteochondritis dissecans has been directed toward the condition as it occurs in the knee joints, not in the elbow. There are three main theories of the etiology of osteochondritis dissecans—ischemia, trauma, and genetic facts.

Ischemia. Because the initial histologic appearance of the involved segment of subchondral bone is that of avascular necrosis, one of the most popular theories suggests that some type of ischemic insult occurs to a very localized area of subchondral bone.[6] The ischemic theory of etiology is based primarily on the histopathologic characteristics of the lesion.

The microscopic changes in the involved area of subchondral bone are typical of those seen in infarction of bone due to interruption of the subchondral terminal arterial vessels.

Initially, the articular cartilage is intact, and the cartilage cells of the most superficial layers continue to receive their nutrition from synovial fluid. Early in the course of disease, hyperemia and edema of the synovium and hyperemia of the metaphysis occur, contributing to the eventual overgrowth of the capitellum and the proximal radius.

Reparative changes characterized by absorption of necrotic bone by vascular granulation tissue occur at the interface between the necrotic subarticular segment and the normal surrounding bone. At this stage a typical zone of rarefaction can be seen around the periphery of the lesion on radiographs.

If the articular cartilage remains intact and the necrotic segment remains in situ, eventual absorption of the avascular segment occurs; it is replaced by viable osseous tissue, and the normal architecture of the articular surface is preserved. This healing process may take several years. If, however, the articular cartilage is fractured during the initial stage of the disease, the necrotic segment is detached and becomes an intra-articular loose body.

Trauma. As far as the elbow is concerned, there is no conclusive evidence that a single traumatic episode produces osteochondritis dissecans of the capitellum.[4, 8] On the other hand, a history of frequent repetitive overuse of the elbow is a common occurrence in this condition. A still unsettled question is whether osteochondritis dissecans occurs in a normal completely ossified capitellar epiphysis or whether it occurs only when there are irregular areas of ossification in the capitellum before complete consolidation of the entire epiphysis occurs. In this situation, repetitive trauma, particularly forceful extension and pronation of the elbow, creates severe compression and shearing forces that are transmitted by the radius to the adjacent articular surface of the capitellum. This results in separation and infarction of an area of subchondral bone and the overlying articular cartilage that has not yet been securely bonded to the rest of the epiphysis by normal bony maturation.

Genetic Factors. There have been numerous but sporadic reports of osteochondritis of the capitellum occurring in the same generation or in several generations of the same family.[2, 5, 10] It has also been reported to occur in more than one joint in the same patient or in more than one family member. In spite of these reports, there is no convincing evidence that osteochondritis dissecans of the capitellum is a heritable disease.

Multiple epiphyseal dysplasia which is a rare heritable condition, superficially has many features that are similar to those of this condition.[1] Multiple epiphyses are involved; the clinical course and prognosis, however, are in no way similar.

TREATMENT

Treatment of osteochondritis is dictated by the clinical findings and the radiographic appearance of the lesion. Routine radiographs, tomograms, arthrograms, and even arthroscopy may all be necessary to determine whether the involved segment is already separated (dissected) or is in the process of being separated from the capitellum.

Type I Lesions

If the lesion appears to be intact with no evidence of displacement from its normal site and no evidence of fracture of the articular cartilage on arthrograms or contrast tomograms, nonoperative treatment is indicated.[8] The elbow should be rested, and all vigorous use of the elbow should be avoided. If pain is a significant complaint, the elbow should be splinted or placed in a cast for 3 to 4 weeks; active range-of-motion exercises are then prescribed to preserve motion. If pain is well controlled and subsequent x-rays every 3 to 6 months show no loss of position of the lesion, protection of the elbow should be continued indefinitely until the affected area gradually revascularizes and heals.

Type II Lesions

If on radiographic evaluation or arthroscopic examination there is evidence of fracture or fissure of the articular cartilage, or even evidence of partial detachment of the lesion, one is faced with two choices—i.e., to try to reattach the area of avascular bone surgically or to excise the loose area to prevent eventual loose body formation.[8]

In this situation, as in the knee, the partially detached lesion is pinned in situ with several fine threaded or unthreaded Kirschner wires under direct vision. The wires are brought out just under the skin in the lateral epicondylar area to facilitate later removal without reentering the elbow joint. The tips of the pins are embedded deep to the articular cartilage so that they do not protrude into the joint. The additional value of repeated drilling of the lesion and its bony bed to stimulate revascularization and healing has never been conclusively established. In general, the pins are not removed for at least 6 to 8 weeks. By this time, there may be early radiographic evidence of healing as shown by resorption of the sclerotic zone at the base of the lesion and preservation of the articular surface.

In some instances, even though there is evidence of successful reattachment of the detached area, the subchondral bone remains sclerotic and avascular, and subsequent collapse and deformation of the capitellar articular surface occur.

Type III Lesions

When the area of osteochondritis dissecans has completely detached from the capitellum and is lying free in the joint, the most effective treatment is to remove the fragment surgically either by open operation or by arthroscopy.[8, 10] In some instances the fragment consists of a large piece of articular cartilage and a small underlying shell of sclerotic subchondral bone, often comprising almost all of the capitellar articular surface.

There have been recent isolated reports of successful reattachment of such a free fragment, but there is still no report of a series of patients in which this method has been uniformly successful.

The usual situation encountered is that of a loose body or bodies that have become rounded and hypertrophied and have been free in the joint for a long time. The crater in the capitellum is often obscured by a layer of fibrous tissue and is much smaller in diameter than the diameter of the loose body.

Removal of the loose body is usually effective in relieving the patient's pain, although there may be no improvement in the range of motion. Late degenerative arthritis may still be the eventual outcome.

If significant radiohumeral degenerative disease is already evident at the time of surgical removal of loose bodies, excision of the radial head should also be considered in the skeletally mature patient.

Summary of Treatment

1. Osteochondrosis of the capitellum (Panner's disease)
   Nonoperative—rest, protection, splinting.
2. Osteochondritis dissecans of the capitellum
   a. Type I lesions: nonoperative—rest, protection, splinting.
   b. Type II lesions: operative
      (1) In situ pinning of the partially detached lesion.
      (2) Excise the partially detached fragment. There is no evidence that drilling or curettage of the crater in the capitellum has any effect in promoting healing of the crater and restoration of a normal capitellar articular surface.
   c. Type III lesions:
      (1) Remove all loose bodies. Smooth the capitellar crater edges (this gives the best results overall).
      (2) If radiocapitellar degenerative arthritis is present and symptoms warrant, and if patient is skeletally mature, excise the radial head.
      (3) Reattachment of the completely loose fragment is still experimental.

References

1. Clanton, T. O., and DeLee, J. E.: Osteochondritis Dissecans. Clin. Orthop. **167**:50, 1982.
2. Gardiner, J. B.: Osteochondritis Dissecans in Three Members of One Family. J. Bone Joint Surg. **37B**:139, 1955.
3. Haraldsson, S.: On Osteochondrosis Deformans Juvenitis, Capituli Humeri Including Investigation of Intraosseous Vasculature in Distal Humerus. Acta Orthop. Scand. Suppl. **38**:1, 1959.
4. Lindholm, T. S., Osterman, K., and Vankka, E.: Osteochondritis Dissecans of Elbow, Ankle, and Hip. Clin. Orthop. **148**:245, 1980.
5. Mitsunaga, M. M., Adishian, D. O., and Bianco, A. J., Jr.: Osteochondritis Dissecans of the Capitellum. J. Trauma **22**(1):53, 1982.
6. Omer, G. E. J.: Primary Articular Osteochondroses. Clin. Orthop. **158**:33, 1981.
7. Panner, H. J.: A Peculiar Affection of the Capitellum Humeri, Resembling Calvé-Perthes Disease of the Hip. Acta Radiol. **8**:617, 1927.
8. Pappas, A. M.: Osteochondritis Dissecans. Clin. Orthop. **158**:59, 1981.
9. Roberts, N., and Hughes, R.: Osteochondritis Dissecans of the Elbow Joint: A Clinical Study. J. Bone Joint Surg. **32B**:348, 1950.
10. Woodward, A. H., and Bianco, A. J., Jr.: Osteochondritis Dissecans of the Elbow. Clin. Orthop. **110**:35, 1975.

CHAPTER 16

Dislocations of the Child's Elbow

MERV LETTS

Dislocations of the elbow in children, in contrast to dislocations of other joints in children, are common, constituting about 6 to 8 percent of elbow injuries.[47, 80] In general, however, because the attachments of ligaments and muscles are stronger than the adjacent growth plate, forces exerted about most joints tend to result in epiphyseal injury rather than dislocation of the adjacent joint. The elbow is unique in children because type I and II fractures through the distal humeral epiphysis are uncommon, and dislocations of the elbow are the most common type of dislocation encountered in the pediatric age group. Indeed, many of the elbow dislocations that occur in the pediatric age group go unrecognized because by the time the child reaches the Emergency Department the elbow has spontaneously reduced, and the only finding on examination is a swollen, tender elbow.

It is the purpose of this chapter to discuss the practical aspects of the cause, recognition, and management of dislocations about the elbow joint in children. Because the elbow is the most common joint injured in childhood it is suggested that the reader be conversant with the various fractures that occur around this joint and that the chapters on fractures about the elbow joint (Chapters 10, 12, 13, and 14) be prerequisite reading for this chapter.

ANATOMIC PREDISPOSING FACTORS TO ELBOW DISLOCATION IN CHILDREN

Although the anatomy of the elbow joint has been thoroughly discussed in Chapter 2, it is important to emphasize some of the anatomic differences that are unique to the pediatric elbow joint.

The Growth Plates, Apophysis, and Secondary Centers of Ossification

To a casual observer, the radiograph of a child's elbow is an enigma—no two ever seem

alike. The reason for this, of course, is that because the child is constantly growing, ossification centers are appearing and fusing and cartilage is calcifying progressively until skeletal maturity is attained.

It is important to emphasize that there is usually a normal contralateral control that can be radiographed and compared with the radiograph of the injured elbow. This is not recommended as a routine practice, but occasionally it is necessary and useful, especially for those who treat elbow injuries in children only occasionally.

In general, the younger the child at the time of injury, the more difficult it is to assess the elbow owing to the larger percentage of cartilage that is present about the elbow joint. For this reason, in the newborn or infant it may be very difficult to diagnose an elbow injury or to determine whether this is a transcondylar fracture or a dislocation of the elbow (the former being much more common at this age). The ossific nuclei about the elbow joint are helpful in radiologic interpretation of elbow dislocation (Chapter 10). The capitellum, whose center of ossification should be present by 6 months of age, facilitates the interpretation of radial head alignment because a line drawn through the radial head should always intersect the capitellium in whatever view the radiograph is taken (Fig. 16–1). This interpretation is improved even further with the appearance of the radial head secondary center of ossification around 5 years of age. The secondary center of ossification of the olecranon, which appears at about 9 years of age, allows a more accurate assessment of the position of the proximal ulna in relation to the distal humerus, an important consideration in the management of dislocations of the elbow in young children.

Both the medial and lateral apophyses of the distal humerus may be injured in dislocations of the elbow in a child. Although many mnemonics have been devised by residents trying to remember the timing of ossi-

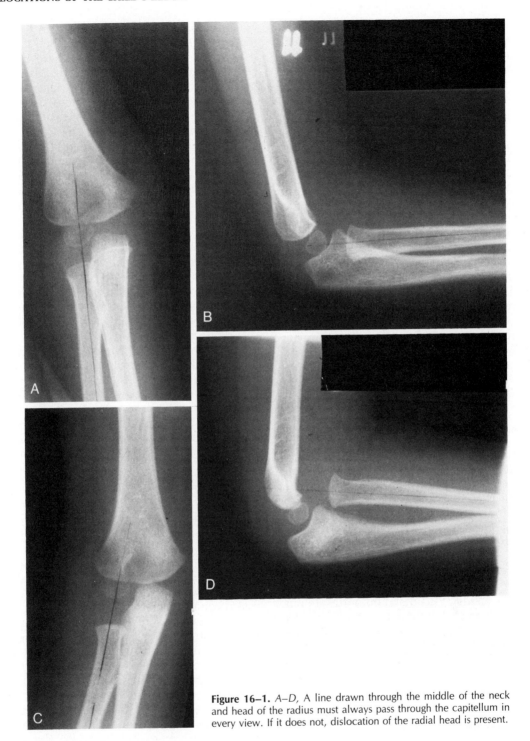

Figure 16–1. A–D, A line drawn through the middle of the neck and head of the radius must always pass through the capitellum in every view. If it does not, dislocation of the radial head is present.

fication of the various centers about the elbow, the most important to remember from a practical standpoint is the medial epicondylar apophysis of the distal humerus. This center is usually present by the age of 5 to 6 years, and because it is not infrequently entrapped within the joint following a dislocation of the elbow, it should always be searched for and identified after this age. If it cannot be iden-

tified it should be assumed that it is within the joint itself. In children under the age of 5 the diagnosis of entrapment must be clinical or by arthrography because the apophysis is entirely cartilaginous.

The lateral epicondylar apophysis is injured less frequently. In posteromedial dislocations it may suffer avulsion owing to a severe varus strain on the elbow. This may necessitate repair at the time of reduction of the dislocation of the elbow if it is unstable. This emphasizes the importance of examining the integrity of the collateral ligaments following reduction of the dislocation.

Elbow Flexibility

The elbow joint in children under 10 years of age is basically a ligamentous joint. There is very little hard tissue and stability is provided almost entirely by cartilage. Because of this there is considerable flexibility in the elbow joint in children. It is not unusual for a child to be able to hyperextend the elbow joint by 10 or 15 degrees and to have a much greater degree of laxity than is seen in an adult or even an adolescent. It is this combination of hyperflexibility and a lack of osseous stability in a joint subjected to considerable trauma that predisposes the elbow joint to dislocation. The major stabilizing ligaments on the medial and lateral sides are attached to the distal humerus through apophyses—structurally weak areas that are prone to avulsion with subsequent loss of joint integrity.

The Olecranon

The proximal ulna provides the greatest osseous stability in the elbow joint. In children the coronoid process, which provides anterior stability, thus resisting posterior dislocation of the ulna, is not well developed until about 12 years of age. Even at this age, this process is largely cartilaginous and when stressed is yielding and resilient. Similarly, the olecranon itself is a largely cartilaginous structure until the early teens. Both the coronoid and olecranon fossae of the distal humerus are not well developed until later in childhood and do not contribute as effectively to the "locking in" phenomenon in flexion or extension that occurs with a well-ossified coronoid process and olecranon that fit snugly into their respective fossae.

The Radial Head and Neck

The radial head and neck in children are cartilaginous but have the same relative diameters as the radial head and neck in adults. Dislocation of the radial head, either as an isolated event or in association with a Monteggia fracture or with dislocation of the elbow joint itself, is encouraged by the resiliency of the cartilaginous component. Children's bones themselves have a consid-

erable amount of plasticity and can be bent like the proverbial greenstick without fracturing. In the type A Monteggia lesion, for instance, it is quite conceivable that the ulna bends to the point of fracture, whereas the radius bends to the point where the radial head slips under the annular ligament and dislocates anteriorly (see Fig. 16–9).

Indeed, in most cases of open reduction of the radial head the annular ligament is intact. A similar situation may be found with the traumatic isolated dislocation of the radial head that occurs in very young children in which the radius bends just enough for the head and neck to slip under the annular ligament. When trauma is less severe, as in a pulled elbow, the head of the radius has simply slipped into the annular ligament and there is no actual dislocation. The supination maneuver simply screws the radial head out of the annular ligament, usually with no actual damage to the ligament itself.

This combination of generalized laxity, the large cartilaginous component, the lack of osseous stability, and the presence of osseous elasticity and of numerous secondary centers of ossification and apophyses all contribute to the anachronism of the pediatric elbow joint—a tendency toward dislocation at a time when dislocations of other joints are uncommon.

TYPES OF DISLOCATION OF THE RADIAL HEAD

Congenital Dislocation

Congenital dislocation of the radial head is a controversial lesion, and indeed some authors maintain that it does not exist and that all so-called congenital lesions are simply traumatic or developmental dislocations that occur for other reasons. This subject is discussed in more detail in Chapter 11. I reserve the diagnosis of congenital dislocation of the radial head for an entity in which congenital malformation of the extremity is obvious (Fig. 16–2). When isolated dislocation of the radial head is not accompanied by other congenital lesions, the congenital basis for the lesion cannot be substantiated. The longstanding nature of the dislocation can be inferred from the marked convexity of the radial head associated with elongation of the radial neck (Fig. 16–3).[19–24] Congenital dislocation of the radial head may be associated with radioulnar synostosis, the synostosis almost always occurring between the proximal radius and the ulna.

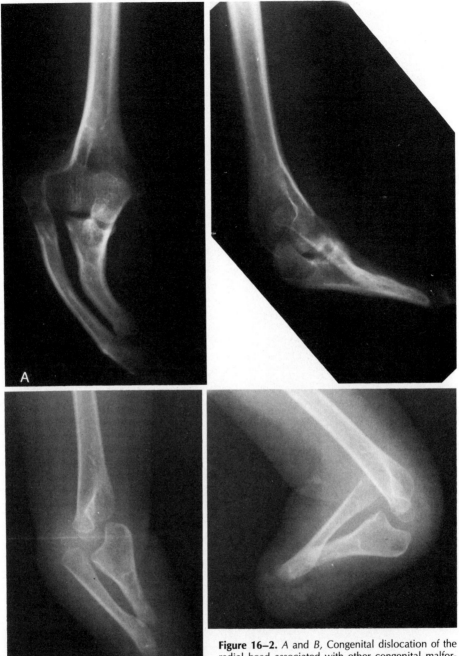

Figure 16–2. *A* and *B,* Congenital dislocation of the radial head associated with other congenital malformations of the forearm. Note the rounded convexity of the radial head.

Developmental Dislocation

Many instances of developmental or secondary dislocation of the radial head are misinterpreted as congenital in origin. Developmental dislocation is defined as any dislocation of the radial head that results from maldevelopment of the forearm. There are many inherited and acquired disease processes affecting the growth plate of the forearm

bones that result in asymmetrical growth between the radius and the ulna and subsequent dislocation of the radial head. These include the nail patella syndrome, Silver syndrome, arthrogryposis, Cornelia de Lange syndrome, and cleidocranial dysostosis. Asymmetrical growth also occurs in multiple exostoses or diaphyseal aclasis. The ulna is most frequently affected at the distal ulnar growth plate, the radius then overgrowing relative to

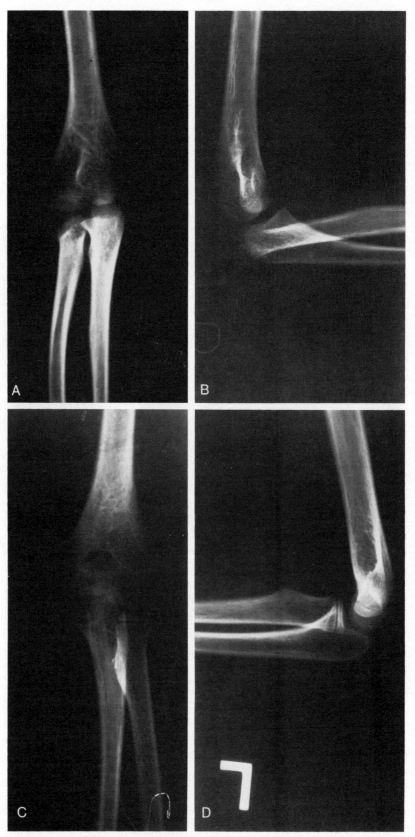

Figure 16–3. Developmental or longstanding dislocation of the radial head. *A–D,* Note rounded appearance of head, convexity of articular surface, and narrow neck typical of this deformity.

Illustration continued on opposite page

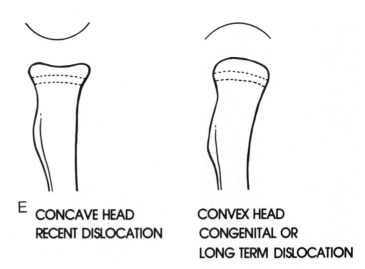

E **CONCAVE HEAD
RECENT DISLOCATION**

**CONVEX HEAD
CONGENITAL OR
LONG TERM DISLOCATION**

Figure 16–3 *Continued. E,* Convexity of head develops if the radius is not in contact with the capitellum.

the ulna (Fig. 16–4). Paralysis of the muscles innervated by the C5–6 nerve root, as in a nerve root palsy, also predisposes to a gradual dislocation of the radial head that occurs over a number of years of growth. Cerebral palsy may also produce isolated dislocation of the radial head through marked spasticity of the muscles attached to the radius (Fig. 16–5).[14] Trauma to the radius or ulna resulting in asymmetrical growth may also produce dislocation of the radial head. Fracture of the neck of the radius that has not been corrected adequately may result in the proximal radial epiphysis growing laterally instead of toward the capitellum (Fig. 16–6).

Developmental dislocation of the radial head is seldom a functional disability. Motion is often full, and impairment, if present, is only minimal. If at skeletal maturity there is limitation of motion of the elbow, the radial head can be excised to improve function. Clinically, the symptoms that occur with a

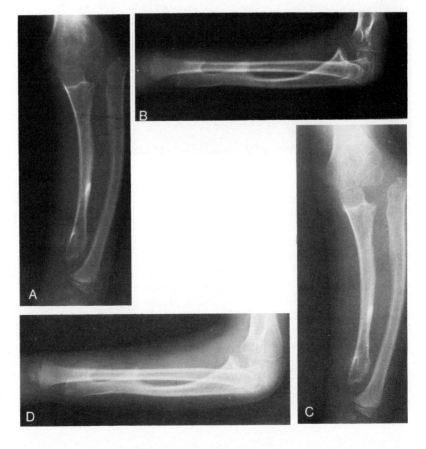

Figure 16–4. *A–D,* Dislocation of the radial head posterolaterally in a patient with multiple exostosis.

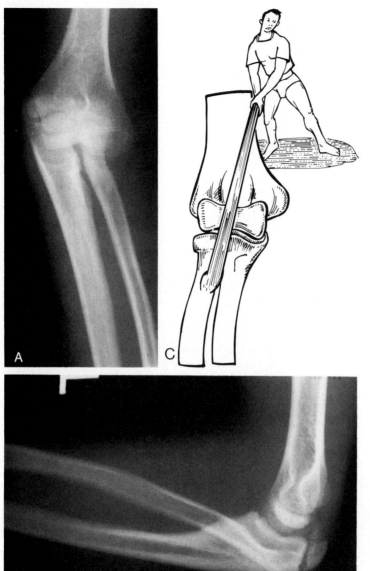

Figure 16–5. *A* and *B*, Longstanding dislocation of the radial head in a child with cerebral palsy. The elongation of the neck and convexity of the head indicates the presence of a prolonged dislocation. *C*, Spasticity or contraction of the biceps tendon may contribute to isolated dislocation of the radial head in children.

gradual dislocation of the radial head seem to be much less severe than those occurring with acute dislocation of the radial head. There is probably little indication for operative treatment of developmental dislocation of the radial head unless it is recognized early. For example, a malunion of the radius and ulna that is obviously directing the head of the radius laterally, posteriorly, or anteriorly should be corrected with an osteotomy to redirect the proximal radius.

In cerebral palsy patients, if the bicipital tendon appears to be subluxating the radial head anteriorly, lengthening the biceps may prevent future dislocation. Once the disloca-

tion is well established, attempts to relocate the radial head should probably not be made, and the dislocation should be accepted. Future resection of the radial head at skeletal maturity can be performed if the head is cosmetically or functionally a problem. The gradual nature of the dislocation and adjacent changes in the surrounding tissues and bone make this type of relocation of the radial head much more difficult than that in the acute traumatic dislocation.

Relocation of the radial head by shortening the radius and reconstitution of the annular ligament is seldom indicated in the developmental dislocation.

Radiographic Appearance

The radiographic appearance of a long-standing dislocated radial head is characterized by a rounded contour or convexity in contrast to the normal concave appearance (Fig. 16–3). The posterior border of the ulna may also be concave rather than slightly convex in anterior dislocations of the radial head. Posterior dislocations result in a longer neck with a typical dome-shaped head. Even an isolated traumatic dislocation of the radial head, when it occurs in a very young child, may take on the appearance of a congenital or developmental dislocation with the passage of time. A relative increase in ulnar length in relation to the radius and the wrist is often noted in patients with developmental dislocation. The capitellum may be hypoplastic or occasionally even absent.

Other factors characteristic of congenital or developmental radial head dislocations have been reported to be bilaterality of involvement, association with other congenital anomalies, familial occurrence, absence of traumatic history, and the presence of the entity in a patient under 6 months of age[12–18] (see Chapter 11).

Natural History

Development dislocation of the radial head seldom causes any serious symptoms. Patients with developmental anterior dislocation of the radial head may complain of clicking or impingement at the radiohumeral joint with flexion of the elbow. This may be associated with some discomfort in teenagers and adults. Posterior dislocation of the radial head sometimes creates a cosmetic protuberance that may also be a source of pain with excessive elbow motion. Aching in the region of the dislocation is not uncommon in the older child. A prominent ulna at the wrist and the resultant radioulnar subluxation at the distal end may result in some limitation of motion at the wrist and occasional discomfort. Most children with this abnormality do not have any complaints in childhood, although some may experience discomfort with excessive

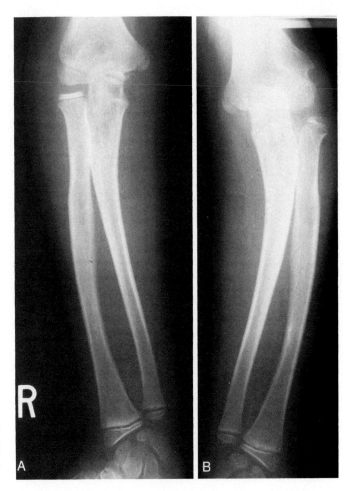

Figure 16–6. A and B, A child sustained a fracture of the ulna and neck of radius that healed in malunion. Four years later the radial head is dislocating laterally due to malposition of the proximal radial epiphyseal plate.

elbow motion in their teens and later as adults. There does not appear to be any progressive loss of motion with further growth, and the joint limitation, if present, remains static.

Traumatic Dislocation

Solitary dislocation of the radial head in children is uncommon but occurs much more frequently in younger children than in teenagers or adults. It is essential to differentiate this entity from a developmental dislocation of the radial head that has been noticed for the first time because of a radiograph that has been taken for a minor elbow injury.

The history may not be of much use in these cases because these children are often young, prone to frequent elbow injuries, and unable to make a reliable contribution to the history. The radiograph, however, is usually diagnostic because it shows the rounded concave appearance of the radial head in the congenital or developmental dislocation (Fig. 16–3).[1–11]

Clinical Features of Isolated Anterior Dislocation

Children who have sustained an anterior dislocation of the radial head usually have a history of trauma associated with inability or unwillingness to use the arm. Careful examination of the extremities and the radiograph may reveal some ulnar bowing. This is somewhat analogous to a Monteggia fracture-dislocation except that the ulna is simply bowed rather than fractured.

Radiographically, a line drawn through the shaft of the radius and the radial head will not intersect the capitellum when the radial head is dislocated (Fig. 16–1). Children who have been subjected to child abuse may present with this particular injury, and again the history will be difficult to elicit.

Treatment of Acute Anterior Dislocation

Closed Reduction. If the child is seen within 3 weeks of the dislocation, a closed reduction may be achieved. Direct pressure over the radial head with gradual flexion of the arm and immobilization in a flexed position of more than 100 degrees is usually successful.

If the radial head has been out of joint for some time or if the annular ligament has fallen back, preventing adequate reduction, an open reduction may have to be performed.

If the radial head can be reduced but is not stable, a Kirschner wire fixation to the ulna may be needed. Driving a pin across the elbow joint through the capitellum into the radial head is *not* recommended because in our experience these Kirschner wires often break, making removal difficult. Breakage occurs because it is virtually impossible to immobilize the elbow completely in a child, and the constant minor motion, even in a cast, may result in a fatigue fracture of the wire. The elbow joint will then have to be opened unnecessarily to remove the fractured pin.

Open Reduction

Triceps Fascial Reconstruction. The technique of open reduction of an anterior dislocation of the radial head in children described by Lloyd-Roberts and Bucknill[13] is one I have used with success. This consists of using the lateral portion of the tendon of the triceps for reconstruction of the annular ligament (Fig. 16–7A).

A posterolateral incision is preferred rather than a posterior incision, which may disorientate the surgeon somewhat to the position of the radial head. The triceps tendon is identified, and a long (10-cm) strip is removed from the lateral margin, ensuring attachment at the distal ulnar insertion. The tendon is increased in length by continuing the dissection through the periosteum of the ulna to a

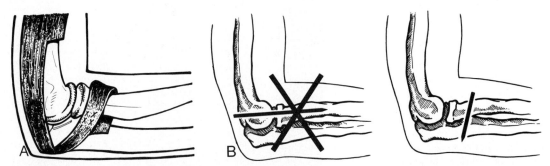

Figure 16–7. *A,* Repair of radial head dislocation by reconstruction of annular ligament using triceps fascia (Lloyd Roberts-Bucknill technique). *B,* A Kirschner wire passed through the capitellum into the radial head (*left*) is not recommended owing to danger of pin fatigue and breakage. The radial head can be safely held in the reduced position by a pin across the radius and ulna (*right*).

point opposite the neck of the radius, where it is then passed around the neck and sutured to itself and the ulnar periosteum with enough tension to hold the radial head in place. A Kirschner wire is then passed through the ulna into the radius to ensure solid fixation until the tendon has healed (Fig. 16–7B). The extremity is kept immobilized in an above-elbow plaster cast for 4 weeks; gradual mobilization is begun 6 weeks after the Kirschner wire has been removed. If there is any difficulty in reducing the radial head, careful inspection of the joint capsule may reveal some infolding, which may have to be excised.

Care must be exercised when exposing the neck of the radius in a child because the normal guidlines that apply to adult anatomy do not apply to the young child. The radial nerve may be only a fingerbreadth below the head of the radius rather than the classic two fingerbreadths that is often used as a standard of measurement for locating the radial nerve in adults.

Fascial Reconstruction of the Annular Ligament.

A method of reconstruction of the annular ligament has been described by Boyd[89] that is also a useful technique. A strip of fascia is dissected off the forearm muscles but is left attached to the proximal ulna. The length of this fascial strip should be about 5 inches by ½ inch. It is passed around the neck of the radius, proximal to the tuberosity and distal to the radial notch of the ulna, and is brought around and fastened to itself with nonabsorbable sutures (Fig. 16–8). Care should be taken to ensure that the length of this fascial strip is adequate. Cross radioulnar pin fixation for 4 weeks is recommended.

Untreated Anterior Dislocation of the Radial Head

A child with a longstanding anterior dislocation of the radial head may actually have

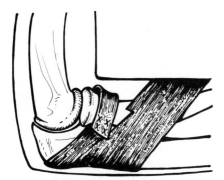

Figure 16–8. Annular ligament reconstruction using forearm fascia (Boyd technique).

good elbow function. The range of motion is usually functional, although the extremes of flexion and extension are usually limited by 20 or 30 degrees, and pain may develop at a later date. The cosmetic deformity is also a concern, and the elbow may appear somewhat grotesque, especially in a small, thin arm. Excision of the radial head at skeletal maturity will relieve most symptoms.

Complications

Relocation of an acute dislocation of the radial head in a child is usually successful, and few cases become recurrent. If the dislocation is not reduced, the child is left with limited motion in the elbow together with a cosmetic deformity. The dislocated radial head may also result in a relative shortening of the radius compared with the ulna with subsequent subluxation at the radioulnar joint at the wrist. As a general rule, the radial head should not be excised in a child because this may further aggravate shortening of the radius by eliminating the proximal radial growth plate, which contributes about 30 percent of the final radial length. If there is pain or a grotesque appearance when the child is near skeletal maturity, the radial head can be removed then. In neglected patients, excision of the radial head may allow improved flexion and rotation and may alleviate complaints of pain and discomfort.

Attempts to reduce a longstanding dislocation of the radial head by shortening the radius and reconstructing the annular ligament are usually unsuccessful and in most instances not indicated.

THE PEDIATRIC MONTEGGIA FRACTURE DISLOCATION

The Monteggia injury is uncommon in children but by no means rare. In the 5-year period from 1978 to 1982 at the Winnipeg Children's Hospital, 33 children were treated for a variety of Monteggia lesions. The true incidence of this fracture-dislocation is unknown, but it is more uncommon than is generally appreciated.

Cause

The most common cause of dislocation of the radial head associated with an ulnar fracture in childhood is a hyperextension injury;[29, 40] less commonly, a hyperpronation injury[30] of the elbow is the cause. In hyperpronation, Bado[25] pointed out that the bicipital tuberosity is most posterior, thus predisposing the proximal radius to the greatest force during violent contraction of the bicipital tendon. In young children the force generated by the biceps is less than that in the adult, and this mechanism probably is significant only in older children.

A direct blow over the posterior proximal ulna will produce a Monteggia lesion with anterior dislocation of the radial head, but this is an uncommon mechanism in children.

In our experience, this lesion is produced by a hyperextension injury. Further support for this theory is the observation that in open type C injuries the proximal ulnar fragment pierces the skin on the volar ulnar aspect of the forearm. This would not be possible if the arm were in full pronation due to imposition of the radius.

Because of the elasticity of the forearm bones, the radial head and neck may slip under the annular ligament and dislocate as the shaft of the radius bends. Indeed, many of the so-called isolated traumatic dislocations of the radial head are undoubtedly variations of the Monteggia lesion[31, 32] (Monteggia equivalent) in which the ulna has simply bent but not fractured. The radial shaft is bent to the extent that the head and neck are slipped

from within the annular ligament, resulting in an apparent isolated dislocation of the radial head.[26, 39]

Classifications

Classifications of the Monteggia lesion are largely based on the injury in adults. Because of differences in the configuration of the injury in childhood, the following classification has been devised to include dislocation of the radial head associated with the elasticity of the forearm bones in childhood (Fig. 16–9).

Classification of Pediatric Monteggia Lesions
Type A: Anterior dislocation of the radial head with anterior bowing of the ulna (Fig. 16–10).
Type B: Anterior dislocation of the radial head with greenstick fracture of the ulna (Fig. 16–11).
Type C: Anterior dislocation of the radial head with transverse fracture of the ulna (Fig. 16–12).
Type D: Posterior dislocation of the radial head with bending or fracture of the ulna (Fig. 16–13).
Type E: Lateral dislocation of the radial head with fracture of the ulna (Fig. 16–14).

Types B and C are the most commonly encountered Monteggia lesions in children.

Clinical Diagnosis

Like Monteggia himself, who explained this injury in a young lady in 1814 long before the advent of x-rays, most physicians today should be able to identify the clinical configuration of this lesion in patients who are seen early before the swelling clouds the clinical signs (Fig. 16–14). The dislocation of the radial head is often evident on inspection of the lateral aspect of the elbow joint. Angulation of the ulna, whether fractured or not necessitates careful appraisal of the position of the radial head. Dislocation of the radial head is frequently missed by those treating pediatric elbow injuries only occasionally.[34, 36] A mental line drawn through the shaft and neck of the radius should intersect the capitellum in all views taken (Fig. 16–1). If it does not, dislocation of the radial head is highly suspect.

In contrast to the lesion in adults, overlap of the ulnar fragments is not a prequisite for dislocation of the radial head in a child. Disruption of the forearm parallelogram may occur as a result of ulnar bend when the radial head slips out of the annular ligament. A good rule of thumb is to obtain adequate films—i.e., anteroposterior and lateral views of the elbow joint in all fractures of the ulna. The apex of the ulnar bend or angulation is

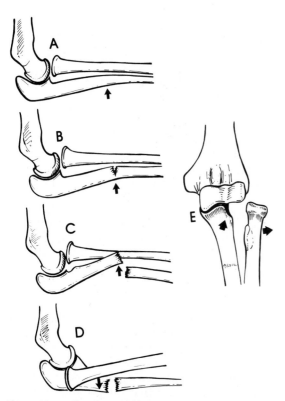

Figure 16–9. Classification of the pediatric Monteggia fracture dislocation: Types A through E.

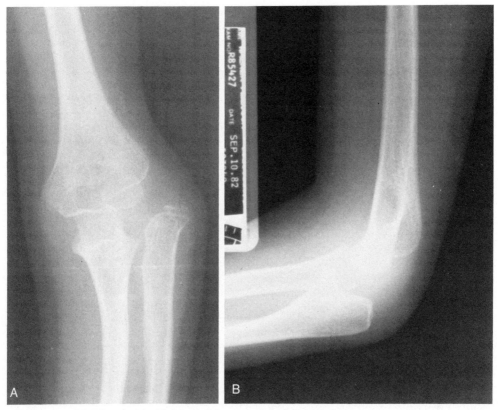

Figure 16–10. *A* and *B,* Ulnar bend with lateral dislocation of the radial head, a type A Monteggia fracture dislocation.

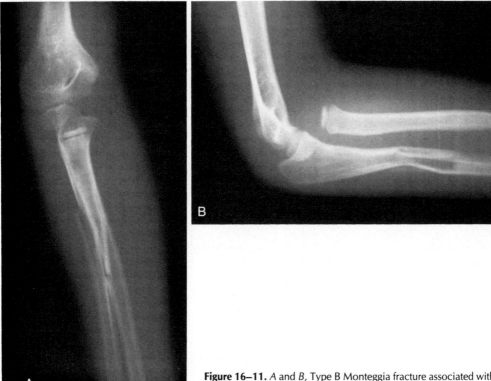

Figure 16–11. *A* and *B,* Type B Monteggia fracture associated with a greenstick fracture of the ulna and anterior dislocation of the radial head.

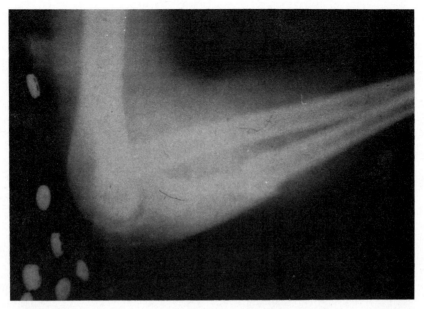

Figure 16–12. Anterior dislocation of the radial head with transverse fracture of ulna.

always in the direction of the radial head dislocation.[41]

The elbow must be carefully examined clinically and radiographically in any child who has an apparently intact radius associated with bowing, greenstick, or complete fracture of the ulna.

Treatment

In contrast to this lesion in adults, the Monteggia injury in children can usually be treated by closed methods.[27] Pressure directed over the dislocated radius will usually result in a stable ulnar reduction provided that im-

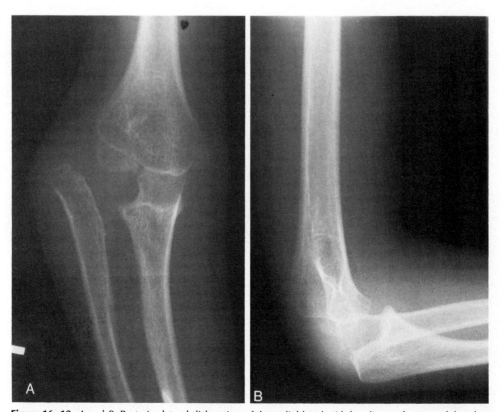

Figure 16–13. A and B, Posterior lateral dislocation of the radial head with bending or fracture of the ulna.

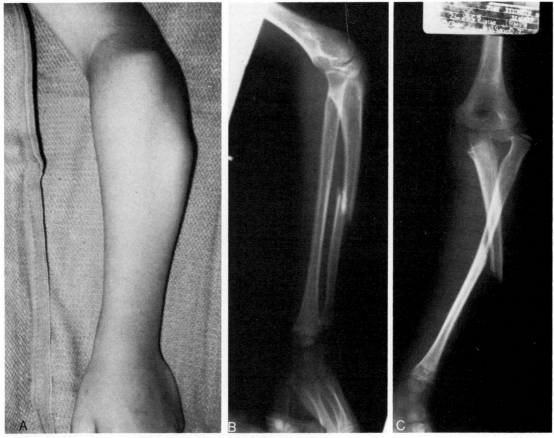

Figure 16–14. Monteggia fracture with lateral dislocation of the radial head. *A*, Clinical appearance. *B* and *C*, Radiologic appearance.

mobilization is imposed with the elbow flexed more than 90 degrees in types A, B, C, and E lesions. Supination assists in minimizing biceps pull. In the uncommon type D Monteggia lesion with posterior dislocation of the radial head, stability is obtained with extension, not flexion, of the elbow.

As long as the radial head is reduced and stable, angulation of the ulna of as much as 15 degrees can be accepted. Remodeling of this angulation will occur with further growth. In children, stable reduction of the radial head is the first priority. A supination-pronation maneuver may facilitate repositioning of the annular ligament, which is seldom completely torn.

If it is impossible to obtain a stable reduction of the radial head, I approach the radial head through a Kocher incision and reapproximate the annular ligament around the neck. If stability is still precarious or if the annular ligament has had to be reconstituted, I recommend internal fixation of the radius to the ulna with a Kirschner wire (Fig. 16–15A). I would caution against maintenance of the

reduction by a wire inserted through the capitellum and into the radial head. No matter how rigid the postoperative immobilization may be there is still a small degree of flexion and extension of the elbow joint that will ultimately result in fatigue breakage of the wire, necessitating re-exploration of the elbow joint (Fig. 16–7B).

If the ulna is unstable in the older child, an open reduction with plate fixation may be necessary, but in my experience this is seldom required in children under 13 years of age.

Nerve Injury Associated with Monteggia Lesions

Anterior dislocation of the radial head may result in stretch injury to the posterior interosseous nerve as it passes dorsolaterally around the proximal radius to enter the substance of the supinator muscle mass between the superficial and deep layers (Fig. 16–15B).[31, 38] Compression of the posterior interosseous nerve may also be aggravated by the fibrous arcade of Frohse, a firm fibrous

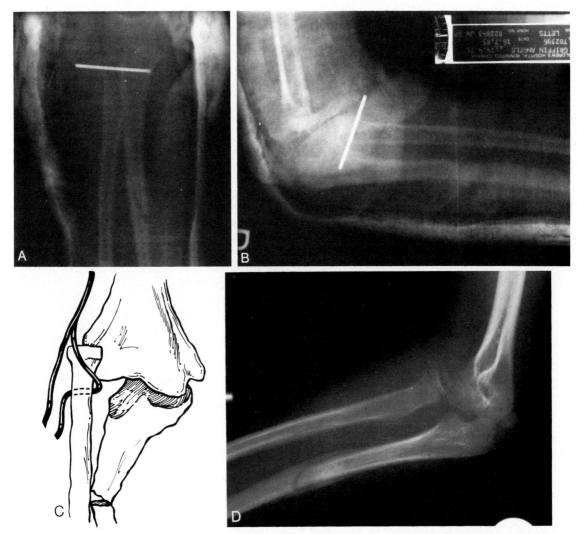

Figure 16–15. *A* and *B*, Preferred radioulnar pinning to hold the radial head in place subsequent to late open reduction of a Monteggia fracture dislocation and annular ligament repair. *C*, Injury to the posterior interosseous nerve may occur in the Monteggia fracture with anterior dislocation of the radial head. *D*, Missed dislocation of the radial head in an unappreciated Monteggia fracture with greenstick fracture of ulna.

band at the proximal edge of the supinator muscle.

In children, nerve injury is less common than in adults, and recovery is the rule in closed injuries.

THE MISSED MONTEGGIA LESION

The missed dislocated radial head that is noticed after the ulna has healed is a common error made by less experienced clinicians. In some instances the dislocated radial head may not be identified for some time, even years later after the initial injury has almost been forgotton (Fig. 16–15C). Some confusion may occasionally arise in connection with the so-called congenital dislocated radial head, but in general the contour of the radial head

should be diagnostic—the congenital lesion having a rounded convex head whereas the recently dislocated radius usually has a concave appearance. It can be appreciated that the younger the child the more difficult it will be to make this interpretation owing to the large cartilaginous component of the proximal radius.

Dislocation-Subluxation of the Radial Head Following Malunion of a Radial Neck Fracture

Fractures of the radial neck in children that have occurred after the age of 6 or 7 may, if unreduced, result in a subluxation (Fig. 16–6). When the angulation is more than 45 to 50 degrees the growth plate becomes redirected laterally or posterolaterally. If there is not enough remodeling to allow the growth plate to reattain its normal transverse anatomy, increased prominence of the radial head results. As the child grows older he will experience pain, irritation, cosmetic deformity, and, to a lesser extent, limitation of supination and pronation. This result can be avoided by ensuring that marked angulation of the radial neck is corrected by closed or open reduction to less than 40 to 45 degrees.

Dislocation of the radial head associated with malunion of the ulna may necessitate osteotomy of the ulna and an open reduction of the radial head. It is of course always prudent to attempt a closed reduction of the radial head if the injury has occurred recently, i.e., within 2 months, because the ulna may still be straightened. Usually, however, in the missed Monteggia lesion an open reduction of the radial head will be necessary, and in this instance it will almost certainly be necessary to reconstitute the annular ligament, either with the ligament itself if possible, with fascia obtained from the triceps, or by utilizing the Bell-Tause procedure.[28, 33] It may also require shortening the radius to permit reduction. Internal fixation with Kirschner wires through the radius to the ulna is advisable. Relocation of the radial head should be attempted in children under 6 years of age. In older children in whom the lesion has been present for more than a year it may be advisable to accept the dislocation since this is quite compatible with excellent function in most instances. If the radial head becomes cosmetically or functionally disabling, excision can be performed when skeletal maturity is attained. Removal of the radial head should not be considered until skeletal maturity is reached because 30 percent of radial growth occurs at the proximal radial epiphysis.

PULLED ELBOW SYNDROME

Nurse maid's elbow or pulled elbow syndrome has been recognized since early in this century.[83] Some children seem to be particularly prone to this injury, and for them even minor pulls on the arm result in the typical pain and failure of elbow motion that is always of concern to parents (Fig. 16–16A).[82, 84]

Etiology

Subsequent to a longitudinal pull on the forearm, the radial head is pulled down into the annular ligament (Fig. 16–16B). This results in inability to rotate the radial head without considerable discomfort. Usually the annular ligament is not torn; however, as the child becomes older the annular ligament is undoubtedly partially torn, which accounts for the persistence of symptoms for several days even after the reduction. At one time it was thought that the radial head in a child was smaller in relation to the neck than in the adults or older children, and thus, subluxation of the radial head into the annular ligament was more common.[84] Studies by Salter[88] and Mehta[86] have shown that even in infants the relative proportion of radial head diameter to neck diameter is similar to that of adults.

A more reasonable explanation for pulled elbow is simply the generalized ligamentous laxity of the elbow that exists at this age and the resiliency imparted to the radial head by the almost entirely cartilaginous structure. The pulled elbow syndrome is most common between the ages of 6 months and 3 years, becoming less common as the radius grows in size and becomes more ossified.[85] A longitudinal pull with accompanying pronation of the forearm screws the radial head down into the annular ligament, and the larger head then becomes caught as if in a Chinese finger trap (Fig. 16–16B).

Clinical Appearance

A child with the pulled elbow syndrome shows primarily pain and failure to move the elbow, and there may or may not be a typical history of a longitudinal pull. The infant may well go about his normal play activities and is comfortable as long as no one attempts to move the elbow. The child keeps the arm in pronation and expresses discomfort and anxiety if anyone attempts to move the elbow or pronate or supinate the forearm. Radiographs are singularly nondiagnostic and are sometimes misinterpreted because it is impossible to position the limb properly.[85] However, the technicians, in attempting to obtain good anteroposterior and lateral films of the elbow, may inadvertently reduce the subluxation by supinating the forearm, and the child returns from the Radiology Department content and moving his elbow quite normally!

Management

Reduction of the pulled elbow is usually simple, consisting of supination motions with the elbow flexed. If the left hand is kept over the radial head a click is often felt and sometimes even heard. As the radial head is screwed up into the annular ligament, the ligament slips down over the head into its normal position around the neck with a snap. In younger children, resumption of normal activity often ensues in minutes; however, in the older child the elbow may still be considerably tender, probably due to small tears within the annular ligament. If persistent pain ensues, immobilization of the arm in a plaster cast or splint for a week or so is indicated and will be curative.

There are no long-term sequelae from the pulled elbow syndrome, although occasionally in some children its frequent recurrence is a cause of concern to the family. In such a

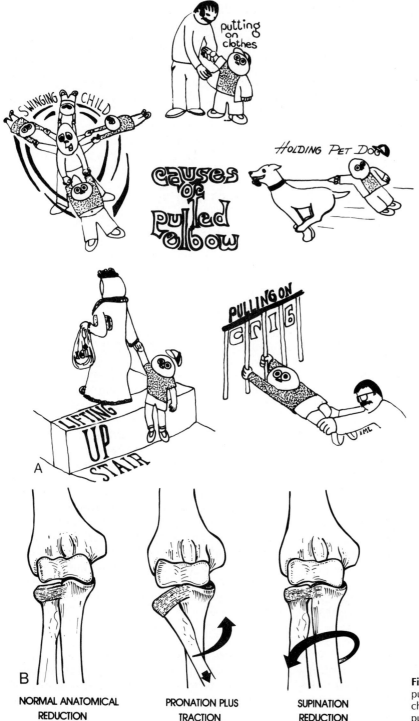

Figure 16–16. *A,* Some causes of pulled elbow syndrome in small children. *B,* Pathophysiology of the pulled elbow syndrome.

NORMAL ANATOMICAL REDUCTION

PRONATION PLUS TRACTION

SUPINATION REDUCTION

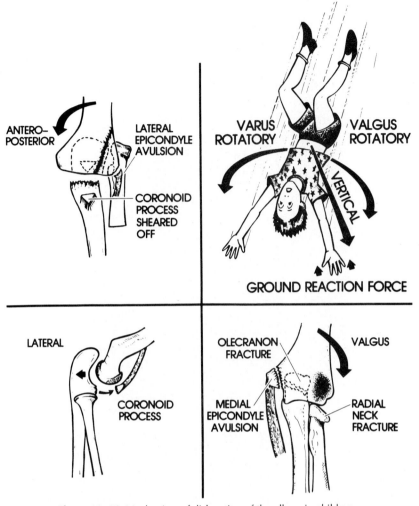

Figure 16–17. Mechanism of dislocation of the elbow in children.

case it is often worthwhile to sit down and explain to the parents what is happening and show them how to reduce recurrence of the pulled elbow to avoid frequent visits to the Emergency Department. Seldom is open repair of the annular ligament necessary, and even in the most recalcitrant recurrent pulled elbow time and growth always diminish and eradicate the instability of the radial head.

TRAUMATIC DISLOCATION OF THE ELBOW

Mechanism of the Dislocation

The elbow joint in a child is basically a ligamentous structure in which only a small portion of cartilaginous stability is imparted by the ulna. The forces about the elbow joint that occur in a fall on the outstretched hand result mainly from the body exerting a downward force on the fixed forearm at its contact

with the ground. Associated with this is a valgus or varus force created by the body falling over the fixed elbow (Fig. 16–17). The forearm is usually in pronation during a fall on the outstretched hand. The coronoid process may be avulsed by the attachment of the brachialis because it is also largely cartilaginous (Fig. 16–18). The valgus force of the body rotating over the fixed elbow often avulses the medial epicondylar apophysis (Fig. 16–19). If the body falls over the elbow medially instead of laterally a varus force is exerted, and the lateral epicondyle of the humerus or the lateral condyle may be avulsed (Fig. 16–20). Occasionally, as in a fall from a height, the forces may be such that the valgus force may disrupt the medial apophysis, and the posterolateral dislocation may also avulse the lateral epicondyle, resulting in elbow instability on both the ulnar and radial sides of the joint. The radius and the ulna seldom separate owing to the strong

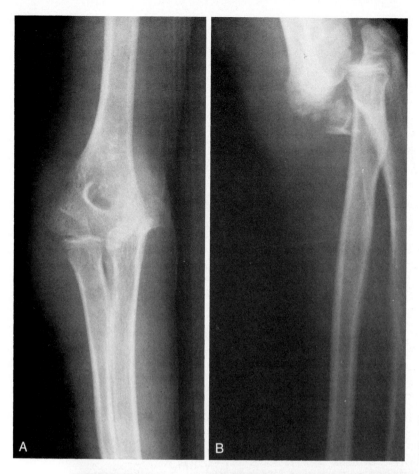

Figure 16–18. *A* and *B,* Fracture of coronoid process of olecranon associated with posterior dislocation of the elbow.

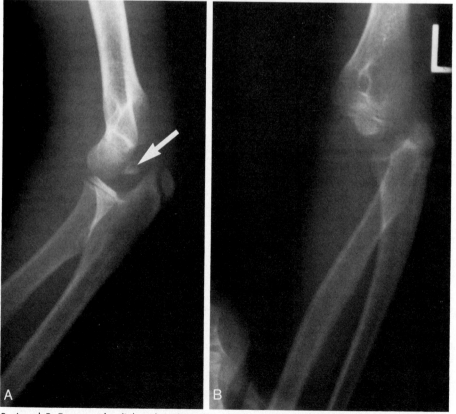

Figure 16–19. *A* and *B,* Fracture of radial neck with avulsion of the medial epicondyle, which has remained intra-articular following spontaneous reduction of the elbow dislocation.

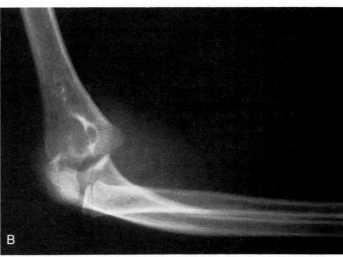

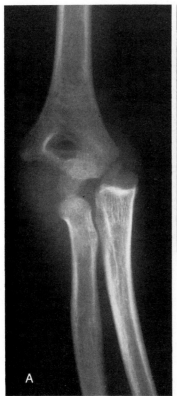

Figure 16–20. *A* and *B*, Dislocation of the elbow associated with fracture of the lateral condyle of the humerus. The radial head maintains its relationship with the displaced capitellum.

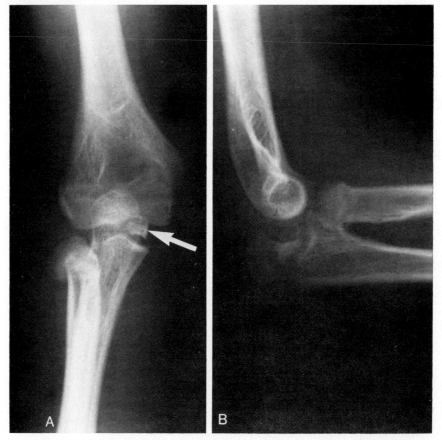

Figure 16–21. *A* and *B*, Dislocation of the elbow with valgus force resulting in fracture of the olecranon, radial neck, and medial epicondyle, which has remained intra-articular following spontaneous reduction.

interosseous membrane, although instances of divergent dislocations with tearing of the interosseous membrane have been reported.[50] Less commonly, traction injuries may result in elbow dislocation.[54]

Occasionally, in falls from a height the valgus force exerted on the elbow joint may result in a fracture of the neck of the radius and the olecranon process (Fig. 16–21). When the arm is in marked extension the capitellum may also be fractured. Associated fractures of the distal radius and ulna occasionally occur (Fig. 16–22).

Capsular tearing is responsible for the prolonged stiffness that often follows dislocation of the elbow. The capsular attachment to the ulna is frequently torn. The posterior capsule may also be torn at its attachment to the humerus.

Spontaneous Reduction of the Dislocated Elbow

Spontaneous reduction of a dislocated elbow in children is common. Often the child will present to the Emergency Department with a history of a fall, the only physical findings being a swollen, boggy elbow and no obvious radiographic evidence of any injury. However, if one looks carefully at the radiograph, signs of previous dislocation may be present

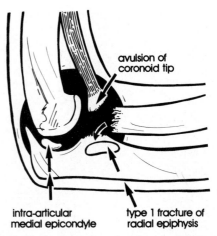

Figure 16–23. Fractures about the elbow in children indicative of spontaneous reduction of an elbow dislocation.

(Fig. 16–23). These include avulsion of the coronoid process (Fig. 16–24). This indicates that the elbow has been transiently out of joint, with the brachialis muscle avulsing the coronoid process.

On reduction, especially when the fracture is associated with vertical body force, the humerus may cause a type I or II fracture through the epiphyseal plate of the proximal radius, resulting in posterior displacement of the radial epiphysis upon reduction (Fig. 16–25).

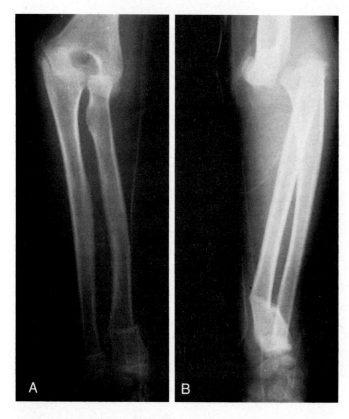

Figure 16–22. *A* and *B,* Fracture of distal radius associated with dislocation of the elbow.

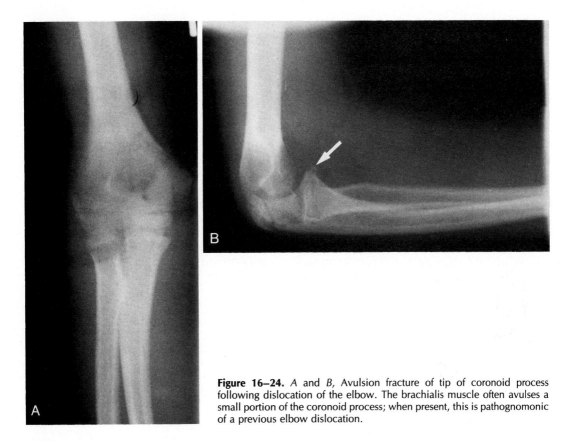

Figure 16–24. *A* and *B*, Avulsion fracture of tip of coronoid process following dislocation of the elbow. The brachialis muscle often avulses a small portion of the coronoid process; when present, this is pathognomonic of a previous elbow dislocation.

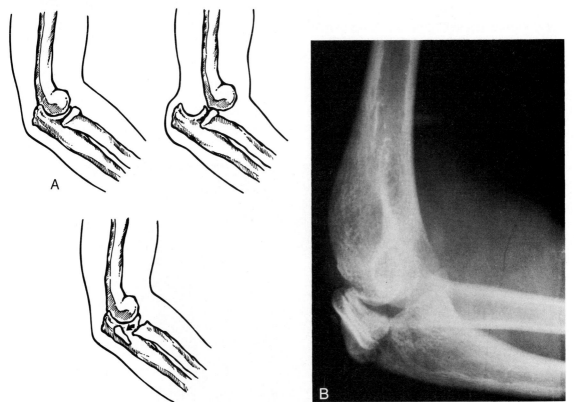

Figure 16–25. *A*, Type I fracture of the proximal radial epiphysis with posterior displacement occasionally occurs in posterior dislocation of the elbow if reduction is forceful. *B*, Fracture of neck of radius secondary to dislocation of the elbow with forceful spontaneous reduction.

Differential Diagnosis of Posterior Dislocation

The child with dislocation of the elbow is severely incapacitated with pain and deformity about the elbow joint. Because fractures are extremely common in childhood, the differential diagnosis basically consists of distinguishing a dislocation from a supracondylar fracture, lateral condylar fracture, and, in the younger child, transcondylar fracture of the humerus (Fig. 16–26). The elbow will be painful and swollen, and, depending on how soon the child is seen after the injury, the posterior deformity may be either obvious or masked by swelling if several hours have passed. The child is always extremely apprehensive and will not allow anyone under any circumstances to move or manipulate the joint.

In my experience the commonly stated rules of lining up the triangular relationship between the medial epicondyle, lateral epicondyle, and olecranon is really not of much practical value in this situation. One can sometimes feel a gap superior to the displaced olecranon indicating that a posterior dislocation has occurred. The humeral condyles can also be palpated anteriorly. The supracondylar fracture is often difficult to differentiate from a posterior dislocation of the elbow, especially if presentation is late and considerable swelling has occurred to obscure the abnormal anatomy. Excessive examination and movement of such an elbow should be avoided as it serves only to make the child more apprehensive and less cooperative.

The neuromuscular examination of the extremity can often be done simply by observation once the confidence and cooperation of the child have been obtained. Sensation then can be gently tested in the three major nerve distributions including the anterior and posterior interosseous divisions. It is essential, of course, to assess the neurologic and vascular condition of the limb in the Emergency Department. The child should be encouraged to make the "O" sign with the index finger and thumb. If this cannot be done, injury to the anterior interosseous nerve has occurred causing paralysis of the flexor pollicis longus, which makes this maneuver impossible. Radiographs are diagnostic in most instances except in the young child under 2 years of age. Dislocation of the elbow is very uncommon at this age, and transcondylar fracture of the humerus should be suspected (Fig. 16–24). This may be difficult to differentiate from a posterior dislocation, and confirmation may require arthrography.[44, 49, 51, 53, 55]

Radiographs should be carefully examined for associated fractures aside from the dislocation. A careful appraisal of the coronoid process, radial neck, olecranon, and medial and lateral epicondyles should be carried out.[43, 60] If the child is over 5 years of age and the medial epicondyle is not present, a radiograph of the other elbow should be inspected to make sure that it is ossified. If it then cannot be found on the radiograph of the dislocated elbow, it must be assumed that it is obscured by its intra-articular position (Fig. 16–19).[42, 47, 59, 64]

An injury to the radial epiphysis may occur when the elbow is forcibly reduced. This may even occur at the time of the injury, the child sustaining the original dislocation by a fall on

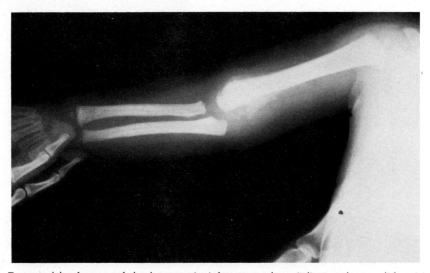

Figure 16–26. Transcondylar fracture of the humerus in infancy may be misdiagnosed as a dislocation of the elbow Arthrography of CT scan is diagnostic.

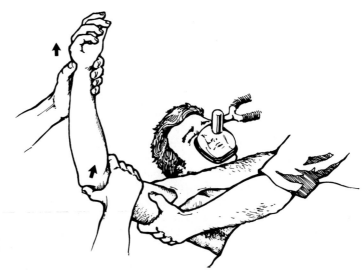

Figure 16–27. The author's preferred technique for reducing a posterior dislocation of the elbow joint in children.

the outstretched hand followed by a direct blow to the elbow as he hits the ground, thus reducing the elbow. The direct force on the radial head results in a type I fracture through the proximal radial epiphysis with posterior displacement (Fig. 16–25).

It is essential to emphasize that many children present to the Emergency Department with simply a swollen, boggy elbow joint and a history of a fall. In such cases one can assume, especially if there is radiographic evidence of avulsion of the coronoid process, that this elbow has been dislocated and has spontaneously reduced.

Treatment of Posterior Dislocation

Posterior dislocation of the elbow is a painful, terrifying experience for a child, and the limb should be put at rest with a splint as soon as possible in the Emergency Department with minimal manipulation of the extremity. No child should ever be sent for radiographs without adequate splintage. The dislocation demands early treatment and of course, if there is any vascular insufficiency, immediate treatment.

Occasionally, in a very cooperative older child the elbow may be reduced in the Emergency Department. The instillation of local anesthetic into the joint itself often facilitates this maneuver. Turning the child prone with the arm dangling over the stretcher facilitates the application of some pressure over the olecranon, and this, combined with gravity or slight traction on the dangling limb, may allow the dislocation to be quickly reduced.[57] If there is an associated fracture of the medial epicondyle, radial neck, or olecranon, this maneuver should probably not be attempted.

In our experience with children under age 12 it is best to proceed with a general anesthetic for complete relaxation, and this should be done within 6 hours of the trauma. It is not appropriate to allow the child to wait overnight because this encourages increased edema and resultant postreduction stiffness as well as being extremely uncomfortable for the child.

Once the child has been anesthetized, it is usually a simple matter to reduce the posterior dislocation of the elbow. Gentle traction on the forearm combined with some anterior pressure over the dislocated olecranon allows the joint to be reduced, usually with an audible and palpable clunk (Fig. 16–27).

Occasionally, in older children the coronoid process becomes locked behind the humerus. In this instance the arm should be put in extension, and again, with traction and good firm thumb pressure over the olecranon the elbow can usually be reduced. Putting the elbow into hyperextension to lever the coronoid process under the humerus is a hazardous procedure, especially if vascular insufficiency is already present because it places more stress on the brachial artery, which is often tented over the distal end of the humerus. Once the elbow is reduced, the integrity of the medial and lateral collateral ligaments should be tested, and the elbow should be moved through a full range of motion to ensure that no fragment, particularly the medial epicondyle, is caught within the joint. If the joint does not move freely or has a spongy feel to it, a mechanical problem with reduction exists. The reduction should always be checked radiographically, especially when a fracture is associated with the injury.[63, 65]

Aspiration of the joint is recommended to

assist in resolving the hematoma and improving joint motion after reduction.

Medial Epicondylar Entrapment

If it is known that the medial epicondyle is indeed trapped within the joint, during the reduction a valgus strain placed on the elbow with flexion of the wrist may allow the attached flexor muscle mass to pull the trapped fragment out of the joint. Occasionally, this may yield an anatomic or near anatomic position. If the medial epicondyle is displaced more than a centimeter, it should be pinned back in place because it will add stability to the elbow subsequent to the dislocation and allow stable elbow motion to occur within 3 to 4 weeks. In children under the age of 5 when the medial epicondyle is not ossified, any springiness in the elbow joint subsequent to the reduction indicates an intra-articular position of the medial epicondyle. If the medial epicondyle cannot be removed from the joint with manipulation, it must be removed surgically. The elbow is approached through a medial incision. The flexor muscle mass initially appears to be anatomically intact as it disappears into the joint; however, with valgus force and gentle pull on the muscle mass, the attached fragment can be removed from the joint and the capsule repaired. The fragment should then be reattached to the distal medial humerus. Care should be taken not to injure the ulnar nerve. If there is any concern about this, the nerve should be identified and retracted with tapes until the repair has been completed.[59, 61]

Postoperative Management

Following reduction of the elbow, the joint should be immobilized at 90 degrees or greater. This is especially important if there has been a coronoid process avulsion. This allows the triceps to tighten posteriorly, acting as a dynamic splint for the elbow, and also helps to prevent the ulna from slipping backward into the dislocated position because of the added stability with flexion.

Other Types of Elbow Dislocation

Anterior Dislocation. Anterior dislocation of the elbow in children is uncommon and usually is the result of severe direct trauma to the posterior aspect of the proximal forearm. This may be associated with a fracture of the olecranon. Reduction should be accomplished by direct pressure anteriorly over the dislocated radius and ulna together with gentle traction on the forearm to allow the olecranon to slide beneath the humerus.[48, 58]

Medial or Lateral Dislocation. Purely medial or lateral dislocations are exremely rare because there is always a posterior element associated with them. Longitudinal traction may be all that is required for reduction. If the joint, however, deviates considerably to either side, appropriate pressure over the medial or lateral aspects to align the elbow prior to reduction often facilitates reduction.[52, 56]

Divergent Dislocation. This is an extremely rare type of dislocation that results from tearing of the interosseous membrane. Although I have never treated one of these dislocations, it seems reasonable to exert medial and lateral pressure over the divergent radius and ulna to try to align the forearm bone prior to reducing it as a simple posterior dislocation.[50]

Complications of Elbow Dislocation

Complications from simple dislocations of the elbow are uncommon in children. This is particularly true when they are compared with the many complications that may occur following dislocation of the elbow in adults.

Joint Stiffness. As in adults, joint stiffness is the most common problem encountered after dislocation of the elbow in children. Clinicians must always counsel the child and his parents that after an elbow dislocation the major difficulty will be regaining full motion in the joint. In older children fully complete extension may never be recovered, although the loss of the last 5 to 10 degrees of extension really is not accompanied by any marked functional deficit. Elbows in children should not be immobilized longer than 4 weeks, and exercises after injury should be primarily active; passive motion should be avoided. Seldom is manipulation or passive physiotherapy required for joint stiffness after a dislocation of the elbow; indeed, this type of treatment often delays recovery because it is accompanied by further joint irritation, capsular tearing, and hematoma formation. A year may be required to regain full motion in the child's elbow, the child being his own best physiotherapist. Unreduced posterior dislocation of the elbow is a rare cause of stiffness in children.[45]

Myositis Ossificans. Myositis ossificans is an uncommon complication of a simple dislocation of the elbow joint in children unless it is accompanied by a crush injury or major trauma. Myositis ossificans may result in bridging across the elbow, usually involving the brachialis muscle. The ossific lesion can be excised once it is mature; however, it is still possible for new myositis ossificans to form.

Nerve Injuries. Nerve injuries are uncommon in simple posterior elbow dislocations in children. The ulnar nerve is most frequently involved.[54] The common posterolateral dislocation of the elbow results in a stretch on the ulnar nerve. The median and rarely the radial nerve may also suffer neuropraxic injuries secondary to posterior dislocation of the elbow.

The median nerve is also vulnerable to occasional entrapment within the joint subsequent to reduction of the elbow dislocation. Although rare, this type of entrapment has been reported only in children, and diagnosis is frequently delayed. It should be suspected when signs of median nerve injury or pain accompany avulsion of the medial epicondyle; in such instances the nerve usually lies "posterior" to the medial epicondyle (Fig. 16–28).

As emphasized by Green[66] in an excellent review of this subject, persistent pain or increasing median nerve dysfunction should alert one to the possibility of nerve entrapment. A late clinical sign of entrapment is persistent limitation of elbow motion; a late radiologic sign of median nerve entrapment is depression of the cortex of the distal humerus, just proximal to the medial epicondyle where the median nerve passes behind the humerus[70] (Fig. 16–29). Median nerve exploration should be undertaken once the diag-

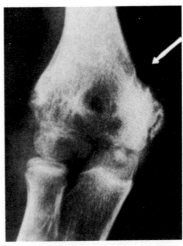

Figure 16–29. Median nerve entrapment 3 months after injury. The arrow points to a cortical depression with interruption of periosteal reaction. (From Matev, I.: Radiological sign of entrapment of the median nerve in the elbow joint after posterior dislocation. J. Bone Joint Surg. 58:353, 1976.)

nosis of nerve entrapment has been made. If the nerve is functionally intact, as demonstrated by nerve stimulation, simple removal of the nerve from the joint is sufficient treatment. If the nerve is obviously severely damaged, crushed or scarred, and nonfunctional, resection of the damaged section with end-to-end reanastomosis is recommended.

Vascular Injury. Injury to the brachial artery to the extent of complete occlusion is not commonly observed in dislocations of the elbow in children. The brachial artery may be stretched over the distal humerus, and if the force is sufficient, damage to the artery may occur. This is evident by the usual signs of vascular impairment, which then demand exploration of the artery. The elbow should always be reduced before making a final assessment of the vascular status of the limb because it may be simply occluded subsequent to the elbow deformity.

In assessing vascular integrity in a child's arm, caution must be advised in putting too much faith in "capillary filling." Collateral circulation may be sufficient to provide excellent capillary filling but insufficient to ensure muscle metabolism (see Chapter 17).

Recurrent Dislocation of the Elbow. Recurrent dislocation of the elbow in children is very uncommon. It may occur after a particularly severe dislocation in which the lateral collateral ligaments have also been torn and healed with resultant ligamentous laxity of the lateral aspect of the elbow.[62] Inadequate treatment in which the elbow has been kept flexed at less than 90 degrees, especially when

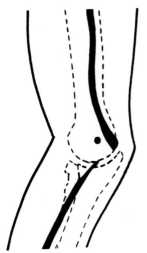

Figure 16–28. Course of median nerve lying entrapped posterior to the medial epicondyle. (From Matev, I.: Radiological sign of entrapment of the median nerve in the elbow joint after posterior dislocation. J. Bone Joint Surg 58:353, 1976.

associated with a fracture of the coronoid process, may result in redislocation of the elbow and reinjury and recurrent dislocation.[75-81]

SUMMARY

Dislocations about the elbow are not uncommon in children. Because they often accompany fractures in the region of the joint, care must be taken to examine the environs of the elbow systematically for evidence of skeletal injury coexisting with the dislocation. Particular care should be exercised to ensure that the radial head is in its proper relationship with the capitellum. Because most problems encountered in elbow dislocations in children are the result of missed diagnoses of associated injuries, the value of a thorough clinical and radiographic examination of the elbow cannot be overemphasized.

References

Traumatic Dislocation of the Radial Head

1. Beddow, F. H., and Corckery, P. H.: Lateral Dislocation of the Radial Humeral Joint with Greenstick Fracture of the Upper End of the Ulna. J. Bone Joint Surg. **42B**:782, 1960.
2. De Lee, J. C.: Transverse Divergent Dislocation of the Elbow in a Child. J. Bone Joint Surg. **63A**:322, 1981.
3. Heidt, R. S., and Stern, P. J.: Isolated Posterior Dislocation of the Radial Head. Clin. Orthop. **168**:136, 1982.
4. Hume, A. C.: Anterior Dislocation of the Head of the Radius Associated with Undisplaced Fracture of the Olecranon in Children. J. Bone Joint Surg. **39B**:508, 1957.
5. Schubert, J. J.: Dislocation of the Radial Head in the Newborn Infant. J. Bone Joint Surg. **47A**:1010, 1965.
6. Stelling, F. H., and Cote, R. H.: Traumatic Dislocation of the Head of the Radius in Children. J.A.M.A. **160**:732, 1956.
7. Storen, G.: Traumatic Dislocation of the Radial Head as an Isolated Lesion in Children. Acta Clin. Scand. **116**:144, 1958.
8. Vesely, D. G.: Isolated Traumatic Dislocation of the Radial Head in Children. Clin. Orthop. **50**:31, 1967.
9. Wiley, J. J., Pegington, J., and Horwich, J. P.: Traumatic Dislocation of the Radius at the Elbow. J. Bone Joint Surg. **56B**:501, 1974.
10. Wright P. R.: Greenstick Fractures of the Upper End of the Ulna with Dislocation of the Radial Humeral Joint or Displacement of the Superior Radial Epiphysis. J. Bone Joint Surg. **45B**:727, 1963.
11. Zivkovic, T.: Traumatic Dislocation of the Radial Head in a 5 Year Old Boy. J. Trauma **18**:289, 1978.

Development Dislocation of the Radial Head

12. Hamilton, W., and Parks, J. C.: Isolated Dislocation of the Radial Head Without Fracture of the Ulna. Clin. Orthop. **97**:94, 1973.
13. Lloyd-Roberts, G. C., and Bucknill, T. M.: Anterior Dislocation of the Radial Head in Children—Etiology, Natural History and Management. J. Bone Joint Surg. **59B**:402, 1977.
14. Pletcher, D., Hofer, M. M., and Koffman, D. M.: Nontraumatic Dislocation of the Radial Head in Cerebral Palsy. J. Bone Joint Surg. **58A**:104, 1976.
15. Peeters, R. L. M.: Radiological manifestations of the Cornelia de Lange Syndrome. Pediatr. Radiol. **3**:41, 1975.
16. Salama, R., Weintroub, S., and Weissman, S. L.: Recurrent Dislocation of the Radial Head. Clin. Orthop. **125**:156, 1977.
17. Silberstein, M. J., Brodeur, A. E., and Graviss, E. R.: Some Vagaries of the Radial Head and Neck. J. Bone Joint Surg. **64A**:1153, 1982.
18. Southmayd, W., and Parks, J. C.: Isolated Dislocation of the Radial Head Without Fracture of the Ulna. Clin. Orthop. **97**:94, 1973.

Congenital Dislocation of the Radial Head

19. Almquist, E. E., Gordon, L. H., and Blue, A. I.: Congenital Dislocation of the Head of the Radius. J. Bone Joint Surg. **51A**:1118, 1969.
20. Carevias, D. E.: Some Observations on Congenital Dislocation of the Head of the Radius. J. Bone Joint Surg. **39B**:86, 1957.
21. Cockshott, W. P., and Omololu, A.: Familial Posterior Dislocation of Both Radial Heads. J. Bone Joint Surg. **40B**:484, 1958.
22. Gunn, D. R., and Pilley, V. K.: Congenital Dislocation of the Head of the Radius. Clin. Orthop. **84**:108, 1964.
23. Kelikian, H.: Dislocations of the Radial Head. In Congenital Deformities of the Hand and Forearm. Philadelphia, W. B. Saunders Co., 1974, pp. 902–938.
24. Mardam-Bey, T., and Ger, E.: Congenital Radial Head Dislocation. J. Hand Surg. **4**:316, 1979.

Monteggia Fracture-Dislocation of the Elbow in Children

25. Bado, J. L.: The Monteggia Lesion. Clin. Orthop. **50**:71, 1967.
26. Beddow, F. H., and Corkeny, P. H.: Lateral Dislocation of the Radiohumeral Joint with Greenstick Fracture of the Upper End of the Ulna. J. Bone Joint Surg. **42B**:782, 1969.
27. Bruce, H. E., Harvey, J. P. W., and Wilson, J. C., Jr.: Monteggia Fractures. J. Bone Joint Surg. **56A**:1563, 1974.
28. Bell-Tause, A. J. F.: The Treatment of Malunited Anterior Monteggia Fractures in Children. J. Bone Joint Surg. **47B**:718, 1965.
29. Eady, J. L.: Acute Monteggia Lesions in Children. J. SC Med. Assoc. **71**:107, 1975.
30. Evans, E. M.: Pronation Injuries of the Forearm with Special Reference to the Anterior Monteggia Fracture. J. Bone Joint Surg. **31B**:578, 1949.
31. Fahmy, N. R. M.: Unusual Monteggia Lesions in Children. Injury **12**:399, 1981.
32. Hume, A. C.: Anterior Dislocation of the Head of the Radius Associated with Undisplaced Fracture of the Olecranon in Children. J. Bone Joint Surg. **39B**:508, 1957.
33. Hurst, L. C., and Dubrow, E. N.: Surgical Treatment of Symptomatic Chronic Radial Head Dislocation: A Neglected Monteggia Fracture. J. Ped. Orthop. **3**:227, 1983.
34. Mullick, S.: The Lateral Monteggia Fracture. J. Bone Joint Surg. **59A**:543, 1977.
35. Peiro, A., Andres, F., and Fernandez-Esteve, F.:

Acute Monteggia Lesions in Children. J. Bone Joint Surg. **59A**:92, 1977.

36. Ramsey, R. H., and Pedersen, H. E.: The Monteggia Fracture-Dislocation in Children. J.A.M.A. **182**:1091, 1962.

37. Spinner, M., Freundlich, B. D., and Teicher, J.: Posterior Interosseous Nerve Palsy as a Complication of Monteggia Fractures in Children. Clin. Orthop. **58**:141, 1968.

38. Stein, F., Grabias, S. L., and Deffer, P. A.: Nerve Injuries Complicating Monteggia Lesions. J. Bone Joint Surg. **53A**:1432, 1971.

39. Theodorou, S. D.: Dislocation of the Head of the Radius Associated with Fractures of the Upper End of the Ulna in Children. J. Bone Joint Surg. **51B**:700, 1969.

40. Tompkins, D. G.: The Anterior Monteggia Fracture. Observations on Etiology and Treatment. J Bone Joint Surg. **53A**:1109, 1971.

41. Wright, P. R.: Greenstick Fracture of the Upper End of the Ulna with Dislocation of the Radiohumeral Joint or Displacement of the Superior Radial Epiphysis. J. Bone Joint Surg. **45B**:727, 1963.

Acute Dislocation of the Elbow in Children

42. Aitken, A. P., and Childress, H. M.: Inter-articular Displacement of the Internal Epicondyle Following Dislocation. J. Bone Joint Surg. **20**:161, 1938.

43. Aufranc, O. E., Jones, W. M., Turner, R. H., and Thomas, W. H.: Dislocation of the Elbow with Fracture of the Radial Head and Distal Radius. J.A.M.A. **202**:131, 1967.

44. Beghin, J. L., Bucholz, R. W., and Wenger, D. R.: Intercondylar Fractures of the Humerus in Young Children. J. Bone Joint Surg. **64A**:1083, 1982.

45. Bilett, D. M.: Unreduced Posterior Dislocation of the Elbow. J. Trauma **19**:186, 1979.

46. Blatz, D. J.: Anterior Dislocation of the Elbow in a Case of Ehlers-Danlos Syndrome. Orthop. Rev. **10**:129, 1981.

47. Blount, W. P.: Fractures in Children. Baltimore, The Williams & Wilkins Co., 1955, pp. 26–75.

48. Caravias, D. E.: Forward Dislocation of the Elbow Without Fracture of the Olecranon. J. Bone Joint Surg. **39B**:334, 1957.

49. D'Ambrosia, R., and Zink, W.: Fractures of the Elbow in Children. Pediatr. Ann. **11**:541, 1982.

50. De Lee, J. C.: Transverse Divergent Dislocation of the Elbow in a Child. J. Bone Joint Surg. **63A**:322, 1981.

51. De Lee, J. C., Wilkens, K. E., Rogers, L. F., and Rockwood, C. A.: Fracture Separation of the Distal Humeral Epiphysis. J. Bone Joint Surg. **62A**:46, 1980.

52. Eppright, R. H., and Wilkins, K. E.: Fractures and Dislocations of the Elbow. *In* Rockwood, C. A., Jr., and Green, D. P. (eds.): Fractures. Vol. I, p. 487. Philadelphia, J. P. Lippincott Co., 1975.

53. Grantham, S. A., and Tietjen, R.: Transcondylar Fracture—Dislocation of the Elbow. J. Bone Joint Surg. **58A**:1030, 1976.

54. Heilbronner, D. M., Manili, A., and Little, R. E.: Elbow Dislocation During Overhead Skeletal Traction Therapy. Clin. Orthop. **147**:185, 1981.

55. Kaplan, S. S., and Reckling, R. W.: Fracture Separation of the Lower Humeral Epiphysis with Medial Displacement. J. Bone Joint Surg. **53A**:1105, 1971.

56. Linscheid, R. L., and Wheeler, D. K.: Elbow Dislocations. J.A.M.A. **194**:1171, 1965.

57. Meyn, M. A., Jr., and Quibley, T. B.: Reduction of Posterior Dislocation of the Elbow by Traction on the Dangling Arm. Clin. Orthop. **103**:106, 1974.

58. Oury, J. H., Roe, R. D., and Laning, R. C.: A Case of Bilateral Anterior Dislocations of the Elbow. J. Bone Joint Surg. **12**:170, 1972.

59. Patrick, J.: Fracture of the Medial Epicondyle with Displacement into the Elbow Joint. J. Bone Joint Surg. **28**:143, 1946.

60. Protzman, R. R.: Dislocation of the Elbow Joint. J. Bone Joint Surg. **60A**:539, 1978.

61. Rang, M.: Children's Fractures. Philadelphia, J. B. Lippincott Co., 1983.

62. Schwab, G. H., Bennett, J. B., Woods, G. W., and Tollos, H. S.: Biomechanics of Elbow Instability—The Medial Collateral Ligament. Clin. Orthop. **146**:42, 1980.

63. Smith, F. M.: Children's Elbow Injuries: Fractures and Dislocations. Clin. Orthop. **50**:7, 1967.

64. Smith, F. M.: Displacement of the Medial Epicondyle of the Humerus into the Elbow Joint. Ann. Surg. **124**:410, 1946.

65. Tachdjian, M. O.: Pediatric Orthopaedics, Vol. 2, p. 1604. Philadelphia, W. B. Saunders Co., 1972.

Complications of Dislocation of the Elbow in Children

66. Green, N. E.: Entrapment of the Median Nerve Following Elbow Dislocation. J. Pediatr. Orthop. **3**:384, 1983.

67. Hallet, J.: Entrapment of the Median Nerve After Dislocation of the Elbow. J. Bone Joint Surg. **63B**:408, 1981.

68. Kerian, R.: Elbow Dislocation and Its Association with Vascular Disruption. J. Bone Joint Surg. **51**:756, 1969.

69. Louis, D. S., Ricciardi, J., and Sprengler, D. M.: Arterial Injuries: A Complication of Posterior Elbow Dislocation. J. Bone Joint Surg. **56A**:1631, 1974.

70. Matev, I.: A Radiological Sign of Entrapment of the Median Nerve in the Elbow Joint After Posterior Dislocation. J. Bone Joint Surg. **58B**:353, 1976.

71. St.Clair-Strange, F. G.: Entrapment of the Medial Nerve After Dislocation of Elbow. J. Bone Joint Surg. **64B**:224, 1982.

72. Stiger, R. N., Larrick, R. D., and Meyer, T. F.: Median Nerve Entrapment Following Elbow Dislocations in Children. J. Bone Joint Surg. **51A**:381, 1969.

73. Tayob, A. A., and Shively, R. A.: Bilateral Elbow Dislocations with Inter-Articular Displacement of the Medial Epicondyle. J. Trauma **20**:332, 1980.

74. Thompson, H. C., and Garcia, A.: Myositis Ossificans After Massive Elbow Injuries. Clin. Orthop. **50**:129, 1967.

Recurrent Dislocation of the Elbow in Children

75. Hall, R. M.: Recurrent Posterior Dislocation of the Elbow Joint in a Boy. J. Bone Joint Surg. **35B**:56, 1953.

76. Hassman, G. C., Brunn, F., and Neer, C. S.: Recurrent Dislocation of the Elbow. J. Bone Joint Surg. **57A**:1080, 1975.

77. Jacobs, R. L.: Recurrent Dislocation of the Elbow; A Case Report and Review of the Literature. Clin. Orthop. **74**:151, 1971.

78. Mantle, J.: Recurrent Posterior Dislocation of the Elbow. J. Bone Joint Surg. **48B**:590, 1966.

79. Nalkawi, H.: Recurrent Dislocation of the Elbow Accompanied by Ulnar Neuropathy. Clin. Orthop. **161**:269, 1981.

80. Osborne, G. B., and Cotterill, P.: Recurrent Dislocation of the Elbow. J. Bone Joint Surg. **48B**:340, 1966.

81. Trias, A., and Comeau, Y.: Recurrent Dislocation of the Elbow in Children. Clin. Orthop. **100**:74, 1974.

Pulled Elbow

82. Blount, W. P.: Fractures in Children. Baltimore, The Williams & Wilkins Co., 1955.
83. Boyette, D. P., Ahoskie, H. C., and London, A. H., Jr.: Subluxation of the Head of the Radius—"Nursemaid's Elbow." J. Pediatr. **32**:278, 1948.
84. Hart, G. M.: Subluxation of the Head of the Radius in Young Children. JAMA **169**:1734, 1959.
85. Magill, H. K., and Aitken, A. P.: Pulled Elbow. Surg. Gynecol. Obstet. **98**:753, 1954.

86. Mehta, L.: Subluxation of Radial Head in Children with Reference to Radial Head and Neck Diameters. J. Ind. Med. Assoc. **166**:220, 1972.
87. Nussbaum, A. J.: The Off-Profile Proximal Radial Epiphysis: Another Potential Pitfall in the X-Ray Diagnosis of Elbow Trauma. **23**:40, 1982.
88. Salter, R. B., and Zaltz, C.: Anatomic Investigations of the Mechanism of Injury and Pathologic Anatomy of "Pulled Elbow" in Young Children. Clin. Orthop. **77**:141, 1971.
89. Speed, J. S., and Boyd, H. B.: Treatment of fractures of the ulna with dislocation of the head of the radius. JAMA **115**:1900, 1940.

CHAPTER 17

Ischemia from Fractures and Injuries About the Elbow

SCOTT J. MUBARAK

Two basic pathologic processes may result from supracondylar fractures or other injuries to the elbow region that can lead to forearm ischemia: (1) compartment syndrome from post-traumatic swelling, and (2) arterial injury that may either lead to a compartment syndrome or result directly in post-traumatic ischemia (Fig. 17–1). The muscles of the extremities are grouped into compartments that are enclosed by a relatively noncompliant osteofascial envelope. Muscle swelling causes increased pressure within the compartment that is not easily dissipated owing to the relatively inelastic nature of the surrounding fascia. If the pressure remains sufficiently high for several hours, loss of function of intracompartmental nerves and muscles due to ischemia may result. A compartment syndrome is a condition in which the high pressure within the compartment compromises the circulation to the nerves and muscles within the involved compartment. In contrast to compartment syndrome, an arterial injury may result from laceration, thrombus, embolus, intimal tear, or pseudoaneurysm (Fig. 17–2). Such an injury may cause nerve and muscle ischemia directly or may result in postischemic swelling or hemorrhage, thereby causing a compartment syndrome. In either event, nerve and muscle ischemia may result, possibly leading to a forearm contracture.

To prevent permanent loss of nerve and muscle function, this condition must be promptly diagnosed and correctly treated. Volkmann's contracture is the popular term that refers to the end-stage of an ischemic injury to the muscles and nerves of the limb (Fig. 17–3). Untreated compartment syndromes or arterial injuries are the primary causes of Volkmann's contracture. The term *Volkmann's ischemia* is nonspecific and probably should not be used.

ANATOMY

The forearm consists of two basic compartments (Fig. 17–4). The volar compartment includes the flexors and pronators of the forearm and wrist, which may be further divided into superficial and deep muscle groups. The superficial muscles include the flexor carpi ulnaris, palmaris longus, flexor carpi radialis, and pronator teres. The deeper group of muscles consists of the flexor digitorum superficialis and profundus, flexor pollicis longus, and pronator quadratus. The median and ulnar nerves traverse the forearm between these two muscle groups (Fig. 17–4). The major arteries about the elbow include the brachial artery, which bifurcates in the region of the radial head to form the radial and ulnar arteries (Fig. 17–5).

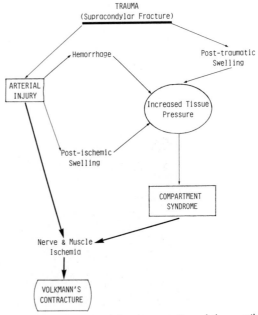

Figure 17–1. Diagrammatic representation of the possible mechanisms of Volkmann's contracture.

289

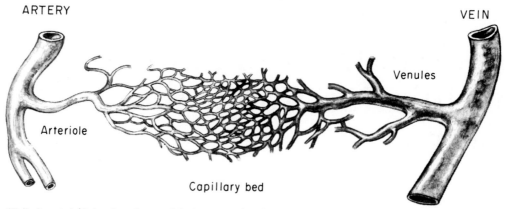

Figure 17–2. An arterial injury is a disease of the large vessels, whereas a compartment syndrome is a disease of small vessels. (From Mubarak, S. J., and Hargans, A. R.: Compartment Syndromes and Volkmann's Contracture. Philadelphia, W. B. Saunders Co., 1981.)

The dorsal compartment consists mainly of the wrist and finger extensors. The "mobile wad" of Henry includes the brachioradialis and the extensor carpi radialis longus and brevis muscles. This group of muscles is physically and functionally distinct; it lies between the dorsal and volar forearm compartments and should probably be considered a separate compartment. The major nerve of the dorsal compartment is the posterior interosseous nerve, a continuation of the radial nerve. The major artery of the dorsal compartment is the posterior interosseous artery.

ETIOLOGY

Trauma is the most common cause of a compartment syndrome or an arterial injury in general (Fig. 17–6). The most common traumatic event that produces one of these problems about the elbow is the supracondylar fracture of the distal humerus (Figs. 17–7 and 17–8). In 1956 Lipscomb noted that supracondylar fractures were the cause of 48 percent of Volkmann's contractures in 92 cases from the Mayo Clinic.[14] In 1967 Ehrlich and Lipscomb, in a review of 32 more cases of Volkmann's contracture, reported that 34 percent were due to supracondylar fractures and 22 percent were due to forearm fractures.[6] In 1979, Mubarak and Carroll, reporting on 58 Volkmann's contractures in children (Fig. 17–9), found that supracondylar fractures had caused only 16 percent of these.[19] In that study, other traumatic events such as elbow dislocations, Monteggia fractures, and radial neck fractures also caused Volkmann's contracture.

Compartment syndromes can result after a soft tissue injury (without fracture) and have been seen after severe burns and arterial injuries (Fig. 17–6).

An arterial injury can produce nerve and muscle ischemia directly or the additional problem of a compartment syndrome by one of two mechanisms (Fig. 17–1).[22] First, if the major vessel is lacerated, hemorrhage into the compartment may produce the syndrome. Second, a compartment syndrome may result from postischemic swelling if there is inade-

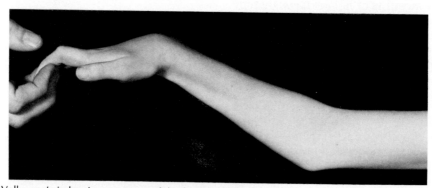

Figure 17–3. Volkmann's ischemic contracture of the forearm. The residual of an untreated forearm compartment syndrome in a 8-year-old boy.

Figure 17–4. Forearm compartments: Transverse sections through the left forearm at various levels. (From Mubarak, S. J., and Hargans, A. R.: Compartment Syndromes and Volkmann's Contracture. Philadelphia, W. B. Saunders Co., 1981.)

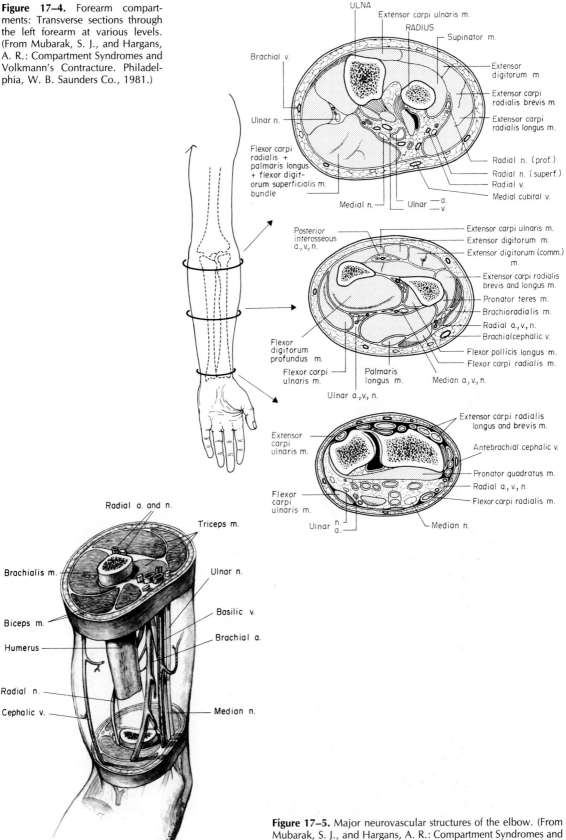

Figure 17–5. Major neurovascular structures of the elbow. (From Mubarak, S. J., and Hargans, A. R.: Compartment Syndromes and Volkmann's Contracture. Philadelphia, W. B. Saunders Co., 1981.)

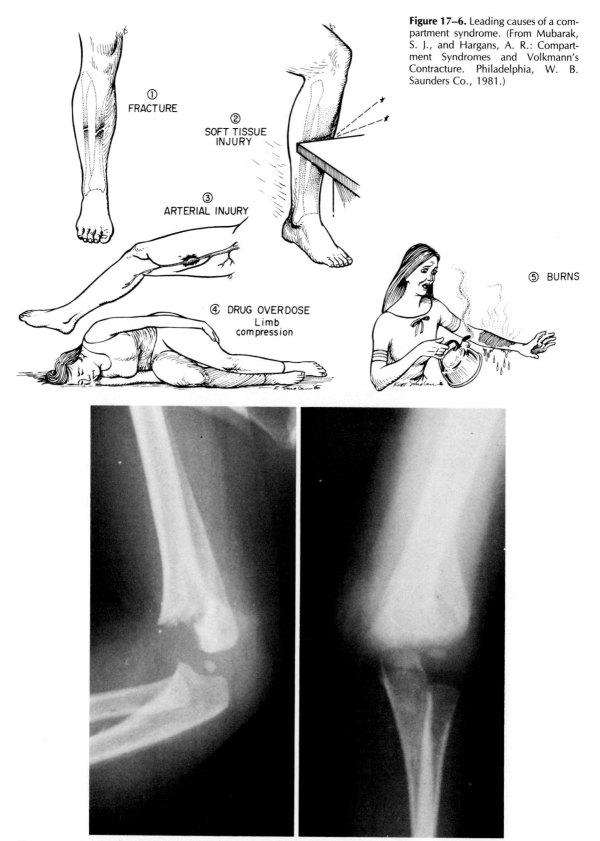

Figure 17–6. Leading causes of a compartment syndrome. (From Mubarak, S. J., and Hargans, A. R.: Compartment Syndromes and Volkmann's Contracture. Philadelphia, W. B. Saunders Co., 1981.)

Figure 17–7. Supracondylar fracture of the distal humerus in a child is the most infamous lesion associated with Volkmann's contracture. (From Mubarak, S. J., and Hargans, A. R.: Compartment Syndromes and Volkmann's Contracture. Philadelphia, W. B. Saunders Co., 1981.)

Figure 17–8. Three-year-old boy whose supracondylar fracture is shown in Figure 17–7. At the time of cast removal, his forearm had poor sensation and was contracted in the pronated and flexed position. (From Mubarak, S. J., and Hargans, A. R.: Compartment Syndromes and Volkmann's Contracture. Philadelphia, W. B. Saunders Co., 1981.)

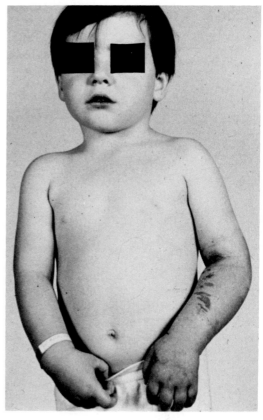

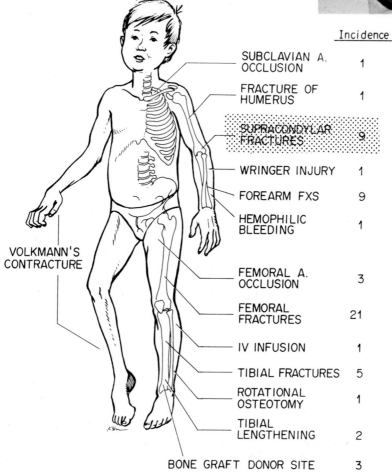

	Incidence
SUBCLAVIAN A. OCCLUSION	1
FRACTURE OF HUMERUS	1
SUPRACONDYLAR FRACTURES	9
WRINGER INJURY	1
FOREARM FXS	9
HEMOPHILIC BLEEDING	1
FEMORAL A. OCCLUSION	3
FEMORAL FRACTURES	21
IV INFUSION	1
TIBIAL FRACTURES	5
ROTATIONAL OSTEOTOMY	1
TIBIAL LENGTHENING	2
BONE GRAFT DONOR SITE	3

VOLKMANN'S CONTRACTURE

Figure 17–9. Causes and incidence of Volkmann's contracture in 58 limbs (55 children). Note that supracondylar fractures account for half of such complications in the upper extremity. (From Mubarak, S. J., and Carroll, N. C.: Volkmann's contracture in children, aetiology and prevention. J. Bone Joint Surg. 61B:285–293, 1979.)

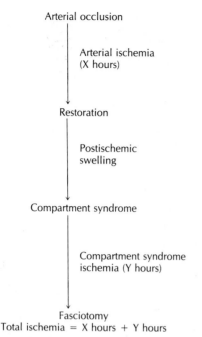

Arterial occlusion

Arterial ischemia
(X hours)

Restoration

Postischemic
swelling

Compartment syndrome

Compartment syndrome
ischemia (Y hours)

Fasciotomy
Total ischemia = X hours + Y hours

Figure 17–10. Pathogenesis of postischemia-initiated compartment syndrome. (From Mubarak, S. J., and Hargans, A. R.: Compartment Syndromes and Volkmann's Contracture. Philadelphia, W. B. Saunders Co., 1981.)

quate collateral circulation or if the vessel is only partially occluded—for example, from an arterial spasm or intimal tear. In this situation, the decreased perfusion and ischemia of both capillaries and muscles will cause an increase in the permeability of the capillary walls. The resulting edema will then cause more ischemia, and a vicious circle may ensue. When there is complete arterial occlusion, a compartment syndrome may develop from postischemic swelling after the circulation is restored (Fig. 17–10). When complete arterial occlusion is secondary to massive emboli or prolonged use of a tourniquet in which the circulation is not restored, gangrene rather than compartment syndrome will result.

CLINICAL DIAGNOSIS

There is an association between supracondylar fractures, absent pulses, and Volkmann's contracture. When the concepts of compartment syndrome as a cause of and fasciotomy as a treatment for Volkmann's contracture became popular, it was only logical that absent pulses, which are associated with arterial injuries, would merge with the signs of compartment syndrome. This misconception has no doubt caused many physicians to delay

treatment for a compartment syndrome while waiting for the pulse to disappear.

Signs of Compartment Syndrome. The early diagnosis of a compartment syndrome depends on recognition of the signs and symptoms of increased intracompartmental pressure. The first and most important symptom of an impending compartment syndrome is pain that is greater than that expected from the primary problem (e.g., the fracture or contusion). The pain is usually described as a feeling of increased pressure and is localized to the affected compartment. It is not relieved by immobilization. Pain may be lacking if a central or peripheral sensory nerve deficit is superimposed.

The earliest and most objective finding is a *tense compartment* that is a direct manifestation of the increased intracompartmental pressure. The tenseness should be evident throughout the involved compartments. To evaluate this, removal of all dressings is required. Although it is not possible, even with experience, to estimate consistently by palpation the degree to which intracompartmental pressures are elevated, the presence of significant tenseness throughout the compartment boundaries suggests a compartment syndrome. Conversely, if the compartment is palpably soft, the examiner may be reassured that, for the moment, compartment pressures are not elevated.

Pain with passive stretch of the muscles in the involved compartment is a common finding usually associated with muscle ischemia. However, direct muscle injury or contusion may elicit this clinical finding.

The volar compartment of the forearm is traversed by nerves (radial, ulnar, and median) that have a distal sensory distribution in the hand. The first sign of nerve ischemia is alteration of sensation, which is manifest early by subjective *paresthesia* in the distribution of the involved nerve, followed by *hypesthesia* and later by anesthesia. Unless there is a superimposed sensory or peripheral nerve deficit, decreased sensation to light touch or pinprick in the distal sensory distribution is a very reliable sign of ischemia. The dorsal compartment of the forearm is not associated with a specific sensory nerve.

Paresis secondary to nerve or neuromuscular junction ischemia and elevated intracompartmental pressure is a common finding. The paresis may be confusing, however, because it may be secondary to proximal nerve injury or guarding secondary to pain rather than to intracompartmental ischemia.

Except in the presence of major arterial

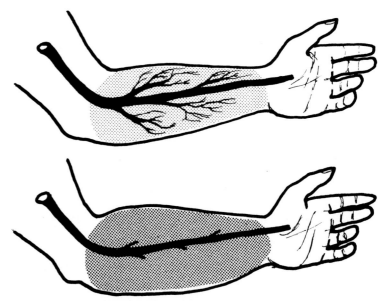

Figure 17–11. Schematic view of forearm compartment syndrome. Intracompartmental pressures are only rarely high enough to occlude the major arteries of the compartment. However, the pressure is sufficient to cause ischemia of muscle and nerve by occluding the microcirculation within the compartment. (From Rang, M.: Children's Fractures. Philadelphia, J. B. Lippincott Co., 1974.)

injury or disease, peripheral *pulses* and capillary filling are routinely intact in compartment syndrome patients. Although intracompartmental pressures may become high enough to cause ischemia of the muscle and nerve by occluding the microcirculation within the compartment, the pressures are rarely high enough to occlude the major arteries (Fig. 17–11). The intracompartmental pressures rarely exceed 80 mm Hg and are more commonly between 40 and 60 mm Hg in our experience. It has been suggested that absent pulses may result from vascular spasm secondary to elevated intracompartmental pressures.[5] In our laboratory, however, pressurization to as high as 80 mm Hg of the entire anterolateral compartment in a number of dogs produced only occasional transient spasm of the midsize vessels on angiography.[10, 21]

Signs of Arterial Injury. As with a compartment syndrome, *pain* out of proportion to that expected for the injury is the earliest symptom of arterial ischemia. The earliest finding for an arterial injury is *pain with passive stretch* of the involved muscles. This will usually be associated with *absent or decreased pulses, poor skin color,* and *decreased skin temperature*. Other early findings are *weakness* and *hypesthesia* in a glovelike distribution.

DIFFERENTIAL DIAGNOSIS

Many traumatic events that precipitate a compartment syndrome or arterial injury can produce by themselves a painful, swollen extremity. The diagnosis of the underlying problem (e.g., fracture or contusion) is obvious; the diagnosis of a superimposed ischemia is more difficult. Pain out of proportion to that expected for the injury and any sensory deficit must be explained. A compartment syndrome or arterial injury must also be differentiated from a nerve injury, which is usually a neurapraxia when it is associated with a closed elbow fracture or dislocation. The clinical findings of these three entities overlap, frequently making the diagnosis difficult, if not impossible, by clinical means. All these problems may be associated with motor or sensory deficits and pain. Careful clinical evaluation is necessary to differentiate these entities (Table 17–1). As noted earlier, an arterial injury usually results in absent pulses, poor skin color, and decreased skin temperature. In contrast, a compartment syndrome routinely presents with intact peripheral circulation unless the underlying etiology is an arterial injury. A nerve injury is usually made by exclusion of the other two entities. Doppler blood-flow studies, arteriography, and pressure measurements are frequently required to aid in the differential diagnosis of these three entities, especially if these problems are present in combination.

Differentiation of these entities is important because therapy for each is radically different. The neurapraxia accompanying a closed fracture is usually best treated by observation. Arterial injuries warrant immediate operative repair of the vessel, and a compartment syndrome necessitates immediate decompressive fasciotomy.

Table 17–1. **Typical Clinical Findings of Compartment Syndrome, Arterial Occlusion, and Neurapraxia**

	Compartment Syndrome	Arterial Occlusion	Neurapraxia
Pressure increased in compartment	+	−	−
Pain with stretch	+	+	−
Paresthesia or anesthesia	+	+	+
Paresis or paralysis	+	+	+
Pulses intact	+	−	+

From Mubarak, S., and Carroll, N.: Volkmann's contracture in children: aetiology and prevention. J. Bone Surg. **61B**:290, 1979.

LABORATORY TESTS

Pressure Measurement. When the patient is cooperative, most compartment syndromes can be diagnosed clinically. In these patients intracompartmental pressure measurement will be only confirmatory. There are three groups of patients in whom difficulties in eliciting or interpreting the physical findings make measurement of intracompartmental pressure particularly valuable as a criterion for decompression:

1. Uncooperative or unreliable patients. A child with an elbow fracture will often be so frightened that careful motor and sensory evaluation is not possible.
2. Unresponsive patients. A patient with a head injury or one that is sedated and on a respirator with a swollen limb needs pressure measurement.
3. Patients with nerve deficits. When a more proximal nerve, brachial plexus, or the spinal cord is injured, evaluation of the forearm and hand is difficult. Also, when there is an associated nerve injury or arterial injury at the elbow, intracompartmental pressure measurement is frequently required to differentiate these problems from a compartment syndrome.

Instrumentation. There are a variety of means of measuring compartment pressure, including the needle technique by Reneman[25] and Whitesides et al.,[28, 29] and the infusion technique advocated by Matsen et al.[16, 18] We have employed the wick catheter technique[21, 23] and more recently the slit catheter technique[26] for tissue pressure measurement. The wick catheter technique was first described in 1968 by Scholander et al.[27] The wick catheter that we used is based on the original design, but instead of cotton a piece of Dacron suture is employed as the wick in the end of the catheter. The development of the clinical wick catheter was initiated in 1973, and the first human studies were begun in 1974. It has since been used to evaluate and diagnose more than 100 compartment sydromes in the past 9 years. The wick technique provides an accurate and reproducible means of determining tissue pressure under equilibrium conditions. The wick in the catheter is designed to prevent blockage of the catheter's tip by tissue and to maximize surface contact between the saline in the catheter and fluids in the tissue. Continuous monitoring of intracompartmental pressures, even during muscular contraction and exercise, is possible.

The slit catheter,* developed by Rorabeck et al.[26] and modified by Mubarak et al.,[20] combines the advantages of the wick catheter and is easier to manufacture (Fig. 17–12). Five 3-mm-long slits (approximately 60 degrees apart) are placed in the tip of a piece of polyethylene tubing. The slits act to maintain continuity between the tissue fluids and saline within the catheter without injection of flushing. Long-term monitoring is feasible. The wick and slit techniques use a pressure transducer and recorder.

Interpretation. Normal intracompartmental pressures measure between 0 and 8 mm Hg.[21] Whitesides suggests that fasciotomy be performed when the intracompartmental pressure approaches a limit of 20 mm Hg less than the patient's diastolic blood pressure.[29] This criterion is based on the use of the needle techique. Matsen et al. suggest fasciotomy at pressures greater than 45 mm Hg.[15, 17] Our initial clinical and animal studies support the conclusion that the threshold intracompartmental pressure at which fasciotomy is desirable is between 30 and 40 mm Hg for an 8-hour pressurization.[10–12, 22, 23] Because the time parameter is usually unknown in most cases of acute compartment syndromes, we recom-

---

*The slit catheter is manufactured by Howmedica Inc., 359 Veterans Boulevard, Rutherford, New Jersey 07070.

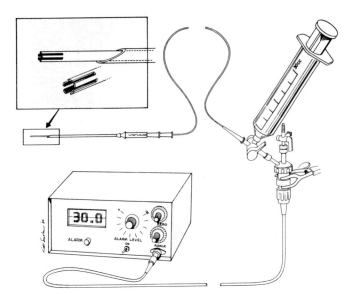

Figure 17–12. Slit catheter technique for continuous measurement of equilibrium, intracompartmental pressure. Prior to insertion into muscle compartment, the sterile slit catheter is connected to the pressure transducer and digital recorder and is then filled with saline by means of a 30-ml syringe. The catheter tip protrudes from the insertion needle during filling so that the tip can be checked for air bubbles (see close-up, upper left). Before insertion into the muscle, the catheter is pulled entirely within the needle. (From Mubarak, S. J., and Hargans, A. R.: Compartment Syndromes and Volkmann's Contracture. Philadelphia, W. B. Saunders Co., 1981.)

mend that any intracompartmental pressure greater than 30 to 35 mm Hg be considered for fasciotomy *if it is combined with the clinical findings* of a compartment syndrome. However, one must remember that any threshold pressure is a relative indication for decompression that should be tempered by the patient's overall condition, blood pressure, and peripheral perfusion, the trend of the symptoms and signs, the trend of the intracompartmental pressures, and the cooperation and reliability of the patient.[22]

Arteriograph and Doppler Studies. Arteriography and Doppler blood-flow studies are employed to evaluate the arterial supply to the limb. The Doppler blood-flow and pulse-reappearance time are very useful for noninvasive documentation of intact pulses in the presence of a markedly swollen distal extremity. Arteriography performed by the radiology department or in the operating room may be helpful in defining the presence and type of arterial injury. With elbow trauma, the level of arterial injuries is known, and if the arteriography study will delay treatment of the arterial injury substantially, one may not be able to obtain that test.

TREATMENT

When evaluating a patient with a traumatized limb and a neurocirculatory deficit, the physician should document carefully the time of injury and examination. A thorough examination should include motor, sensory, and circulatory evaluation. When a neurologic deficit is observed in a painful, traumatized, and swollen limb, the physician must evaluate

and treat the patient promptly. Initially, cast splitting should be performed. If the neurologic deficit persists without improvement for more than an hour, removal of the cast and all circular dressings is mandatory. If the compartments are observed to be tense, measurement of pressure is necessary. At this stage, one must differentiate the troublesome problems of compartment syndrome, neurapraxia, and arterial injury.

Forearm Fasciotomy. Bardenheuer was the first to report on fasciotomy in the forearm.[1] Eichler and Lipscomb described an approach to a patient with a forearm compartment syndrome that included a division of forearm skin, subcutaneous tissue, and fascia.[6] In 1972, Eaton and Green described a specific operative technique in which their skin incision began distal to the elbow flexion crease and medial to the bicipital tendon and extended distally in the longitudinal axis of the midforearm to the transverse flexion crease at the wrist.[4] The forearm fascia was incised longitudinally along its full length. The epimysium of all poorly vascularized muscles was sectioned. The fascia was left open, and delayed closure with split-thickness skin grafts and relaxing incisions was performed 48 to 72 hours later.

Neumeyer and Kilgore's incision began adjacent to the medial epicondyle, extended obliquely across the antecubital fossa over the volar mobile wad, and returned to the midline in the distal forearm.[24] It continued in a curvilinear fashion across the carpal canal to the midpalm. This report recommended wide exposure of all three possible areas of involvement—the volar and dorsal compartments of the forearm and the intrinsic compartments of the hand. Closure was accomplished by split-thickness skin grafts after several days.

Whitesides and associates described another operative approach in which their incision began above the elbow laterally and was carried transversely across the antecubital fossa to the proximal-medial forearm.[30] The incision was continued distally along the ulnar border of the forearm to the wrist, where it curved laterally in the flexor crease of the wrist and extended into the palm in the thenar crease. The fascia was opened from above the elbow to the midpalm. The carpal tunnel and all neurovascular and muscular envelopes were opened fully. They noted that subcutaneous fasciotomy should never be performed in the forearm. The fascia was left open and was closed by split-thickness skin grafts 48 to 72 hours later. Similarly, Matsen and associates used the volar-ulnar approach.[15] They frequently performed carpal tunnel release and epimysiotomy as recommended by Eaton and Green.[4] The advantage of this volar-ulnar approach is that the flexor tendons and median nerve are not left exposed in the distal forearm.

The effectiveness of the volar forearm fasciotomy was evaluated initially in a series of cadaver experiments.[9] The incisions used were the volar-ulnar incision described by Whitesides et al.[30] and the curvilinear midline volar incision. Both incisions were effective in lowering pressures in the volar forearm and both also lowered pressure within the mobile wad and dorsal regions in approximately half of the limbs. However, the curvilinear incision allowed easier exposure of the arteries and nerves of the forearm and the mobile wad. The volar forearm pressure generally fell to normal values when the antebrachial fascia had been divided from the lacertus fibrosus to the junction of the middle and distal thirds of the forearm. When the dorsal pressures remained elevated following volar fasciotomy, a dorsal fasciotomy was performed.

RESULTS AND COMPLICATIONS

The results of early decompression of forearm compartment syndromes are related to a number of variables:

1. Type and severity of the injury.
2. Magnitude of pressure elevation.
3. Duration of the ischemia.

Gelberman et al. reported no cases of Volkmann's contracture in a recent study of su-

pracondylar fractures.[8] However, they noted that crush injuries or severe open injuries, when associated with compartment syndromes, resulted in considerable disability with decreased strength and limitation of forearm and hand motion. In these cases, much of the functional loss can be attributed to the crush injury alone; the compartment syndrome is an additional insult.[8]

A Volkmann's contracture is the major complication of a compartment syndrome. Fortunately, the incidence of that complication following supracondylar fractures as pointed out earlier in this chapter, has declined signifcantly in the past 25 years (48 percent to 16 percent). With proper treatment of the elbow injury and early recognition and treatment of ischemia, a Volkmann's contracture is rarely seen.

Many large series on the treatment of supracondylar fractures report no cases of Volkmann's contracture when treated by Dunlap's traction,[3] overhead pin traction,[2] or percutaneous pinning.[7] In these series the complication rate for nerve injuries ranged from 9 to 13 percent, and for injury to the brachial artery, from 8 to 18 percent (see Chapter 12).

A complete discussion of the treatment of an established contracture is covered by Gelberman and others[22] and is beyond the scope of this discussion.

AUTHOR'S PREFERRED METHOD

Fasciotomy Technique. We prefer a single longitudinal curvilinear incision for decompression of the volar forearm (Fig. 17–13). This incision allows an easy approach to the antebrachial fascia and transverse carpal ligament as well as to the neurovascular structures of the forearm and the mobile wad (Fig. 17–14). The incision is nearly identical to McConnell's combined exposure of the median and ulnar neurovascular bundles as described by Henry.[13] A straight longitudinal incision is used for the dorsal compartment of the forearm (Fig. 17–13). Technique and postoperative care are described in detail elsewhere.[8, 9, 22] The adequacy of this technique has been confirmed by intraoperative pressure monitoring in more than 20 patients to date.[8]

Elbow Fractures and Compartment Syndromes. Elbow fractures associated with acute forearm compartment syndromes should, in nearly all cases, be treated by internal fixation at the time of fasciotomy. This approach allows for ease of handling the fasciotomy wounds and for earlier rehabilitation and motion of the extremity.

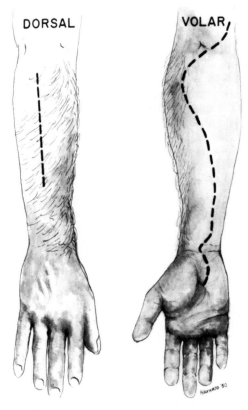

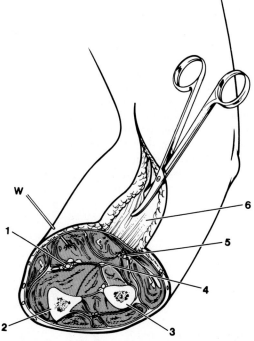

Figure 17–13. Dorsal and volar forearm incisions. (From Gelberman, R. H.: Compartment syndromes of the forearm: Diagnosis and treatment. Clin. Orthop. 161:252–261, 1981.)

Figure 17–14. Cross-section of left forearm with wick catheter illustrating its position and fasciotomy incision. W, Wick catheter; 1, ulnar nerve; 2, ulna; 3, radius; 4, median nerve; 5, radial artery; 6, forearm fascia. (From Mubarak, S. J., and Hargans, A. R.: Compartment Syndromes and Volkmann's Contracture. Philadelphia, W. B. Saunders Co., 1981.)

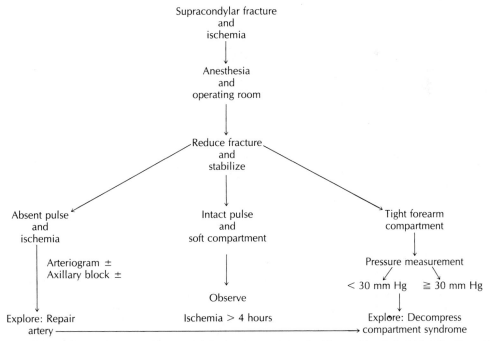

Figure 17–15. Scheme for management of supracondylar fractures associated with upper extremity ischemia. (From Mubarak, S. J., and Hargans, A. R.: Compartment Syndromes and Volkmann's Contracture. Philadelphia, W. B. Saunders Co., 1981.)

Elbow Fractures, Compartment Syndromes and Arterial Injury. Arterial injuries associated with compartment syndromes most often occur following supracondylar fractures. If an arterial injury associated with a compartment syndrome and supracondylar fracture is suspected, the patient should be taken immediately to the operating room. The fracture should be reduced and stabilized by percutaneous pinning or by open reduction and internal fixation. It is extremely important in this situation to stabilize the fracture so that all attention can be directed toward the vascular problems and the ischemia (Fig. 17–15).

After fracture reduction and stabilization, the circulation should be reassessed. If the compartments are tense, intracompartmental pressures should be obtained for the volar,

dorsal, and hand compartments. If the pressures are elevated above 35 mm Hg, fasciotomy should be carried out. The brachial, radial, and ulnar arteries should be explored at the time of decompression. if a segment of the artery is in spasm, it should be cleansed meticulously. Topical paraverine (2½ percent) or lidocaine (1 percent) or an axillary block is often helpful in clearing the spasm. It may take 20 to 30 minutes for the spasm to improve significantly. If a segment of the artery is irreparably damaged or lacerated, it should be repaired. The surgeon must be certain that the hand circulation is adequate before leaving the operating room.[22]

If a forearm compartment syndrome is not present but the pulses and the hand circulation are poor, the physician should consider

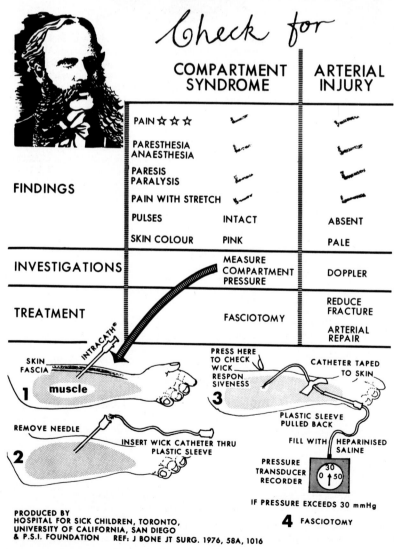

Figure 17–16. Poster outlining the clinical findings, investigations, and treatment of compartment syndromes that is used to alert medical and nursing staff to the diagnosis and prevention of Volkmann's ischemic contracture. (From Mubarak, S. J., and Hargans, A. R.: Compartment Syndromes and Volkmann's Contracture. Philadelphia, W. B. Saunders Co., 1981.)

obtaining a transfemoral-brachial arteriogram depending on the ease with which that study can be obtained. Subsequently, exploration and repair of the artery should be performed.

Prophylactic fasciotomy of the forearm should be considered after brachial artery repair if the period of ischemia is more than 4 hours.

It is clear that many factors influence the result of an elbow injury associated with ischemia. However, a physician who carefully assesses the clinical findings, promptly achieves the correct diagnosis with objective methods such as intracompartmental pressure measurements (for compartment syndrome) or an arteriogram (for an arterial injury), and promptly treats the problem will achieve the best results (Fig. 17–16).

References

1. Bardenheuer, L.: Die Entstehung und Behandlung der ischamischen Muskelkontractur und Gangran. Dtsch. Z. Chir. **108**:44, 1911.
2. D'Ambrosia, R. D.: Supracondylar Fractures of the Humerus: Prevention of Cubitus Varus. J. Bone Joint Surg. **54A**:60, 1972.
3. Dodge, H. S.: Displaced Supracondylar Fractures of the Humerus in Children: Treatment by Dunlop's Traction. J. Bone Joint Surg. **54A**:1408, 1972.
4. Eaton, R. G., and Green, W. T.: Epimysiotomy and Fasciotomy in the Treatment of Volkmann's Ischemic Contracture. Orthop. Clin. North Am. **3**:175, 1972.
5. Eaton, R. G., and Green, W. T.: Volkmann's Ischemia. A Volar Compartment Syndrome of the Forearm. Clin. Orthop. **113**:58, 1975.
6. Eichler, G. R., and Lipscomb, P. R.: The Changing Treatment of Volkmann's Ischemic Contractures from 1955 to 1965 at the Mayo Clinic. Clin. Orthop. **50**:215, 1967.
7. Flynn, J. C., Matthews, J. G., and Benoit, R. L.: Blind Pinning of Displaced Supracondylar Fractures of the Humerus in Children. J. Bone Joint Surg. **56A**:263, 1974.
8. Gelberman, R. H., Garfin, S. R., Hergenroeder, P. T., Mubarak, S. J., and Menon, J.: Compartment Syndromes of the Forearm: Diagnosis and Treatment. Clin. Orthop. **161**:252, 1981.
9. Gelberman, R. H., Zakaib, G. S., Mubarak, S. J., Hargens, A. R., and Akeson, W. H.: Decompression of Forearm Compartment Syndromes. Clin. Orthop. **134**:225, 1978.
10. Hargens, A. R., Akeson, W. H., Mubarak, S. J., Owen, C. A., Evans, K. L., Garetto, L. P., Gonsalves, M. R., and Schmidt, D. A.: Fluid Balance Within the Canine Anterolateral Compartment and Its Relationship to Compartment Syndromes. J. Bone Joint Surg. **60A**:499, 1978.
11. Hargens, A. R., Romine, J. S., Sipe, J. C., Evans, K. L., Mubarak, S. J., and Akeson, W. H.: Peripheral Nerve-Conduction Block by High Muscle-Compartment Pressure. J. Bone Joint Surg. **61A**:192, 1979.
12. Hargens, A. R., Schmidt, D. A., Evans, K. L., Gonsalves, M. R., Garfin, S. R., Mubarak, S. J., Hagan, P. L., and Akeson, W. H.: Quantitation of Skeletal-Muscle Necrosis in a Model Compartment Syndrome. (In press, J. Bone Joint Surg., 1984.)
13. Henry, A. K.: Extensile Exposure, 2nd ed. Edinburgh, Churchill Livingstone, 1973.
14. Lipscomb, P. R.: The Etiology and Prevention of Volkmann's Ischemic Contracture. Surg. Gynecol. Obstet. **103**:353, 1956.
15. Matsen, F. A.: Compartmental Syndromes. New York, Raven Press, 1980.
16. Matsen, F. A., III, Mayo, K. A., Sheridan, G. W., and Krugmire, R. B., Jr.: Monitoring of Intramuscular Pressure. Surgery **79**:702, 1976.
17. Matsen, F. A., III, Winquest, R. A., and Krugmire, R. B.: Diagnosis and Management of Compartmental Syndromes. J. Bone Joint Surg. **62A**:286, 1980.
18. Matsen, F. A., III, Wyss, C. R., and King, R. V.: The Continuous Infusion in the Assessment of Clinical Compartment Syndromes. In Hargens, A. R. (ed.): Tissue Fluid Pressure and Composition. Baltimore, The Williams & Wilkins Co., 1981, pp. 255–259.
19. Mubarak, S. J., and Carroll, N. C.: Volkmann's Contracture in Children: Aetiology and Prevention. J. Bone Joint Surg. **61B**:285, 1979.
20. Mubarak, S. J., Hargens, A. R., Lee, Y. F., Lundblad, A. K., Castle, G. S. P., and Rorabeck, C. H.: Slit Catheter—A New Technique for Measuring Tissue Fluid Pressure and Quantifying Muscle Contraction. 27th Annual Meeting, Orthopaedic Research Society, Las Vegas, 1981.
21. Mubarak, S. J., Hargens, A. R., Owen, C. A., Akeson, W. H., and Garetto, L. P.: The Wick Technique for Measurement of Intramuscular Pressure: A New Research and Clinical Tool. J. Bone Joint Surg. **58A**:1016, 1976.
22. Mubarak, S. J., and Hargens, A. R.: Compartment Syndromes and Volkmann's Contracture. Philadelphia, W.B. Saunders Co., 1981.
23. Mubarak, S. J., Owen, C. A., Hargens, A. R., Garetto, L. P., and Akeson, W. H.: Acute Compartment Syndromes: Diagnosis and Treatment with the Aid of the Wick Catheter. J. Bone Joint Surg., **60A**:1091, 1978.
24. Neumeyer, W. L., and Kilgore, E. S., Jr.: Volkmann's Ischemic Contracture due to Soft Tissue Injury Alone. J. Hand Surg. **1**:221, 1976.
25. Reneman, R. S.: The Anterior and the Lateral Compartment Syndrome of the Leg. The Hague, Mouton, 1968.
26. Rorabeck, C. H., Castle, G. S. P., Hardie, R., and Logan, J.: Compartmental Pressure Measurements. An Experimental Investigation Using the Slit Catheter. J. Trauma **21**:446, 1981.
27. Scholander, P. F., Hargens, A. R., and Miller, S. L.: Negative Pressure in the Interstitial Fluid of Animals. Science **161**:321, 1968.
28. Whitesides, T. E., Jr., Haney, T. C., Hirada, H., Holmes, H. E., and Morimoto, K.: A Simple Method for Tissue Pressure Determination. Arch. Surg. **110**:1311, 1975a.
29. Whitesides, T. E., Jr., Haney, T. C., Morimoto, K., and Hirada, H.: Tissue Pressure Measurements as a Determinant for the Need of Fasciotomy. Clin. Orthop. **113**:43, 1975b.
30. Whitesides, T. E., Jr., Hirada, H., and Morimoto, K.: Compartment Syndromes and the Role of Fasciotomy, Its Parameters and Techniques. In The American Academy of Orthopedic Surgeons: Instructional Course Lectures, Vol 26. St. Louis, The C. V. Mosby Co., 1977, pp. 179–194.

PART III

Trauma to the Adult Elbow

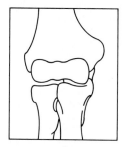

CHAPTER 18

Fractures of the Distal Humerus

R. S. BRYAN and B. F. MORREY

Little or nothing is gained by attempting to reassemble the fragments and contain them by some form of internal fixation. Even the classical T and Y fractures are best left alone; the results of operative treatment with internal fixation in perfect anatomical reposition are disappointing almost invariably; in fact, I will go further and say that usually they are extremely bad.[45]

Manipulative reduction usually fails .... Olecranon traction, exerted through the collateral ligaments, actually seems to increase the rotational pull upon the condyles ... [The results of] collar and cuff sling followed by early joint mobilization ... in our experience ... have been poor.[48]

Probably no matter what treatment is used one must expect some limitation of motion at the elbow.[71]

These quotations, although taken out of context, illustrate the strong controversy that exists concerning the treatment of distal humeral fractures. Obviously, if good results

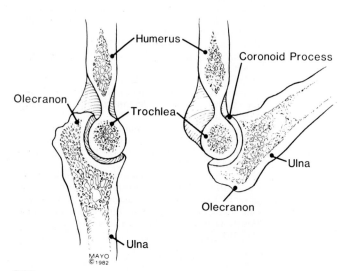

Figure 18–1. Transverse section of the supracondylar bone demonstrating the greater cross-sectional area of the lateral compared with the medial supracondylar bony columns.

302

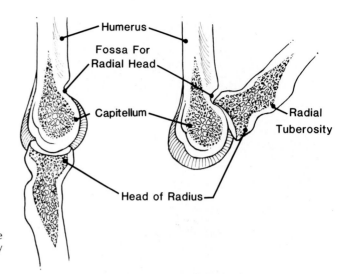

Figure 18–2. A sagittal view showing the more substantial supracondylar bone present laterally compared with the medial side. (See Figure 18–1.)

were readily obtainable there would be no disagreement. Why are some fractures of the distal humerus so difficult to treat? The answer lies in the congruency of the joint, the sensitivity of the capsule and soft tissue to trauma, and the relationship of the muscles and ligaments to the articular surface. The fossae that permit the extremes of flexion and extension are responsible for the configuration that, because of exacting tolerances, causes much of the difficulty in fracture treatment. Figure 18–1 shows a section through

the trochlear notch at 90 degrees to the coronal plane and demonstrates the precise relationships that are often grossly disturbed and that must be recreated after fracture. A similar view through the radial head and capitellar articulation (Fig. 18–2) further illustrates the close tolerances involved.

To fully understand the difficulty of managing fractures of the distal humerus, the pathologic anatomy must be precisely understood. Supracondylar fractures are not only difficult to reduce but may also compromise

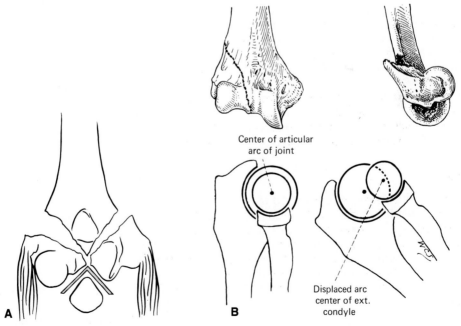

Figure 18–3. Fractures across the articular surface demonstrate deformity in the frontal plane due to internal rotation brought about by the muscle attachments. This gives rise to the so-called inverted V-sign *(A)*, and the lack of bone stock makes reduction and fixation difficult. Malalignment of the humeral condyles causes obliteration of the axis of rotation, which will limit both flexion and extension motion *(B)*. *(B,* from Magnuson, P. B., and Stack, J. K.: Fractures, 5th ed. Philadelphia, J. B. Lippincott Co., 1949.)

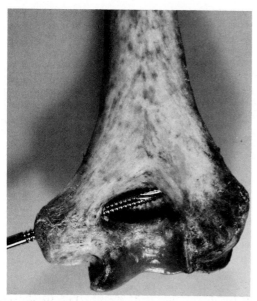

Figure 18–4. Motion is lost if internal fixation devices violate the coronoid fossa anteriorly or the olecranon fossa posteriorly.

Table 18–1. **Fractures of the Distal Humerus**

Extra-articular Fractures
Supracondylar
Transcondylar (dicondylar)
Epicondylar
Medial
Lateral
Supracondylar process
Intra-articular Fractures
T and Y condylar
Lateral condylar
Medial condylar
Articular
Capitellum
Trochlea
Massive Trauma

the neurovascular status of the extremity. Fractures across the supracondylar columns cause serious difficulty with alignment because of the deforming forces of the muscles and the inadequacy of the fracture surface in providing stability. Fractures involving the articulation may demonstrate rotational deformity as well as displacement in the frontal and sagittal planes (Fig. 18–3). Healing callus or fixation devices (Fig. 18–4) may encroach on the fossae, limiting motion. Thus, either the quality of the reduction or the healing callus or fixation device may contribute to limitation of motion after healing has taken place.

Finally, the lack of soft tissue attachment of the intra-articular fragments further complicates these fractures, making management difficult and the prognosis unfavorable.

Incidence

Fractures about the elbow are not uncommon but are not considered frequent compared with other fractures. Several large series suggest that elbow fractures account for about 7 percent of all fractures treated.[17, 39, 104] About a third involve the distal humerus—thus distal humeral fractures account for about 2 percent of all fractures.

Classification

The classification of these fractures is logically grouped into intra-articular and extra-articular types (Table 18–1). Extra-articular fractures include supracondylar and transcondylar, epicondylar and supracondylar process fractures. Intra-articular injuries are composed of T or Y condylar fractures, those involving a single condyle, and those that violate the articulation only, usually the capitellum. Finally, the elbow may be involved in massive trauma, traditionally called the "sideswipe" injury.

EXTRA-ARTICULAR FRACTURES

Supracondylar and Transcondylar Fractures

Supracondylar fractures are uncommon after the physes have closed,[41] about 20 percent occurring in patients over 20 years of age.[101] The transcondylar fracture is less common[2, 24, 46] but occurs more commonly in the older age group.[88, 17, 101] These two fractures, supracondylar and transcondylar, account for 5[47] to 33 percent[39] of fractures of the distal humerus in adults. The transcondylar fracture is only about one-tenth as common as the supracondylar injury.[39]

Classification and Mechanism of Injury

Supracondylar and transcondylar fractures may both be classified as extension or flexion fractures. The more common *extension* injury results from a fall on the outstretched hand. In the lateral view, the fracture line passes from distal anterior to proximal posterior, and the distal fragment is displaced posteriorly (Fig. 18–5). The distal end of the proximal fragment extends anteriorly and may cause damage to vessels or nerves. In the anteroposterior view the fracture line may be directed upward and laterally or upward and medially,

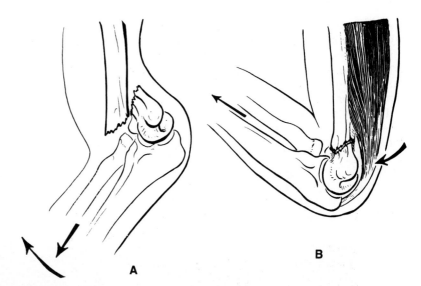

Figure 18–5. *A,* Supracondylar extension fractures result in posterior displacement and proximal migration of the distal fragment. *B,* Reduction is usually readily accomplished by longitudinal traction and flexion of the elbow. (From Van Gorder, G. W.: Dislocations and fractures of the elbow. *In* Cave, E. F. (ed.): Fractures and Other Injuries. Copyright © 1958 by Year Book Medical Publishers, Inc., Chicago.)

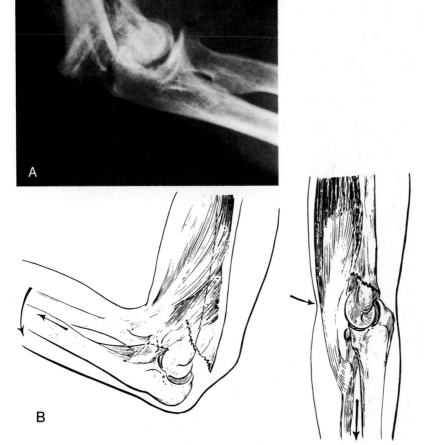

Figure 18–6. Flexion supracondylar fractures usually demonstrate a more transverse fracture line and, as a rule, less displacement. The degree of displacement shown in *A* is unusual. Reduction is accomplished by extension of the elbow, but this may be more difficult in the more severely displaced fractures (*B*). (From Van Gorder, G. W.: Dislocations and fractures of the elbow. *In* Cave, E. F. (ed.): Fractures and Other Injuries. Copyright © 1958 by Year Book Medical Publishers, Inc., Chicago.)

leading some[32] to subclassify this fracture as an abduction or adduction type. We feel this distinction has little merit and will ignore it. Proximal and posterior displacement of the distal fragment is secondary to the pull of the triceps muscle.

The *flexion* injury is much less common. The distal fragment is carried forward by a force directed against the posterior aspect of the flexed elbow (Fig. 18–6). Because considerable violence may be required to produce this injury, the fracture is sometimes compounded.[7] In our experience supracondylar and transcondylar fractures are more frequent in the elderly, in whom the bone is often osteoporotic (Fig. 18–7). Falls often occur in an unprotected manner in the older person, whereas younger people with quicker reaction times instinctively cushion and position a fall in a more protective way.

Because the fracture line extends across the supracondylar columns, the transcondylar fracture is both intra-articular and potentially unstable. Both of these features require special treatment considerations, which will be discussed below.

Diagnosis. Obvious deformity is readily apparent. Examination of the relationship be-

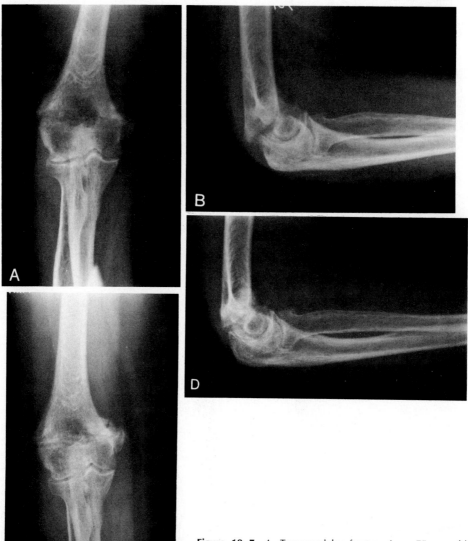

Figure 18–7. *A,* Transcondylar fracture in a 75-year-old woman. *B,* Note the transverse fracture line and the minimal displacement. *C, D,* After cast immobilization for 10 days in extension and then 5 days in flexion, there was a minimal amount of displacement, and solid bony union occurred at 4 months. (From Bryan, R. S.: Fractures about the elbow in adults. *In* The American Academy of Orthopaedic Surgeons: Instructional Course Lectures, Vol. 30. St. Louis, The C. V. Mosby Co., 1981.)

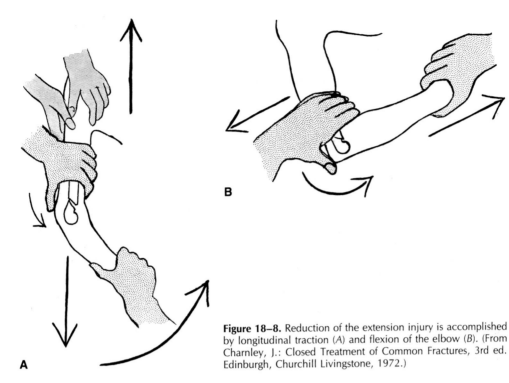

Figure 18–8. Reduction of the extension injury is accomplished by longitudinal traction (A) and flexion of the elbow (B). (From Charnley, J.: Closed Treatment of Common Fractures, 3rd ed. Edinburgh, Churchill Livingstone, 1972.)

tween the tip of the olecranon and the epicondyles reveals that the normal alignment is maintained. Careful examination of the neurovascular status is important because the brachial artery and the median and radial nerves are all at risk.[58] The diagnosis is confirmed by the radiograph, but the precise character of the fracture is sometimes difficult to define accurately. In the extension injury the fracture line is more oblique in adults and more transverse in children.[46]

Treatment

Closed Manipulation. Both supracondylar and transcondylar fractures can usually be treated without surgery, but adequate anesthesia and muscle relaxation are necessary. The principles of closed fracture reduction are important in the management of this fracture. For extension injuries, longitudinal traction is used to overcome the pull of the triceps and biceps; the forearm should be slightly extended, and the physician's thumb manipulates the distal humeral fragment into place (Fig. 18–8). To maintain a stable reduction, the elbow should be flexed to the extent allowed by swelling and the need to maintain circulation. Early authors[32, 36, 68, 102] recommended extreme flexion as the desirable position for immobilization, but currently only that degree necessary for stability is recommended. The position of the forearm during immobilization is debatable, but because the

pronator and supinator muscles both originate from the fracture fragment, we do not think this is critical in the adult and prefer to place the forearm in neutral rotation.

Reduction of the supracondylar and transcondylar flexion injury is more difficult to attain and maintain than the extension type. Milch[68] recommends converting the fracture to an extension type with the distal fragment displaced posteriorly. If this cannot be done, longitudinal traction is exerted with the elbow flexed at 90 degrees to release the deforming force of the forearm muscles. The distal fragment is pushed posteriorly, and the distal humerus is displaced anteriorly (Fig. 18–6).

An additional method of closed reduction for the flexion supracondylar fracture requires the application of traction along the axis of the humerus with the forearm in supination and the elbow flexed at 85 degrees.[93] Plaster is then applied to the arm, which is lifted forward as the elbow is flexed to 95 to 100 degrees. The cast is then extended below the elbow as pressure is exerted along the line of the ulna. Others have recommended traction to attain close alignment without regard to the radiographic appearance of the fracture.[91] After reduction most authors recommend placing the elbow in full extension,[14, 102] but some advocate holding this fracture in about 90 degrees of flexion.[39, 46] The difficulty of regaining flexion in the older person has also influenced Eppright and Wilkins[24] to avoid immobilization in the fully extended position.

The elbow is immobilized for 2 to 6 weeks depending on the inherent stability of the fracture. A posterior splint, long arm cast, hanging arm cast, or simple coaptation splint can be used during this period.[2]

Skeletal Traction. Traction using an olecranon pin and overhead suspension, which is so popular for children's fractures, is much less utilized in adults. The use of traction is indicated (1) if reduction cannot be achieved by manipulation (it may be particularly helpful for distal fragment alignment);[90] (2) if excessive swelling prevents maintenance of reduction owing to circulatory compromise; (3) if the fracture is inherently unstable and reduction cannot be maintained; or (4) if significant associated trauma precludes closed reduction and cast application. In the adult, bedrest is not as well tolerated, and prolonged traction is very expensive;[23] problems with pin site infection can also be troublesome.[17]

Surgical Stabilization. Percutaneous or limited open pinning has been used much more frequently in these fractures in recent years, although the technique was suggested almost 50 years ago.[70] This method does pose some danger of nerve or vessel injury, but it is usually quite safe after reduction, especially with the use of image intensification and if swelling is not excessive. This makes unnecessary the acute flexion often needed to maintain reduction of the extension type fracture without fixation.

Internal fixation by reduction and the use of screws or plates may be indicated rarely. External fixing devices have also been used but pose some risk to the ulnar and radial nerves and do introduce a slightly increased risk of infection along the pin tract. If the flexion fracture cannot be reduced by closed methods, a modification of the anterior approach of Henry has been recommended.[44] However, a posterior medial triceps-sparing approach as described by Bryan and Morrey,[9] the lateral approach of Kocher,[49] or the bilateral triceps reflection technique of Alanso Llames[3] are usually adequate if the displacement and obliquity of the fracture are appropriate.

Treatment of Transcondylar Fractures. This fracture, also called dicondylar, is really a variant of the supracondylar fracture except that it occurs transversely across the olecranon fossa and thus technically may be an intra-articular injury. The mechanism of fracture is identical to that in the supracondylar injury, and both flexion and extension types can occur. This is a rare fracture, accounting for about 10 percent of supracondylar fractures in adults and about 0.1 percent of all fractures. Often the injury will be minimally displaced or undisplaced.[37] A rare flexion type of transcondylar fracture, the so-called Posadas fracture,[24] consists of complete anterior displacement of the articular condyles while the ulna is displaced posteriorly.

Treatment is similar to that described for the supracondylar injury except that the transcondylar fracture line is more transverse in the lateral plane (Fig. 18–9), and if dis-

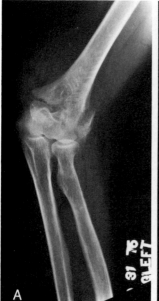
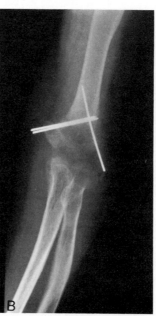
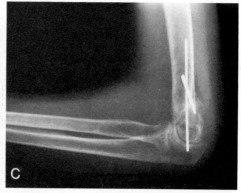

Figure 18–9. Transcondylar fracture in a 65-year-old woman. A, Closed reduction could not be maintained, and under a limited open procedure, the fracture was fixed with percutaneous Kirschner wires (B and C). Final motion was 35 to 145 degrees. (From Bryan, R. S.: Fractures about the elbow in adults. In The America Academy of Orthopaedic Surgeons: Instructional Course Lectures, Vol. 30. St. Louis, The C. V. Mosby Co., 1981.)

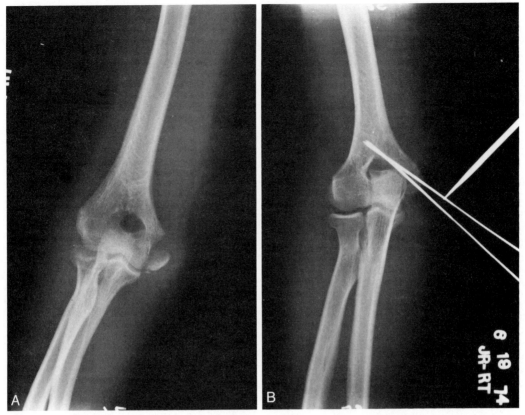

Figure 18–10. A, Medial epicondylar fracture displaced more than 3 mm in a 35-year-old woman. B, Open reduction and internal fixation anatomically reduced the fracture.

placement has occurred, reduction may be difficult to achieve and maintain. Because the fracture occurs across the supracondylar bony columns, exuberant callus may encroach on the olecranon and coronoid fossae, thus limiting motion. Great care must therefore be exercised to secure as accurate a reduction as possible. Occasionally pin fixation may be beneficial if the fracture shows unacceptable instability (Fig. 18–9), but open reduction is rarely indicated. The intra-articular nature of the fracture may also retard the healing time if displacement has taken place.

Fractures of the Epicondyles

Fracture of either epicondyle as an isolated injury in the adult is quite rare because ossification is complete by the end of adolescence. The medial epicondyle is most frequently involved because it is a much more prominent structure.

Medial Epicondylar Fracture

The fracture may be caused by avulsion from a valgus stress in children but more often results from a direct blow in adults. In a series of 143 consecutive fractures of the medial epicondyle, Smith[88] found only six instances of this injury in the adult, and only two were unassociated with other fractures or dislocations. Both of these were due to a direct blow, a mechanism described by others.[34] The diagnosis is suggested by the mechanism of injury and by local tenderness at the epicondyle. Because of the proximity of the ulnar nerve careful sensory and motor examination should be carried out before and after treatment. The radiograph is diagnostic if significant displacement has occurred (Fig. 18–10), but the diagnosis can be difficult if the fracture is minimally displaced in the older adolescent because the physis may still be open. If significant displacement has occurred, particularly if the fragment is lodged in the joint, associated elbow dislocation must be suspected because the medial collateral ligament is attached to the fragment.

Treatment is symptomatic if no displacement or minimal displacement has occurred; usually immobilization for 1 to 2 weeks[2, 24, 46] is sufficient. The elbow is flexed to 90 degrees, the forearm pronated to relax the pronator teres muscle, and the wrist mildly flexed to relax the common flexor muscle group that originates from the avulsed fragment. If the fracture is trapped in the medial joint or displaced to the level of the joint, closed reduction is usually unsuccessful, but good results have been reported even with marked displacement.[78] Generally, open reduction and pin or screw fixation are recommended in this setting. Treatment of fractures with intermediate displacement of about 3 mm is the subject of some disagreement. Smith reviewed more than 100 fractures treated nonoperatively, concluding that the results of fibrous union were comparable with those of bony union, and only one instance of ulnar nerve injury was recorded.[88] Hence, he recommended closed treatment of these fractures. It has been suggested that displacement of the medial epicondyle can cause grip weakness because of distal displacement of the flexor origin muscle group. Ulnar nerve dysfunction has also been reported with this fracture.[69] Thus, Anderson recommends open reduction and internal fixation for fractures with displacement of more than 1 mm.[2]

One additional consideration that has not been emphasized influences our treatment of this fracture. Because the ulnar collateral ligament originates from the undersurface of the medial epicondyle, displacement can potentially cause elbow instability. Clinically, this

association has been noted by Linscheid and Wheeler[57] and is yet another consideration that might prompt open reduction and fixation for mildly (2 to 3 mm) displaced fractures (Fig. 18–10).

Lateral Epicondylar Fracture

Because the lateral epicondyle is much less prominent it is not subject to fracture from a direct blow. Isolated fractures of this structure due to varus stress in adults are so rare that some authors have questioned whether the fracture can occur in adults at all.[14, 37, 102] Because the lateral ulnar collateral ligament maintains elbow stability and because displacement is usually minimal, treatment is by immobilization of the elbow in 90 degrees of flexion with the forearm in supination and the wrist extended to relax the muscles that originate from the fractured fragment. Rarely, a large fragment will justify fixation (Fig. 18–11).

Fracture of the Supracondylar Process

The supracondylar process is a curiosity that has captured the fancy of anatomists[96] and radiologists[62] and is occasionally of importance to the orthopedic surgeon. The supracondylar process is a bony projection of variable size, often with a curve or hooked shape,

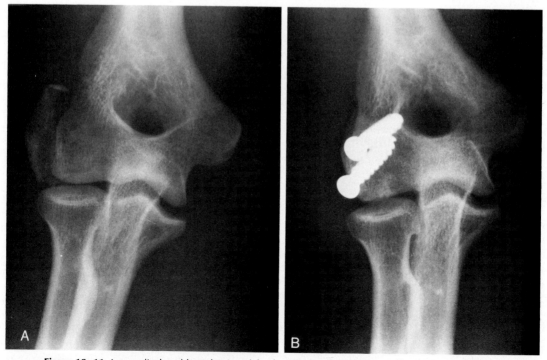

Figure 18–11. Large, displaced lateral epicondylar fracture (*A*) fixed anatomically with AO screws (*B*).

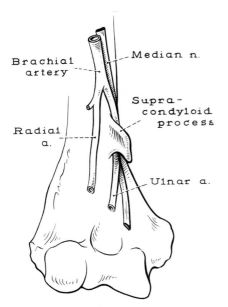

Figure 18–12. The brachial artery and the median nerve are in close proximity to the supracondylar process, which is found on the anterior medial aspect of the humerus approximately 7 cm above the medial epicondyle. (From Marquis, J. S., et al.: Supracondyloid process of the humerus. Proc. Staff Mayo Clin. 37:691, 1957.)

that arises 5 to 7 cm above and anterior to the medial epicondyle. Its size and length vary, ranging from 2 to 20 mm[31] in length, and a fibrous band sometimes connects the tip of the structure to the medial epicondyle. Through this arcade the brachial artery and median nerve may pass (Fig. 18–12), and the structure serves as an attachment to an anomalous origin of the pronator teres as well as a site of insertion for the coracobrachialis muscle. The supracondylar process is present in about 1 percent of Caucasians[96] and is clinically significant because occasionally it may fracture from a direct blow. Of the few reports of injury to the process two have been in military personnel.[4, 31] The injury presents with marked pain and possibly median nerve irritation. Routine radiographs may not show the pathologic lesion because the process is located on the anterior medial aspect of the distal humerus, so oblique films may be necessary.[21] If pain is persistent, surgical excision is recommended.[4, 21, 31, 50, 59]

Authors' Preferred Treatment of Extra-Articular Fractures

Supracondylar and Transcondylar Fractures

Most supracondylar and transcondylar fractures occur in elderly patients with osteopo-

rotic bones. We prefer to utilize closed reduction and casting or splinting if the fracture is stable after reduction and the circulation is unimpaired (Fig. 18–7). The technique has been discussed earlier. If the fracture is unstable or displaces after reduction, limited open reduction or percutaneous pinning under fluoroscopic control (Fig. 18–9) permits splinting with the joint in less flexion and earlier return of motion. Percutaneous pinning is done with power drive and threaded Kirschner wires that are inserted with the aid of the image intensifier to avoid injury to the nerves. The pins are cut off beneath the skin, and usually only three or four are necessary to prevent slippage as long as splinting is maintained. Usually the swelling and pain have ceased 2 to 3 weeks later, and active gentle motion in flexion can be started with a gradual increase in extension. The results of inadequate treatment are shown in Figure 18–13.

Injuries of the Medial Epicondyle

We prefer immobilization for 1 to 2 weeks followed by gentle motion in minimally displaced fractures. Open reduction and fixation with two smooth pins or a small screw (Fig. 18–10) is performed if the fracture is displaced more than 2 to 3 mm. We do not feel that percutaneous pinning offers any significant advantage over limited exposure and it does carry an increased risk of injury to the ulnar nerve.

Injuries of the Supracondylar Process

If a fracture of the supracondylar process does not heal and persistent pain is present for more than 3 or 4 months or median nerve symptoms are present, excision of the fragment is the treatment of choice. This should be undertaken, however, with an awareness of the proximity of the median nerve and brachial artery and knowledge that myositis ossificans has been reported after removal of a fractured process.[50]

INTRA-ARTICULAR FRACTURES

Intra-articular fractures can pose a most difficult problem for the clinician. Unlike extra-articular injuries, these fractures frequently require open reduction and internal fixation. Included among intra-articular fractures of the distal humerus are T and Y condylar, lateral and medial condylar, capitellar, and trochlear fractures.

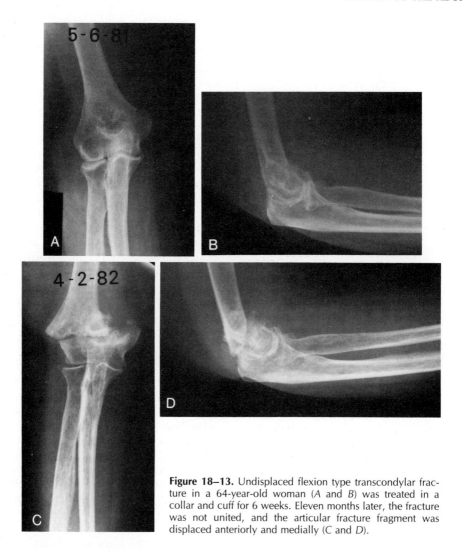

Figure 18–13. Undisplaced flexion type transcondylar fracture in a 64-year-old woman (*A* and *B*) was treated in a collar and cuff for 6 weeks. Eleven months later, the fracture was not united, and the articular fracture fragment was displaced anteriorly and medially (*C* and *D*).

T and Y Condylar Fractures

The late Sir John Charnley in 1961 stated that "the elbow almost invariably does badly after operative treatment. Particularly disappointing is open reduction and internal fixation for Y fractures in the adult."[15] On the other hand, the prognosis appears to be so poor with closed treatment that the older textbooks recommend simply casting the elbow in a position of function and waiting for ankylosis to occur.

Incidence

Because not all investigators include the same injuries in their reports, a precise estimate of the frequency of the T and Y condylar fracture is difficult to establish. Eppright and Wilkins[24] refer to the fracture as rare, whereas Smith considers it a common fracture in the adult.[88] Hitzrot reported that 4 of 34 (12 percent) distal humeral fractures in the adult were of this variety.[39] Lecestre and colleagues reported

503 fractures of the humerus, among which 25 percent were simple T and Y condylar fractures and 37 percent were comminuted intracondylar fractures.[54] Knight places the incidence at about 5 percent of all distal humeral fractures in the adult.[47] Fortunately, in absolute terms this fracture does not occur in large numbers, as shown by most reports in the literature, which contain fewer than 30 to 40 cases.

Mechanism of Injury

The common denominator of all split fractures of the condyles is the wedge effect of the longitudinal groove of the proximal ulna across the trochlea. This occurs with longitudinal loading to the extended elbow[88] with the coronoid serving as the wedge. Reich in 1936 stated that the cause of this fracture was usually a blow to the flexed elbow.[79] The olecranon thus acted as a wedge, splitting off the medial and lateral condyles with or without comminution of the humeral articular surface. The fracture begins in the groove of the trochlea and continues to the fossa; it is completed by shearing across both supracondylar columns or up the shaft of the humerus. In severe injuries, the fracture is completed by internal rotation of each portion of the articulation owing to the effect of the flexor and extensor muscle groups originating from the fracture fragments (Fig. 18–3). Rotation and displacement give rise to the so-called inverted V deformity (Fig. 18–14).

Inspection of the injured extremity reveals variable deformities depending on the amount of displacement. The posterior triangular relationship of the bony landmarks is violated, and the disposition of the injury is readily confirmed by radiographs.

Classification

Riseborough and Radin in 1969 provided a classification of this fracture that aids not only in understanding the mechanism but also, more importantly, in managing the injury (Fig. 18–15).[82]

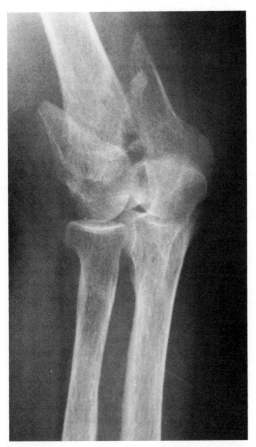

Figure 18–14. Classic Y-condylar fracture with external rotation of both condylar components creating the inverted V appearance.

Type I: Undisplaced.
Type II: Displacement between the trochlea and the capitellum; no rotation
Type III: Separation of fragments proximally and rotation distally by the pull of the forearm muscles
Type IV: Wide separation, comminution, and rotation of the articular surfaces

One should keep in mind that each type of fracture occurs with a commensurate amount of energy, which is dissipated to the soft tissue structures—the capsule, muscle, and occasionally the nerve and artery. The prognostic value of the classification is due in part to the fact that displacement and rotation of the fracture fragments also reflect, to some extent, the amount of soft tissue injury.

Treatment

The treatment of the T–Y condylar fracture is obviously directed toward attaining as great a degree of function as possible. Rarely does the fracture interfere with pronation and supination regardless of the treatment modality. At times there is a very satisfactory radiographic appearance although the joint is stiff or painful. On the other hand, considerable radiographic deformity may be present in a joint with surprisingly good function. Not surprisingly, a number of treatment modalities have been employed through the years, but unless the fracture type is specified, assessment and comparison of the various methods are difficult. We feel that there has been a marked improvement in the understanding of the fracture since Riseborough and Radin contributed their workable classification in 1969. Since this time, improved surgical technique has resulted in greater emphasis on the surgical management of the fracture. This is ironic because Riseborough and Radin recommended nonoperative treatment for most fractures. Most disagreement occurs about the treatment of type III and IV injuries. Any meaningful comparison of results should discuss the treatment according to the fracture type.

Nonoperative Treatment. "Manipulation and closed reduction are always the method of choice."[99] Nonoperative treatment was the early standard. The various possibilities include closed reduction and casting for variable periods, use of skeletal traction initially or as a prolonged treatment modality, and early use of motion without regard to the radiographic appearance—the so-called bag-of-bones treatment.

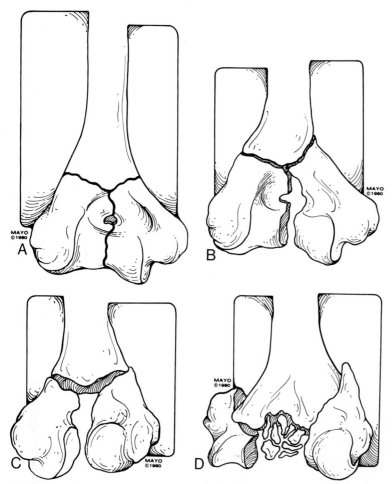

Figure 18–15. *A,* Type I undisplaced T-condylar fracture of the elbow. *B,* Type II displaced but not rotated T-condylar fracture. *C,* Type III displaced and rotated T-condylar fracture. *D,* Type IV displaced, rotated, and comminuted T-condylar fracture. (From Bryan, R. S.: Fractures about the elbow in adults. *In* American Academy of Orthopedic Surgeons: Instructional Course Lectures, Vol. 30. St. Louis, The C. V. Mosby Co., 1981.)

Closed Reduction and Immobilization. Longitudinal traction with the elbow held at 90 degrees and molding of the condylar fragments is the common manipulative technique used to achieve reduction. Several attempts to obtain reduction may be required. Reich recognized the rotational force of the flexor and extensor muscle groups and utilized modified ice tongs to press the condyles together while applying traction to align the supracondylar fracture.[81] Others have used a carpenter's clamp to mold the fragments.[99] Mobilization with the elbow at 90 degrees with splints[39] or a cast for 4 to 6 weeks was the accepted treatment in the past. Although closed reduction and immobilization remain the accepted mode of treatment for type I and II fractures, prolonged immobilization markedly compromises elbow function and should be avoided.

Traction. Traction is the treatment of choice for many severe injuries that cannot be fixed by surgery[71, 103] and is often recommended for the less comminuted type III fractures as well.[95] There is much variation in the technique of traction treatment. Probably the most effective and commonly used means is that of overhead skeletal traction with an olecranon pin (Fig. 18–16). Dunlop traction with the arm to the side is also sometimes recommended (Fig. 18–17). Because of the occasional pin tract infection,[17, 39] skin traction using a flat sling across the proximal forearm with the elbow held at 90 degrees has also been employed.[83]

Traction is continued for about 2 weeks and is followed by an additional period of 2 to 3 weeks of immobilization in a splint or cast.[95, 103] Intermittent motion is permitted depending on the alignment, stability of the fracture, and compliance of the patient. Traction may be time-consuming, and hospitalization is occasionally required for periods of up to 6 weeks.[88]

Satisfactory results with an average arc of flexion of 47 degrees in 7 of 11 patients were reported by Miller[71] in 1964 using skeletal traction techniques. Three recent reviews report a combined result of 4 excellent, 4 good, and 7 poor results with traction.[40, 52, 95] The

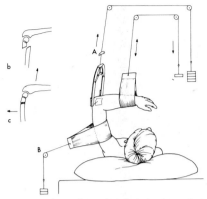

Figure 18–16. Balanced overhead skeletal traction with a pin through the olecranon. This technique helps to achieve and maintain reduction of distal humeral fractures, and the elevation overhead helps to decrease edema. (From Smith, F. M.: Traction and suspension in the treatment of fractures. Surg. Clin. N. Am., April, 1951.)

technique is reported to give excellent or good results in about 60 percent of type III and type IV fractures (Fig. 18–18).[95]

Bag-of-Bones (Conscientious Neglect). This time-honored treatment gives surprisingly better results than might be expected in the patient who is unable to endure prolonged anesthesia or in whom excessive comminution makes open reduction impossible.

Eastwood in 1937[22] first advocated traction at 90 degrees of flexion, under general anesthesia, if tolerable, combined with compressive manipulation of the condyles followed by collar and cuff with the elbow flexed as much as possible within the limits imposed by swelling and the need to maintain circulation. Motion in flexion is begun at 2 weeks, and at 4 weeks the elbow should have from 90 degrees to full flexion. The hand and wrist are mobilized from the day of fracture and the shoulder within 2 weeks.

Brown and Morgan reported 10 type III or type IV fractures that were treated with collar

and cuff in 120 degrees of flexion with early motion in flexion and gradual loosening of the sling every few days, until the elbow was extended beyond 90 degrees.[6] The sling was discarded at 6 weeks. The group obtained an average range of motion of 95 degrees, and the authors noted that flexion must be gained by 3 weeks if it is to be gained at all. Evans observed that although the bag-of-bones treatment was satisfactory in the elderly, it resulted in a weak and unstable elbow that was unsatisfactory in the younger patient.[25] The uncertainty of the technique and the residual performance deficit noted by Evans continues to limit this modality to older patients with severely comminuted fractures.

Surgical Treatment. Treatment by surgery may be divided into pin fixation or open reduction with internal fixation, usually with rigid devices. "While reasonably good function may be obtained in many elbows which have been permitted to unite with varying degrees of condylar deformity, one should not be satisfied as a routine plan of treatment with a method attended with so much uncertainty."[94]

The rising popularity of internal fixation is related to improved technique and clinical results using the ASIF technique of fracture fixation. Advocates of this option have increased in recent years.

Indications. A displaced type II or type III fracture in the young active adult provides an ideal indication for surgical treatment.[7, 8, 54] If the injury is complicated by vascular embarrassment requiring surgery, the fracture should also be surgically stabilized at the time of exploration for the vascular injury. The type IV injury is less amenable to surgery because the multiple fragments can rarely be adequately reassembled, and rigid fixation is almost impossible. Cassebaum,[13] however, a staunch advocate of surgical treatment, states that he has not seen a fracture so comminuted

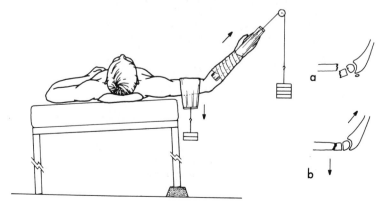

Figure 18–17. Side arm or Dunlop's traction is used to treat supracondylar fractures with displacement or circulatory embarrassment. Countertraction is obtained by tilting the bed opposite to the traction weights. (From Smith, F. M.: Traction and suspension in the treatment of fractures. Surg. Clin. N. Am., April, 1951.)

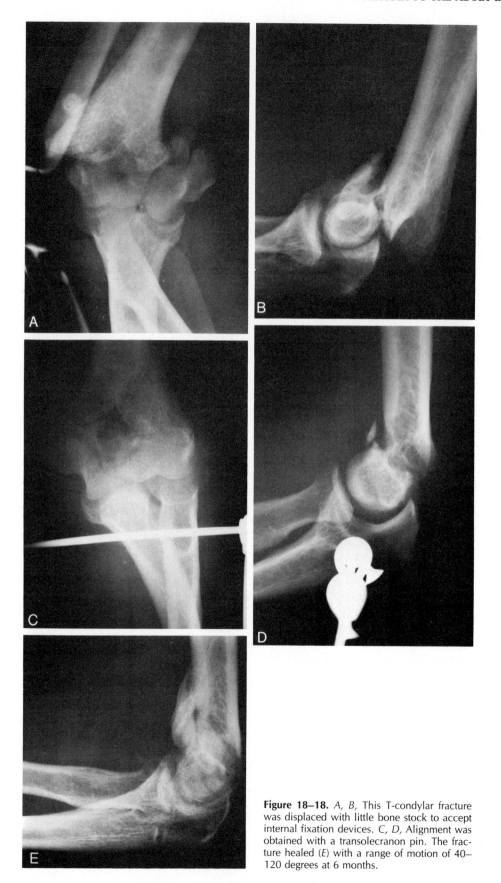

Figure 18–18. *A, B,* This T-condylar fracture was displaced with little bone stock to accept internal fixation devices. *C, D,* Alignment was obtained with a transolecranon pin. The fracture healed (*E*) with a range of motion of 40–120 degrees at 6 months.

that it could not be treated by proper reduction and internal fixation.

Limited Exposure and Pinning. This technique is used in an attempt to restore the anatomy without adding excessive trauma to the soft tissue by a formal surgical exposure of the distal humerus.[70] The fracture is reduced and fixed first with Kirschner wires inserted to stabilize the reduction and then with additional pins to secure the fixation. Introduced in 1936, this approach appears to have limited application today. Occasionally, however, the use of transfixing pins and external support is effective if the fracture cannot otherwise be adequately reduced or circumstances preclude an open reduction. Such was the case with the patient depicted in Figure 18–19. We have also used such means of fixation with good results in patients with badly devitalized muscle or open wounds. The surgeon must be careful that the pins do not block motion by intruding in the fossa (Fig. 18–4). Half pins may prove useful to fix the distal fragment. Extreme care must be used to avoid injury to the ulnar nerve with this technique, which, again, should be reserved for very unusual circumstances.

Open Reduction and Fixation—Technique. Several operative techniques have been described, but all have one feature in common. The articular surface is reassembled and fixed with smooth or threaded wires or screws. The supracondylar extremity is treated in one of several ways (Fig. 18–20). Evans[25] stopped here, converting the injury to a supracondylar fracture and then treating it as such with a pressure bandage in flexion; motion was begun in 3 weeks. He reported that five of six patients obtained excellent results, but three were teenagers.

Because early motion is felt to be a major goal of surgery, rigid fixation of the fracture is the current treatment of choice. It is generally felt that less dissection is preferable, and screw fixation, if possible, has been a favored type of treatment.[7, 43] The Y-shaped plate has been useful, but because the medial condyle is not on the same plane as the lateral condyle, it may have to be bent if it is to fit the contour of the bone properly (Fig. 18–21). Further, the plate may limit motion by its bulk under the triceps, and periosteal stripping is necessary for its placement. Use of the Y plate also usually requires translocation of the ulnar nerve anteriorly. Malleable side plates contoured to the medial and lateral columns may be used in some cases (Case 6,

Fig. 18–22). These present less threat to limitation of motion both because the area of bone exposed is smaller and because any ossification that occurs is less likely to impede motion. As the exposure is carried proximally, there is danger to both the ulnar and radial nerves as they cross the intermuscular septum, so they must be carefully protected.

Bryan in 1981 reaffirmed his belief in operative reduction and demonstrated some cases that illustrated the principles of treatment.[8] The surgical principles described by Speed[94] in 1950 and elaborated by Eppright and Wilkins[24] in 1975 are worthy of emphasis and may be summarized as follows:

1. The articular surface must first be assembled and stabilized.
2. Loss of articular surface can be accepted; incongruity cannot.
3. Any large separate fragments from the epitrochlear ridges should be fixed to the proximal shaft before an attempt is made to stabilize the articular condyles because they act as buttresses to restore the height of the fossa.
4. Proximally directed screws must engage the opposite cortex to achieve fixation; the cancellous bone of the distal humeral shaft will not adequately hold a screw.
5. Screws are preferable to Kirschner wires; plates increase soft tissue dissection and should be used only when necessary.
6. The fossae must be clear of apparatus, bone, and debris. The entire bone of the olecranon fossa and even the tip of the olecranon may be excised with impunity and even benefit. This principle emphasizes that stability depends on two stable columns of bone, the medial and lateral condyles.
7. Restoration of the alignment of the axis of motion through the center of the capitellum and trochlea and in line with the anterior cortex of the humerus is necessary to prevent loss of motion due to impingement.

Open Reduction and Fixation—Surgical Exposure. To accomplish these goals the surgical approach is obviously of extreme importance. Limited medial or lateral exposure is not adequate (see Fig. 18–24). Posterior exposures of the elbow have been the choice of most surgeons, and each has its advantages (Fig. 18–23). The MacAusland approach popularized by Cassebaum[12] affords perhaps the best view of the trochlea. It introduces an osteotomy site opposite the trochlea and can be a

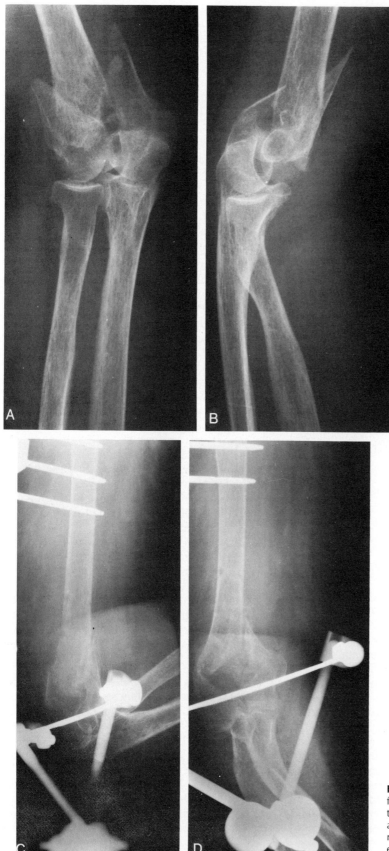

Figure 18–19. Type III Y-condylar fracture with rotation of the fracture fragments in both frontal (*A*) and sagittal (*B*) planes. Satisfactory reduction was obtained with an external skeletal fixator (*C* and *D*). *Illustration continued on opposite page*

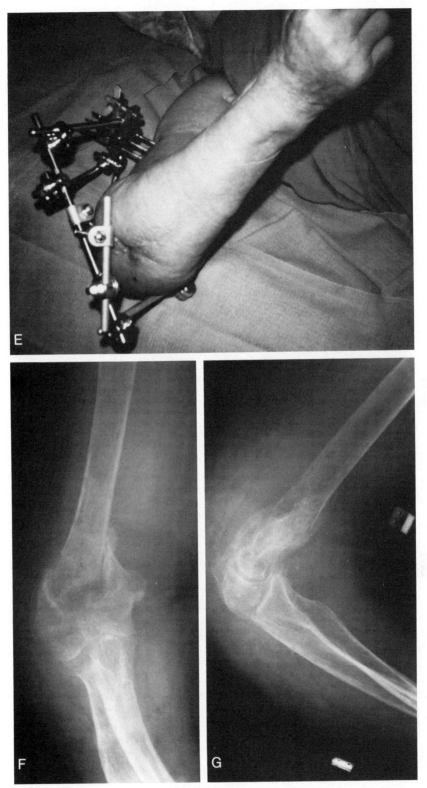

Figure 18–19 *Continued.* At 1 year the fracture was well healed with mild varus and posterior displacement (*E*). The patient had an arc of motion of 35 to 125 degrees and was pleased with the result (*F* and *G*).

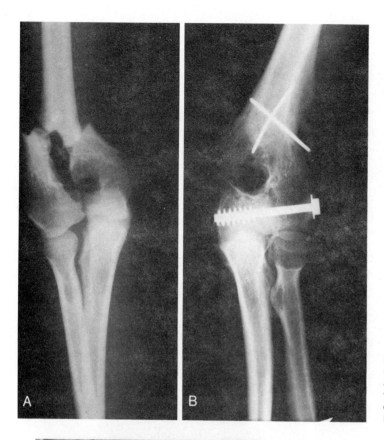

Figure 18–20. *A,* Displacement without significant rotation of a Y-condylar fracture in a 13-year-old boy. *B,* The articular surface was anatomically restored; the supracondylar component was treated with cross Kirschner wires as an "internal suture."

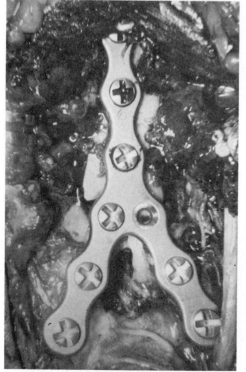

Figure 18–21. Y-plate for comminuted T-condylar fracture. Notice that the ulnar nerve is in close proximation to the plate (lower right) requiring anterior translocation of the nerve. (From Bryan, R. S., and Bickel, W. H.: T condylar fractures of the distal humerus. J. Trauma 11(10):830–835, 1971.)

source of adhesions and excess callus formation as well as nonunion.[95] An oblique osteotomy across the tip of the olecranon as described by Miller is equally efficacious but possibly risks the triceps a bit more. Van Gorder in 1940[100] popularized an approach first described for arthroplasty by Willis Campbell in 1932.[11] This gives a good view of the fossa but not as good a view of the trochlea and capitellum and limits early motion due to soft tissue healing. Added exposure and improved extension postoperatively may be obtained by excision of the tip of the olecranon.[48] Reflection of the triceps in continuity from medial to lateral, as described by Bryan and Morrey,[9] or lateral to medial, as described by Kocher,[49] gives excellent exposure without removing the olecranon against which the comminuted trochlea can be assembled and tested prior to closure. Alonso-Llames[3] has introduced a technique of medial and lateral release of the triceps from the humerus, leaving it attached to the ulna. Although effective for supracondylar fractures, this will not provide adequate visualization for fixing most type III fractures.

In any of these approaches, the surgeon should consider the specific injury and utilize the approach that least traumatizes normal

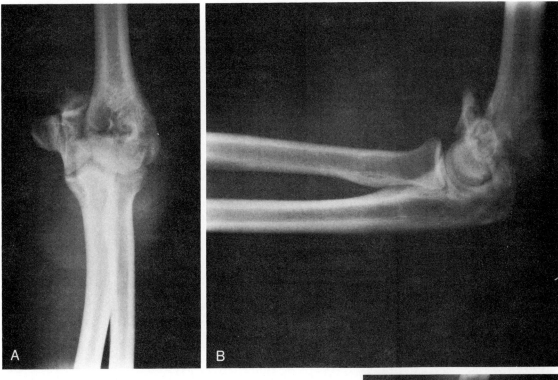

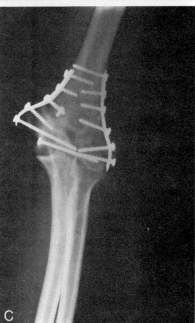

Figure 18–22. *A, B,* Type III T-condylar fracture in a 20-year-old man involved in a motor vehicle accident. A type I compound wound was present. *C,* The patient was treated with medial and lateral buttress plates.

tissue. For example, many fractures are open with a wound that needs cleansing and debridement. Often there is a rent in the triceps that directly connects with the joint and can be incorporated with one of the above approaches to gain exposure. The posterior exposures are described in detail in Chapter 8.

Postoperative Management. After the fracture has been repaired postoperative management is extremely important. In fact,

Henderson[35] states, ". . . the after care is more often the cause of poor results than the primary or active care." Toward this end Cassebaum advocated early motion in balanced suspension beginning 2 to 10 days after operation for a minimum of 20 minutes a day.[13] Early postoperative motion is emphasized as an essential ingredient in the planning of surgery.[8, 94, 107] This appears to be confirmed by Horne's experience of poor results in 50

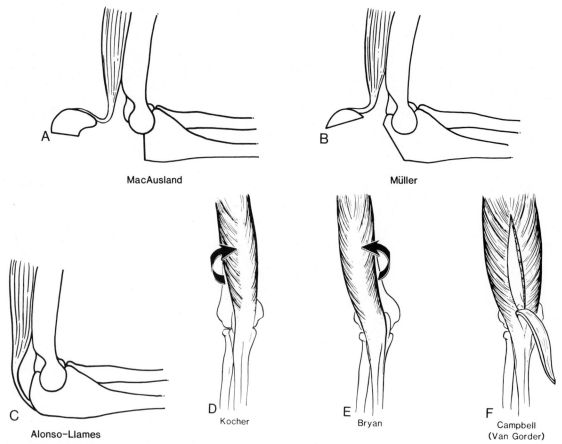

Figure 18–23. Posterior exposure of the distal humerus can be obtained by osteotomizing the proximal ulna (*A* and *B*), by releasing the triceps medially and laterally from the humerus (*C*), by reflecting the triceps mechanism medially (*D*) or laterally (*E*), or by distal reflection of the triceps fascia and medial and lateral retraction of the muscle and tendon (*F*).

percent of six patients treated by internal fixation followed by immobilization for 1 to 4 weeks after surgery.[40] Horne concluded that comminuted fractures are best treated with closed reduction and traction. Occasionally, a patient will also improve after the hardware is removed if this is the demonstrable source of pain or motion limitation.[43]

Results

A meaningful comparison of results reported from different sources is always a difficult task, and few studies have addressed the question of comparable fractures treated with operative and nonoperative modalities.

For all subsequent discussions on the results of treatment, we will employ the scale used by Bickel and Perry[5] comprising the following categories: excellent (stable, pain-free, nearly normal range of motion); good (stable, no deformity, 60 degrees of flexion-extension in a usable range, rotation at least 50 percent of normal, no more than mild aching with heavy use); fair (stable, mild pain with normal use, significant loss of motion, moderate deformity); and poor (any one of instability, pain, deformity, or greatly restricted range of motion).

Results of treatment with traction have led some[87] to recommend it alone as the treatment of choice. In general, satisfactory results have been reported in about 50 to 60 percent[40, 52, 54] of those treated by traction or by open reduction and fixation followed by traction.[40, 52] Most fractures so treated are of types III and IV. The mean arc of motion among 29 patients treated by traction alone by several investigators was 57 degrees.[52, 71, 76, 92]

On the other hand, excellent or good results have been tabulated in 84 percent of 104 patients compiled from the literature[5, 10, 43, 107] in whom ASIF principles and early motion were employed. These fractures covered a broad range including types II, III, and IV.

The average arc of flexion in these series was 91 degrees.

Complications

Although complications are reviewed in general below, a discussion of those associated with both the injury and the treatment of T and Y condylar fractures is appropriate because this is one of the most difficult fractures to manage.

Other than predictable loss of motion, nerve injury is probably the most common complication of the T–Y condylar fracture. The ulnar nerve is most commonly injured, reportedly in as much as 15 percent of cases.[10] Nieman reported two radial and two median nerve palsies after 24 fractures with two ulnar palsies occurring in a group of 18 patients who underwent surgery.[76] Similar experiences have been reported by Bryan[7] and others.[5] A most comprehensive assessment of complications and their treatment has been presented by Lecestre and colleagues.[54] Among 388 fractures about the elbow, 110 of which were open injuries, there were 15 aseptic nonunions (4 percent), 21 deep infections (5.4 percent), postoperative paralyses (16 percent), and 31 loosened or broken inserts (21 percent). These are sobering data considering that this experience is from a group experienced in trauma surgery and well versed in the ASIF technique. We feel that wide exposure crossing natural tissue planes, meticulous hemostasis, and excellent soft tissue technique is mandatory if the fracture is to be effectively treated by surgical modalities.

Condylar Fractures

Fractures of the condyles are uncommon and account for 3[54] to 5[47] percent of distal humeral fractures, which in turn account for only about 2 percent of all fractures.[17] The lateral condyle is fractured more frequently than its medial counterpart.[34, 37, 69] This intra-articular fracture can pose significant difficulties for the clinician unless the pathologic anatomy and precise nature of the fracture are appreciated. A clear distinction should be made between the lateral condylar and the capitellar fracture (Fig. 18–24). The condylar fracture occurs in the sagittal plane; it involves the epicondyle and thus possesses some soft tissue attachment. Capitellar fractures, on the other hand, occur in the coronal plane and although varying portions of the trochlea may be involved, there is no soft tissue attachment.

The medial margin of the radial head initiates the fracture of the lateral condyle as it strikes the sulcus between the capitellum and the trochlea from an axially directed force. The longitudinal groove of the sigmoid notch compresses the sulcus of the trochlea, causing a fracture of the trochlea. The energy is dissipated proximally either medially or laterally, giving rise to the medial or lateral condylar fracture. This fracture has been extensively studied and discussed by Milch,[67, 68, 69] who has provided the basis of our present understanding and treatment of this injury.

Mechanism of Injury

Each condyle is subject to one of two disruptive forces that determine whether the medial or the lateral condyle is fractured and whether proximal or distal displacement occurs (Fig. 18–25).

1. An avulsion fracture is caused by an indirect force, and the fracture rotates distally.[40]
2. A shearing fracture is caused by an axial force and the fragment is displaced proximally.

Classification

The nature of the fracture is an important factor in determining whether the injury is stable and hence whether surgery is necessary. A type I fracture involves the capitellum laterally or the medial lip of the trochlea medially. A type II fracture involves the capitellum and the lateral trochlea laterally or the entire trochlea medially (Fig. 18–26). In the type II fracture, the ulna articulates with the displaced fractured fragment, technically

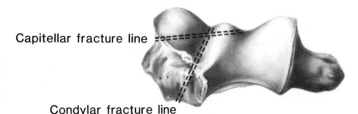

Capitellar fracture line

Condylar fracture line

Figure 18–24. Transverse view of the distal humerus demonstrating the fracture line of the condylar fracture compared with the type I capitellar fracture in which the fracture line is limited to the sagittal plane.

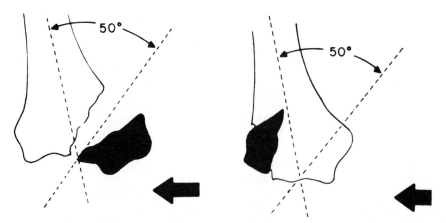

Figure 18–25. Medial or lateral condylar fracture results from longitudinal shearing force of the lateral condyle or a tension fracture of the medial condyle. Abduction force reverses the fracture pattern. (From Milch, H.: Fractures and fracture dislocations of the humeral condyles. J. Trauma 4:592–607, 1964.)

rendering the injury a fracture dislocation. This is a very unstable injury; without adequate treatment, permanent deformity will result. In the lateral type II injury, the medial collateral ligament is often torn, giving rise to marked displacement and the possibility of ulnar nerve injury.[88]

Treatment

Nonoperative. Undisplaced fractures may be splinted or casted for 4 to 5 weeks but must be closely monitored because loss of reduction may occur, and any displacement at all is likely to produce subsequent problems with limitation of motion and arthritis.

Displaced medial and lateral type I fractures may be treated by closed reduction (Fig.

18–27). For the lateral condylar fracture the joint is adducted, the forearm supinated, and the wrist and fingers extended. The type I medial injury is reduced using the opposite maneuver—that is, abduction, pronation, and wrist and finger flexion. If the maneuver is successful, the extremity is immobilized in moderately acute flexion for about 4 weeks.[88] The type II fracture is unstable and is not amenable to nonoperative management.

Operative. Early open reduction and internal fixation are employed for displaced type I fractures and for all type II fractures with even the most minimal displacement because of the unstable nature of this fracture. Delayed reduction and fixation or reconstruction is generally not successful.[34] Exposure for the

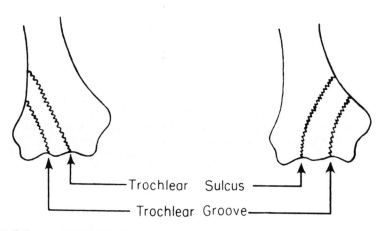

Trochlear Sulcus

Trochlear Groove

LATERAL CONDYLE FRACTURES

MEDIAL CONDYLE FRACTURES

Figure 18–26. Milch classification of condylar fractures. The type II fracture involves the lateral lip of the trochlea; thus its inherent instability. (From Milch, H.: Fractures and fracture dislocations of the humeral condyles. J. Trauma 4:592–607, 1964.)

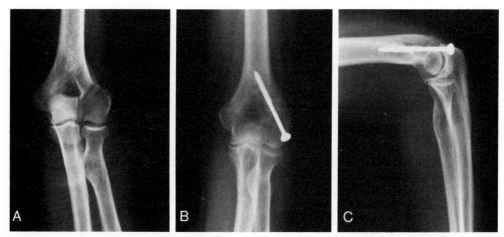

Figure 18–27. *A,* Undisplaced lateral condylar fracture occurring in a 64-year-old woman. *B, C,* Fixed with single screw. (From Bryan, R. S.: Fracture about the elbow in adults. *In* American Academy of Orthopaedic Surgeons: Instructional Course Lectures, Vol. 30. St. Louis, The C. V. Mosby Co., 1981.)

lateral condylar injury is readily obtained by using the Kocher approach, which can be extended proximally if necessary (see Chapter 8). Screw fixation is adequate, but care must be taken to assure perfect congruity of the joint and avoid violating the fossa with screws that may limit motion; in lateral fractures be wary of proximal dissection, which may injure the radial nerve. For medial condylar fractures, the approach of Bryan and Morrey is preferred because complete visualization of the joint is assured. The ulnar nerve is exposed and may be transposed if necessary to fix the fracture properly.

Long-term follow-up reports of untreated type II fractures 50 to 84 years after injury have appeared,[51, 89] and we have treated a bilateral fracture 56 years after injury (Fig. 18–28). A functional arc of motion but painful deformity and tardy ulnar nerve palsy were present in all cases. The consistent pattern of deformity is well illustrated by the virtual mirror-image injury that occurred in both extremities in the bilateral case.

Nonunion and Malunion

Malunited type I lateral condylar fractures cause a cosmetically unacceptable, mechanically unsound, deformed elbow that jeopardizes ulnar nerve function. The deformity may be readily corrected with a laterally based open wedge osteotomy. The varus deformity from the medial condylar fracture is similarly treated with a medially based open wedge osteotomy. The type II fracture poses a more complex problem because the ulnohumeral joint is not congruous and the joint is subluxed. Angular correction with translatory realignment of the distal fragment may

be considered if the deformity is relatively recent.[69] Total elbow arthroplasty has also been successfully employed (Fig. 18–29).

Fractures of the Capitellum

Incidence

Hahn is credited with the first description of the fracture in 1853.[55] A prominence palpable in the anterolateral aspect of the elbow was confirmed at autopsy to be the capitellum, which had healed in this displaced position. This fracture accounted for 6 percent of the 503 fractures of the distal humerus reported by Lecestere,[54] an incidence similar to that reported by Knight.[47] It has been estimated to account for 1 percent of all elbow injuries.[24] By 1942 approximately 100 cases had been reported.[80] The fracture is possibly more common in females[33] and usually occurs in adults because similar trauma in a child will result in a supracondylar fracture.

Classification

The classic description of the fracture includes two types, but a third category should probably be added. It is unfortunate that a recent comprehensive study of this fracture has reclassified the injury.[33] To avoid confusion, we will discuss this fracture according to the generally accepted classification.

Type I. This fracture is the most common type and involves a majority of the capitellum and sometimes a lateral portion of the trochlea.[30] This complete fracture of the capitellum was first described by Hahn and Stenthal and is thus termed the Hahn-Stenthal fracture.[55]

Type II. This fracture is less common and

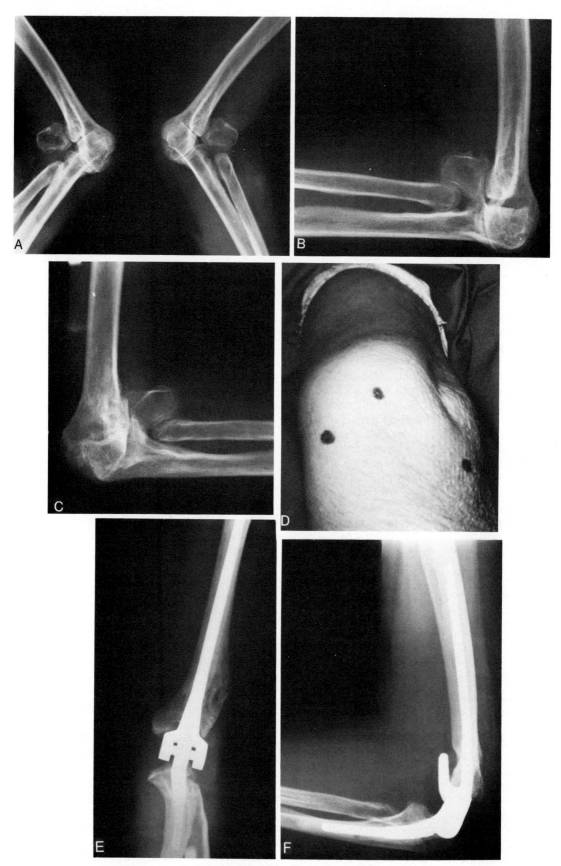

Figure 18–28. *See legend on opposite page*

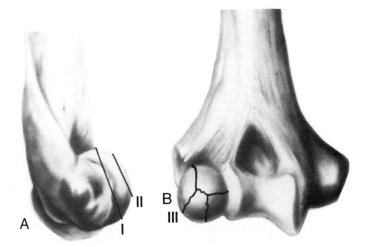

Figure 18–29. The type I capitellar fracture involves a large portion of bone, often the entire structure. Type II is a shear fracture, often with minimal subchondral bone, and may displace posteriorly (A). A type III fracture is a comminuted fracture with varying amounts of displacement of the fracture fragments (B).

involves a variable amount of the articular surface sometimes with very minimal subchondral bone. The partial or slice fracture was first described by Kocher and Lorenze—hence the eponym Kocher-Lorenze fracture.[55]

Type III. A comminuted or compression fracture of the articular surface[33, 45, 102] is sometimes discussed as a variant to the type II injury, but we think it is appropriate to consider it a distinct fracture.

Mechanism of Injury

The most common fracture, the type I, involves the majority of the capitellum and is due either to direct trauma[55] or to a fall on the outstretched hand. According to Lee, the partially flexed, partially pronated elbow joint exposes the capitellum, making it vulnerable to a fracture from a direct blow. A fall on the partially flexed, abducted, pronated forearm[30] or simply on the outstretched hand[64] has been implicated as a cause of this fracture. This is currently the most commonly accepted mechanism of injury. In either instance, displacement occurs usually anteriorly and superiorly. The less common type II slice fracture is most frequently a result of an indirect force transmitted across the joint. This fracture may occur with hammering, lifting, and similar activities. The fragment is usually small and may displace posteriorly. The mechanism of injury is analogous to that for the osteochon-

dral fracture described by Matthewson and Dandy of the lateral femoral condyle secondary to shearing forces.[63] The type III fracture is caused by a fall on the outstretched hand as exemplified by the report of Milch,[66] who described a case in which there was impaction of the capitellum into a fractured radial head. The relationship between radial head injuries and capitellar fractures has been noted by Watson-Jones[102] and emphasized by Reich.[81] Palmer[77] observed that 31 percent of capitellar fractures have a concomitant radial head injury, and Wilson[104] has suggested that the impacted fracture of the capitellum be considered a distinct category.

Diagnosis

Examination of the elbow is extremely important in the diagnosis of these intra-articular fractures. T or Y condylar fractures cause significant swelling, and the normal triangular relationships of the epicondyles and olecranon are distorted. Supracondylar fractures present an angular deformity proximal to the joint. With an intra-articular fracture, on the other hand, the form is preserved and swelling is often minimal. Careful palpation over the posterolateral joint at about 45 degrees of flexion from full extension while gently rotating the forearm and flexing and extending the joint a few degrees is often helpful in localizing the injury and detecting effusion. The

Figure 18–28. Interesting case of bilateral type II lateral condylar fractures that occurred when the patient was 6 years old (A). At 62 years of age, the patient had painful limitation of motion and developed bilateral tardy ulnar nerve palsy. B, C, Lateral view demonstrates the almost identically altered anatomy. Bilateral injury nicely demonstrates a predictable and almost perfect mirror image deformity that results from the internal muscle forces and is common following lateral condylar type II injuries. Gross disruption of the posterior triangle is obvious (D). This patient was treated with total elbow arthroplasty (E and F) and is currently asymptomatic.

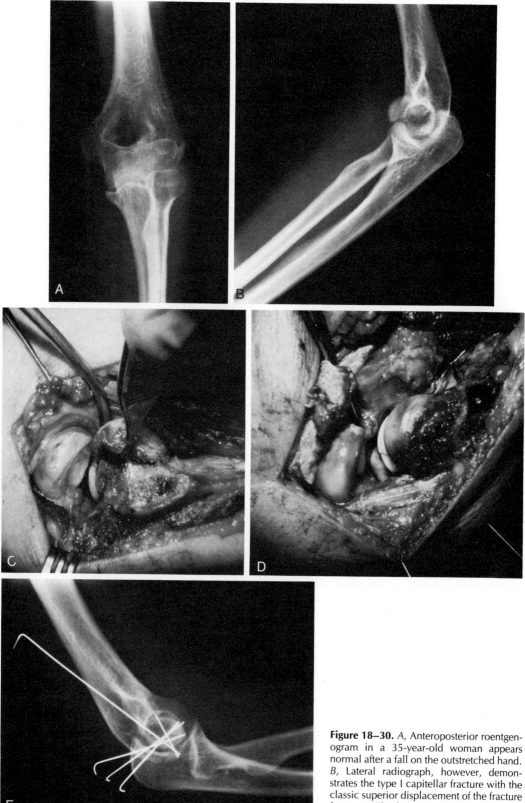

Figure 18–30. *A,* Anteroposterior roentgenogram in a 35-year-old woman appears normal after a fall on the outstretched hand. *B,* Lateral radiograph, however, demonstrates the type I capitellar fracture with the classic superior displacement of the fracture fragment. The fracture was reduced (*C*) and stabilized with Kirschner wires (*D* and *E*).

contact of the capitellum with the radial head may cause painful crepitus, especially with valgus stress. In the absence of gross swelling, the medial and lateral collateral ligaments can be palpated and should be tested for stability even in obese patients. Aspiration of the joint may aid in diagnosis of the more subtle type II or type III injuries after the radiographs have been taken. Should the aspirate contain no blood, fracture is, of course, less likely.

Several characteristic features of the fracture have been described:[56, 64] (1) pain independent of position, (2) maintenance of the normal, gross anatomic landmarks, (3) progressive loss of motion, (4) palpable mass in the antecubital fossa, (5) crepitus, particularly with flexion and extension, and (6) disability exceeding that expected from the gross findings.

This fracture, especially the type II injury, may be difficult to diagnose or accurately describe even with radiographs. The antero-posterior view is usually of little help (Fig. 18–30A). The radiographic fat pad sign is important as a diagnostic clue.[86] Corbett found that the posterior fat pad displaced by intra-articular effusion was always accompanied by fracture, but the anterior fat pad might be visible normally and without injury.[19] Smith and Lee, in a series of 89 injuries, found that 61 with a negative fat pad sign had no effusion and no bony injury but 28 with a positive fat pad sign did have effusion.[86] Twenty-three of these had fractures, nine of which could not be seen on the first radiograph. On the lateral view, the type I fracture is often apparent with anterior-superior displacement (Fig. 18–30B). The type II fracture frequently has only a small amount of bone, thus making diagnosis difficult even with the aid of a radiograph. Because the mechanism of the injury is often a force transmitted across the radial head, the roentgenogram must be carefully scrutinized to be sure that the fragments are from the capitellum and not from the radial head. As a rule, if the fracture is proximal to the radial head, the fragment is unlikely to have arisen from the radius, and capitellar fracture should be suspected.[66] Tomography may disclose an undisplaced fracture in patients with a positive fat pad sign. If there is marked swelling and radiographs have been taken at varied positions, comparison films of the opposite elbow in the same positions may be helpful. It should be stressed that the physical and radiographic examination in every severe elbow injury should include the wrist and the shoulder joint as well.

Treatment

Nonoperative. Closed reduction and immobilization can result in a successful outcome for the large fragments of the type I fracture. An anteriorly displaced fracture is most amenable to this treatment modality. Reduction must be accurate; if it is not, poor results or even ankylosis may occur.[16] Assessment of the quality of the reduction cannot always be accurately determined from the radiograph. Mazel has reported an instance of apparent reduction that was accompanied by restriction of flexion and forearm rotation.[64] When the fracture fragment was removed, full range of motion returned.

To perform closed manipulation the arm is grasped and longitudinal traction is exerted with the elbow extended. Direct pressure in the antecubital fossa as the elbow is supinated and flexed completes the reduction.[16] The joint is then immobilized from 3 to 6 weeks, although there has been a recent tendency to lessen this period of time.

Operative. Although nonoperative treatment has been the standard for other fractures about the elbow, operative intervention has long been the treatment of choice for this particular fracture.[20] The early recommendation was for complete excision of the type I or type II fragment,[26, 56] the rationale being that this was mechanically comparable to excision of the radial head.[55] The theory was tested by Darrach, who replaced the fragment only to find that this resulted in marked limitation of motion with healing. In 1934, Lee and Summey[55] published an excellent description of the injury and documented the universally poor results achieved in 10 patients who were treated with closed reduction or fragment replacement, whereas all 22 treated by excision of the fracture fragments had a good result. Fowles and Kassab[27] have noted that the better results may be expected for early but not necessarily for late excision.

Alvarez et al.,[1] in summarizing the literature, found good or excellent results in 63 percent of 38 patients treated with closed reduction, 51 percent of 41 treated by open reduction and internal fixation, and 78 percent of 94 treated by excision. In their series of 14 patients, 10 were treated by excision.

With improved surgical technique treatment options for type I fractures include not only excision of the fragment but also open reduction and internal fixation.[53] Several recent articles have reviewed the results of both surgical modalities.

Collert in 1977[18] reported on 20 cases, of which 13 involved a portion of the trochlea. Of these 13, 6 had an open reduction with 4 good or excellent results, and 7 had excision with 4 good and no excellent results. The remaining five (38 percent) had a poor result. In those seven cases in which only the capitellum was involved excision was done in one and open reduction and internal fixation was performed in six; all had excellent results. There were three attempts at closed reduction in this series, all of which failed. No late instability from excision was found.

Lansinger and Mare in 1981[53] reported 12 patients with capitellar fractures, of whom 10 were treated by operation with internal fixation. Nine of these had good results, achieving 30 to 115 degrees of motion. All wore a plaster splint for 2 to 8 weeks. The authors reported avascular necrosis in one patient that ended with a good result. Grantham et al.[33] studied 29 fractures and documented the results in 17. The study showed one excellent, eight good, four fair, and four poor results.

The reported data support the following recommendations: Early resection of the osteochondral slice fracture (type II) and the comminuted fracture (type III). The anteriorly rotated and displaced fracture (type I), which occurs most frequently, should be treated by open reduction and internal fixation in the young or by early resection if fixation cannot be attained. If experience has been gained with closed reduction, then this technique combined with early motion is also probably acceptable.

The postoperative care of this injury is determined by its treatment. If the capitellum is excised, early motion is permitted and the patient is encouraged to do as much as possible without discomfort. If the capitellum is reduced and securely fixed, early motion is also permitted and the patient's progress is carefully monitored. If fixation is undertaken, a short period of immobilization of about 2 to 3 weeks is appropriate.

Complications

Limitation of flexion and extension and residual pain are the most common sequelae of this fracture. Forearm rotation is usually not affected. Disruption of the medial collateral ligament can occur with fractures due to falls on the outstretched hand,[18] but this is rare. More commonly, the fracture may be complicated by a fracture of the ipsilateral radial head. Avascular necrosis has also been reported but appears to be rare even though the fragment is void of soft tissue attachment.

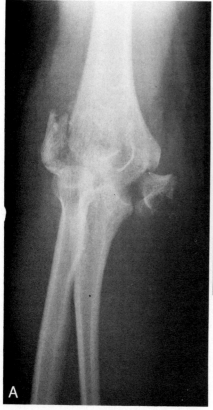

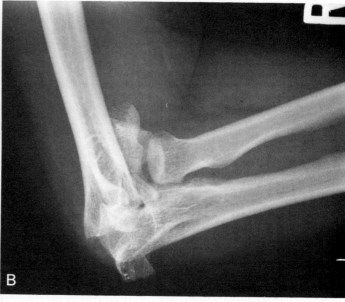

Figure 18–31. *A* and *B,* A 26-year-old woman sustained a comminuted fracture of the articular surface of the trochlea with involvement of the capitellum.

Illustration continued on opposite page

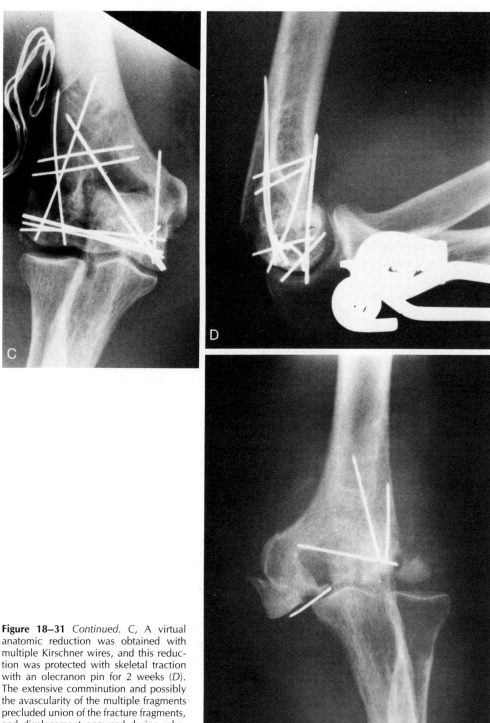

Figure 18–31 *Continued. C,* A virtual anatomic reduction was obtained with multiple Kirschner wires, and this reduction was protected with skeletal traction with an olecranon pin for 2 weeks *(D).* The extensive comminution and possibly the avascularity of the multiple fragments precluded union of the fracture fragments, and displacement occurred during rehabilitation *(E).*

Fractures of the Trochlea

Isolated fractures of the trochlea are extremely rare because this bone has no capsular, muscular, or ligamentous attachments and is supported on half of its circumference by the ulna. Forces that are sufficient to cause frac-

ture usually also disrupt the ulna, fracture the condyles in the supracondylar area, or dislocate the elbow. Nonetheless, fractures can occur with the capitellum sometimes involved as well (Fig. 18–31). If displacement occurs, the joint must be explored to restore congruity. Very small fragments often cannot be replaced or fixed anatomically and are best excised as suggested by Smith.[88] Because of the lack of bone substance, stability of this fracture may be very difficult to attain.

Small defects in the articular surface fill with fibrous tissue and may be well tolerated if motion is begun early at 3 to 5 days, but they form dense, adhesive bands to the ulna if motion is delayed. Linear irregularities in the sagittal plane are also well tolerated. Coronoid displacement alters the mechanics and stability of the ulnohumeral articulation and can lead to disastrous results if the fragment size or displacement is significant.

Authors' Preferred Method of Treatment of Intra-Articular Fractures

T and Y Condylar Fractures

Type I. These fractures are extremely rare, are relatively stable, and have little soft tissue injury. Hence, we feel they may very well be treated by plaster immobilization for 3 weeks followed by splinting with intermittent active mobilization for another 2 to 3 weeks.

Type II. These fractures are often amenable to fixation with screws as shown in Figure 18–20, and because displacement occurs without rotation, a good reduction can be obtained by simple compression and held by Kirschner wires. If reduction has been obtained by manipulation, screws may be inserted, usually through medial and lateral approaches. Postoperatively, the elbow is splinted for 3 to 5 days. The drain is removed at 24 hours. When acute postoperative swelling has subsided at 3 to 5 days, gentle active motion is begun. The elbow is not forced or used for lifting weights for 6 weeks or until the fracture appears to be healed on radiographs. Use of the extremity for normal personal care and feeding is encouraged during this period.

Because of the current emphasis on internal fixation and cartilage nutrition aided by early continuous motion,[84] we can look forward to a new era in elbow surgery in which controlled, early passive motion will help to eliminate edema and fibrosis and improve results. This has certainly been our experience with the knee, and we expect it to be the same with elbow surgery. It seems logical that mobilization of a T condylar fracture should begin as soon as swelling has diminished and pain permits.

Type III. Because these fractures are much more difficult to treat, we prefer internal fix-

ation. A full exposure through one of the posterior approaches is employed. Because of the frequency of involvement of the ulnar nerve, we prefer the medial-to-lateral triceps reflection with unroofing of the ulnar nerve and translocation if necessary. The articular surfaces are most easily assembled with one or two Kirschner wires or one screw, and we prefer the use of medial and lateral plates contoured to the bone. The double plate technique is the most rigid type of fixation and is best employed in the comminuted fracture. Threaded Kirschner wires inserted with one of the newer power drives have proved extremely useful in the assembly of the columns and the articular surface, thus facilitating fixation of the condyles to the shaft. We must remember that at the time most of the pessimistic articles regarding surgical intervention were written this ancillary equipment was not available.

It is usually easiest to fix the lateral condyle first. Dissection must be very carefully done at the origin of the brachioradialis muscle because the radial nerve crosses the interosseous membrane at that point. To avoid the nerve either a plate contoured to the posterior humerus or a short plate can be used. We usually excise the bone of the fossa and any adjacent portion of the trochlea that is not anatomically reducible. The wound is copiously irrigated, usually with propulsive irrigation, and hemostasis is obtained before closure. A suction drain is inserted for 24 hours. The arm is splinted with the elbow in 45 degrees of flexion to improve circulation to the posterior tissue, and it is continuously elevated. When the surgical reaction has subsided in 3 to 5 days motion is begun as in the type II injury.

Type IV. We treat these fractures the same way as type III fractures unless the patient is a poor surgical risk. The articular contour is assembled with multiple K wires because the comminution does not allow the use of screws. In this poor-risk patient treatment begins with traction through an olecranon pin with perhaps some gentle molding of the fracture fragments for 1 to 3 weeks; the institution of a collar and cuff with motion in flexion for the next 2 to 3 weeks followed by gradual extension is sometimes the best we can do.

Medial and Lateral Condylar Fractures

Lateral Condylar Fractures. Displaced fractures are treated surgically. Usually it is safer to perform an open reduction using a Kocher posterolateral approach. Once the skin incision has been made, the fracture line is readily identified, and by careful dissection the lateral condyle can be retracted to expose the joint and the trochlea. Clotted blood can best be removed by irrigation and the use of a small suction tip. This allows inspection of the capitellum, trochlea, and olecranon, and any loose fragments of cartilage or bone can be removed without creating obstacles to the anatomic reduction of the fracture. The radial head may be visualized by opening the posterior capsule along the anconeus interval. This exposure permits direct observation of the fracture line after reduction. When satisfactory reduction has been obtained, the fracture is fixed by either a screw, as in Figure 18–10, or threaded Kirschner wires inserted from the lateral condyle along the lateral supracondylar column to engage the opposite cortex of the humerus. If the opposite cortex is not reached, fixation is considered inadequate. A transverse wire or screw may also be necessary to prevent subluxation. The screws and wires must not in any circumstances intrude upon the fossa because motion must be regained very early. Active range of motion exercises should begin in 5 to 10 days when inflammation and pain have lessened. The arm is usually splinted between exercise periods for 3 to 6 weeks. This may not be necessary if fixation is very secure. Periodic radiographs to help diagnose any loss of reduction before the situation becomes nonsalvagable are recommended. Late recognition of proximal displacement may lead to ulnar neuropathy as well as arthritis changes and an unstable, weak, and painful elbow.

Medial Condylar Fractures. These fractures are much rarer than fractures of the lateral condyle. They are generally managed in the same way as lateral fractures. A posteromedial surgical approach is used because it permits identification and protection of the ulnar nerve and can be extended to visualize the trochlea by retraction of the ulnar nerve and division of the thin superior portion of the medial collateral ligament and the capsule. It also permits good visualization of the fossa and of the medial trochlea. Rigid fixation must be obtained, and this may necessitate the use of a plate if the supracondylar bone is comminuted. It is probably advisable to translocate the ulnar nerve anteriorly if it cannot be replaced in a smooth bed, and it should be left unroofed in either instance.

Capitellar Fractures. Displaced type I or total capitellar fractures with or without a portion of the trochlea are treated by open anatomic reduction and internal fixation. The posterior portion of the lateral condyle is not articular, and fixation can be maintained by small screws or threaded Kirschner wires inserted just beneath the chondral surface as shown in Figure 18–31. Smillie nails may be countersunk, but these tend to drift as do smooth Kirschner wires. Reduction and fixation can be easily tested at the time of surgery if the posterolateral Kocher approach has been utilized, releasing the extensor muscles and the capsule from the lateral condyle as necessary to visualize the capitellum. Postoperatively, it is very important to begin motion as soon as inflammation has subsided, which often occurs in only 2 to 3 days in these less traumatic intra-articular injuries. If necessary, fixation that has been introduced from posterior to anterior is readily removed without violating the cartilage.

Type II or slice fractures contain cartilage with little if any bone and are unlikely to be reducible by any means. The cartilage will continue to grow and impede motion, and thus the preferred treatment is excision.

Similarly, type III or comminuted fractures of the capitellum are not anatomically reducible because of the small size of the fragments. Hence, small fragments are best excised, but if there is a large fragment including a portion of the trochlea, this may be reduced and fixed with threaded Kirschner wires or a screw and Kirschner wire. Defects in the articular surface will be filled with fibrous tissue and are usually well tolerated, but protuberances and off-set edges can cause pain, impingement, and severe limitation of function.

MASSIVE TRAUMA TO THE ELBOW

The elbow is generally no more vulnerable to extensive injury than the other peripheral joints and is less frequently involved than the weight-bearing joints of the ankle or knee. Massive trauma is characterized by involvement of all the major tissue systems—bone, joint, vessels, nerve, muscle, and skin. The most common causes of this type of injury in today's society is the gunshot wound in metropolitan areas, various war injuries in the military population, and auger injuries in the rural setting (Fig. 18–32). The latter injury is usually complicated by gross contamination, which adds to the complexity of management.

The massively traumatized elbow was in-

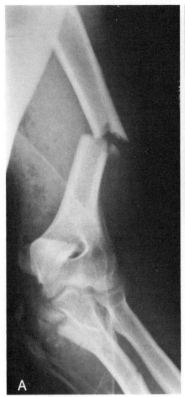
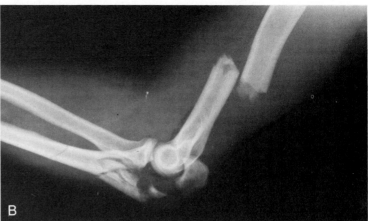

Figure 18–32. Massive elbow trauma sustained in a snowmobile accident. An aggressive management program with rigid fixation of the humeral fracture and excision or fixation of the olecranon fracture is recommended, but such severe injuries portend a poor prognosis.

troduced into the orthopedic literature as the "sideswipe" or "car window" injury that was so common in the 1940s[38, 75] before the advent of car air conditioning, turn signals, and wider roads. This injury characteristically involves the left elbow as it rests on the rolled-down window ledge that is struck by an oncoming car. The pathologic findings usually consist of a compound, comminuted fracture of the proximal ulna, dislocation at the elbow, and fracture of the distal humerus. The devastating nature of the event is obvious by the 50 percent amputation rate reported with this injury.[105]

The specifics of this entity today are of academic or historical interest only because the principles of management of the massively traumatized limb have been refined. In the 1940s initial treatment recommendations included limited debridement and traction. More extensive debridement and fixation of the ulnar fracture might be performed later. Immediate arthroplasty has even been recommended.[106] Sepsis was common, and ankylosis or a flail joint was anticipated. Today, such an injury is more common with gunshot wounds, auger injuries, or recreational pursuits (Fig. 18–32). The principles of management have changed as follows:

1. Judicious debridement of bone and soft tissue
2. Extensive lavage, ideally with a pulsating stream
3. Reduction and fixation of the intra-articular fractures if they are not grossly contaminated. Wound is left open
4. Delayed closure when the chance of sepsis is minimized
5. Motion as soon as possible

Rogers et al.[83] have recently characterized the "floating elbow" as yet another variant of this type of injury. They recommend rigid fixation of the humeral and forearm fractures and early mobilization as the optimum treatment goal.

A particular effort should be made to avoid the development of sepsis, which will preclude the possibility of late reconstruction with a prosthetic implant. In our experience the chances of successful prosthetic treatment in a traumatized joint with a history of sepsis are indeed limited.

COMPLICATIONS

Several serious complications are associated with fractures of the distal humerus. Because

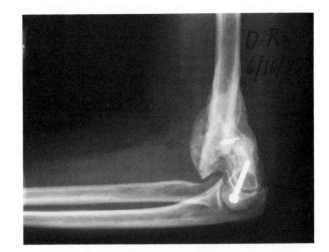

Figure 18–33. Posterior proximal displacement of a healed T-condylar fracture precludes flexion past 90 degrees due to impingement of the anterior distal aspect of the proximal fragment.

of their complex pathophysiology and the difficulty of treatment, many have been dealt with in separate chapters.

Loss of Motion

Loss of motion is probably the most common complication of fractures about the elbow. Several distinct but related factors that lead to motion loss may be identified: (1) soft tissue fibrosis and scarring, (2) articular malalignment, (3) excessive callus formation, (4) improper placement of the internal fixation device, and (5) development of myositis ossificans.[79]

Soft tissue contracture may be significant with intra-articular fractures if the anterior capsule is damaged. Surgical trauma and prolonged immobilization are treatment factors that also contribute to soft tissue fibrosis.

Articular malalignment or supracondylar fractures may interfere with the arc but not usually with the range of motion. Intra-articular malalignment due to rotation in the frontal or sagittal plane is a common source of motion loss (Fig. 18–33).

Malunion and excessive callus formation may compromise the close tolerances characteristic of this joint (Fig. 18–34). These usually involve the supracondylar bone and fossa. Improperly placed internal fixation devices can also cause mechanical destruction of the normal motion of the joint. Myositis ossificans involves the soft tissue envelope of the joint[98] and can be a source of severe motion loss leading to ankylosis. This topic is discussed in detail below (Chapter 26). The characteristic pattern of motion limitation is considerable loss of extension but usually mild limitation of rotation.

Treatment of ankylosis or motion loss is discussed in detail in Chapter 24. In general, we prefer to operate on patients with greater than 60 degrees fixed flexion contracture or those in whom a discrete mechanical cause is identified as the offending agent.

Nerve Injury

Injuries to all three nerves can occur with distal humeral fractures.[58] The insult can orig-

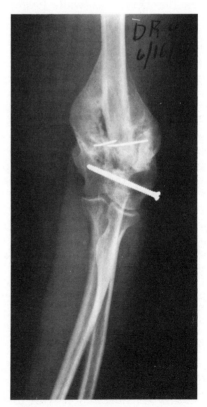

Figure 18–34. Osseous overgrowth of the olecranon and coronoid fossa due to marked callus proliferation limits full extension in this 56-year-old woman after healing of a T-condylar fracture.

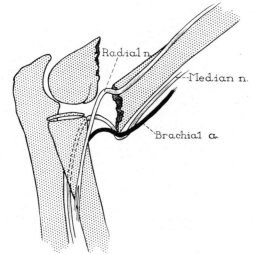

Figure 18–35. Posterior displacement of the distal humerus places the brachial artery as well as the radial and median nerves in jeopardy from the prominent distal humeral bone fragment. (From Lipscomb, P. R., and Burleson, R. J.: Vascular and neural complications in supracondylar fractures of the humerus in children. J. Bone Joint Surg. 37A:468, 1955.

inate at the time of the injury, with manipulation, or during surgery (Fig. 18–35). Massive trauma violates all tissue planes and certainly involves the nerves as well. Postoperative nerve dysfunction is a constant concern and most commonly involves ulnar nerve injury after treatment of a T or Y condylar fracture (Fig. 18–21).[7, 54, 76]

Tardy ulnar nerve palsy is a late sequela that is classically associated with increased valgus angulation at the elbow, especially after lateral type II condylar fractures as described in detail by Milch et al.[89] In a review of 100 tardy ulnar nerve palsies conducted by Gay and Love at the Mayo Clinic,[29] 57 percent resulted from a previous elbow fracture. The usual symptoms were parasthesia (85 percent), atrophy (81 percent), paralysis of some motor function (62 percent), pain (39 percent), and anesthesia (25 percent). Physical examination revealed atrophy and weakness in 96 percent of patients with anesthesia in 77 percent. In this series 70 percent obtained a satisfactory result with surgical treatment, usually anterior intramuscular transplantation. Treatment of nerve entrapment injuries is discussed in detail in Chapter 45.

Malunion

Malunion is not uncommon with distal humeral fractures but usually does not necessitate additional surgery. Supracondylar osteotomy is indicated, however, when the articulation is intact and an ulnar nerve palsy

has developed or when improvement of the arc of motion is desirable. An intracondylar fracture can also cause an unstable joint and an incongruous distal humerus; osteotomy has been recommended by Milch[69] to correct this deformity. The cosmetic appearance of a varus or valgus deformity is also an indication for surgical intervention in the selected patient (Chapter 19).

Instability

Most distal humeral fractures are complicated by stiffness, not instability. Instability about the elbow following fractures is due either to articular surface loss[67] or to ligament injury.[42] The type II condylar fracture is the only fracture characterized by instability, and this can be avoided by immediate open reduction and internal fixation. The mechanism of injury in capitellar fractures is similar to that for radial head fractures, and consequently the ulnar collateral ligament can be torn. It is unusual to perform ligamentous repair with either of these fractures, but this has occasionally been recommended.[42, 88] In general, symptomatic joint laxity does not occur.

Vascular Injuries

Vascular injury is probably the most worrisome and devastating of all complications occurring with distal humeral fractures.[65] It occurs more often after supracondylar and T–Y condylar injuries. The intense pain with ischemia and the unreliable peripheral pulse are familiar to everyone. The clinical features are supplemented by compartment pressure measurements. This complex problem is discussed in detail in Chapter 17.

Myositis Ossificans

This complication is most often seen following fracture-dislocation,[60, 73] especially that involving the radial head.[97] Proximal radial and lateral condylar fractures are less common etiologic events. Heterotopic ossification has even been reported after excision of the supracondylar process.[50] Development of this entity has been related to massage and passive motion of the injured joint.[73] As with exuberant callus, myositis ossificans can cause limitation of motion but is not so readily treated, although Mohan[73] reported successful results after excision in 66 of 70 patients. Passive motion and manipulation are, of course, to be condemned, but early active motion probably does not contribute to the development of this complication. The diagnosis and treatment of myositis ossificans has been discussed in detail in Chapter 26.

Nonunion

Nonunion of the distal humerus is quite uncommon, occurring in less than 5 percent of all distal humeral fractures, and is often related to failed surgical fixation. This complication and the experience of Mitsunaga et al.[72] are discussed in detail in Chapter 19.

References

1. Alvarez, E., Patel, M. R., Nimberg, G., and Pearlman, H. S.: Fracture of the Capitulum Humeri. J. Bone Joint Surg. **57A**:1093, 1975.
2. Anderson, L. D.: Fractures. In Crenshaw, A. H. (Ed.): Campbell's Operative Orthopedics, 5th ed. St. Louis, C. V. Mosby Co., 1921, pp. 645–651.
3. Alonso Llames, M.: Bilaterotricipital Approach to the Elbow. Acta Orthop. Scand. **43**:479, 1972.
4. Barnard, L. B., and McCoy, S. M.: The Supracondyloid Process of the Humerus. J. Bone Joint Surg. **28**(4):845, 1946.
5. Bickel, W. H., and Perry, R. E.: Comminuted Fractures of the Distal Humerus. J.A.M.A. **184**:553, 1963.
6. Brown, R. F., and Morgan, R. G.: Intercondylar T-Shaped Fracture of the Humerus. J. Bone Joint Surg. **53**:425, 1971.
7. Bryan, R. S.: Fracture About the Elbow in Adults. In American Academy of Orthopedic Surgeons: Instructional Course Lectures, Vol. 30. St. Louis, C.V. Mosby Co., 1981.
8. Bryan, R. S., and Bickel, W. H.: T Condylar Fractures of the Distal Humerus. J. Trauma **11**(10):830, 1971.
9. Bryan, R. S., and Morrey, B. F.: Extensive Posterior Exposure of the Elbow—A Triceps-Sparing Approach. Clin. Orthop. **166**:188, 1982.
10. Burri, C., Henkelmeyer, H., and Spier, W.: Results of Operative Treatment of Intra-Articular Fractures of the Distal Humerus. Acta Orthop. Belgica **41**(2):227, 1975.
11. Campbell, W. C.: Arthroplasty of the Elbow. Ann. Surg. **76**:615, 1932.
12. Cassebaum, W. H.: Operative Treatment of T and Y Fractures of the Lower End of the Humerus. Am. J. Surg. **83**:265, 1952.
13. Cassebaum, W. H.: Open Reduction of T and Y Fractures of the Lower End of the Humerus. J. Trauma, **9**:915, 1969.
14. Cave, E. F.: Fractures and Other Injuries. Chicago, Year Book Medical Publishers, 1958, pp. 314–333.
15. Charnley, J.: Closed Treatment of Common Fractures. Baltimore, The Williams & Wilkins Co., 1961, pp. 70–71.
16. Christopher, F., and Bushnell, L. F.: Conservative Treatment of Fracture of the Capitellum. J. Bone Joint Surg. **17**:489, 1935.
17. Conn, J., and Wade, P. A.: Injuries of the Elbow: A Ten Year Review. J. Trauma **1**:248, 1961.
18. Collert, S.: Surgical Management of Fractures of the Capitulum Humeri. Acta Orthop. Scand. **48**:603, 1977.
19. Corbett, R. H.: Displaced Fat Pads in Trauma to the Elbow. Injury **9**(4):297, 1978.
20. Darrach, W.: Transactions of the New York Surgical Society: Open Reduction of Fractured External Condyle of Humerus; Open Reduction of Fracture of the Capitellum; Fractures of the Neck of the Scapula. Ann. Surg. **63**:486, 1916.
21. Doane, C. P.: Fractures of the Supracondylar Process of the Humerus. J. Bone Joint Surg. **18**:757, 1936.
22. Eastwood, W. J.: The T-Shaped Fracture of the Lower End of the Humerus. J. Bone Joint Surg. **19**:364, 1937.
23. Edman, P., and Lohr, G.: Supracondylar Fractures of the Humerus Treated with Olecranon Traction. Acta Chir. Scand. **126**:505, 1963.
24. Eppright, R. H., and Wilkins, K. E.: Intracondylar T or Y Fracture. In Rockwood, C. A., and Green, D. P. (Eds.): Fractures, Vol. 1. Philadelphia, J. B. Lippincott Co., 1975, pp. 501–509.
25. Evans, E. M.: Supracondylar Y Fracture of the Humerus. J. Bone Joint Surg. **35B**:381, 1953.
26. Flint, C. P.: Fracture of the Eminentia Capitata. Surg. Gynecol. Obstet. **7**:342, 1908.
27. Fowles, J. V., and Kassab, M. T.: Fracture of the Capitulum Humeri. Treatment by Excision. J. Bone Joint Surg. **56A**:794, 1974.
28. Garceau, G. J.: Fractures of the Lower End of the Humerus. J.A.M.A. **112**:623, 1939.
29. Gay, J. R., and Love, J. G.: Diagnosis and Treatment of Tardy Paralysis of the Ulnar Nerve. J. Bone Joint Surg. **29**:1087, 1947.
30. Gejrot, W.: An Intra-Articular Fracture of the Capitellum and Trochlea of the Humerus with Special Reference to Treatment. Acta Chir. Scand. **71**:253, 1932.
31. Genner, B. A.: Fracture of the Supracondylar Process. J. Bone Joint Surg. **41A**:1333, 1959.
32. Gilcreest, E. L.: Fractures of the Elbow Joint and of the Lower End of the Humerus. Surg. Gynecol. Obstet. **37**:452, 1923.
33. Grantham, S. A., Norris, T. R., and Bush, D. C.: Isolated Fracture of the Humeral Capitellum. Clin. Orthop. **161**:262, 1981.
34. Hasner, E., and Husby, J.: Fracture of Epicondyle and Condyle of Humerus. Acta Chir. Scand. **101**:195, 1951.
35. Henderson, M. S.: Studies in Treatment of Fractures. Collected Papers of the Mayo Clinic, Vol. 6. Philadelphia, W. B. Saunders Co., 1914.
36. Henderson, M. S.: Fractures Considered as Potential Deformities. Collected Papers of the Mayo Clinic, Vol. 2. Philadelphia, W. B. Saunders Co., 1919.
37. Heppenstall, R. B.: Fracture Treatment and Healing. Philadelphia, W. B. Saunders Co., 1980.
38. Highsmith, L. S., and Phalen, G. S.: Side Swipe Injuries. Arch. Surg. **52**:78, 1941.
39. Hitzrot, J. M.: Fractures at the Lower End of the Humerus in Adults. Surg. Clin. North Am. **12**:291, 1932.
40. Horne, G.: Supracondylar Fracture of the Humerus in Adults. J. Trauma **20**(1):71, 1980.
41. Hoyer, A.: Treatment of Supracondylar Fracture of the Humerus by Skeletal Traction in an Abduction Splint. J. Bone Joint Surg. **34A**:623, 1952.
42. Johansson, O.: Capsular and Ligament Injuries of the Elbow Joint. Acta Chir. Scand. Suppl. **287**, 1962.
43. Johansson, H., and Olerud, S.: Operative Treatment of Intercondylar Fractures of the Humerus. J. Trauma **11**(10):836, 1971.
44. Kelly, R. P., and Griffin, T. W.: Open Reduction of T-Condylar Fractures of the Humerus Through an Anterior Approach. J. Trauma **9**:901, 1969.
45. Keon-Cohen, B.: Fractures at the Elbow. AAOS Instructional Course Lectures. J. Bone Joint Surg. **48A**:1623, 1966.

46. Key, A. J., and Conwell, H. E.: Management of Fractures, Dislocations and Sprains, 7th ed. St. Louis, C. V. Mosby Co., 1961.

47. Knight, R. A.: Fractures of the Humeral Condyles in Adults. South. Med. J. **48**:1165, 1955.

48. Knight, R. A.: The Management of Fractures About the Elbow in Adults. In American Academy of Orthopedic Surgeons: Instructional Course Lectures, Vol. 14. Ann Arbor, J. W. Edwards, 1957, pp. 123–141.

49. Kocher, T.: Text Book of Operative Surgery, 3rd ed. Transl. by H. Stiles and C. Paul. London, A & C Book Co., 1911.

50. Kolb, L. W., and Moore, R. D.: Fractures of the Supracondylar Process of the Humerus. J. Bone Joint Surg. **49A**:532, 1967.

51. Kolenak, A.: Ununited Fracture of the Lateral Condyle of the Humerus. A 50 Year Follow-up. Clin. Orthop. **124**:181, 1977.

52. Lansinger, O., and Mare, K.: Intercondylar T Fractures of the Humerus in Adults. Acta Orthop. Traumatal. Surg. **100**:37, 1982.

53. Lansinger, O., and Mare, K.: Fracture of the Capitulum Humeri. Acta Orthop. Scand. **52**:39, 1981.

54. Lecestre, R.: Round Table on Fractures of the Lower End of the Humerus. Societe Francaise de Chirurgie Orthopedique et Traumatologie. Ortho. Trans. **4**(2):123, 1980.

55. Lee, W. E., and Summey, T. J.: Fracture of the Capitellum of the Humerus. Am Surg. **99**:497, 1934.

56. Lindem, M. C.: Fractures of the Capitellum and Trochlea. Ann. Surg. **76**:78, 1922.

57. Linscheid, R. L., and Wheeler, D.: Elbow Dislocations. J.A.M.A. **194**:1171, 1965.

58. Lipscomb, P. R., and Burleson, R. J.: Vascular and Neural Complications in Supracondylar Fractures of the Humerus in Children. J. Bone Joint Surg. **37A**:468, 1955.

59. Lund, H. J.: Fracture of the Supracondyloid Process of the Humerus. Report of a Case. J. Bone Joint Surg. **12**:925, 1930.

60. McLaughlin, H. L.: Some Fractures With a Time Limit. Surg. Clin. North Am. **35**:553, 1955.

61. Magnuson, P. B., and Stack, J. K.: Fractures, 5th ed. Philadelphia, J. B. Lippincott Co., 1949.

62. Marquis, J. W., Bruwer, A. J., and Keith, H. M.: Supracondyloid Process of the Humerus. Proc. Staff Mayo Clin. **37**:691, 1957.

63. Matthewson, M. H., and Dandy, D. J.: Osteochondral Fractures of the Lateral Femoral Condyle. J. Bone Joint Surg. **60B**:199, 1978.

64. Mazel, M. S.: Fracture of the Capitellum. J. Bone Joint Surg. **17**:483, 1935.

65. Meyerding, H. W.: Volkmann's Ischemic Contracture Associated With Supracondylar Fracture of the Humerus. J.A.M.A. **106**:1138, 1936.

66. Milch, H.: Unusual Fracture of the Capitulum Humeri and Capitulum Radii. J. Bone Joint Surg. **13**:882, 1931.

67. Milch, H.: Fracture of the External Humeral Condyle. J.A.M.A. **160**:641, 1956.

68. Milch, H.: Fracture Surgery; A Textbook of Common Fractures. New York, Hoeber, 1959.

69. Milch, H.: Fractures and Fracture Dislocations of the Humeral Condyles. J. Trauma **4**:592, 1964.

70. Miller, O. L.: Blind Nailing of the T Fracture of the Lower End of the Humerus Which Involves the Joint. J. Bone Joint Surg. **21**:933, 1936.

71. Miller, W. E.: Comminuted Fractures of the Distal End of the Humerus in the Adult. AAOS Instructional Course Lectures. J. Bone Joint Surg. **46A**:644, 1964.

72. Mitsunaga, M. M., Bryan, R. S., and Linscheid, R. L.: Condylar Nonunions of the Elbow. J. Trauma **22**(9):787, 1982.

73. Mohan, K.: Myositis Ossificans Traumatica of the Elbow. Internat. Surg. **57**:475, 1972.

74. Muller, M. E., Allgower, M., and Willenegger, H.: Manual of Internal Fixation. New York, Springer-Verlag, 1970.

75. Nicholson, J. T.: Compound Comminuted Fractures Involving the Elbow Joint. J. Bone Joint Surg. **28**:565, 1946.

76. Nieman, K.: Condylar Fractures of the Distal Humerus in Adults. South. Med. J. **70**(8):915, 1977.

77. Palmer, I.: The Validity of the Rule of Alternativity in Traumatology. Acta Chir. Scand. **21**:481, 1961.

78. Patrick, J.: Fracture of the Medial Epicondyle with Displacement into the Elbow Joint. J. Bone Joint Surg. **28**:143, 1946.

79. Reich, R. S.: Treatment of Intracondylar Fractures of the Elbow by Means of Traction. J. Bone Joint Surg. **18**:997, 1936.

80. Rhodin, R.: On the Treatment of Fracture of the Capitellum. Acta Chir. Scand. **86**:475, 1942.

81. Riech, P. L.: Fractures of the Radial Head—Associated with Chip Fracture of the Capitellum in Adults; Surgical Considerations. Southern Surgeon **14**:154, 1948.

82. Riseborough, E. J., and Radin, E. L.: Intracondylar T Fractures of the Humerus in the Adult. J. Bone Joint Surg. **51A**:130, 1969.

83. Rogers, J., Bennett, B., and Tullow, H. S.: Management of "Floating Elbow" Injuries. Orthop. Trans. **6**:359, 1982.

84. Salter, R. B., Simmonds, D. F., Malcolm, B. W., Rumble, E. J., MacMichael, D., and Clements, N. D.: The Biologic Effect of Continuous Passive Motion on the Healing of Full Thickness Defects in Articular Cartilage. J. Bone Joint Surg. **62A**:1232, 1980.

85. Shorbe, H. B.: Car Window Elbows. South. Med. J. **34**:372, 1941.

86. Smith, D. N., and Lee, J. R.: The Radiological Diagnosis of Post Traumatic Effusion of the Elbow Joint and the Clinical Significance of the Displaced Fat Pad Sign. Injury **10**(2):115, 1978.

87. Smith, F. M.: Traction and Suspension in the Treatment of Fractures. Surg. Clin. North Am. **3**:545, 1951.

88. Smith, F. M.: Surgery of the Elbow. Philadelphia, W. B. Saunders Co., 1972, p. 102.

89. Smith, F. M.: An 84-Year Follow-up on a Patient with Ununited Fracture of the Lateral Condyle of the Humerus. J. Bone Joint Surg. **55A**:378, 1973.

90. Smith, L.: Deformity Following Supracondylar Fractures of the Humerus. J. Bone Joint Surg. **42A**:235, 1960.

91. Smith, L.: Supracondylar Fracture of the Humerus Treated by Direct Observation. Clin. Orthop. **50**:37, 1967.

92. Sotgiu, F., Melis, G. C., and Tolu, S.: Classification and Treatment of Intercondyloid Fracture of the Humerus. Ital. J. Orthop. Traumatol. **2**(2):281, 1976.

93. Soltanpur, A.: Anterior Supracondylar Fracture of the Humerus (Flexion Type). A Simple Technique for Closed Reduction and Fixation in Adults and the Aged. J. Bone Joint Surg. **60B**(3):383, 1978.

94. Speed, J. S.: Surgical Treatment of Condylar Fracture of the Humerus. In American Academy of Orthopedic Surgeons: Instructional Course Lectures, Vol. 7. St. Louis, C. V. Mosby Co., 1950, pp. 187–194.

95. Suman, R. K., and Miller, J. H.: Intercondylar Frac-

tures of the Distal Humerus. J. Roy. Coll. Surg. Edinburgh **27**:276, 1982.

96. Terry, R. J.: New Data on the Incidence of the Supracondyloid Variation. Am. J. Phys. Anthropol. **9**:265, 1926.

97. Thompson, H. E., III, and Garcia, A.: Myositis Ossificans. Clin. Orthop. **50**:129, 1967.

98. Thorndike, A.: Myositis Ossificans Traumatica. J. Bone Joint Surg. **22**:315, 1940.

99. Trynin, A. H.: Intercondylar T Fracture of Elbow. J. Bone Joint Surg. **23**:709, 1941.

100. Van Gorder, G. W.: Surgical Approach in Supracondylar T Fracture of the Humerus Requiring Open Reduction. J. Bone Joint Surg. **22**:278, 1940.

101. Wade, F. V., and Batdorf, J.: Supracondylar Fractures of the Humerus: A Twelve Year Review with Follow-up. J. Trauma **1**:269, 1961.

102. Watson-Jones, R.: Fractures and Joint Injuries, Vol. 2, No. 4, 4th ed. Baltimore, The Williams & Williams Co., 1955, pp. 534–536.

103. Wickstrom, J., and Meyer, P. R., Jr.: Fractures of the Distal Humerus in Adults. Clin. Orthop. **50**:43, 1967.

104. Wilson, P. D.: Fracture and Dislocations in the Region of the Elbow. Surg. Gynecol. Obstet. **56**:335, 1933.

105. Wood, C. F.: Traffic Elbow. Kentucky Med. J. **39**:78, 1941.

106. Young, A.: Primary Elbow Arthroplasty. Arch. Surg. **101**:78, 1970.

107. Zagorski, J. B., Jennings, J. J., and Burkhalter, W. E.: Comminuted Intra-Articular or Bicondylar Fractures of the Distal Humerus. Orthop. Trans. **5**(3):403, 1981.

CHAPTER 19

Nonunion and Delayed Union of Distal Humeral Fractures

FRANKLIN H. SIM

NONUNION

Despite recent advances in operative treatment, nonunion of fractures of the distal humerus in close proximity to the elbow continue to pose a challenging problem to the surgeon. Although debate continues with regard to the initial treatment of these fractures (see Chapter 18), nonunion in the supracondylar region and between the condylar fragments of the distal humerus occurs after both open and closed treatment methods. When a nonunion does occur there is significant disability because of pain, instability, and periarticular fibrosis.

Fortunately, nonunion of these uncommon fractures is rare. Horne did not mention pseudarthrosis as a complication among 50 distal humeral fractures.[12] Even when early motion was begun "a few days" after injury, nonunion was rare and did not occur after 10 fractures so treated and reported by Brown and Morgan.[6] A comprehensive survey of fractures using several epidemiologic sources excluded the supracondylar region of the humerus from among the 12 most common sites for development of nonunion.[24] Only 1 of 55 nonunions reported by Solheim and Daagev involved the distal humerus, and no comment was made about this one case.[21] A similar incidence was documented in a Russian experience describing 4 nonunions of the distal humerus among 197 nonunions of the long bones[19] and by Wilson, who reported a 2 percent incidence of nonunion among 50 such fractures.[23] Knight has indicated that nonunion occurs very rarely between the condylar fragments but may occur in the supracondylar region.[14] In the Mayo Clinic series of 30 surgically treated T condylar fractures, 2 (7 percent) developed pseudarthrosis.[8] The literature suggests that approximately 2 percent of fractures involve the supracondylar or distal humeral region (Chapter 18). Of these, approximately 2 percent will go on to nonunion. Hence, this is not a frequent complication, which accounts for the dearth of literature on the subject. It is not surprising that there is hardly a word in any orthopedic source discussing the management of this entity. Mitsunaga et al. recently reported on 32 patients with delayed union and nonunion of the distal humeral fractures in close proximity to the elbow who were treated at the Mayo Clinic.[17]

Predisposing Factors

As in nonunions of other fractures several factors may play a causative role. Infection, comminution, or inappropriate initial treatment may influence the development of this complication.[2] A pseudarthrosis may occur because effective primary surgical fixation was not achieved due to comminution, multiple associated injuries, or excessive damage to the soft tissues. In addition, overdistraction from skeletal traction may be a factor if this modality of treatment is not carefully supervised. In our experience, however, inadequate internal fixation is the most common contributory factor.

The primary treatment goal with any acute fracture is both to achieve union and to restore function. The technique selected to achieve these goals should complement and not compete with each other. Loosening or breakage of the internal fixation device occurs when the initial reduction is not anatomic and fixation is insecure. In our experience, Kirschner wires and Steinmann pins are often inadequate to maintain reduction and provide the stability that is needed to allow early motion. It must also be remembered that any exposure further compromises the blood supply to the fracture fragments.

Evaluation

Distal humeral nonunions involving the elbow present difficult treatment problems that require a great deal of judgment. Evaluation requires a very careful assessment of the patient, including his age and functional demands, the status of the soft tissues, and the presence of infection. Smith has reported an 84-year follow-up of a lateral condylar nonunion in an individual with a near-painless extremity who pursued a 35-year career as a professional musician—possibly as good or better a result than could have been produced by reconstructive surgery.[20]

The status of the elbow joint itself is an important consideration. The amount of post-traumatic arthritis, the extent of joint stiffness, and the functional demands must be carefully considered. Radiographs and tomograms should be studied preoperatively to best understand the components and characteristics of the nonunion, paying particular attention to the quality of the articular surface. It is also important to assess the bone quality of the distal fragments to decide if it is possible to achieve reduction and fixation of the articular surfaces. The classification and distribution of nonunions seen at the Mayo Clinic over a period of 10 years is shown in Figure 19–1.

Just as in the acute fracture, each nonunion will have its own character, and the treatment of each case must be individualized. In our experience the major complaints of 32 patients at presentation were pain in 25, instability in 6 who had symptoms of a flail elbow, significant limitation of elbow motion in 7. In this experience the time from the original fracture to the treatment of the delayed union or nonunion ranged from 4 months to 41 years (average, 3.3 years). Supracondylar nonunions predominated, occurring in 17 patients, followed by T condylar nonunions, which occurred in 9. There were three lateral condylar nonunions, two transcondylar nonunions, and one nonunion of the medial condyle.

Treatment Options

Several treatment programs may be considered. Leaving a painless pseudarthrosis alone is appropriate if reasonable motion and stability are present. If function is severely compromised or significant pain exists, achieving stable osteosynthesis by internal or external fixation and bone grafting are the techniques most commonly employed. Resectional arthroplasty or total joint arthroplasty are additional options if joint salvage in unobtainable due to marked osteoporosis, insufficient bone for stable fixation, marked traumatic changes of the elbow articular cartilage, or joint stiffness. Distraction arthroplasty may also be an effective alternative treatment.[11] In elderly patients whose demands on the extremity may not be great, resection of the nonunion as described by Anderson[2] or total elbow arthroplasty[17] are certainly viable options.

In most instances, particularly in the younger, active person, internal fixation with bone grafting is the preferred mode of treatment. The goal is to achieve total anatomic

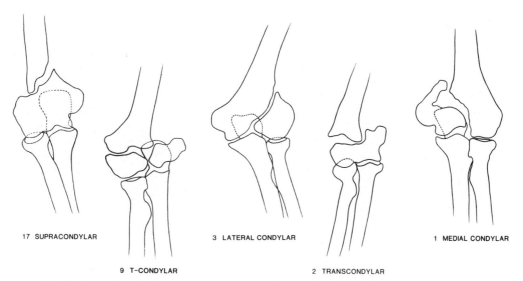

Figure 19–1. Classification and distribution of nonunions as treated at the Mayo Clinic. (From Mitsunaga, M., et al.: Condylar nonunions of the elbow. J. Trauma 22:787, 1982. © 1982, The Williams & Wilkins Co., Baltimore.)

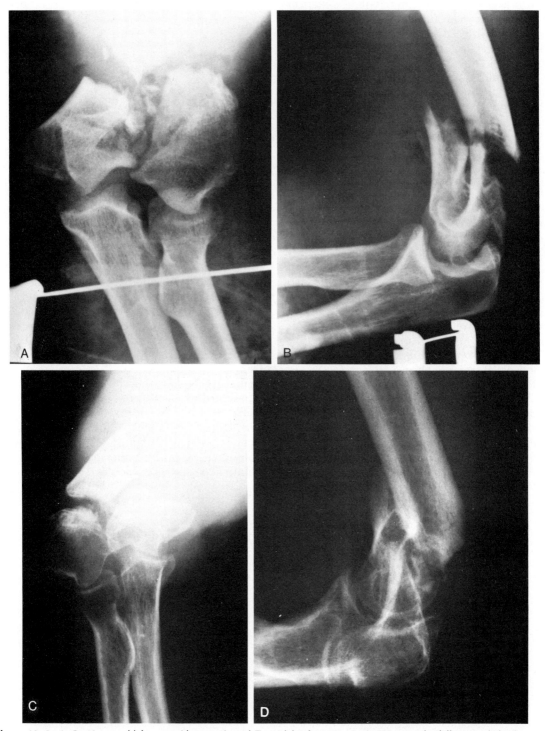

Figure 19–2. *A, B,* 49-year-old farmer with comminuted T-condylar fracture. *C, D,* Five months following skeletal traction and subsequent casting, a nonunion with only 20 to 60 degrees of elbow flexion is present.

Illustration continued on opposite page

restoration of the distal humerus with fixation that is secure enough to allow early motion designed to attain a functional arc. In some patients with extensive joint damage and periarticular fibrosis, residual disability is certain, yet open reduction and fixation can restore the contour of the elbow and preserve the bone stock and the collateral ligaments, thus allowing a more satisfactory resection, distraction, or replacement at a later date (Fig. 19–2).

Although electrical stimulation has been demonstrated to be effective in the treatment of many nonunions[3, 5] the elbow tolerates the necessary duration of immobilization poorly. Hence, surgical treatment of nonunions about the elbow is necessary to restore stability, alignment, and function of the joint.

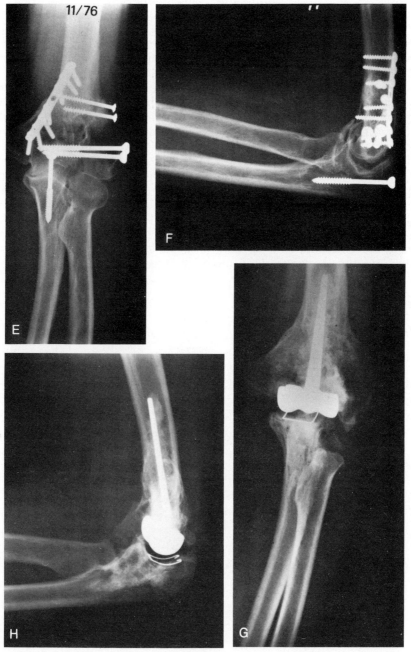

Figure 19–2 *Continued. E, F,* Eight months following internal fixation, supracondylar but not intercondylar union is present. *G, H,* Two years following total elbow arthroplasty, elbow motion ranges from 57 to 106 degrees of flexion.

Surgical Technique of Osteosynthesis

Treatment of nonunions in the elbow region varies according to the nature of the fracture and the status of the articular surface. Because the technique of surgical fixation of the nonunion depends largely on the type of fracture and because each fracture is different, there is no one standard method of treatment. A variety of equipment for internal fixation must be available, and the same basic principles outlined for surgical treatment of acute fractures should be followed. The articular surface must first be restored as well as possible and then secured by interfragmentary compression if necessary. Rigid fixation of the condylar to the diaphyseal portion of the humerus is then completed with condylar screws, lateral or medial compression plates, or a Y plate (Fig. 19–3).

Selection of the surgical approach is based largely on the amount of scarring of the soft tissues from previous surgery and the amount of dissection needed to expose the distal humerus.[7, 8] For gross deformity of the distal fragments a transolecranon approach is reasonable. For proximal lesions, medial or lateral reflection of the triceps may be the optimal approach. In the Mayo series, the posterolateral triceps reflection approach of Kocher[7] was utilized in 11 patients, the Campbell posterior triceps-splitting technique in 9, the Mayo posterior approach in 9,[9] and the transolecranon approach, popularized by Cassebaum, in 3.[10]

The major fracture fragments are exposed, and the fragments are freshened, removing sclerosed bone and fibrous tissue. In achieving reduction an attempt must be made to restore angulation to maintain the proper alignment of the condyles with the shaft in the anterior, posterior, and mediolateral planes. Ideally, the axis of rotation should be along a line extending from the anterior cortex of the distal humerus.[18] Regardless of the fixation device, the distal humeral fossa must not be obliterated.

In the Mayo Clinic experience, *supracondylar nonunion* was the most frequent type of nonunion (Fig. 19–1), and this was most commonly treated by either a Y or a compression plate with autogenous iliac bone grafting (Fig. 19–4). Moreover, in four supracondylar fractures an external fixator was necessary to obtain rigid stabilization because of poor bone stock due to osteoporosis or previous internal fixation (Fig. 19–5).

The *transcondylar nonunion* is usually too distal for plate or external fixation techniques, but crossed compression lag screws with bone grafting are usually effective. If periarticular

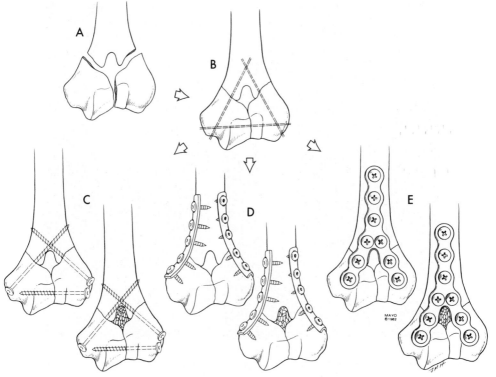

Figure 19–3. Techniques of internal fixation of T-condylar fractures.

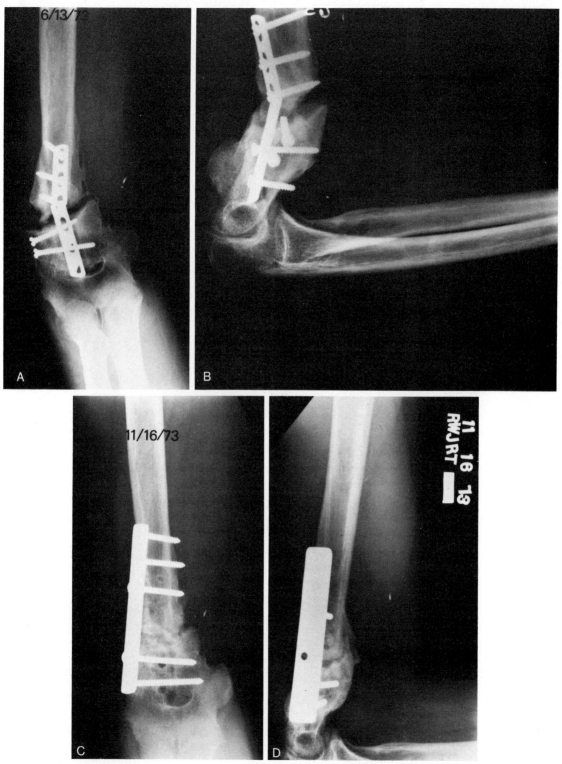

Figure 19–4. *A, B,* 24-year-old man with a 2-year-old supracondylar nonunion that had been treated previously with three failed surgical procedures. *C, D,* Radiographs 5 months after application of compression plate and bone grafting show solid union but also residual posterior position of the articular surface referable to the humeral shaft.

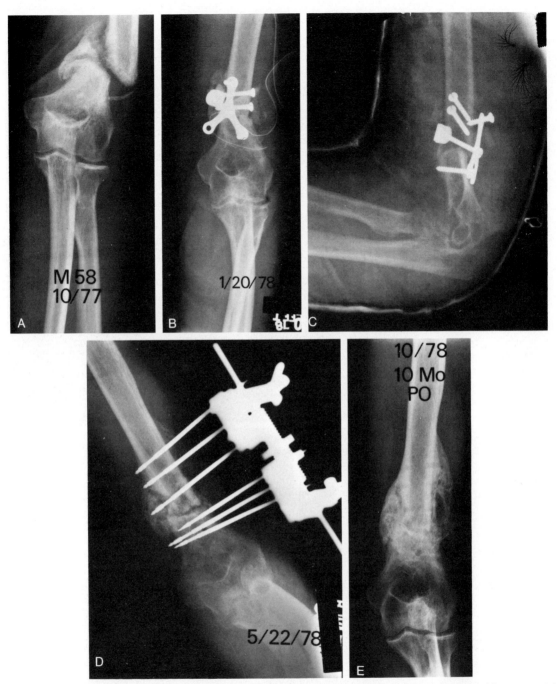

Figure 19–5. A, Anteroposterior roentgenogram of the elbow of a 58-year-old man with a 6-month old supracondylar nonunion. B, C, Initial Y plate fixation was inadequate. D, Revision with a Hoffman external fixator and bone graft. E, Healing was complete at 10 months following the initial operation. (From Mitsunaga, M., et al.: Condylar nonunions of the elbow. J. Trauma 22:787, 1982. © 1982, The Williams & Wilkins Co., Baltimore.)

soft tissue contraction is not extensive, the prognosis is better in these fractures because there is no disruption of the intercondylar articular surface (Fig. 19–6).

Lateral or medial condylar nonunions are best treated by transfixing compression screws to the remaining bone stock and bone

grafting. Solid screw fixation usually allows early motion and restores the articular contour (Fig. 19–7). If the fracture is neglected or badly displaced, osteotomy[16] or artificial joint replacement surgery (see Chapter 18) is required.

T condylar nonunions present the most

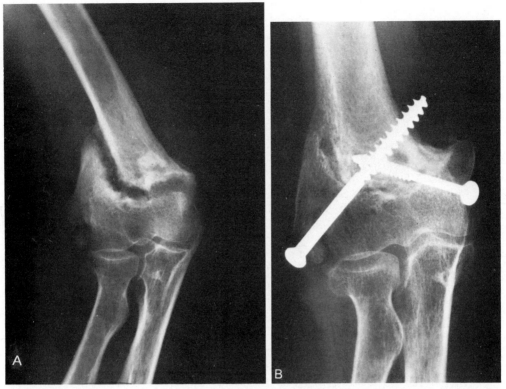

Figure 19–6. *A*, 45-year-old woman with 4-month-old transcondylar fracture with gross motion at the fracture site. *B*, Five months after a lag screw fixation across the fracture site the fracture has united.

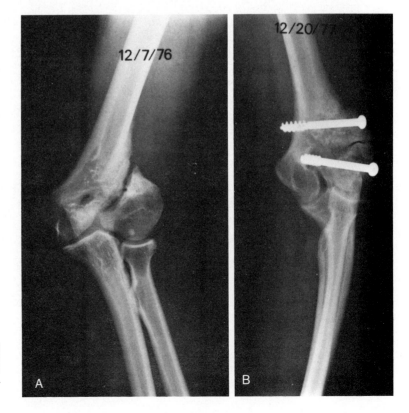

Figure 19–7. *A*, 24-year-old man with established nonunion of the lateral condyle. A solid union occurred 1 year following the use of a compression cancellous screw (*B*).

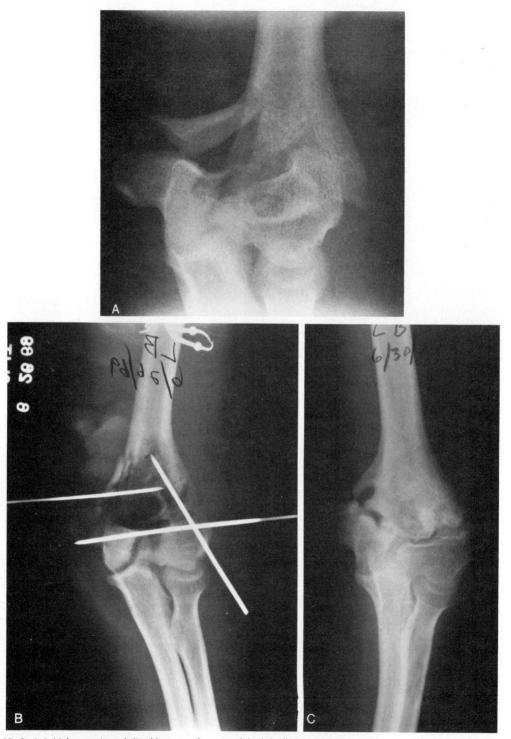

Figure 19–8. *A,* Initial comminuted distal humerus fracture of the left elbow of a 21-year-old male. Although initially anatomic reduction was achieved, inadequate Kirschner wire fixation was used with cast immobilization (*B*). *C,* One year following inadequate fixation painful nonunion occurred.

Illustration continued on opposite page

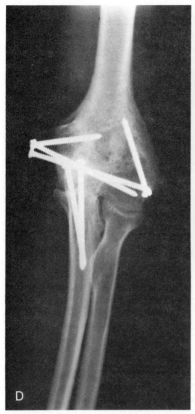

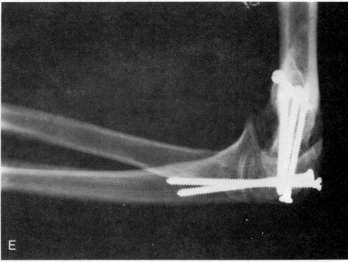

Figure 19–8 *Continued. D, E,* At 19 months' follow-up there is solid union following cross-screw technique and bone grafting using the transolecranon posterior exposure.

difficult problems of management because of the intra-articular component. The joint surface of the condyles must be accurately reduced to avoid incongruity, which limits motion. This is difficult because of the fragment rotation that is often present in the anteroposterior as well as in the sagittal plane (see Chapter 18). When there is a bony defect in the intercondylar area after the fixation is achieved, cancellous autogenous bone grafts are sometimes used to fill the defect. Once the condyles are reduced and stabilized with a transverse mediolateral screw as described by Bickel and Perry,[4] the condylar fragments are then transfixed to the supracondylar segment of the distal humerus (Fig. 19–8). If the medial or lateral epicondylar ridge has been fractured, forming a separate piece, these must be accurately reattached to the proximal fragment with a proximally directed screw to reestablish the buttress to which the condyles are attached. Following reduction of the fracture fragments and restoration of the articular surface with secure fixation of the condylar fragments, rigid proximal fixation may be achieved utilizing a Y type of plate (Fig. 19–9) or dual compression plates along both medial and lateral supracondylar ridges. The fracture lines are packed with autogenous iliac bone

grafts, and the wound is closed over a suction drain.

Postoperative Management

Postoperative management of the elbow depends on the stability of fixation achieved at surgery. In supracondylar or isolated lateral-medial condylar nonunions, solid fixation with compression plates and compression lag screws allows early active elbow motion within the first 10 days following surgery if there are no wound problems and swelling is minimal. In intra-articular T condylar nonunions and when fixation is suboptimal because of osteoporosis and multiple previous surgical procedures, active elbow motion is best delayed for 3 weeks. When wound healing has occurred and when swelling and pain are diminished, active elbow motion may begin, supplemented by a hinged splint if necessary (see Chapter 9).

Results

Although much has been written about open or closed treatment of acute fractures, there is no clear documentation of the relationship between the initial treatment and a failed

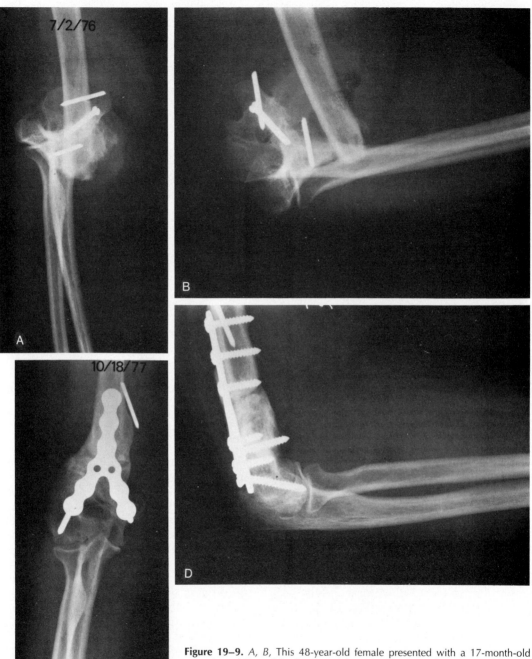

Figure 19–9. *A, B,* This 48-year-old female presented with a 17-month-old comminuted T-condylar fracture of the right elbow. Inadequate initial fixation using Kirschner wires and Steinmann pins resulted in gross instability, pain, and elbow motion of only 35 to 60 degrees of flexion. Fifteen months following fixation with a Y plate and bone graft, solid union was achieved. Because of rigid fixation, casting was not necessary, and elbow motion now ranges from 45 to 145 degrees of flexion (*C* and *D*).

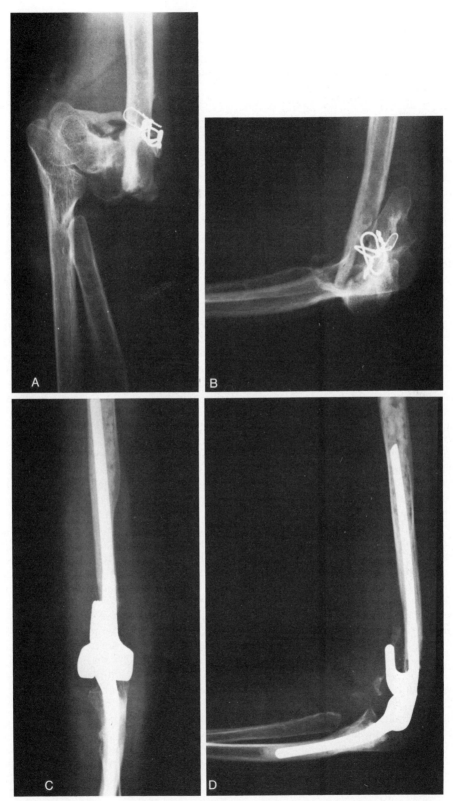

Figure 19–10. *A, B,* Nonunion of supracondylar fracture with a 2-year history of painful limited motion in 60-year-old woman. *C, D,* Two years after total elbow arthroplasty, the patient has 40 to 130 degrees of painless motion.

union.[4, 6, 7, 12, 15, 21] In the Mayo series of 32 nonunions, 19 fractures had been initially treated open and 13 had been treated closed. Of those fractures that were initially fixed operatively, material failure of the internal fixation occurred in 11. Moreover, we have found no reference discussing the management or results of these problem cases.

Mitsunaga et al. reviewed the Mayo experience with 32 patients, of whom 25 were treated with open reduction and internal fixation of the nonunion and 7 with excision of the distal fragments and total elbow arthroplasty[17] (Fig. 19–10). Of the patients with a total elbow arthroplasty Coonrad devices were used in six and a Pritchard-Walker device in one. This group of patients was older (mean, 60 years) than that undergoing osteosynthesis (mean, 43 years). Moreover, the nonunions in the group with joint replacement had persisted longer (average, 5.7 years) than those in the group treated with open reduction and fixation (average, 2.1 years). Of the 25 patients who had nonunions treated with open reduction and fixation, 22 achieved union after an average period of 7.7 months. However, 6 of the 22 patients required a second or third operation before union occurred at an average of 12 months after the first procedure. In two of the three patients in whom union did not occur, the failure was related to infection. Of the 22 patients that achieved osteosynthesis after surgery, the overall motion averaged 71 degrees, representing a gain of 9 degrees from the preoperative examination. In the group with total elbow arthroplasty, motion averaged only 74 degrees before operation and 103 degrees after surgery, a gain of 29 degrees.

Postoperatively, 14 of the 22 (64 percent) who had open reduction and internal fixation had no symptoms or mild residual symptoms, whereas 6 of the 7 patients (85 percent) who had total elbow arthroplasty had no symptoms or mild symptoms.

Complications

Eight patients had complications. Two patients with open reduction and fixation had infection, and both developed persistent painful nonunions. Three patients had postoperative radial nerve injuries; one of these had a Hoffman external fixator, one had a compression plate, and the other underwent a prosthetic elbow replacement. In addition, two patients in the total elbow arthroplasty group had loosening of the humeral components and required revision, and one other patient in this group had significant heterotrophic bone formation.

MALUNION

There is a paucity of information in the literature on the treatment of elbow malunion. In 1938 Tyler reported the 15-year result of treatment of a malunion.[22] Supracondylar malunions in children with either a cubitus varus or valgus deformity or malunion occurring after a Milch type II condylar fracture[16] most commonly come to osteotomy (see Chapters 12 and 18).

Assessment of malunion of the distal humerus must be predicated on the goals attainable with corrective surgery. For a functional arc of motion, flexion is more desirable than extension. Alteration in the varus-valgus angle or the carrying angle, is usually primarily of cosmetic interest. However, tardy ulnar nerve palsy seen with severe valgus angulation or after lateral condylar displacement is a consideration with this particular deformity. Intra-articular osteotomy may rarely be considered when the patient is seen early and secondary arthritis is not yet present. Preoperative evaluation should include biplanar radiographs and tomograms to assess the intra-articular malunion. More recently, computed tomography has been helpful in assessing the position of the intra-articular malunion.

Osteotomy to restore the distal humeral alignment to provide a more useful arc of motion is a legitimate indication for surgery. However, when the malunion is of long duration, secondary post-traumatic arthritis may preclude this treatment. If arthritis is present it is probably best to defer osteotomy and consider some form of arthroplasty depending on the age of the patient (see Chapters 32, 33, and 34).

The technique of correcting a malunion with wedge osteotomy has been described previously by French[13] and Amspacher and Messenbaugh.[1] It is emphasized that corrective osteotomy should be performed in patients with a reasonably normal joint articulation. For malunion of the medial or lateral condyle, Milch has demonstrated a complex osteotomy to restore function (Chapter 18). The radial head may be sacrificed on occasion to attain forearm rotation in association with supracondylar osteotomy, but as a rule combined procedures should be avoided and a staged approach used instead. Rigid fixation is desirable just as with nonunion, and early motion is usually recommended. These prin-

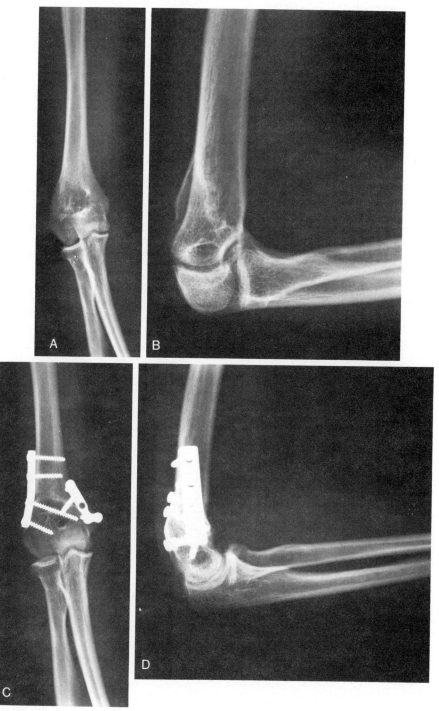

Figure 19–11. *A,* 25-year-old woman who had sustained a supracondylar fracture 13 years previously developed a gun stock deformity that was obvious clinically. *B,* The most significant feature was an inability to flex past 90 degrees owing to the posterior rotation of the articular surface. A biplanar osteotomy was performed using a small plate medially to serve as a hinge. *C,* The osteotomy was closed laterally. *D,* In order to attain functional motion, the articular surface was rotated anteriorly. Notice that the anterior border of the distal humerus transects the midportion of the trochlea, indicating that the axis of rotation of the ulnohumeral joint has been restored to normal. The postoperative range of motion was from 20 to 140 degrees. The osteotomy healed in 3 months.

ciples were carried out in a 25-year-old woman who had sustained a supracondylar fracture 13 years previously (Fig. 19–11).

SUMMARY

Nonunion and malunion of the distal humerus cause significant disability due to pain and elbow dysfunction. In nonunions reconstructive joint salvage and bony union can be achieved with rigid fixation and bone grafting, and this is usually the preferred method of treatment in patients less than 60 years of age with a reasonably normal joint articulation. Union of these fractures usually achieves relief of pain and good functional motion of the elbow. A variety of fixation devices and techniques can be used depending on the type of articular nonunion and the amount and quality of the remaining bone. We consider total elbow arthroplasty a salvage procedure and reserve it for older, less active patients. With improved devices and surgical technique, this option may become more viable in time (see Chapter 34). Distraction arthroplasty may also prove helpful in younger patients.

Acknowledgement

The author wishes to express appreciation to Dr. Morris Mitsunaga (Honolulu, Hawaii) for use of the cases in his study[17] and his assistance in preparation of the manuscript.

References

1. Amspacher, J. C., and Messenbaugh, J. R.: Supracondylar Osteotomy of the Humerus for Correction of Rotational and Angular Deformities of the Elbow. South. Med. J. **57**:846, 1964.
2. Anderson, L. D.: Fractures. In Campbell's Operative Orthopedics, Vol. 1. St. Louis, C. V. Mosby Co., 1977.
3. Bassett, C. A., Mitchell, S. N., Norton, L., Caulo, N., and Gaston, S. R.: Electromagnetic Repairs of Nonunions. In Brighton, C. T., Black, J., and Pollack, S. R. (Eds): Electrical Properties of Bone and Cartilage. Experimental Effects and Clinical Applications. New York, Grune & Stratton, 1979, pp. 605–630.
4. Bickel, W. E., and Perry, P. E.: Comminuted Fractures of the Distal Humerus. J.A.M.A. **184**:553, 1963.
5. Brighton, C. T.: Current Concepts Review: The Treatment of Nonunions with Electricity. J. Bone Joint Surg. **63A**:5, 1981.
6. Brown, R. F., and Morgan, R. G.: Intra-Condylar "T" T-shaped Fractures of the Humerus. J. Bone Joint Surg. **53B**:425, 1971.
7. Bryan, R. S.: Fractures About the Elbow. In American Academy of Orthopedic Surgeons: Instructional Course Lectures, Vol. 38. St. Louis, The C. V. Mosby Co., pp. 200–223.
8. Bryan, R. S., and Bickel, W. H.: "T" Condylar Fractures of the Distal Humerus. J. Trauma **11**:830, 1971.
9. Bryan, R. S., and Morrey, B. F.: Extensive Posterior Exposure of the Elbow: A Triceps Sparing Approach. Clin. Orthop. **166**:188, 1982.
10. Cassebaum, W. H.: Open Reduction of "T" and Y Fractures of the Lower End of the Humerus. J. Trauma **9**:915, 1969.
11. Ewald, F.: Distraction Arthroplasty. In American Academy of Orthopedic Surgeons: Instructional Course Lectures, Atlanta, February, 1984.
12. Horne, G.: Supracondylar Fractures of the Humerus in Adults. J. Trauma **20**:71, 1980.
13. French, P. R.: Varus Deformity of the Elbow Following Supracondylar Fractures of the Humerus in Children. Lancet **1**:439, 1959.
14. Knight, R. A.: The Management of Fractures About the Elbow in Adults. American Academy of Orthopedic Surgeons: Instructional Course Lectures, Vol. 14. St. Louis, The C. V. Mosby Co., 1957, pp. 123–141.
15. Lecestre, P.: Roundtable: Fractures of the Lower End of the Humerus. Orthop. Trans. **4**:123, 1980.
16. Milch, H.: Fractures and Fracture Dislocations of the Humeral Condyles. J. Trauma **4**:592, 1964.
17. Mitsunaga, M. S., Bryan, R. S., and Linscheid, R. L.: Condylar Nonunions of the Elbow. J. Trauma **22**:787, 1982.
18. Morrey, B. F., and Chao, E. Y.: Passive Motion of the Elbow Joint. J. Bone Joint Surg. **58A**:501, 1976.
19. Okhotsky, V. T., and Souvalyana, G.: The Treatment of Nonunion and Pseudarthrosis of Long Bones with Thick Nails. Injury **10**:92, 1978.
20. Smith, F. M.: An 84-Year Follow-up on a Patient with Ununited Fracture of the Lateral Condyle of the Humerus. J. Bone Joint Surg. **55A**:378, 1973.
21. Solheim, K., and Daagev, F.: Delayed Union and Nonunion of Fractures: Clinical Experience with the ASIF Method. J. Trauma **13**:121, 1973.
22. Tyler, G. T.: Malunion in Supracondylar Fracture of Humerus. Result 15 Years After Operation. Am. J. Surg. **39**:652, 1938.
23. Wilson, P. D.: Fractures and Dislocations in the Region of the Elbow. Surg. Gynecol. Obstet. **56**:335, 1933.
24. Wood, A. M., Calandruccio, R. A., Brighton, C., Wyman, E., and Dassetta, L.: Incidence of Fractures and Fracture Nonunion: United States. Orthop. Trans. **5**:441, 1981.

CHAPTER 20

Radial Head Fracture

B. F. MORREY

Historical Review

The history of the radial head fracture has been well summarized by Schwartz and Young.[88] The first description was probably made by Paul of Aegina (625–690 A.D.) "The ulna and radius are sometimes fractured together and sometimes one of them only, either in the middle or at one end as at the elbow or the wrist."[2] Early difficulty in making the diagnosis was encountered because of "thick muscle covering."[29, 78] Sir Astley Cooper (1844) stated that he never saw this fracture.[25] The variable and often disappointing results were noted as early as 1897 by Helferich, who recommended resection of the radial head for late deformity.[45]

Three to four weeks of immobilization,[101] passive motion, avoidance of "operative interference,"[41] removal of the fracture fragment,[82] and excision of the entire head for severe comminution[47] were all recommended in the early 1900s. Other pertinent contributions include a classification by Cutler[27] and the suggestion that surgery is not a matter of *election* but rather of *selection*.[47] Although much has subsequently been written about this fracture, the controversy about treatment is far from over.

Incidence

The frequency of radial head and neck fracture has been variously reported as 1.7 to 5.4 percent of all fractures. [24, 51, 72] Radial head fractures occur in about 17 to 19 percent of elbow trauma[106, 109] and account for about 33 percent of elbow fractures.[64]

Age and Sex

Fracture of the proximal end of the radius occurs at any age. In general, about 15 to 20 percent of these fractures involve the neck,[72, 101] usually in children in whom the physis has not closed.[9] Approximately 85 percent of fractures occur in persons between 20 and 60 years of age,[18, 24] with a mean age of 30[19, 27, 44] to 40 years.[51] The fracture tends to occur more frequently in females in a ratio of approximately 2:1.[4, 19, 51]

MECHANISM OF FRACTURE

The experimental work of Thomas clearly demonstrated that an axial load on the pronated forearm consistently produces a fracture of the radial head similar to that seen in clinical experience (Fig. 20–1).[101] Odelberg observed precisely the same effect, noting that the fracture (1) occurred with posterior subluxation of the "forearm as far as the ligaments allowed," and (2) involved the most anterior portion of the radial head when the forearm was pronated.[77] Because the head of the radius is eccentric to the central axis of the neck,[93] the posterior-lateral aspect of the radial head comes into intimate contact with the capitellum during pronation. Further, this part of the radial head lacks subchondral bone and is therefore weaker. The common occurrence of an anterior-lateral fracture fragment supports this theory.[27, 30, 51] The possibility of an associated valgus stress component in some instances[50] is supported by the occasional medial collateral ligament injury, but this does not appear to be the primary mechanism of fracture. A direct blow is another uncommon cause of this fracture.[27, 37]

CLASSIFICATION

The most commonly used classification of this fracture is that proposed by Mason and consists of three types:
    Type I: undisplaced
    Type II: displaced (often a single fragment)
    Type III: comminuted
Because elbow dislocation occurs in about 10 percent of all radial head fractures and implies different treatment and prognostic features,[11] we feel that this injury should be considered a type IV injury (Fig. 20–2).

Radial neck fracture may be either included in this scheme[50] or placed in a separate category.[19, 27] More complex subclassifications

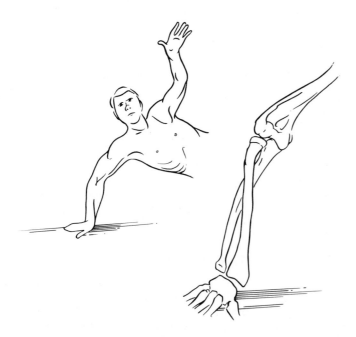

Figure 20–1. Mechanism of injury of most radial head fractures is a fall on the outstretched hand with the elbow partially flexed and supinated. A variable amount of valgus force accounts for the associated injuries that are occasionally seen.

based on different degrees of displacement of comminution have also been proposed.[72, 80, 94] We feel that these systems are of little value because excessive detail can be cumbersome. As with most classifications, there may be some difficulty in distinguishing between fracture types. The most vexing question is what percentage of involvement of the radial head or what degree of displacement should constitute the type II fracture.

ASSOCIATED INJURIES

Associated injuries to the neurovascular, muscular, osseous, and ligamentous structures play a significant role in the management and prognosis of this fracture.

Other Fractures

Fracture of the olecranon and radial head has been analyzed in detail by Scharplatz et al.,

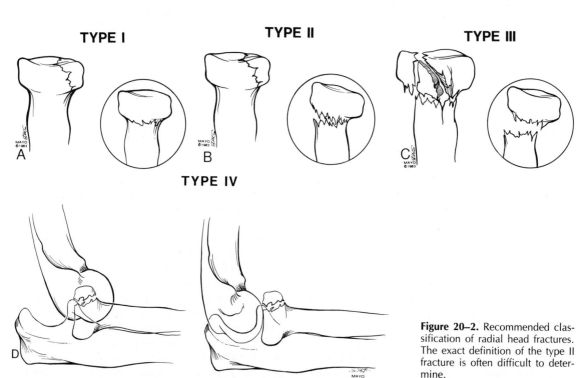

TYPE I

TYPE II

TYPE III

TYPE IV

Figure 20–2. Recommended classification of radial head fractures. The exact definition of the type II fracture is often difficult to determine.

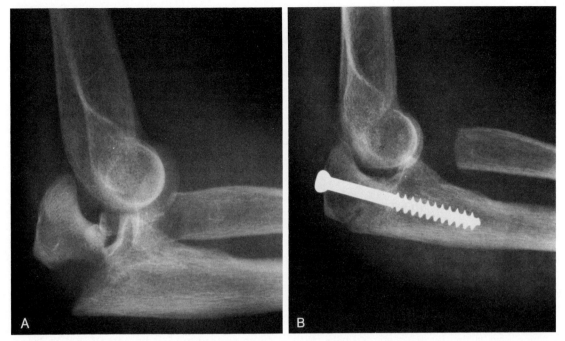

Figure 20–3. *A,* A Monteggia fracture involving the proximal ulna as well as a radial head fracture. *B,* Perfect reduction of the proximal ulna is necessary to allow the proximal radius to maintain its alignment.

who concluded that the mechanism of this complex injury is that of a transverse or lateral force probably combined with an axial load;[85] it may be considered a Monteggia variant and should be so managed (Fig. 20–3).

Fractures of the coronoid suggest a type IV injury. If the fragment is large, significant elbow instability may occur.[42] Fractures or cartilage injuries of the capitellum are common,[84, 105] although not always appreciated. Violence to the capitellum can cause adhesions and may result in painful limitation of motion even when the radiograph is reasonably normal.

Ligamentous Injury at the Elbow

Although some degree of ligamentous injury may well occur with many radial head fractures, this association may not be fully appreciated.[44, 48, 50, 77, 105] Wagner, in 1955, observed 24 patients with calcification in the medial collateral ligament,[104] and Arner et al. described a 12 percent incidence of ulnar collateral ligament calcification in 1957.[4] Arvidsson et al. found ligament or capsular disruption by arthrogram with various types of radial head fractures.[5] Johansson demonstrated positive arthrograms in 4 percent of type I, 21 percent of type II, and 85 percent of type III injuries.[50]

The experimental data suggest that an increased carrying angle, occasionally observed

after radial head fractures,[18, 72, 87, 88, 99, 100] is probably associated with an incompetent or at least a stretched ulnar collateral ligament (see Chapter 3). Finally, a ligamentous injury sustained at the distal radioulnar joint at the time of the radial head fracture[14, 26, 33, 91] is uncommon but important in respect to the treatment and prognosis and is discussed in detail below.

Neurovascular Complications

The uncomplicated fracture of the radial head is rarely associated with any neurovascular symptoms. If a type IV injury is present, vascular injury may occur rarely, as discussed in Chapter 17. Alteration of the local vascular structures about the elbow has been postulated as an explanation for the unpredictable but frequent occurrence of stiffness following radial head fracture.[74] There are really no data, however, to substantiate this thesis.

Muscular Injury

By definition the type IV injury must violate the brachialis muscle (Fig. 20–4), and this factor is thought to be an important variable in the development of myositis ossificans.[60, 102] The significance and management of this complication are discussed later in this chapter as well as in Chapter 26.

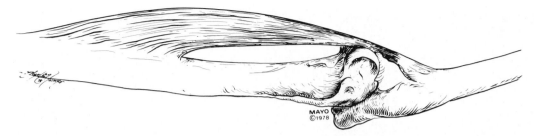

Figure 20–4. The brachialis muscle is in intimate contact with the anterior capsule and crosses the joint more as muscular than as tendinous tissue, thus making it vulnerable to injury with type IV fracture-dislocations.

FRACTURE MANAGEMENT

Most clinicians have personally experienced disappointment with the treatment of this fracture, as evident by the following remarks:

> The fracture of the head of the radius is a serious injury, and while the prognosis is good for recovery of a useful elbow, rarely is it a normal elbow.[106]

> In none of these cases should a too optimistic prognosis be given, for traumatic arthritis with painful restricted rotation may follow an apparently minor injury with or without displacement, regardless of treatment.[32]

In general, the treatment of radial head fractures is based on the fracture type and the presence of any associated injury.

Undisplaced Fracture—Type I

There is little question that the type I fracture (Fig. 20–5), because of its good prognosis and lack of concurrent soft tissue or other osseous injury, should be managed without surgery.

Treatment

The recommended period of immobilization is 2 to 3 weeks,[6, 40, 72] but a longer period has been recommended by some[19, 30, 44, 83, 101] to allow the soft tissues to heal and to avoid the possibility of displacement. Early motion is probably the more popular current practice,[1, 4, 6, 19, 21, 38, 48, 80, 105] although the precise temporal definition is not always clear. To facilitate immediate motion, a concept long

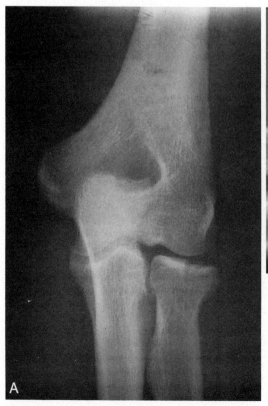

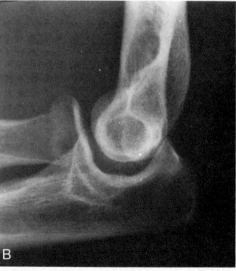

Figure 20–5. A, Type I fracture involving approximately 50 percent of the head but with less than 2 mm displacement. B, Minimally angulated neck fracture is also considered a type I fracture.

advocated by Dehna and Torp,[28] aspiration of the joint is recommended by some[21, 79, 81] even without specific protection after operation.[74]

Results

Although the ultimate result may be independent of the treatment program, early mo-

tion compared with prolonged immobilization does appear to offer advantages of early return of function. Mason and Schutkin, reporting a military experience, found a mean period of disability of 4 weeks in 18 patients treated with early motion compared with 7 weeks of disability in 7 individuals treated

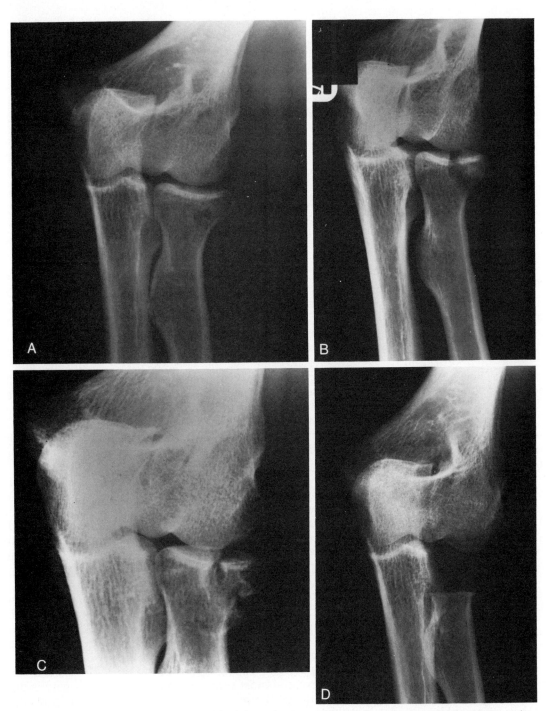

Figure 20–6. *A,* Type I undisplaced fracture of the left nondominant extremity in a 49-year-old male. Treatment by early motion as tolerated resulted in displacement of the fragment *(B),* which went on to a nonunion *(C). D,* Treatment by late excision of the radial head 4 months after the fracture decreased the pain and improved pronation and supination 6 months after the procedure. (Courtesy of E. T. O'Brien, San Antonio, Texas.)

with 3 weeks of immobilization.[63] The major residua is loss of extension rather than pain.[27] Adler reports 23 excellent and 3 good results in 26 patients treated with early motion.[1] No poor results among 79 patients were reported by Gaston et al.[38] or in 55 patients reported by Johnson[51] when treated by early motion. In spite of these optimistic accounts this fracture may be associated with an inexplicable poor outcome, in 5[6, 80] to 13 percent of patients.[83] Mason reported that about one third of his 62 patients with this fracture lost an average of 7 degrees of extension.[64] Displacement following early motion was implicated as a factor in some of these treatment failures (Fig. 20–6), and this may occur more often than is appreciated.

Displaced Fracture Fragment—Type II

Most of the controversy dealing with radial head fractures is focused on the proper management of type II fractures. A large part of the problem results from the lack of a clear definition of what constitutes this type of fracture.

Nonoperative Treatment

Nonoperative treatment for this fracture is similar to that described for the type I fracture—that is, early motion as tolerated, but if displacement is considered possible, 2 to 3 weeks of immobilization is recommended. Some clinicians have treated a majority of type II fractures with nonoperative methods.[1, 6] Because of the rather broad spectrum of pathology that may exist even within this one fracture type, the surgeon may elect to employ a nonoperative program varying from a few days[1] to 3 to 4 weeks of immobilization (Fig. 20–7).[19, 51, 64, 83] The spectrum of possibilities is presented by Paulson and Tophoj. They reported that among 23 fractures,[80] nine (39 percent) were treated without the use of plaster and with early motion, six (26 percent) were managed with 1 to 2 weeks of immobilization, six (26 percent) were treated with 2 to 3 weeks of immobilization, and two (9 percent) were immobilized for more than 4 weeks.

Operative Treatment

Four surgical treatment options have been recommended for the management of type I fractures. In uncomplicated fractures, excision of the fracture fragment or the entire radial head or open reduction with internal fixation may be considered. The fourth option, prosthetic replacement, is usually re-

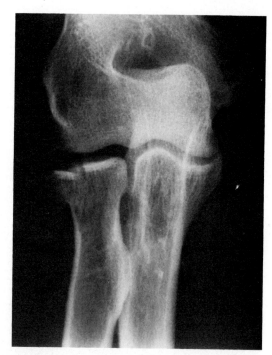

Figure 20–7. Type II fracture treated by early motion. Produced a satisfactory result.

served in our practice for individuals with associated injuries related to instability after the radial head has been excised.

Fracture Fragment Excision. In the early literature, simple excision of the fragment was recommended for limitation of pronation or supination (Fig. 20–8).[40, 41, 89] In the largest study of partial excisions, 82 percent of 33 patients had a satisfactory result.[18] In general, however, simple excision of the displaced fracture fragment is not advocated and is strongly discouraged by some.[21, 72, 104, 105] Obviously, patient selection is an important part of this type of treatment.

Excision of the Radial Head. Radial head excision is a most controversial topic; for example, "when in doubt, resect,"[64, 68] or "when in doubt, leave alone."[21, 51, 80] Indications for surgical excision generally include significant displacement (2 to 3 mm) of at least one large fragment (<30 percent) or several smaller fragments comprising a large (30 to 50 percent) portion of the radial head with considerable forearm rotation (40 degrees) or extension loss (30 degrees) due to impingement of the fracture fragments.[8, 51, 53, 64, 72, 92, 104]

Timing. If resection is to be carried out, most surgeons agree that early surgery is preferable.[53, 72] According to some, the procedure should be performed in the first 24 hours[15, 20, 38, 51] at least within the first 7 to 10 days.[18, 30, 48, 64, 106] Charnley recommends exci-

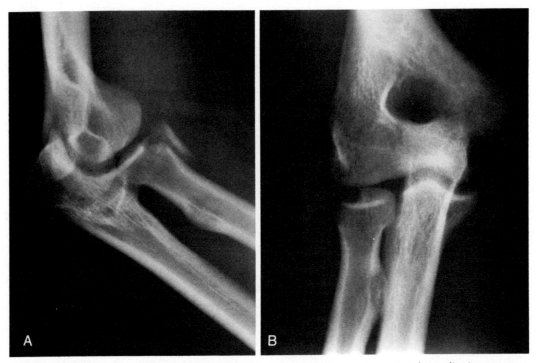

Figure 20–8. A, Type II fracture treated by simple fragment excision (B). Because no associated complication was present, a good result was obtained.

sion after about 2 weeks if displacement or loss of motion has occurred.[21] Some prefer to delay surgery for at least one month to allow the acute trauma to heal.[56] Others have assumed the rather agnostic position that the timing of excision is less important than other factors.[1, 4, 13]

Techniques. Although an anterior[4, 89] or anterior-lateral[48, 104] approach has been recommended, the safer Kocher incision between the anconeus and the extensor carpi ulnaris is the most frequently used exposure of the radiocapitellar joint.

Surgical technique is rather straightforward (Chapter 8), but certain aspects are worthy of emphasis. (1) All fragments should be removed and reassembled to ensure that no fracture fragments have been left behind. (2) A Gili saw can spread bone in the soft tissues,[91] so a sharp, oscillating saw is probably the most frequently employed technique today. Care must be taken to remove the bone dust. (3) An axial load is exerted on the radius at the wrist after the head is removed to assess distal radioulnar stability. We place Gel-Foam between the proximal radius and the capitellum to try to eliminate adhesion formation as well. (4) An attempt is made to restore the integrity of the radiocollateral ligament and accessory ligaments when closing the wound to avoid late instability.

Probably the most controversial feature of the surgical technique is the amount of bone removed. A generous resection to ensure adequate forearm rotation has been suggested[18, 30, 38, 47, 92] even to the level of the radial tuberosity[13] (Fig. 20–9), but removal of the radial head at the level of the annular ligament[92, 104] is most frequently recommended today. The only study found to support either position was presented by Carstam, who showed that with 14 proximal resections, five good, six fair, and three poor results were obtained.[18] In contrast, one excellent, five good, one fair, and one poor result were observed after eight more extensive excisions of the head and neck. We do not feel that these data are adequate to support the recommendation of a more generous resection; in practice, the level of the fracture will often dictate the level of the resection.

Postoperative Care. Postoperative management consists of immobilization in 90 degrees of flexion and in neutral rotation. Motion is begun as soon as it can be done comfortably or as determined by associated injuries, ideally less than 5 and usually less than 10 days.

Results

The results of nonoperative treatment have been very good. Conn and Wade described "excellent motion and no deformity" in 61 of

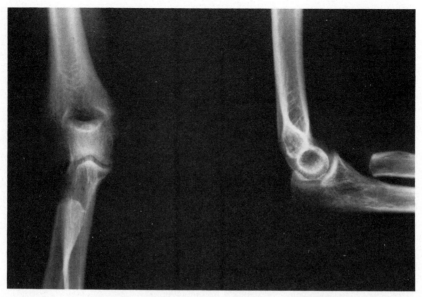

Figure 20–9. Excessive bone removed at the time of fracture. Residual pain at the elbow is a difficult problem to manage without the presence of adequate bone stock. No currently available prosthesis is adequate in this setting.

63 type II fractures treated without surgery.[24] Additional reports of 85[51] to 95 percent[6, 80, 108] good results argue strongly in favor of this treatment modality.

When more than 25 percent of the radial head is involved, however, Mason reported that 9 of 15 had some pain an average of 11.5 years after injury and consequently advocated a more aggressive surgical approach.[64] More precise documentation of radial head excision of type II fractures suggest that this is a satisfactory option.[14, 24, 48, 106, 109] Gaston et al. reported excellent motion and minimal pain in 19 patients with resection less than 1 week after fracture, but 4 (21 percent) developed mild valgus laxity of about 5 degrees.[38] Carstam graded 26 patients an average of 8 years after surgery and found that 35 percent had perfect results, 19 percent had good, 31 percent fair, and 15 percent poor.[18] Better results were obtained if less displacement had occurred, but the size of the fracture fragment was felt to be unimportant.

A few studies have actually compared operative and nonoperative management of the type II fracture. Adler and Shaftan found roughly comparable short-term good results in 17 of 20 patients without surgery and in 13 of 18 undergoing resection.[1] Because selection factors had dictated the treatment choice, these two groups were not strictly comparable. Murray compared 30 nonoperative with 16 surgically treated cases.[72] Full motion was obtained in about 35 percent of both groups. Less than 10 degrees of motion loss was present in 16 percent of the conservatively

treated group and in 12 percent of the surgically treated group. The operatively treated patients included 5 with total excision and 11 with partial excision. The former group appeared to have slightly better results. The retrospective survey of Radin and Riseborough included 16 nonoperatively treated patients, 6 of whom were managed with early radial head excision.[83] The motion in these patients was "far greater" than that in the conservatively treated group, but if surgery was delayed, the success rate decreased. In addition, if the fracture involved more than two thirds of the radial head, those treated conservatively did poorly. In Burton's experience, only 2 of 9 nonoperatively treated patients had a good result compared with 22 of 25 after excision of the radial head.[14]

Wagner feels that an anatomic classification is unreliable for determining whether surgery is indicated and instead prefers to make treatment decisions based on the amount of motion present after the joint has been aspirated and injected with local anesthetic.[104] If a good range of motion without a catch or grating sound is present, a conservative course is followed. At 1 year, 31 of 42 (74 percent) of the nonoperatively treated patients had "normal" motion, and only 2 (5 percent) had 20 degrees loss of extension and 20 degrees loss of pronation and supination. Among the 24 surgically treated patients, 16 (67 percent) had full motion and 3 (12 percent) had loss of 20 degrees of extension, 20 degrees of pronation, and 20 degrees of supination.

To summarize, radial head excision is justified but not clearly superior to nonoperative treatment. The precise basis of selection remains unclear. Resection is generally recommended if the degree of involvement of the radial head is significant (30 percent) and the amount of displacement of the single or comminuted fracture fragments (2 to 3 mm) causes considerable (30 degrees) motion loss.

Type III (Comminuted) Fracture of the Radial Head

This fracture is generally associated with a more severe injury and hence a worse prognosis than fractures of types I and II. Capitellar involvement is common, and arthrography has demonstrated that up to 85 percent of these injuries have capsular or ligamentous disruption.[50] In addition, the degree of comminution is commonly more extensive than is suggested by the radiographic appearance (Fig. 20–10). [6, 21, 105]

Treatment

There is relatively uniform agreement that the comminuted radial head fracture is best

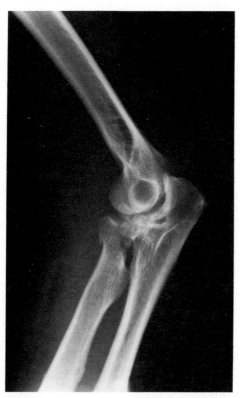

Figure 20–10. Type III fracture demonstrating comminution, which was more extensive at surgery than this radiograph suggests.

treated by complete excision,[4, 18, 19, 27, 30, 44, 47, 48, 51, 53, 64, 72, 109] which is preferred over simple removal of the more displaced fragments.[21, 72]

Early excision is more critical in this fracture than in the type II injury. [18, 19, 27, 30, 50, 64, 86] Yet, because of delayed changes at the wrist and an increased valgus angulation seen in a few patients, a more conservative attitude toward this fracture may be emerging.[103] Closed reduction with early motion can provide good results in comminuted type III fractures,[6] and if early motion is too painful or if motion limitation is unacceptable with this treatment, resection may be carried out at a later date.

Results

Because there is greater comminution in the type III fracture, less satisfactory results might be anticipated than after the type I or II injury. In Mason's 18 patients, extension loss averaged 25 degrees, pronation 15 degrees, and supination 15 degrees.[64] Return to work was observed in 17 of the 18 patients within 9.5 weeks. Yet Conn and Wade reported good results in 28 of 33 with simple excision.[24] Radin and Riseborough observed satisfactory results in six of seven patients that underwent early excision, but there was a poor outcome with nonoperative treatment or late excision.[83] The difference betwen objective and subjective results has been noted by Carstam who reported satisfactory subjective results in 85 percent but objective satisfactory results in only 55 percent.[18]

There have been few attempts to compare different treatments. Cutler reported that the early results of nonoperative treatment were better than those of operative treatment; however, at 1 year, the two groups were comparable.[27] Johnson presented five patients treated nonoperatively who had approximately 16 degrees of rotation loss and 5 degrees of extension loss.[51] The six undergoing surgery, on the other hand, had 10 degrees of extension loss but full pronation-supination. Arner et al. followed ten patients treated nonoperatively and found eight excellent, one good, and one fair result.[4] After radial head excision only 6 of 13 had a satisfactory outcome.

We have reported objective functional results in six patients undergoing radial head excision for type III fractures an average of 21 years after surgery.[69] The mean range of motion was 5 to 137 degrees of flexion-extension, 63 degrees of pronation, and 66 degrees supination. Losses of 12 percent of flexion strength, 8 percent of extension strength, 24

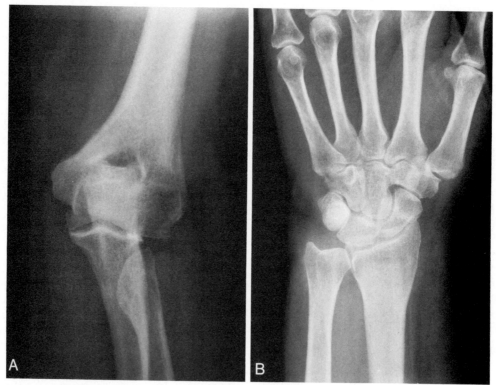

Figure 20–11. *A,* With long-term follow-up of 10 years, there is osteophyte formation at the ulnohumeral joint after radial head excision, but symptoms are mild. Patient had no wrist symptoms *(B).*

percent of pronation, 13 percent of supination, and 11 percent of grip strength were reported. The radiographic findings of these six patients revealed that five of the six had

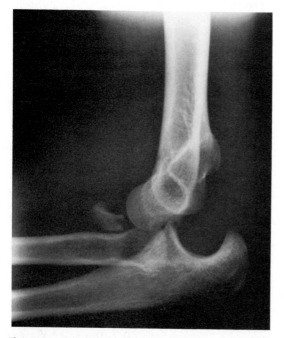

Figure 20–12. Fracture-dislocation of the radial head. This may be considered a type IV injury.

minimal and one had moderate degenerative changes at the ulnohumeral articulation. The disparity between the radiographic and clinical results was reported by Castberg and Thing, who observed that half of their patients had radiographic changes at the ulnohumeral joint (Fig. 20–11).[19]

Type IV (Fracture-Dislocation)

Elbow dislocation with radial head fracture is a rather common associated injury. A review of several series[1, 6, 18, 23, 38, 43, 51, 72, 109] reveals 119 elbow dislocations complicating 1459 fractures, an incidence of about 8 percent.

The inverse relationship—that is, a radial head fracture with elbow dislocation, averages about 12 percent.[23, 59, 73, 109] Simply stated, approximately 10 percent of those sustaining an elbow dislocation will have an associated radial head fracture, and similarly, about 10 percent of radial head fractures will be complicated by an elbow dislocation, that is, a type IV fracture. Most radial head fractures are displaced[44] type II or type III fractures (Fig. 20–12).[11]

Treatment

Treatment usually consists of an immediate reduction of the dislocation and treatment of the fractured radial head on its own merit. Some clinicians do not alter the treatment plan because of the dislocation.[1, 18] The most common tratment recommendation is early excision of the radial head to avoid the development of myositis ossificans. McLaughlin recommends immediate excision with a degree of urgency "to be measured in hours."[67] Even Adler, a rather staunch advocate of nonoperative management of radial head fracture, emphasizes that if surgery is necessary, it should be done within the first 24 hours.[1] After excision, immobilization of the elbow in the neutral position for 3 or 4 weeks has been recommended.[1, 24] This has been shown to be an excessively long period of immobilization, so we begin motion after about 1 week or sooner with a hinged splint.[11]

Results

More than half of all poor results associated with radial head fractures have been attributed to this type of fracture.[1] Flexion contracture of 15 to 30 degrees and 25 to 50 degrees of forearm rotation can be expected.[1, 43, 51] Early motion, beginning by the sixth day, has improved the outcome,[38] resulting in motion of 10 to 140 degrees of flexion in most patients. In our experience, no good outcome occurred if immobilization lasted for more than 4 weeks,[11] and early motion yielded results that were nearly as good as those achieved with uncomplicated fractures (Fig. 20–13).[11]

Delayed Excision of the Radial Head

One of the most striking features of the voluminous literature on fractures of the radial head is the absence of information on late excision. A distinction must be made between planned excision for displacement, the intentional delay of 5 or 6 weeks to allow the soft tissues to heal,[56, 16] and excision for treatment of established residual pain or loss of motion. Speed stated in 1941 that late excision is "of great help" but suggested that the results were not as good as those obtained by early surgery.[91] If delayed more than 6 weeks, surgical excision is said to give poor results.[95]

Delayed excision is reportedly more effective for relieving pain than for restoring motion[76] and should be done before arthritis has developed (Fig. 20–14).[53] We have observed both improved motion and pain relief after this procedure.[10]

Results

Cutler mentions four cases of late excision; he describes no specific results but recommends this treatment if the initial management fails.[27] Radin and Riseborough observed that all three individuals undergoing late excision of the radial head had a poor result,[83] and a similar experience was reported by Gaston.[38] In six individuals with late excision 3 months to 16 years after fracture, the range of motion averaged 5 to 100 degrees of flexion, 63 degrees of pronation, and 66 degrees of supination a mean of 20 years after surgery. Decrease in strength averaged 12 percent in flexion, 8 per cent in extension, 24 percent in pronation, 13 percent in supination, and 11 percent in grip strength.[69]

From the limited data available it appears that delayed excision of the radial head can be worthwhile in appropriately selected patients. In general, some improvement in flex-

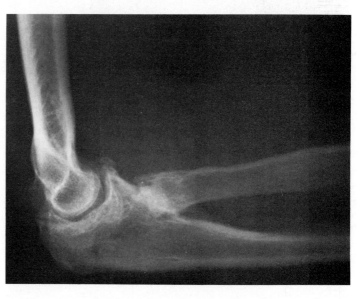

Figure 20–13. The comminuted radial head fracture was excised in a patient with elbow dislocation. The patient has a good result 15 years after surgery but has x-ray evidence of arthritis.

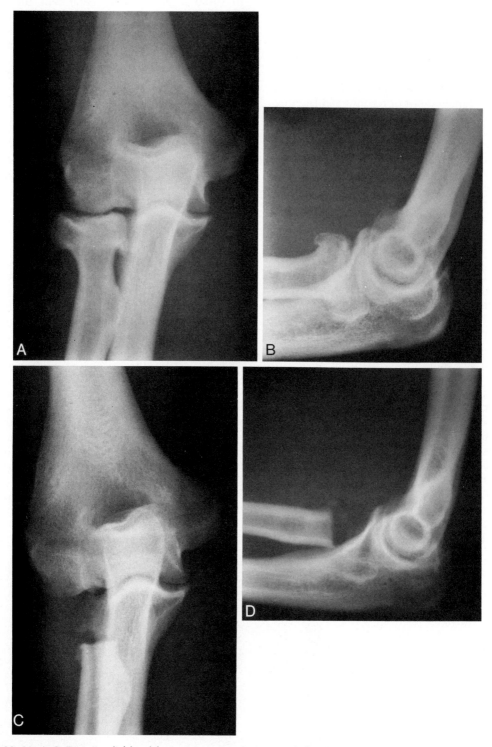

Figure 20–14. *A, B,* Type II radial head fracture was treated nonoperatively. *C, D,* Persistent pain and limitation of motion resulted in a delayed excision of the radial head. The patient appreciated a satisfactory result with less pain and 20 to 135 degrees of motion.

ion and forearm rotation and moderate relief of pain may reasonaably be expected.[10] If secondary arthrosis has intervened, the chances of a satisfactory result will be compromised.

COMPLICATIONS

Nonoperative Management

The most frequent complication of type I fracture is displacement of the fracture fragment (see Fig. 20–6). If this occurs, nonunion may ensue, and delayed excision of the entire head must be considered. Late excision of the displaced fragment alone is of little value.

Complications occurring with the nonoperatively managed type II or type III fracture include residual pain and motion loss. Proximal radial migration may occur even in this group, as observed in 3 of 48 instances reported by Radin and Riseborough.[83] The radiographic findings usually are those of a deformed radial head without subsequent arthrosis, lack of heterotopic bone, and a striking lack of correlation with the clinical results.[19]

Surgical Excision

Several significant complications are associated with radial head excision.

Symptoms at the Wrist

Pain at the wrist is common if a concurrent disruption of the distal radioulnar joint has occurred. This uncommon injury was first reported in two patients by Brockman[12] in 1930 and later by Speed[91] and Curr and Coe.[26] In 1951 two additional cases were described by Essex-Lopresti,[33] and the injury has subsequently been associated with him. Given the frequency of radial head fracture and the relatively rare reports of concurrent wrist injury, this condition is uncommon, probably occurring in about 1 to 2 percent of fractures.[57]

Concurrent wrist injury is not to be confused with the delayed process that occurs after radial head excision (Fig. 20–15).[34, 58] In a carefully studied series of 94 cases, McDougall and White demonstrated that proximal radial migration ranging from 1 to 5 mm was present in 25 percent.[66] Only about one half of these patients had symptoms. If such migration occurs, it usually does so within the first or second year after excision, but late symptoms have been reported.[18, 46] Many investigators have noted an increase of 2 to 3 mm in proximal radial migration with a frequency of 8,[18] 12,[6] 27,[57] and even 54 percent.[100] Symptoms of the wrist are reported variously as insignificant[6, 18, 54] or to occur with a frequency of 12[83] or even 87 percent.[100]

Arthrosis of the wrist is not a common finding and was not felt to be significant in 13 patients who had an average proximal radial migration of 1.9 mm and were followed for an average of 20 years by Morrey et al.[69]

In summary, proximal migration does occur as a result of radial head excision. Unless distal radial ulnar ligamentous support is compromised at the time of injury, the amount of migration is usually only 1 or 2 mm, and wrist symptoms, usually mild, ensue only in a relatively small number of patients. This particular sequela is not in itself a contraindication to radial head excision.

Instability

Increased elbow valgus (increased carrying angle) following radial head excision was recognized early (Fig. 20–16).[88] The degree of change varies from 5 to 20 degrees and occurs in about 5 percent of patients.[6, 38, 72] The largest and most carefully conducted study reports an average increase of 8 degrees valgus in 31 of 71 patients after total excision and 5.5 degrees if the fracture fragment alone had been removed.[18] We found no consistent increase in the carrying angle among 13 patients with long-term follow-up and noted that the measurement is not valid if more than about 15 degrees of flexion contracture are present.[69] Stress analysis of the elbow joint suggests that the elbow is stable to valgus stress[71] if the ulnar collateral ligament is intact even if the radial head has been removed (Fig. 20–17). Hence, it seems likely that the valgus instability that occurs in some patients is related in part to an associated injury to the ulnar collateral ligament at the time of fracture.

Instability in pronation and supination is uncommon,[30, 38, 104] and its clinical relevance has not been generally recognized.

Strength

Loss of strength has rarely been quantitated after this injury or its treatment. Carstam noted that 25 of 69 patients had a measurable strength loss of about 5 to 10 percent.[18] Torque dynamometer measurements of 13 patients conducted in our laboratory demonstrated an average loss of grip, pronation, and supination strength of about 18 percent. Flexion strength loss averaged 9 percent and extension weakness 6 percent.[69] No comparable data are available in a group treated nonoperatively,

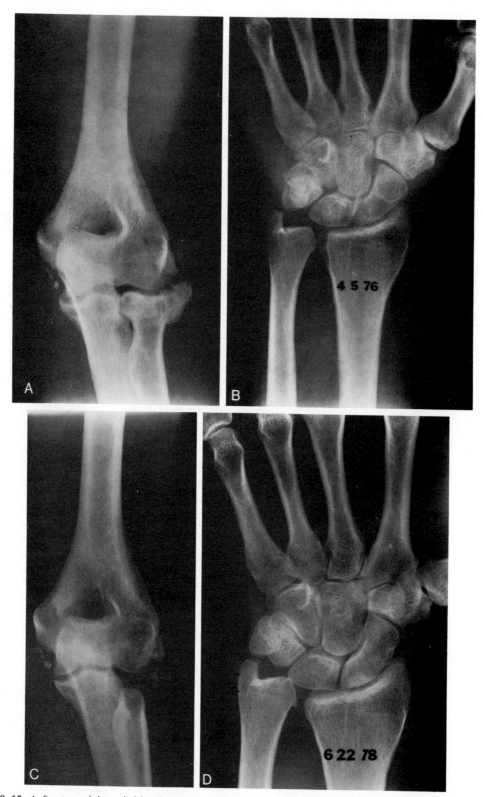

Figure 20–15. *A,* Fracture of the radial head treated without surgery. *B,* Widening of the distal radioulnar joint was present after the fracture had healed. *C,* The radial head was removed, and 5 mm of proximal migration occurred during the next 2 years *(D).*

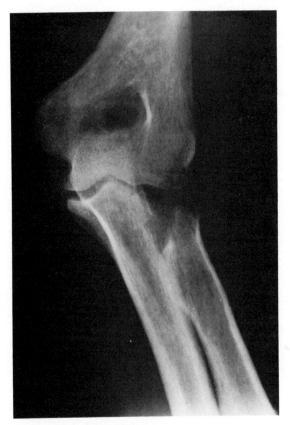

Figure 20–16. Radial head excision resulting in significant increase of carrying angle. Yet the radiograph shows only mild widening of the medial ulnohumeral joint.

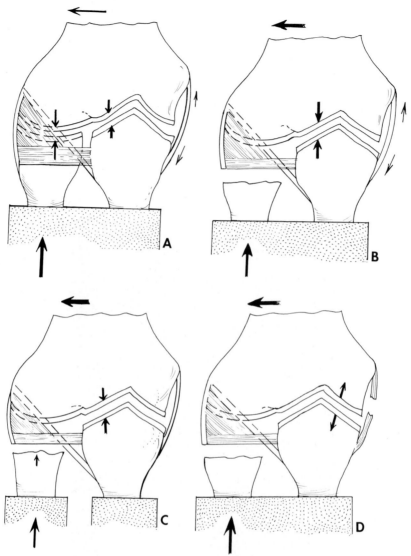

Figure 20–17. *A,* Elbow stability requires articular and ligamentous integrity. *B,* Absence of the radial head does not cause instability if the ulnar collateral ligament and distal radioulnar joint are intact. *C,* Proximal migration can occur if distal ligaments are ruptured. *D,* Valgus laxity may be present if the ulnar ligament is violated.

and consequently the specific functional loss due to the absent radial head compared to the direct effect of trauma is open to speculation.

Degenerative Arthritis

Arthritis at the ulnohumeral joint is observable radiographically after radial head excision, but unfortunately, no good studies are available for comparison with a similar, nonoperative group (see Fig. 20–11). Although Mason found no arthrosis in 18 patients[64] and Wagner none in 26,[104] elbow arthritis has been reported by others.[4, 6, 95] Radiographic arthritis was reported in 28 of 69 patients (41 percent) who were followed an average of nine years

by Carstam.[18] Little significance has been attributed to these changes, but we correlated elbow pain with the more extensive roentgenographic changes seen in 13 patients who were followed for 10 to 30 years. The data suggest that mild but definite symptoms of arthrosis occur with longer follow-up. Poor radiographic correlation with the final result was observed by Broberg and Morrey after type IV fractures.[11]

Heterotopic Calcification

The presence of calcification after radial head excision has been variably reported (Fig. 20–18)[14, 54] In fact, Sutro indicates that the

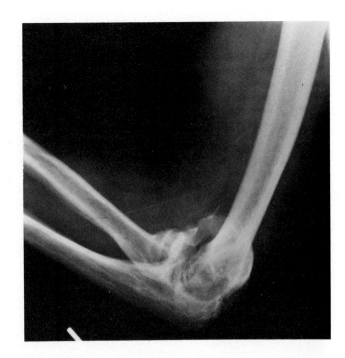

Figure 20–18. Heterotopic ossification occurred in this elbow after radial head excision was performed approximately 5 days after a type IV injury occurred.

process can be so extensive that reformation of a radial head results.[97] Rather significant calcification about the osteotomy site has been reported in 10[38] to 30 percent of patients.[104] However, there is relatively little clinical correlation with the presence and extent of such heterotopic bone.[64] Proximal radioulnar synostosis due to extensive heterotopic bone is most frequently seen in the pediatric age group.[54]

Myositis Ossificans

Certainly the most dreaded complication of this fracture is that of myositis ossificans, as stressed by McLaughlin.[67] Thompson and Garcia found that the complication developed most commonly in radial head fractures with associated elbow dislocation.[102] Of the seven instances in which myositis ossificans was observed in the 110 patients reported by Adler,[1] five had a type IV fracture. Gaston observed no instances of myositis ossificans in 12 patients treated with excision and early motion.[38]

OPEN REDUCTION AND INTERNAL FIXATION

Treatment of radial head fractures by open reduction and internal fixation has recently gained some popularity, especially in Europe. Although this technique had been employed sporadically in the past, the perception that it had "not proved successful in anyone's

hands" limited its use.[83] The poor earlier results were probably due to an inadequate understanding of anatomy, less refined techniques for effective internal fixation, and possibly, the perception of universal satisfaction with simple excision. Because today's standards probably demand a greater degree of satisfactory function, internal fixation of radial head fractures should be considered in selected instances.

Anatomy and Indications

The fracture fragment frequently has a periosteal hinge, indicating that its viability is possible.[43] The ideal fracture for fixation is a simple, large (comprising 30 percent of the head) fragment that involves the anterolateral margin of the head (Fig. 20–19). Because this aspect of the head does not articulate with the lesser sigmoid notch, fixation of this fragment will not result in impingement. If there are multiple but large fragments, open reduction is still performed by some,[43] but the technique is more demanding. If distal radioulnar disruption has occurred or if ulnar collateral ligament injury has been diagnosed, fixation rather than excision of the radial head is a viable option, particularly in younger, more active individuals.[90] In addition, fractures distal to the annular ligament in which excision would possibly result in instability of the proximal radius are considered amenable to reduction and fixation. When these

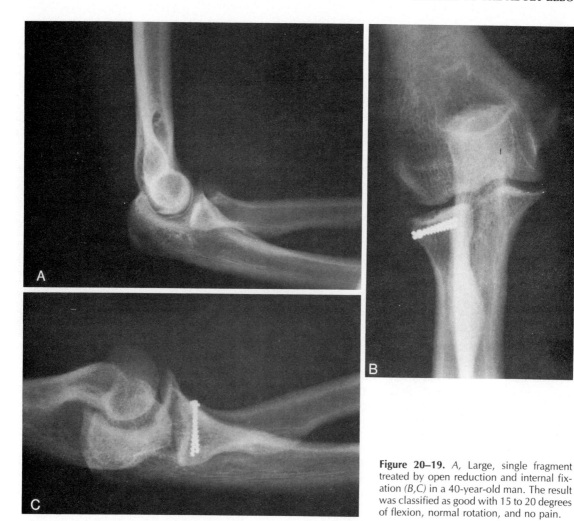

Figure 20–19. *A,* Large, single fragment treated by open reduction and internal fixation *(B,C)* in a 40-year-old man. The result was classified as good with 15 to 20 degrees of flexion, normal rotation, and no pain.

indications are employed, 5[90] to 16 percent[86] of patients with radial head fractures are candidates for internal fixation.

Results

In the recent experience with open reduction and internal fixation there has been a satisfactory outcome in more than 90 percent.[86, 90]

Technique

The technique used for reduction and fixation of radial head fractures has been outlined in detail by Heim and Trub.[43] The Kocher approach is regularly employed and the annular ligament entered through a posterolateral capsular incision. In some instances, a loose fragment will be impacted in the midportion of the radial head; it should be retrieved if present. If a single fragment or large fragments are present, they should be reduced and secured with a towel clip. Kirschner wires or

compression screws are more commonly used[36, 43, 86, 90] than circulage wire[55] or small plates. The annular ligament is repaired, and if no associated injuries are present, immediate motion is begun. Immobilization for 3 to 4 weeks is usually recommended if associated injuries are present.[35, 36, 75]

Present data suggest that open reduction and internal fixation does have a role in the management of radial head fractures. The precise indications for this modality will become clearer in time as more experience with it is obtained. A sound understanding and familiarity with the principles of surgical fracture treatment are still necessary to obtain the optimum results from fracture fragment fixation.

PROSTHETIC REPLACEMENT

Background

The first English reference to prosthetic replacement of the radial head is that of Speed in 1941.[91] After extensive experimentation and several design modifications, Vitallium ferrule caps were implanted in three patients. A decade later, Cherry[22] discussed a limited experience with an acrylic implant. The concept was later popularized by Swanson,[98] who used a silicone prosthesis.

Indications

Indications for the use of the prosthetic radial head are generally related to some form of instability. Distal radioulnar separation that occurs at the time of fracture causes an unstable radius. In this setting some consideration must be given to the additional pathology. This may be done by distal stabilization, proximal stabilization with a radial head implant, or both.

Late migration is a controversial issue, as discussed above. Swanson has demonstrated that dynamic proximal radial migration occurs during active grip and that the true incidence or significance of the complication cannot be appreciated with the routine radiographic examination.[99] Distal ulnar resection is sometimes required to treat pain after radial head fracture. Among 60 cases, Albert reported that the distal ulna was removed in ten patients with radial head fracture.[3] Of these ten, five had had a prior radial head resection. However, the other five patients who had wrist pain after fracture of the radial head had been treated nonoperatively. Hence, this secondary procedure as an indication of the clinical relevance of proximal migration and wrist symptoms fails to resolve the issue.

In addition to wrist pain, significant proximal migration narrows the interosseous distance, thus decreasing forearm rotation.[66] We were, however, unable to demonstrate a direct correlation between loss of forearm rotation due to proximal radial migration and the presence of the wrist symptoms in a long-term follow-up study.[70]

Ulnohumeral instability is another indication for prosthetic radial head replacement. A careful analysis of the subject was presented by Harrington and Tountas,[42] who listed four clinical settings in which such instability was observed:

1. Dislocation of the elbow with radial head fracture (type IV fracture)

2. Monteggia variant with olecranon and radial head fracture

3. Concurrent medial collateral ligament disruption

4. Fracture of a major portion of the coronoid

In the type IV injury, if the radial head fracture is excised, replacement with a radial head prosthesis might be considered if it enhances stability and allows early motion (Fig. 20–20). Increased valgus angulation, probably due to concurrent medial ligament injury[5, 50, 87] may be obtained with use of the spacer.[61, 98] Instability of the proximal radius associated with severe fractures or excessive excision[61, 91, 100] may be lessened with the use of an implant. Finally, when large coronoid fractures are displaced, the prosthesis may provide some element of stability, allowing early rehabilitation.

Other Indications. The implant has also been used occasionally at the time of delayed excision of the radial head. Unless instability is present, the rationale for this treatment option is unclear. Occasionally, pain after radial head removal will respond to delayed insertion of a prosthesis (Fig. 20–21).

The primary consequence of the development of ectopic bone is the loss of motion, particularly forearm rotation. This bothersome complication is considered by some[49, 91, 99] to be an indication for prosthetic replacement, but a comparative series is not currently available to confirm this impression.

Results

An accurate assessment of the long-term results of radial head implants is not possible at this time. Most reports are of few cases with limited data and follow-up.[22, 57, 107] The early prostheses were made of Vitallium[91] or acrylic,[22] but that made of Silastic and designed by Swanson is probably the most commonly used in this country[65, 70, 99] and abroad.[61, 62]

The Vitallium replacement provided satisfactory results in 12 instances of "uncomplicated" radial head fractures.[17] A careful and detailed description of the use of 15 Vitallium and 2 Silastic replacements for unstable elbow joints due to associated fractures was reported by Harrington and Tountes.[42] A rating system of results based on pain, motion, strength, and stability documented eight excellent, six good, two fair, and one poor. These investigators recommend use of the implant in complicated but not in uncomplicated radial head fractures. Experience with 18 Silastic implants for types II, III, and IV radial head fractures showed 7 excellent, 10 good, and 1 poor result after an average of 26 months follow-up.[61] No increase in carrying angle was present in this group, but four patients had as much as 4 mm of distal

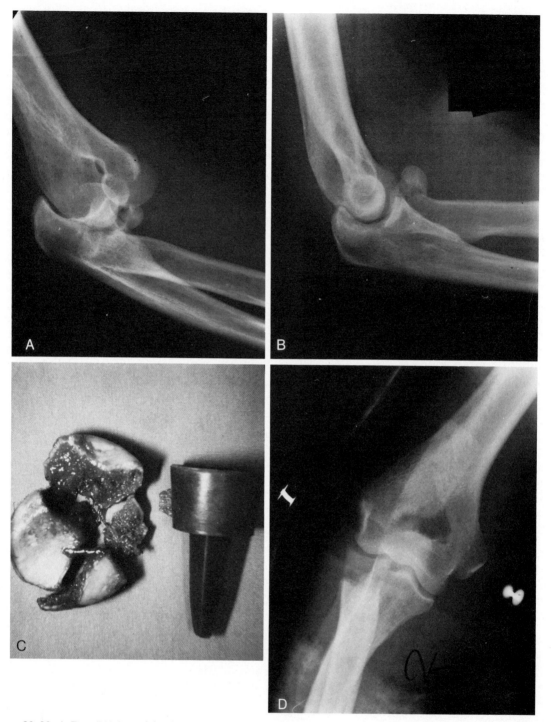

Figure 20–20. *A,* Type IV injury of the dominant elbow in 48-year-old man. *B,* A residual type III fracture was present after reduction. *C,* A Silastic implant was used to replace the radial head *(D).*

subluxation, and one of these had pain and tenderness at the wrist. Of interest is the fact that five reported wrist symptoms with heavy work even though roentgenograms were normal. The use of the Silastic implant was reported in six patients with an average follow-up period of 2.6 years by Swanson et al.[99]

Of these six, three had sustained type III fractures, and three had type IV fractures. All six returned to full activity without significant elbow pain or wrist symptoms. Shortening of 2 mm was present in one patient, and the prosthesis was intact at follow-up in all.

Comparison of groups with and without an

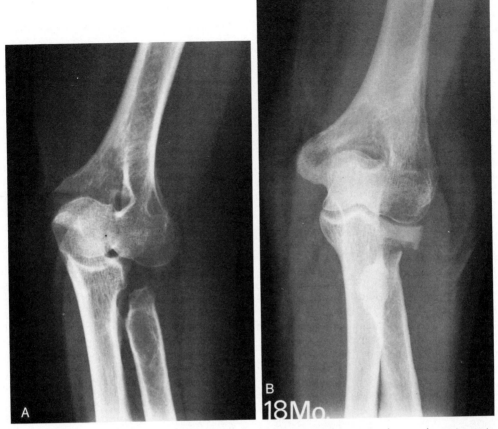

Figure 20–21. *A,* Patient was treated by immediate simple radial head excision for a type II fracture, but pain persisted after excision. *B,* A radial head prosthesis was inserted. The patient complained of some weakness but was essentially pain-free at 18 months. (From Morrey, B. F., et al.: Silastic prosthetic replacement for the radial head. J. Bone Joint Surg. 63A:454, 1981.)

acrylic prosthesis has also been done. Fourteen patients with simple radial head fractures treated by excision and prosthetic replacement were compared with 11 patients with simple fractures treated by excision alone; the average follow-up time was 3.5 years.[31] A clear advantage was demonstrated

Table 20–1. **Results of Radial Head Resection**

	Simple Radial Head Excision (11)	Radial Head Prosthesis (14)
Patient's evaluation of operation		
Excellent	37%	57%
Good	37%	29%
Fair	9%	14%
Poor	18%	0%
Able to work as well after as before accident	55%	79%

Edwards, G. E., and Rostrup, O.: Radial head prosthesis in the management of radial head fractures. Can. J. Surg. 3:153, 1960.

for the group with the prosthesis (Table 20–1); they had less elbow and wrist pain and greater elbow motion.

In contrast, we studied 13 patients with simple radial head excision[69] and 6 with acute fractures and a Silastic implant who were followed for an average of 7 years.[70] No difference in pain, motion, strength, and patient satisfaction was demonstrated between the two groups. Hence, the routine use of the spacer was not advocated.

In summary, the present data are limited but suggest that the prosthesis is valuable in fractures associated with elbow or wrist instability. Its value in uncomplicated fractures is unclear. As greater clinical experience is obtained and reported the exact role of the prosthesis will emerge with time.

Complications

A distinction must be made between complications arising from the injury and those originating from the treatment. Complications of the fracture have been discussed earlier. Specific problems with the prosthesis are fracture, dislocation, or reaction to the implant. The cause of these failures may be broadly considered as related to patient selection, surgical technique, or material failure of the implant.

Patient Selection

The use of a prosthesis when the radial head is not well oriented with the capitellum may predispose to dislocation.[98] The instability associated with the Monteggia fracture is sometimes managed with an implant.[31, 42, 62, 70] If used in this situation, a perfect reduction of the olecranon fracture is imperative to ensure proper alignment of the proximal radius. Failure to do so could result in dislocation.

Surgical Technique

Inadequate bone resection may cause an improper fit of the prosthesis and can predispose to dislocation or shear fracture at the stem (Fig. 20–22).[42, 98] Failure to repair the annular ligament may allow the prosthesis to dislocate. Improper handling of the Silastic implant may damage the surface and lead to material failure from fatigue fracture.[98]

Material Properties of the Prosthesis

Few detailed reports of the metallic prosthesis are available. Carr and Howard reported no complications in 12 patients with the Vitallium cap.[17] Harrington observed one dislocation among 15 with the metal prosthesis.[42] Adverse bone reaction has been reported to occur with the metal and Silastic prostheses.[99]

The prosthesis is used to absorb force. This implies that the material must withstand the repetitive forces that are generated at this joint. Fatigue failure has occurred with both the acrylic[31] and the Silastic[65, 70] prostheses. Edwards and Rostrup reported two fractures among 12 patients' acrylic prostheses with a mean follow-up time of 3.5 years.[31] In the report by Morrey et al.[70] three of six Silastic implants showed fracture of the prosthesis (Fig. 20–23). All patients were doing well, and the results were rated as good despite this radiographic finding. Mayhall et al.,[65] however, reviewed a community experience with the Silastic prosthesis and reported that 4 of 12 patients had symptomatic fractures of the device requiring revision of the prosthesis 9 to 36 months after surgery. Because the Silastic device is radiolucent, special imaging techniques may be necessary to assess the integrity of the implant properly.[7] Swanson demonstrated minimal radiographic alteration in one of six prostheses 7.4 years after the implant was inserted;[98] he emphasizes that better results should be anticipated with the more durable, "high-performance" Silastic. Although technique may be responsible for some prosthetic failures, fatigue failure of the implant appears to account for some poor results. The development of the high-performance Silastic prosthesis may lessen the likelihood of fracture, but material failure remains a concern and is a major reason why, in our opinion, the routine use of the prosthesis for uncomplicated fractures is not indicated.

Finally, the occasional synovitis reported to occur with Silastic implants can and does occur at the elbow.[39, 110] This complication has been observed to respond readily and completely to the removal of the Silastic implant. Worsing et al. observed two patients with radial head implants who had recurrent painful synovitis.[110] An experimental model developed by these investigators revealed a histologic process of foreign-body giant cell reaction elicited by particulate Silastic debris that was similar to the clinical pathologic

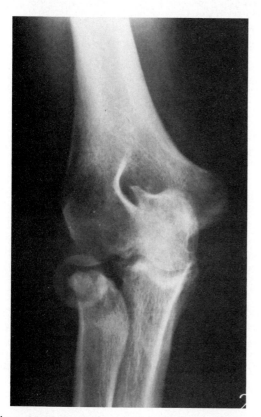

Figure 20–22. An implant was inserted for persistent pain after excision of a fractured radial head. Inadequate bone was removed, and the implant was dislocated 2 weeks after surgery.

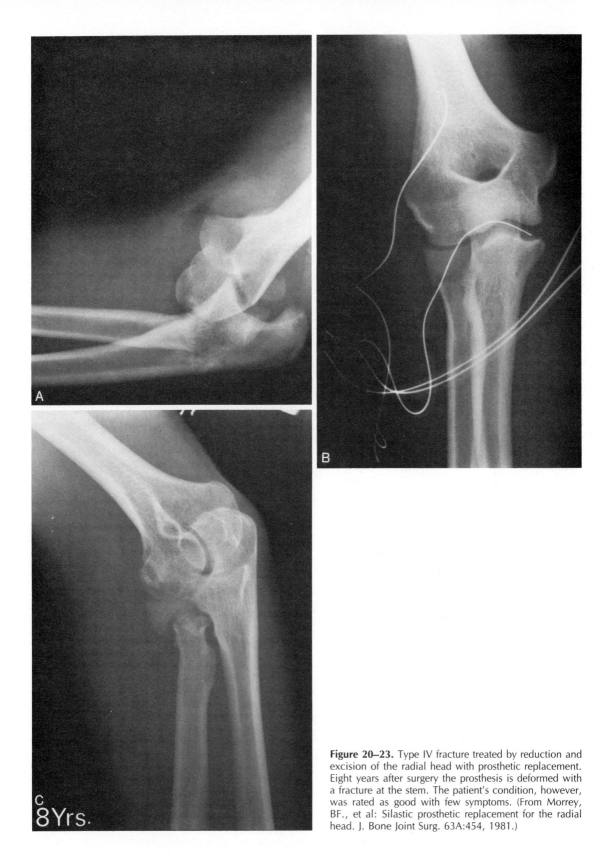

Figure 20–23. Type IV fracture treated by reduction and excision of the radial head with prosthetic replacement. Eight years after surgery the prosthesis is deformed with a fracture at the stem. The patient's condition, however, was rated as good with few symptoms. (From Morrey, BF., et al: Silastic prosthetic replacement for the radial head. J. Bone Joint Surg. 63A:454, 1981.)

process. They speculated that the mechanism of the synovitis may be due to debris that occurs from abrasion of the prosthesis. A careful analysis of the question of silicone-induced synovitis in six patients by Gordon and Bullough.[39] revealed a "hyperplastic chronic inflammatory synovitis induced by a foreign-body giant cell reaction to silicone rubber." Considering the great number of implants used, the incidence of this reaction is probably low and appears to be tissue dependent[110] but should be considered a possibility when any implant is used as a replacement arthroplasty against cartilage.

AUTHOR'S PREFERRED TREATMENT

For all fracture types, treatment is initiated by a word of caution to the patient to expect some loss of motion. If motion loss does not occur, so much the better. If motion is lost, concern about it is lessened by the early admonition of its possibililty.

Type I Fractures

These fractures are treated by joint aspiration, a collar and cuff, and immediate motion is tolerated. We use a local anesthetic at the time of aspiration. If the fracture is stable, we see the patient in about 7 to 10 days; if it is unstable, reevaluation is done at 3 to 5 days and at regular intervals for up to 3 months. We do not routinely use physical therapy in such patients.

Type II Fractures

Management of the type II fracture varies depending on the nature of the fracture and the presence or absence of complications (Fig. 20–24).

If displacement is less than 2 mm and if less than one third of the head is involved, the joint is aspirated and injected with a local anesthetic. If no significant block to extension (less than 10 degrees) or forearm rotation (less than 30 degrees) is present, a collar and cuff with a removal night splint and early motion are prescribed. This patient is followed on a weekly basis to ensure that the fragment does not displace.

If the displacement is more than 2 mm and more than 30 percent of the head is involved, surgery is performed. In the young person with a large fragment, open reduction and internal fixation is carried out. In uncomplicated cases, surgical excision is the treatment of choice if the fragment cannot be fixed. If, however, complications that compromise stability are present—for example, rupture of the medial collateral ligament or elbow or distal radioulnar dislocation—simple excision is not performed. If possible, internal fixation is carried out. If the fracture does not allow this, a prosthetic implant is employed. The distal radioulnar joint may require surgical stabilization by an open procedure or percutaneous cross-pinning in order to maintain radial length. Elbow flexion and extension are allowed within the first week, usually on the third or fourth day after surgery.

The surgical technique basically follows that described above. The Kocher approach is used, and an attempt is made to close the remnants of the annular ligament; the distal end of the radius is covered with Gel-foam, and the elbow and radius are carefully tested for stability before closing.

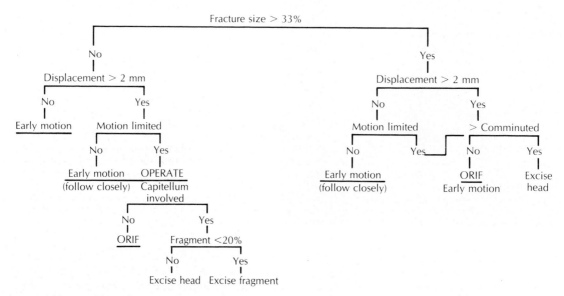

Figure 20–24. Example of treatment logic that might be employed for the management of the uncomplicated radial head fracture.

Type III Fractures

In uncomplicated injuries we prefer complete and early excision (within 24 hours of such a fracture), followed by active motion in 3 to 5 days. If circumstances preclude this treatment, then early active motion is recommended with intent to perform an excision if pain or motion limitation occurs.

Type IV Fractures

Type IV fractures require urgent management. The elbow dislocation is reduced immediately. A long-term follow-up study of 50 type IV fractures treated at the Mayo Clinic[11] has provided our guidelines of treatment.

Partial radial head removal has little advantage, especially as a late procedure. Late residual instability is very rare, and immobilization should not exceed 4 weeks in any instance. If increased stability required for early, active rehabilitation is provided only by an implant, then a radial head prosthesis is employed. Large, single fragments are fixed with small compression screws. Immobilization is continued for only 3 to 5 days, after which a hinged splint is helpful to provide stability as well as early active motion.

References

1. Adler, J. B., and Shaftan, G. W.: Radial Head Fracture, Is Excision Necessary? J. Trauma 4:115, 1964.
2. Aegina, P.: Fractures and dislocations. Translation by F. Adams. New Sydenham Society, 1846, p. 464.
3. Albert, S. M., Wohl, M.A., and Rechtman, A. M.: Treatment of the Disrupted Radio-Ulnar Joint. J. Bone Joint Surg. 45A:1373, 1963.
4. Arner, O., Ekengren, K., and Von Schreeb, T.: Fractures of the Head and Neck of the Radius. A Clinical and Roentgenographic Study of 310 Cases. Acta Chir Scand. 112:115, 1957.
5. Arvidsson, H., and Johansson, O.: Arthrography of the Elbow-Joint. Acta Radiol. (Stockh.). 43:445, 1955.
6. Bakalim, G.: Fractures of Radial Head and Their Treatment. Acta Orthop. Scand. 41:320, 1970.
7. Bohl, W. R., and Brightman, E.: Fracture of a Silastic Radial Head Prosthesis: Diagnosis and Localization of Fragments by Xerography. J. Bone Joint Surg. 63A:1482, 1981.
8. Bohler, L.: The Treatment of Fractures, Vol. 1. New York, Grune & Stratton, 1956.
9. Bohrer, J. V.: Fractures of the Head and Neck of the Radius. Ann. Surg. 97:204, 1933.
10. Broberg, M., and Morrey, B. F.: Late Excision of Radial Head Fractures. In press, 1985.
11. Broberg, M., and Morrey, B. F.: Treatment of Radial Head Fracture and Elbow Dislocation. A Long-Term Follow-up Study. In preparation.
12. Brockman, E. P.: Two Cases of Disability at the Wrist Joint Following Excision of the Head of the Radius. Proc. R. Soc. Med. 24:904, 1930.
13. Buffington, C. B.: Treatment of Simple and Comminuted Fractures of Head of the Radius. West Virginia Med. J. 43:198, 1947.
14. Burton, A. E.: Fractures of the Head of the Radius. Proc. R. Soc. Med. 35:764, 1942.
15. Bush, L. F., and McLain, E. J., Jr.: Operative Treatment of Fractures of the Elbow in Adults. In American Academy of Orthopedic Surgeons: Instructional Course Lectures, Vol. 16. St. Louis, C. V. Mosby, 1959, pp. 265–277.
16. Buxton, St., J. D.: Ossification in the Ligaments of the Elbow Joint. J. Bone Joint Surg. 20:709, 1938.
17. Carr, C. R., and Howard, J. W.: Metallic Cap Replacement of Radial Head Following Fracture. West J. Surg. 59:539, 1951.
18. Carstam, N.: Operative Treatment of Fractures of the Upper End of the Radius. Acta Orthop. Scand. 19:502, 1950.
19. Castberg, T., and Thing, E.: Treatment of Fractures of the Upper End of the Radius. Acta Chir. Scand. 1051:62, 1953.
20. Cave, E. F. (ed.): Fractures and Other Injuries. Chicago, Year Book Medical Publishers, 1958, pp. 329–331.
21. Charnley, J.: The Closed Treatment of Common Fractures, 3rd ed. Baltimore, The Williams & Wilkins Co., 1961, p. 78.
22. Cherry, J. C.: Use of Acrylic Prosthesis in the Treatment of Fracture of the Head of the Radius. J. Bone Joint Surg. 35B:70, 1953.
23. Cohn, I.: Fractures of the Elbow. Am. J. Surg. 55:210, 1942.
24. Conn, J., and Wade, P.: Injuries of the Elbow: A Ten Year Review. J. Trauma 1:248, 1961.
25. Cooper, A.: Dislocations and Fractures of the Joints. Cooper, R. B. (ed.) Boston, T. R. Marvin, 1844, p. 412.
26. Curr, J., and Coe, W.: Dislocation of the Inferior Radio-Ulnar Joint. Br. J. Surg. 34:74, 1946.
27. Cutler, C.: Fractures of the Head and Neck of the Radius. Ann. Surg. 8:267, 1926.
28. Dehna, R., and Torp, R. P.: Treatment of Joint Injuries by Immediate Mobilization. Clin. Orthop. 77:218, 1981.
29. Desault, P. J.: A Treatise on Fractures, Luxations and Affections of the Bones, 2nd ed. Bichat, Xav. (ed.) Translated by C. Caldwell. Philadelphia, Kimber & Conrad, 1811, pp. 165–168.
30. Dickson, F. D.: Fractures of the Upper End of the Radius and Ulna. Surg. Gynecol. Obstet. 88:69, 1949.
31. Edwards, G. E., and Rostrup, O.: Radial Head Prosthesis in the Management of Radial Head Fractures. Can. J. Surg. 3:153, 1960.
32. Elison, E. L., and North, J. P.: Fractures About the Elbow. Am. J. Surg. 44:88, 1939.
33. Essex-Lopresti, P.: Fractures of the Radial Head with Distal Radio-Ulnar Dislocation. J. Bone Joint Surg. 33B:244, 1951.
34. Fairbank, H. A. T.: Discussion of Two Cases of Disability at the Wrist Joint Following Excision of the Head of the Radius. Proc. R. Soc. Med. 24:904, 1930.
35. Firicia, A., and Troianescu, O.: Fractures Comminutives de la Tet Radiale: Technique de Reconstruction Chirurgicale. Rev. Chir. Orthop. 65 (Suppl. 2):66, 1979.
36. Fischer, L. P., Gonon, G. P., Carret, J. P., Dimnet, J., and DeMourgues, G.: Possibilities de Vissage dans Certaines Fractures Simples de la Tet Radiale (avec Considerations Anatomo-Physiologiques sur l'Articulation Radio-Cubitale Superieure). Rev. Chir. Orthop. (Suppl.) 2:90, 1976.

37. Fleming, C.: Fractures of the Head of the Radius. Proc. R. Soc. Med. **25**:1011, 1932.
38. Gaston, S. R., Smith, F. M., and Baab, O. D.: Adult Injuries of the Radial Head and Neck. Am. J. Surg. **78**:631, 1949.
39. Gordon, M., and Bullough, P. G.: Synovial and Osseous Inflammation in Failed Silicone-Rubber Prostheses. J. Bone Joint Surg. **64A**:574, 1982.
40. Grossman, J.: Fracture of the Head and Neck of the Radius. N.Y. J. Med. **17**:472, 1923.
41. Hammond, R.: Fracture of the Head and Neck of the Radius. Ann. Surg. **53**:207, 1910.
42. Harrington, I. J., and Tountas, A. A.: Replacement of the Radial Head in the Treatment of Unstable Elbow Fractures. Injury **12**:405, 1981.
43. Heim, U., and Trub, H. J.: Erfahrungen mit der Primaren Osteosynthese von Radius-Kopfchenfrakturen. Helv. Chir. Acta **45**:63, 1978.
44. Hein, B.: Fractures of the Head of the Radius. An Analysis of 52 Cases with Specific Reference to Disabilities. Indust. Med. **6**:529, 1937.
45. Helferich, H.: Fractures and Dislocations. Translated by J. Hutchinson. New Sydenham Society, 1899, p. 96–97.
46. Hergenroeder, T. P., and Gelberman, R. H.: Distal Radioulnar Joint Subluxation Secondary to Excision of the Radial Head. Orthopedics **3**:649, 1980.
47. Hitzrot, J.: The Treatment of Simple Fractures: A Study of Some End Results. Ann. Surg. **55**:338, 1912.
48. Jacobs, J., and Kernodle, H.: Fractures of the Head of the Radius. J. Bone Joint Surg. **28**:616, 1946.
49. Jeffrey, C. C.: Fracture of the Head of the Radius Treated by Excision and Substitution of an Acrylic Head. J. Bone Joint Surg. **35B**:486, 1953.
50. Johansson, O.: Caspular and Ligament Injuries of the Elbow Joint. Acta Chir. Scand. (Stockh.) Suppl. 287, 1962.
51. Johnson, G.: A Follow-up of One Hundred Cases of Fractures of the Head of the Radius With a Review of the Literature. Ulster Med. J. **31**:51, 1962.
52. Keon-Cohen, B. T.: Fractures at the Elbow. J. Bone Joint Surg. **48B**:1623, 1966.
53. Key, J.: Treatment of Fractures of the Head and Neck of the Radius. J.A.M.A. **96**:101, 1931.
54. King, B.: Resection of the Radial Head and Neck. An End-Result Study of Thirteen Cases. J. Bone Joint Surg. **21**:839, 1939.
55. Kopp, P.: Zur Problematik der Operativen Therapie von Radiuskopfchen und Olecranonfrakturen. Beitr. Orthop. Traumatol. **22**:483, 1975.
56. Lassen, E.: Frakturerne Icatitulumog Collum Radii. Hospitalstidende **36**:909, 1929.
57. Levin, P. D.: Fracture of the Radial Head With Dislocation of the Distal Radio-Ulnar Joint: Case Report. Treatment by Prosthetic Replacement of the Radial Head. J. Bone Joint Surg. **55A**:837, 1973.
58. Lewis, R. W., and Thibodeau, A. A.: Deformity of the Wrist Following Resection of the Radial Head. Surg. Gynec. Obstet. **64**:1079, 1937.
59. Linscheid, R. L., and Wheeler, D. K.: Elbow Dislocation. J.A.M.A. **194**:1171, 1965.
60. Loomis, L. K.: Reduction and After-Treatment of Posterior Dislocation of the Elbow. Am. J. Surg. **63**:56, 1944.
61. Mackay, I., Fitzgerald, B., and Miller, J. H.: Silastic Replacement of the Head of the Radius in Trauma. J. Bone Joint Surg. **61B**:494, 1979.
62. Martinelli, B.: Fractures of the Radial Head Treated by Substitution With the Silastic Prosthesis. Bull. Hosp. Joint Dis. **36**:61, 1975.
63. Mason, J. A., and Shutkin, N. M.: Immediate Active Motion in the Treatment of Fractures of the Head and Neck of the Radius. Surg. Gynec. Obstet. **76**:731, 1943.
64. Mason, M. B.: Some Observations on Fractures of the Head of the Radius with a Review of One Hundred Cases. Br. J. Surg. **42**:123, 1954.
65. Mayhall, W. S. T., Tiley, F. T., and Paluska, D. J.: Fractures of Silastic Radial Head Prosthesis. J. Bone Surg. **63A**:459, 1981.
66. McDougall, A., and White, J.: Subluxation of the Inferior Radio-Ulnar Joint Complicating Fracture of the Radial Head. J. Bone Joint Surg. **39B**:278, 1957.
67. McLaughlin, H. L.: Some Fractures With a Time Limit. Surg. Clin. North Am. **35**:553, 1955.
68. Meekson, D. M.: Fractures of the Head of the Radius. J. Bone Joint Surg. **27**:82, 1945.
69. Morrey, B. F., Chao, E. Y., and Hui, F. C.: Biomechanical Study of the Elbow Following Excision of the Radial Head. J. Bone Joint Surg. **61A**:63, 1979.
70. Morrey, B. F., Askew, L., and Chao, E. Y.: Silastic Prosthetic Replacement for the Radial Head. J. Bone Joint Surg. **63A**:454, 1981.
71. Morrey, B. F., and An, K. N.: Articular and Ligamentous Contributions to the Varus/Valgus Stability of the Elbow. J. Sports Med. **11**:315, 1983.
72. Murray, R.: Fractures of the Head and Neck of the Radius. Br. J. Surg. **28**:106, 1940.
73. Naviaser, J. S., and Wickstrom, J. K.: Dislocation of the Elbow: A Retrospective Study of 115 Patients. South Med. J. **70**:172, 1977.
74. Neuwirth, A. A.: Nonsplinting Treatment of Fractures of Elbow Joint. J.A.M.A. **118**:971, 1942.
75. Odenheimer, K., and Harvey, J. P., Jr.: Internal Fixation of Fractures of the Head of the Radius. J. Bone Joint Surg. **61A**:785, 1979.
76. Ogilvie, W. H.: Discussion of Minor Injuries of the Elbow. Proc. R. Soc. Med. **23**:306, 1930.
77. Odelberg-Johnsson, G.: On Fractures of the Proximal Portion of the Radius and Their Causes. Acta Radiol. **3**:45, 1924.
78. Petit, J. L.: A Treatise of the Disease of the Bones; Containing an Extract and Complete Account of All Their Various Kinds. Vol. 6. London, T. Woodward, 1720, p. 288.
79. Postethwait, R. W.: Modified Treatment for Fracture of the Head of the Radius. Am. J. Surg. **67**:77, 1945.
80. Paulsen, J. O., and Tophoj, K.: Fracture of the Head and Neck of the Radius. Acta Orthop. Scand. **45**:66, 1974.
81. Quigley, T. B.: Aspiration of the Elbow Joint in the Treatment of Fractures of the Head of the Radius. N. Engl. J. Med. **240**:915, 1949.
82. Rabourdin, A. N.: Fractures of the Head of the Radius. Paris, Steinheill, 1910, p. 11.
83. Radin, E. L., and Riseborough, E. J.: Fractures of the Radial Head. J. Bone Joint Surg. **48A**:1055, 1966.
84. Reith, P. L.: Fractures of the Radial Head Associated with Chip Fracture of the Capitellum in Adults; Surgical Considerations. South. Surgeon **14**:154, 1948.
85. Scharplatz, D., and Allgower, M.: Fracture-Dislocations of the Elbow. Injury **7**:143, 1976.
86. Shmueli, G., and Herold, H. Z.: Compression Screwing of Displaced Fractures of the Head of the Radius. J. Bone Joint Surg. **63B**:535, 1981.
87. Schwab, G. H., Bennett, J. B., Woods, G. W., and Tulloos, H. S.: The Biomechanics of Elbow Stability: The Role of the Medical Collateral Ligament. Clin. Orthop. **146**:42, 1980.
88. Schwartz, R., and Young, F.: Treatment of Fractures

of the Head and Neck of the Radius and Slipped Radial Epiphysis in Children. Surg. Gynecol. Obstet. **57**:528, 1933.

89. Sever, J.: Fractures of the Head and Neck of the Radius. A Study of End Results. J.A.M.A. **84**:1551, 1925.

90. Soler, R. R., Tarela, J. P., and Minores, J. M.: Internal Fixation of Fractures of the Proximal End of the Radius in Adults. Injury **10**:268, 1979.

91. Speed, K.: Ferrule Caps for the Head of the Radius. Surg. Gynecol. Obstet. **73**:845, 1941.

92. Speed, K.: Fracture of the Head of the Radius. Am. J. Surg. **38**:157, 1924.

93. Spinner, M., and Kaplan, E. B.: The Quadrate Ligament of the Elbow—Its Relationship to the Stability of the Proximal Radioulnar Joint. Acta Orthop. Scand. **41**:632, 1970.

94. Stankovic, P.: Über die Operative Versorgung von Frakturen des Proximalen Radiusendes. Chirurg. **49**:377, 1978.

95. Stephen, I. B. M.: Excision of the Radial Head for Closed Fracture. Acta Orthop. Scand. **52**:409, 1981.

96. Strachan, J. C. H., and Ellis, B. W.: Vulnerability of the Posterior Interosseous Nerve During Radial Head Resection. J. Bone Joint Surg. **53B**:320, 1971.

97. Sutro, C. J.: Regrowth of Bone at the Proximal End of the Radius Following Resection in this Region. J. Bone Joint Surg. **17**:867, 1935.

98. Swanson, A. B.: Flexible Implant Resection Arthroplasty in the Hand and Extremities. St. Louis, C. V. Mosby Co., 1973.

99. Swanson, A. B., Jaeger, S. H., and LaRochelle, D.: Comminuted Fractures of the Radial Head. The Role of Silicone-Implant Replacement Arthroplasty. J. Bone Joint Surg. **63A**:1039, 1981.

100. Taylor, T. K. F., and O'Connor, B. T.: The Effect Upon the Inferior Radio-Ulnar Joint of Excision of the Head of the Radius in Adults. J. Bone Joint Surg. **46B**:83, 1964.

101. Thomas, T. T.: Fractures of the Head and the Radius. Univ. Pa. Med. Bull. **18**:184–197, June; **18**:221–234, July, 1905.

102. Thompson, H. C., III, and Garcia, A.: Myositis Ossificans: Aftermath of Elbow Injuries. Clin. Orthop. **50**:129, 1967.

103. Vertongen, P.: Displaced Fractures of the Radial Head. J. Bone Joint Surg. **43B**:191, 1961.

104. Wagner, C.: Fractures of the Head of the Radius. Am. J. Surg. **89**:911, 1955.

105. Watson-Jones, R.: Discussion of Minor Injuries of the Elbow Joint. Proc. R. Soc. Med. **23**:323, 1930.

106. Watson-Jones, R.: Fractures and Other Bone and Joint Injuries. 2nd ed. Baltimore, 1941, The Williams & Wilkins Co., p. 336.

107. Weingarden, T. L.: Prosthetic Replacement in the Treatment of Fractures of the Radial Head. J. Am. Osteopath. Assoc. **77**:804, 1978.

108. Weseley, M. S., Barenfeld, P. A., and Eisenstein, A. L.: Closed Treatment of Isolated Radial Head Fractures. J. Trauma **23A**:36, 1983.

109. Wilson, P. D.: Fracture and Dislocation in the Region of the Elbow. Surg. Gynecol. Obstet. **56**:335, 1933.

110. Worsing, R. A., Engber, W. D., and Lange, T. A.: Reactive Synovitis from Particulate Silastic. J. Bone Joint Surg. **64A**:581, 1982.

CHAPTER 21

Fractures of the Proximal Ulna and Olecranon

MIGUEL E. CABANELA

FRACTURES OF THE OLECRANON

The olecranon process forms the proximal and posterior portions of the ulna. Its articular surface joins that of the coronoid process to form the sigmoid (semilunar) notch of the ulna, which articulates with the trochlea of the humerus. The layer of cartilage covering the sigmoid notch is usually interrupted by a transverse streak of uncovered bone situated between the olecranon and the coronoid process; because of this, anatomic reconstruction of a fracture through this area is not necessary for optimal function. Elbow stability is secured primarily by the joint surfaces, which allow motion only in one plane. Stability is supplemented by the collateral ligaments, both of which have insertions in the proximal ulna. Posteriorly, the triceps tendon inserts into the olecranon and its fascia has a medial and lateral expansion similar to that of the quadriceps retinacula in the knee. Because of its subcutaneous position the olecranon is particularly vulnerable to direct trauma. Most olecranon fractures are intra-articular and therefore can compromise the stability of the elbow joint. If the triceps fascial expansions are torn, the fractures are displaced; if not, the displacement may be minimal. The ossification center for the olecranon appears at age 9 and consistently fuses at the age of 14 to 14½ years. Persistent physeal lines, usually bilateral, have been reported and are easily differentiated from fractures.[37] They are often partial, are perpendicular to the ulnar shaft, and are not accompanied by soft tissue swelling. Patella cubiti,[29] an accessory ossicle in the triceps tendon adjacent to the olecranon, is also bilateral when present (see Chapter 47).

Historical Aspects

Early treatises on fractures of the proximal ulna recommended splinting in extension for a period of 4 to 6 weeks. The usual result, a stiff elbow in a nonfunctional position, led to a change in the position of immobilization to one of midflexion, which discouraged union by allowing separation of the fragments. Sachs in 1894 advised treatment solely by massage and reported good functional results.[46a] Because this treatment was reported before the advent of radiography, it is not certain but is suspected that many of these cases represented nonunion or fibrous union with resultant weakness of extension. Elliot in 1934 advised no splint, massage starting on the second day, and active motion at 2½ weeks.[21] He reported complete restoration of function at 5 weeks and observed uniformly good functional results in 20 to 30 cases in which bony or fibrous union ultimately occurred. As long ago as 1879 surgical fixation was reported by Shelton.[46b] Lister in 1884 utilized a wire loop to fix the fractured fragments,[30a] and this technique was also utilized by Berger[8] in 1902 and later adopted by Bohler[10] in 1929.

Daland in 1933 reported the first important series of olecranon fractures and treated the majority of them with surgery.[19] He used different materials, including wire, nails, bone pegs, kangaroo tendon, and fascia lata, but preferred the latter. Rombold in 1934 reported four excellent results in four fractures treated with a new technique utilizing triceps fascial strips.[45] Hey-Groves in 1939 advised open reduction and wiring of the fragments,[26] and MacAusland in 1942 introduced the use of longitudinal screw or nail fixation.[32] Since then a vast array of internal fixation devices (e.g., flexible screws, hook plate, among others) have been tried with varying degrees of success.

Excision of the fractured proximal fragment and repair of the triceps tendon was first reported by Fiolle[23a] in 1918 and by Perkins in 1936.[40] Dunn in 1939 described two cases using this technique and observed excellent results.[20] Wainwright in 1942 reported 17 excellent results in 20 cases treated by excision

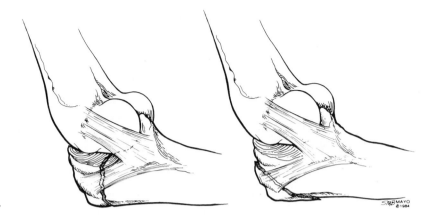

Figure 21–1. Avulsion fracture.

of the olecranon fragment;[54] he felt that the advantages of this procedure were its technical ease, the rapid rehabilitation period, and the lack of arthritis on follow-up. Its disadvantages include limitation of elbow extension, loss of triceps power, loss of the point of the elbow, and the possibility of anteroposterior instability of the joint. This technique was popularized in the United States by McKeever and Buck,[34] who in 1947 reported good strength and excellent range of motion in 10 patients treated with this method. They were the first to point out that 80 percent of the olecranon can be removed without fear of elbow joint instability, and they believed that this technique was indicated in (1) ununited fractures, (2) fractures in the elderly, (3) fractures that do not involve the trochlear notch, and (4) very comminuted fractures. Because some patients complained of frequent injury to the "crazy bone," they suggested anterior translocation of the ulnar nerve at the time of excision of the olecranon fragment.

During the last thirty years better techniques of internal fixation have produced improvement in the quality of results, but de-spite this the indications for olecranon excision remain those suggested by McKeever and Buck.

Classification and Mechanisms of Injury

Olecranon fractures have been classified as displaced, undisplaced, transverse, oblique, and comminuted. The classification presented here (modified from that of Colton[16]) is based on the anatomy of the fracture and can serve as a basis for selection of the appropriate therapy.

Undisplaced Fractures

These are usually the result of a direct blow to the elbow. Fragments are separated by less than 2 mm, and the separation does not increase with elbow flexion. In addition, active elbow extension against gravity is preserved.

Displaced Fractures

Avulsion Fractures. In this pattern (Fig. 21–1), a transverse or oblique fracture line separates a small, often nonarticular fragment of the olecranon process that can be displaced

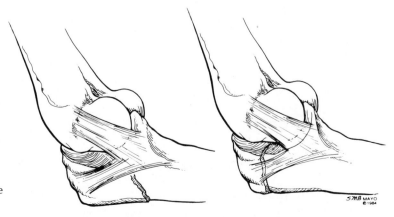

Figure 21–2. Oblique or transverse fracture.

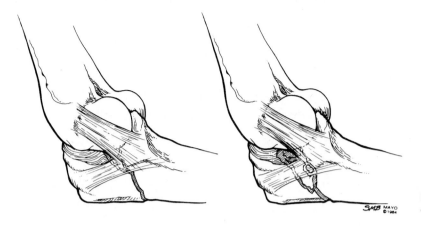

Figure 21–3. Oblique fracture with comminution.

by the pull of the triceps fibers that are inserted on this fragment. This fracture is commonly the result of an indirect mechanism such as a fall on the hand with the elbow in flexion accompanied by a strong contraction of the triceps.

Transverse or Oblique Fractures. Often resulting from an indirect mechanism or, more likely, a bending movement about the trochlear fulcrum caused by the sudden synergistic contraction of the elbow flexors and extensors, the fracture line (Fig. 21–2) runs from the deepest part of the semilunar notch transversely or obliquely to the subcutaneous crest of the ulna. If the violence of the injury is not exhausted in producing a single fracture line, the trochlea can be driven into the olecranon and split off a wedge-shaped central fragment that, in more severe injuries, can be depressed and comminuted (Fig. 21–3). This is the most common form of olecranon comminution.

Comminuted Fractures. These fractures (Fig. 21–4) are the result of direct severe trauma to

the posterior aspect of the elbow. The fracture lines run in multiple planes, and the fragments may be severely crushed. Associated fractures of the distal end of the humerus, of the radial head, and even of the forearm bones are often encountered.

Fracture-Dislocation. When the fracture line is near the level of the tip of the coronoid process, and the injury was caused by a blow to the posterior aspect of the elbow, anterior subluxation or dislocation of the ulna (Fig. 21–5) and radius can result, producing a variant of the Monteggia lesion.[9, 49, 56]

Radiologic Evaluation

An anteroposterior view delineates the fracture in the sagittal plane, but a true lateral view is essential to assess precisely the degree of comminution, the amount of articular disruption, and the displacement, if any, of the radial head. Failure to obtain a true lateral view is the most common pitfall in the initial evaluation.

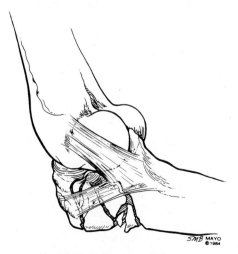

Figure 21–4. Comminuted fracture.

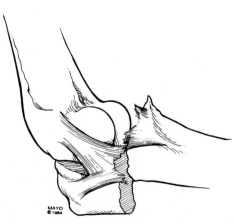

Figure 21–5. Fracture-dislocation.

Treatment Methods

The goals of treatment in olecranon fractures are (1) avoidance of articular incongruity, (2) preservation of motor power, (3) restoration of stability, (4) prevention of stiffness of the joint, and (5) avoidance or lessening of complications. With this in mind, it is obvious that all these fractures but especially undisplaced fractures should be handled by surgical means. Only in the elderly patient who makes decreased demands on the joint is masterly neglect and early motion a reasonable alternative.[46]

Undisplaced Fractures

Undisplaced fractures can be easily handled by immobilization for a short time with a long arm cast or a simple posterior splint. The best position is one of midflexion. Full extension should be avoided because it may be conducive to significant loss of flexion.

Repeat roentgenograms should be obtained 6 to 8 days after the initial treatment to rule out displacement. Generally, sufficient stability is present at 3 weeks to allow early motion; in the elderly patient motion should be started even earlier. Flexion beyond 90 degrees should be avoided until bony union is complete, usually by 6 to 8 weeks.

Displaced Fractures

The two accepted methods of treatment are (1) open reduction and internal fixation and (2) excision and reconstruction of the triceps mechanism.

If the goals of treatment are kept in mind it is evident that open reduction and internal fixation should be sufficiently rigid to allow early motion. The history of olecranon fracture treatment shows that many failures were due to inadequate methods of internal fixation. This led to the early interest in olecranon excision. However, if anatomic reconstruction can be achieved and maintained, particularly in young persons, this clearly has the best chance to achieve an optimal result. But because in many fractures anatomic reconstruction may be technically impossible, primary excision offers a better alternative in this situation. Primary excision may also be indicated because of other reasons arising from the injured extremity (multiple injuries) or because of the age and general condition of the patient.

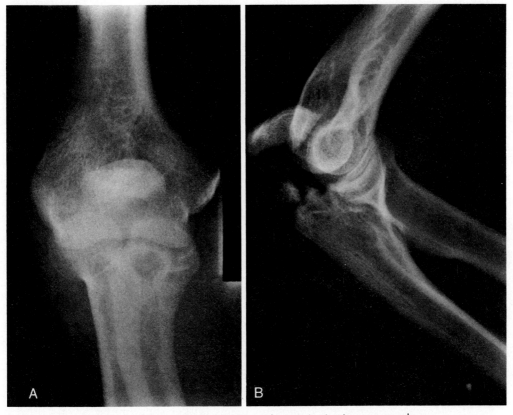

Figure 21–6. *A, B,* Oblique fracture with comminution in a young male.

Current Methods of Internal Fixation

Wiring

Approximation of the fragments with a loop of various materials is now obsolete.[2, 22, 31, 40, 53, 54] Even with wire, the fixation that can be achieved with a simple loop is not rigid enough, and failure often occurs if early motion is attempted unless the fracture anatomy provides some stability.

Circlage wire has been superseded today by tension band wiring introduced by the AO group.[16, 36] The principle of this method (the tension band principle) is based on the transformation of distraction forces at the fracture site into compression forces across the fracture. After reduction the fragments are temporarily fixed with two parallel intramedullary Kirschner wires. Then a figure-of-eight loop of stainless steel wire is advanced through a coronal drill hole in the distal fragment. The wire is then crossed over on the posterior surface of the olecranon, passed around the protruding end of the pins, which can be then bent slightly inward, and tightened and secured with a twist (Figs. 21–6, 21–7). When the wire is tightened some gapping at the articular aspect of the fracture can be seen occasionally; however, early active flexion will create enough compression across the fracture to close the gap. Weber has suggested that both sides of the figure-of-eight wire loop should be twisted.[36] This improves the rigidity of the fixation and may equalize the compression forces on the medial and lateral aspects of the fracture. However, it also complicates the necessary removal of the Kirschner pins and the wire after fracture healing has occurred.

Tension band wiring can be difficult when there is a central cuneiform or comminuted fragment. Careful repositioning of the articular fragments is essential and may necessitate

the use of a small cancellous graft to fill the void left after articular reconstruction. If central comminution is such that reconstruction is impossible but there is still a large intact proximal fragment, it may be possible to discard the comminuted fragments, produce smooth surfaces in the intact proximal and distal fragments by careful osteotomies, and fix them with the proximal fragment in a distally advanced position. This requires very accurate preservation of the trochlear curve to avoid articular incongruity.

Longitudinal Intramedullary Fixation

The problem with this type of fixation is that adequate fixation may not be obtained either in the proximal fragment or distally into the ulnar shaft. Rush rods, threaded Steinmann pins, long wood screws,[25, 32] and especially designed devices have been utilized. One of the screws commonly used, the Leinbach screw, is long enough to obtain adequate distal fixation, but unfortunately we have observed fractures of the screw at the shank-screw junction. Another device, the McAtee olecranon device,[18] uses a long, flexible intramedullary bolt that crosses the fracture site and engages distally with a perpendicular compression nut. It is said to allow controlled accurate compression of the fracture fragments and to provide strong fixation. Its almost completely intramedullary position is an advantage, but insertion is not easy, and it is possible to fail to engage the distal compression nut. Cancellous AO screws have been also used in association with tension band wiring, but they do not provide as rigid fixation, particularly control of rotation, as the two parallel pins, especially if comminution is present. In general, intramedullary devices perform best with simple fractures in which the fracture anatomy itself gives some stability after reduction.

Bicortical Screw Fixation

Interfragmentary compression with a bicortical screw has been advised for transverse or oblique fractures that occur near the coronoid process. Once the fracture is reduced, the fracture surfaces themselves provide some stability, and the strong fixation achieved with a bicortical compression screw allows early motion and enhances functional recovery.

Plates

The AO manual[36] recommends the use of plates (either semitubular or one third tubu-

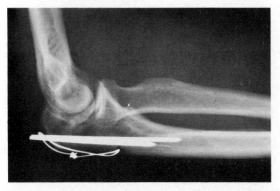

Figure 21–7. Same elbow after treatment with tension band wiring.

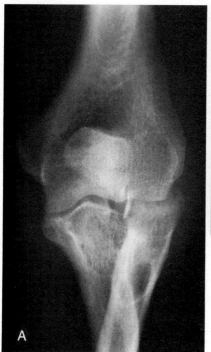
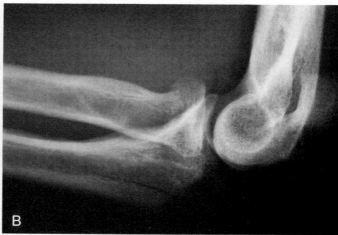

Figure 21–8. *A, B,* Transverse fracture in an elderly male.

lar) to protect the reduction of comminuted fractures after careful reconstruction of the joint surface. In general, because of the subcutaneous location of the bone plates, they are frequently not advisable (Figs. 21–8, 21–9). Modified plates have been designed that function according to the tension band principle. One such device, the Zuelzer hook plate, adds a built-in buttressing effect at the fracture site that is allegedly useful when there is obliquity of comminution of the fracture or in patients with osteoporotic bone. Weseley et al. reported uniformly excellent or good results using a modified Zuelzer hook

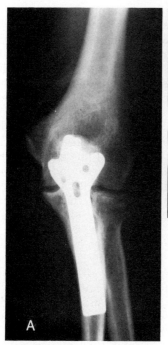
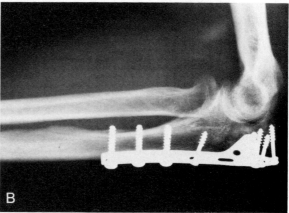

Figure 21–9. *A, B,* Postoperative x-ray of same patient treated with AO cobra plate; excellent result, although mild extension lag was present.

plate in 25 patients with fractures of the olecranon without associated lesions of the elbow joint.[55]

External Fixation

Recently Burghele and Serban reported on the use of an external fixation device based on two Kirschner wires passed transversely through the proximal and distal fragments and applied to either side of the olecranon.[15] The device has been used in 50 open and closed fractures as well as in a case involving a dislocation or subluxation of the elbow (in this instance, however, one or two additional axial Kirschner wires were necessary to maintain the reduction of the dislocation). Because of the excellent fixation obtained, mobilization with this device can commence in 2 to 3 days, and, unlike internal fixation devices, no second intervention is necessary for removal of the fixation material. Consolidation occurred in 30 to 40 days, and the functional results reported were excellent.

Excision

Loss of fixation resulting from the poor fracture stability that was achieved with early materials and methods of internal fixation led to removal of the fracture fragments as the primary treatment for certain olecranon fractures. Proponents of this method of treatment suggest the following advantages: (1) the possibility of imperfect articular surface reduction and post-traumatic arthritis is eliminated; (2) early motion can be allowed; (3) elbow stability is not affected if the coronoid process and anterior tissues are intact; (4) there is no risk of failure of an internal fixation device; (5) the need for a second operation to remove hardware is eliminated; and (6) the healing time is reduced because fascial healing occurs faster than bone healing.

However, instability after excision of the olecranon has occurred, and loss of extension power and range of motion has been a concern. The indications for primary excision set forth by McKeever and Buck[34] in 1947 have been by and large followed since then. MacAusland suggested the following guidelines for olecranectomy:[1, 33] (1) The entire olecranon process can be excised as long as the coronoid process and anterior soft tissues are intact; (2) secure reattachment of the triceps tendon must be achieved with nonabsorbable sutures; (3) active motion is permitted immediately after surgery, but active flexion must be guarded against for several weeks.

A review of several reports on olecranectomy[1, 17, 20, 24, 34, 41, 54] shows that, of a total of more than 100 such procedures, excellent results were achieved in more than 90 percent. These results are better than those generally reported with open reduction and internal fixation, with which failure of fixation, discomfort due to the subcutaneous location of the fixation devices, and incongruity of the joint surfaces are the most commonly reported problems.[17, 22, 24, 31, 44] However, it must be pointed out that patients treated by excision are generally older and obviously make fewer demands on the elbow joint. Nevertheless, Gartsman et al., in an excellent follow-up study of 29 olecranon fractures treated by open reduction and internal fixation in 15 instances and by excision in 14, found no significant difference between both groups of patients in regard to pain, range of motion, or presence of instability on clinical or radiographic examination.[24] More important, no significant differences between the two groups were encountered when objective measurements of static and dynamic strength of elbow extensors were made. Complications were encountered more frequently in patients treated by internal fixation than in those treated by excision, a fact that was also noted by Wainwright[54] and Rettig et al.[44]

Complications

Complications include decreased range of motion, ulnar neuropathy, post-traumatic arthritis, instability, and nonunion. Nonunion is discussed in Chapter 22.

Rigid internal fixation or excision followed by early mobilization should diminish the incidence of late stiffness.[28, 52] However, even with excellent internal fixation extension losses of up to 30 degrees are not uncommon, although functionally they are not disabling. An incidence of decreased motion has been reported in up to 50 percent of cases[22, 24, 44, 52] and seems to occur as often in patients treated by excision as in those treated by internal fixation. The highest incidence of stiffness occurs, as expected, after fracture-dislocation.[9]

Symptoms of ulnar neuropathy have been reported by Rettig in 2 percent of patients,[44] and by Eriksson in 10 percent.[22] Careful operative technique and occasional anterior transposition of the ulnar nerve when it seems to be in jeopardy may help to minimize or prevent this problem.

Anterior instability after excision of the

olecranon has been infrequently noted* and occurs only after an unrecognized fracture-dislocation has been treated by this method. Gartsman reported no instances of instability following excision in 53 patients.[24]

Radiologic evidence of post-traumatic arthritis occurs rather frequently (in 20 to 35 percent) and correlates with the severity of the original injury[53] and with the quality of the reduction.[22] Gartsman reported a similar incidence of radiologic degenerative changes in patients treated by internal fixation and by excision.[24] Symptoms of degenerative disease in the elbow are not as common as they are in a weight-bearing joint, but Eriksson found a certain correlation between their presence and the extent of radiologic findings.[22]

Author's Preferred Method of Treatment

Undisplaced Fractures

We generally use a posterior splint in a position of midflexion and start gentle range of motion after 7 to 10 days. Full flexion is discouraged for 4 to 6 weeks, and roentgenograms are obtained weekly for the first 3 weeks.

Avulsion Fractures

If the fracture fragment is extra-articular, we prefer excision and reattachment of the triceps mechanism. If it is larger and involves the joint surface, we usually prefer tension

---

*Coonrad, R. Personal communication, 1983.

band wiring. We like the posteromedial approach described by Taylor and Scham.[50]

Transverse or Oblique Fractures

Pure transverse fractures are well suited for accurate open reduction and internal fixation with tension band wiring, and pure oblique fractures may be handled with bicortical lag screw fixation. The joint surface must be visualized to ensure anatomic reduction. If a wedge-shaped central fragment is present it must be carefully repositioned, but if it is comminuted this may be difficult (Figs. 21–6, 21–7). When the central comminution is significant, we prefer excision of the proximal fragments and triceps reattachment. In general, we do not like fixation of these fractures with intramedullary single screws or similar devices because rotational stability may be unsatisfactory, and we have seen failures of long slender intramedullary screws.

Comminuted Fractures

By and large, we handle these injuries by excision of the comminuted fragments and triceps reattachment (Figs. 21–10, 21–11). This is our treatment of choice in elderly patients. Only when there are associated injuries to the elbow that would compromise joint stability if olecranon excision were performed do we attempt accurate joint reconstruction by carefully "reassembling the joint surface puzzle." Defects in the cancellous bone should be filled with cancellous bone graft, and rigid fixation should be achieved, usually by using a plate. In this situation

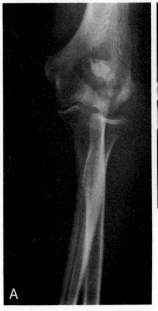
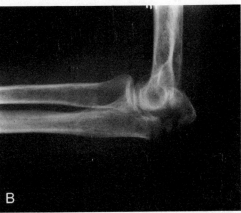

Figure 21–10. A, B, Comminuted fracture in an elderly person.

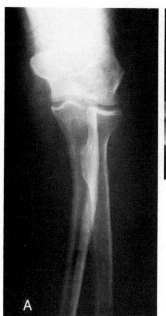

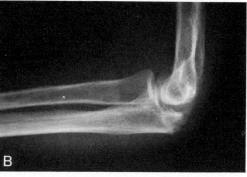

Figure 21–11. *A, B,* Treatment of the above injury by excision.

stability is usually attained at the expense of motion.

Fracture-Dislocations

Fracture-dislocations are the most difficult injuries to treat owing to the associated anterior soft tissue damage. Accurate reduction and rigid fixation are essential to prevent compromising joint stability. Olecranon excision is therefore contraindicated. If the fracture comminution is minimal or nonexistent, tension band wiring is our first choice (Figs.

21–12, 21–13, 21–14). If comminution is significant we prefer plate fixation, but an alternative procedure is to maintain the reduction by external means until soft tissue healing has occurred and then proceed with excision of the comminuted fragments.

Rehabilitation

Regardless of the method of treatment, gentle active range of motion should begin when

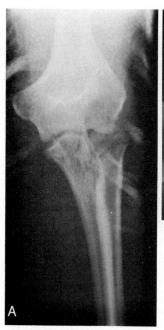

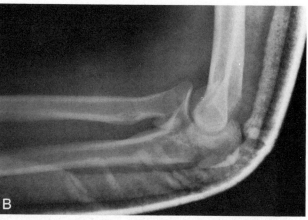

Figure 21–12. *A, B,* Fracture subluxation with associated radial head fracture in a young tennis player.

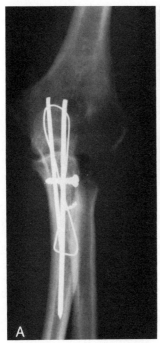

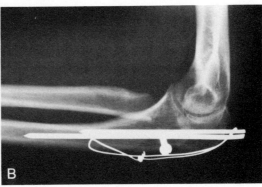

Figure 21–13. *A, B,* Treatment by rigid open reduction and internal fixation with tension band wiring plus interfragmentary screw and excision of the radial head, all done through a Boyd approach.

postoperative pain has subsided, usually between 3 and 7 days after the operation. Extremes of motion, particularly flexion, are discouraged, at least during the first 4 weeks. Strengthening exercises should not be started until union is firm when internal fixation has been the treatment used, or until 8 weeks postoperatively when excision has been carried out.

When tension band wiring is used range of motion exercises may be uncomfortable owing to the protruding ends of the Kirschner wires against the triceps tendon or the subcutaneous tissues. In fact, maximum extension may not be achieved until the wires are removed, but removal should obviously be delayed until firm radiologic union is present and in any case never before 8 weeks.

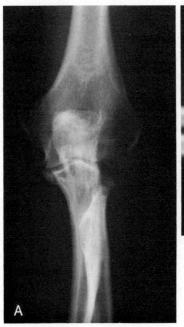

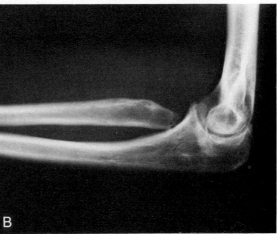

Figure 21–14. The result 3 years postoperatively—minimal range of motion and excellent function.

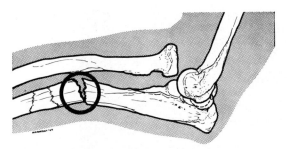

Figure 21–15. Monteggia lesion type I. (From Reckling, F. W., and Cordel, L. B.: Unstable fracture-dislocations of the forearm. The Monteggia and Galeazzi lesions. Arch. Surg. 96:999, 1968.)

MONTEGGIA FRACTURE

Giovanni Battista Monteggia of Milan first described this injury in 1814,[35a] the same year that Colles described his fracture. He initially reported on a fracture of the ulna associated with anterior dislocation of the radial head, which is today recognized as the most common of the Monteggia lesions, a term coined by Bado,[6] which includes all ulnar fractures associated with dislocations of the radiocapitellar articulation. These lesions are uncommon (7 percent of ulnar fracture, 0.7 percent of elbow injuries[7]), but are potentially very serious.

Classification

Although three distinct types of injuries were recognized early, depending on the type of dislocation of the radial head (anterior, posterior, and lateral), it was Bado[6] who first proposed a classification that encompasses the entire spectrum of these injuries. This classification is now universally accepted.

Type I. This is an anterior dislocation of the radial head associated with a fracture of the ulnar diaphysis at any level with anterior

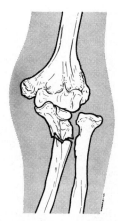

Figure 21–17. Monteggia lesion type III. (From Reckling, F. W., and Cordell, L. B.: Unstable fracture-dislocations of the forearm. The Monteggia and Galeazzi lesions. Arch. Surg. 96:999, 1968.)

angulation (Fig. 21–15). This is the most common type of lesion (55 to 78 percent of Monteggia fractures, depending on the series) and is most common in children.

Type II. This is a posterior or posterolateral dislocation of the radial head associated with a fracture of the ulnar diaphysis with posterior angulation (Fig. 21–16). It usually is more proximal. The lesion occurs most commonly in adults, with a frequency of about 10 to 15 percent of cases.

Type III. This injury is a lateral or anterolateral dislocation of the radial head associated with a fracture of the ulnar metaphysis (Fig. 21–17). More common in children, it occurs with a frequency of 6.7 to 20 percent of cases.

Type IV. This fracture, the most rare type (5 percent of cases), consists of an anterior dislocation of the radial head associated with a fracture of the proximal third of the radius and a fracture of the ulna at the same level (Fig. 21–18).

In addition, Bado described equivalents to types I and II injury as follows; according to him, types III and IV have no equivalents.

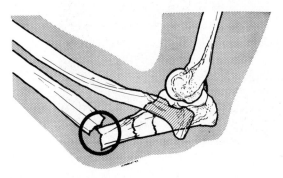

Figure 21–16. Monteggia lesion type II. (From Reckling, F. W., and Cordell, L. B.: Unstable fracture-dislocations of the forearm. The Monteggia and Galeazzi lesions. Arch. Surg. 96:999, 1968.)

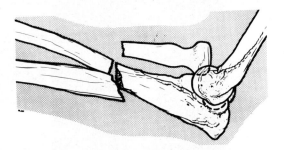

Figure 21–18. Monteggia lesion type IV. (From Reckling, F. W.: Unstable fracture-dislocation of the forearm (Monteggia and Galeazzi lesions). J. Bone Joint Surg. 64A:857, 1982.)

Type I Equivalents

1. Isolated anterior dislocation of the radial head in children (nursemaid's elbow).

2. Fracture of the ulnar diaphysis with fracture of the neck of the radius in adults.

3. Isolated fracture of the neck of the radius.

4. Fracture of the ulnar diaphysis with a more proximal fracture of the radial diaphysis.

5. Fracture of the ulnar diaphysis with anterior dislocation of the radial head and fracture of the olecranon.

6. Posterior dislocation of the elbow and fracture of the ulnar diaphysis with or without fracture of the proximal radius.

Type II Equivalents

1. Epiphyseal fractures of the dislocated radial head.

2. Fractures of the neck of the radius.

Mechanism of Injury

Different theories have been proposed to explain the mechanism of injury, which of course varies according to the type of lesion.

The greatest controversy concerns the type I lesion. A direct blow to the posterior aspect of the ulna would seem to be the likely mechanism in those cases, in which hematomas are encountered over the ulnar fracture site. However, a fall on the outstretched hand with the forearm in pronation may be the most common mechanism. Evans postulated that on such a fall, in which the hand is fixed to the ground by the weight of the body, the full pronation of the forearm is exaggerated by external rotation of the arm on the hand, and an oblique fracture of the ulna occurs.[23] At the same time, the radius, forced into extreme pronation, crosses the ulna at the junction of the middle and proximal thirds. This contact acts as a fulcrum, forcing the proximal radius anteriorly to dislocate its head or to fracture, or, exceptionally, to do both (type IV). Evans carried out cadaver experiments that produced Monteggia type I or equivalent lesions 17 times out of 18, confirming his hypothesis. Tompkins, on the other hand, postulated that on a fall on the outstretched hand the radial head is dislocated by a violent reflex contraction of the biceps;[51] this causes all the weight to be borne by the ulna, and, owing to the longitudinal compressive force combined with the pull of the interosseous membrane and the simultaneous contracting brachialis, the ulna fractures and angulates anteriorly. Thus, the mechanism is one of hyperextension. This theory, if correct, would have implications in treatment, because flexion of 100 to 110 degrees would be necessary after reduction to avoid redislocation of the radial head. It is likely that all three mechanisms (direct blow to the ulna, hyperpronation, and hyperextension) can play a role in the generation of type I injuries.

Type II injuries were studied by Penrose,[39] who found that they occurred more often among middle-aged women in whom ligamentous attachments of the proximal ulna are stronger than the ulna itself. This explains the mechanism of injury, which is similar to that in a posterior elbow dislocation and was also proved by Penrose in cadaver experiments. Bado felt that these injuries are caused by a direct and rotational force—supination,[6] but this has not been proved.

Bado states that the mechanism of injury in type III fractures is a direct blow on the inner side of the elbow with or without rotation.[6]

Symptoms and Signs

Clinically, Monteggia lesions have different presentations depending on the type. Pain and marked tenderness and functional incapacity of the elbow are common to all types.

In type I lesions the forearm and hand remain in a fixed attitude of pronation. Shortening of the forearm, swelling, and anterior angulation of the fractured ulna are present, and the radial head can be palpated in the antecubital fossa. If the fracture is compound, the skin lesion is usually anterior.

In type II lesions, the ulnar fracture is more proximal, and the angulation is posterior. The radial head (often fractured), can be palpated posteriorly, and if the fracture is open, the wound is usually posterior.

In type III lesions there is a lateral angulation of the ulna at the level of the fracture, the forearm is usually in midposition, and the radial head can be felt laterally.

In type IV lesions the findings are similar to those in type I injuries, but there is usually tenderness over the radial shaft fracture.

The most common associated injury is paralysis of the deep branch of the radial nerve (posterior interosseous nerve). This appears to occur more commonly after types I and III injuries.[12, 13, 14, 27, 35, 48, 57] The prognosis for spontaneous recovery is quite favorable. Associated injuries to the median[27] and ulnar nerves[14, 35] have been rarely reported.

Radiologic Findings

Adequate roentgenograms in two planes including the elbow and wrist joints are essential. The ulnar fracture is easy to recognize, but the dislocation of the radial head may be missed in poor quality views, particularly if the displacement is mild or if the dislocation has been reduced inadvertently by a previous examiner or at the time of positioning the patient for the x-ray examination.[3] Thus, the pitfall here is to miss the radial head injury. Speed and Boyd reported in 1940 that 52 percent of the injuries were not diagnosed until 4 weeks after injury;[47] this incidence of delayed discovery of the radial head dislocation had decreased to 24 percent when Boyd and Boals reported on an expanded series of 159 lesions in 1965.[12] Mobley and Janes reported that 5 of 15 patients (33 percent) had old lesions,[35] and Reckling and Cordell found that 4 patients of 25 (16 percent) had old lesions.[42] Diagnosis remains a problem with Monteggia lesions, much as Monteggia pointed out 170 years ago.

Treatment

It is generally agreed that these lesions can be treated satisfactorily in children by closed methods. It is also agreed that closed treatment produces usually unsatisfactory results in adults.

Monteggia used closed reduction in his two cases and found the results unsatisfactory with persistent dislocation of the radial head.[35a] Watson-Jones observed that myositis ossificans and ankylosis of the radioulnar joint occurred frequently with immediate operative reduction of the radial head.[54a] He also stated that end results from this injury lead to permanent disability in 95 percent of cases. Speed and Boyd in 1940 concluded that closed treatment is unsatisfactory and advocated open reduction and internal fixation of the ulna and reconstruction of the annular ligament with a fascial loop.[47] In 1969, Boyd and Boals recommended open reduction and internal fixation of the ulna with a compression plate or an intramedullary nail, but suggested that closed reduction of the radial head was usually adequate and open reduction usually unnecessary.[12] If a fracture of the radial head was present, they suggested excision. They found the Boyd[11] approach to the ulna and proximal third of the radius very satisfactory and obtained excellent or good results in 77 percent of acute lesions.

Evans in 1949 carried out a clinical and experimental study of the anterior Monteggia fracture and pointed out that immobilization in full supination is the surest safeguard against the recurrence of the deformity.[23]

Bado advised closed treatment for type I injuries.[6] Manipulation with gentle traction in pronation followed by supination corrects the dislocation and the deviation of the ulnar fracture. This is followed by immobilization of the elbow in 90 degrees of flexion and supination.

Penrose in 1951 advised open reduction and internal fixation of the ulnar fracture combined with partial or total radial head excision (if the radial head was fractured) for type II injuries.[39] Pavel et al., however, reported poor results after early radial head excisions for these injuries.[38] Bryan and Reckling reported also a lower incidence of satisfactory results with type II injuries.[14, 43]

Bado suggested closed treatment for type II injuries with manipulation by gentle traction and pronation to reduce the dislocation.[6] If the ulnar fracture is not reduced, he advised intramedullary nailing. He also mentioned that results of treatment are less satisfactory with this type of injury.

Reckling, in a study reported in 1968[42] and expanded in 1982[43] showed that the results of treatment of Monteggia lesions in adults were uniformly worse than those in children and that the best results were obtained with open anatomic reduction of the ulnar fracture, internal fixation, and complete closed reduction of the radial head dislocation. Yet only 9 of 40 adult patients obtained an excellent result.

Type III injuries are almost exclusively found in children. Bryan, however, reported on three such lesions in adults, two treated surgically with good results and one by closed means with a poor result.[14]

Type IV injuries are clearly surgical lesions. Both fractures should be managed by open reduction and internal fixation, and the radial head dislocation can often be reduced by closed manipulation (supination).

The worst problem is the undiagnosed or inadequately treated Monteggia lesion that is seen late (after 4 weeks). The radial head has remained subluxed or redislocated, and the ulna may be healing in an anteriorly angulated position or may simply be ununited. Minor degrees of angulation of the ulna and minimal subluxation of the radial head are best left alone. Excellent function can result in this situation. Moderate angulation of the ulna and dislocation of the radial head is best treated by ulnar realignment osteotomy and plating if a malunion is present, or by realignment and plating of a nonunion, and by resection of the radial head.

Five out of Mobley and Janes' 15 cases were old lesions,[35] and in Boyd's experience 52 percent of the injuries before 1940[12] but only 24 percent of those after 1940[47] were old lesions. It is hoped that the incidence of missed radial head dislocations and of inadequate ulnar reductions and fixations is decreasing.

Complications

Radial neuropathy, particularly that involving the posterior interosseous branch, has been reported rather frequently.[13, 14, 27, 35, 57] Causes of the deficit are direct trauma, compression of the nerve in the arcade of Frohse, or stretching of the nerve by a laterally dislocated radial head (the nerve lesion that is most common with type III Monteggia lesions). Its incidence has been as high as 20 percent of acute lesions, but its prognosis is usually good; complete recovery is the rule, and it begins,

according to Jessing, by 6 to 8 weeks. Exploration of the posterior interosseous nerve is advisable when no evidence of recovery is present by 8 to 10 weeks. Tardy palsy of the radial nerve after a Monteggia fracture has been rarely reported[5, 30] and always occurs after an old unreduced lesion with longstanding dislocation of the radial head. Improvement has occurred after exploration of the radial nerve and excision of the radial head, which compresses the nerve during movements of pronation and supination.

Median[27] and ulnar[14, 35] nerve palsies are very rare in association with Monteggia lesions.

Malunion of the ulna is seldom seen today, because diagnosis of the lesion is less frequently missed. Late redislocation or subluxation of the head of the radius may be the result of poor internal fixation of the ulna or postoperative immobilization of the elbow in a poor position or for too short a period of time.

Cross-union between the radius and ulna has been reported and may be the result of a high energy injury with significant commi-

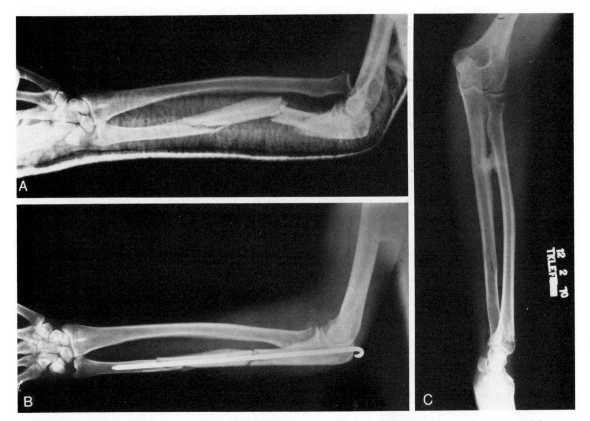

Figure 21–19. A, Type I Monteggia fracture with segmental comminuted ulna fracture. B, Same lesion treated by open reduction and internal fixation of the ulna by Rush rod and closed reduction of the radial head. C, End result with a cross union at the level of proximal ulna fracture; significant restriction of pronation and supination exists.

nution (Fig. 21–19). The Boyd approach has also been implicated in some instances of cross-union.

Nonunion of the ulna is most commonly related to infection but is also the result of inadequate internal fixation.[4] Compression plating, properly executed, produces the lowest rate of nonunion. We have found external fixation useful in the treatment of one infected ununited Monteggia fracture.

Author's Preferred Method of Treatment

We think that the following principles of treatment of Monteggia lesions in adults must be respected to achieve satisfactory results:

1. Accurate Diagnosis. Missing the dislocation of the radial head will result in inadequate treatment, and a poor outcome is likely (but a lucky good outcome can occur if the dislocation reduces spontaneously and remains reduced).

2. Accurate Reduction of the Ulnar Fracture and Maintenance of the Reduction. This is best achieved today by compression plating, sup-

plemented by cancellous bone graft if there is significant comminution (Figs. 21–20, 21–21, 21–22). In type IV injuries, compression plating of the radial and ulnar shaft fractures is the treatment of choice.

3. Restoration of the Radiohumeral Joint. Usually the radial head reduces spontaneously when the ulnar fracture is reduced. In those rare instances when it fails to do so, open reduction with incision of the annular ligament is necessary. When fracture of the radial head is present, as in some type II injuries, partial or complete excision of the radial head may be necessary. In the rare instances when the radial head needs to be exposed, we prefer the Boyd approach to the proximal radius and ulna. In type IV injuries the radial head dislocation usually reduces with closed methods.

4. Adequate Postoperative Immobilization. For types I, III, and IV injuries, flexion of at least 90 degrees, maintained for 4 weeks in moderate supination if the internal fixation achieved is rigid, usually suffices. Lateral roentgenograms should be rechecked at 1 and 2 weeks to assess the position of the radial

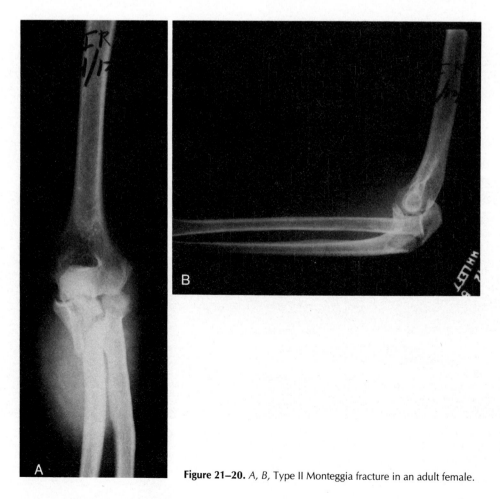

Figure 21–20. *A, B,* Type II Monteggia fracture in an adult female.

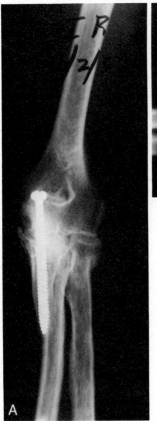

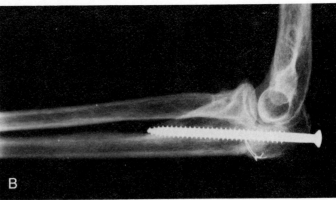

Figure 21–21. *A, B,* Radiographic result 6 months after operation. Good range of motion; no pain; internal fixation of the ulna by a wood screw.

head. In type II lesions, immobilization should be maintained in about 70 degrees of flexion.

5. Active Rehabilitation. After the immobilization has been discontinued, active range of motion exercises are begun. Improvement occurs slowly, but passive stretching is not advisable.

The advent of rigid internal fixation methods has improved the prognosis for these potentially treacherous injuries.

References

1. Adler, S., Fay, G. D., and MacAusland, W. R., Jr.: Treatment of Olecranon Fractures. Indications for

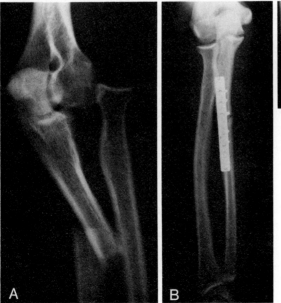

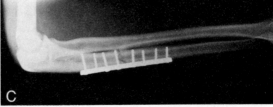

Figure 21–22. *A,* Type I Monteggia lesion in an 18-year-old boy. *B, C,* Postoperative x-ray view after open reduction of ulna with AO compression plate and closed reduction of radial head. Full recovery occurred in 3 months.

Excision of the Olecranon Fragment and Repair of the Triceps Tendon. J. Trauma **2**:597, 1962.

2. Aldredge, G. H., Jr., and Gregory, C. F.: Triceps Advancement in Olecranon Fractures. J. Bone Jt. Surg. **51A**:816, 1969.

3. Anderson, L. D.: Fractures of the Shaft of the Radius and Ulna. In Rockwood, C. A., and Green, D. P.: Fractures. Philadelphia, J. B. Lippincott Co., 1975.

4. Anderson, L. D., Sisk, T. D., Tooms, R. E., and Park, W. I.: Compression-Plate Fixation in Acute Diaphyseal Fractures of the Radius and Ulna. J. Bone Jt. Surg. **57A**:287, 1975.

5. Austin, R.: Tardy Palsy of Radial Nerve From a Monteggia Fracture. Injury **7**:202, 1976.

6. Bado, J. L.: The Monteggia Lesion. Clin. Orthop. **50**:71, 1967.

7. Beck, C., and Dabezies, E. J.: Monteggia Fracture-Dislocation. Orthopedics **7**:329, 1984.

8. Berger, P.: Le Traitement de Fractures de l'Olecrane et Particulierement la Sutur de l'Olecrane par un Procede. Ga. 2, Hebd. de Med., 193–199, 1902.

9. Biga, N., and Thomine, J. M.: la Luxation Trans-olecranienne du Coude. Rev. Chir. Orthop. **60**:557, 1974.

10. Bohler, L.: The Treatment of Fractures. Vienna, Wilhelm Mandrich, 1929.

11. Boyd, H. B.: Surgical Exposure of the Ulna and Proximal Third of the Radius Through One Incision. Surg. Gynecol. Obstet. **71**:86, 1940.

12. Boyd, H. B., and Boals, J. C.: The Monteggia Lesion. A Review of 159 Cases. Clin. Orthop. **66**:94, 1969.

13. Bruce, H. E., Harvey, J. P., and Wilson, J. C.: Monteggia Fractures. J. Bone Jt. Surg. **56A**:1563, 1974.

14. Bryan, R. S.: Monteggia Fracture of the Forearm. J. Trauma **11**:992, 1971.

15. Burghele, H., and Serban, N.: Fractures of the Olecranon: Treatment by External Fixation. Ital. J. Orthop. Traumatol. **8**:159, 1982.

16. Colton, C. L.: Fractures of the Olecranon in Adults: Classification and Management. Injury **5**:121, 1973.

17. Conn, J., and Wade, P. A.: Injuries of the Elbow: A Ten Year Review. J. Trauma **1**:248, 1961.

18. Coughling, N. J., Slabaugh, P. B., and Smith, T. K.: Experience With the McAtee Olecranon Device in Olecranon Fractures. J. Bone Jt. Surg. **61A**:385, 1979.

19. Daland, E. N.: Fractures of the Olecranon. J. Bone Jt. Surg. **15**:601, 1933.

20. Dunn, N.: Operation for Fracture of the Olecranon. Br. Med. J. **1**:214, 1939.

21. Elliot, E., Jr.: Fracture of the Olecranon. Surg. Clin. North Am. **14**:487, 1934.

22. Eriksson, E., Sahlen, O., and Sandohl, U.: Late Results of Conservative and Surgical Treatment of Fractures of the Olecranon. Acta. Chir. Scand. **113**:153, 1957.

23. Evans, E. M.: Pronation Injuries of the Forearm with Special Reference to the Anterior Monteggia Fracture. J. Bone Jt. Surg. **31B**:578, 1949.

23a. Fiolle, 1918: As quoted by Perruello, N. N., 1955.

24. Gartsman, G. M., Sculco, T. P., and Otis, J. C.: Operative Treatment of Olecranon Fractures. J. Bone Jt. Surg. **63A**:718, 1981.

25. Harmon, P. H.: Treatment of Fractures of the Olecranon by Fixation with a Stainless-Steel Screw. J. Bone Jt. Surg. **27**:328, 1945.

26. Hey-Groves, E. W.: Fractures of the Olecranon. Br. Med. J. **1**:296, 1939.

27. Jessing, P.: Monteggia Lesions and Their Complicating Nerve Damage. Acta Orthop. Scand. **46**:601, 1975.

28. Kiviluoto, O., and Santavirta, S.: Fractures of the

Olecranon: An Analysis of 37 Consecutive Cases. Acta Orthop. Scand. **49**:28, 1978.

29. Kohler, A., and Zimmer, E. A.: Borderlands of the Normal and Early Pathologic in Skeletal Roentgenology. New York, Grune & Stratton, 1968.

30. Lichter, R. L., and Jacobsen, T.: Tardy Palsy of the Posterior Interosseous Nerve With a Monteggia Fracture. J. Bone Jt. Surg. **57A**:124, 1975.

30a. Lister: As quoted by Elliot, 1934.

31. Lou, I.: Olecranon Fractures Treated in the Orthopedic Hospital, Copenhagen, 1936–1947. A Follow-up Examination. Acta Orthop. Scand. **19**:166, 1949–1950.

32. MacAusland, W. R.: The Treatment of Fractures of the Olecranon by Longitudinal Screw or Nail Fixation. Ann. Surg. **116**:293, 1942.

33. MacAusland, W. R., Jr., and Wyman, E. T.: Fractures of the Adult Elbow. In American Academy of Orthopedic Surgeons: Instructional Course Lectures, Vol. 24, St. Louis, C. V. Mosby Co., 1975, pp. 169–181.

34. McKeever, F. M., and Buck, R. N.: Fracture of the Olecranon Process of the Ulna. Treatment by Excision of Fragment and Repair of Triceps. J.A.M.A. **135**:1, 1947.

35. Mobley, J. E., and Janes, J. M.: Monteggia Fractures. Proc. Staff Meet. Mayo Clin. **30**:497, 1955.

35a. Monteggia, G. B.: Instituzioni Chirurgiche, Vol. 5. Milan, Maspero, 1814.

36. Muller, M. E., Allgower, M., Schneider, R., and Willenegger, H.: Manual of Internal Fixation. Techniques Recommended by the AO Group, 2nd ed. New York, Springer-Verlag, 1979.

37. O'Donoghue, D. H., and Sell, L. S.: Persistent Olecranon Epiphysis in Adults. J. Bone Jt. Surg. **24**:677, 1942.

38. Pavel, A., Pitman, J. M., Lance, E. M., and Wade, P. A.: The Posterior Monteggia Fracture: A Clinical Study. J. Trauma **5**:185, 1965.

39. Penrose, J. H.: The Monteggia Fractures with Posterior Dislocation of the Radial Head. J. Bone Jt. Surg. **33B**:65, 1951.

40. Perkins, G.: Fractures of the Olecranon. Br. Med. J. **2**:668, 1936.

41. Perruelo, N. N., and Platigorsky, H.: Fractura de Olecranon-Olecranectomia. Acta Ortoped.-Traumatol. Iberica **3**:12, 1955.

42. Reckling, F. W., and Cordell, L. B.: Unstable Fracture-Dislocations of the Forearm. The Monteggia and Galeazzi Lesions. Arch. Surg. **96**:999, 1968.

43. Reckling, F. W.: Unstable Fracture-Dislocation of the Forearm (Monteggia and Galeazzi Lesions). J. Bone Jt. Surg. **64A**:857, 1982.

44. Rettig, A. C., Waugh, T. R., and Evanski, P. M.: Fracture of the Olecranon: A Problem of Management. J. Trauma **19**:23, 1979.

45. Rombold, C.: A New Operative Treatment for Fractures of the Olecranon. J. Bone Jt. Surg. **16**:947, 1934.

46. Rowe, C. R.: The Management of Fractures in Elderly Patients is Different. J. Bone Jt. Surg. **47A**:1043, 1965.

46a. Sachs, 1898: As quoted by Elliot, 1934.

46b. Shelton: As quoted by Van der Kloot, 1964.

47. Speed, J. S., and Boyd, H. B.: Treatment of Fractures of the Ulna With Dislocation of Head of Radius (Monteggia Fracture). J.A.M.A. **115**:1699, 1940.

48. Spinner, M., Freundlich, B. D., and Teicher, J.: Posterior Interosseous Nerve Palsy as a Complication of Monteggia Fractures in Children. Clin. Orthop. **58**:141, 1968.

49. Strug, L. H.: Anterior Dislocation of the Elbow with

Fracture of the Olecranon. Am. J. Surg. **75**:700, 1948.

50. Taylor, T. K. F., and Scham, S. M.: A Posteromedial Approach to the Proximal End of the Ulna for Internal Fixation of Olecranon Fractures. J. Trauma **9**:594, 1969.

51. Tompkins, D. G.: The Anterior Monteggia Fracture. Observations on Etiology and Treatment. J. Bone Jt. Surg. **53A**:1109, 1971.

52. Van der Horst, M. A. M., and Keeman, J. N.: Treatment of Olecranon Fractures. Netherlands J. Surg. **35**:27, 1983.

53. Van de Kloot, J. F. V. R.: Results of Treatment of Fractures of the Olecranon. Arch. Chir. Neerlandicum **16**:237, 1964.

54. Wainwright, D.: Fractures of the Olecranon Process. Br. J. Surg. **29**:403, 1942.

54a. Watson-Jones: As quoted by Mobley and Janes, 1955.

55. Weseley, M. S., Barenfeld, P. A., and Eisenstein, A. L.: The Use of the Zuelzer Hook Plate in Fixation of Olecranon Fractures. J. Bone Jt. Surg. **58A**:859, 1976.

56. Wilppula, E., and Bakalim, G.: Fractures of the Olecranon. III: Fractures Complicated by Forward Dislocation of the Forearm. Ann. Chir. Gynaecolog. Fenniae **60**:105, 1971.

57. Yamamoto, K., Yanase, Y., and Tomihara, M.: Posterior Interosseous Nerve Palsy as Complication of Monteggia Fractures. Arch. Japanische Chir. **46**:46, 1977.

CHAPTER 22

Nonunion of the Olecranon and Proximal Ulna

RALPH W. COONRAD

Nonunion of displaced fractures of the olecranon has become relatively uncommon in adults and rare in children since the abandonment of earlier forms of treatment by extension immobilization or token internal fixation with figure-of-eight catgut, nonabsorbable soft suture material, or single circumferential approximating wire.[8, 26] Appreciation for the significant tension exerting distraction force of the triceps on proximal fragments has led to the present accepted forms of treatment which are (1) fragment excision, and (2) rigid internal fixation.

In a review of current world literature, two factors stand out in relation to nonunion of the proximal ulna. First, nonunion of the olecranon usually results from inadequate primary internal fixation or loss of reduction. Second, early functional restoration of motion at the elbow is important if stiffness or contracture is to be minimized. This is particularly true when the articular surface is involved in a nonunion.[2, 16, 22, 28, 33, 43, 53, 55]

INCIDENCE

Nonunion of fractures of the proximal ulna and olecranon has been reported to occur in 5 percent of all olecranon fractures.[32] This figure has been put in perspective by Boyd, who reported that the incidence of nonunion in the ulna was 6 percent of that of the larger long ones in the body.[9, 10] In numerical frequency, nonunions occur more commonly in the femur, tibia, humerus, and radius than in the ulna, according to Crenshaw's study of 964 patients.[18] An estimated 6 percent of all fractures undergoing treatment are located about the elbow.[10] Hence, nonunions of this region are approximately equal to the expected rate based on the incidence of this fracture.

SOME GENERAL REMARKS ABOUT NONUNION

Definition

A definitive clinical diagnosis of nonunion cannot be determined until a pseudarthrosis is evident. The temporal difference between slow union, delayed union, and nonunion as defined by various authors is not arbitrary because fracture healing time is variable from bone to bone in various parts of the body. In fractures of long bones, 6 months is usually the minimum accepted time before a definite diagnosis of nonunion may be considered. However, a precise and understandable method of describing the fracture healing process has been described by Mayer and Evarts.[32] According to these authors, a *slow union* is an indolent union that maintains the appearance of the early stages of a healing fracture; the fracture line is visible, and no decalcification or sclerosis is present at the bone ends. *Delayed union* is described as fracture healing in which evidence of attempted union is present roentgenographically. Microscopically, granulation rather than scar tissue formation is present between the fracture fragments. Reactive hyperemia, early resorption of bone ends, and some widening of the fracture site are usually associated with delayed union. *Nonunion* is assumed when all evidence of bone healing has ceased. Pathologically, in a nonunion the bone ends and medullary canals are capped, the endosteal blood supply does not extend across the fracture site, and sclerosis of the bone ends is present in at least 25 percent of patients.[25] Scar tissue rather than granulation tissue is present between the bone ends at the fracture site (unless motion is occurring), and characteristically, a bursal sac usually develops with much movement. Clinically, tender-

Table 22–1. **Causes or Predisposing Factors Contributing to Nonunion of the Olecranon**

Inadequate, non-rigid internal fixation
Inadequate immobilization
Distraction
Compounding of fracture
Wound infection
Comminution
Impairment of blood supply
Defects between bone fragments
Interposition of soft tissue
Abnormalities of electrochemical or cellular physiologic mechanisms involved in fracture healing

ness is a consistent complaint. Other characteristics may include some degree of false motion and a varying radiographic defect between the bone ends.

CAUSES

Ossification in the olecranon begins at two or more centers that may then fuse together before uniting with the parent bone. The normal characteristics of the growing epiphysis may thus be misinterpreted or confused radiographically with a fracture line or nonunion. The reader is referred to an excellent treatise on the subject by Silberstein et al.[42]

The actual cause of nonunion is unknown, although predisposing factors that are frequently implicated in delay of the fracture healing process of any bone include inadequate fixation or immobilization, distraction, compounding of the fracture, wound infection, comminution, impairment of the blood supply, bone defects or interposition of soft tissue, and abnormalities of the normal electrochemical and cellular physiologic mechanisms involved in fracture healing[1, 2, 32] (Table 22–1). Boyd's classic review of fractures with delayed union and nonunion revealed that nonunion was four times more common in males than in females in all bones studied except the clavicle.[9, 10] This ratio may be related to a generally higher frequency of fractures in males. Nonunion of the olecranon is rare in children but may occur when displaced fractures are unrecognized or when inadequate internal fixation results in redisplacement.[31, 36] Nonunion of the olecranon has been reported in an infant following a birth injury and in an adolescent stress fracture.[29, 47] Although children have a higher rate of periosteal response, Boyd et al. showed by their studies that the prognosis for fracture healing in patients in the older age groups is good despite the fact that their fractures tend to heal at a slower rate than those in the younger patient.[10] Iron deficiency anemia has been shown experimentally to retard fracture healing in mice, and fracture healing may also be slowed in the diabetic or in the patient undergoing irradiation treatment.[17, 24, 40]

Possibly the most important factor in the treatment of either fresh fractures or nonunion of the olecranon is the need to convert the tensile forces arising from the forearm flexors and the triceps acting across the fracture or nonunion site to a compressive force (Fig. 22–1).[14]

Distraction produces a tension force in bone

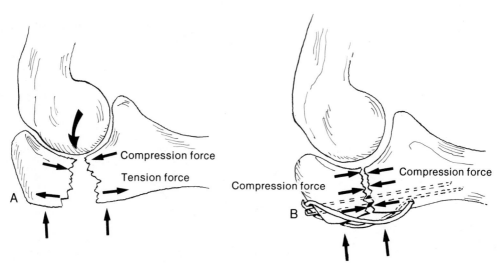

Figure 22–1. *A*, Diagram of the location of compression forces present near the articular surface of the olecranon and tension forces near the posterior surface produced by either an impacting fracture force of the lower end of the humerus, or the force of the elbow flexors and extensor force in nonunions. *B*, The use of tension band wiring (or similar fixation) converts the tension force to a compression or impacting force. Kirschner wires should be placed closer to the posterior surface when possible.

as well as in soft tissue locally at the fracture site and in turn is more likely to inhibit the healing process. In tissue culture experiments with bone explants, Bassett has shown that tension forces may prevent ossious precursors from forming cartilage or bone and promote the growth of fibrous tissue.[4, 5] Tension forces tend to produce an osteoclastic-induced positive electrical potential that may interfere with bone healing. Compression forces, on the other hand, tend to effect an osteoblastic-induced negative electrical potential that produces an enhancing effect on fracture healing.[6, 32]

CLASSIFICATION

Nonunions have been classified by Judet, Muller, and Weber and Cech into two types, hypervascular and avascular, according to the biologic activity at the ends of the fracture fragments. The *hypervascular* type has rich blood supply at the ends of the fragments and may be confirmed by increased strontium-85 or technetium-99 uptake on bone scanning. The *avascular* type has nonviable ends of the fracture fragments and may also be confirmed by a decreased strontium-85 or technetium-99 uptake in the bone.[27, 35, 52]

No classification of olecranon nonunions has been been described in the orthopedic literature I have reviewed; however, it can be assumed that such a classification would be quite similar to that of displaced olecranon fractures because the principles of treatment are nearly identical. Colton in 1973,[3, 14] and Wadsworth in 1976,[51] proposed anatomic classifications of olecranon fractures. Diagramed below is my minor modification of Colton's classification applied to five anatomic types of nonunion (Fig. 22–2).

Type 1 generally includes transverse nonunions involving less than 50 percent of the articular surface of the olecranon notch. Type 2 consists of nonarticular nonunions through the proximal olecranon, usually from avulsion-type injuries. Type 3 comprises nonunions extending transversely through 50 percent or more of the articular surface of the olecranon notch. Type 4 includes stable nonunions extending obliquely from the distal articular surface of the olecranon notch through the proximal ulnar shaft. Type 5 nonunions are unstable Monteggia-type injuries with disruption of the medial collateral ligament and a nonunion either just proximal at or distal to the coronoid process extending through the shaft of the proximal ulna. A sixth type of nonunion results from a comminuted fracture usually due to direct trauma that can be classified with any of the other five types, depending on the location and degree of articular surface involvement (Fig. 21–2). Nonunion of the proximal ulna distal to the insertion of the medial collateral ligament carries a better prognosis for reconstruction because the articular surface of the trochlear notch is intact. Tullos has stressed the importance of the medial collateral ligament as the stabilizing structure that must be torn or separated if anterior displacement and dislocation of the radial head is to occur in an articular fracture adjacent to the coronoid process.[48] Any reconstruction for nonunion in an unstable injury at this level may need medial collateral ligament repair or reconstitution in *addition* to rigid internal fixation.

TREATMENT AND TREATMENT OPTIONS FOR OLECRANON NONUNION

The goals of treatment of olecranon nonunion are the same as those of primary treatment for any displaced fracture. These goals are (1) to restore congruity of the trochlear notch surface, (2) to restore or retain ligamentous stability, particularly of the medial collateral

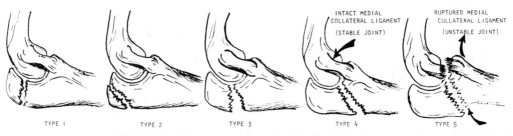

Figure 22–2. Author's minor modification of Colton's classification of olecranon fractures into five types of nonunion. A sixth type is not shown; this is comminuted nonunion that would be subclassified with any of the other five types depending on location and degree of articular involvement. Note the medial collateral ligament disruption in type 5 with an unstable nonunion.

ligament, (3) to restore good triceps extensor function, and (4) to restore mobility of the joint. Historically, the most important principle in the treatment of nonunion of the olecranon is the conversion of tensile forces acting across the joint or nonunion site to a compressive force (Fig. 22–1B).[14] The indications for treatment, however, also require separation of olecranon nonunions into two groups: (1) those in which the articular surface of the trochlear notch has not been severely damaged and should be salvaged, and (2) those in which articular cartilage has been severely damaged by arthritis or traumatic loss of the joint surface. Treatment options under these two broad classifications are described from an historical standpoint below.

Treatment of Nonunion in Which Articular Cartilage Has Not Been Severely Damaged

Fortunately, nonunion of the olecranon is rare, and treatment of large series of isolated instances of this complication has not been reported. Varied methods of treatment have generally been reported in both large and small series of olecranon fractures. However, in the older patient with a nonunion of a small avulsion fragment or of a fragment involving less than 50 percent of the trochlear articular surface, excision of the fragment and meticulous triceps reattachment, or internal fixation with tension band technique, has produced about equally satisfactory results.[28, 33, 53]

Foille in 1918 and Dunn in 1939 gave early descriptions of the results of proximal fragment excision.[19, 21] In 1947, McKeever and Buck reported that 80 percent of the trochlear notch could be excised without producing instability of the elbow joint (Fig. 22–3).[33] Excision of nonunited fracture fragments is contraindicated in the growing child with an open proximal epiphysis. In a series of 107 olecranon fractures treated almost equally by internal fixation and fragment excision, Gartsman found that restoration of elbow extensor function was equal in the two groups as measured by static and dynamic strength testing.[22] In the young patient or in the older patient with a nonunion involving more than 50 percent of the trochlear notch, satisfactory results have been achieved by taking down the pseudarthrosis, excising the intervening scar tissue, realigning the fragments, and carrying out rigid internal fixation. Some of the more frequently used techniques include those that follow:

Tension Band Wiring

This technique is described in Chapter 21, and the reader is also referred to Colton's description and the AO manual for details.[14, 35] Barford has described a modification of this procedure when there is a large central depressed fragment or several comminuted fragments involving the articular surface of the trochlear notch. Because a satisfactory reduction is often precluded in this setting, segmental excision of the middle third of the trochlear notch can be carried out and the proximal and distal segments of the olecranon rigidly fixed with a shallower and shorter articular surface of contact. If tension band wiring is to be used for nonunion in which central portions of the olecranon notch are missing, pin fixation should always be placed toward the posterior rather than the articular side of the proximal ulna. This will allow more compression toward the posterior surface and tend to prevent constriction of the notch. When compression is placed close to the articular surface, narrowing of the trochlear notch may result in later arthritic changes (Fig. 22–4). The tension band wiring technique can be applied in some nonunions with fragments that involve up to 50 percent of the trochlear notch and has been used for oblique fragments that extend further distally. Generally, however, this technique is best applied to acute fractures. Comminuted or unstable fragments with anterior subluxation or instability warrant consideration of other techniques listed below.

Plating

Many types of plates with screw fixation have been described for olecranon nonunions. The most common type of plate and screw fixation currently used is the AO tubular plate, particularly for oblique or transverse fractures involving the mid or distal portion of the articular surface. Plating may be the only available method of salvaging a comminuted fracture and of achieving rigid stability in unstable fractures that involve the coronoid process with rupture of the medial collateral ligament. The AO group recommends a six-hole rather than four-hole plate. Anatomic visualization and reconstitution of the joint surface is mandatory; the fracture type may limit the size of plate that can be used. With dislocation of the radial head and longstanding subluxation or dislocation of the ulnohumeral joint, excision of the radial head is usually necessary (Fig. 22–5). Sufficient bone must be removed to regain not only normal alignment of the

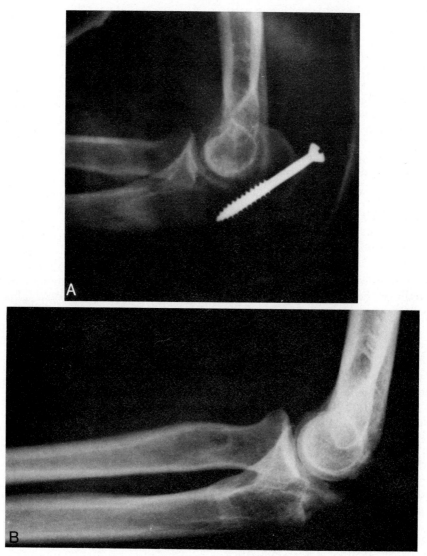

Figure 22–3. *A,* Preoperative radiograph of a nonunion in a 60-year-old woman. The original fracture was treated by a lag screw of inadequate length. *B,* The elbow after excision of the olecranon fragment (involving 50 percent of the articular surface). Satisfactory function resulted.

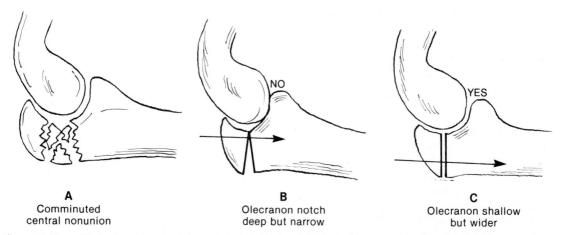

Figure 22–4. *A,* Diagram of a central comminuted nonunion of the articular surface. *B,* Shows tendency toward constriction of the trochlear notch when tension band wires are placed adjacent to the articular surface. *C,* The reverse tendency to maintain a more obtuse notch when tension band wires are placed more posteriorly.

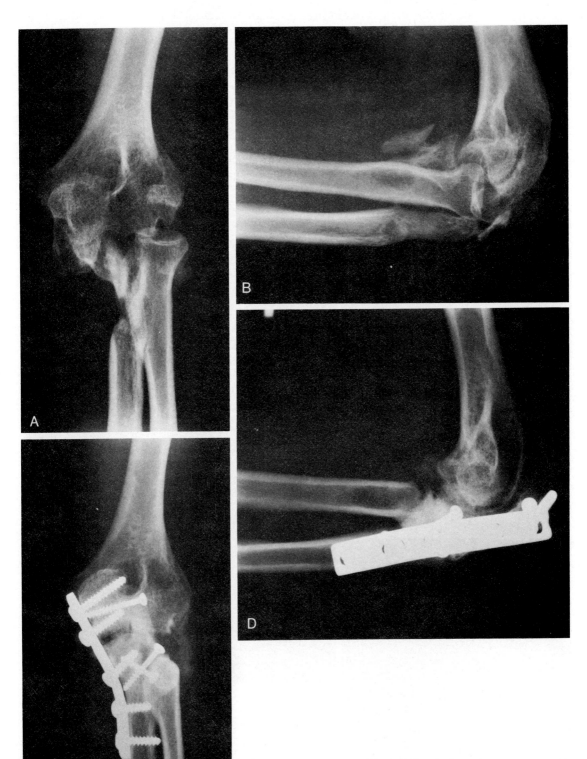

Figure 22–5. *A, B,* AP and lateral elbow radiographs in a 19-year-old woman with nonunion after segmental loss of the proximal ulna and dislocation of the radial head. *C, D,* Healed result after cortical-cancellous iliac graft with a compression plate. Motion was improved from 45–90 degrees to 45–125 degrees with loss of pain (Mayo Clinic Case).

olecranon itself but also an adequate contour of the joint surface of the ulna articulating with the trochlea. Repair or reconstruction of the medial collateral ligament should be carried out if instability persists when stress testing is carried out at the operating table.[48]

The use of hooked-type plates such as the Zuelzer hook plate have not been reported with any series of nonunions of the olecranon; however, the principle of their use should be kept in mind when nonunion with comminution of the fragments makes ordinary tubular plating difficult.[55]

Lag Screw Fixation

Single fragment transverse or oblique nonunions of the olecranon or proximal ulna can be rigidly fixed internally with an intramedullary, axially directed lag screw. Sufficient length to engage the metaphysis of the ulna adequately and overdrilling of the proximal fragment to achieve compression are required (Fig. 22–6). A washer may be used beneath the head of the screw proximally, and the screw should be of the AO cancellous type or one with large threads. If used with an avulsion-type, small, proximal ununited fragment,

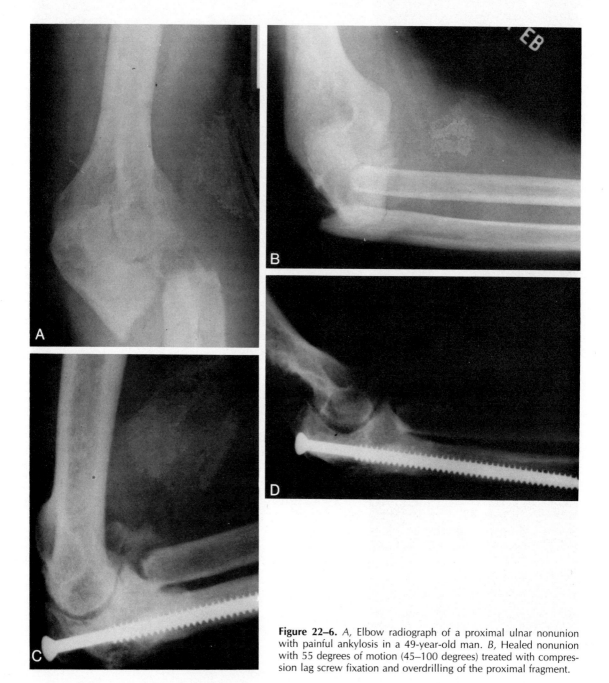

Figure 22–6. A, Elbow radiograph of a proximal ulnar nonunion with painful ankylosis in a 49-year-old man. B, Healed nonunion with 55 degrees of motion (45–100 degrees) treated with compression lag screw fixation and overdrilling of the proximal fragment.

the screw head may penetrate or pull through the triceps tendon attachment if a washer is not used. Nonunions with smaller fragments generally give more predictable results with excision rather than with screw fixation.[22, 35, 39]

Nonunion of an oblique or transverse fracture is also well suited to "bicortical screw fixation," which was described first in 1969 by Taylor and Scham and later reported by Wadsworth in 1976; it involves the use of a washer beneath the screw head.[45, 51] Use of either the oblique or an axially directed screw without overdrilling the proximal fragment may fail to compress the fragments or even hold them apart, causing recurrent nonunion or failure of the fixator.

The use of Rush rods, Knowles pins, or Kirschner wires with smooth surfaces is not recommended because fixation is often inadequate, resulting in displacement.

Malleable or Flexible Screw Fixation

The use of a malleable or flexible screw has resulted in a large percentage of fatigue fractures of the device, according to reports in the literature and in our own personal observation. The use of such devices cannot be recommended for either primary or reconstructive surgery of olecranon fractures or nonunions.

Bone Grafting

The olecranon consists of cancellous bone with a good blood supply and sufficient vascularity to make the addition of cancellous or cortical grafting usually unnecessary.[23] However, every effort possible should be made to obtain union with a single operation if nonunion has already occurred. Supplementary cancellous grafting from the ilium with fragments placed in and about a nonunion defect or to buttress a comminuted articular fragment may be effective. With Monteggia-type nonunions, cancellous grafting is indicated with whatever type of internal fixation is used. Defects of the proximal ulna can be bridged with single or dual onlay grafts with a technique described by Crenshaw.[18]

Electrical Stimulation

When nonunion has occurred without significant fragment separation or trochlear articular surface disruption and when the overall alignment is acceptable, consideration should be given to electrical stimulation of osteogenesis (Fig. 22–7). Bassett and co-workers have achieved an overall success rate of 80 percent with the use of noninvasive pulsing electromagnetic fields with nonunited fractures of many types (including the olecranon) and failed arthrodeses.[6] Direct current stimulation of the fracture site as described by Brighton and by Paterson has achieved comparable results.[11, 38]

A definite healing effect of electrical stimulation has also been noted with co-existing low-grade infections. The technique for the use of either the invasive or the noninvasive method should be obtained from the commercial manufacturer. The noninvasive method can be used on an outpatient basis and has been successful in a failed olecranon nonunion as long as 4 years from the time of prior bone grafting.[41] The disadvantages of prolonged immobilization of a joint, which is often already compromised by injury and fibrosis, must be considered when selecting this modality because cast immobilization for extended periods is generally recommended with this technique.

Treatment of Nonunions of the Olecranon When Articular Cartilage Has Been Severely Damaged

This group of nonunions requires an entirely different approach from that used in the first group. The patient's overall functional and occupational goals as well as the level of function in the opposite upper extremity and the ipsilateral shoulder, wrist, and hand must be considered in the decision-making process. If the olecranon nonunion is an isolated problem and if the ulnohumeral articular surface is destroyed beyond restoration from recent or old trauma, the factors of pain, malalignments, infection, age, and instability all become important. Each patient's problem, the type of fracture, and the other factors listed above must be evaluated on an individual basis. When dislocation or instability is not present and limited motion is acceptable and when pain relief is a prime consideration, the use of induced electromagnetic fields or direct current sitmulation of osteogenesis as described above warrants an initial trial. It must be remembered, however, that plaster immobilization is necessary throughout the period of electrical stimulation.

If the nonunion is associated with articular distortion or loss of motion, excision of the loose fragments, if it comprises less than 50 to 60 percent of the joint, may be the most reliable option. The postoperative rehabilita-

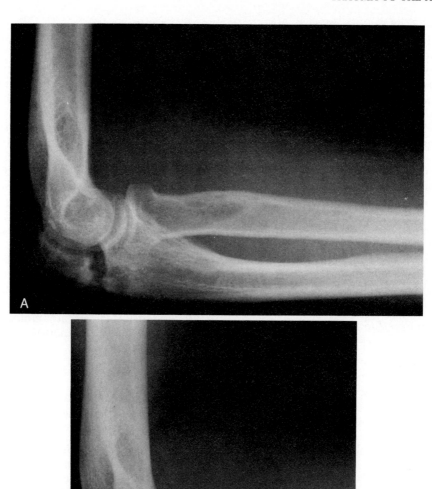

Figure 22–7. *A,* Elbow radiograph of a 19-year-old man with olecranon nonunion at 9 months from open reduction and internal fixation with two threaded and one unthreaded Kirschner wires without tension band wiring. Motion was initiated after Kirschner wire removal at 6 weeks. *B,* Healing of the nonunion 11 months later after noninvasive electrical stimulation. (Courtesy of Dr. Frank Logue.)

tion is shortened as well (see below, Fig. 22–8).

In a salvage situation and when articular surface destruction, the patient's pain, instability, and the overall assessment preclude lesser procedures, arthrodesis, total joint replacement, or allograft replacement are additional options. In a salvage situation when stressful use of the elbow mandates a stable joint such as in a laborer, arthrodesis is still a consideration. A number of techniques have been described in Chapter 36. The elbow is one of the most difficult joints in the body in

which to achieve arthrodesis, and concomitant bone grafting of nonunions for elbow fusion may be necessary. We feel that this option is rarely indicated today.

In a salvage situation when pain and instability are paramount and only sedentary activity is acceptable, total joint replacement has been successful, using the semiconstrained types of prosthetic replacement described in Chapter 34. Similarly, composite frozen cadaver bone allograft replacement, either of the total elbow joint or of the olecranon, has been successful. However, the series reported are small, and complications of repeat nonunion and delayed union have occurred; these require bone grafting but often without compromising the early results. Late "charcot-like" traumatic or degenerative arthritic changes can be anticipated, yet with allograft replacement, the bone stock is preserved and the possibility for total joint replacement as a secondary salvage procedure in the future remains an option. The complication of infection in this situation is the major risk requiring consideration.

AUTHOR'S PREFERRED METHOD OF TREATMENT FOR OLECRANON NONUNIONS

Nonunion of Proximal Avulsion Fractures

Nonunited avulsion fragments are usually small, and best results have been obtained in the author's hands by simple excision and meticulous repair or advancement of the triceps tendon to the olecranon. Care must be taken to repair the medial and lateral retinacular portions of the triceps tendon, using nonabsorbable suture material. Stay sutures should be placed directly through drill holes extending through the posterior cortex of the distal olecranon fragment (Fig. 22–8). The tendon margin is preferably placed adjacent to the articular surface rather than to the posterior cortex. This improves the stability at the expense of a slightly decreased lever

arm. Stainless steel wire is avoided because it is likely to break when motion is initiated. Postoperative immobilization is achieved at 90 degrees of flexion. Early active motion is permitted and encouraged 5 days after surgery through a range of 0 to 90 degrees, but flexion beyond 90 degrees should not be permitted for 4 to 6 weeks, depending on the extent of tendon advancement.

Nonunion of Transverse and Oblique Fractures

Nonunion of transverse and oblique fractures usually results from inadequate or failed primary repair. My best treatment results have been obtained with the use of a large threaded lag screw. Care is taken to overdrill the proximal fragment and to use a sufficiently long screw extending in the axial direction into the medullary canal of the ulnar metaphysis. The length of the screw should be at least twice or three times the length of the nonunited fragment. A washer has been used occasionally to improve the compressive force. Particular care should be taken to avoid having the thread cross the nonunion site because this can result in failure of the procedure owing to distraction.

Alternatively, I have had equally satisfactory results with tension band wiring or bicortical screw fixation with more oblique fractures.

Postoperative care with either of the rigid forms of internal fixation mentioned above

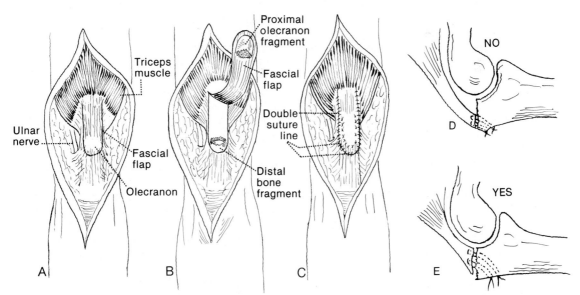

Figure 22–8. *A,* Type of U-shape incision made over the proximal avulsion fragment from the olecranon. *B,* The proximal fragment is elevated with the flap and excised. *C,* The flap is turned down against the bone defect, and heavy sutures of nonabsorbable suture material are used to maintain the tendon reattachment at the articular level *(E)* rather than at the posterior cortex *(D).*

includes immobilization after surgery at 90 degrees of flexion, with early active motion at 4 to 5 days in a range of from 0 to 90 degrees. If rigid fixation is not achieved, immobilization for 6 to 10 weeks or longer is necessary.

When motion is a serious consideration postoperatively, the Mayo Clinic Group has been using dynamic splints similar to those used by hand surgeons.[34] If the triceps is repaired or the olecranon rigidly fixed, active flexion is not a concern, but active extension may be; thus, an extension night splint, which allows the patient to flex against resistance, is prescribed. This should tend only to close the fracture if the appropriate procedure has been carried out; the distracting activity of the triceps is avoided by rubber band extension.

Nonunion of Comminuted Fractures

When comminuted fragments of the olecranon are large enough to permit restoration of the articular surface of the trochlear notch, and even when dislocation of the proximal ulna and radial head has occurred with disruption of the medial collateral ligament, my best results have been obtained with a six- to eight-hole tubular AO plate with cancellous or bicortical screw fixation. Immobilization should be at 90 degrees, and early active motion should be initiated in the range of 0 to 90 degrees a few days after surgery, provided fixation is rigid; otherwise, 6 to 10 weeks of protection is required.

In the older patient in whom comminution and damage to the articular surface preclude restoration and when the joint is stable, best results have been obtained by excising the olecranon fragments, reattaching the triceps tendon with nonabsorbable sutures through drill holes in the posterior cortex, and placing the tendon attachment adjacent to the articular surface. Concurrent repair of the lateral expansion of the triceps to the olecranon periosteum is important and will permit early active motion. The elbow is immobilized at 90 degrees of flexion for 4 to 5 days before initiating active motion through a range of 0 to 90 degrees. Care must be taken to test the elbow for instability and document this radiographically, if necessary, because this factor will influence the postoperative management.

Nonunion with Anterior Fracture Dislocation

Nonunion with anterior fracture dislocation is the most severe and most difficult injury of the olecranon to treat, and my preferred method of treatment is divided into two groups: (1) injuries with a restorable articular surface, and (2) those in which articular surface damage precludes restoration.

In the first group, accurate realignment and restoration of the articular surface is mandatory. After taking down and repositioning or shortening the fragments, rigid internal fixation must be achieved. More than 2 mm offset of the articular surface will probably produce later arthritic changes. The subluxed distal ulnar segment must be reduced, and care must be taken to dissect the anterior capsule from the coronoid process and tubercle to protect the vital anterior neurovascular structures. Exposure is generally achieved by the posterior all-purpose approach described by Bryan.[13] The olecranon periosteum and the triceps attachment and expansion can be kept intact and dissected free from single or comminuted fragments. Preliminary identification and protection of the ulnar nerve are mandatory with this exposure. The medial collateral ligament is identified and repaired or reconstructed before closure. Shortening of the ulna may be necessary to prevent pressure of the ulnar articular surface against the trochlea of the humerus. Internal fixation is best achieved with either a long lag screw or with a 6- to 8-hole tubular AO plate and screws. Early motion is initiated either a few days after surgery or at 3 weeks through a range of 0 to 100 degrees. Initially, immobilization is at 90 degrees of flexion. The complication of an infected wound precludes the use of internal fixation, and maintenance of the elbow in a position of flexion and stability, usually a little greater than 90 degrees, is required to maintain reduction.

When the trochlear notch articular surface is destroyed and dislocation has existed so long that the articular surface of the lower humerus has been destroyed, assessment of the age and overall functional level of the patient is determined in order to choose the appropriate treatment for the olecranon nonunion (Fig. 22–9). If stressful use of the extremity is demanded, arthrodesis is still a consideration, and the technique is determined by the amount of bone stock present.

When chronic nonunion is associated with anterior dislocation and joint destruction, when pain or instability warrant reconstruction, and when sedentary use of the extremity is acceptable, total joint replacement with a semiconstrained prosthesis, preferably with a long stem model for both the ulna and the humerus, has been a more satisfactory ap-

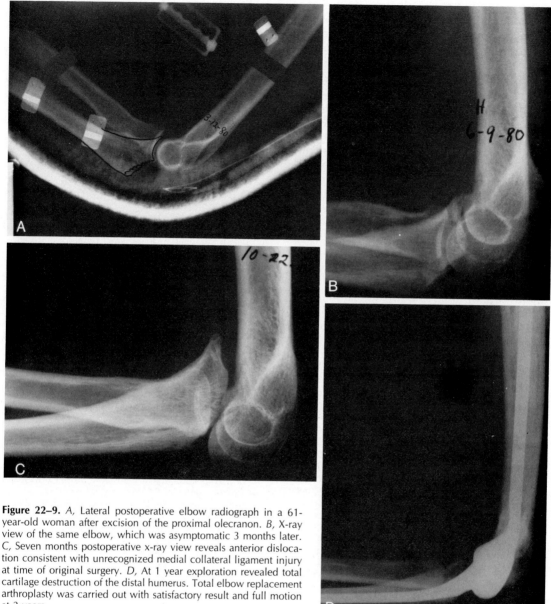

Figure 22–9. *A,* Lateral postoperative elbow radiograph in a 61-year-old woman after excision of the proximal olecranon. *B,* X-ray view of the same elbow, which was asymptomatic 3 months later. *C,* Seven months postoperative x-ray view reveals anterior dislocation consistent with unrecognized medial collateral ligament injury at time of original surgery. *D,* At 1 year exploration revealed total cartilage destruction of the distal humerus. Total elbow replacement arthroplasty was carried out with satisfactory result and full motion at 2 years.

proach than resection or interposition arthroplasty in my hands.

COMPLICATIONS OF TREATMENT OF NONUNIONS

The complications of treatment for nonunion of olecranon fractures are primarily diminished range of motion, traumatic arthritic changes, and pain. Extension is often restricted after open reduction of fresh fractures, but both flexion and extension ranges of motion are more likely to be limited after reconstruction for nonunion.[30] When rigid internal fixation is achieved and early motion is initiated at 5 to 7 days in the functional range of 30 to 130 degrees, less permanent contracture may be anticipated. Associated ossification and calcification of the soft tissues about the elbow joint are common and unpredictable factors. Unless this occurs in the brachialis muscle or anterior capsule, ectopic calcification is usually of no consequence.

The incidence of ulnar nerve paresis with treatment for olecranon nonunion is unknown but is probably greater than the 10 percent with fresh fractures reported by Eriksson et al.[20] Certainly routine preliminary operative isolation and protection of the nerve are warranted with virtually all reconstructive surgery for nonunion at the elbow. The use of a nerve stimulator and high power loops for dissection of scar tissue about the ulnar nerve is helpful.

RESULTS

In a review of 60 olecranon fractures at Durham General Hospital during a 20-year period (1960–1980), only one nonunion resulted from inadequate internal fixation.* However, after excision of the proximal fragment involving 50 percent of the articular surface, good function was restored. A follow-up of olecranon fractures at the Mayo Clinic between 1977 and 1983 revealed only two nonunions; one occurred after placement of a bicortical screw across an oblique type 4 fracture, and the other occurred after a proximal osteotomy of the olecranon to expose a lower humeral comminuted fracture. Excision of the small olecranon fragment in the latter instance and tension band fixation in the former produced satisfactory results.†

References

1. Adler, S., Fay, G. F., and McAusland, W. R., Jr.: Treatment of Olecranon Fractures. J. Trauma **2**:597, 1962.
2. Bakalim, G., and Wilppula, E.: Fractures of the Olecranon I, II, III. Ann. Chir. Gynaecolog. Fenn. **60**:95, 1971.
3. Barford, B.: quoted in personal communication with drawing by Colton, C. L.: Fracture of the Olecranon in Adults: Classification and Management. Injury **5**:121, 1973.
4. Bassett, C. A., et al.: Contributions of Endostium, Cortex and Soft Tissue to Osteogenesis. Surg. Gynecol. Obstet. **112**:145, 1961.
5. Bassett, C., and Andrew, L.: Pulsing Electromagnetic Fields: A New Method to Modify Cell Behavior in Calcified and Noncalcified Tissues. Calcified Tissue International **34**:1–8, 1982.
6. Bassett, C., Andrew L., Valdes, M. G., and Hernandez, E.: Modification of Fracture Repair with Selected Pulsing Eelctromagnetic Fields. J. Bone Joint Surg. **64A**(6):888, 1982.
7. Becker, R., et al.: Bioelectric Factors Controlling Bone Structure. In Frost, H. M. (ed.): Bone Biodynamics. Boston, Little, Brown & Co., 1964.
8. Berger, P.: Le Traitement de Fractures de l'Olecrane et Particilurement la Sutur de l'Olecrane pa un Procede (Cedarg de l'Olecranon). Ga. 2 Hebd. de Med. 193, 1902.
9. Boyd, H. B., and Boles, J. C.: The Monteggia Lesion. A Review of 159 Cases. Clin. Orthop. **66**:94, 1969.
10. Boyd, H. B., Lipinski, S. W., and Wiley, J. H.: Observations on Nonunions of the Shafts of the Long Bones, with a Statistical Analysis of 842 patients. J. Bone Joint Surg. **43A**:159, 1961.
11. Brighton, C. T., Black, J., Friedenberg, Z. B., et al.: A Multicenter Study of the Treatment of Non-union with Constant Direct Current. J. Bone Joint Surg. **63**:1, 1981.
12. Brooks, M.: The Blood Supply of Bone. New York, Appleton Century-Crofts, 1971.
13. Bryan, R. S., and Morrey, B. F.: Extensive Posterior Exposure of the Elbow. Clin. Orthop. **166**:188, 1982.
14. Colton, C. L.: Fractures of the Olecranon in Adults: Classification and Management. Injury **5**:121, 1973.
15. Conn, J., and Wade, P. A.: Injuries of the Elbow (A Ten-Year Review). J. Trauma **1**:248, 1961.
16. Coughlin, M. J., Slabaugh, P. B., and Smith, T. K.: Experience with the McAtee Olecranon Device in Olecranon Fractures. J. Bone and Joint Surg. **61A**:385, 1979.
17. Cozen, L.: Does Diabetes Delay Fracture Healing? Clin. Orthop. **82**:134, 1972.
18. Crenshaw, A. H.: Delayed Union and Nonunion of Fractures. In Edmonson A., and Crenshaw, A. H. (eds.): Campbell's Operative Orthopedics, 5th ed.
19. Dunn, N.: Operation for Fracture of the Olecranon, Br. Med. J. **1**:214, 1939.
20. Eriksson, E., Sahlen, O., and Sandohl, U.: Late Results of Conservative and Surgical Treatment of Fracture of the Olecranon. Acta Chir. Scand. **113**:153, 1957.
21. Foille, D. J.: Note Sur les Fractures de l'Olecrane Par Projectiles de Guerre. Marseille Medical **55**:241, 1918.
22. Gartsman, G. M., Sculco, T. P., and Otis, J. C.: Operative Treatment of Olecranon Fractures. J. Bone Joint Surg. **63A**:718, 1981.
23. Green, D. P., and Rockwood, C. A.: Fractures. Philadelphia, J. B. Lippincott Co., 1975.
24. Green, N.: Radiation Induced Delayed Union of Fractures. Radiology **93**:635, 1969.
25. Heppenstall, R. B.: Fracture Treatment and Healing. Philadelphia, W. B. Saunders Co., 1980, pp. 83–84.
26. Howard, J. L., and Urist, M. R.: Fracture Dislocation of Radius and Ulna at the Elbow Joint. Clin. Orthop. **12**:276, 1958.
27. Judet, J., and Jude, R.: L'Osteogenese et les Retards de Colsolidation et les Pseudarthroses des Os Longs. 196 Hutieine Congres SICOT, pp. 315.
28. Kiviluoto, O., and Santauirta, S.: Fractures of the Olecranon. Analysis of 37 Consecutive Cases. Acta Orthop. Scand. **49**:28, 1978.
29. Lehman, M. A.: Nonunion of an Olecranon Fracture Following Birth Injury. Bull. Hosp. Joint Dis. **26**(2):187, 1965.
30. Levy, R. N., and Sherry, H. S.: Complications of Treatment of Fractures and Dislocations of the Elbow. In Epps, C. H. (ed.): Complications in Orthopedic Surgery. Philadelphia, J. B. Lippincott Co., 1975, pp. 237.
31. Mathews, J. G.: Fractures of the Olecranon in Children. Injury **12**:207, 1980.
32. Mayer, P. J., and Evarts, C. M.: Nonunion, Delayed Union, Malunion, and Avascular Necrosis. In Epps, C. H. (ed.): Complications in Orthopedic Surgery. Philadelphia, J. B. Lippincott, 1975, 159.
33. McKeever, F. M., and Buck, R. M.: Fracture of Olecranon Process of the Ulna. J.A.M.A. **135**(1):1, 1947.
34. Morrey, B. F., and Kai-New, A.: Functional Anatomy of the Ligaments of the Elbow. Dept. of Orthopedics, Mayo Clinic, Rochester, Minn. 55905. Submitted for publication, 1984.
35. Muller, M. E., Allgower, M., and Willenegger, H.: Manual of Internal Fixation. Berlin, Springer-Verlag, 1970.

---

*Bugg, E. I., Jr. Personal communication, 1982.
†Cabanella, M. E. Personal communication, 1983.

36. Muller, M. E.: Treatment of Nonunion by Compression. Clin. Orthop. 43:83, 1965.
37. Newell, R. L. M.: Olecranon Fractures in Children. Injury 37:33, 1975.
38. Paterson, D. C., Lewis, G. N., and Cass, C. A.: Treatment of Delayed Union and Nonunion with an Implanted Direct Current Stimulator. Clin. Orthop. 148:117, 1980.
39. Rettig, A. C., Waugh, T. R., and Evanski, P. M.: Fracture of the Olecranon: A Problem of Management. J. Trauma 12:23, 1979.
40. Rothman, R.: The Effect of Iron Deficiency Anemia on Fracture Healing. Clin. Orthop. 77:276, 1971.
41. Sharrard, W. J. W., Sutcliffe, M. S., Robson, M. J., and Maceachern, A. G.: The Treatment of Fibrous Nonunion of Fractures by Pulsing Electromagnetic Stimulation. J. Bone Joint Surg. 64B(2):189, 1982.
42. Silberstein, M. J., Bradeur, A. E., Graviss, E. R., and Luisiri, A.: J. Bone Joint Surg. 63:722, 1981.
43. Smith, F. M.: Surgery of the Elbow. Philadelphia, W. B. Saunders Co., 1972, pp. 260–261.
44. Srivastava, K. P., Vyas, O. N., Varshney, A. K., and Singh, C. P.: Compression Osteosynthesis in Fractures of the Olecranon. Int. Surg. 63(1):20, 1978.
45. Taylor, T. K. F., and Scham, S. M.: A Postero-medial Approach to the Proximal End of the Ulna for the Internal Fixation of Olecranon Fractures. J. Trauma 9:594, 1969.
46. Tonna, E. A.: The Cellular Complement on the Skeletal System Studied Autoradiographically Tritiated Thymidine (HDTR) During Growth and Aging. J. Biophys. Biochem. Cytol. 9:813, 1961.
47. Torg, J. S., and Moyer, R. A.: Nonunion of a Stress Fracture Through the Olecranon Epiphyseal Plate Observed in an Adolescent Baseball Pitcher. J. Bone Joint Surg. 59A:264, 1977.
48. Tullos, H. S., Schwab, G., Bennett, J. B., and Woods, W. G.: Factors Influencing Elbow Instability. In American Academy of Orthopedic Surgeons: Instructional Course Lectures, Vol. 30. St. Louis, C. V. Mosby Co., 1981, p. 193.
49. Urbaniak, James R., Personal Communication, November, 1982.
50. Waddell, G., and Howat, T. W.: A Technique of Plating Severe Olecranon Fractures. Injury 5:135, 1973.
51. Wadsworth, T. G.: Screw Fixation of the Olecranon after Fracture of Osteotomy. Clin. Orthop. 119:197, 1976.
52. Weber, B. G., and Cech, O.: Pseudarthrosis—Pathology, Biomechanics, Therapy, Results. Berne, Hans Huber Medical Publ., 1976.
53. Weber, B., and Vasey, H.: Osteosynthese bei Olecranon Fraktur. Z. Unfallmed. Berufskr. 2:90, 1963.
54. Weisband, I. D.: Tension Band Wiring Technique for Treatment of Olecranon Fractures. J. Am. Osteopath. Assoc. 77:390, 1978.
55. Weseley, M. S., Barnfield, P. A., Einstein, A. I.: The Use of the Zuelzer Hook Plate in Fixation of Olecranon Fractures. J. Bone Joint Surg. 58A(6):859, 1976.

CHAPTER 23

Elbow Dislocations

RONALD L. LINSCHEID

The diagnosis of dislocation of the elbow as distinct from fractures or fracture-dislocations of the elbow evolved with the development of modern roentgen techniques. In children under 10, dislocation of the elbow is the most common dislocation seen; it is the second most common dislocation of a major joint after that of the shoulder in adults. Despite the prevalence of this injury, there are few analyses of series of this dislocation in the literature.[5, 34, 41, 48, 55, 61, 82] There has been considerable interest in the complications of elbow dislocation.

MECHANISM OF INJURY

Falls on the outstretched upper extremity account for the large majority of dislocations; motor vehicle accidents, direct trauma, and miscellaneous causes account for a minority. Injury to the nondominant upper extremity occurs in about 60 percent of cases, perhaps as a result of employment of the dominant arm or unconscious protection of it at the time of injury.

There are two primary theories of the mechanism of dislocation—hyperextension of the elbow and direct posterior orientation of the resultant force dislocation occurring with the elbow in slight flexion.

The hyperextension theory postulates that the olecranon at the termination of extension impinges on the olecranon fossa (Fig. 23–1).[20, 74, 77] Further extensor force acts on the fulcrum of the olecranon, which levers the ulna and radius from their capsular constraints. The anterior capsule is avulsed from or avulses a small bony component of the

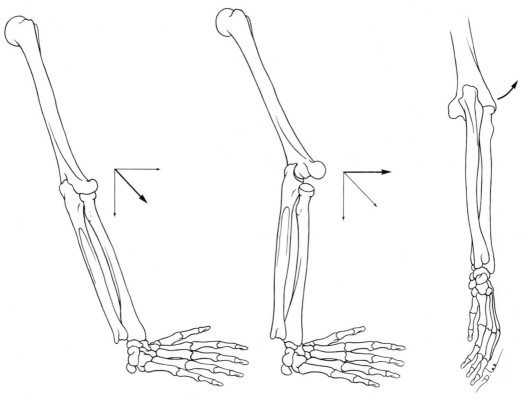

Figure 23–1. The mechanism of dislocation. Hyperextension theory postulates that the olecranon impinges within the olecranon fossa, and the joint is levered out in hyperextension.

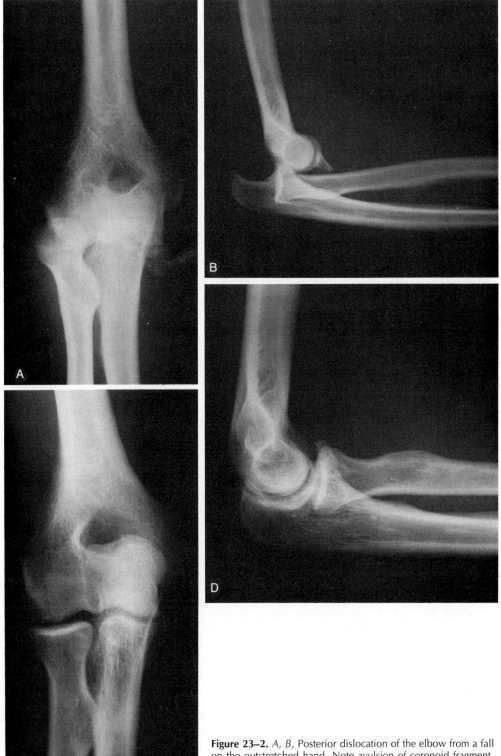

Figure 23–2. *A, B,* Posterior dislocation of the elbow from a fall on the outstretched hand. Note avulsion of coronoid fragment. *C, D,* Coronoid fragment has healed.

coronoid.[24] At the same time, the collateral ligament attachments are strained, usually at their condylar attachments. The anterior fibers are torn or avulsed first, followed by the more posterior attachments.[47, 63] Rotational forces may act to pivot the dislocation about an intact posterior portion of a collateral ligament. Because of its greater strength and mechanical advantage in relation to the fulcrum of dislocation, some component of the medial collateral ligament is felt to be the pivot focus. In the adolescent the medial epicondyle is particularly vulnerable to avulsion through its physis, and occasionally the lateral epicondyle or a fragment of it may be avulsed. As it continues, hyperextension places the anteriorly located neurovascular structures and musculotendinous units under tension. Tearing of the fleshy brachialis with resultant intramuscular hematoma has consequences later relating to heterogeneous bone formation and joint contracture. Stretching of the median nerve or brachial artery may lead to injury of both these structures.[8] The ulnar nerve is at risk from stretch when significant valgus deformity occurs during the dislocation sequence. Thomas noted that violent compression of the elbow in extension with the forearm pronated and the palm in contact with the floor resulted in elbow flexion.[77] He believed that this was due to the morphology of the elbow, which resulted in offsetting of the lines of force through the humerus and radius. He further noted that the force in the radius was transmitted to the ulna through the interosseous membrane, thus driving the ulna posteriorly. Interestingly, most patients with elbow dislocation insist that in falling, they struck the elbow over the point of the olecranon, a fact that may be accounted for by the suddenness of the dislocation or by actually striking the olecranon at the completion of flexion-dislocation.

The resultant force theory of Osborne and Cotterill[52] suggests that dislocation occurs with the elbow slightly flexed, in which position it is subject to axial compression loading. This force acts on the slight lateral obliquity of the trochlear surface, producing a force that effects a posterolateral displacement of the radius on the capitellum. In consequence, the radial collateral ligament and the lateral capsule are torn, allowing posterior escape of the forearm on the humerus. These investigators suggested a method of repair for recurrent dislocation based on this theory of mechanism (see later, Recurrent Dislocation).

The forces acting on the joint, besides producing tensile forces that avulse the ligamentous constraints, also produce substantial compressive and shear forces on the articular surfaces. Adjunctive fractures such as those occurring in the radial head and neck or capitellum are, therefore, frequent.[1, 11] There is evidence from reports of dislocations treated by open means that chondral injuries to the capitellar and trochlear surfaces are probably much more common than was previously believed.[7, 17]

In the child, late nucleation and closure of the physes alter the response to dislocation forces and certainly increase the difficulty of radiographic interpretation. This is covered separately in Chapter 14.

Understanding the mechanism of injury is obviously important for appreciating a classification, interpreting the clinical and radiographic findings, instituting treatment, anticipating complications, and providing adequate follow-up care.

CLASSIFICATION

Elbow dislocations are classed as posterior, anterior, recurrent, and divergent.

Posterior Dislocations. By far the most common dislocation occurs posteriorly (Fig. 23–2). The position of the forearm medial or lateral to the trochlea determines whether the dislocation is posterolateral or posteromedial. The forearm is also usually deviated into a varus or valgus position.

Lateral Dislocations. These dislocations are quite rare (Fig. 23–3). This type of dislocation usually implies extensive tearing of all the medial soft tissues.[10, 12, 82] Isolated radial head dislocations occur rarely and frequently require open reduction.[21, 38, 62]

Anterior Dislocations. Anterior dislocations are also extremely rare and are usually seen in younger individuals (Fig. 23–4).[3] The forearm bones are displaced anterior to the distal humerus. The mechanism of injury may be similar to that described above for posterior dislocations, but there is a forward rebounding response that allows the anterior projections after extensive hyperextension has allowed the olecranon to slide under the trochlea.

Recurrent Dislocations. Recurrent dislocations are also uncommon. They result from failure of the capsular and ligamentous constraints to heal sufficiently to prevent the joint being levered out in response to forces that are considerably less than those responsible for the initial dislocation (Fig. 23–5). Weak-

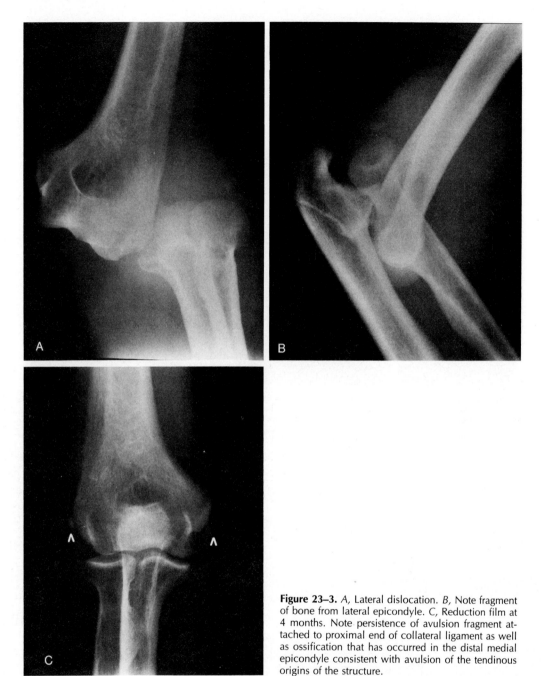

Figure 23–3. *A,* Lateral dislocation. *B,* Note fragment of bone from lateral epicondyle. *C,* Reduction film at 4 months. Note persistence of avulsion fragment attached to proximal end of collateral ligament as well as ossification that has occurred in the distal medial epicondyle consistent with avulsion of the tendinous origins of the structure.

ness of the posterolateral capsule has been suggested as the primary problem, but an ununited coronoid process with weakness of the anterior capsule has been noted as well.[43] It is also unlikely that recurrent dislocation could occur unless there was attenuation of at least the anterior aspect of the ulnar collateral ligament.

Divergent Dislocations. Displacement of the radius from the ulna with concomitant dislocation is a rare injury associated with energetic trauma.[6, 37] The interosseous membrane, annular ligament, and distal radioulnar joint capsule are necessarily torn.

TREATMENT

The principles of treatment are to restore the articular alignment of the elbow with due promptness without causing further damage or overlooking neurovascular complications or associated musculoskeletal injuries. The reduction should optimize the chances for restoration of the joint anatomy and an early return to a functional capacity.

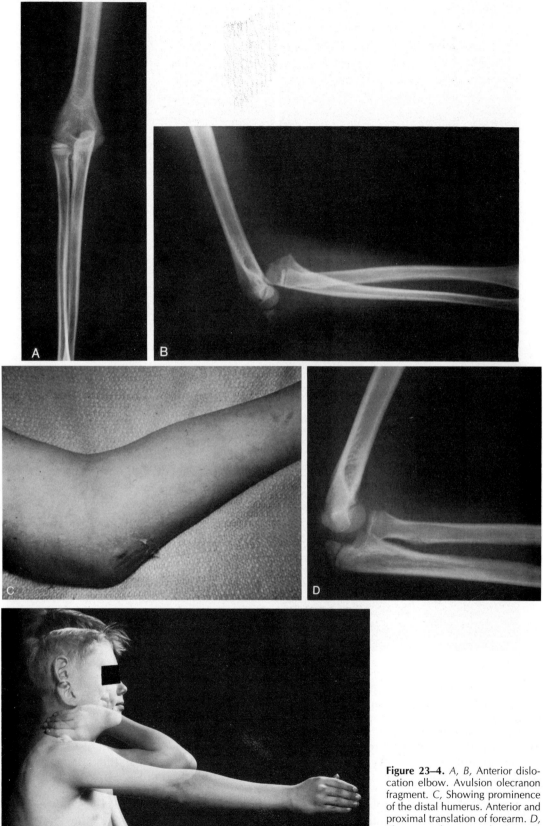

Figure 23–4. *A, B,* Anterior dislocation elbow. Avulsion olecranon fragment. *C,* Showing prominence of the distal humerus. Anterior and proximal translation of forearm. *D,* Three weeks postreduction. *E,* Normal range of motion at 1 year.

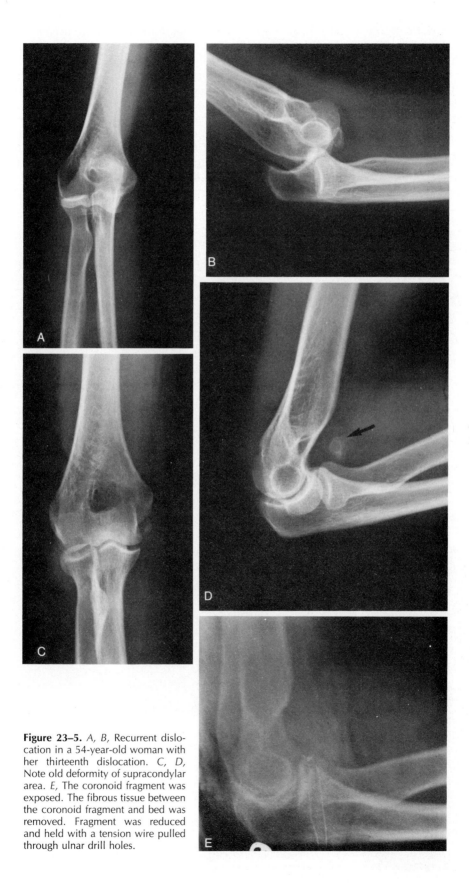

Figure 23–5. *A, B,* Recurrent dislocation in a 54-year-old woman with her thirteenth dislocation. *C, D,* Note old deformity of supracondylar area. *E,* The coronoid fragment was exposed. The fibrous tissue between the coronoid fragment and bed was removed. Fragment was reduced and held with a tension wire pulled through ulnar drill holes.

A careful and systematic prereduction evaluation is essential to achieve these goals and need not jeopardize prompt reduction if it is adeptly performed. Vascularity can be duly assessed by feeling the radial pulse and judging the capillary filling of the nails. The ulnar nerve may be quickly tested by resisting finger spread, which assesses the function of the first dorsal interosseous and abductor digiti quinti. The median nerve is evaluated by having the patient flex the flexor pollicis longus and index profundus, and abduct the thumb toward the palm against resistance.

The radial nerve is assessed by having the patient extend the wrist, finger, and thumb against resistance. Sensory testing is often unreliable immediately after injury unless it is very carefully performed, preferably at the autonomous zones of each of the three nerves. If adequate neurologic examination is omitted in the prereduction assessment and a neurologic deficit is observed subsequent to reduction, the surgeon may face the dilemma of whether or not to explore a nerve entrapped by the reduction. Additionally, one must consider the liability of the surgeon should there

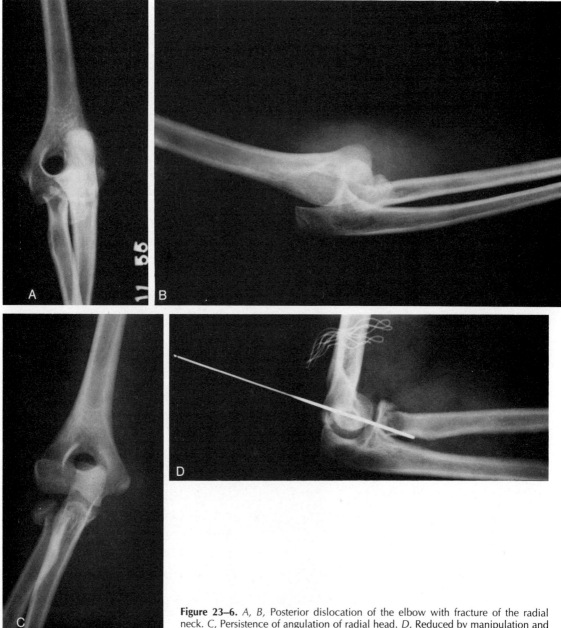

Figure 23–6. *A, B,* Posterior dislocation of the elbow with fracture of the radial neck. *C,* Persistence of angulation of radial head. *D,* Reduced by manipulation and transfixed with Kirschner wire.

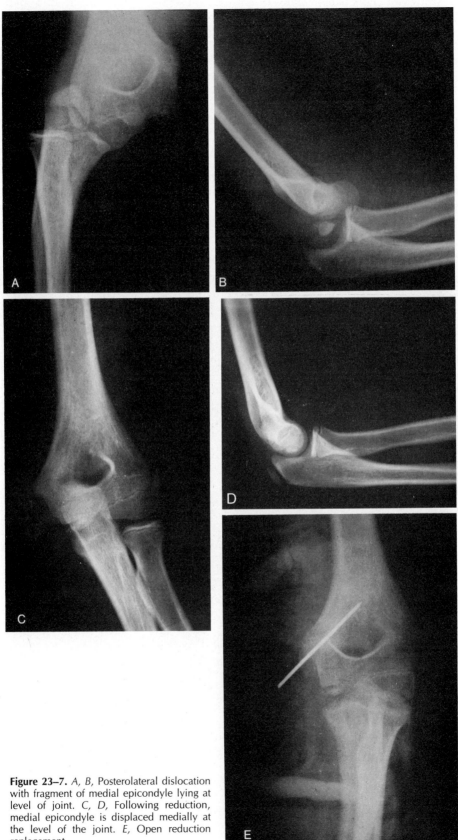

Figure 23–7. *A, B,* Posterolateral dislocation with fragment of medial epicondyle lying at level of joint. *C, D,* Following reduction, medial epicondyle is displaced medially at the level of the joint. *E,* Open reduction replacement.

be an untoward result. This is especially true of median nerve entrapment within the joint (see later, Complications).

Accessory injuries with elbow dislocation are common.[25, 28, 50, 51, 63, 66, 81, 83] Radial head and neck fractures occur in about 5 to 10 percent of cases secondary to compressive loading at the radiocapitellar joint (Fig. 23–6). Avulsion of fragments from either the medial or lateral epicondyles occurs in approximately 12 percent of cases, and avulsion of the coronoid process occurs in 10 percent of dislocations (Fig. 23–2).

Displacement of the medial epicondyle in adolescents ranges from minimal to incarceration of the epicondyle within the joint (Fig.

23–7).[34, 56, 65, 84] The latter, if undetected, results in significant traumatic arthrosis (Figs. 23–8 and 23–9). Interestingly, previous medial epicondylar fracture with subsequent displacement probably rendered four adults in our original series more susceptible to late secondary dislocation.[34] This vulnerability may be explained by the loss of medial collateral ligament integrity with this injury.

Intra-articular fracture, as in the capitellum, occurs occasionally, but osteochondral injuries are probably much more common than standard roentgenograms would lead one to suspect.[117]

Associated injuries are also common with elbow dislocations, occurring in approxi-

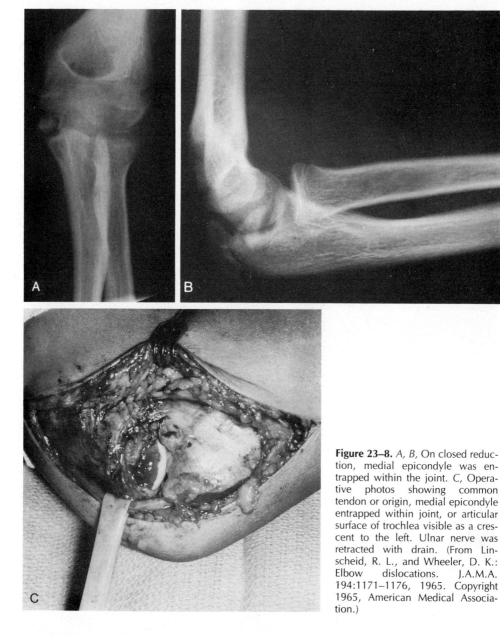

Figure 23–8. A, B, On closed reduction, medial epicondyle was entrapped within the joint. C, Operative photos showing common tendon or origin, medial epicondyle entrapped within joint, or articular surface of trochlea visible as a crescent to the left. Ulnar nerve was retracted with drain. (From Linscheid, R. L., and Wheeler, D. K.: Elbow dislocations. J.A.M.A. 194:1171–1176, 1965. Copyright 1965, American Medical Association.)

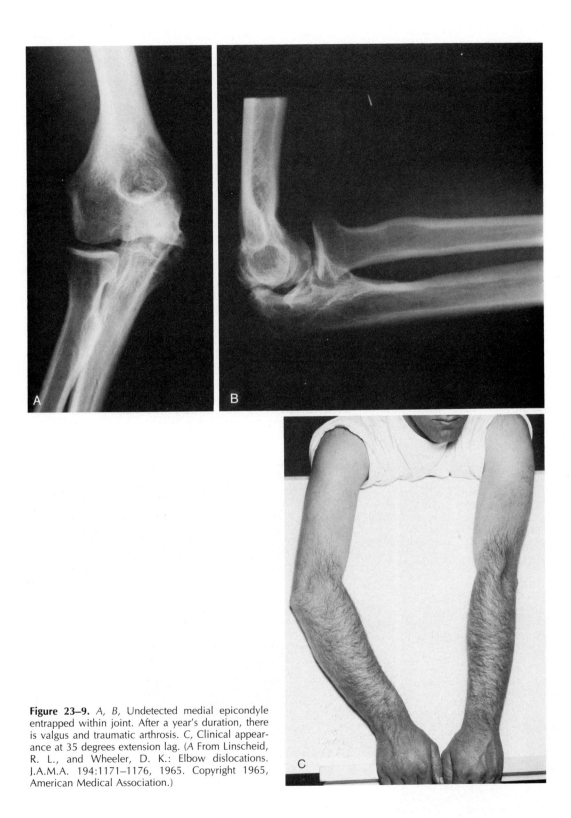

Figure 23–9. *A, B,* Undetected medial epicondyle entrapped within joint. After a year's duration, there is valgus and traumatic arthrosis. *C,* Clinical appearance at 35 degrees extension lag. (*A* From Linscheid, R. L., and Wheeler, D. K.: Elbow dislocations. J.A.M.A. 194:1171–1176, 1965. Copyright 1965, American Medical Association.)

mately 12 percent of the cases.[34, 48, 80] Fracture of the distal radius, ulnar styloid, perilunar dislocations, and shoulder injuries of the same extremity are the most common of these injuries, with multiple injuries of other areas secondary to severe trauma accounting for the rest (Fig. 23–10).

When the elbow is dislocated, the extensive soft tissue damage results in marked swelling. The intact structures in the area such as the forearm fascia, the biceps tendon, and the lacertus fibrosus may exert a marked constricting effect, resulting in increased compartmental pressures. Volkmann's ischemic contracture may result on occasion if this condition is left unrecognized and must be differentiated early from neurologic stretch injuries if it is to be adequately treated. Intracompartmental pressure measurements in the proximal forearm should not take precedence over early reduction, but they should be monitored as early as possible and after reduction if indicated clinically (see Chapter 17).

Preanesthetic evaluation includes a history of the recency of food ingestion, alcohol intake, cardiovascular status, other medical conditions, and the overall status of trauma.

It is occasionally possible to reduce the elbow without an anesthetic while the elbow region is insensitive to trauma, especially if it is seen before there is marked swelling or the dislocation is not badly displaced. Prudence suggests transport to a suitable facility for anesthetic coverage and support facilities except in unusual circumstances. General or regional block anesthetic is preferable for muscular relaxation and pain relief. Although reduction may be possible with a narcotic-tranquilizer combination, the extra force that is occasionally necessary and the possibility of adding complications make this a less desirable method.

Reduction

Reduction may occur by inadvertent manipulation during evaluation, x-ray positioning, or examination, but most often preparations must be made for manipulative reduction in a suitable area. Chronic elbow dislocations that are of weeks to years duration are rare and will not ordinarily be confused with acute dislocations but should be considered, especially in undeveloped countries (Fig. 23–11).[2]

Closed reduction is successful in most instances.[33] Methods include:

1. Application of traction to the forearm, which is flexed at 90 degrees over the edge of the table with the patient prone. A 2- to 5-kg weight may be attached at the wrist as a substitute for manual traction.

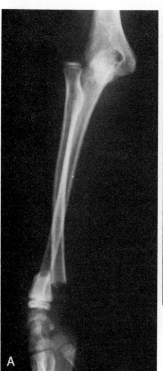

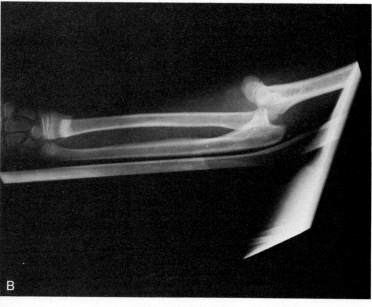

Figure 23–10. *A, B,* Posterolateral elbow dislocation with displaced fracture. Dislocation of the distal radius.

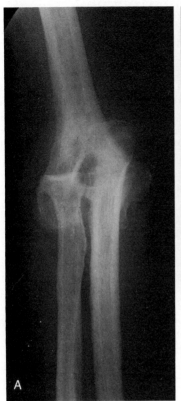
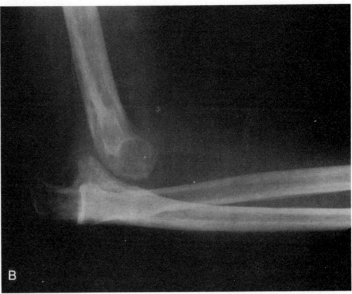

Figure 23–11. *A,* Persistent dislocation unreduced for a 3-month period. Note secondary osteoporosis. *B,* Reduction was accomplished by lateral exposure, clearing the joint surfaces and exerting prolonged traction.

2. Manual reduction with forearm traction and brachial countertraction. This allows the physician to palpate and manipulate the elbow.

3. Manual reduction using the operator's knee as a fulcrum against which to apply traction to the forearm.

4. Hyperextension to unlock the coronoid followed by traction, medial or lateral translation, and flexion until the joint is felt and heard to reduce.

Open reduction may be indicated for a problem situation that has been neglected for more than 10 days when firm but gentle manipulation fails.[31] Rarely, closed reduction is prevented by interposition of the annular ligament or a collateral ligament.[53] A laterally placed Kocher incision is preferred, especially if there are concomitant intra-articular fractures or loose fragments at the radiocapitellar joint.[8] Buttonholing of the radial head through the capsule may be recognized readily with this approach.

Open reduction is more commonly used to retrieve an incarcerated medial epicondyle from within the ulnotrochlear joint,[56] a situation that usually occurs in the pediatric patient. If this is necessary, the ulnar nerve should be identified beneath the deep fascia posterior to the medial intermuscular septum for protection during the procedure. The medial collateral ligament attached to the epicondyle may have been avulsed also from the proximal area of the medial humeral condyle. It should be reapproximated and tacked into position with sutures as necessary to maintain its position and ensure better medial stability. If there has been obvious ulnar nerve injury or clinical neuropraxia, anterior translocation may be considered simultaneously before reattaching the medial epicondyle. In many instances, moderate displacement of the epicondyle may be present without significant neurovascular problems. Accurate anatomic reduction and fixation are, however, desirable.

POSTREDUCTION CARE AND REHABILITATION

The elbow is generally held in a padded dressing with a posterior plaster splint at 90 degrees of flexion because this is the position of stability. The pulses should be checked frequently during the first 24 hours, and the dressings must be open enough at the wrist to encourage accurate assessment by the nursing staff. Persistent or increasing pain or loss or diminution of the pulse requires wide release of the dressing anteriorly, inspection of the antecubital space, and a check of the neuromuscular status for signs of impending ischemia. Continuous compartment monitoring or arteriography is indicated if there is reasonable doubt of the forearm's vascularity. Positive findings are an indication for anterior soft tissue release and arterial inspection and repair (see later, Complications, and Chapter 17). The neurologic status should be thoroughly checked at 24 hours and appropriately thereafter during recovery (see later, Complications).

Shoulder and hand exercises may commence the day after reduction and should progess as tolerated. Gentle active flexion from the splint with the forearm dressings split may start the first week. As the swelling subsides, the plaster splint is changed or replaced by an Orthoplast splint the second week, allowing the elbow to assume a −60-degree extension position with gentle, active, assisted flexion four times daily for 10 to 15 days until the third week.

In an otherwise uncomplicated situation, the splint is removed at three weeks, and active unprotected flexion-extension exercises are encouraged. The need for supervised therapy is usually apparent at this time.[16] Flexion is generally regained early, with extension being slower. The involuntary inhibition of extension activity by the para-articular soft tissue receptors generally occurs at a specific angle of extension that decreases with resolution of post-traumatic inflammation.[4] Overly enthusiastic passive stretching at this point may be detrimental (see later, Complications). Muscle strengthening, particularly of the triceps, is encouraged.

If at 10 to 12 weeks the extension lag appears to have become static, an Orthoplast static night splint is fabricated to be placed anteriorly on the arm. A broad, padded olecranon strap with Velcro fixation is tightened to a tolerable level for sleep. An alternate approach is to use a dynamic extension splint at night. Significant heterotopic bone formation may be a contraindication to passive stretching.[15, 78] On rare occasions a "fall away" cast is used to encourage extension. This is applied in as much extension as is readily tolerated by the patient. The posterior aspect of the forearm portion of the cast is removed, and active extension is encouraged. Felt shims may be inserted anteriorly at the wrist to maintain progress. The cast is usually changed at 1- to 2-week intervals. Patient toleration for this cast varies.

RECURRENT DISLOCATION

Recurrent dislocation is sufficiently uncommon that few surgeons obtain wide experience with it.[23, 27, 74, 76] Patients with a lax ligamentous body habitus are at greater risk. Osborne and Cotterill felt attenuation of the posterolateral capsule and radial collateral ligament allowed recurrent dislocation and proposed imbrication and repair of this lateral pocket.[52] Mobilization before healing of the capsule has progressed satisfactorily has been suggested as a factor. Hassman emphasized the desirability of débridement of osteochondral debris during this repair.[20] This has largely superseded other methods of repair, which include (1) transfer of the biceps tendon to the soft tissue at the coronoid[59] or inserting it through a drill hole in the coronoid process;[27] (2) deepening the semilunar notch of the ulna by resecton,[22] lengthening osteotomy of the coronoid,[39] or insertion of an anterior bone block;[42] (3) posterior olecranon bone block;[67, 70] (4) anterior capsule repairs or augmentation;[29, 32, 58, 69] and (5) transhumeral ligament construction using strips of triceps or biceps.[26, 70] Osteosynthesis of a large coronoid fragment with a cancellous bone screw or tension band wiring has been satisfactory in our series as well (Fig. 23–5). There is evidence that attenuation of the medial collateral ligament is a significant factor in recurrent dislocations.[7, 44, 45, 46, 49, 64] Repair or reconstruction of this structure, particularly the strong anterior component, may prove to be the most efficacious procedure for this problem.

RESULTS

Uncomplicated dislocations generally have very satisfactory results. Excellent results with full range of motion, normal strength, absent pain, and good stability may be expected in 55 percent of unselected dislocations (Fig. 23–12). Good results with a loss of no more than 15 degrees of either flexion or extension, minimal discomfort, and normal stability is anticipated in an additional 30 percent of cases. Fair or poor results are generally associated with complications (discussed below) and may be expected in 15 percent of dislocations. Fair or poor results are generally seen in the more severe original injuries.[34]

Most patients note continuing improvement for at least 6 months and some for as long as 18 months.

Limitation of extension is probably the most common problem. In the statistics listed

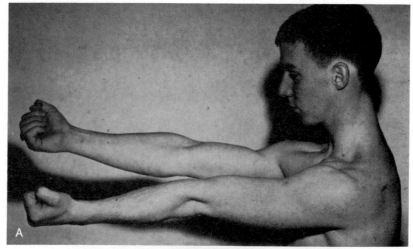

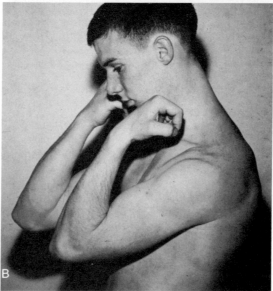

Figure 23–12. *A, B,* One year following otherwise uncomplicated posterior dislocation. Right elbow extends to neutral, left elbow to +10 degrees. Flexion limited by 5 degrees on right.

above most patients were immobilized for 3 to 5 weeks at 90 degrees of flexion. A more progressive rehabilitation program as outlined below may improve extension, although the extensive soft tissue injury associated with dislocation produces induration and scarring anteriorly that is inherently limiting.[16, 18]

Interestingly, instability of the elbow to varovalgus stress is quite uncommon.[7, 44, 64, 84] Presumably this is due to the monaxial joint configuration that provides considerable geometric stability to the joint in the healing phase. It may also attest to the fact that the collateral ligaments are seldom markedly displaced following reduction.[44, 49]

Neurologic problems occur in approximately 20 percent of dislocations. The ulnar nerve is the most susceptible major nerve.[34]

Symptoms vary from transient paresthesias in the ulnar distribution to a rare permanent ulnar palsy. Median nerve symptoms are less common and also range from a transient to a complete palsy.

Combined median-ulnar nerve injuries are usually associated with severe injuries that frequently involve the brachial artery as well. Vascular injuries usually result in significant long-term disabilities[31] (see Complications).

COMPLICATIONS

Neurovascular

Neurovascular problems have already been discussed in the section on treatment, but they deserve additional emphasis.[14, 28, 76, 79] Stretching and distortion of the anterior struc-

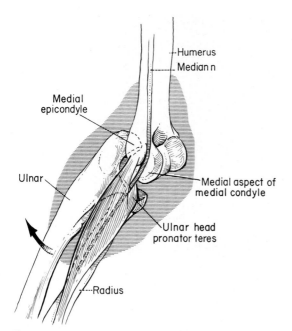

Figure 23–13. Entrapment of the median nerve within the elbow joint may occur as the nerve slips around the medial condyle and is stretched across the posterior aspect of the trochlea. During reduction the nerve may be caught in the sulcus of the trochlea and imprisoned by the ulnar articular surface. (From Pritchard, D. J., et al.: Intra-articular median nerve entrapment with dislocation of the elbow. Clin. Orthop. 90:100–103, 1975.)

tures may result in spasm, intimal damage, thrombosis, or rupture of the brachial artery.[10, 34, 36, 68, 72] Because dislocation often is also disruptive of collateral circulation, the forearm is at risk in this instance. Ischemic myositis, impaired vascularity, or later claudication may result (see Chapter 17).

Median nerve symptoms are apt to be associated with arterial injury because of the close proximity of nerve and artery in their course between the brachialis and the pronator teres. Stretch injuries to the nerve occur at the time of dislocation.[57] These must be differentiated from secondary compressive injuries, which may occur with increased intracompartmental pressure in the flexor space or intra-articular entrapment. The latter may be suspected if median paresthesias occur shortly after reduction, if there is widening of the medial joint space, or if reduction has an "incomplete feel."[64] This complication is more common in children (Fig. 23–13). There have been several explanations of the mechanism of intra-articular entrapment of the median nerve. The nerve may be displaced posteriorly through a space created by avulsion of the medial epicondyle or the common flexor origin.[71] Tension of the nerve across the

margin of the epicondylar flare may "notch" the bone to produce a late roentgenologic sign known as Matev's sign after the investigator who described it.[40] The nerve has also been seen to have slipped through the space between the medial condyle and the collateral ligament, and then became entrapped between the trochlea and the semilunar notch on reduction.[54] Traction with the elbow in extension and correction of lateral displacement before effecting reduction may help to prevent this complication.

The ulnar nerve is the nerve most frequently injured in elbow dislocations, primarily because of valgus stretching.[31, 65] The induration, hypertrophy, and ossification present within the cubital tunnel may compress the nerve and diminish gliding, causing persistent symptoms. For this reason anterior translocation may be considered if progressive resolution of paresthesias and paresis is not apparent.

Compartment Syndrome

Intramuscular bleeding and edema formation within the flexor compartment of the forearm may lead to ischemic myositis, especially if it is associated with a concomitant vascular injury. Pain, pallor, paralysis, and pulselessness are important indications of this problem, but impending problems should be recognized even earlier if there is marked induration of the proximal forearm and passive finger or wrist extension is difficult and painful. Compartment pressure measurements are indicated, and arteriography is necessary if arterial injury is suspected. Adequate anterior decompression with special emphasis on sectioning of the lacertus fibrosus and the lower brachial and forearm fascia should not be delayed. The brachial, radial, and ulnar arteries should be carefully visualized with the tourniquet tight and their patency then checked with it deflated. Arterial repair follows the established procedures for rupture, intimal damage, and so on. The wound margins are left open for later closure. (This complication of elbow trauma in general is covered in Chapter 17.)

Articular Injuries

Loose flecks of bone within the joint following reduction usually represent inclusion of an avulsed fragment of the medial epicondyle or a fragment of the articular surface.[17] In the latter case the fragment is usually significantly larger than the roentgenographic appearance suggests owing to the radiolucent chondral layer. Such fragments should be removed or replaced as indicated by the findings. If the joint is explored, débridement, irrigation, and soft tissue replacement should be accomplished as soon as possible.[8]

Fractures of the radial head or neck if displacement is minimal are best ignored during the initial period.[1, 13, 15, 45] Greater displacements may require open reduction or, if comminution and capitellar injury are present, excision of the radial head.[23] If radial head excision is performed, a valgus instability can result from failure of the medial collateral ligament to heal at its normal length. Repair of the ulnar collateral ligament may be considered, and use of a hinged elbow orthosis during the healing period helps to protect the ulnar collateral ligament.

Excision of the radial head induces longitudinal instability of the radius on the ulna in persons with lax ligaments and in patients with sufficient injury to the distal radioulnar joint and interosseous membrane. If this complication is suspected, temporary Kirschner wiring of the radius to the ulna with the radius distracted for 4 to 6 weeks allows the injured structures to tighten. The value of radial head replacement in the acute injury to prevent proximal migration of the radius has received mixed reviews.[9, 19, 45, 73]

Late Limited Motion

Limitation of extension is common following dislocation. Bracing and physical therapy probably have little effect after 6 months to a year. If there is sufficient limitation of 30 degrees or more at that time, capsulolysis may be considered. The anterior capsule is often thickened and shortened. It usually can be released through a lateral incision, although extreme care needs to be exercised if flexion contracture persists owing to tightening at the ulnar side of the joint. The capsule can usually be released from the proximal humeral attachment. An ulnar incision and clearing of the olecranon fossa may be necessary.

Heterotopic Bone Formation

This occurs at three primary locations following dislocation. Ossification in the lateral and medial collateral ligaments occurs frequently but is seldom sufficient to cause marked functional impairment. Obviously it does, however, affect the suppleness of the ligaments. Ossification also occurs in the anterior capsule above the coronoid process (Fig. 23–14). Occasionally marked heterotopic ossification occurs in the brachialis muscle, seriously impairing flexion and extension of the elbow.[30, 35, 60, 78] Excision is delayed until the reactive bone mass is mature, usually at 1

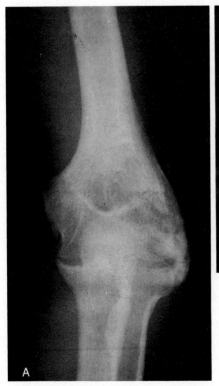

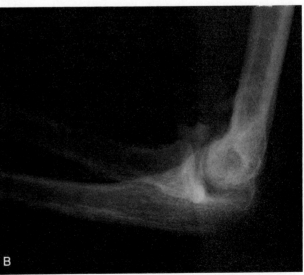

Figure 23–14. A, One year following posterior dislocation. B, Anterior and lateral ossification consistent with mild myositis ossificans. (From Linscheid, R. L., and Wheeler, D. K.: Elbow dislocations. J.A.M.A. 194:1171–1176, 1965. Copyright 1965, American Medical Association.)

year. Excision at that time usually allows substantial improvement in motion after excitation of the osteoblastic response has subsided (see Chapter 26).

AUTHOR'S PREFERRED TREATMENT METHOD

After suitable anesthesia with satisfactory muscle relaxation and with the patient lying supine on the operating table, the arm is abducted, and gentle longitudinal traction is applied. If an assistant is available, he can provide counteraction and posteriorly directed pressure over the midbrachium. Direct pressure over the humeral articulation is avoided, particularly if there is concern about the neurovascular status. A broad strap with a 5- to 10-kg weight attached may be substituted for an assistant. The forearm is gently displaced medially or laterally until alignment is effected. The prereduction radiographs should be illuminated directly in front of the operator for easy and frequent reference. It is desirable to have an image intensifier in place beneath the elbow during reduction. This helps to achieve alignment and shows when adequate distraction has been achieved. At this point, gentle elbow flexion, anteriorly directed pressure on the olecranon, or anterior pressure on the humerus should bring about reduction. If reduction has not been achieved, the joint should be reobserved under the image intensifier, or radiographs should be made in several planes with traction maintained. If subsequent manipulations fail, open reduction should be considered.

After reduction the elbow is held in 45 to 90 degrees of flexion, and stability is checked with gentle varus-valgus stress. The antecubital area is palpated for excessive induration. The radial and ulnar pulses should be checked as well. The elbow is placed in a posterior plaster shell about 45 degrees over a nonconstricting bandage such as cast cotton batting and held with a bias-cut stockinette. The forearm is placed in neutral rotation. The neural status is rechecked as soon as feasible, and the vascular status is checked hourly during the first 12 to 24 hours.

For lateral and medial dislocations the positioning is similar. It may be necessary to pull the arm and forearm apart before applying lateral or medial pressure to obtain realignment. Pronating or supinating the forearm may be helpful. The reduction is usually not difficult.

Anterior dislocation presents a different problem. Gentle flexion of the forearm helps to unlock the olecranon from its position in front of the trochlea. Traction followed by posterior displacement of the forearm results in prompt reduction. Postreduction clinical and radiographic examinations are important. Palpation of the triceps to assess possible avulsion or tearing is performed.

Divergent dislocation requires separate reduction of each bone, and because of the disruption of the interosseous membrane and other soft tissue damage, greater instability may be expected.

Under special circumstances postreduction positioning may be held in nearly full extension if prevention of flexor limitation, as in some athletic professions, is a factor. Careful follow-up to prevent redislocation, however, is essential. For all dislocations special care is taken to inform the patient of the possible loss of motion that frequently occurs as a natural consequence of this injury.

References

1. Adler, B., and Shaftan, G. W.: Radial Head Fractures, Is Excision Necessary? J. Trauma **4**:115, 1964.
2. Billett, D. M.: Unreduced Posterior Dislocation of the Elbow. J. Trauma **19**:186, 1979.
3. Blatz, D. J.: Anterior Dislocation of the Elbow. Findings in a Case of Ehlers-Danlos Syndrome. Orthop. Rev. **10**:129, 1981.
4. Blockey, N. J.: An Observation Concerning the Flexor Muscles During Recovery of Function After Dislocation of the Elbow. J. Bone Joint Surg. **36A**(4):833, 1954.
5. Conn, J., and Wade, P.: Injuries of the Elbow: A Ten Year Review. J. Trauma **1**:248, 1961.
6. DeLee, J. C.: Transverse Divergent Dislocation of the Elbow in a Child. J. Bone Joint Surg. **63A**:322, 1981.
7. Dryer, R., Buckwalter, J., and Sprague, B.: Treatment of Chronic Elbow Instability. Clin. Orthop. **100**:254, 1974.
8. Durig, M., Muller, W., Ruedi, T. P., and Gauer, E. F.: The Operative Treatment of Elbow Dislocation in the Adult. J. Bone Joint Surg. **61A**:23, 1979.
9. Edward, G. E., and Rostrup, O.: Radial Head Prosthesis in the Management of Radial Head Fractures. Can. J. Surg. **3**:153, 1960.
10. Eliason, E. L., and Brown, R. B.: Posterior Dislocation at the Elbow with Rupture of the Radial and Ulnar Arteries. Ann. Surg. **106**:1111, 1937.
11. Eppright, R. H., and Wilkins, K. E.: Fractures and Dislocations of the Elbow. In Rockwood, C. A., and Green, D. P. (eds.): Fractures, Vol I, Philadelphia, J. B. Lippincott Co., 1975.
12. Exarchou, E. J.: Lateral Dislocation of the Elbow. Acta Orthop. Scand. **48**:161, 1977.
13. Gaston, S. R., Smith, M., and Orren, D.: Adult Injuries of the Radial Head and Neck. Am. J. Surg. **78**:631, 1949.
14. Galbraith, K. A., et al.: Acute Nerve Injury as a Complication of Closed Fractures or Dislocations of the Elbow. Injury **11**(2):159, 1979.
15. Garland, D. E., and O'Hollaren, R. M.: Fractures and

Dislocations About the Elbow in the Head-Injured Adult. Clin. Orthop. **168**:38, 1982.

16. Glissan, D. J.: The After-Treatment of Dislocations of the Elbow, With a Note on Treatment of Stiff Elbows. Aust. N. Z. J. Surg. **5**:134, 1935.

17. Grant, I. R., and Miller, J. H.: Osteochondral Fracture of the Trochlea Associated With Fracture-Dislocation of the Elbow. Injury **6**(3):257, 1976.

18. Gutierrez, L. S.: A Contribution to the Study of the Limiting Factors of Elbow Extension. Acta Anat. **56**:146, 1964.

19. Harrington, I. J., and Tountas, A. A.: Replacement of the Radial Head in the Treatment of Unstable Elbow Fractures. Injury **12**(5):405, 1980.

20. Hassmann, G. C., Brunn, F., and Neer, C. S.: Recurrent Dislocation of the Elbow. J. Bone Joint Surg. **57A**(8):1080, 1975.

21. Heidt, R. S., Jr., and Stern, P. J.: Isolated Posterior Dislocation of the Radial Head. Clin. Orthop. **168**:136, 1982.

22. Heusner, L.: Ein Fall von habitueller Luxation des Ellenbogen. *In* Fetschrift zur Feier des funfzigjahrigin Jubilamus des Vereins der Aertze des Regierungsberzirks Dusseldorf. Weisbaden, 1894.

23. Jacobs, R. L.: Recurrent Dislocation of the Elbow Joint. A Case Report and a Review of the Literature. Clin. Orthop. **74**:151, 1971.

24. Johanson, O.: Capsular and Ligamentous Injuries of the Elbow Joint. A Clinical and Arthrographic Study. Acta Chir. Scand. (Suppl.) **287**:1, 1962.

25. Johnston, G. W.: Follow-Up of 100 Cases of Fracture of the Head of the Radius. Ulster Med. J. **31**:51, 1962.

26. Kapel, O.: Operation for Habitual Dislocation of the Elbow. J. Bone Joint Surg. **33A**:707, 1951.

27. King, T.: Recurrent Dislocation of the Elbow. J. Bone Joint Surg. **35B**:50, 1953.

28. Kini, M. G.: Dislocation of the Elbow and Its Complications. J. Bone Joint Surg. **22**:107, 1940.

29. Knoflach, J. G.: Zur Operation der habituellen Elbogenluxation. Zbl. Chir. **62**:2897, 1935.

30. Krishan, M.: Myositis Ossificans Traumatic of the Elbow. Int. Surg. **57**:475, 1972.

31. Krishnamoorthy, S., Bose, K., and Wong, K. P.: Treatment of Old Unreduced Dislocation of the Elbow. Injury **8**(1):39, 1976.

32. Lahz, J.: Recurrent Dislocation of the Elbow. Case Report. Australian Orthopedic Association Meeting. J. Bone Joint Surg. **42B**:406, 1960.

33. Lavine, L.: A Simple Method of Reducing Dislocations of the Elbow Joint. J. Bone Joint Surg. **35A**:785, 1953.

34. Linscheid, R. L., and Wheeler, D. K.: Elbow Dislocations. J.A.M.A. **194**:1171, 1965.

35. Loomis, L. K.: Reduction and After-Treatment of Posterior Dislocation of the Elbow. With Special Attention to the Brachialis Muscle and Myositis Ossificans. Am. J. Surg. **63**:56, 1944.

36. Louis, A., Ricciardi, J., and Spengler, D.: Arterial Injury: A Complication of Posterior Elbow Dislocation. J. Bone Joint Surg. **56A**:1631, 1979.

37. MacSween, W. A.: Transposition of Radius and Ulna Associated With Dislocation of the Elbow in a Child. Injury *10*(4):314, 1979.

38. Manske, P. R.: Unreduced Isolated Radial Head Dislocation in a Child. A Case Report. Orthopedics **5**(10):1327, 1982.

39. Mantle, J. A.: Recurrent Posterior Dislocation of the Elbow. J. Bone Joint Surg. **48B**:590, 1966.

40. Matev, I.: A Radiological Sign of Entrapment of the Median Nerve in the Elbow Joint After Posterior Dislocation. A Report of Two Cases. J. Bone Joint Surg. **58B**(3):353, 1976.

41. Maylahn, D. J., and Fahey, J. J.: Fractures of the Elbow in Children: Review of Three Hundred Consecutive Cases. J.A.M.A. **166**:220, 1958.

42. Milch, H.: Bilateral Recurrent Dislocation of the Ulna at the Elbow. J. Bone Joint Surg. **18**:777, 1936.

43. Mink, J. H., Eckardt, J. J., and Grant, T. T.: Arthrography in Recurrent Dislocation of the Elbow. Am. J. Roentgenol. **136**(6):1242, 1981.

44. Morrey, B. F., and An, K. N.: Articular and Ligamentous Contributions to the Stability of the Elbow Joint. Am. J. Sports Med. **11**:315, 1983.

45. Morrey, B. F., Askew, L., and Chao, E. Y.: Silastic Implant for the Radial Head. J. Bone Joint Surg. **63A**:454, 1981.

46. Morrey, B. F., and Chao, E. Y.: Biomechanical Study of the Elbow Following Excision of the Radial Head. J. Bone Joint Surg. **61A**:63, 1979.

47. Murray, R. C.: Fractures of the Head and Neck of the Radius. Br. J. Surg. **29**:106, 1940.

48. Neviaser, J. S., and Wickstrom, J.: Dislocation of the Elbow: A Retrospective Study of 115 Patients. South. Med. J. **70**(2):172, 1977.

49. Norwood, L., and Shook, D.: Acute Medial Elbow Ruptures. Am. J. Sports Med. **9**:16, 1981.

50. Odenheimer, K., and Harvey, J. P.: Internal Fixation of the Head and Neck of the Radius. J. Bone Joint Surg. **61A**:785, 1979.

51. O'Hara, J. P., Morrey, B. F., Johnson, E. W., and Johnson, K. A.: Dislocations and Fracture-Dislocations of the Elbow. Fracture Conference. Minn. Med. **58**:697, 1975.

52. Osborne, G., and Cotterill, P.: Recurrent Dislocation of the Elbow. J. Bone Joint Surg. **48B**:340, 1966.

53. Pawlowski, R. F., Palumbo, F. C., and Callahan, J. J.: Irreducible Posterolateral Elbow Dislocation: Report of a Rare Case. J. Trauma **10**:260, 1970.

54. Pritchard, D. J., Linscheid, R. L., and Svein, H. J.: Intra-Articular Median Nerve Entrapment With Dislocation of the Elbow. Clin. Orthop. **90**:100, 1973.

55. Protzmann, R. R.: Dislocation of the Elbow Joint. J. Bone Joint Surg. [Am.] **60**(4):539, 1978.

56. Purser, D. W.: Dislocation of the Elbow and Inclusion of the Medial Epicondyle in the Adult. J. Bone Joint Surg. **36B**:247, 1954.

57. Rana, N. A., Kenwright, J., Taylor, R. G., and Rushworth, G.: Complete Lesion of the Median Nerve Associated With Dislocation of the Elbow Joint. Acta Orthop. Scand. **45**:365, 1974.

58. Rehn, E.: Gelenkkapselplastik bei habitueller Ellbogenluxation. Neue Deutsch. Chir. **26B**:522, 1924.

59. Reichenheim, P. P.: Transplantation of the Biceps Tendon as a Treatment for Recurrent Dislocation of the Elbow. Br. J. Surg. **35**:201, 1947.

60. Roberts, J. B., et al.: The Surgical Treatment of Heterotopic Ossification at the Elbow Following Long-Term Coma. J. Bone Joint Surg. **61A**(5):760, 1979.

61. Roberts, P. H.: Dislocation of the Elbow. Br. J. Surg. **56**(11):806, 1969.

62. Salama, R., Wientroub, S., and Weissman, S. L.: Recurrent Dislocation of the Head of the Radius. Clin. Orthop. **125**:156, 1977.

63. Scharplatz, D., and Allgower, M.: Fracture-Dislocations of the Elbow. Injury **7**(2):143, 1975.

64. Schwab, G. H., Bennett, J. B., Woods, G. W., and Tullos, H. S.: Biomechanics of Elbow Instability: The Role of the Medial Collateral Ligament. Clin. Orthop. **146**:42, 1980.

65. Sharma, R. K., et al.: An Unusual Ulnar Nerve Injury Associated With Dislocation of the Elbow. Injury **8**(2):145, 1976.

66. Smith, D. N., et al.: The Radiological Diagnosis of Posttraumatic Effusion of the Elbow Joint and Its

Clinical Significance: The "Displaced Fat Pad" Sign. Injury **10**(2):115, 1978.

67. Sorel, E.: Luxation Recidivante due Caude Operation. Guerison Bull. Mem. Soc. Nat. Chir. **61**:790, 1935.

68. Spear, H. C., and Janes, J. M.: Rupture of the Brachial Artery Accompanying Dislocation of the Elbow or Supracondylar Fracture. J. Bone Joint Surg. **33A**:889, 1951.

69. Spring, W. E.: Report of a Case of Recurrent Dislocation of the Elbow. J. Bone Joint Surg. **35B**:55, 1953.

70. Staplemohr, S. von: Über Luxation Habitualis Cubiti Posterior. Acta Chir. Scand. **98**:511, 1949.

71. Strange, F. G. St. Clair: Entrapment of the Median Nerve After Dislocation of the Elbow. J. Bone Joint Surg. **64B**:224, 1982.

72. Sturm, J. T., Rothenberger, D. A., and Strate, R. G.: Brachial Artery Disruption Following Closed Elbow Dislocation. Trauma **18**(5):364, 1978.

73. Swanson, A. B., Jaeger, S. H., and LaRochelle, D.: Comminuted Fractures of the Radial Head. The Role of Silicone Implant Replacement Arthroplasty. J. Bone Joint Surg. **63A**:1039, 1981.

74. Symeonides, P. P., Paschaloglou, C., Stavrou, Z., and Pangalides, T.: Recurrent Dislocation of the Elbow. J. Bone Joint Surg. **57A**(8): 1084, 1975.

75. Tayob, A. A., et al.: Bilateral Elbow Dislocations With Intra-Articular Displacement of the Medial Epicondyles. J. Trauma **20**(4):332, 1980.

76. Trias, A., and Comeau, Y.: Recurrent Dislocation of the Elbow in Children. Clin. Orthop. **100**:74, 1974.

77. Thomas, T. T.: A Contribution to the Mechanism of Fractures and Dislocations in the Elbow Region. Ann. Surg. **89**:108, 1929.

78. Thompson, H., and Garcia, A.: Myositis Ossificans: Aftermath of Elbow Injuries. Clin. Orthop. **50**:129, 1967.

79. Van Rossum, J., Buruma, O. J. J., Kamphuisen, H. A. C., and Onolee, G. J.: Tennis Elbow—A Radial Tunnel Syndrome? J. Bone Joint Surg. **60B**:197, 1978.

80. Walker, R. H., and Tanner, J. B.: Fracture of the Proximal Shaft of the Radius Associated with Posterior Dislocation of the Elbow. Clin. Orthop. **168**:35, 1982.

81. Wheeler, D. K., and Linscheid, R. L.: Fracture-Dislocations of the Elbow. Clin. Orthop. **50**:95, 1967.

82. Wiley, J. J., Pegington, J., and Horwich, J. P.: Traumatic Dislocation of the Radius at the Elbow. J. Bone Joint Surg. **56B**(3):501, 1974.

83. Wilson, P. D.: Fractures and Dislocations in the Region of the Elbow. Surg. Gynecol. Obstet. **56**:335, 1933.

84. Woods, W., and Tullos, H.: Elbow Instability and Medial Epicondyle Fractures. Am. J. Sports Med. **5**:23, 1977.

CHAPTER 24

Contractures and Burns

W. P. Cooney, III

As a result of its specific anatomy, its high potential for serious injury, and a high incidence of inappropriate treatment, the elbow joint, more than any other in the body, may develop ankylosis from intrinsic (intra-articular) or extrinsic (extra-articular) causes. In this chapter, we will review the natural history of elbow ankylosis, classify the most frequent types, and discuss the reported as well as the author's preferred methods of treatment.

Historical Aspects

Historically, the elbow joint has long been known to be vulnerable to post-traumatic ankylosis as well as ankylosis from arthritis, burns, and birth deformities. Early recognition of post-traumatic ankylosis was described by Jones.[26] Blount admonished the orthopedist to allow the child to regain his own useful range of motion rather than to force physiotherapy.[2] Soft tissue fibrosis associated with supracondylar and intra-articular elbow fractures and dislocations in children was recognized by Campbell,[6] who considered that this was a self-limiting process and that elbow motion would return to normal given time and the absence of forced manipulation. In adult elbow fracture-dislocations, the importance of accurate reduction, solid fracture fixation, and early joint motion was emphasized by Watson-Jones,[59] Campbell,[5, 6] and Green.[17]

Incidence and Etiology

Post-traumatic contractures are related to the initial force of injury, the extent of periosteal stripping, and the degree of intra-articular involvement. Supracondylar and transcondylar fractures are particularly associated with flexion contracture secondary to anterior capsular stripping and brachialis muscle injury. Johanson reported a 5 percent incidence of ankylosis after elbow injuries,[25] and Campbell stated that "fractures about the elbow more frequently cause permanent disability

than do those of any other joint."[6] The development of ankylosis was particularly high in the mid-Eastern world,[38, 55, 56] where local bone setters and masseurs are common. Ankylosis, with or without myositis ossificans, is the most frequent complication after elbow injury. The relative incidence of ankylosis was noted in a series by Mohan,[38] in which supracondylar fractures accounted for 6 percent, T condylar fractures for 2 percent, condylar fractures for 12 percent, dislocations for 20 percent, fracture-dislocations for 38 percent, and fractures of the proximal radius for 10 percent of 200 instances of elbow ankylosis.

Congenital contractures of the elbow fortunately represent a much less frequent cause of elbow ankylosis (see Chapter 11). These contractures are primarily caused by arthrogryposis[34, 62] but may represent other conditions.[21, 36, 40, 44, 49] Most congenital contractures are muscular in origin, and joint contracture occurs secondarily. Flexion or extension contractures can occur based on the muscle group involved and the physiologic basis of the pathologic process (neurogenic or myopathic). The relative incidence of arthrogryposis is 1 per 500,000 live births. Its exact etiology remains unknown, but it probably represents a failure of differentiation of parts.

Major contractures of the elbow are also found as paralytic conditions in adults (spastic hemiplegia)[30] or children (cerebral or obstetrical palsy).[37, 46] Cerebral palsy flexion contracture is the most common involvement of this type.[46] These are more properly called acquired conditions, although they present early and can be confused with congenital lesions (see Chapter 38).

The final major group of contractures includes those acquired from rheumatoid arthritis,[48] burns,[12, 23] hemophilia,[10] or infection.[16] Intra-articular response to inflammation leads to synovitis, capsule edema, muscle contracture, and eventual loss of motion. Many patients with rheumatoid arthritis who have elbow involvement will develop a contracture by this mechanism, and in some,

Table 24–1. **Classification and Types of Elbow Contracture**

Pathology
Intra-articular
Extra-articular
Position
Extension
Flexion
Etiology (mechanism)
Traumatic
Dislocation
Fracture
Intra-articular
Periarticular
Mixed
Congenital
Arthrogryposis
Larsen's syndrome
Meiten's syndrome
Acquired
Osteoarthritis
Inflammatory arthritis (rheumatoid)
Burn
Septic
Paralytic

usually children, bony ankylosis may accompany the intra-articular process. Burn contractures of the elbow are frequent when there are deep partial- and full-thickness burns of the upper extremity that primarily involve the soft tissues. Hemophiliacs are subject to recurrent elbow joint hemorrhages. Too often a vicious cycle of bleeding, immobilization, muscle atrophy, weakness, and synovitis develops. This situation leads to recurrent bleeding, chronic synovitis, and ultimately cartilage and bone destruction (see Chapter 43).[9] Infectious arthritis due to suppurative or tuberculous organisms are notorious for causing joint ankylosis or spontaneous fusion.

Classification

Contractures about the elbow may be classified as intra-articular or extra-articular in origin or primarily flexion or extension by position (Table 24–1). The most convenient classification is based on mechanism and etiology—traumatic, congenital, and acquired.

GENERAL MECHANISMS

Traumatic

The elbow joint is closely guarded by muscle on all sides. The brachialis and biceps muscles sweep anteriorly, the common wrist extensors and brachioradialis bridge it laterally, the flexor pronator group guard it medially,

and the tendinous aponeurosis of the triceps muscle expands it posteriorly. The complex anatomy of the joint surface comprises the radiocapitellar, ulnohumeral, and radioulnar joint articular surfaces. Further, the joint is tightly constrained by medial and lateral collateral ligaments in continuity with the anterior capsule and adjacent periosteum. It is convenient, therefore, to think of stiffness at the elbow joint as (1) extra-articular, arising from the soft tissue, or (2) intra-articular, secondary to joint incongruity or fibrosis.

The mechanism of extra-articular (soft tissue) contracture after trauma is explained in part by pain and hemarthrosis.[54] With injury, the periarticular muscle, capsule, and periosteum are torn, contused, or ruptured. The elbow joint flexes to accommodate the hemarthrosis. Hemorrhage into the muscles congeals into a hematoma, fibrous degeneration, or sometimes muscle calcification.[52] If the injured tissues are not splinted or additional trauma occurs during treatment, pain, swelling, limited motion, and contraction will then lead to the irreversible changes comprising extra-articular ankylosis.

Collateral ligament injuries can contribute to elbow ankylosis from permanent contracture.[4, 18a, 25] The details of the ligament-flexion and stabilizing relationship have been variously reported by Gutierrez,[18] Morrey and An,[39a, 39b] and Tucker.[54] Fibrosis and shortening of these collateral ligaments is considered a primary cause of elbow stiffness.[25]

The third element in extra-articular or soft tissue contractures of the elbow is the joint capsule. With many elbow fracture-dislocations,[61] in particular, anterior dislocations,[29, 47] the joint capsule and adjacent brachialis muscle are violently torn (Fig. 24–1). In the absence of early joint motion, fibrosis within the healing capsule and muscle envelope produces a firm restriction to movement (Fig. 24–2).

Intra-articular injuries[48, 61] lead to elbow ankylosis by somewhat different mechanisms than those described above. The presence of articular incongruity may offer a mechanical limitation to elbow motion (Fig. 24–3). On the lateral side of the joint, this is most commonly caused by either radial head enlargement due to unreduced childhood[2] or congenital dislocations[31] or by fracture or osteochondritis. Medially, where a more congruous relationship of articular surfaces exists, any intra-articular fracture may cause adhesions, bone incongruity, and stiffness. Fracture fragments may restrict extension be-

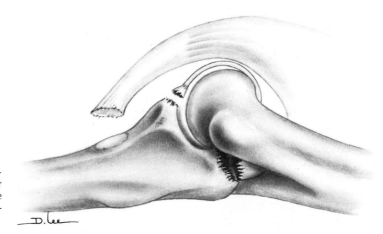

Figure 24–1. Close application of the brachialis muscle and capsule to the articular surface of the extended elbow place these structures at jeopardy with elbow dislocation.

cause of loose bodies within the olecranon fossa or limit flexion from posterior pericapsular fibrosis.

The type of restrictive pathology is related to the mechanism of injury.[43, 51] For example, T condylar fractures are notorious for causing incongruity and soft tissue damage (Fig. 24–4). Posterior dislocations rupture the anterior capsule, and one or both collateral ligaments, often resulting in a loss of extension (Fig. 24–1).[16] Forces that cause a radial head or capitellum fracture may also disrupt the medial collateral ligament. When there are combined injuries, soft tissue fibrosis and calcification, bone block, obliteration of the fossae, or intra-articular incongruity may coexist, producing severe or complete joint ankylosis (Fig. 24–4).

Congenital

Ankylosis in most congenital deformities appears to be caused by a primary muscle or

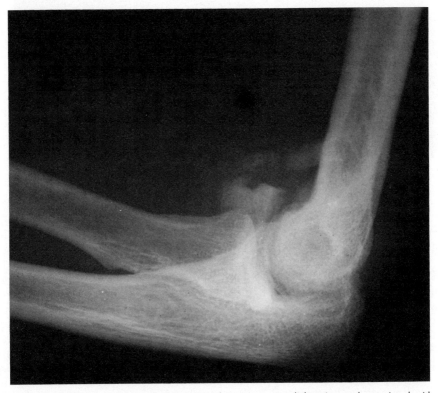

Figure 24–2. Anterior capsule heterotopic ossification secondary to anterior dislocation and associated with overaggressive passive stretching and the use of heavy weights.

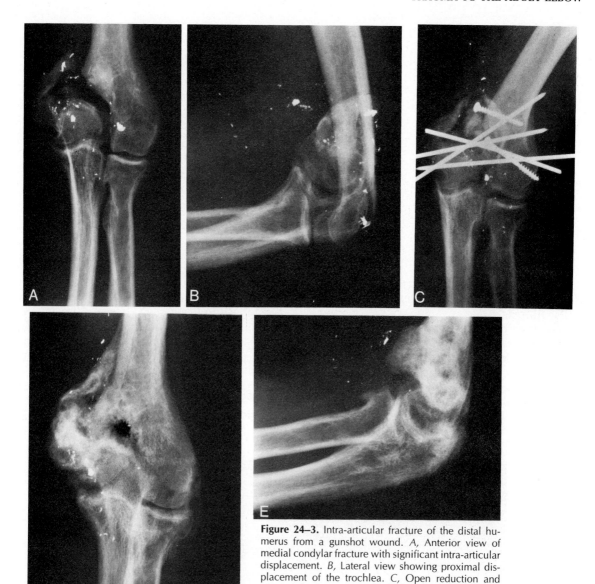

Figure 24–3. Intra-articular fracture of the distal humerus from a gunshot wound. *A,* Anterior view of medial condylar fracture with significant intra-articular displacement. *B,* Lateral view showing proximal displacement of the trochlea. *C,* Open reduction and internal fixation was performed. *D,* Elbow ankylosis was associated with both extra-articular and intra-articular ossification, here involving both the lateral and medial collateral ligaments. *E,* Anterior capsule.

nerve deficiency.[34] Arthrogryposis, originally thought to represent a type of joint ankylosis, is now known to be secondary to muscle weakness of a myopathic or neurogenic type.[34, 45] The process begins in the intra-uterine stage and probably does not progress during life. Muscles are hypoplastic with fibrous and fatty degeneration and a decrease in the size and quality of the muscle fibers. The potential for active contraction of muscle fibers is often lacking. Flexion or extension contracture develops most commonly, the latter being the most difficult to treat.[11, 60] The pathology in most cases varies from a completely extra-articular contracture to a grossly deformed joint with limited movement based on articular incongruity and only a secondary contribution from extra-articular sources.

Congenital conditions in which there are elbow contractures similar to those due to arthrogryposis include Larsen's syndrome (multiple joint dislocations with secondary contractures),[22, 53] Meiten's syndrome (mental retardation, growth failure, dislocation of the radius with bilateral elbow contractures),[40] and arachnodactyly.[36] The conditions are similar to arthrogryposis in that there is a primary muscle deficiency or disease that leads to the secondary failure of joint development (see Chapter 11).

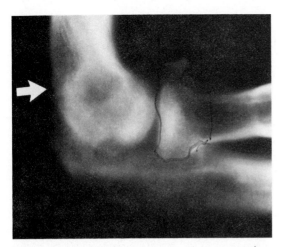

Figure 24–4. Radial head impingment with heterotopic bone blocking elbow extension. Lateral tomogram (arrow).

Acquired

In the adult, the nontraumatic elbow contractures are usually caused by a primary inflammatory process. In osteoarthritis, a mild inflammatory synovitis occurs with periarticular fibrosis and osteophytic new bone formation.[41] In rheumatoid conditions, the primary mechanism for loss of elbow motion is usually related to synovitis, effusion, and muscle spasm. With time the flexed position becomes permanent, and the joint space becomes narrowed. Intra-articular abnormalities in rheumatoid arthritis generally are not major causes of elbow contracture because cartilage loss is accompanied by bone resorption that allows surprisingly good function. Hemophilia,[10] juvenile rheumatoid arthritis, acute and chronic septic arthritis, and periarticular new bone formation after head injury[15, 30, 33] may each produce ankylosis of the elbow. These conditions are discussed in detail in the chapters dealing with these conditions.

TREATMENT

Principles of Treatment

The goal of treatment of elbow ankylosis is to provide a functional and, ideally, a painless arc of motion. To obtain this, four principles must be considered: (1) pain must be controlled or prevented; (2) the contractile tissues should be mature; (3) early and sustained motion should be obtained; and (4) recurrence should be avoided by prolonged splinting.

Pain Control. Pain may be present from either intra- or extra-articular causes. The treatment of contracted tissues is effective only after pain has been controlled, and this often implies control of inflammation (see Chapter 9). Because with intra-articular pathology there is usually some extra-articular component, treating the pain from both sources is essential.

Tissue Maturation. For successful excision the collagenous or osseous elements must be mature. No reliable tests for measuring maturity are available. Radioactive isotopic scanning (Fig. 24–5) may be of some help, but it is not absolutely reliable in showing when the maturation process is complete.[12]

Early Motion. After acute injuries, early return of elbow motion is helpful for preventing secondary joint contracture. Similarly, after surgical treatment of fibrosis or bony ankylosis, early joint motion is essential for maintaining the achieved range of motion and preventing recurrence. Passive static or active dynamic splints[18] can be used effectively in this situation to avoid the excessive force that causes an inflammatory fibrotic response.

Splinting. Finally, protective splinting, particularly at night, to maintain the improved motion and joint position is essential. Premature relaxation of splinting programs unfortunately leads to loss of correction. What is gained dynamically, actively or isometrically during the day must be maintained by static, fixed-position splinting at night.

Treatment Alternatives

The selection of treatment for elbow ankylosis is related to patient age, occupation, and extremity dominance as well as to the type of disease or injury process. The technique of passive stretch, for example, might be well tolerated by an adult but poorly by a child. The response to treatment varies according to the degress of involvment of the elbow. The surgeon must explore all conservative measures and base any surgical intervention on these factors tempered by his experience.

Nonoperative Treatment

Conservative treatment measures are preferred in the initial management of elbow joint contractures that are less than 1 year old. These modalities include local heat, active gentle assisted stretch, ultrasound, dynamic orthoplast splinting, and occupational modulation. Physical therapy should be directed at gentle active assisted motion with muscle strengthening and avoidance of inflammation. When a joint contracture is com-

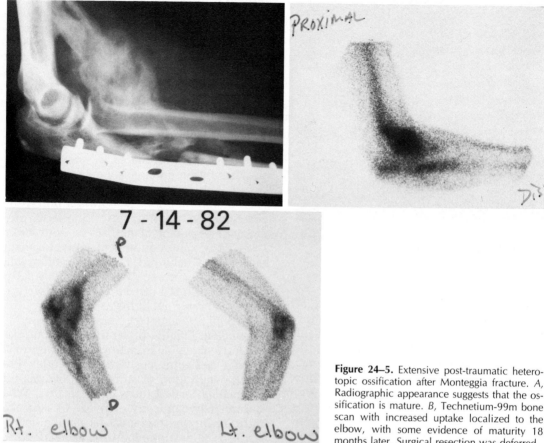

Figure 24–5. Extensive post-traumatic heterotopic ossification after Monteggia fracture. *A,* Radiographic appearance suggests that the ossification is mature. *B,* Technetium-99m bone scan with increased uptake localized to the elbow, with some evidence of maturity 18 months later. Surgical resection was deferred.

plicated by muscle weakness, muscle stimulation techniques may be effective.

Dynamic splinting is also an effective means of preventing the development of elbow contractures. Current choices include a turnbuckle orthosis in which there is a gradual increase in the static stretch of tight structures.[17, 32] Although turnbuckle devices have been used for many years, the effectiveness of this device for the elbow has been reintroduced by Green and co-workers (Fig. 24–6).[17] The turnbuckle is placed upright on the out-

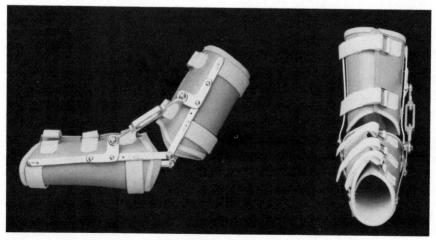

Figure 24–6. Turnbuckle orthosis for static stretch of developing contractures. (From Green, D. P., and McCoy, H.: Turnbuckle orthotic correction of elbow flexion contractures after acute injuries. J. Bone Joint Surg. 61A:1092, 1979.)

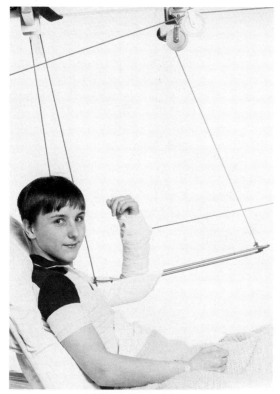

Figure 24–7. Reversed dynamic sling attached to Thomas splint. (From Dickson, R. A.: Reversed dynamic slings: A new concept in the treatment of post-traumatic elbow flexion contractures. Injury 8:35, 1976).

side, and the patient is instructed to increase the force applied by the turnbuckle to the point of discomfort but not pain.

A reversed dynamic sling is especially indicated for post-traumatic contractures,[9] but, like the turnbuckle, it is not applied in long-standing conditions (Fig. 24–7). With this system, dynamic traction by weights is applied to the elbow through a combination of longitudinal traction and passive stretch. As with the dynamic splint, active flexion can be maintained during the period of passive stretch, which is an advantage over static devices such as the turnbuckle. This system uses skin traction, which can limit the amount of force applied.

Goller and Enders have used a thermoplastic brace that provides an extension moment about the elbow based on proximal and distal force couples.[18] A cast is molded into a model, reheated to give approximately 20 additional degrees of extension, and applied to the patient.

Polycentric cast brace hinges can be used to gain early elbow motion and prevent contractures; they are aligned with the lateral and medial epicondyles of the elbow.[32] We have used a hinged orthosis with a rubberband traction pull to achieve the same goal as that gained with the turnbuckle splint. The degree of stretch can be altered by the patient by increasing or decreasing the tension on the rubberbands or tubing (Fig. 24–8). The device is usually worn only during the day, and the position is maintained by a static splint at night.

The concept of continuous passive motion has recently been applied to the elbow (Fig. 24–9), and, while promising, is still an investigative technique at this time.

Operative Treatment

Indications for surgical management of elbow ankylosis are applied after conservative treatment has failed. When a contracture is fixed and mature, and renders a nonfunctional arc of motion, surgical treatment is necessary. Basically, three types of surgical intervention are available: (1) excision and release, (2) release and muscle transfer, and (3) joint excisional arthroplasty with or without distraction and early motion.

Excision and Release. This form of treatment (excisional arthroplasty) is recommended by some for ankylosis secondary to infectious arthritis and rheumatoid arthritis and after trauma.[5] Excessive extra-articular scarring and significant muscle weakness are contraindications. The details of interposition arthroplasty are reported in Chapter 32.

When contractures are caused by extra-articular factors, excision of fibrotic portions of the capsule and removal of heterotopic bone are required. Wilson advocated this approach, reporting good results following anterior capsulectomy.[63] Glynn and Niebauer have reviewed their experience with capsulectomy for both flexion and extension contractures.[16] These authors use an anterior approach for flexion contractures, transecting the brachialis muscle and lengthening the biceps tendon to expose the anterior capsule, which is then generously excised. Release of the anterior half of the collateral ligaments is usually needed. The brachialis muscle and the lengthened biceps tendon are repaired, and the elbow is then splinted in a position short of maximal extension. Postoperative evaluation of pulses and neurologic status is important.

In extension contractures, a posterior approach through a Van Gorder V-type incision has been recommended.[63] A wide posterior capsulectomy, removal of osteophytes, and a 1-cm removal of the olecranon process com-

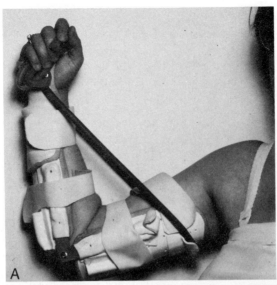

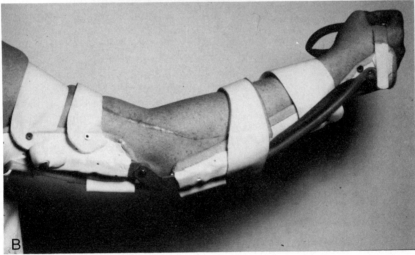

Figure 24–8. Dynamic hinged elbow joint with rubberband traction and outriggers to increase leverage after postoperative lateral release. *A*, Flexion. *B*, Active assisted extension.

plete the release. The triceps is closed in a V-Y fashion without tension, and the elbow is placed in 90 degrees of flexion. Early postoperative mobilization follows both procedures.

The role of the collateral ligaments in elbow contractures is not fully understood, although the anatomic studies of Gutierrez have suggested the implication.[18a] A hinged orthoplast splint, if the collateral ligaments were released, would appear to be necessary to prevent elbow instability.[33] When bony ankylosis (with heterotopic bone) accompanies fibrotic contracture, excision of the heterotopic bone, when mature, combined with release of the associated contracted tissues is indicated.[20] It is important to remember that surgical excision of heterotopic bone in children is con-

traindicated because it is invariably followed by recurrence and usually will resolve given sufficient time (see Chapter 12).

When joint ankylosis follows elbow fracture-dislocation, excision and release may include resection of the radial head, anterior capsulectomy, and adhesion release.[51] This is usually accomplished using a lateral approach[6, 38, 47, 61] (see Chapter 8).

Burn contractures mainly affect the antecubital fossa and can produce severe contractures of the skin and underlying soft tissues.[12, 20] In these cases, Millard advocates lengthening the shortened tendons, neurolysis, and capsule release (if required).[35] He found that split-thickness skin grafting is rarely adequate and preferred flap coverage of a tubed pedicle type (Fig. 24–10). Evans concurred with this approach, adding that three-point splinting in extension and early motion are important (Fig. 24–11).[13] Evans also emphasized preventive splinting, dynamic traction, and suspension and maintenance of joint excursion and mobility.

Release and Muscle Transfer. Muscle transfer has been thoroughly addressed in Chapter 37 and will be discussed only briefly here. Transfer of the pectoralis major[21] or latissimus dorsi[28] muscles can be effective in restoring elbow flexion only after fixed or dynamic contractures have been treated. Occasionally, if these muscles are not strong enough, the flexor pronator origin (Steindler) or triceps muscle[7] can be transferred[21] (see Chapter 37).

In patients with arthrogryposis, Doyle et al. reported 18 procedures in 15 patients to gain elbow flexion.[11] These included pectoralis major transfer (seven cases), triceps transfer (seven cases), and Steindler flexor-plasty (two cases). Better motion and strength and single-handed feeding were observed following pectoralis or triceps muscle transfer. The need to

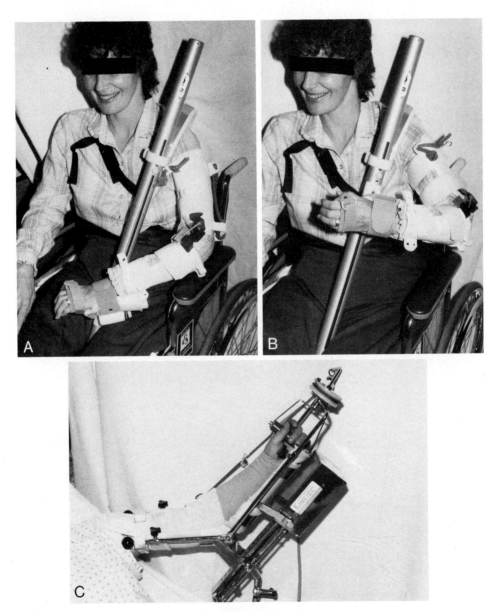

Figure 24–9. Passive elbow exercises. *A, B,* Elbow flexion-extension passive motion used with a custom hinged elbow splint. Range of motion is controlled by stops. Note orthoplastic splints with rubber cord flexion and extension assists. *C,* Cam-driven exerciser for pronation and supination during flexion-extension. Continuous or intermittent motion is obtained with adjustable speed.

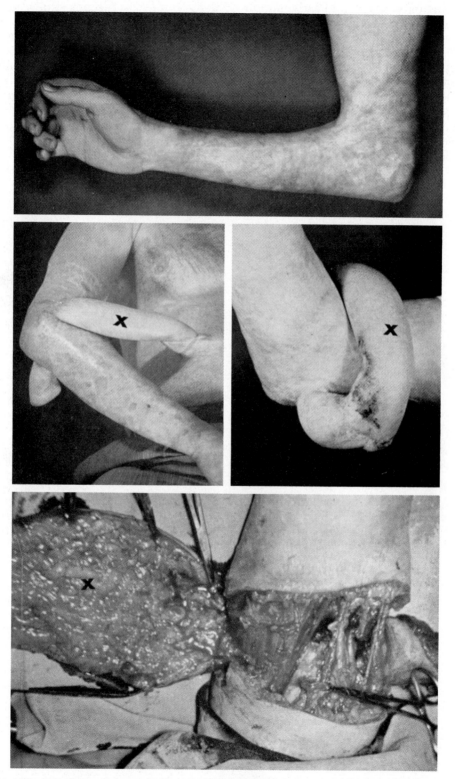

Figure 24–10. Millard has designed a bipedicle flap that can be applied for direct coverage of severe elbow burn contractures. *A,* Right elbow burn contracture with limited motion. *B,* Second tubule pedicle (x). *C,* Larger pedicle attached to the stub of the first pedicle. *D,* Pedicle opened and elbow contracture released. This included division of the joint capsule and biceps-tendon lengthening. (From Millard, D. R., Jr., and Ortiz, A. C.: Correction of severe elbow contractures. J. Bone Joint Surg. 47A(7):1347, 1965.)

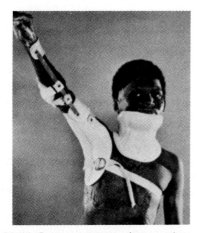

Figure 24–11. Burn contracture splinting utilizing the principle of three point fixators about the distal radius (dorsal), posterior elbow, and proximal humerus. (From Evans, E. B., et al.: Prevention and correction of deformity after burns. Surg. Clin. North Am. 50:1361, 1970.)

first release the extension contracture in this condition was emphasized by Meyn and Ruby.[34] These investigators found that skin and capsular tightness was associated with radial head dislocation and other joint abnormalities. The recommended procedure includes posterior capsulotomy, triceps lengthening, and soft tissue release combined with tendon transfer (tendons of triceps or flexor pronator origin). Radial head excision was deferred.

Spastic flexion contracture, which is commonly observed in cerebral palsy and is occasionally seen in arthrogryposis, congenital arachnodactyly, Larsen's syndrome, and Meiten's syndrome, requires procedures to overcome the flexion forces. Mital described his treatment of 32 spastic contracted elbows.[37] This consisted of excision of the lacertus fibrosus, lengthening of the biceps tendon, and incision of the aponeurologic fibers covering the brachialis muscle (at two or more levels). In severe deformities the skin and anterior capsule may need release.[46] Although good return of elbow motion and power was obtained by these authors, the results can be somewhat unpredictable (see Chapter 38).

To maintain hygiene and facilitate nursing care with severe fixed flexion and supination deformities of the elbow in tetraplegics, Freehafter recommends biceps tenotomy and splinting.[14] Correction in these patients allows independent transfer, wheelchair propulsion, and prehensile function.

Arthroplasty with Distraction. With the resurgence of external fixation devices, flexion-extension hinge distractors have been devel-

oped to improve the results in treating elbow contractures. In principle, these devices should work more efficiently than cast brace or orthotic devices because they are centered precisely at the axis of rotation and thus can exert forces directly to the skeleton.

An elbow hinge-distractor was popularized by Volkov and Oganesian in 1977 (Fig. 24–12).[58] This device employed transosseous pins, an artificial external joint, and an external fixation frame. Because correct centering of the fixator and pin tract drainage have been problems, a more simple elbow-hinged distractor (Fig. 24–13) was recently reported by Deland and co-workers.[8] These authors emphasize the importance of replicating the correct axis of rotation. Distraction is obtained by a screw that separates the ulnar from the humeral side plate. Both lateral and medial sides can be adjusted independently. Early reports are encouraging.[13] More rigid hinge distraction fixators are currently being developed that will allow half-pin fixation to the humerus and ulna.

Distraction is also an effective adjunctive aid when it is combined with excisional arthroplasty of the elbow[5, 44, 48] and with external cast brace or splints. The advantages of distraction across the elbow joint to reduce compressive loads are attractive and should improve the results of excisional arthroplasty.

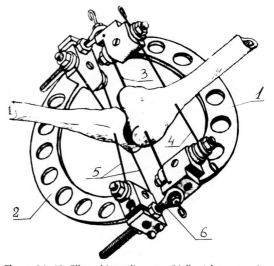

Figure 24–12. Elbow hinge distractor (Volkov) for restoration of elbow motion. It is applied to mobilize joint contractures, reduce old dislocations, and immobilize para-articular fractures. K-wire loosening with pin tract drainage and proper centering have been clinical problems. (From Volkov, M. V., and Oganesian, O. V.: Restoration of function in the knee and elbow with a hinge-distractor apparatus. J. Bone Joint Surg. 57A(5):591, 1975.)

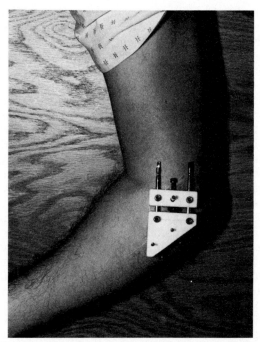

Figure 24–13. Simplified external hinge distractor designed for accurate location of center of rotation. Limited clinical experience but definite potential for correcting ankylosis. (From Deland, J. T., et al.: Treatment of post-traumatic elbows with a new hinge-distractor. Orthopedics 6:732, 1983.)

Elbow instability with this technique has not been a problem.

COMPLICATIONS

Complications associated with elbow ankylosis are recurrence of the contracture and secondary arthrosis. These complications are not usually discussed in the few series that have been reported on the results of elbow ankylosis treatment. In our own experience, these problems are common. A partial recurrence of the contracture, especially in extension, is typical. Lack of prolonged splinting or, more likely, incomplete excision or inappropriate timing may be important factors. Waiting at least 6 months after injury or until there is no clinical tenderness or pain on

stress of the contracted tissues (i.e., subsidence of inflammation) is a helpful temporal standard. Further, accepting a flexion deformity of more than 25 degrees appears to lead to recurrence of deformity to 45 or 50 degrees more readily than will a 10- to 15-degree contracture progress to 20 or 25 degrees. Therefore, complete resection of all involved tissues without sacrificing function is most important.

Neurovascular perioperative complications may also occur. Carefully planned, adequate exposure is essential to avoid injury to these structures. Hence, both medial and lateral incisions may be needed to identify nerves and vessels proximal and distal to the lesion so that the contracted tissue may be safely released (Fig. 24–14). Vessel injury is uncommon with lateral or posterior approaches, but the release may need to be a gradual one to avoid excessive stretch of the anterior structures. A preoperative arteriogram is useful in cases of deformity after fracture. Radial and ulnar pulses and capillary refill must be observed following release to prevent overstretching of the brachial artery when applying passive extension splinting.

Wound healing may be impaired after many previous procedures or may result from use of poorly supervised passive motion machines, dynamic flexion or extension splinting, or aggressive physical therapy. Occasionally, upper limb dystrophy can occur. Infection is no more common in these procedures than in other operations about the elbow, and therefore prophylactic antibiotics are not routinely recommended unless the operative procedure is prolonged or other risk factors obtain.

AUTHOR'S PREFERRED TREATMENT METHOD

Flexion Contractures

Dynamic Splinting

Flexion contractures of less than 6 months duration are treated with dynamic splints or

Figure 24–14. Fracture-dislocation of the elbow. A, Internal fixation of the proximal ulna fracture (radial head fracture). B, C, Status after radial head resection, elbow reduction, and long arm cast application. Note ossification of the medial collateral ligament, joint space narrowing with capsular ankylosis, and synostosis between the proximal radius and the ulna (arrows). Elbow motion was 80 to 115 degrees of flexion, no pronation-supination. D, Surgical treatment consisted of resection of proximal synostosis resection with Silastic interposition; resection of heterotopic bone from the medial and lateral elbow approaches, and Volkov hinge distractor external fixation. Postoperative low-dose radiation was given on days 10 to 20. E, F, Improved joint space; elbow motion was 30 to 125 degrees flexion, 50 degrees pronation, and 60 degrees supination. There was mild recurrence of heterotopic bone. The elbow was stable and painless 1 year later. This particular case exhibits many principles of treatment for osseous and soft tissue components of flexion and forearm rotation contracture. Two incisions, distraction, Silastic interposition, irradiation, and postoperative splinting were used to provide a gratifying result.

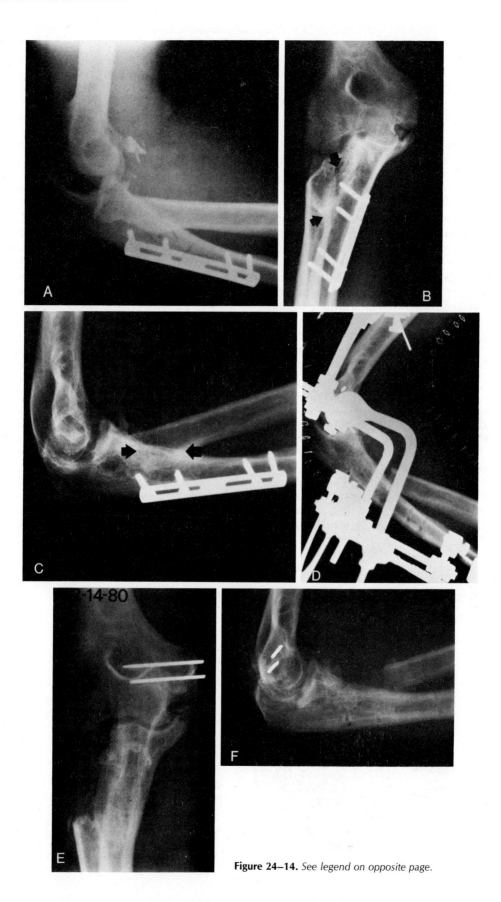

Figure 24–14. *See legend on opposite page.*

hinged elbow traction for deformities of up to 90 degrees. Ultrasound is used to reduce collagen stiffness and may be applied in conjunction with the dynamic splints. Adjustable static night splints maintain the motion gained during the day. Muscle spasms are controlled by medication.

For difficult or longer existing flexion contractures that are resistant to dynamic splinting, we use the turnbuckle arthrosis to provide a constantly applied force.

Surgical Release

Extension beyond 30 degrees is unpredictable, so we generally do not offer an anterior release in patients with a flexion contracture of less than 45 degrees.

Lateral Approach. For mild to moderate flexion contractures (45 to 60 degrees) associated with radial head fractures or following anterior fracture-dislocations, infection, or acquired disease (hemophilia, rheumatoid arthritis), a direct lateral or Kocher-type approach is preferred. With this procedure, the entire lateral side of the elbow joint is exposed with or without an epicondylar osteotomy (Fig. 24–15). The anterior capsule is dissected free with periosteal elevators, and if necessary the lateral intramuscular septum and brachialis muscle are elevated away from the bone. A radial head excision is often required. Capsular excision and limited medial joint debridément can be performed with this approach. The olecranon fossa can also be examined, and fibrous tissue or bone can

be excised. Passive manipulation of the joint is then performed. Motion to within 15 to 20 degrees of full extension requires a more complete capsule release with a scalpel and occasionally release of the brachialis muscle.

A medial approach has been found useful only in cases in which there has been recurrence of the contracture, primary injury to the medial side of the elbow joint, a need to apply associated ulnar nerve symptoms, or the distraction arthroplasty device.

Following closure, the elbow is splinted in extension for 5 to 7 days, and then dynamic extension splinting is started with early active motion.

Anterior Approach. For more significant elbow flexion contractures, particularly those that are extra-articular, a sterile tourniquet and an anterior (Henry) approach is preferred (Chapter 8). The cubital fossa is incised by a lazy-S or -Z incision with the upper limb of the incision placed laterally (Fig. 24–16). The lacertus fibrosus is released or excised and a fasciotomy performed. With the lateral antebrachial cutaneous nerve retracted, the biceps tendon is lengthened by Z-plasty. The brachialis muscle is examined, and if contracted, it is released near its insertion, dividing through both fascia and muscle. Alternatively, infraction or serial incisional lengthening of the brachialis aponeurosis in one or more places can be performed, with capsulectomy as required if any residual flexion contracture exists (Fig. 24–16). The biceps tendon is reconstituted at a new resting length, and the

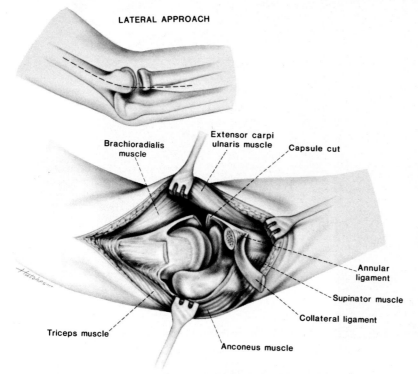

LATERAL APPROACH

Brachioradialis muscle

Extensor carpi ulnaris muscle

Capsule cut

Annular ligament

Supinator muscle

Collateral ligament

Triceps muscle

Anconeus muscle

Figure 24–15. Lateral approach to the elbow. Skin incision line follows the interval along the brachioradialis, over the lateral epicondyle, and distally between the radial wrist extensor and the finger extensors (A). Lateral epicondylectomy of release of collateral ligament and elevation of the anterior capsule is done. If needed, resection of the radial head and anterior capsule can be carried out. Complete exposure of the elbow, including the medial joint, can be obtained if débridement is necessary.

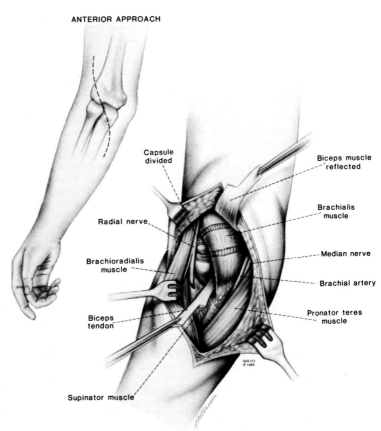

ANTERIOR APPROACH

Capsule
divided

Radial nerve

Brachioradialis
muscle

Biceps
tendon

Supinator muscle

Biceps muscle
reflected

Brachialis
muscle

Median nerve

Brachial artery

Pronator teres
muscle

MAYO
©1984

Figure 24–16. Anterior approach to the elbow. This approach is preferred for extra-articular ankylosis within the brachialis muscle and anterior capsule. *A,* A lazy S or Z-plasty approach through the antecubital fossa with release of the lacertus fibrosus is done. The biceps tendon is lengthened by Z-plasty. The brachialis muscle is released by interaction of the aponeuroses. *B,* Anterior capsule release and radial head excision.

vascular supply to the extremity is examined in the new position of elbow extension. Electrical stimulation of the median and radial nerve can be performed if these appear to be excessively tight or seem to limit elbow extension. This is rarely the case in adults but can occur in children.

After 5 days of splinting in extension, a dynamic elbow extension splint for daytime use and a static extension night splint are applied. If heterotopic bone was removed, low-dosage radiation therapy is started in the patient who is over 50 years of age. Alternatively, passive elbow motion exercises offer great promise of maintaining the improved motion. Our experience with these exercises has been excellent with the exception of congenital contractures such as those due to arthrogryposis. Physiotherapy under direct supervision is continued during this time until 8 weeks following surgery. A resting (extension) night splint is continued for 6 months, because late recurrence of contractures has occurred.

Most flexion contractures are post-traumatic in origin, and treatment other than release or excision of the affected tissues is rarely indicated. Entrapment of both radial and median nerves has been encountered,

however, and, if scarring is extensive, neurolysis, or rarely, nerve grafting may be required. In congenital or cerebral palsy-related elbow contractures, elbow release alone is preferred. In cases of tetraplegia in which elbow contracture develops secondary to lack of splinting and physiotherapy, tendon transfer to restore elbow extension[37a] has been our preference.

Extension Contractures

Contractures of the elbow joint in extension result from congenital or hereditary disorders such as arthrogryposis;[62] from post-traumatic conditions,[38] such as olecranon fracture, dislocation, forced manipulation, and burns; or from acquired disease, such as hemophilia[10] or tetanus.[24] The preferred surgical treatment of these less common types of ankylosis should be based on an individual approach.

Posterior Approach. For post-traumatic conditions, a posterior Campbell (Van Gorder) approach to the elbow has been preferred (see Chapter 8). This approach provides excellent exposure to the olecranon fossa, posterior capsule, and collateral ligaments and has the additional advantage of lengthening the triceps aponeurosis by a V-Y technique. The triceps aponeurosis and muscle are freed from bone where it may be adherent, and the aponeurosis is divided longitudinally in the midline, leaving a distally based flap attached to the olecranon process. Subperiosteal dissection may be needed both medially and laterally to free the posterior capsule and posterior portions of the collateral ligaments. The medial and lateral collateral ligaments can be released completely from their respective epicondyles if necessary. From this exposure, radial head resection and intra-articular adhesions can be released as necessary.

Following release of the posterior capsule and ligaments and lengthening of the triceps mechanism, the elbow is positioned in flexion, taking care to be certain that the joint moves passively without hinging on soft tissue and without anterior obstruction. Immobilization at more than 90 degrees of flexion should be attempted so that the elbow flexors have a mechanical advantage for active, assisted motion. Supportive splints postoperatively are essential; dynamic flexion splints are utilized if there is residual resistance to full flexion.

Procedures for Static and Dynamic Dysfunction

Although some authors prefer a staged procedure for stiff joints associated with inadequate motor power,[11] we believe that in some cases it might be advantageous to use a combined procedure. For example, in arthrogryposis, transfer of a strong triceps anteriorly would best be performed at the time of posterior release. Alternatively, if a second motor to provide elbow flexion is available, such as the pectoralis major or the latissimus dorsi, we would stage the reconstruction. First the contracture would be released posteriorly and full motion gained with physiotherapy and dynamic splinting (using passive elbow motion exercise or dynamic splints), and then, once motion is obtained, transfer of an appropriate muscle should be performed. We do not favor a Steindler flexorplasty as recommended by some,[62, 34] because this provides weak elbow flexion and is associated with anterior capsular scarring. We also avoid elbow arthrodesis in "a more functional position" as suggested by Kelikian or closing wedge osteotomies that improve forearm position without gaining elbow motion.

Burn Contractures

Ankylosis of the elbow secondary to burn contractures is a difficult management prob-

lem. Soft tissue scarring, loss of protective substances (skin and subcutaneous tissues), and tendon, muscle, and joint contractures require the combined skills of several disciplines.

An aggressive preventive treatment program will help the majority of burn contractures. Following primary treatment of the burned extremity, we utilize static three-point splinting to maintain the elbow in extension (Fig. 24–11). If the injury is associated with fractures or joint injuries, we have employed skeletal traction to maintain alignment and also allow for adequate wound treatment. Olecranon or radius pins can be used for balanced traction to allow joint mobilization without loss of fracture stability. Orthoplast splinting and bracing, both static and dynamic, are judiciously applied early in the burn treatment program. Compressive garments (Jobst or foam padding) are placed beneath the splints to control hypertrophic scarring. Splints are continued until the skin and soft tissue are supple and until further danger of scar contraction has passed.

Surgical treatment of burn contractures must address anterior, posterior, or generalized involvement. Posterior contracture is less common but is usually more severe. Ossification within the triceps muscle occurs and acts as a block to elbow extension. Surgical treatment requires excision of the heterotopic ossification when mature. We recommend that the surgical excision be performed through a longitudinal posterior incision without skin flaps. The heterotopic bone, posterior capsule, and olecranon process are removed, and the raw bone surfaces are covered with bone wax, Gelfoam or local fat. The ulnar nerve is always identified and if necessary transferred anteriorly. The anterior capsule, tendon, and muscles may undergo secondary contracture as a result of posterior heterotopic ossification. If they require tenoloysis and capsular release, this should be performed at the same operation as the excision of the heterotopic ossification.

Anterior full-thickness contractures are the more common type of injury, involving skin, fascia, tendon, and muscle elements. The major problem is providing muscle and tendon release while maintaining adequate skin coverage because split-thickness skin grafts will not cover or heal over these structures. Both orthopedic and plastic surgical techniques are required to solve this problem. After skin Z-plasty and muscle and capsule release, the resultant soft tissue and skin defects are covered by an extended groin or thoracoepigastric flap. We have had less success with local muscle pedicle flaps using the brachioradialis or flexor carpi ulnaris muscles. We prefer the bipedicle tube flap described by Millard,[35] which involves a delayed procedure. The ability to splint the elbow in the desired position is certainly easier with such a flap than it is with the standard or tubed groin flap.

Ectopic Ossification

The topic of elbow ankyloses from ectopic ossification is covered elsewhere (Chapter 26) but will be discussed briefly here for completeness.

Our approach to ectopic bone formation is based primarily on the specific functional needs of the patient and the feasibility of surgical intervention. A painless stiff elbow in 90 to 100 degrees of flexion may be acceptable. Curiously, we find more patients concerned with the loss of forearm rotation as a consequence of heterotopic bone than with the loss of elbow flexion-extension. Guidelines for surgical treatment of these disorders include the following:

1. Heterotopic bone must be mature as determined by technetium bone scan.
2. Pain should be a significant component of the patient's complaint.
3. Neurologic function in the extremity should be near normal including functional motor nerves to the joint.
4. Surgical resection of heterotopic bone is feasible without causing neurovascular compromise.

Assuming that these factors are present, surgical excision of heterotopic bone to regain flexion and forearm rotation should be performed at a single procedure. Our approach to this problem is exemplified in Figure 24–14. Both anterior and posterior incisions can be performed simultaneously if needed. Anteriorly, the Henry approach is preferred. Posteriorly, a Campbell approach is usually adequate. Freeing the ulnar nerve is required, with anterior transposition if posteromedial bone excision associated with subperiosteal stripping is needed. The radial nerve will be involved more commonly with anterolateral heterotopic ossification and must be identified and protected. The median nerve and brachial artery are rarely directly involved in the ossification process but require exposure to be certain of a "safe" excision.

Dynamic splints are helpful to maintain motion gained at surgery. Problems of wound healing, pressure sores, pain, and muscle contraction must be evaluated during the treatment program, and occasionally motion assists should be used but only after a trial period of active assisted motion.

To help prevent the recurrence of heterotopic bone, preoperative, intraoperative, and postoperative modalities have been tried. Preoperative diphosphonates are administered for 3 weeks before and 3 months after surgery at a dose of 20 mg per kg per day. Interposition of Silastic membranes, fascia lata, and local fat or dermis between the radius and ulna or between the trochlear and olecranon articular surfaces has been performed. Silastic is best for small surfaces and appears to prevent bone overgrowth (Fig. 24–14). Fascia lata and fat are less predictable materials for preventing heterotopic ossification but do work well in fibrous arthroplasties with larger surfaces.

Our experience with low-dose radiation at the elbow has been limited to only a few patients, but the results have been gratifying. The theoretical limitation of this modality is late calcification of the osseous matrix. Concern about malignant transformation discourages irradiation in the younger patient. Whether long-term results will justify the continued use of these or other agents remains to be seen.

Arthrogryposis

Our personal experience with the treatment of arthrogryposis of the elbow has not been completely satisfactory. The approach to patients with this problem must be divided into those who have the appearance of a near-normal joint with absence of certain muscles and those without elbow articular surfaces and greatly restricted passive motion. In the former, even when there is some loss of passive motion, usually in flexion, improved function and strength can be anticipated through posterior capsule release and anterior muscle transfer (triceps or pectoralis major being preferred).

The lack of joint articular surfaces requires a more extensive program. A joint is first created, passive motion attained, and active function provided. To gain an effective joint, shortening of the humerus by 2 to 3 cm may be needed, and fascial interposition over both proximal and distal bone ends is helpful to ensure maintenance of the "joint" space. The triceps is lengthened (V-Y technique, using a Van Gorder approach) to reestablish an elbow extensor, and muscle transfers are necessary for active flexion. Finally, soft tissue closure using rotation flaps may be required.

Postoperative programs using static splinting to maintain elbow flexion stance and dynamic assisted flexion with hinged splints or passive elbow motion machines have been implemented to complement the results obtained from surgery. Cautious expectation in patients who lack an elbow joint is advised, and the long-term goals of obtaining motion to provide better hand use for self-care must be remembered in recommending reconstructive surgery, both before and after surgery.

References

1. Bankov, S.: A Test for Differentiation Between Contracture and Spasm of the Biceps Muscle in Post-Traumatic Rigidities of the Elbow Joint. Hand 7(3):262, 1975.
2. Blount, W. P.: Fractures in Children. In Injuries About the Elbow. Baltimore, The Williams & Wilkins Co., 1954.
3. Bowers, R. F.: Myositis Ossificans Traumatic. J. Bone Joint Surg., 19(1):215, 1937.
4. Buxton, J. D.: Ossification in the Ligaments of the Elbow. J. Bone Joint Surg., 20:709, 1938.
5. Campbell, W. C.: Arthroplasty of the Elbow. Ann Surg. 76:615, 1922.
6. Campbell, W. C.: Mobilization of Joints With Bony Ankylosis. J.A.M.A. 83:976, 1924.
7. Carroll, R. E., and Hill, N. A.: Triceps Transfer to Restore Elbow Flexion. J. Bone Joint Surg. 52A(2):239, 1970.
8. Deland, J. T., Walker, P. S., Sledge, C. B., and Farberov, A.: Treatment of Post-Traumatic Elbows With a New Hinge-Distractor. Orthopedics 6:732, 1983.
9. Dickson, R. A.: Reversed Dynamic Slings: A New Concept in the Treatment of Post-Traumatic Elbow Flexion Contractures. Injury 8:35, 1976.
10. Dietrich, S.L.: Rehabilation and Nonsurgical Management of Musculoskeletal Problems in the Hemophilic Patient. Ann. N.Y. Acad. Sci. 240:328, 1975.
11. Doyle, J. R., James, P. M., Larsen, L. J., and Ashley, R. K.: Restoration of Elbow Flexion in Arthrogryposis Multiplex Congenita. J. Hand Surg. 5:149, 1980.
12. Evans, E. B., Larson, D. L., and Yates, S.: Preservation and Restoration of Joint Function in Patients With Severe Burns. J.A.M.A. 204(10):91–96, June, 1968.
13. Evans, E. B., Larson, D. L., Abston, S., and Willis, B.: Prevention and Correction of Deformity Ater Burns. Surg. Clin. North Am., 50:1361, 1970.
13a. Ewald, F.: Reconstruction of the Elbow. In American Academy of Orthopedic Surgeons: Lectures. Atlanta, 1984.
14. Freehafter, A. A.: Flexion and Supination Deformities of the Elbow in Tetraplegics. Paraplegia 15:221, 1977–1978.
15. Garland, D. E. and O'Hollarin, R.M.: Fractures and Dislocations About the Elbow in the Head Injury Adult. Clin. Orthop., 168:38, 1982.
16. Glynn, J. J., and Niebauer, J. J.: Flexion and Extension Contractures of the Elbow. Clin Orthop. 117:289, 1976.
17. Goller, H., and Enders, M.: A Dynamic Plastic Elbow—Extension Orthosis for Reduction of Flexion and Contractures. Orthotics and Prosthetics, 30:44, 1976.
18. Green, D. P., and McCoy, H.; Turnbuckle Orthotic Correction of Elbow Flexion Contractures After Acute Injuries. J. Bone Joint Surg. 61A:1092, 1979.
18a. Gutierrez, L. S.: A Contribution to the Study of the Limiting Factors of Elbow Extension. Acta Anat. 56:146, 1964.
19. Hassmann, G. C., Brunn, F., and Neer, C. S.: Recurrent Dislocations of the Elbow. J. Bone Joint Surg. 57A:1080, 1975.
20. Hoffer, M. M., Brody, G., and Ferlic, F.: Excision of Heterotopic Ossification About Elbows in Patients With Thermal Injury. J. Trauma 18(9):667, 1978.
21. Holtmann, B., Wray, R. C., Lowrey, R., and Weeks, P.: Restoration of Elbow Flexion. Hand, 7(3):256, 1975.
22. Houston, C. S., Reed, M. H., and DeSautels, J. E.: Separating Larsen Syndrome from the "Arthrygryposis Basket." J. Can. Assoc. Radiol. 32(4):206, 1981.
23. Huang, T. T., Blackwell, S. J., and Lewis, S. R.: Ten Years of Experience in Managing Patients with Burn Contractures of Axilla, Elbow, Wrist, and Knee Joints. Plast. Recons. Surg. 61(1):70, 1978.
24. Jajic, I., and Rulnjevic, J.: Myositis Ossificans Localisata as a Complication of Tetanus. Acta Orthop. Scand. 50:547, 1979.
25. Johanson, O.: Capsular and Ligament Injuries of the Elbow Joint: Clinical and Arthrographic Study. Acta Chir. Scand Suppl. 287:124, 1962.
26. Jones, R.: Injuries to the Elbow Joint. Clin. J. 25:17, 1904.
27. Kalisman, M., Wexler, M. R., Yeschua, R., and Neuman, Z.: Comparison Between the Early Use of Skin Flap and Skin Graft for the Correction of Large Tissue Loss at the Elbow. Ann. Plast. Surg. 1(5):474, 1978.
27a. Kelikian, H.: Congenital Deformities of the Hand and Forearm. Philadelphia, W.B. Saunders, 1974.
28. Landra, A. P.: The Latissimus Dorsi Musculocutaneous Flap Used to Resurface a Defect on the Upper Arm and Restore Extension to the Elbow. Br. J. Plast. Surg. 32(4):275, 1979.
29. Linscheid, R. L., and Wheeler, D. K.: Elbow Dislocations. J.A.M.A. 194:1171, 1965.
30. Lusskin, R., Grynbaum, B. B., and Dhir, R. S.: Rehabilitation Surgery in Adult Spastic Hemiplegia. Clin. Orthorp. 63:132, 1969.
31. Mardam-Bey, T., and Ger, E.: Congenital Radial Head Dislocation. J. Hand Surg. 4(4):316, 1979.
32. McMaster, W. C., Tivnon, M. C., and Waugh, T. R.: Cast Brace for the Upper Extremity. Clin. Orthop. 109:126, 1975.
33. Mendelson, L., Grosswassner, Z., Najenson, T., Sandbank, U., and Solzi, P.: Periarticular New Bone Formation in Patients Suffering From Severe Head Injuries. Scand. J. Rehab. Med. 7:141, 1975–1976.
34. Meyn, M., and Ruby, L.: Arthrogryposis of the Upper Extremity. Orthop. Clin. North Am. 7(2):501, 176.
35. Millard, D. R., Jr. and Ortiz, A. C.: Correction of Severe Elbow Contractures. J. Bone Joint Surg. 47A(7):1347, 1965.
36. Mirise, R. T., and Shear, S.: Congenital Contractual Arachnodactyly. Arth. Rheum. 22(5):542, 1979.
37. Mital, M. A.: Lengthening of the Elbow Flexors in Cerebral Palsy. J. Bone Joint Surg. 61A:516, 1979.
37. Mital, M. A.: Lengthening of the Elbow Flexors in Cerebral Palsy. J. Bone Joint Surg. 61A:516, 1979.
37a. Moberg, E.: Upper Limb Tetraplegia. A New Approach to Surgical Rehabilitation. Stuttgart, Georg Theime, 1978.
38. Mohan, K.: Myositis Ossificans Traumatica of the Elbow. Int. Surg. 57(6):475, 1972.
39. Morrey, B. F., Askew, L. J., and An, K. N.: Biomechanical Study of Normal Elbow Motion. J. Bone Joint Surg. 63A:872, 1981.

39a. Morrey, B. F., and An, K. N.: Articular and Ligamentous Contributions to the Stability of the Elbow Joint. Am. J. Sports Med. 11:315, 1983.

39b. Morrey, B. F., and An, K. N.: Functional Anatomy of the Ligaments of the Elbow. COKR, in press.

40. Nagano, A., Kurokawa, T., Tachibana, S., and Tsuyama, N.: Meiten's Syndrome. Arch. Orthop. Unfallchir. 89(1):81, 1977.

41. Newton, D. R. L.: The Management of Non-Articular Rheumatism. Practitioner 8:64, 1972.

41a. Norwood, L. A., Shook, J. A., and Andrews, J. R.: Acute Medial Elbow Ruptures. Am. J. Sports Med. 9:16, 1981.

42. Oh, I., Smith, J. A., Spencer, G. E., Jr., Frankel, V. H., and Mack, R. P.: Fibrous Contracture of Muscles Following Intramuscular Injections in Adults. Clin. Orthop., 127:214, 1977.

43. Roberts, P. H.: Dislocation of the Elbow. Br. J. Surg. 56(11):806, 1969.

44. Shahriaree, H., Sajadi, K., Silver, C. M., and Sheikholeslamzadeh, S.: Excisional Arthroplasty of the Elbow. J. Bone Joint Surg. 61A(6):922, 1977.

45. Sheldon, W.: Amoplasia Congenita. Arth. Dis. Child. 7:117, 1932.

46. Sherk, H. H.: Treatment of Severe Rigid Contractures of Cerebral Palsied Upper Limbs. Clin. Orthop. 125:151, 1977.

47. Silva, J. F.: The Problems Relating to Old Dislocations and the Restriction on the Elbow Movement. Acta Orthop. Belg. 41(4):399, 1975.

48. Smith, F. M.: Surgery of the Elbow. Philadelphia, W. B. Saunders Co., 1972.

49. Steindler, A.: Arthrogryposis. J. Int. Coll. Surg. 12:21, 1949.

50. Stern, P.: Latissimus Dorsi Musculocutaneous Flap for Elbow Flexion. J. Hand Surg. 7:25, 1982.

51. Thompson, H. C., and Garcia, A.: Myositis Ossificans: Aftermath of Elbow Injuries. Clin. Orthop. 50:129, 1967.

52. Thorndike, A., Jr.: Myositis Ossificans Traumatica. J. Bone Joint Surg. 2(2):315, 1940.

53. Trigueros, A. P., Vazquez, V., and DeMiguel, G. F.: Larsen's Syndrome. Report of Three Cases in the One Family, Mother and Two Offspring. Acta Orthop. Scand. 49(6):582, 1978.

54. Tucker, K.: Some Aspects of Post-Traumatic Elbow Stiffness. Injury 9:216, 1977.

55. Varma, B. P., and Chandra, U.: Bilateral Ankylosis of the Elbows in Extension Due to Contracture of the Triceps. Int. Surg. 52:337, 1969.

56. Varma, B. P.: Localized Myositis Ossificans Traumatica. Int. Surg., 49(4):452, 1968.

57. Vas, W., Cockshott, W. P., Martin, R. F., Pai, M. K., and Walker, I.: Myositis Ossificans in Hemophilia. Adv. Orthop. Surg. 7(1):11, 1983.

58. Volkov, M. V. and Oganesian, O. V.: Restoration of Function in the Knee and Elbow with a Hinge-Distractor Apparatus. J. Bone Joint Surg. 57A(5):591, 1975.

59. Watson-Jones, R., and Roberts, R. E.: Calcification, Decalcification and Ossification. Br. J. Surg. 21:461, 1933.

60. Weeks, P. M.: Surgical Correction of Upper Extremity Deformities in Arthrogrypotics. Plast. Reconst. Surg. 36(4):459, 1965.

61. Wheeler, D. K., and Linscheid, R. L.: Fracture-Dislocations of the Elbow. Clin. Orthop. 50:95, 1967.

62. Williams, P. F.: The Elbow in Arthrogryposis. J. Bone Joint Surg. 55B(4):834, 1973.

63. Wilson, P. D.: Capsulectomy for the Relief of Flexion Contractures of the Elbow. J. Bone Joint Surg. 267:1, 1944.

CHAPTER 25

Tendon Injuries About the Elbow

B. F. MORREY

Other than epicondylitis, injury to the muscles or tendons about the elbow as an isolated event is rather uncommon.[3, 9, 13, 25, 58] Distal biceps tendon avulsion from the radial tuberosity and detachment of the triceps from its insertion on the olecranon, although rare, are the two most common tendinous injuries in this region.

DISTAL BICEPS TENDON RUPTURE

Rupture of the distal biceps tendon is infrequent, but the correct diagnosis and appropriate treatment is essential to avoid significant disability.

Incidence

Avulsion at its distal insertion was reported in 3 of 100 patients with biceps tendon rupture studied by Gilcreest.[25] The European literature suggests that the distal avulsion injury accounts for 3 to 10 percent[27] of all biceps tendon ruptures. The rarity of the condition is exemplified by the fact that only 24 cases were reported in the 43-year period from the original descriptions by Johnson in 1897[31] and Acquaviva in 1898[1] to the survey by Dobbie in 1941.[17] Three hundred and fifty-five surgeons responded to a questionnaire and added only 51 cases. In addition, only three of this group had experience with as many as three cases. By 1956 the world's literature contained 152 reported cases.[23]

In spite of the uncommon nature of the injury, its typical features have allowed it to be well characterized. To date, we have not encountered a single case report in the English literature, nor have we personally experienced the injury occurring in a female. In addition, more than 80 percent of the reported cases have involved the right dominant upper extremity, usually in a well-developed male,[6, 48] who has an average age of about 50 years.[4, 17, 42] The youngest individual reported with this injury was 21,[48] and the oldest was 70[17] years of age.

Mechanism of Injury

In virtually every reported case,[5, 17, 42, 54] a single traumatic event, often of 40 kg or more against resistance with the elbow in about 90 degrees of flexion has been implicated. Preexisting degenerative changes in the tendon predispose to the rupture.[14, 15] Acute pain, as in the antecubital fossa, is noted immediately. Rarely, a patient will complain of a second episode of acute pain several days later. Such a history suggests the possibility of secondary failure of the lacertus fibrosus.[10] Forearm pain has been reported occasionally and has been experienced in one of our cases but is considered rather uncommon.

Presentation

Subjective Complaints

The common symptom of distal biceps tendon rupture is a sudden, sharp tearing-type pain followed by discomfort in the antecubital fossa or in the lower anterior aspect of the brachium. The intense pain usually subsides in several hours, but a dull ache persists for weeks. In fact, if surgical repair is not performed, chronic pain with activity is common in the antecubital fossa and proximal forearm.[30] Flexion weakness is inevitably present but tends to decrease with time.[34] Loss of supination strength has been reported as the source of variable dysfunction, and diminution of grip strength has been recognized as well.[34, 42]

Objective Findings

Ecchymosis is present in the antecubital fossa[17, 47] and occasionally over the proximal ulnar aspect of the elbow joint.[6] With elbow flexion the muscle contracts proximally, and

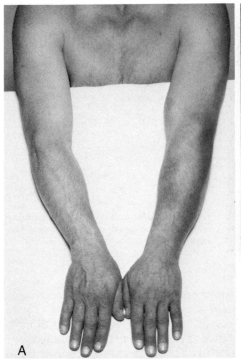

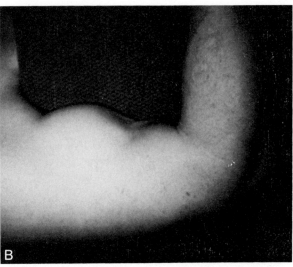

Figure 25–1. The left forearm ecchymosis is vaguely seen in this patient, who presented 10 days after injury (A). However, the proximal retraction of the biceps muscle is obvious and should allow the diagnosis to be readily made (B).

a visible, palpable defect of the distal biceps muscle is obvious (Fig. 25–1). This finding alone is not diagnostic because a similar diagnosis may be suggested by a space-occupying lesion such as lipoma or fibrosis of the biceps muscle.[21] Hence, assessment of strength alteration is essential to substantiate the diagnosis. Local tenderness is present in the antecubital fossa. The defect may be palpable, but if not, and symptoms are otherwise consistent with the diagnosis, a partial rupture may have occurred. Motion is not altered except possibly that due to pain at the extremes of flexion, extension, and supination. Flexion weakness is usually detectable by routine clinical examination. The loss of strength may be profound,[17] especially immediately after injury. Curiously, near-normal flexion strength has been claimed to return occasionally when not treated.[29] Loss of supination function is more variably altered,[46] being reported by some to be minimally affected[16] but is often not even mentioned in the report.[34, 47, 55] Interestingly, loss of grip strength has been noted in one of the instances reported by Lee[34] and was also evident in 1 of the 10 patients evaluated by us.[42]

Roentgenographic Changes

The etiology of the injury has been discussed by several authors and is considered in detail by Davis and Yassine.[14] Degeneration of the biceps tendon found at the time of surgery[17, 29, 48] is consistent with the roentgenographic changes that are often observed on the volar aspect of the radial tuberosity (Fig. 25–2). During pronation and supination, inflammation and subsequent attenuation of the biceps tendon are initiated by irritation from the irregularity of the radial tuberosity (Fig. 25–3).

Surgical Findings

If explored early, local hemorrhage is present in the antecubital space but usually is not extensive. The tendon is found to lie loosely curled in the antecubital fossa. Invariably, the tendon has been observed to separate cleanly from the radial tuberosity,[6, 17, 34, 38, 42, 47] supporting the hypothesis and observation of Davis and of Chevallier that the underlying pathology is degeneration occurring at the site of attachment.[10, 14] The lacertus fibrosus may be attenuated but is not always completely torn. After several months, the tendon has usually retracted into the substance of the biceps muscle, making retrieval and reattachment impossible. In this instance, the lacertus fibrosus is usually torn and retracted. We have noted attenuation or a tear in continuity of the biceps tendon in one instance. Disruption of the musculotendinous junction has also been reported by Steindler.[56] Usually, however, because this injury and the tear in con-

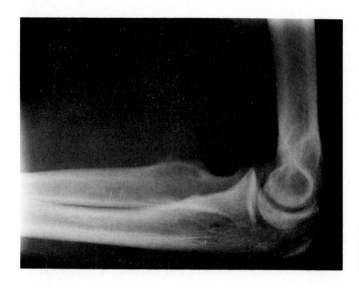

Figure 25–2. Irregularity of the biceps tuberosity is frequently observed, suggesting that a degenerative process may be implicated, at least in part, in the etiology of this condition.

tinuity are not considered surgical lesions, frequency of such pathology is difficult to ascertain.

Treatment

Acute Disruption

The literature suggests that some latitude may be permissible in the treatment of this entity in the acute stage. Nonoperative management has been reported to provide satisfactory results in approximately 50 per cent of cases,[29] although this author did not recommend nonoperative treatment. For complete ruptures, the functional superiority of surgical treatment is obvious when the results of cases treated with and without surgical intervention are reviewed.[42] With a partial rupture there is

less functional loss, and hence operative management may not be necessary.

Thus, although there is little question about the cause of the injury, there is considerable uncertainty about the specific procedure to be followed for its repair. After reviewing 51 cases reported by 41 of 355 surgeons responding to his questionnaire, Dobbie recommends against anatomic reattachment.[17] This conclusion is supported by others.[22, 33, 48, 54] The rationale for this recommendation rests on the impression that a universally good result is attained by inserting the tendon into the brachialis muscle, thus avoiding the risk of injuring the radial nerve during reimplantation—"[because] . . . the biceps is not essential for forearm supination . . . reattachment of the radial tuberosity is not essential."[33]

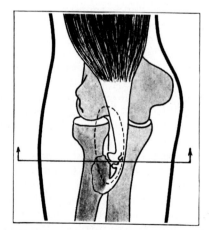
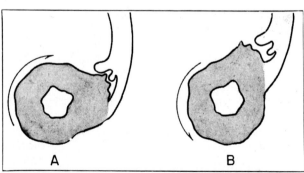

Figure 25–3. Illustration showing the pathophysiology of distal biceps rupture. Hypertrophic changes at the radiotuberosity cause irritation of the tendon, thus predisposing this structure to undergo degenerative changes and rupture during pronation and supination. (From Davis, W. M., and Yassine, Z.: An etiologic factor in the tear of the distal tendon of the biceps brachii. J. Bone Joint Surg. 38A:1368, 1956.)

Table 25–1. **Strength of Various Functions After Different Treatments for Distal Biceps Tendon Rupture**

Treatment (No. of Patients)	Follow-Up per Month	Strength (Percent)[a]				
		Flexion	Extension	Pronation	Supination	Grip
None (2)	15	61	100	93	63	86
Reattachment early (2)	17	97	117	99	95	114
Reattachment late (1)	36	85	74	94	64	77
Insertion into brachialis (1)	20	87	105	113	43	100

[a]Percent difference from opposite extremity, corrected for effect of the dominant side.

Most investigators do not share this opinion. Reattachment to the radius by any one of several techniques[4, 6, 29, 32, 47] is considered the treatment of choice. The specific technique varies widely from direct reimplantation[6, 29, 42, 47] to inserting a loop of fascia graft about the proximal radius.[32] The difficulty of the exposure needed to avoid nerve injury has prompted the development of a second incision placed over the dorsal aspect of the forearm.[8] Curiously, this technique appears to have been first employed in 1937 by Plummer to reattach the biceps tendon to the proximal ulna.[17] Our experience strongly suggests that immediate reattachment of the radial tuberosity is the treatment of choice for this condition. If done early, the tract of the biceps tendon is still present and is easily identified. If performed late (more than 2 weeks after injury), this tract may be obliterated, making the exposure more difficult.[28] Thus, the optimum treatment of direct reattachment into the radial tuberosity has been recommended by Baker in a recent review of 14 cases and has been and probably is the most commonly performed procedure.[21, 29, 34, 50]

Results

Questionnaire data have reported 97.8 percent excellent or good results with surgery.[17] Accurate objective reports of functional capability are, however, lacking. Among those recommending insertion into the brachialis, the result of "full function of the forearm,"[33] including adequate supination,[17, 48] has been reported. Such comments must, however, be carefully considered. The restoration of normal or near-normal supination strength without anatomic reinsertion of the biceps tendon is incomprehensible. The result may be surprisingly good, but it is *not normal*. We have conducted strength assessment tests on seven patients at least 15 months after treatment using a technique that has been demonstrated to be reliable and reproducible in previous

clinical studies.[42] The results are depicted in Table 25–1. Nontreated distal biceps rupture results in a loss of about 40 percent of both flexion and supination strength (Fig. 25–4A). Attachment into the brachialis or late reattachment may improve function but does not make it normal. Immediate reattachment into the radial tuberosity can provide near-normal strength in both flexion and supination (Fig. 25–4B). Based on this experience, the treatment of choice is clearly immediate reattachment to the tuberosity.

Complications

There are no individual reports of complications of surgical treatment of distal biceps tendon rupture in the English literature. Transient radial nerve palsy with reattachment to the tuberosity has been occasionally noted.[17, 40] As mentioned above, reattachment to the tuberosity is avoided by some to prevent injury to the nerve. Ectopic bone (Fig. 25–5A) has been reported in one instance,[17] and we have treated another such case in which there was proximal radioulnar synostosis.[42] This occurred after the two-incision technique in both cases. After excision (Fig. 25–5B), near-normal return of flexion strength as well as supination strength and motion followed (Fig. 25–5C.)

Author's Preferred Treatment Method

If the diagnosis of disruption of the distal biceps tendon is made within the first 7 to 10 days, reattachment to the radial tuberosity using the two-incision technique is recommended. The procedure is as follows:

With the patient in the supine position, the extremity is prepared and draped in the usual fashion. A sterile tourniquet is applied to the arm but is removed if greater exposure is necessary. An anterior lateral incision is begun over the distal aspect of the brachium and turned transversely in the antecubital fossa (Fig. 25–6A.) The dissection is carried

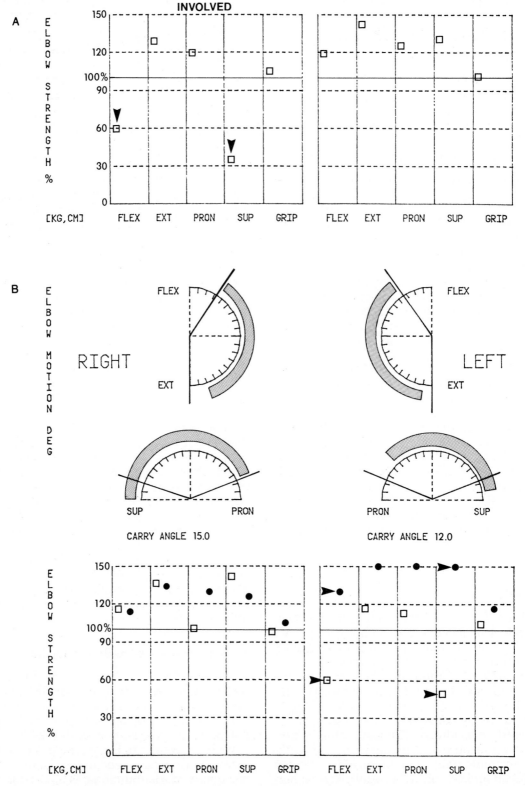

Figure 25–4. *A,* Biomechanical evaluation form of an individual 8 months after injury without undergoing repair. It is noted that a loss of approximately 50 percent in flexion and supination strength has occurred (arrows). The 100 percent reference line relates to 100 normal subjects. *B,* This individual was evaluated 1 year after reattachment of the biceps to the radial tuberosity. The profound weakness that was present on the left preoperatively (open squares) has been restored to normal (solid dots) with the reattachment. Arcs of motion and two normal studies of the right side are included.

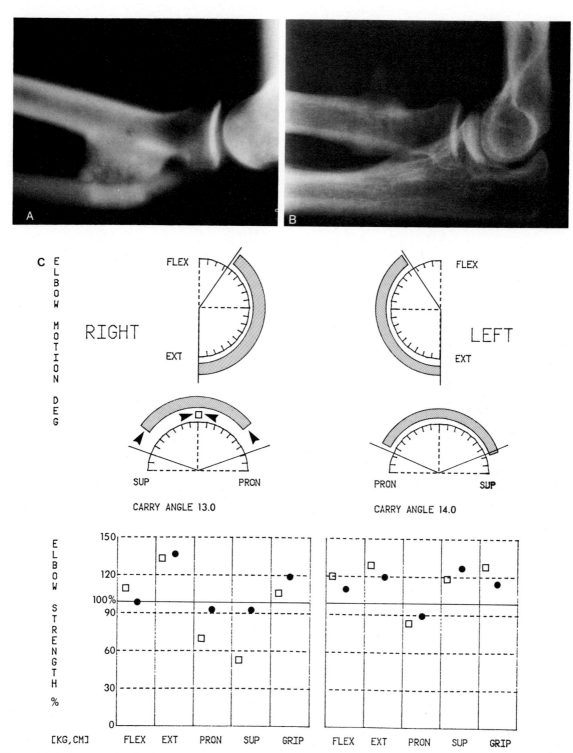

Figure 25–5. *A,* Proximal radioulnar synostosis resulted from reattachment of an avulsed right biceps tendon to the radial tuberosity using the two-incision technique of Boyd and Anderson. *B,* Three months after removal, the radioulnar synostosis has not recurred. Computer printout of functional examination shows the patient had improved pronation and supination strength by 20 to 40 percent, and the arc of motion had improved from 5 degrees to 50 degrees pronation and 60 degrees supination (C).

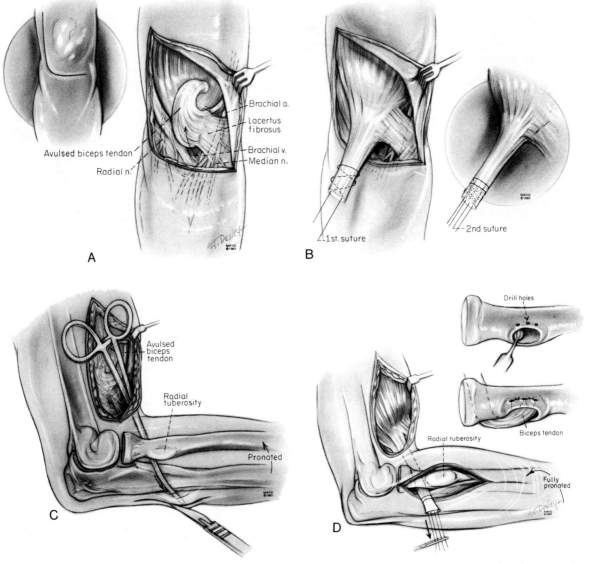

Figure 25–6. *A,* The proximal portion of a Henry incision is used to expose the antecubital space proximally. The retracted biceps tendon is identified, taking care to avoid injury to the brachial artery and median and radial nerves and their branches. *B,* Two Bunnel sutures are placed in the end of the tendon. *C,* A blunt instrument is introduced in the tract of the biceps tendon, and the skin is indented on the volar aspect of the proximal forearm. An incision is made over this instrument, exposing the radial tuberosity, which comes into view with full pronation in the forearm. *D,* The radial tuberosity is excavated using a high-speed bur. The biceps tendon is then brought through its previous tract and reinserted into the radial tuberosity.

through the subcutaneous tissue, exposing the hematoma, which is evacuated. The biceps muscle with the tendon is readily observed. The tendon is inspected and is found invariably to have avulsed cleanly from the radial tuberosity; it is then retracted. The distal end of the torn biceps tendon is minimally debrided, and two nonabsorbable Bunnell sutures are placed in the torn tendon (Fig. 25–6B). A blunt, curved hemostat is carefully inserted into the space previously occupied by the biceps tendon so that the tip of the

instrument may be palpated on the dorsal aspect of the proximal forearm between the ulna and radius (Fig. 25–6C). A second incision is made over the instrument, exposing the proximal ulna and radial tuberosity. The forearm is then maximally pronated, and a highspeed bur is used to evacuate a 5- to 7-mm defect in the radial tuberosity (Fig. 25–6D.) Three holes are then placed through this window to the opposite side of the tuberosity. The sutures are delivered through the second incision and placed through the holes in the tuberosity. The tendon is carefully introduced into the window formed in the tuberosity, and the sutures are pulled tight and secured. The wounds are closed in layers with a suction drain inserted in the depths of the wound both anteriorly and posteriorly. The elbow is placed in 90 degrees of flexion and in full supination, and a compressive dressing is applied.

Postoperative Care

The drains are removed within 24 hours and the surgical dressing at 4 to 5 days. The elbow is maintained in 90 degrees of flexion using a static splint for an additional 3 weeks. A hinged orthoplast splint is then applied with a dynamic flexion component that provides for passive flexion. Active extension is allowed and encouraged (Fig. 25–7). The use of this splint is continued for 4 to 6 weeks. Approximately 10 weeks after surgery, if flexion strength has returned to near normal, as determined clinically or by biomechanical functional strength assessment, the splint is discarded, and gradual resumption of normal activity is encouraged. Full activity is not recommended for 6 months after the surgical repair.

Late Reconstruction

The individual needs of the patient as well as the goals of any late surgical procedure must be carefully balanced. If the patient's occupation and residual strength do not re-

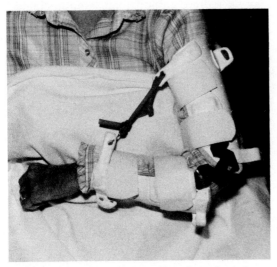

Figure 25–7. A dynamic flexion splint allows the patient to begin motion at approximately 3 to 4 weeks. Active extension and passive flexion protect the repair.

quire improvement of supination strength, simple reinsertion into the brachialis muscle is recommended. This surgical procedure is easy, improves flexion strength, and is essentially free of complications. Postoperative rehabilitation is similar to that previously described except that no limitation is placed on pronation and supination in the early postoperative course. If, after careful discussion with the patient, improved supination strength is found to be required, then a fascia lata graft as described by Hovelius and Josefsson might be considered.[29]

RUPTURE OF THE TRICEPS TENDON

Incidence

Tendinous rupture is a more common injury in the upper extremity than in the lower. Anzel et al. reported that 85 percent of the 1015 tendon injuries treated at the Mayo Clinic involved the upper extremity.[3] Of this group of 856, only 8 instances of triceps injury were reported, and 4 of these were due to laceration. These data support the clinical observation of others that injury to the triceps tendon is the most rare or among the most rare of tendon ruptures.[13, 58] Since the first report of Partridge in 1868,[45] fewer than 30 instances have been recorded in the English literature. The injury occurs two to three times more commonly in males. A wide range of patient age has been reported, with a mean of 33 years (range, 7 to 67).

Mechanism of Injury

Rupture of the triceps tendon may occur either spontaneously or after trauma. Two types of traumatic episodes may be implicated. The most common event is a deceleration force imparted to the arm during extension as the triceps muscle is contracting. This usually occurs during a fall, but avulsion has been reported due to simple, uncoordinated triceps muscle contraction against a flexing elbow.[38] A direct blow to the posterior aspect of the triceps at its insertion in varying positions has also been reported in several instances[2, 46, 59] but is probably an uncommon mechanism of injury. Disruption of the triceps may also occur spontaneously with minimal trauma in individuals who are compromised by a systemic disease process.[49] Tendon ruptures in general have become increasingly recognized in association with renal osteodystrophy and secondary hyperparathyroid-

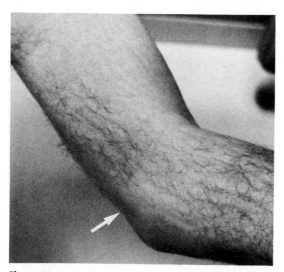

Figure 25–8. On gross examination of the lateral aspect of the elbow, a depression just proximal to the olecranon is noted (arrow) that demonstrates proximal retraction of the triceps. (From Farrar, E. L., and Lippert, F. G.: Avulsion of the triceps tendon. Clin. Orthop. 161:240, 1981.)

Diagnosis

Either complete or partial tears of the tendon may occur, but the latter is much less common.[19, 57] The history is commonly that of a fall on the outstretched hand. Swelling and pain are nonspecific but obvious early findings; ecchymosis appears after a couple of days. A palpable defect is present in some instances, depending on the extent of triceps retraction (Fig. 25–8). Some loss of extension power is universally observed. If no active elbow extension is present, a complete rupture has occurred. The roentgenogram is of considerable benefit for diagnosis of this injury because in approximately 80 percent of the patients flecks of avulsed bone will be apparent on the lateral radiograph (Fig. 25–9).[19, 57]

Pathology

Experimentally, the substance of a normal tendon rarely ruptures. Three sites of failure have been demonstrated experimentally as well as clinically—the muscle belly, the musculotendinous junction, and at the osseous tendon insertion.[39] For this particular injury, the failure has almost universally occurred at the site of insertion, although failure at the musculotendinous junction has occasionally been reported.[21, 41] Thus, a more proper designation of this injury might be triceps avulsion rather than triceps rupture.

Associated injuries have also been reported. Several instances of fracture of the radial head have been noted,[44, 49] and a recent report of six such injuries suggests that the association may be more common than is appreciated.[36] We have not diagnosed this combination in

ism[12, 20, 43] and with Marfan's syndrome.[53] Ruptures have also been reported in association with steroid treatment for lupus erythematosus[59] and chronic acidosis,[43] and in individuals with osteogenesis imperfecta tarda.[37] Although the pathophysiology of this association has not been completely explained, an increased amount of elastic fibers in the tendons of patients with renal osteodystrophy undergoing dialysis has been reported.[43] Calcification due to the chronic hypercalcemia of secondary hyperparathyroidism may be yet another explanation for the associated tendon ruptures in this group of patients.[49]

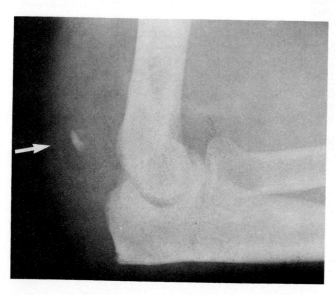

Figure 25–9. Radiograph of a patient with triceps rupture. Avulsed osseous fragments posterior and proximal to the olecranon are visualized in both the right and left arms. (From Farrar, E. L., and Lippert, F. G.: Avulsion of the triceps tendon. Clin. Orthop. 161:240, 1981.)

our practice. A single report of fracture of the wrist[35] along with fracture of the radial head supports the case for the mechanism of injury being a fall on the outstretched hand.

Treatment

Immediate surgery is the treatment of choice for complete rupture. At the time of exploration, the tendinous portion of the triceps is often found to be retracted within the muscle, a situation similar to that seen in rupture of the distal aspect of the biceps.[35, 49]

Several techniques may be employed, but reattachment with a nonabsorbable suture through drill holes placed in the olecranon or through a subperiosteal flap is quite effective in the acute injury. If the lesion has been overlooked or the treatment delayed by several months, the repair may need to be supplemented. Bennett has described reinforcing the repair with a 6- by 3-cm tongue of forearm fascia.[7] The attachment to the epicondylar region is maintained, and the flap is raised from distal to proximal and sutured to the distal triceps. Farrar and Lippert suggest that such a reinforcement may be beneficial in a patient with a systemic disease that compromises the quality of the tissue and, hence, the quality of the repair. After surgery, the arm is immobilized in less than 90 degrees of flexion for 3 weeks, and gentle active motion is begun.

Partial ruptures may be diagnosed by incomplete loss of extension and the close proximity of the osseous flecks of bone to the olecranon. This lesion can be treated without surgery but requires very close observation to ensure that no increase in fragment separation occurs.[19]

Results

The results of immediate or delayed repair have been universally good. In most instances normal strength and full motion have been restored. A loss of approximately 5 degrees of terminal extension has been noted in about 20 percent of patients and appears to be the only demonstrable residual of the injury. Surprisingly, good results have been observed with repair or reconstruction that has been delayed for up to a year.

Complications

There has not been a single complication reported to date after surgical repair of the avulsed or ruptured triceps tendon. Panta-

zopoulous et al. did observe olecranon bursitis, apparently secondary to the sutures in the proximal portion of the ulna,[44] but this was the source of minimal problems.

Author's Preferred Method of Treatment

Immediate repair with a posterior-based incision just lateral to the midline is the treatment of choice in our opinion. Number 0 nonabsorbable sutures are placed in Bunnell fashion in the torn tendon and then through holes in the proximal ulna. We have no experience with reinforcement using forearm fascia as recommended by Bennett,[7] but this could be considered to obtain a solid repair if the tissue appears to be of inadequate quality.

SNAPPING TRICEPS TENDON

The perception of a snapping elbow may sometimes be localized posteriorly and medially. The cause of such symptoms may be due to a subluxing ulnar nerve[11] or to dislocation of a portion of the triceps mechanism. An anomalous slip of the triceps tendon may cause these symptoms, but the most common etiology is subluxation of the medial head of the triceps over the medial epicondyle, usually occurring spontaneously in the second decade of life.[18, 51]

A common associated finding with this condition is chronic irritation of the ulnar nerve causing an ulnar neuritis.[18, 51] Other than this

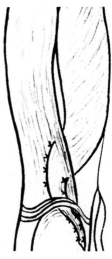

Figure 25–10. The most common cause of snapping elbow is dislocation of the medial head of the triceps, which subluxes over the medial epicondyle. (From Dryfuss, U.: Snapping elbow due to dislocation of the medial head of the triceps. J. Bone Joint Surg. 60B:57, 1978.)

feature, however, the snapping is generally well tolerated. Until more cases are reported, the etiology of the problem will remain unclear.

Treatment consists of detaching and rerouting the offending portion from the medial attachment under the triceps mechanism to its lateral attachment (Fig. 25–10). Of the three reported cases, recurrence has developed in one. Management of the ulnar nerve symptoms depends on the stability of the ulnar nerve and its particular status at the time of surgery.

RUPTURE OF THE BRACHIALIS MUSCLE

A single case report describes rupture of the brachialis muscle at the musculotendinous junction following direct trauma to the muscle.[26] Diagnosis was made by demonstrating a palpable defect at the musculotendinous junction. Treatment by direct suture was reported as successful.[26]

References

1. Acquaviva: Rupture du Tendon Inferieur du Biceps Brachial Droit a son Insertion sur la Tuberosite Bicipitale. Tenosuture Succes Operatoire. Marseilles Med. 35:570, 1898.
2. Anderson, K. J., and LeCoco, J. F.: Rupture of the Triceps Tendon. J. Bone Joint Surg. 39A(2):44, 1957.
3. Anzel, S. H., Covey, K. W., Weiner, A. D., and Lipscomb, P. R.: Disruption of Muscles and Tendons. An Analysis of 1,014 Cases. Surgery, 45:406, 1959.
4. Baker, B. E.: Operative vs. Non-Operative Treatments of Disruption of the Distal Tendon of Biceps. Orthop. Rev. 11(10):71, 1982.
5. Bauman, B. S.: Triceps Tendon Rupture. J. Bone Joint Surg. 44A:741, 1962.
6. Bauman, G. I.: Rupture of the Biceps Tendon. J. Bone Joint Surg. 16:966, 1934.
7. Bennett, B. S.: Triceps Tendon Ruptures. J. Bone Joint Surg. 44A:741, 1961.
8. Boyd, H. B., and Anderson, M. D.: A Method for Reinsertion of the Distal Biceps Brachii Tendon. J. Bone Joint Surg. 43A:1041, 1961.
9. Brickner, W. M., and Milch, H.: Ruptures of Muscles and Tendons. Int. Clin. 2:94, 1928.
10. Chevallier, C. H.: Sur un Cas de Desinsertion du Tendon Bicipital Inferieur. Mem. Acad. Chir. 79:137, 1953.
11. Childress, H. M.: Recurrent Ulnar-Nerve Dislocation at the Elbow. Clin. Orthop. 108:168, 1975.
12. Cirincione, R. J., and Baker, B. E.: Tendon Ruptures With Secondary Hyperparathyroidism. A Case Report. J. Bone Joint Surg. 57A:852, 1975.
13. Conwell, H. E., and Alldredge, R. H.: Ruptures and Tears of Muscles and Tendons. Am. J. Surg. 35(1):22, 1937.
14. Davis, W. M., and Yassine, Z.: An Etiologic Factor in the Tear of the Distal Tendon of the Biceps Brachii. J. Bone Joint Surg. 38A:1368, 1956.
15. Debeyre, J.: Desinsertion du Tendon Inferieur du Biceps Brachial. Mem. Acad. Chir. 74:339, 1948.
16. Delarue, J., and Denoix, P.: L'Alteration Degenerative des Tendons. Cause de Rupture—Amorce de Tumeurs. Presse Med. 54:869, 1946.
17. Dobbie, R. P.: Avulsion of the Lower Biceps Brachii Tendon. Analysis of Fifty-One Previously Reported Cases. Am. J. Surg. 51:661, 1941.
18. Dreyfuss, U.: Snapping Elbow Due to Dislocation of the Medial Head of the Triceps. J. Bone Joint Surg. 60B:57, 1978.
19. Farrar, E. L., III, and Lippert, F. G., III: Avulsion of the Triceps Tendon. Clin. Orthop. 161:242, 1981.
20. Fery, A., Sommelet, J., Schmitt, D., and Lipp, B.: Avulsion Bilaterale Simultanee des Tendons Quadricipital et Rotulien et Rupture du Tendon Tricipital Chez un Hemodialyse Hyperparathyroidien. Rev. Chir. Orthop. 64:175, 1978.
21. Gilcreest, E. L.: Rupture of Muscles and Tendons. J.A.M.A. 84:1819, 1925.
22. Gimbal, T., and Genteir, R.: Traumatic Disinsertion of the Lower Tendon of the Brachial Biceps. Surg. Gynecol. Obstet. 51:505, 1930.
23. Giugaro, A., and Proscia, N.: Le Rotture del Tendine Distale e del Tendine del Capo Breve del Bicipite Brachiale. Min. Orthop. 8:57, 1957.
24. Granato, F., and Marcacci, G.: Su Tre Casi di Lacerazione Traumatic della Inserzione Distale del Bicipite Brachiale. Clin. Orthop. 9:254, 1957.
25. Haldeman, K. O., and Soto-Hall, R.: Injuries to Muscles and Tendons. J.A.M.A. 104(26):2319, 1935.
26. Hamilton, A. T.: Subcutaneous Rupture of the Brachioradialis Muscle. Surgery 23:806, 1948.
27. Hempel, K., and Schwenke K.: Über Abrisse der Distalen Bizepssehne. Arch. Orthop. Unfallchir. 79:313, 1974.
28. Hook, F. R., and Mazet, R., Jr.: Avulsion of the Biceps Tendon from Its Radial Insertion. U.S. Nav. Med. Bull. 40:409, 1942.
29. Hovelius, L., and Josefsson, G.: Rupture of the Distal Biceps Tendon. Acta Orthop. Scand. 48:280, 1977.
30. Jaslow, I. A., and May, V. R.: Avulsion of the Distal Tendon of the Biceps Brachii Muscle. Guthrie Clin. Bull. 15:124, 1946.
31. Johnson, A. B.: Avulsion of Biceps Tendon From the Radius. N.Y. Med. J. 66:261, 1897.
32. Kalnberzs, W. K., and Veisman, J. A.: Zur Röntgendiagnostik und Operativebehandlung Geschlossener Verletzungen der Distalen Bizepsschne. Z. Orthop. 113:956, 1975.
33. Kron, S. D., and Satinsky, V. P.: Avulsion of the Distal Biceps Brachii Tendon. Am. J. Surg. 88:657, 1954.
34. Lee, H. G.: Traumatic Avulsion of Tendon of Insertion of Biceps Brachii. Am. J. Surg. 82:290, 1951.
35. Lee, M. L. H.: Rupture of Triceps Tendon. Br. Med. J. 2:197, 1960.
36. Levy, M., Fishel, R. E., and Stern, G. M.: Triceps Tendon Avulsion With or Without Fracture of the Radial Head—A Rare Injury? J. Trauma 18:677, 1978.
37. Match, R. M., and Corrylos, E. V.: Bilateral Avulsion Fracture of the Triceps Tendon Insertion from Skiing with Osteogenesis Imperfecta Tarda. Am. J. Sports Med. 11:99, 1983.
38. Maydl, K.: Ueber Subcutane Muskel und Sehnenzerreissungen, sowie Riss-Fracturen mit Berucksichtigung der Analogen, durch Directe Gewalt Enstandenen und Offenen Verletzungen. Deut. Zschr. Chir. 17:306, 1882, 18:35, 1883.
39. McMaster, P. E.: Tendon and Muscle Ruptures. Clinical and Experimental Studies on Causes and Loca-

tions of Subcutaneous Ruptures. J. Bone Joint Surg. **15**:705, 1933.

40. Meherin, J. H., and Kilgore, B. S., Jr.: The Treatment of Rupture of the Distal Biceps Brachii Tendon. Am. J. Surg. **99**:636, 1960.

41. Montgomery, A. H.: Two Cases of Muscle Injury. Surg. Clin. Chic., **4**:871, 1920.

42. Morrey, B. F., Askew, L. J., An, K. H., and Dobyns, J. H.: Rupture of the Distal Biceps Tendon: Biomechanical Assessment of Different Treatment Options. Submitted for publication, J. Bone Joint Surg. (In press, 1984.)

43. Murphy, K. J., and McPhee, I.: Tears of Major Tendons in Chronic Acidosis with Elastosis. J. Bone Joint Surg. **47A**:1253, 1965.

44. Pantazopoulos, T., Exarchou, E., Stavrou, Z., and Hartofilakidis-Garofalidis, G.: Avulsion of the Triceps Tendon. J. Trauma **15**:827, 1975.

45. Partridge: A Case Report of Rupture of the Triceps Cubiti. Med. Times and Gaz. **1**:175, 1868.

46. Penhallow, D. P.: Report of a Case of Ruptured Triceps due to Direct Violence. N.Y. Med. J. **91**:76, 1910.

47. Platt, H.: Observations of Some Tendon Ruptures. Br. Med. J. **1**:611, 1931.

48. Postacchini, F., and Puddu, G.: Subcutaneous Rupture of the Distal Biceps Brachii Tendon. J. Sports Med. **15(2)**:81, 1975.

49. Preston, F. S., and Adicoff, A.: Hyperparathyroidism with Avulsion at Three Major Tendons. N. Engl. J. Med. **266**:968, 1961.

50. Rogers, S. P.: Avulsion of Tendon of Attachment of Biceps Brachii. J. Bone Joint Surg. **21:1**:197, 1939.

51. Rolfsen, L.: Snapping Triceps Tendon with Ulnar Neuritis. Acta Orthop. Scand. **41**:74, 1970.

52. Schlossbach, T.: Avulsion of the Lower Biceps Brachii Tendon. J. Med. Soc. N.J. **47(4)**:166, 1950.

53. Schutt, R. C., Powell, R. L., and Winter, W. G.: Spontaneous Ruptures of Large Tendons. American Academy of Orthopedic Surgeons Annual Meeting, New Orleans, January 25, 1982.

54. Seneque, J., and Berthe, R.: Ruptures et Desinsertions du Tendon Distal du Biceps Brachial. J. Chir. **46**:347–354, 1935.

55. Sonnenschein, H. D.: Rupture of the Biceps Tendon. J. Bone Joint Surg. **14**:416, 1932.

56. Steindler, D.: Traumatic Deformities of the Upper Extremities. Springfield, Ill., Charles C Thomas, 1946.

57. Tarsney, F. F.: Rupture and Avulsion of the Triceps. Clin. Orthop. **83**:177, 1972.

58. Waugh, R. L., Hathcock, T. A., and Elliott, J. L.: Ruptures of Muscle and Tendons. Surgery **25**:370, 1949.

59. Wener, J. A., and Schein, A. J.: Simultaneous Bilateral Rupture of the Patello Tendon and Quadriceps Expansions in Systemic Lupus Erythematosus. A Case Report. J. Bone Joint Surg. **56A**:823, 1974.

60. Witvoet, J., Robin, B., and Charbrol, J.: A Propos d'une Desinsertion de l'Extremite Inferieur du Biceps Brachial. Presse Med. **74**:389, 1966.

CHAPTER 26

Ectopic Ossification About the Elbow

MARK B. COVENTRY

Three terms are used more or less interchangeably when one speaks of bone forming around a joint or, indeed, even in muscle distant from a joint. The term *ectopic* bone is derived from the Latin meaning "out (of) place," *heterotopic* means "other or different place," and *myositis ossificans* means "ossified inflammatory muscle." *Ectopic* bone and *heterotopic* bone have a similar connotation, and for the purposes of this chapter, the term *ectopic bone* (EB) will be used. Myositis ossificans connotes a different situation, usually bone formation in the muscle itself, and is found most commonly after an injury in which a severe contusion to the thigh muscles occurs or after a fracture-dislocation of the elbow.[25] In addition, the term is commonly used to describe patients who have formed massive periarticular EB following an injury to the central nervous system.

One must be aware of the distinction between "calcification" and bone. Calcific deposits do occur in tendons, articular cartilage, synovium, and articular capsule, and consist of calcium pyrophosphates for the most part. The appearance is amorphous. Calcifications are more circumscribed than ossifications. They are usually globular, although they can be linear. They have no trabecular structure, however, and this is their main distinguishing feature. They should always be distinguished from bone itself, and this can easily be done by a critical review of the roentgenogram.

Ectopic bone passes through a formative cycle. Radiographically, it is seldom seen before 3 weeks after injury (or surgery). At this time, it can usually be detected if one looks critically for it. The soft density on the roentgenogram must be visualized under a bright light. In a study of 224 consecutive total hip arthroplasties,[11] we could detect by roentgenogram, in retrospect, 89 percent of all EB formation at 3 weeks. By 6 weeks, all formation was obvious, and no additional bone was seen to develop after 8 weeks. The bone matures further after this and will show increased density and increased trabecular pattern, but its total volume is usually complete by 8 weeks from the time of inception. Early detection by measurement of the alkaline phosphatase serum levels has not proved helpful. Detection by technetium scanning, however, is showing some promise. In a preliminary study[26] we have found (with one exception) that we were able to demonstrate by technetium scanning 7 days after surgery the presence or absence of later visible EB. It appears likely that technetium scanning will allow detection of EB within a week after injury or surgery.

There are those who feel that inordinate pain, especially with motion, might be due in part to early EB formation, but no correlative studies have confirmed this. This opinion is an "impression," usually a retrospective one. What we do know, however, is that once EB has formed and matured, pain is not usually a problem. Restriction of motion is the subjective and objective finding. Our overall Harris hip score, which measures pain, motion, and daily activities for total hip arthroplasty, for example, was 89. But when EB was present it dropped to 73. This decrease was due almost entirely to diminished motion. The presence of EB about the elbow following fracture, dislocation, or both, or following surgical intervention will likewise impair an otherwise good result by limitation of motion. Unlike the hip, this limitation may be painful when it involves the elbow joint.

The reasons for formation of EB in certain individuals are still obscure. The hip joint forms EB after injury more frequently and to a greater degree than any other joint. In fact, almost 80 percent of patients show some soft tissue density after hip replacement, but only in 5 percent might it be classified as extensive.[16] It has been postulated that such densities occur because of the increased bulk of mesenchymal tissue about the hip. Primitive

464

mesenchymal cells are the progenitors of osteoblasts and osteocytes. What causes the primitive mesenchymal cell to differentiate into an osteocyte? We do know that differentiation is incited by injury, but beyond this there is a certain amount of conjecture. Craven and Urist, publishing their early research on rats, demonstrated a morphogenic movement of primitive mesenchymal cells to form osteoblasts.[4] This movement may be stimulated by bone morphogenic protein (BMP). In the rat this movement of cells in response to BMP takes place during an interval of 2 to 4 days after injury. Urist[25] thinks that the BMP is transferred from the host bone to the surrounding soft tisues, especially perivascular mesenchymal cell-types, which then differentiate into bone. Thus, the BMP might be transferred locally from the surrounding radius, ulna, and humerus in patients who are particularly susceptible. A systemic BMP level that increases the risk of heterotopic osteogenesis in the patient with central nervous system injury has also been postulated.[25] Whatever the specific inciting cause, certain patients seem to be more susceptible to developing the condition than others. In general, the development of EB cannot be diagnosed until it becomes visible on the roentgenogram (unless technetium scanning proves to be an earlier method of detection). Once EB is visible it continues to mature in both the amount of calcium deposition and the number and size of trabeculae. Yet the total volume probably does not increase after 6 to 8 weeks from the time of inciting injury.

What is the incidence of EB about the elbow? Statistics are few, and the lack of a common standard for classifying the appearance makes comparisons of limited value. The distribution of ectopic bone and calcification has been discussed by Broberg and Morrey (Fig. 26–1).[2] Thompson and Garcia reported

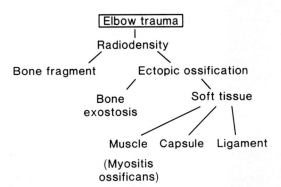

Figure 26–1. Distribution of possible roentgenographic densities about the elbow after trauma.

35 patients with EB in 447 dislocations.[24] Three hundred and eleven had dislocations without fracture, and among these only 11 developed EB. Their data also show that dislocation produces a five times greater chance of myositis than fracture alone and that young people are less prone to develop myositis after injury than older persons. It was also demonstrated that if patients are treated for fracture or dislocation early (i.e., within 24 hours), they develop less EB than if treated later.

This experience had been reported previously by McLaughlin, who related the development of ectopic ossification to delay in removing the radial head when fracture was complicated by dislocation.[14] If fracture reduction is accomplished early but mobilization is delayed beyond a week, an increase in the amount of ectopic bone is observed.[24] As would be expected, repeated manipulations of the elbow tend to increase the amount of EB.

Roberts reported 60 patients with dislocation of the elbow.[21] Twenty-three had accompanying fractures. In 28 patients with dislocations of the elbow without fracture who were followed by roentgenogram, some new bone formation in the capsule and collateral ligaments was seen in 12, but none showed motion limitation due to the EB. In an additional patient, EB was found in the brachialis muscle somewhat distant from the joint itself. Of the 15 patients sustaining dislocation and fracture involving the joint surfaces, roentgenograms showed EB in the brachialis muscle in two elbows. Linscheid and Wheeler reported four patients with EB in the anterior capsule of the elbow in 110 cases of dislocation, but no mention was made of whether or not there was an accompanying fracture.[12]

By far the largest experience with EB formation following trauma to the elbow has been reported from India.[15] Among 700 patients with stiff elbows due to trauma, usually dislocations or fracture-dislocations,[15] no bony injury could be demonstrated in almost one third of the patients. Two hundred and fifteen of these 700 cases were supracondylar fractures, but of the 215 only 12 developed EB. Yet two thirds of those with dislocations and fracture-dislocations developed EB. Massage is a common form of treatment by "bone setters" in India, and a relationship between the use of early massage after injury and the development of what the author termed *traumatic ossification*, (that is, ectopic bone) was established. In these studies the bone was seen in the triceps, biceps, and brachialis muscles, was more common anteriorly than posteriorly, and was found most commonly in the collateral ligament.

It has long been observed that EB (myositis ossificans, para-osteoarthropathy) occurs with high frequency in the spinal cord and in the head-injured patients.[22] Garland and O'Hollaron recently documented the incidence of fractures and dislocations about the elbow in the head-injured adult.[10] Five hundred and forty-eight patients admitted to the adult head trauma service at Rancho Los Amigos had a total of 18 fractures and dislocations about the elbow. When combined with a head injury, fractures and dislocations of the elbow showed an 89 percent incidence of EB. This is in contrast to a 5 percent incidence reported by Garland, a 3 percent incidence reported by Thompson and Garcia, and a 4 percent frequency reported by Broberg and Morrey[2] in patients with fracture-dislocations of the elbow without head injury. In the head-injured patient, ectopic ossification is not necessarily associated with spasticity or neurologic residuals, and the bone is usually found in the collateral ligaments. Supracondylar fractures, and elbow dislocations with or without fracture, developed the most significant amounts of new bone. The severity of the injury and the length of delay in treatment seemed to be the determining factors.

Thus, the incidence of EB about the elbow is relatively low (unless there is head or spinal cord injury), and the combination of disloca-tion and fracture is more likely to produce EB than dislocation alone. Early reduction infrequent manipulations, and early elbow motion will decrease the chance of EB formation. The younger the patient, the less EB is apt to occur.

PATHOLOGY

Ectopic bone about the elbow forms in both the ligaments and the capsule and only rarely in the muscle (Fig. 26–2).

The histology of EB reveals that it is similar to normal bone. It is similarly calcified, and the bone matrix-forming cells produce a highly organized bone containing secondary Haversian systems as evidence of bone remodeling. When bone from the iliac cortex of a normal 12-year-old boy is compared with a bony plaque from a patient with myositis ossificans progressiva, they appear alike (Fig. 26–3).

TREATMENT

Not all EB about the elbow requires treatment, but a severe handicap results if there is marked limitation of motion. To mobilize the elbow joint in these instances it is necessary to excise the EB. Thus, although the goal of treatment is to obtain better motion, just how much limitation of motion must exist before surgery is indicated is a moot question (Fig. 26–4).

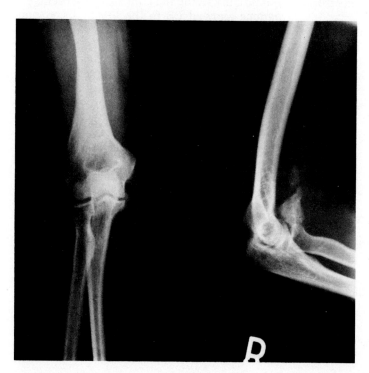

Figure 26–2. A 52-year-old woman suffered a posterior dislocation of the elbow. It was reduced within 12 hours, and active exercise started at 6 days. Two months following injury, there was mature-appearing ectopic bone, mostly anterior.

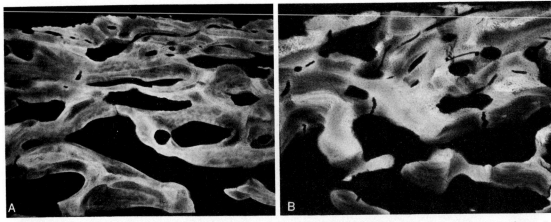

Figure 26–3. *A,* Iliac crest cortex of a 12-year-old boy shows well-organized trabecular pattern with resorption surfaces. *B,* A similar histologic appearance is demonstrated in this biopsy from a patient with myositis ossificans progressiva.

If surgery is considered, the timing of the procedure is probably important, but there are no definite guidelines. Traditionally, delay until the process has "matured"—usually at 9 to 12 months—is recommended. In our experience, the use of technetium-99 bone scans does not allow accurate interpretation of a "mature" process.

The association of a tardy ulnar palsy may be an additional indication for removal of EB if there is definite evidence of nerve involvement.

PROPHYLAXIS

Our work with the use of radiation to inhibit the transfer of the primitive mesenchymal cell to the active osteocyte, published in relation to the hip[3, 7] and confirmed more recently by Parkinson et al.,[18] applies to the elbow as well. It may be reasonable to administer roentgen therapy prophylactically in patients with fracture-dislocations about the elbow whose epiphyses have closed if there is some delay in treatment or if repeated manipulations are required. These patients are at higher risk of developing EB. But how long a "delay" between injury and treatment, and how many manipulations constitute an increased risk (and how great a risk) is unknown. If there is an associated head injury, the risk is much greater, as noted above. But to date we have used radiation only in the patient in whom, in an effort to mobilize the elbow, EB has been excised. Here the radiation should be administered at an early date, preferably 3 or 4 days postoperatively. This, however, poses a dilemma, because irradiation ports to the elbow may include the incision and thus possibly delay wound healing. In the past we have waited until 10 days after surgery to give the roentgen therapy, and this is clearly too late to alter the mesenchymal cells and prevent their transformation to osteoblasts as illustrated in Figure 26–5. Two thousand rads in 10 fractions is given in 10 increments. The smaller dimensions of the elbow mean that a smaller dose should be administered, but the tissue dose at the midplane would be the same.* In the patient with open physes, however, radiation is inappropriate, because the dosage may cause premature closure of the physes.

Experimentally, diphosphonates (EHDP)[7, 8, 9, 13] help to prevent calcification of the forming EB callus,[19] but do not inhibit bone induction.[19] Yet the multicenter study of Finerman et al.,[6] seemed to demonstrate less overall production of EB in operated hips at 1 year than in controls who were not given diphosphonates.[6] It would seem to be especially appropriate to administer this medication in cases of excision of EB from the elbows of head-injured patients in whom the incidence of recurrence is so great or in other high-risk patients (Fig. 26–6).

Indomethacin has been shown to inhibit bone growth and delay fracture healing.[23] In addition, Dahl[5] and Almasbakk and Roysland[1] found less EB formation after indomethacin was administered to patients undergoing total hip arthroplasty. In a recent report on his experience with indomethacin in attempts to prevent EB after total hip arthroplasty, Ritter showed a reduction from 63 percent EB for-

---

*Scanlon, P. W.: Personal communication.

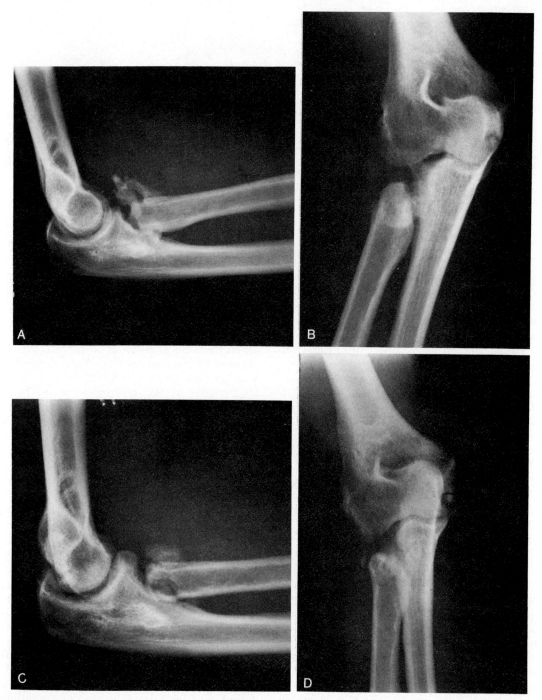

Figure 26–4. A 26-year-old male had a posterior dislocation of the elbow with radial head fracture. Delayed resection of the radial head was carried out at another clinic, but stiffness increased because of ectopic bone shown in the lateral (A) and anteroposterior (B) roentgenograms. The ectopic bone was removed, a further partial head resection was done, and Silastic sheeting was sutured over the proximal radius. Follow-up 5 years later showed excellent motion, no pain, and about one-third reformation of ectopic bone on the lateral (C) and anteroposterior (D) radiographs.

Figure 26–5. A 42-year-old male with a history of severe injury to his right elbow, probably a Monteggia fracture-dislocation. Open reduction and internal fixation and resection of the radial head with a Silastic radial head replacement was done elsewhere. When first seen at the Mayo Clinic, he had extensive heterotopic bone about the elbow with complete ankylosis of pronation and supination. His range of motion was 65 to 115 degrees of flexion (A). He underwent surgical resection of the proximal radius, release of ankylosis involving the proximal radioulnar joint, anterior capsulorrhaphy, and medial epicondylectomy with resection of ectopic bone from the right elbow. Bony ankylosis of the radius and ulna recurred. Additional surgery was performed 17 months later consisting of a fascia lata arthroplasty of the proximal radioulnar joint followed in 13 days by a 10-day course of radiotherapy of 2000 rads. Eight weeks later the patient had 30 to 125 degrees of flexion, 15 degrees of supination, and 50 degrees of pronation (B). This patient later went on again to complete ankylosis of the radioulnar joint. The radiation was ineffective because it was started 13 days postoperatively rather than within the first few days.

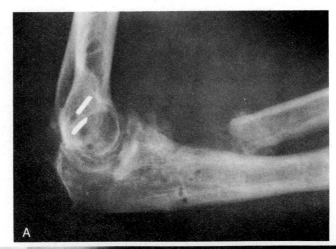

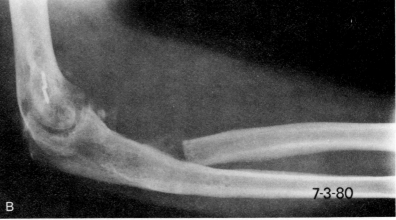

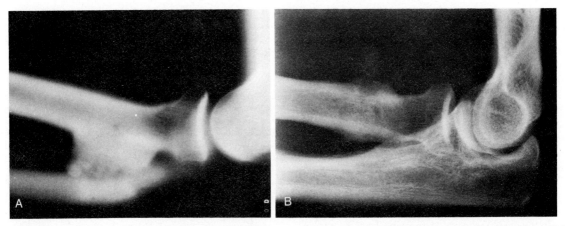

Figure 26–6. This 47-year-old man underwent repair of a spontaneous rupture of the insertion of the biceps to the radial tuberosity using the two-incision technique of Boyd. He was in a cast for approximately 4 weeks; 1 year after injury he had bony ankylosis of the proximal radius and ulna with approximately 10 degrees of pronation and supination (A). He was placed on diphosphonates for 3 weeks, and surgical excision was then performed. At 3-month follow-up there was approximately 35 degrees of supination and approximately 30 degrees of pronation (B). Eighteen months later he had lost only a few degrees of motion.

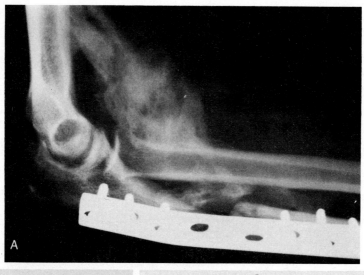

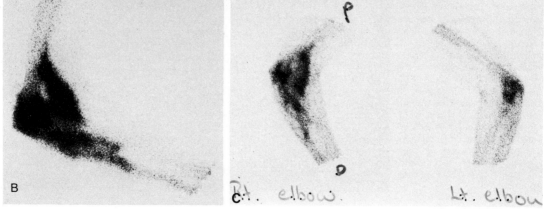

Figure 26–7. This 26-year-old man was involved in a motor vehicle accident and sustained a dislocation of his right elbow with a proximal ulnar fracture. Open reduction and internal fixation of the ulna was done 3 weeks after his injury. He was first seen at the Mayo Clinic 4 months later with extensive (A) ectopic bone. B, The technetium-99m scan marked uptake at 4 months, which persisted for 18 months (C).

mation (of any amount) in a control group to 17 percent in a similar group treated with indomethacin.[20] His present regime consists of 25 mg of indomethacin daily for 6 weeks after surgery. It seems reasonable to use a similar program in patients with elbow injuries at high risk of EB formation, although further clinical confirmation of the effects of indomethacin on EB formation is necessary. Delay in fracture healing and even nonunion might be expected when a fracture accompanies a dislocation of the elbow.

In certain patients it may be best to accept the partial or complete ankylosis, depending on the degree of impairment and disability caused by the EB and the real chances for success by surgical intervention (Fig. 26–7).

References

1. Almasbakk, K. H. and Roysland, P.: Does Indomethacin Prevent Postoperative Ectopic Ossification in Total Hip Replacement? (Abstract) Acta Orthop. Scand. **48:**556, 1977.
2. Broberg, M., and Morrey, B. F.: Type Four Radial Head Fracture. Long-Term Results. Read at AAOS, Annual Meeting, Atlanta, 1984.
3. Coventry, M. B., and Scanlon, P. W.: The Use of Radiation to Discourage Ectopic Bone. A Nine-Year Study in Surgery About the Hip. J. Bone Joint Surg. **63A(2)P:**201, 1981.
4. Craven, P. L., and Urist, M. R.: Osteogenesis by Radioisotope Labelled Cell Populations in Implants of Bone Matrix Under the Influence of Ionizing Radiation. Clin. Orthop. **76:**213, 1971.
5. Dahl, H. K.: Clinical Observations. In Symposium on Artrose: Proceedings of a Conference, October, 1974,

Blinder, Norway. MSD, 1975. Translated from Kliniske Observasjoner, pp. 37–46, The Language Service, Inc., P.O. Box 8, 135 South Side Avenue, Hastings-on-Hudson, NY 10706.

6. Finerman, G. A. M., Brooker, A. F., Coventry, M. B., Krengel, W. F., Jr., McRoberts, R. L., Salvati, E. A., and Volz, R. G.: Symposium: Heterotopic Ossification Following Total Hip Replacement. Contemp. Orthop. **5(4)**:95, 1982.

7. Finerman, G. A. M., Krengel, W. F. Jr., Lowell, J. D., Murray, W. R., Volz, R. G., Bowerman, J. W., and Gold, R. H.: Role of Diphosphonate (EHDP) in the Prevention of Heterotopic Ossification After Total Hip Arthroplasty: A Preliminary Report. *In* The Hip. Proceedings of the Fifth Open Scientific Meeting of the Hip Society. St. Louis, C. V. Mosby Co., 1977.

8. Fleisch, H., Russell, R. G. G., Bisaz, S., Muhlbauer, R. C., and Williams, D. A.: The Inhibitory Effect of Phosphonates on the Formation of Calcium Phosphate Crystals *In Vitro* and on Aortic and Kidney Calcification *In Vivo*. Eur. J. Clin. Invest. **1**:12, 1970.

9. Francis, M. D., Russell, R. G. G., and Fleisch, H.: Diphosphonates Inhibit Formation of Calcium Phosphate Crystals *In Vitro* and Pathological Calcification *In Vivo*. Science **165**:1264, 1969.

10. Garland, D. E., and O'Hollaren, R. M.: Fractures and Dislocations About the Elbow in the Head-Injured Adult. Clin. Orthop. **168**:38, 1982.

11. Jowsey, J., Coventry, M. B., and Robins, P. R.: Heterotopic Ossification: Theoretical Considerations, Possible Etiologic Factors, and a Clinical Review of Total Hip Arthroplasty and Patients Exhibiting This Phenomenon. The Hip Society. *In* The Hip. Proceedings of the Fifth Open Scientific Meeting of the Hip Society. St. Louis, C. V. Mosby Co., 1977.

12. Linscheid, R. L., and Wheeler, D. K.: Elbow Dislocations. J.A.M.A. **194**:1171, 1965.

13. Lowell, J. D.: *In* Scheller, A., and Turner, R. (eds.): Revision Total Hip Arthroplasty. New York, Grune & Stratton, 1982, pp 359–378.

14. McLaughlin, H. L.: Some Fractures With a Time Limit. Surg. Clin. North Am. **35**:553, 1955.

15. Mohan, K.: Myositis Ossificans Traumatic of the Elbow. Int. Surg. **57(6)**:475, 1972.

16. Morrey, B. F., Adams, R., and Cabanela, M. E.: Heterotopic Bone After Total Hip Replacement: A Comparison of Three Surgical Approaches. Clin. Orthop. 1984, forthcoming.

17. Nolan, D. R., Fitzgerald, R. H. Jr., Beckenbaugh, R. D., and Coventry, M. B.: Complications of Total Hip Arthroplasty Treated by Reoperation. J. Bone Joint Surg. **57A(7)**:977, 1975.

18. Parkinson, J. R., Evarts, C. M., and Hubbard, L. F.: Radiation Therapy in the Prevention of Heterotopic Ossification After Total Hip Arthroplasty. *In* The Hip. Proceedings of the Fifth Open Scientific Meeting of the Hip Society. St. Louis, C. V. Mosby Co., 1982.

19. Plasmans, C. M. T., Kuypers, W., and Slooff, T. J. J. H.: The Effect of Ethane-1-Hydroxy-1, 1-Diphosphonic Acid (EHDP) on Matrix Induced Ectopic Bone Formation. Clin. Orthop. **117**:209, 1978.

20. Ritter, M. E. and Gioe, T. J.: The Effect of Indomethacin on Para-Articular Ectopic Ossification Following Total Hip Arthroplasty. Clin. Orthop. **167**:113, 1982.

21. Roberts, P. H.: Dislocation of the Elbow. Br. J. Surg. **56**:806, 1969.

22. Rossier, A. B., Bussat, Ph., Infante, P. F., Zender, R., Courvoisier, B., Muheim, G., Donath, A., Vasey, H., Taillard, W., Lagier, R., Gabbiani, G., Baud, C. A., Pouezat, J. A., Very, J. M., and Hachen, H. J.: Current Facts on Para-Osteo-Arthropathy. Paraplegia **2**:38, May, 1973.

23. Sudmann, E., and Hagen, T.: Indomethacin-Induced Delayed Fracture Healing. Arch. Orthop. Unfallchir. **85**:151, 1976.

24. Thompson, H. C. and Garcia, A.: Myositis Ossificans: Aftermath of Elbow Injuries. Clin. Orthop. **50**:129, 1967.

25. Urist, M. R.: New Bone Formation Induced in Postfetal Life by Bone Morphogenic Protein. *In* Becker, R. O. (ed.): Mechanisms of Growth Control. Springfield, Ill. Charles C Thomas, 1981.

26. Wahner, H. W., and Coventry, M. B.: Unpublished data.

CHAPTER 27

Replantation About the Elbow

MICHAEL B. WOOD

Since the first successful human limb reattachment in 1962,[16, 17] replantation of severed parts has become a relatively common surgical procedure. Nonetheless, limb replantation about the elbow is infrequent because there have been few appropriate candidates. Although the term *replantation* is restricted to reattachment of a completely severed part, there is probably a larger group of patients with physiologic rather than anatomic amputations about the elbow for which much of the following discussion applies.

Classification

The American Academy of Orthopaedic Surgeons Committee on Upper Extremity[33] has recently defined ten anatomic zones of amputation pertaining to replantation (Table 27–1). Three of these levels (6, 7, and 8) occur about the elbow and will be discussed in this chapter.

Zone 8 is an amputation through the upper limb above the elbow (i.e., transhumeral at any level). In this group of patients a plausible and worthwhile surgical goal may be the conversion of an above-elbow amputation to a functioning below-elbow level. Depending

Table 27–1. **Classification of Upper Extremity Amputation Levels**

Zone	Level
1	Finger distal to insertion of superficialis tendon
2	Finger proximal to insertion of superficialis tendon
3	Through the metacarpal
4	Through the wrist
5	Through the forearm distal to the muscle-tendon junction
6	Through the forearm proximal to the muscle-tendon junction
7	Through the elbow joint
8	Through the arm above the elbow
9	Through the thumb (specify level)
10	Amputation of multiple digits

on other factors, additional function may result, including the use of the wrist and hand, which would augment the success of the procedure.

Zone 7 is an amputation level through the elbow joint. In this group of patients it is implied that replantation will require sacrifice of the elbow joint. Hence, at this level the goal of converting an above-elbow amputee to a functioning below-elbow level is less likely. The possibility remains, however, of regaining function to the wrist and hand, and this should be considered along with the proper position of the fused or ankylosed joint.

Zone 6 involves the forearm below the elbow but above the musculotendinous junction. In this group it is generally implied that a functioning below-elbow amputation already exists, so the success of the procedure will depend on recovery of function to the wrist and hand.

Incidence

It is difficult to determine the true incidence of replantation about the elbow. Most reports on this topic involve only a few cases or a large series without clear differentiation of the level of injury or whether the injury was a complete or incomplete amputation. My review of the literature yielded 257 reported apparent major limb replantations.[1, 8, 23, 33, 37] Of this number, 47 were above-elbow (zone 8), 12 were trans-elbow (zone 7), and 33 were proximal forearm amputations (zone 6). Thus, 36 percent of reported major limb replantations are about the elbow region (Fig. 27–1).

MECHANISM OF INJURY

There is, of course, great variation in the mechanism of all traumatic amputations at any level; however, certain trends are apparent with this particular group of patients. In

472

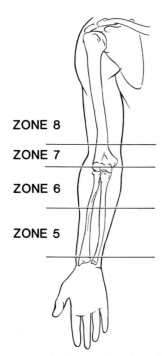

Figure 27–1. Levels of amputation about the elbow.

general, above-elbow amputations (zone 8) are usually violent avulsions frequently associated with other major injuries. In our practice they are most often an agricultural injury produced by a tractor power take-off or an auger device.

Trans-elbow amputations (zone 7) by contrast are most often sharp, guillotine-type injuries, perhaps with some local crushing. The literature and our own experience suggest that these are more commonly nonagricultural industrial injuries or the result of vehicular accidents.

The proximal forearm group (zone 6) does not appear to be associated with a clear pattern of injury. Sharp severance, frank avulsion, and crush amputations have all been reported resulting from industrial and recreational activities.

GOALS OF TREATMENT

The goals of limb replantation about the elbow should be the restoration of limb function in excess of that possible at the level of injury by presently available limb prostheses. It cannot be overemphasized that this goal must be commensurate with the patient's medical condition, age, economic resources, wishes, and realistic expectations.

In zone 8 (above-elbow level) the minimum expectation should be conversion of an above-elbow amputation to a functional below-el-bow level. In zones 7 and 6 the minimum expectations should be a functioning hand unit that permits at least simple hook-grasp and prehension with protective sensibility.

INDICATIONS FOR REPLANTATION

The ideal candidate for limb replantation about the elbow is a sharp, guillotine-type transsection that occurred as an isolated event without direct injury to the elbow joint, with minimum contamination and minimum ischemic time in a young, emotionally stable patient. Unfortunately, the potential candidate most of us deal with strays from this description to a greater or lesser extent. Therefore, the indications for limb replantation about the elbow will depend on a composite consideration of a number of factors including the age and general medical condition of the patient, the presence of associated major injuries, the degree of damage within the amputated part, the length of normothermic and hypothermic ischemia, the degree of wound contamination, and the mechanism of injury.

Age. In general, age is a factor in that it relates to the general medical state of the patient and to his economic state in terms of a prolonged recovery and rehabilitation period. Limb replantation at this level is a major undertaking associated with prolonged anesthetics, considerable blood loss, possible metabolic acidosis, myoglobinemia and renal complications, and frequently multiple post-replantation procedures. Maximum recovery is primarily influenced by the speed and adequacy of recovery of peripheral nerve function and may require a minimum of 2 or 3 years. Most authors agree that age 50 or 60, if the general health is excellent, is the upper range for consideration of replantation at this level.[33]

Medical Condition of the Patient. For the reasons mentioned above, a patient's medical condition may modify his candidacy for this procedure. Cardiopulmonary, peripheral vascular, renal, and metabolic factors require careful scrutiny. Not to be overlooked also is the psychiatric stability of the patient and his ability to deal with a prolonged rehabilitation program.

Associated Injuries. Associated injuries, particularly to the thorax and brachial plexus, are common. The appropriate management of open chest wounds should never be compromised by a zealous replantation effort and may be an absolute contraindication to the procedure. Brachial plexus avulsion should also be regarded as a contraindication[27] unless it is probably postganglionic and occurs in the very young patient. Head, abdominal, and other injuries require individual consideration and should be assigned appropriate priority.

Degree of Damage Within the Amputated Part. Injury distal to the site of amputation within the part is common. Although segmental vascular and nerve injuries can be successfully managed, they should be regarded as relative contraindications to replantation. Distal fractures should be evaluated and managed on their own merits and usually are not contraindications in themselves. Extreme distal crushing and shredding militates against consideration of replantation.

Ischemic Time. In any major limb amputation the duration of normothermic and hypothermic ischemic time is critical.[7, 10, 12, 14, 18, 27, 42] Myonecrosis resulting in late irreversible loss of muscle function and immediate myoglobinemia and metabolic acidosis may become significant after 6 hours at room temperature and 12 hours with appropriate cooling. In general, revascularization of the part beyond these time limits is not advised.[33]

Degree of Wound Contamination. Because sepsis is one of the most common causes of failure with these cases,[21] the degree and type of wound contamination merits scrutiny. However, it is important to realize that radical debridément at the level of amputation with considerable skeletal shortening is both possible and advisable.[27] For this reason, a contaminated wound at the level of transsection can frequently be rendered quite tidy by appropriate debridément.

Mechanism of Injury. With any replantation procedure sharp transsection is most ideal. Limited crush at the level of amputation is acceptable and can be managed by skeletal shortening. Massive crush is a definite contraindication to the procedure.[12, 24] Avulsion is a relative contraindication, depending on the extent of injury within the vascular structures. If limited, resection of the damaged structures and replacement by autogenous vein grafts may be possible.

MANAGEMENT

The initial management problem in these patients concerns general resuscitation. Control of bleeding at the level of amputation is generally not a major problem provided that the transsected vessels can retract. Bleeding is usually amenable to direct pressure with a sterile compressive dressing. Direct clamping of the vessels in the proximal stump is to be avoided if at all possible because it may further damage the vessels more proximally. Ensuring an adequate airway if it is compromised, volume and blood replacement as necessary, tetanus prophylaxis, and extreme care to avoid overlooking additional associated injuries are standard but occasionally neglected aspects of initial management.

The amputated part should be inspected to assess the level of injury, the presence of additional, more distal injury in the limb, the degree of contamination, and, if possible, the mechanisms of injury. The transsected end should be thoroughly irrigated and a saline or Ringer's moist dressing applied, and the amputated part should be placed in a clean or preferably sterile container. For amputations about the elbow, a sterile, surgical x-ray cassette polyethylene bag is convenient for this purpose. The wrapped limb should then be placed on ice in preparation for replantation.

The time period following injury until reestablishment of circulation to the limb is critical for amputations about the elbow because of the large bulk of skeletal muscle within the severed part. These are true emergencies and every effort should be made to minimize the period of ischemia and to cool the limb prior to reperfusion as efficiently as possible.[7, 12, 25, 27]

Surgical Technique

Once the patient and limb arrive in the operating room the initial procedure is thorough and radical debridément of all obvious foreign material and contused or crushed skeletal muscle, both at the amputated part and proximally at the stump. Skeletal shortening is always carried out, at times for as much as 8 or more cm. Shortening is usually carried out in the amputated segment unless this will compromise the integrity of the elbow joint or make internal skeletal fixation difficult. In the process of debridément the major arteries, veins, nerves, tendons, and muscle bellies are identified. Although there is not uniform agreement about this, most authors believe that perfusion of the amputated part prior to replantation helps to dilute accumulated toxic metabolites and lactic acid within the part.[16, 34] We prefer routinely to perfuse the limb by gravity drip with 3 liters of Ringer's lactate solution containing 1 ampule of sodium bicarbonate per liter.

Once the above measures are accomplished, the process of reattachment begins with rigid osteosynthesis. Although the choice of tech-

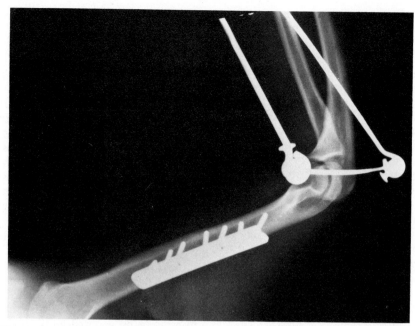

Figure 27–2. Midhumeral replantation—immediate postoperative x-ray. (Note skeletal traction pin in olecranon for elevation and stable internal fixation plate.)

nique for internal fixation will vary with the injury, we prefer humeral or radial and ulnar osteosynthesis by compression plates. Trans-elbow injuries (zone 7) are not amenable to compression plate fixation and require Stein-mann pins or Rush rods, often in conjunction with an exoskeletal fixation device. For amputations above the elbow (zone 8), bony fixation may be sufficiently stable to permit elevation of the limb by a skeletal traction pin in the postoperative period (Fig. 27–2). This detail is extremely important for facilitating management of the wound and soft tissue defect, for minimizing postoperative lymphedema and fluid and protein losses, and for general nursing care.

Following stabilization, repair of the remaining structures follows a sequential order from deep to superficial. Muscle bellies and tendons are repaired in a conventional manner according to the surgeon's preference. We prefer large whip-stitch coaptation of the muscle bellies, Bunnell criss-cross or Kessler side-locking sutures for cylindrical tendons (i.e., biceps), and multiple horizontal mattress sutures for flat tendons (i.e., triceps).

Nerve repairs should be carefully executed because they will have a major influence on the ultimate functional result. The initial requirement in this regard is proper isolation and correct anatomic identification of the various nerves. No nerve length is debrided prior to the time of actual coaptation. At the time of neurorrhaphy the nerve ends are resected,

both proximally and distally, to a length that will permit repair without tension. An epineural neurorrhaphy under magnification is then carried out. We prefer to accomplish this with multiple sutures of 8–0 nylon. There is no evidence to suggest that a group fascicular neurorrhaphy improves the quality of repair with this type of injury because it is impossible to be certain that the nerve ends are uninjured. Thus, extra surgical time expended on fascicular nerve repairs is not justified.

The vascular repairs are, of course, of crucial importance in the immediate success of the procedure. In contrast to more distal replantations, in which the sequence of vascular repair is unimportant, in major limb reattachments arterial repair should always precede the venous anastomoses. This is necessary because the reperfusion of the limb is urgent and the initial venous effluent containing high concentrations of lactic acid, myoglobin, and other myonecrotic products must be prevented from entering the central circulation. After arterial reperfusion of the limb is accomplished, multiple venous anastomoses should be carried out relatively swiftly to minimize blood loss and to curtail the massive swelling of the limb that characteristically occurs. In general, the more venous anastomoses there are, including both deep and superficial systems, the fewer are the problems related to swelling and fluid and protein losses from the limb in the postoperative period.[12] It is imperative that arteries and veins, both proximally and distally, be resected until the vessel wall and lumen appear pristine. Vein grafts may be necessary depending on the extent of vessel resection. At this level both the arterial and venous repairs are usually accomplished with interrupted, full-thickness, simple sutures of 8–0 nylon.[6]

A partial closure of the wound is desirable to achieve skin or subcutaneous tissue coverage over the neurovascular structures. However, complete closure of the wound should be avoided at the initial procedure. Volar and distal forearm fasciotomy as well as decompression of the hypothenar, interossei, and thenar compartments of the hand is routine. If there is no evidence of sepsis, a delayed primary skin closure or, more commonly, closure by skin grafting is carried out in the first postoperative week. Occasionally a distant or local pedicle skin flap may be necessary to achieve coverage over bone or neurovascular structures.

Postoperative Care

Postoperatively, the limb is elevated to decrease edema and venous congestion. The ideal position of splinting is with the elbow in 45 degrees of flexion, the forearm in neutral rotation, the wrist in 40 degrees of extension, the thumb in palmar abduction, and the fingers in an intrinsic-plus position with metacarpophalangeal joint flexion and nearly complete interphalangeal joint extension. A skeletal traction pin through the olecranon and a forearm plaster or thermoplastic splint is ideal for maintaining both elevation and proper positioning. Frequent dressing changes are usually required postoperatively. The patient is usually returned to the operating room 48 hours postoperatively for assessment of the need for further débridement. As soon as possible but after complete débridement of all nonviable tissue is ensured, wound closure by whatever means necessary should be accomplished.

Antibiotics consistent with the results of wound culture obtained at the time of surgery are routinely employed. There is no agreement about the value or choice of anticoagulants, but all authors agree that systemic heparinization should be avoided. To minimize the risks of myoglobinemia and resultant renal complications, a high-fluid turnover and alkalinization of the urine are recommended. Finally, during the postoperative period emotional depression of varying severity may occur and should not be overlooked. The initial euphoria of a "successful" reattachment soon gives way to the realization that a long period of continued medical treatment is necessary and that a permanent, profound functional deficit of the upper limb will result.

REHABILITATION

Rehabilitation considerations begin in the early postoperative period and continue often for years thereafter. As soon as compatible with wound healing, gentle passive range of motion exercises are initiated for the distal joints. After the first month these efforts are augmented by the use of dynamic splints and other modalities including ultrasound and galvanic stimulation. Edema may be a problem for several months. As soon as compatible with stable wound healing, antilymphedema pumps or garments should be utilized. In the late phase, sensory and motor reeducation, assistive orthoses, and secondary procedures of tendon transfers, tenolysis, and capsulotomies may be a consideration. Vocational retraining may be necessary in many cases. In all instances the ultimate goal of replantation is to return the patient to a productive, independent, and dignified position in society with the maximum upper extremity function.

RESULTS

The results of replantation about the elbow requires evaluation, both in terms of immediate survival and long-term functional outcome. For the reasons mentioned previously, it is difficult from a literature review to glean accurate information in this regard. Moreover, a distinction between survival and functional success is often vague because follow-up reports in many cases are relatively brief. Our recent review of the literature on this subject yielded 257 reports of major limb replantations or revascularizations with an overall limb survival rate of 73.4 percent.[33] Of this group only a relatively small number of reports of complete replantations present sufficient detail to assess the functional result at a given level.

At above-elbow levels (zone 8) we collected 36 cases in which there was a limb survival rate of 50 percent.[5, 9, 11, 13, 16, 18, 22, 26, 30, 32, 35, 41, 43, 45] Of the 18 failures, sepsis was the cause in 8 and thrombosis of the vascular anastomoses in 5, and death occurred from intra- or postoperative complications in 4. One additional failure was a patient who underwent elective amputation after survival of a useless, painful limb.[29] Of the 18 successful cases there was adequate follow-up (mean, 3.2 years) in 11. In this group a mean of 1.78

secondary procedures was necessary after the initial replantation effort. Functionally, results in 9 of the 11 were rated good, and 2 were rated poor.

At the trans-elbow level (zone 7) only eight cases have been reported in detail[5, 9, 13] with survival of the limb in seven. The one failure was due to sepsis. Of the seven surviving limbs, five had sufficient follow-up for evaluation, and these required a mean of one additional secondary procedure. Of the five, two were rated functionally good, one was fair, and two were poor.

At proximal forearm levels (zone 6) we collected 20 cases with an overall limb survival rate of 65 percent.[2, 3, 4, 9, 13, 16, 26, 29, 31, 36, 40, 44] Of the seven failures most were due to vascular thrombosis, and only one was the result of sepsis. Only eight of the survivors have been reported with sufficient follow-up, and these required a mean of 2.0 secondary procedures. Of the eight, one was rated functionally excellent, three were good, two were fair, and two were poor.

My experience with replantations about the elbow consists of 10 cases with follow-up of over 1 year. Overall, the limb survival rate is 60 percent. All the survivors have been rated functionally good to fair, although multiple secondary procedures are nearly always required for maximum function (mean, 2.0 procedures). Of the four surviving above-elbow replanted limbs, two have achieved useful hand function in excess of that possible with a conventional prosthetic terminal device. The other two patients have regained good elbow control but do not have useful hand function.

COMPLICATIONS

Perioperative and postoperative complications in this group of patients include those complications seen with any major mutilating extremity injury. At this level sepsis and vascular thrombosis are probably the chief complications leading to ultimate failure of the replantation effort. If survival occurs, poor recovery of neurologic function is the chief reason for an unsatisfactory functional outcome.

In addition, a spectrum of complications called replantation toxemia[7, 14, 18, 20, 38, 39, 42] may occur in this group, particularly in above-elbow (zone 8) amputations. This term refers to a number of metabolic disturbances associated with the reperfusion of a significant bulk of ischemic skeletal muscle and is relatively unique to major limb replantations and revascularizations. Included among these disturbances are metabolic acidosis from lactic acid accumulation in the limb,[20] hyperkalemia from excessive potassium losses from the limb,[15, 19, 28] and protein and fluid losses from edema of the replanted part.[7] Which of these factors, if any, are most important in terms of systemic effects is unclear. However, a number of deaths following major limb replantation have been attributed to "toxemia."[8, 9, 26, 30] In addition, the renal complications occurring from myoglobinemia following replantation of a large amount of muscle undergoing rhabdomyolysis are perhaps of greater significance. Decreased limb ischemic time and effective cooling of the amputated part are thought to minimize the problems of toxemia as well as myoglobinemia.[7, 9, 14, 18, 20] In addition, preoperative perfusion of the amputated part, anastomosis of the arteries before veins, volume diuresis, alkalinization of the urine, and meticulous attention to serum electrolyte balance are all helpful measures in preventing complications of this type.

AUTHOR'S PREFERRED TREATMENT METHOD

The author's preferred technique of limb replantation about the elbow has been discussed above. However, in addition, our group places all replantation candidates with injuries above the proximal forearm on a prescribed protocol of monitoring and management. Preoperatively, all patients undergo baseline serum lactate and myoglobin determinations in addition to the usual laboratory studies. Immediately postoperatively and daily for 5 days thereafter, serum electrolytes, myoglobin and lactate, arterial blood gases, and urine myoglobin levels are monitored. Depending on the results of these studies, a high fluid diuresis is maintained by intravenous fluid and mannitol as necessary. Urine pH is monitored every 4 to 6 hours for the first 5 postoperative days. Sodium bicarbonate is added to the intravenous intake as necessary to maintain a urine pH above 6.0. Albumin may be necessary because of serum protein sequestration and losses. Blood loss may be excessive, and replacement should be liberal.

Both an aminoglycoside and a cephalosporin antibiotic, provided there is no allergic history to these, are given intravenously preoperatively and maintained postoperatively until wound culture results become available. Antibiotics are then modified consistent with the culture sensitivity report.

Anticoagulation is usually limited to a combination of aspirin (10 grains) and dipyridamole (50 mg) three times a day postoperatively. In the absence of any bleeding difficulties, this regimen is continued for 2 to 4 weeks.

The principles of management may be synthesized as applied in the following case report.

D.S., a 23-year-old farmer, presented with a traumatic amputation of the right (dominant) upper limb at the supracondylar level of the humerus

(Fig. 27–3A). The injury was the result of an avulsion from a tractor power take-off device. At surgery, following extensive debridément of the limb, perfusion with Ringer's lactate, and skeletal shortening, fixation was accomplished with an AO T-plate and seven screws (Fig. 27–3B). Triceps, biceps, and brachioradialis muscles or tendons, radial, ulnar, and median nerves, brachial artery, and four major veins were repaired in a 10-hour procedure. Revascularization was accomplished by 12.5 hours postinjury with effective interim cooling. Volar forearm fasciotomy was done intraoperatively (Fig. 27–3C). The wounds were left open

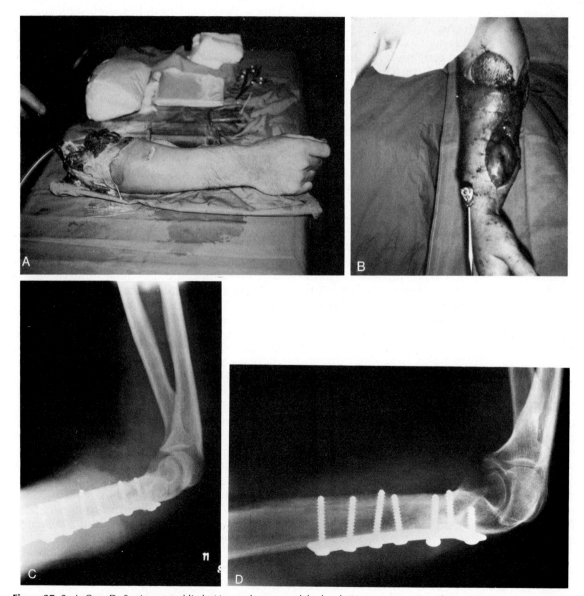

Figure 27–3. *A,* Case D. S.: Amputated limb. Humeral supracondylar level. (Note compression plate application and perfusion catheter in preparation for replantation.)
  B, Immediate postoperative view. (Note open fasciotomy wounds and skeletal traction pin for elevation.)
  C, Six days postoperative. (Note stable internal fixation device.)
  D, Six months postoperative. (Note bone union at replantation site.)

Illustration continued on opposite page

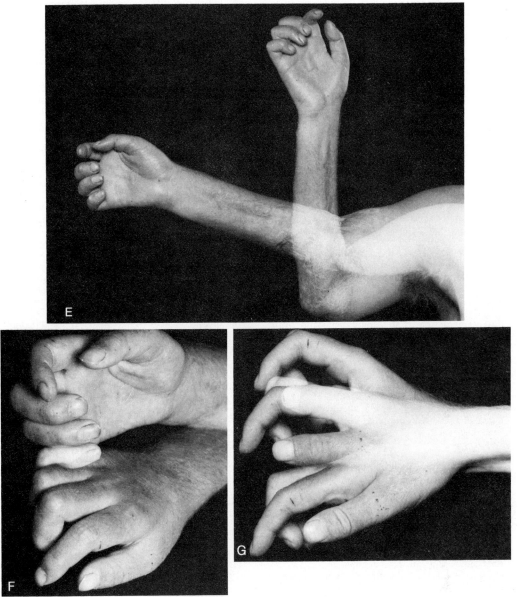

Figure 27–3 *Continued. E,* Range of active elbow flexion and extension. (There was no interim surgery after replantation.)
  F, Range of active forearm pronosupination.
  G, Range of active wrist extension and flexion.

and the limb suspended in skeletal traction post-operatively. A high fluid output by intravenous fluid infusion and mannitol with alkalinization of the urine to maintain a urinary pH above 6.0 was carried out for the first 5 postoperative days. Serum myoglobin peaked at 25,000 ng/ml on the first postoperative day, but urinary myoglobin was negligible at 120 μg/ml. Serum myoglobin levels gradually decreased during the first postoperative week. Skin grafting was carried out 1, 3 and 4 weeks postoperatively. Joint mobilization was initiated 3 weeks postoperatively, and the patient was dismissed at 6 weeks. No subsequent hospital admissions or surgical procedures were carried out. He returned to active farming but without

actual use of the right upper extremity 3 months postoperatively. Bone union was confirmed at 6 months (Fig. 27–3D). At last evaluation, 22 months after the injury, the patient was an independent farmer, had good elbow and wrist control, was capable of light grasp activity, and had good protective tactile sensibility in the hand but poor pinch prehension (Figs. 27–3E–G). Functionally, the limb was used primarily in an assistive manner.

References

1. Balas, P.: The Present Status of Replantation of Amputated Extremities. Vasc. Surg. **4**:190, 1970.
2. Ch'en, C. W., Ch'ien, Y. C., and Pao, Y. S.: Further

Experiences in the Restoration of Amputated Limbs. Chinese Med. J. **82**:633, 1963.

3. Ch'en, C. W., Ch'ien, Y. C., and Pao, Y. S.: Further Experiences in the Restoration of Amputated Limbs. Chinese Med. J. **84**:225, 1965.

4. Ch'en C. W., Qian, Y. Q., and Yu, Z. J.: Extremity Replantation. World J. Surg. **2**:513, 1978.

5. Christeas, N., Balas, P., and Giannikas, A.: Replantation of Amputated Extremities. Am. J. Surg. **118**:68, 1969.

6. Carrel, A.: Results of Transplantation of Blood Vessels, Organs and Limbs. J. A. M. A. **51**:1662, 1908.

7. Eiken O., Nabseth, D. C., Mayer, R. F., and Deterling, R. A.: Limb Replantation. Arch. Surg. **88**:70, 1964.

8. Engber, W. D., and Hardin, C. A.: Replantation of Extremities. Surg. Gynecol. Obstet. **132**:901, 1971.

9. Ferriera, M. C., Marques, E. F., and Azze, R. J.: Limb Replantation. Clin. Plast. Surg. **5**:211, 1978.

10. Fukunishi, H.: Studies on Cause of Shock Following Replantation of Amputated Extremity. J. Nara. Med. Assoc. **19**:127, 1968.

11. Halmagyi, A. F., Baker, C. B., Campbell, H. H., Evans, J. G., and Mahoney, L. J.: Reimplantation of a Completely Severed Arm Followed by Reamputation Because of Failure of Reinnervation. Can. J. Surg. **12**:222, 1969.

12. Herbsman, H., Lafer, D. J., and Shaftan, G. W.: Successful Replantation of an Amputated Hand. Ann. Surg. **163**:137, 1966.

13. Ikuta, Y.: Method of Bone Fixation in Reattachment of Amputations in the Upper Extremities. Clin. Orthop. **133**:169, 1978.

14. Kleinert, H. E., Jablon, M., and Tsai, T. M.: An Overview of Replantation and Results of 347 Replants in 245 Patients. J. Trauma **20**:390, 1980.

15. Kohama, A.: Changes Following Recirculation of Ischemic Leg. Cent. Jap. J. Orthop. Trauma **12**:555, 1969.

16. Malt, R. A., and McKhann, C. F.: Replantation of Severed Arm. J.A.M.A. **189**:114, 1964.

17. Malt, R. A., Remensynder, J. P., and Harris, W. H.: Long-Term Utility of Replanted Arms. Ann. Surg. **176**:334, 1972.

18. McNeill, I. F., and Wilson, J. J. P.: The Problems of Limb Replacement. Br. J. Surg. **57**:356, 1970.

19. Meer, D. C., Valkenburg, P. W., Ariens, A. T., and Benthem, R. V.: Cause of Death in Tourniquet Shock in Rats. Am. J. Physiol. **21**:513, 1966.

20. Mehl, R. L., Paul, H. A., Shorey, W., Schneewind, J., and Beattie, E. J.: Treatment of "Toxemia" After Extremity Replantation. Arch. Surg. **89**:871, 1964.

21. Morrison, W. A., O'Brien, B. M., and Macleod, A. M.: Major Limb Replantation. Orthop. Clin. North Am. **8**:343, 1977.

22. Nasseri, M., and Voss, H.: Late Results of Successful Replantation of Upper and Lower Extremities. Ann. Surg. **177**:121, 1973.

23. O'Brien, B. M.: Replantation Surgery. Clin. Plast. Surg. **1**:405, 1974.

24. O'Brien, B. M., Miller, G. D. H., Macleod, A. M., and Newing, R. K.: Saving the Amputated Digit and Hand. Med. J. Aust. **1**:558, 1973.

25. O'Brien, B. M.: Replantation Surgery in China. Med. J. Aust. **2**:255, 1974.

26. O'Brien, B. M., Macleod, A. M., Hayhurst, J. W., Morrison, W. A., and Ishida, H.: Major Replantation Surgery in the Upper Limb. Hand, **6**:217, 1974.

27. O'Brien, B. M., and Macleod, A. M.: *In* Daniller, A. I., and Strauch, B. (eds.): Symposium on Microsurgery. St. Louis, C. V. Mosby Co., 1976.

28. Onji, Y., Kohama, A., Tamai, S., Fukunishi, H., and Komtsui, S.: Metabolic Alteration Following Replantation of an Amputated Extremity. J. Jap. Orthop. Assoc. **41**:55, 1967.

29. Paletta, F. X., Willman, V., and Ship, A. G.: Prolonged Tourniquet Ischemia of Extremities. J. Bone Joint Surg. **42A**:945, 1960.

30. Peking Trauma Hospital: Replantation of Severed Limbs. Chinese Med. J. **1**:265, 1975.

31. Ramirez, M. Z., Duque, M., Hernandez, L., Londono, A., and Cadvid, G.: Reimplantation of Limbs. Plast. Reconstr. Surg. **40**:315, 1967.

32. Rosenkrantz, J. G., Sullivan, R. C., Welch, K., Miles, J. S., Salder, K. M., and Paton, B. C.: Replantation of an Infant's Arm. N. Engl. J. Med. **276**:609, 1967.

33. Results of Microsurgery in Orthopaedics. Committee on the Upper Extremity, American Academy of Orthopaedic Surgeons. Publication No. 665–1981. June 4–5, 1981.

34. Shaftan, G. W., Herbsman, H., and Malt, R. A.: Replantation of Limbs. Minn. Med. **48**:1645, 1965.

35. Shaftan, G. W., and McAlvanah, M. J.: *In* Daniller, A. I., and Strauch, B. (eds.): Symposium on Microsurgery. St. Louis, C. V. Mosby Co., 1976.

36. Shorey, W. D., Schneewind, J. H., and Paul, H. A.: Significant Factors in the Reimplantation of an Amputated Hand. Bull. Soc. Int. Chir. **24**:44, 1965.

37. Shanghai Sixth Peoples Hospital: Extremity Replantation. Chinese Med. J. **4**:5, 1978.

38. Shaw, R. S.: Treatment of the Extremity Suffering Near or Total Severance with Special Consideration of the Vascular Problem. Clin. Orthop. **29**:56, 1963.

39. Snyder, C. C., Knowles, R. P., Mayer, P. W., and Hobbs, J. C.: Extremity Replantation. Plast. Reconstr. Surg. **26**:251, 1960.

40. Tamai, S., Hori, Y., Tatsumi, Y., Okuda, H., Nakamura, Y., Sakamoto, H., and Takita, T.: Major Limb, Hand and Digital Replantation. World J. Surg. **3**:17, 1979.

41. Ts'ui, C., Feng, Y., T'ang, C., Li, C., Yu, Y., Ch'en, H. P. and Shih, Y.: Microvascular Anastomosis and Transplantation. Chinese Med. J. **85**:610, 1966.

42. Usui, M., Ishii, S., Muramatsu, J., and Takahata, N.: An Experimental Study on "Replantation Toxemia." J. Hand. Surg. **3**:589, 1978.

43. Williams, G. R., Carter, D. R., Frank, G. R., and Price, W. E.: Replantation of Amputated Extremities. Ann. Surg. **163**:758, 1966.

44. Worman, L. W., Darin, J. C., and Kritter, A. E.: The Anatomy of a Limb Replantation Failure. Arch. Surg. **91**:211, 1965.

45. Wright, P. E.: Convention Reporter 67th Annual Meeting of the Clinical Orthopaedic Society **3**:1, 1979.

PART IV

Sports—and Overuse Injuries to the Elbow

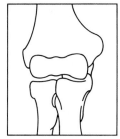

CHAPTER 28

Muscle and Tendon Trauma: Tennis Elbow

ROBERT P. NIRSCHL*

Tennis elbow, which was originally coined as *lawn-tennis elbow* in 1883,[22,39] is a popular term. Over the years it has been used to describe a variety of maladies that occur in and about the elbow.[5] To eliminate confusion, it is important to define terms accurately. On the basis of clinical and surgical experience,[26,27,31] it can be stated with confidence that the pathology of classic tennis elbow is that of a tendinitis.

INCIDENCE

A random study of 200 tennis players in three tennis clubs revealed that 50 per cent of players over the age of 30 had experienced symptoms of characteristic tennis elbow at one time or another.[30] Of this group, 50 per cent noted minor symptoms with a duration of less than 6 months, and the remaining 50 per cent had had major symptoms with an average duration of 2½ years. A larger statistical analysis of 2500 patients performed by Priest at the Vic Braden Tennis Camps re-

vealed similar data.[36] Not restricted to tennis, the malady is commonly noted in other sports including baseball, field events involving throwing, swimming, and fencing. Occupational activity that requires stressful forearm use such as carpentry, plumbing, meat cutting, and textile production can also cause tennis elbow.

CLASSIFICATION

Elbow tendinitis may be simply classified on an anatomic basis.

Lateral Tennis Elbow. Lateral tendinitis primarily involves the origin of the extensor carpi radialis brevis, occasionally the anterior edges of the extensor communis and the underside of the extensor carpi radialis longus, and rarely the origin of the extensor carpi ulnaris.

Medial Tennis Elbow. Medial tennis elbow primarily involves the flexor pronator origin at the medial epicondyle. An additional complicating factor of medial tennis elbow is the commonly associated finding of compression neuropraxia of the ulnar nerve (discussed below).

*Appreciation is expressed to E. Stay, M.D., for the discussion of the pathologic changes of tennis elbow.

Posterior Tennis Elbow. Tendinitis of the triceps at its attachment to the olecranon is relatively uncommon.

ASSOCIATED ABNORMALITIES AND DIFFERENTIAL DIAGNOSIS

Associated problems can and do appear either independently or in combination with tennis elbow tendinitis. The most common examples include the following:

Ulnar Nerve Neurapraxia. Ulnar nerve neurapraxia is commonly associated with tennis elbow and is discussed below.

Carpal Tunnel Syndrome. In our experience, about 10 per cent of surgical patients have signs and symptoms of carpal tunnel syndrome.[31] This association has led to the conclusion that a constitutional factor may play a significant role in certain tennis elbow patients.[29]

Radial Nerve Entrapment. Entrapment of the motor branch of the radial nerve in the radial tunnel can cause symptoms similar to those seen with lateral epicondylitis. Roles and Maudsley reported a surgical experience with 33 cases in 1972.[38] Specific care was taken to decompress the radial tunnel by releasing the origin of the extensor carpi radialis brevis. Thus, the success of the reported operation may be due to an alteration of the origin of the extensor brevis. Entrapment of the posterior interosseous nerve has also been implicated as the cause of lateral elbow pain by Werner[41] and Dobyns* (see Chapter 45). Yet a random sample of 20 electromyographic studies in patients with the classic signs of clinical lateral tennis elbow failed to reveal any radial nerve abnormality.[33] In our opinion, although radial nerve entrapment may occur, it is not associated in a major statistical way with classic lateral tennis elbow.

Cervical Osteoarthritis and Nerve Root Compression. Gunn has reported relieving the pain of tennis elbow in 53 cases by directing treatment to osteoarthritis of the cervical spine.[16] It should be noted that the greatest incidence of tennis elbow is in the fourth and fifth decades, and because the findings of lateral tennis elbow are usually specific, it is unlikely that osteoarthritis in the cervical spine is anything but a coincidental finding.

Intra-Articular Abnormalities and Joint Laxity. Individuals who use the arm with high torque and shearing forces as in the aggressive activities of baseball or javelin throwing are vulnerable to associated intra-articular problems.[19,42] This generally takes the form of traumatic osteoarthritis and osteocartilaginous loose bodies present in the lateral (Newman) or, more rarely, medial elbow compartments, as well as in the posterior olecranon fossa.[19,25,42] When associated with ligamentous laxity of the medial collateral ligamentous structures, ulnar neuropathy may also complicate the clinical picture.

ETIOLOGY

Age, Sex. The characteristic age of onset is between 35 and 50 with a median of 41 years.[26,31,32,36,37] Although most common in the third, fourth, and fifth decades, we have diagnosed the condition in patients as young as 12 and as old as 80. Depending on a given patient population, the overall male-female ratio is usually equal.

Overuse. It is quite clear that the overall intensity and duration of arm use is the ultimate cause of this tendinitis. In this regard, younger patients such as competitive tennis or professional baseball athletes characteristically place high demands on the upper extremities. An inadequate, marginal, or compromised musculoskeletal condition also appears to play a role in the etiology of medial or lateral elbow tendinitis.

Lateral tennis elbow is directly related to activities that increase the tension and hence the stress of the wrist extensor and supinator muscles.

Medial tennis elbow characteristically occurs with wrist flexor activity and active pronation as in baseball pitching, the tennis serve and overhead strokes, and the pull-through strokes of swimming.

Posterior tennis elbow consists of intrinsic overload of the triceps attachment that occurs in such sports as javelin throwing and baseball pitching, which cause a sudden snap of elbow extension.

It should be appreciated that the primary overload abuse in tendinitis is caused by intrinsic concentric muscular contraction (see Chapter 5). Tensile extrinsic overload is more likely to cause excessive joint torque forces leading to ligamentous rupture and traumatic osteoarthritis. In sports activities both factors are likely to obtain.

Traumatic Etiology. Excessive forearm use is clearly associated with the development of tennis elbow.[33,37,38] A typical patient is an active recreational tennis player who plays at least three or four times per week.[33,37,38] The most common onset of symptoms is insidious and gradual, usually appearing after a fairly

---

*Dobyns, J.: Personal communication.

vigorous activity sequence. Less commonly, the onset may be associated with a direct blow to one of the epicondylar areas or a sudden extreme effort or activity with acute onset of pain.

Constitutional Factors. We have observed that the etiologic factors of tennis elbow also involve a distinct, albeit small, subgroup of patients who have a tendency to develop generalized tendinitis. This observation was initially reported in 1968 and termed the *mesenchymal syndrome*.[29] In the extreme case, the mesenchymal abnormalities may include bilateral rotator cuff tendinitis, medial and lateral tennis elbow, carpal tunnel syndrome, triggering tenovaginitis of the finger flexors, and DeQuervain's syndrome all in the same patient. In almost all instances, routine rheumatologic work-up is normal. These observations have led to the conclusion that some individuals have a heritable constitutional factor that predispose to profuse or generalized tendinitis.

PATHOLOGY

Gross Abnormalities

Before 1960, some confusion existed about the precise pathologic anatomy of this condition. In 1922 Osgood[34] and in 1932 Carp[9] related the condition to radiohumeral bursitis. Goldie, in his classic study of 1964, was the first to describe evidence of pathology in the tendinous areas adjacent to the lateral elbow as an etiologic explanation of lateral tendinitis.[13] Unlike previously described operative procedures using transverse incisions at the tendon level that obliterated or bypassed the pathology, Goldie used longitudinal incisions and binocular magnification for more thorough assessment of the tissues. The popular techniques described by Bosworth[6] and Hohmann[17] are characterized by failure to observe pathologic abnormalities. Unfortunately, lack of clear pathologic identification has resulted in substantial confusion and inappropriate conclusions about the success obtained with these operative techniques. It is clear that careful clinical examination of the classic lateral tennis elbow patient usually localizes symptoms over the tendinous origin of the extensor carpi radialis brevis. Formulation of a surgical technique to explore this area of maximum tenderness logically follows.

Careful, gross surgical inspection of the abnormal specimen reveals a characteristically grayish color and homogeneous and generally quite edematous tissue (Fig. 28–1).

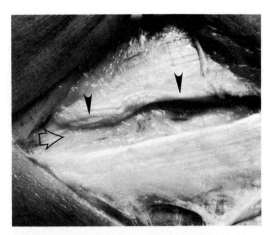

Figure 28–1. Gross pathologic appearance. The brevis origin is exposed by retracting the extensor longus anteriorly (closed arrows). Characteristic visual appearance of angiofibroblastic hyperplasia (open arrow) is a grayish, homogeneous, edematous, and friable tissue. This appearance has led us to coin the phrase "thick unhappy gray tendon, weeping with edema."

This typical gross pathologic appearance is present at all affected anatomic sites in lateral, medial, and posterior tendinitis. Indeed, similar visual characteristics are present in tendinitis involving the rotator cuff and the patellar and Achilles tendons, and even in plantar fasciitis. In our surgical series of lateral tennis elbow, 97 per cent of cases demonstrated varying degrees of this pathologic tissue at the origin of the extensor brevis tendon (which was ruptured in 35 per cent).[31] Roentgenographic examination revealed that 22 per cent of patients had some form of calcification at the lateral epicondyle.

Microscopic Pathology

An understanding of the dense connective tissue that comprises the fiber makeup of the tendon is necessary for better appreciation and definition of the pathologic process that is present in tennis elbow.* In tendons, collagen fibers and primary tendon bundles run parallel courses (Fig. 28–2). Fibroblasts are the only type of cell present; in longitudinal sections they are lined in rows between collagen fibers. Surrounding the primary bundles, a small amount of loose connective tissue termed *endotendineum* is identified. Groups of primary bundles form secondary bundles or fascicles, which in turn are surrounded by a coarse type of connective tissue, the peritendineum. The tendon thus is com-

---

*Stay, E.: Personal communication.

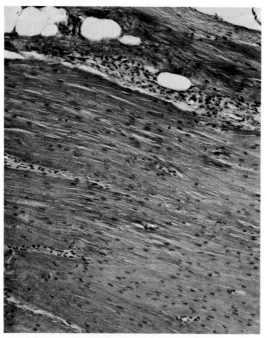

Figure 28–2. Normal tendon. Parallel collagen fibers lined longitudinally by fibroblasts.

posed of a variable number of fascicles and is sheathed by a thick connective tissue covering called the epitendineum. In normal tendons, nerves and blood vessels extend through the major connective tissue septa but do not invade the fascicles. On gross examination, the tendon appears firm, taut, and tan or beige in color.

In tendinitis, the abnormal tissue ordinarily can be easily identified by its appearance and is distinct from the normal tendon.[33] Visual examination usually reveals gray, shiny, sometimes edematous and friable, immature appearing tissue that closely resembles scar tissue.[31] Microscopically, the normal orderly tendon fibers are disrupted by a characteristic invasion of fibroblasts and vascular granulationlike tissue which may be described as an angiofibroblastic hyperplasia (Fig. 28–3). Adjacent to this early proliferating vascular reparative tissue, the tendon appears hypercellular, degenerative, and microfragmented. The degree of angiofibroblastic infiltration appears to correlate generally with the duration of symptoms.[33] In advanced lesions, fibroadipose, connective, and even musculoskeletal tissue can reveal infiltration by this pathologic proliferative tissue. Degeneration of skeletal muscle fibers, fibrosis and degeneration of fat, and vascular sclerosis may be seen. A mild sprinkling of chronic inflammatory cells may be seen scattered about in these supportive

tissues, but it is highly unusual to detect inflammatory cells in the tendinous tissue itself, even in cases of long duration. Evidence of acute inflammation is virtually absent in all cases. Occasional concomitant lesions may include mild osteoarthritis, a nonspecific chronic synovitis, or intra-articular rice bodies. Again, however, inflammatory cells are scarce.

In cases treated by steroid injection, a clear distinction can be made between the characteristic angiofibroblastic proliferation and the injection site. At the injection site, nonpolarizable amorphous eosinophilic material can be identified, often without any foreign body response and usually without evidence of calcification (Fig. 28–4). Indeed, the proliferating vascular reparative tissue often insinuates itself between normal and abnormal tissue in regions very close to the injection site.*

CLINICAL CORRELATIONS OF PATHOLOGY

It is most helpful to have an appreciation of the nature and magnitude of the pathology when formulating a treatment plan. Our observations during the years have resulted in the formation of the following pathologic cat-

---

*Stay, E.: Unpublished data.

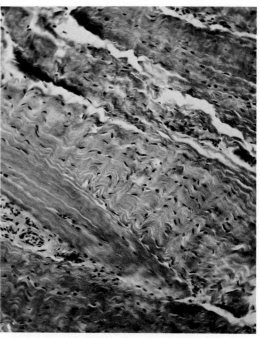

Figure 28–3. Angiofibroblastic hyperplasia (see text).

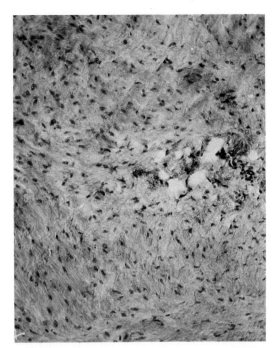

Figure 28–4. Cortisone injection site. Microscopic photograph demonstrates nonpolarizable amorphous eosinophilic material.

egories with corresponding clinical and therapeutic implications.[26]

Category I

Pathology. Acute, reversible inflammation but no angiofibroblastic invasion.

Clinical Signs. Minor aching pain is evident, usually after heavy activity.

Treatment. There is a quick response to simple anti-inflammatory measures followed by future avoidance of force overload or overuse.

Category II

Pathology. There is a partial angiofibroblastic invasion. The process is irreversible, but the response varies depending on the biologic maturation of the pathologic process and the extent of involvement.

Clinical Signs. Often, there is intense pain with activity as well as symptoms at rest. However, after periods of rest, most routine activities can be accomplished without significant discomfort.

Treatment. If less than 50 per cent of the tendon is involved, treatment concepts that promote healing will gradually bring about resolution, and this process can be managed nonoperatively. Anti-inflammatory and rest (antiabuse) treatment programs are recom-

mended. Occasionally, however, these patients will undergo surgery.

Category III

Pathology. Extensive angiofibroblastic invasion with partial or complete rupture of the tendon.

Clinical Signs. Significant functional defects that include pain at rest as well as night pain make routine daily activities difficult or impossible.

Treatment. The condition invariably requires surgery because this advanced stage does not usually respond to nonoperative measures.

NONSURGICAL TREATMENT

Relief of Pain and Inflammation

The general concepts of elbow rehabilitation are covered in detail in Chapter 9. A brief overview is appropriate, however, at this time.[26, 31] The tennis elbow patient most commonly presents for evaluation and treatment because of pain rather than a mechanical functional disability. It is important, therefore, to control pain, but this does not necessarily imply enhancement of healing. The time-honored modalities of rest and application of cold are appropriate. Activity that aggravates the condition should be eliminated. The utilization of aspirin as an anti-inflammatory agent is our first choice, but nonsteroidal, anti-inflammatory medications including indomethacin and Butazolidin certainly are helpful in some patients. The popularity of DMSO among the lay population has prompted one prospective, double-blind study of its effectiveness in tennis elbow. This topical medication, surprisingly, offered no greater relief than did a placebo.[35] The physical therapy modality of high-voltage galvanic stimulation has been helpful in relieving pain and inflammation.

If the process does not respond to this treatment program and the patient is incapable of doing the prescribed exercises, a cortisone injection is appropriate. We use 2.5 ml of 0.5 per cent Xylocaine mixed with 20 mg of triamcinolone, instilled below the extensor brevis just anterior and slightly distal to the lateral epicondyle into a triangular fatty recess that occupies this area. The repeated use of cortisone injections (more than three in one year) is inappropriate and probably harmful because they will cause cellular death and potentially weaken the surrounding normal

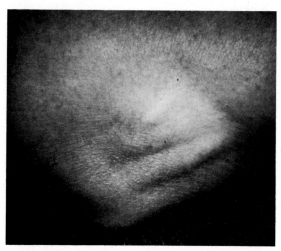

Figure 28–5. Subcutaneous atrophy following cortisone injection.

tissues.[40] Indeed, some patients are extremely sensitive to local instillation of cortisone, and subcutaneous atrophy (Fig. 28–5), occasionally after only one injection, may be noted when the injection is placed superficial to the tendon. Thus, no more than three injections should be instilled in any one area and certainly direct intratendinous injections should be avoided.[1, 32]

Promotion of Healing

The healing process may be hastened by three general measures: rest, galvanic stimulation, and rehabilitation.

Rest

The injured part may be rested by (1) alteration of activity to avoid abuse, (2) alteration of inappropriate technique or activity, (3) selection of proper equipment, and (4) counterforce bracing.

Absence of Abuse. Rest attained by casting has not been effective in controlling pain when activities are resumed. In addition, significant disuse atrophy of the surrounding tissues compromise rehabilitative efforts. Partial immobilization by wrist extension splints have little value except in the early, fully reversible inflammatory phase of category I injuries. Overall, therefore, modification or elimination of abusive activities is a more appropriate and useful interpretation of the term *rest* than formal immobilization.

A graduated activity program for the injured part coupled with an aggressive activity program for the adjacent normal uninjured tissues should be emphasized.

Alteration of Technique. A careful history and observation are fundamental for identification of faulty technique that may be causing the problem. Some physicians may find this aspect beyond their expertise. Under these circumstances it is appropriate to have the patient observed by someone who is knowledgeable in the sport or the occupational activity (e.g., coach, trainer). There is accumulating evidence that the correct technique of a sport not only enhances performance but is less likely to cause injury.[26, 32] The sports most likely to be causally related to tennis elbow include tennis, baseball throwing, swimming, track and field events, golf, and weight lifting. The occupational activities commonly associated with tennis elbow include meat cutting and handling, carpentry, plumbing, repetitive assembly line activity, typing, writing, and hand shaking (e.g., politicians at campaign time). Even so, it is of course recognized that anyone may be afflicted, and the specific abusive activity may not always be obvious or detectable.

Equipment Alteration. Equipment (especially in the racquet sports) may play an important role in imparting forces and thus alter the overuse syndrome.[26,32] Racquets are available in a wide variety of sizes, weight, materials, and frame design. Stringing materials and string tension are also instrumental in force load control. Biomechanically, it is most appropriate to hit the ball at the "center of percussion" (sweet spot) because the increased torsion of off-center hits increases the stresses at the joint and plays a great role in initiating tennis elbow.

Activities that cause forearm impact or stress necessitate the proper size, weight, balance, and grip to avoid excessive forces.[26, 30, 32] In general, the larger the handle of the device, the greater the leverage for torsion control, but the handle must be molded to hand size.[5] We have found that the distance from the midpalmar crease to the ring finger is helpful in selecting the proper handle size (Fig. 28–6).[30]

Finally, the weight and dimension of the equipment should match the available strength of the individual. In general, with racquets or impact implements, we have found it better to utilize a device that is somewhat lighter to ensure proper positioning of the equipment at the time of impact. This consideration is certainly true in individuals who do not have great upper body strength or are lacking in skills or experience.

Counterforce Bracing. The concepts of elbow bracing for tennis elbow were initially

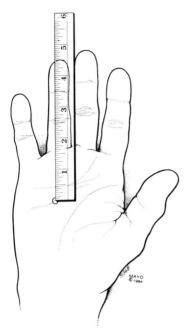

Figure 28–6. Nirschl technique for proper handle size. Measure from proximal palmar crease to tip of ring finger. Place measuring rule between ring and long fingers for proper ruler placement on palmar crease. The measurement obtained is the proper handle size—that is, if this distance is 4½ inches, the proper grip size is 4½ inches.

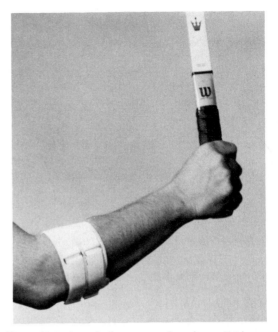

Figure 28–7. Lateral elbow counterforce brace. Wide nonelastic support is curved to fit conical forearm shape. Dual tension straps extend the width of the brace for full adjustments.

introduced by Ilfeld in 1965.[18] Froimson published a paper concerning a forearm band in 1971.[11] Influenced by both investigators, in 1972 we introduced a wide nonelastic support that was curved for better fit and support of the conical shape of the forearm.[30] Simply stated, the counterforce concept constrains full muscular expansion, thereby decreasing intrinsic muscular force to sensitive or vulnerable areas: the forearm extensors for lateral tennis elbow and the forearm flexors for medial tennis elbow (Fig. 28–7). In medial tennis elbow an additional support just distal to the medial epicondyle is sometimes helpful (Fig. 28–8).

Rigid types of immobilization at the elbow or wrist, as noted previously, will relieve pain but at the price of atrophy and immobility and thus are not recommended.

High-Voltage Galvanic Stimulation

It has been the practice of our sports medicine unit to utilize high-voltage galvanic stimulation in the treatment of both acute and chronic tendinitis. It is my definite clinical impression

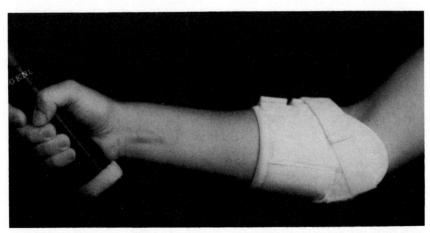

Figure 28–8. Medial elbow counterforce brace. Extended projection of brace provides additional counter force support to a key pathologic area.

that this modality of physical therapy has the capacity to diminish pain and inflammation and to promote the healing process. Unfortunately, we have no objective way of visualizing tendon tissue, and thus it is not possible to state with scientific certainty that a biologic stimulus to healing does occur. In any event, the progress of patients treated with galvanic stimulation appears to be hastened. This observation certainly is consistent with the enhancement of bone healing observed with use of electrical stimulation.[2,3] Our standard practice is to employ four to six sessions of high-voltage galvanic stimulation during a 2- to 3-week period.

Rehabilitative Exercise Program

This topic has been discussed in detail in Chapter 31. Once the inflammatory response and the pain have been controlled, an orderly progression of the graduated strength and endurance exercise is started. Force overloads are controlled by decreasing the intensity and duration of daily and sports activity. This is particularly important in the early return to sports or occupational activity. The patient is protected in the early going by use of the appropriate elbow counterforce brace, which is generally eliminated after the patient has obtained approximately 30 percent of the exercise goals. If, during this exercise program, pain and inflammatory symptoms recur, it is appropriate to return to the anti-inflammatory phases of the treatment plan. The capacity of the patient to tolerate exercise is extremely variable and depends upon the intensity and magnitude of the original injury and the pathological process as well as individual pain tolerance.

Graduated Exercise and Full Strength Training. After the patient has reached his early rehabilitative strength and flexibility goals, objective strength testing is monitored until it has returned to near normal levels of strength, endurance, and flexibility. When this goal is reached, it is then appropriate to continue the strength training program to even higher conditioning levels than the pre-injury state. This is important, since a return only to the pre-injury level still offers the potential for significant force overload.

Continuation of the strength and endurance exercise program includes either isokinetic and/or isotonic interspaced with the isoflex system of exercises. Prior to a final return to a sport or occupational activity, the patient should be capable of anaerobic sprint repetitions to fatigue without major activity pain. As the patient returns to his previous sport

or occupational activity, initial modifications of intensity and duration are recommended and gradual resumption of normal activity is encouraged.

SURGICAL TREATMENT

Historical Review. The recent literature concerning the surgical treatment of tennis elbow might be considered to have begun with Hohmann in 1927, who described release of the extensor aponeurosis at the level of the lateral epicondyle,[17] a technique now commonly referred to as a muscle slide procedure.[21] Modifications of Hohmann's procedure have included percutaneous approaches as well as destruction of the extensor aponeurosis by electrical cautery. Actual pathologic changes were not recognized or described by Hohmann.

Cyriax published an extensive review article in 1936,[10] correctly concluding that the origin of the extensor brevis was the major site of pathology. Interestingly, he theorized that the extensor brevis origin was often partially torn, and he reported success in treating it by closed manipulation of passive forceful elbow extension and forearm supination, thereby presumably converting a partial to a complete tear.

Bosworth in 1955 reported a series of 27 elbows utilizing four different techniques.[6] He suggested that this third technique, which included a release of the extensor aponeurosis as well as the orbicular ligament in and about the radial head, was seemingly curative, although only four patients had been so treated. Bosworth also correctly observed the intimate relationship between the orbicular ligament and the subtendinous layers of the finger and wrist extensors. With release of the extensor aponeurosis and generous removal of the orbicular ligament, he undoubtedly released or removed the origin of the extensor brevis. Curiously, Bosworth performed the Hohmann-type operation in 17 instances, but "all" still had some complaints.

After surgery, "the duration of disability postoperatively extended from 8 days to 6 weeks except in two cases." Although the definition of "disability" is vague, such a statement is difficult to accept by present standards or observations.

In a fascinating application of the conviction that the origin of the extensor brevis was the source of pathology, Garden reported 50 instances in which the extensor brevis tendon was lengthened in the *distal forearm*.[12] He concluded, as had others,[10] that active muscular contraction of the extensor carpi radialis brevis causes pain, but he theorized that the intimate relationship of the origin of the brevis to the orbicular ligament may also be part of the problem. He appreciated the potential of a much higher morbidity with the Bosworth technique of resecting a portion of the annular ligament than was reported by Bosworth.[6] In 44 cases treated by open Z-plasty lengthening at the musculotendinous junction, no operative site problems occurred. In six cases the ECRB was lengthened at wrist level with significant postoperative wrist pain. Full relief was apparently obtained in all cases, a result not duplicated by others.* Obtaining grip and wrist extensor dynamometer data, Garden concluded: "This operation causes diminution neither of the power of wrist dorsiflexion nor in the efficiency of the grip." However, a critical review of his data reveals 20 cases (40 per cent) in which strength had not returned to normal.

Goldie in 1964 presented a comprehensive thesis that for the first time detailed pathologic changes in the subtendinous tissue in and about the lateral epicondyle in 49 patients.[13] He described tendinous tissue that was invaded in "many places" by cellular infiltration of round and fibroblastic cells as well as vascular infiltrates. He described this tissue as granular in nature.

Kaplan reported three cases of resection of the radial nerve to the lateral epicondyle and lateral articular areas with no attempt to identify or remove pathologic tissues.[20] He noted excellent pain relief, but, interestingly, denervation of a motor branch to the extensor brevis probably occurred with this technique. The length of the surgical incision was approximately 6 inches, and the hospital stay was 5, 6, and 7 days in the three cases. Roles and Maudsley described 33 patients who responded to surgical decompression of the radial nerve.[38] The surgery was performed by 11 different surgeons over a 10-year period. Careful review of the article reveals that the origin of the extensor brevis may possibly have been released in these cases as a necessary component of decompression of the distal canal of the radial nerve as it enters the forearm.

Surgical Pathology

A basic principle of any orthopedic surgery is that a clear definition of the pathology is essential for a well-conceived surgical proce-

dure that will provide consistently reliable results. In many of the prior surgical procedures described, with the exception of those reported by Goldie and Coonrad, this principle has not been strictly followed. Because the extensor brevis origin is largely covered by the muscle belly of the extensor carpi radialis longus, a thorough release of the common extensor origin may correct the pathology even if it is not directly visualized.

Coonrad described gross pathologic changes (including tears) in and about the tendinous structures in both medial and lateral tennis elbow but did not comment on histologic changes.[7] Blazina et al. have suggested that the major pathological tendon changes in chronic tendinitis occur by moderate but repetitive overload that results in microrupture of the normal tendinous tissue and secondary replacement by the resulting pathologic healing process.[4] Although this theory is attractive, I believe that a more likely sequence of events is similar to that described by McNab in the rotator cuff region of the shoulder[23, 24]—namely, a vascular compromise, an altered nutritional state, and force overload cause angiofibroblastic changes and then ultimate rupture of these vulnerable tissues.[32] In any event, actual disruption of tissue, usually incomplete, occurs in approximately 35 per cent of cases.

Postoperative Rehabilitation

The postoperative rehabilitation of either lateral or medial tennis elbow follows the treatment principles outlined for conservative care and detailed in Chapter 31. The elbow is maintained in an elbow immobilizer in the immediate postoperative period for 8 days. Limbering activities are thereafter undertaken, generally by working the arm actively in a warm shower for a period of 1 week followed by a gradual return to a strength-training exercise (usually isoflex exercise) with protection by a medial or lateral counterforce brace (usually for the first week of strength training).[27] For recreational tennis, it is usual to start easy strokes approximately 6 weeks from the time of surgery. For return to competitive athletics or occupation, the increase in intensity should be gradual and gentle with counterforce brace protection until full strength has returned to the extremity as measured by cybex or dynamometer tests and circumferential girth plus satisfactory completion of the exercise program. Full strength return for competitive athletics, even at the world class level, averages 4 to 5

---

*Carroll, R. E.: Personal communication.

months for lateral elbow tendinitis and 5 to 6 months for medial elbow tendinitis.

Surgical Results

Eighty-five per cent of patients in our experience and that of others can expect full return to all prior activities without pain.[7,31] In 12 per cent improvement has occurred with some pain during aggressive activities, but often the patient is able to participate in sports. In about 3 per cent no improvement is obtained, and the surgery is considered a failure. The failures may be related to entrapment of the posterior interosseous nerve as the cause of symptoms.[41]

AUTHOR'S PREFERRED TREATMENT METHOD

Selection Factors for Surgery

Duration of Symptoms. Patients who have undergone a high-quality conservative treatment program but have symptoms lingering for more than 1 year are more likely to have category 3 pathologic changes.

Calcification. Calcification in or about the tendinous attachment is present in about 20 per cent of those undergoing surgery and suggests a refractory process (Fig. 28–9).

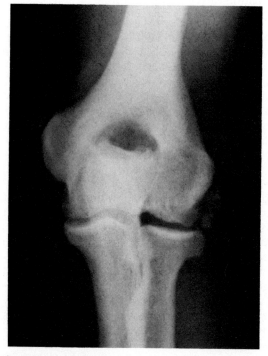

Figure 28–9. Calcification in and about the lateral epicondyle occurs in 22 per cent of surgical cases.

Multiple Cortisone Injections. Patients who have received three or more cortisone injections in or about the same area are surgical candidates. Considerations in this group are twofold. First, the patient's symptoms were of such severity that cortisone injection was warranted and may have indicated a higher pathologic category at the time the patient sought clinical help. Second, the studies of Unverferth suggest that large amounts of cortisone infiltration do have a deleterious effect on the quality of the tendon that is different from the true pathologic changes of angiofibroblastic hyperplasia.[40]

Pain (Constant) Without Activity. Pain that alters the routine daily function suggests the need for surgery.

Ease of Injection Flow. It has been my observation that easy injection flow into the triangular recess under the extensor brevis origin, just distal and anterior to the lateral epicondyle, invariably indicates loosened edematous tissue. This injection "feel" is a clear indication that category 3 pathologic changes are present.[33]

Patient Frustration. Patients with chronic tendinitis are well aware that the situation is not a major threat to "life or limb" and have the option to modify their work or recreational activities. Those unwilling to modify their activity level are likely candidates for surgical intervention. This type of patient usually is highly motivated and is likely to be an excellent patient in terms of postoperative rehabilitation.

Technique

Identification of Pathology. Identification and excision of all pathologic tendinous tissue generally includes most, if not the entire origin, of the extensor carpi radialis brevis (Fig. 28–10). On occasion, this also includes the anterior aspects of the extensor aponeurosis and rarely, the removal of pathologic tissue from the underside of the extensor longus. When the extensor brevis origin is excised, the intimate relationship between the fascia of the extensor brevis and the orbicular ligament eliminates any retraction of the extensor brevis distally. Maintenance of normal muscle length ensures a normal leverage length of the remainder of the musculotendinous unit of the extensor brevis and increases the potential for a return to normal strength.

Vascular Enhancement. Once the pathologic tissue has been removed, a tissue defect is present in varying degrees. Because this region of the lateral elbow is completely housed

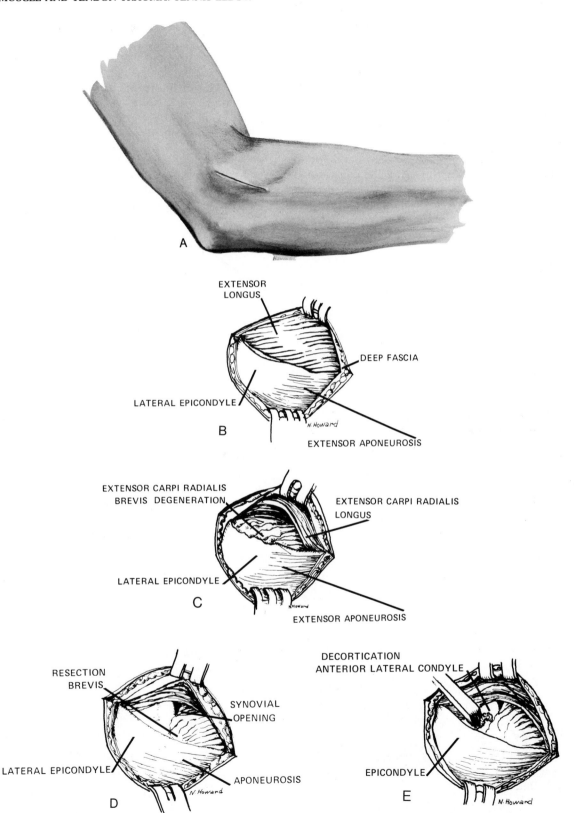

Figure 28–10. A, Skin incision. B, Incision at interface of extensor longus and aponeurosis. C, Anterior retraction of extensor longus exposing the origin of the extensor brevis. D, Excision of pathologic tissue, usually of extensor brevis origin. A small incision may be made through the synovium for visual inspection of the lateral compartment. E, Vascular enhancement is accomplished by osteotome decortication as shown, or three to four holes (five sixty-fourths inch) are drilled through cortical bone to cancellous areas to enhance vascular supply. Drilling causes less postoperative pain. (From Nirschl, R. P., and Pettrone, F.: Tennis Elbow. The Surgical Treatment of Lateral Epicondylitis. J. Bone Joint Surg. 61A:832, 1979).

on one side by hard cortical bone, it is appropriate to attempt to enhance the blood supply by decortication or by drilling four or five small holes through the cortical bone into the cancellous area, thereby encouraging extravascular ingrowth (Fig. 28–10).

Tissue Repair. Simply imbricating the extensor longus over the anterior edge of the extensor aponeurosis tends to block full elbow extension. Restoration of the normal anatomic position, by sewing the posterior edge of the extensor longus to the anterior edge of the extensor aponeurosis, has been quite success-

ful in relieving pain without causing loss of motion. Surgical scar tissue has a different microscopic character than the histologic appearance of the pathologic angiofibroblastic hyperplasia of tendinitis and also has much different healing, pain, and maturation characteristics.

Because all the incisions are made longitudinally and in most cases do not disturb the extensor aponeurosis attachment to the lateral epicondyle, the surgery provides a very firm anchoring point for prompt initiation of the postoperative rehabilitative exercises.

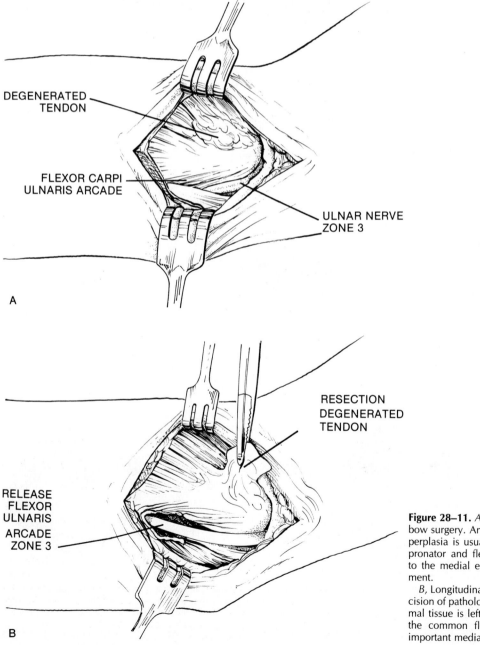

Figure 28–11. *A,* Medial tennis elbow surgery. Angiofibroblastic hyperplasia is usually located in the pronator and flexor radialis close to the medial epicondylar attachment.

B, Longitudinal and elliptical excision of pathologic tissue. All normal tissue is left attached because the common flexor origin is an important medial stabilizer.

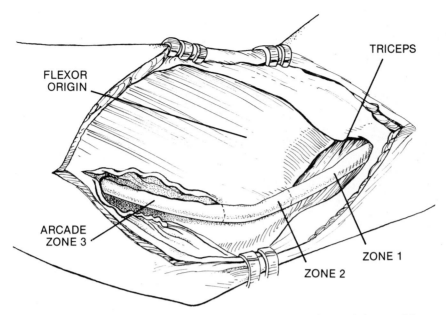

Figure 28–12. Ulnar nerve zones at medial epicondylar groove. Zone 1: proximal to medial epicondyle; zone 2: at medial epicondyle; zone 3: distal to medial epicondyle. Zone 3 includes penetration of the nerve through the flexor ulnaris arcade and is the most common site for compression neurapraxia of the ulnar nerve.

Associated Considerations

In approximately 22 per cent of cases there is some calcification in either the extensor brevis origin or, more commonly, at the tip of the lateral epicondyle, which is often noted after a direct blow to the lateral epicondyle. On occasion, a partial peelback of the origin of the extensor aponeurosis and removal of the calcification is undertaken. Routine reattachment of the aponeurosis to the posterior edge of the extensor longus is then instituted. It is rarely necessary to remove a major portion of the aponeurosis from the lateral epicondyle.

Tears in the extensor brevis occur in 35 per cent of cases and occasionally may extend through the synovium and into the lateral compartment of the joint. This associated finding is also of no basic consequence. In the performance of the operation, we routinely make a small opening in the synovium to inspect the lateral articular compartment. During inspection of the lateral compartment in many elderly patients (e.g., those in the fifth and sixth decades), an occasional small erosion of the hyaline cartilaginous surface may be detected on the radial head.[25] It is extremely rare to find any other pathologic changes in the lateral compartment without additional unrelated trauma or disease such as osteochondritis dissecans, traumatic ar-

thritis, osteocartilaginous loose bodies, rheumatoid arthritis, and the like.

Medial Tennis Elbow

Medial tennis elbow may occur independently or may on occasion be associated with lateral tennis elbow. Using longitudinal incisions, the area of pathology is generally found to be at the interface between the pronator teres and the flexor carpi radialis but has also been noted on the underside of the flexor sublimus origin as well as in the palmaris longus and the flexor carpi ulnaris (Fig. 28–11). Major rupture in any of these areas may occur from time to time but is not nearly as common as in lateral tennis elbow. Elliptical incisions are used to remove the pathologic tissue (Fig. 28–11). It should be appreciated that the common flexor origin is a very important stabilizer for the medial elbow, and previously suggested operations of complete transverse release carry a significant hazard of medial elbow instability that is catastrophic in the racquet and throwing sports.

Ulnar Nerve at the Medial Elbow. In cases of medial tennis elbow that have been operated upon, 60 per cent have had symptoms of ulnar nerve neurapraxia.[28] We have divided the medial epicondylar groove into three zones (Fig. 28–12):

Zone 1: Proximal to the medial epicondyle

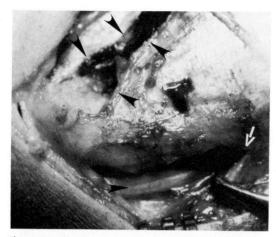

Figure 28–13. Ulnar nerve decompression of left elbow. In most cases decompression of the ulnar nerve in zone 3 is the recommended treatment for compression neurapraxia associated with medial tennis elbow. Surgical photograph after decompression (white arrow) of the ulnar nerve (closed arrow) and resection of *medial* pathologic tissue (black arrows).

Zone 2: At the medial epicondyle
Zone 3: Distal to the medial epicondyle
In patients surgically treated for medial involvement, 60 per cent had some signs and symptoms of ulnar nerve neurapraxia.[28] Similar clinical findings were present in 15 per cent of those with mixed medial and lateral tendinitis.[31]

The symptoms of ulnar nerve neurapraxia are usually localized to the zone 3 level of the medial epicondylar groove and generally are mild, intermittent, and primarily sensory.

They extend to the small and ring fingers without major distortion of ulnar nerve motor function. Tinel's sign is often positive with the signs and symptoms that characteristically occur at times of heavy forearm activity. When symptoms are quiescent, electromyographic and conduction studies are commonly normal.

In the classic case of neurapraxia compression in zone 3, decompression without transfer of the nerve is highly successful and is the recommended procedure (Fig. 28–13).

Indications for Ulnar Nerve Transfer. Ulnar nerve transfer is not to be considered lightly. A proper relaxed anterior transfer requires wide dissection for release and often compromises the vascular supply to the nerve. Additional tissue dissection also increases morbidity and prolongs postoperative rehabilitation. Our criteria for anterior ulnar nerve transfer include the following:

1. Congenital or iatrogenic subluxation or dislocation of the nerve with elbow flexion (Fig. 28–14).
2. Symptomatic tension neurapraxia secondary to abnormal skeletal valgus (such as old fracture) or major ligamentous valgus instability.
3. Necessary transfer for surgical exposure of the medial elbow compartment or for ligament reconstruction.
4. Intractible hostile environment (such as a scar from a prior injury or surgery).

Most symptomatic ulnar nerve neurapraxia is, however, secondary to zone 3 compression. Simple surgical decompression without an-

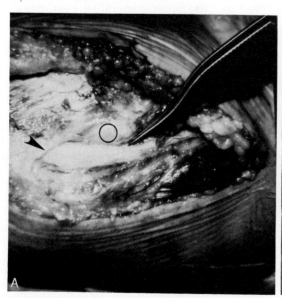
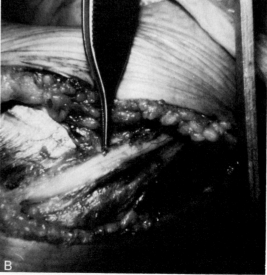

Figure 28–14. *A,* Medial epicondylitis with bursa over right medial epicondyle (circle). Forceps is on ulnar nerve. Arrow at flexor ulnaris arcade. With flexion, the ulnar nerve subluxes over the epicondyle (*B*).

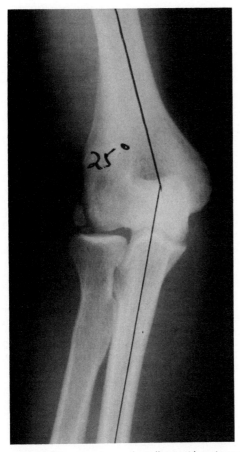

Figure 28–15. Roentgenogram of an elbow with an increased valgus angle. Ligamentous instability or skeletal deformity may cause tension neurapraxia of the ulnar nerve and is an indication for anterior nerve transfer. Ligamentous instability causes compression of the lateral compartment, as suggested by calcification.

collateral ligament reconstruction as with the palmaris longus free tendon graft. Osteocartilaginous loose bodies are best removed when present, especially if joint locking occurs.

If ulnar nerve tension neurapraxia occurs in association with valgus instability, anterior transfer may be indicated (Fig. 28–15).

terior transfer will suffice in this patient group. It is emphasized that accurate clinical evaluation should be made preoperatively and a limited early exposure be performed to avoid iatrogenic dislocation.

Medial Elbow Instability. The classic case of medial tennis elbow may occasionally have associated medial instability. The usual cause is major ligamentous injury from aggressive valgus overload as occurs in baseball or javelin throwing. Such instability often results in compression of the lateral compartment and olecranon shift with secondary formation of osteocartilaginous loose bodies in the lateral and posterior compartments. Stretch neuropraxia of the ulnar nerve may also occur under these circumstances.

With sudden ligamentous rupture, primary repair is indicated (see Chapter 30). Chronic medial instability may benefit from medial

References

1. Balasubramaniam, P., and Prathap, K.: The Effect of Injection of Hydrocortisone into Rabbit Calcaneal Tendons. J. Bone Joint Surg. **54B**:729, 1972.
2. Bassett, C. A. L.: Pulsing Electromagnetic Fields: A New Method to Modify Cell Behavior in Calcified and Noncalcified Tissues. Calcif. Tissue Int. **34**:1, 1982.
3. Bassett, C. A. L., Choksh, H. R., Hernandez, E., Pawlik, R. J., and Strap, M.: The Effect of Pulsing Electromagnetic Fields on Cellular Calcium and Calcification of Non-unions. In Brighton, C. T., Black, J., and Pollack, S. R. (eds.): Electrical Properties of Bone and Cartilage, Experimental Effects and Clinical Applications. New York, Grune & Stratton, 1979.
4. Blazina, H. E., Kerlan, R. K., Jobe, F. W., Carter, J. S., and Carlson, G. J.: Jumper's Knee. Orthop. Clin. North Am. **413**:665, 1973.
5. Bernhang, A. M.: The Many Causes of Tennis Elbow. N.Y. State J. Med. **79(9)**:1363, 1979.
6. Bosworth, D. H.: The Role of the Orbicular Ligament in Tennis Elbow. J. Bone Joint Surg. **37A**:527, 1955.
7. Coonrad, R. W., and Hooper, W. R.: Tennis Elbow. Its Course, Natural History, Conservative and Surgical Management. J. Bone Joint Surg. **55A**:1177, 1973.
8. Carroll, R. E.: Personal communication.
9. Carp, L.: Tennis Elbow Caused by Radiohumeral Bursitis. Arch. Surg. **24**:905, 1932.
10. Cyriax, J. H.: The Pathology and Treatment of Tennis Elbow. J. Bone Joint Surg. **18(4)**:921, 1936.
11. Froimson, A. I.: Treatment of Tennis Elbow with Forearm Support Band. J. Bone Joint Surg. **53A**:183, 1971.
12. Garden, R. S.: Tennis Elbow. J. Bone Joint Surg. **43B**:100, 1961.
13. Goldie, I.: Epicondylitis Lateralis Humeri (Epicondylalgia or Tennis Elbow). A Pathogenetical Study. Acta Chir. Scand. Suppl. **339**, 1964.
14. Groppel, J. L., Nirschl, R. P., Pfantsch, E., and Greer, N.: A Mechanical and Electromyographical Analysis of the Effects of Various Joint Counterforce Braces on the Tennis Player. Unpublished data, 1984.
15. Groppel, J. L., Nirschl, R. P., Sholes, J., and Sobel, J.: A Mechanical Comparison of an Iso-Flex Exercise Device to the Use of Free Weights. Unpublished data, 1984.
16. Gunn, C. C., and Milbrandt, W. E.: Tennis Elbow and the Cervical Spine. Can. Med. Assoc. J. **114**:803, 1976.
17. Hohmann, G.: Das Wesen und die Behandlung des Sogenannten Tennissellenbogens. Munch. Med. Wehnschr. **80**:250, 1933.
18. Ilfeld, F. W., and Field, S. M.: Treatment of Tennis Elbow: Use of Special Brace. J.A.M.A. **195(2)**:67, 1966.
19. Indelicato, P. A., Jobe, F. W., Kerlan, R. K., Carter, V. S., Shields, C. L., and Lombardo, S. J.: Correctable

Elbow Lesions in Professional Baseball Players. A Review of 25 Cases. Am. J. Sports Med. **7(1)**:72, 1979.

20. Kaplan, E. B.: Treatment of Tennis Elbow (Epicondylitis) by Denervation. J. Bone Joint Surg. **41A**:147, 1959.

21. Michele, A. A., and Krueger, F. J.: Lateral Epicondylitis of the Elbow Treated by Fasciotomy. Surgery **39**:277, 1956.

22. Major, H. P.: Lawn-Tennis Elbow. Br. Med. J. **2**:557, 1883.

23. McNab, I.: Rotator Cuff Tendinitis. Ann. R. Coll. Surg. Engl. **53(5)**:271, 1973.

24. Moseley, H. F., and Goldie, I.: The Arterial Pattern of the Rotator Cuff of the Shoulder. J. Bone Joint Surg. **45B**:780, 1963.

25. Newman, J. H., and Goodfellow, J. W.: Fibrillation of the Head of the Radius: One Cause of Tennis Elbow. J. Bone Joint Surg. **57B**:115, 1975.

26. Nirschl, R. P.: Arm Care. Arlington, Va., Med. Sprts Pub., 1983.

27. Nirschl, R. P.: Isoflex Exercise System. Arlington, Med. Sports Pub., 1983.

28. Nirschl, R. P.: Medical Tennis Elbow. The Surgical Treatment. Read at the Annual Meeting of the American Academy of Orthopedic Surgeons, Atlanta, Ga., March 1, 1980.

29. Nirschl, R. P.: Mesenchymal Syndrome. Virginia Med. M. **96**:659, 1969.

30. Nirschl, R. P.: Tennis Elbow. Orthop. Clin. North Am. **4(3)**:787, 1973.

31. Nirschl, R. P., and Pettrone, F.: Tennis Elbow. The Surgical Treatment of Lateral Epicondylitis. J. Bone Joint Surg. **61A**:832, 1979.

32. Nirschl, R. P., and Sobel, J.: Conservative Treatment of Tennis Elbow. Phys. Sports Med. **9**:42, 1981.

33. Nirschl, R. P.: Unpublished data, 1982.

34. Osgood, R. B.: Radiohumeral Bursitis, Epicondylitis, Epicondylalgia (Tennis Elbow). A Personal Experience. Arch. Surg. **4**:420, 1922.

35. Percy, C., and Carson, J. D.: Use of DMSO in Tennis Elbow and Rotator Cuff Tendinitis: Double Blind Study. Med. Sci., Sports Exercise **13**:215, 1981.

36. Priest, J. D., Braden, V., and Gerberich, J. G.: The Elbow and Tennis (Part I). Phys. Sports Med. **8(4)**:80, 1980.

37. Priest, J. D., Braden, V., and Gerberich, J. G.: The Elbow and Tennis (Part II). Phys. Sports Med. **8(5)**:77, 1980.

38. Roles, N. C., and Maudsley, R. H.: Radial Tunnel Syndrome, Resistant Tennis Elbow as a Nerve Entrapment. J. Bone Joint Surg. **54B**:499, 1972.

39. Runge, F.: Zur Genese und Behandlung des Schreibekrampfes. Berl. Klin. Wnschr. **10**:245, 1873.

40. Unverferth, L. J., and Olix, M. L.: The Effect of Local Steroid Injection on Tendon. J. Sports Med. **1(4)**:31, 1973.

41. Werner, C. O.: Lateral Elbow Pain and Posterior Interosseous Nerve Entrapment. Acta Orthop. Scand. Suppl. **174**:1, 1979.

42. Woods, G. W., Tullos, H. S., and King, J. W.: The Throwing Arm. Elbow Joint Injuries. J. Sports Med. **1(4)**:43, 1973.

CHAPTER 29

Nerve Injuries

FRANK W. JOBE and GARY S. FANTON

Ulnar neuritis at the elbow, which has been well described in the literature, may be related to a number of etiologic factors.[1, 20, 21] Among these are direct trauma, traction, recurrent subluxation or dislocation, congenital or developmental soft tissue anomalies, bony changes secondary to fracture or degenerative disease, cubital tunnel compression, metabolic or endocrine abnormalities, inflammatory conditions, and tumors. The athlete, of course, is susceptible to any of these injurious conditions, and frequently more than one pathologic process is encountered. Because of the intensity of his activities and the biomechanical forces at play, however, the athlete is more likely to develop ulnar nerve irritation on a mechanical basis, i.e. from stretch, friction, or compression.

This chapter will focus on the events that lead to ulnar neuritis in the athlete, who is best exemplified by the player involved in throwing or racquet sports, and will emphasize the anatomic and biomechanical forces that predispose to this problem.

ANATOMY

The ulnar nerve enters the arm as a continuation of the medial cord of the brachial plexus. As it passes from the anterior compartment of the brachium into the posterior compartment, it penetrates a thick fibrous raphe, which was first described by Struthers in 1854.[18] This arcade of fibrous tissue is formed by components of the medial intermuscular septum, superficial muscular fibers of the medial head of the triceps, and the deep investing fascia of the arm.[17] The arcade of Struthers is located approximately 8 cm above the medial epicondyle and may present a source of ulnar nerve entrapment either primarily or as a result of tethering after ulnar nerve transposition surgery.

As the ulnar nerve courses behind the medial epicondyle, it enters the cubital tunnel, whose boundaries are the ulnar collateral ligament of the elbow, the medial edge of the trochlea, and the medial epicondylar groove.[21]

The roof of this tunnel is formed by the triangular arcuate ligament that extends from the medial epicondyle to the medial border of the olecranon process and acts as the tendinous origin of the flexor carpi ulnaris muscle. The nerve then continues into the forearm between the humeral and ulnar heads of this muscle.

During the normal course of elbow motion several changes take place in the surrounding soft tissue. For each 45 degrees of flexion the arcuate ligament must stretch nearly 5 mm, and at 90 degrees of flexion the proximal edge becomes taut.[20] The ulnar collateral ligament, on the other hand, tends to relax and bulge slightly with elbow flexion.[4] Combined, these changes can significantly reduce the volume of the cubital tunnel. In addition, Apfelberg and Larson have shown that the ulnar nerve elongates an average of 4.7 mm during elbow flexion and that the medial head of the triceps can push the nerve 7 mm medially.[1] Thus, the ulnar nerve is not normally a fixed structure at the elbow but requires freedom to move both longitudinally and medially during elbow motion.

PATHOPHYSIOLOGY

In the athlete ulnar neuritis appears to be one syndrome in a spectrum of disorders that affect the medial side of the elbow. During the act of pitching, for example, considerable tensile forces are generated on the medial side of the elbow, whereas compressive forces are predominant at the radiocapitellar articulation. In one overhead baseball pitch, the time from forward arm swing to release takes less than 400 msec and may generate ball velocities of up to 130 feet per second.[2] Concomitantly, the elbow rapidly progresses from a 90-degree flexed position to full extension, and the forearm is swung into strong pronation. The harder the ball is thrown, the more the forearm lags behind the brachium at ball release and the greater the valgus stresses applied at the elbow.

With chronic activity adaptive physical

changes may become evident.[10, 11] King et al., in an analysis of the pitching arms of 50 professional baseball players, found such changes as bony hypertrophy of the humerus, enlargement of the olecranon and olecranon fossa, fixed flexion contracture of the elbow, and muscle hypertrophy when compared with the nondominant arm.[10] An increased incidence of valgus deformity at the elbow also was noted. Similar changes have been described in the serving arm of top-level tennis players.

Ulnar neuritis in the athlete therefore can result from physiologic as well as from pathologic responses to specific activity. The thrower may develop traction neuritis from an attenuated ulnar collateral ligament that allows the medial side of the joint to "open up" or from progressive fixed flexion and valgus deformity. The nerve may become tethered by scar formation, traction spurs, calcific deposits in or around the medial collateral ligament, or from an irregular ulnar groove secondary to degenerative changes or an old medial epicondylar separation.[5, 8, 9]

Especially common is entrapment of the nerve beneath a thickened arcuate ligament, the so-called Osborne lesion.[14, 15] This may be seen in conjunction with hypertrophy of the flexor musculature of the forearm. Pechan and Julis demonstrated elevation of intraneural pressures by direct measurement in the ulnar nerve with flexion of the elbow at 90 degrees and extension of the wrist.[16] This is probably caused by both the physiologic stretch of the nerve and external compression from the overlying aponeurosis of the flexor carpi ulnaris muscle. Further flexion of the elbow, extension of the wrist, and abduction of the shoulder, such as occurs in the early stages of the overhead pitch, can elevate the pressure up to six times higher than it is in the relaxed nerve.[16] Compression of this magnitude not only may lead to fibrosis from direct injury but actually may exceed the capillary perfusion pressures, and if prolonged or continually repeated, it may lead to a localized ischemic insult.

Another common finding is friction neuritis from recurrent dislocation of the nerve anterior to the medial epicondyle. Childress noted that 16.2 per cent of the population demonstrates recurrent dislocation of the ulnar nerve as the elbow is taken from complete extension to full flexion.[3] This hypermobility of the nerve is secondary to congenital or developmental laxity of the soft tissue constraints that normally hold it anatomically in the epicondylar groove. He found that those nerves that

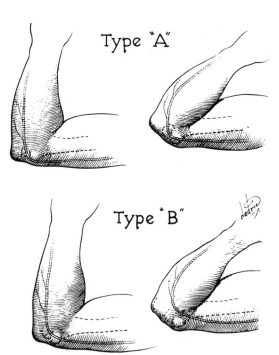

Figure 29–1. Ulnar nerve instability may be incomplete, type A, or complete, type B. (From Childress, H. M.: Recurrent ulnar nerve dislocation at the elbow. Clin. Orthop. Rel. Res. 108:168–173, 1975.)

incompletely dislocate over the medial epicondyle (type A) are more susceptible to direct trauma, whereas those that completely dislocate anterior to the epicondyle (type B) are more prone to develop friction neuritis (Fig. 29–1).

Finally, compression of the ulnar nerve may be seen in association with hypertrophy of the medial head of the triceps or anconeus epitrochlearis muscle.[14, 20] This condition is occasionally encountered in the top-level pitcher or weight lifter.[4]

Thus, any one of a number of pathologic changes may lead eventually to ulnar neuritis in the athlete. Compression in the soft tissues above the elbow or in the cubital tunnel, friction secondary to hypermobility of the nerve, tethering of its normal gliding motion as a result of adhesions, inflammation, bony alterations, muscle hypertrophy, and direct trauma can all play a role and must be considered before proper treatment can be rendered.

CLINICAL PRESENTATION

The clinical findings of ulnar neuritis at the elbow in the athlete are not unlike those seen in the general population. Numbness and tingling in the little and ring fingers are encountered early and usually precede any detectable

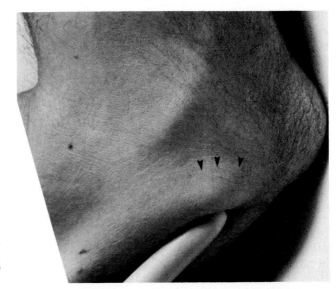

Figure 29–2. Subluxed ulnar nerve (arrows) occurring bilaterally suggests congenital predisposition. Symptoms were intermittent and usually related to direct pressure.

motor weakness of the hand. Weakness of the flexor carpi ulnaris and flexor digitorum profundus is rarely encountered because the nerve fibers to these muscles are the most deeply situated in the cubital tunnel and therefore are usually spared.[19] Pain in the elbow with radiation down the ulnar aspect of the forearm to the hand is particularly common. Clumsiness or heaviness of the hand and fingers, especially after pitching a few innings, may be the major complaint. In most athletes these symptoms are significantly improved or absent with rest but recur with increasing frequency when activity is resumed. A diagnosis of "elbow strain" or "medial epicondylitis" is often entertained, and a course of anti-inflammatory medications or local injections is tried with little or no relief. The athlete with recurrent dislocation of the ulnar nerve may complain of a painful snapping or popping sensation when the elbow is rapidly flexed and extended, with sharp pains radiating into the forearm and hand. The nerve may feel thickened or "doughy" and can often be manually subluxed or dislocated from the groove (Fig. 29–2).

The diagnosis, therefore, requires a strong clinical suspicion when the player is first seen in the office. Physical findings of hypesthesia or motor weakness of the intrinsic musculature of the hand are subtle at best and are usually absent. Tinel's sign, however, is frequently positive at the epicondylar groove or just below the epicondyle. As mentioned, associated pathology such as ligament laxity, loose bodies, or degenerative changes of the elbow must also be considered, not only as possible sources of nerve irritation but also because treatment should address the entire

spectrum of changes that can take place from sports participation. Electromyography and nerve conduction studies, although helpful when positive, are often nonconfirmatory because of the intermittent nature of the problem.[5] A complete series of elbow roentgenograms including a cubital tunnel view[21] should be performed (Fig. 29–3).

Important also is consideration of nerve compression lesions at other levels.[21] Cervical

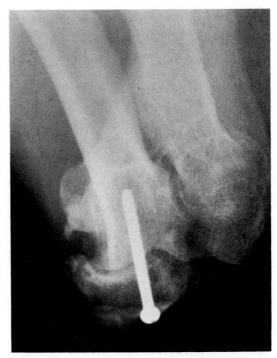

Figure 29–3. Cubital tunnel view showing post-traumatic encroachment of the cubital tunnel from osteophytes occurring at the medial epicondyle and medial margin of the olecranon (arrow).

rib, scalenus anticus syndrome, superior sulcus tumor, cervical disc protrusion with radiculopathy, compression at Guyon's canal, or compression of the deep branch of the ulnar nerve in the hand can all produce symptoms along the ulnar nerve distribution and should be specifically ruled out.

TREATMENT

The management of ulnar neuritis at the elbow usually requires surgical intervention. In an acute situation rest, anti-inflammatory agents, and occasionally immobilization with a plaster splint for 2 to 3 weeks will provide some relief. Throwing is discouraged, and if the neuropathy appears to be traumatic in origin, ample padding is recommended. However, in most athletes conservative management fails to provide significant improvement. Anterior transposition of the ulnar nerve deep to the flexor muscle group allows ample protection from the direct and indirect trauma that occurs during athletic activity. Simple decompression alone, as advocated by others,[6, 15] will not suffice.

Surgical Technique

The surgical technique is similar to that described by Learmonth in 1942.[12, 13] A curved medial incision is made on the ulnar side of the elbow, centered at the medial epicondyle. The medial antebrachial cutaneous nerve branches are always identified and protected. The soft tissues overlying the ulnar nerve are dissected free proximally, up to the arcade of Struthers, which must be released. The arcuate ligament is divided, and the interval

between the heads of the flexor carpi ulnaris muscle is developed distally to the muscular branches of the nerve. The ulnar nerve is then lifted with a Penrose drain and dissected from the epicondylar groove. The distal portion of the intermuscular septum is resected where it forms a thick band above the epicondyle. This prevents kinking or tethering of the nerve after anterior transposition. When considerable scarring or hour-glass constriction of the nerve is encountered, a neurolysis should be performed.

The flexor-pronator muscle group is then detached at the epicondyle. The underlying ulnar collateral ligament can be inspected and, if necessary, the posterior compartment explored by extending the incision proximally along the ulnar border of the olecranon. This affords an extensile approach to the medial side of the elbow and is useful in dealing with other problems that are often encountered in athletes, such as calcific deposits in the ulnar collateral ligament, traction spurs, loose bodies, synovitis, or posterior compartment osteophytes.

The ulnar nerve is then transferred anteriorly to lie on a thin carpet of muscle fibers on the ligamentous structures beneath the flexor muscle mass (Fig. 29–4). These muscles are reattached to the epicondyle by direct suture to a soft tissue cuff or through drill holes made in the bone, and, after skin closure, the elbow is splinted at 90 degrees for 10 days. Range of motion exercises are begun 2 weeks postoperatively, following which gradual strengthening exercises are instituted. About 2 months after surgery, the player is usually ready to start tossing, gradually increasing his throwing speed and power over

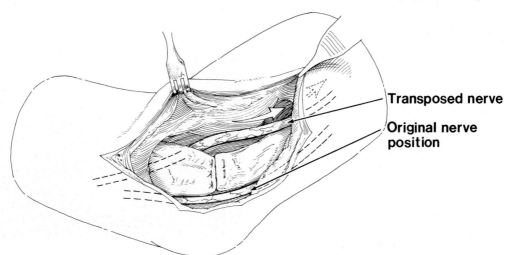

Transposed nerve

Original nerve position

Figure 29–4. Ulnar nerve path, showing its original and transposed positions. Arrows indicate area of arcade of Struthers, which is divided during the surgical procedure.

the next 3 to 4 months, when full activities are allowed.

Elevation and reattachment of the flexor muscle origin has not been a problem, even in top-level pitchers or tennis players. Reattachment has been secure in all cases, and rerupture or tearing near the epicondyle has not been encountered.

The prognosis for players to return to their preoperative level of competition is good, especially when nerve transposition has been performed early. Patients with mild sensory deficits and no detectable motor weakness of the hand usually recover fully, whereas those with more severe lesions and intrinsic muscle paralysis have a less favorable outcome.[6] In nearly all patients the progression of the neuropathy is halted. The severity of the neurologic findings, rather than the duration of the condition or etiology, appears to be the best prognostic indicator. However, one must remember that in athletes, particularly those involved in throwing sports, the prognosis may be related more directly to other associated pathologic conditions encountered at the time of surgery. Ulnar neuritis is but one component in a spectrum of disorders that affects the medial side of the elbow in athletes, and proper functional rehabilitation requires the physician to consider these other problems closely.

References

1. Apfelberg, D. B., and Larson, S. J.: Dynamic Anatomy of the Ulnar Nerve at the Elbow. Plast. Reconstr. Surg. **51**:76, 1973.
2. Atwater, A. E.: Biomechanics of Overarm Throwing Movements and of Throwing Injuries. Exerc. Sport Sci. Rev. **7**:43, 1979.
3. Childress, H. M.: Recurrent Ulnar Nerve Dislocation at the Elbow. Clin. Orthop. **108**:168, 1975.
4. Dangles, C. J., and Bilos, Z. J.: Ulnar Neuritis in a World Champion Weight Lifter. Am. J. Sports Med. **8**:443, 1980.
5. Del Pizzo, W., Jobe, F. W., and Norwood, L.: Ulnar Nerve Entrapment Syndrome in Baseball Players. Am. J. Sports Med. **5**:182, 1977.
6. Foster, R. J., and Edshage, S.: Factors Related to the Outcome of Surgically Managed Compressive Ulnar Neuropathy at the Elbow Level. J. Hand Surg. **6**:181, 1981.
7. Fromison, A. I., and Sahrawi, F.: Treatment of Compression Neuropathy of the Ulnar Nerve at the Elbow by Epicondylectomy and Neurolysis. J. Hand Surg. **5**:391, 1980.
8. Godshall, R. W., and Hansen, C. A.: Traumatic Ulnar Neuropathy in Adolescent Baseball Pitchers. J. Bone Joint Surg. **53A**:359, 1971.
9. Hang, Y.: Tardy Ulnar Neuritis in a Little League Baseball Player. Am. J. Sports Med. **9**:244, 1981.
10. King, J. W., Brelsford, H. J., and Tullos, H. S.: Analysis of the Pitching Arm of the Professional Baseball Pitcher. Clin. Orthop. **67**:116, 1969.
11. Larson, R. L., et al.: Little League Survey: The Eugene Study. Am. J. Sports Med. **4**:201, 1976.
12. Learmonth, J. R.: A Technique for Transplanting the Ulnar Nerve. Surg. Gynecol. Obstet. **75**:792, 1942.
13. Leffert, R. D.: Anterior Submuscular Transposition of the Ulnar Nerves by the Learmonth Technique. J. Hand Surg. **7**:147, 1982.
14. MacNicol, M. F.: The results of operation for ulnar neuritis. J. Bone Joint Surg. **61B**:159, 1979.
15. Osborne, G. V.: The Surgical Treatment of Tardy Ulnar Neuritis. J. Bone Joint Surg. **39B**:782, 1957.
16. Pechan, J., and Julis, I.: The Pressure Measurement in the Ulnar Nerve. A Contribution to the Pathophysiology of the Cubital Tunnel Syndrome. J. Biomechanics **8(1)**:75, 1975.
17. Spinner, M., and Kaplan, E. B.: The Relationship of the Ulnar Nerve to the Medial Intermuscular Septum in the Arm and Its Clinical Significance. Hand **8**:239, 1976.
18. Struthers, J.: On Some Points in the Abnormal Anatomy of the Arm. Br. Foreign Med. Chir. Rev. **14**:170, 1854.
19. Sunderland, S.: Intraneural Topography of the Radial, Median, and Ulnar Nerves. Brain **68**:243, 1945.
20. Vanderpool, D. W., et al.: Peripheral Compression Lesions of the Ulnar Nerve. J. Bone Joint Surg. **50B**:792, 1968.
21. Wadsworth, T. G.: The External Compression Syndrome of the Ulnar Nerve at the Cubital Tunnel. Clin. Orthop. **124**:189, 1977.

CHAPTER 30

Ligamentous and Articular Injuries in the Athlete

JAMES B. BENNETT and HUGH S. TULLOS

Athletes at all levels of sports competition are involved in diverse activities such as throwing, catching, hammering, pushing, and pulling. These activities produce significant stresses about the elbow joint. Chronic stress overuse syndromes as well as acute trauma may involve the ligaments, capsule, muscles, and articular surfaces of the joint and subsequently impair elbow function.[1, 5, 6] Acute and chronic elbow pain and instability in the young athlete[39, 50] has been nonspecifically referred to as Little League elbow;[7] in the college athlete acute muscle and ligament rupture and in the professional chronic instability are common pathologic patterns. Fractures about the elbow in conjunction with ligamentous instability are uncommon in competitive athletics and occur with equal regularity in the general population.[3, 8, 10]

Instability about the elbow is primarily a manifestation of valgus stress. Pain, weakness, recurrent posterior, or posterior lateral elbow dislocations may occur as a result. Although varus instability may be present with bone defects at the ulnohumeral articulation, it is associated with major skeletal trauma and bone loss and is rarely seen in the competitive athlete. Likewise, anterior dislocation is associated with massive elbow trauma resulting in fracture of the olecranon with displacement and rupture of the supporting collateral ligaments.[3, 13, 48] Acute neurovascular compromise may occur with massive trauma but rarely occurs in athletic injuries,[26; 32, 40] whereas chronic neurovascular changes are often diagnosed.[53]

FUNCTIONAL ANATOMY

The anatomy of the elbow joint has been discussed in detail in Chapter 2, but the pertinent features are reviewed here.

Ligaments

The lateral or radial collateral ligamentous complex offers varus stability, but this is rarely stressed in the athlete. The radial collateral ligament arises from the lateral epicondyle and inserts not on the radius but on to the annular ligament, which surrounds the head of the radius. An accessory collateral ligament inserts into the ulna (see Chapter 2). The anconeus muscle is a dynamic structure that transverses the radiocapitellar articulation laterally (Fig. 30–1). Both the anconeus muscle and the lateral collateral ligaments form a complex that serves as a static and dynamic lateral stabilizer to the elbow. The broad, fan-shaped medial collateral ligament is composed of three basic parts: an anterior oblique, a posterior oblique, and a transverse ligament (Fig. 30–2). The transverse band is probably of little or no significance. The anterior oblique portion of the medial collateral ligament is a substantial structure originating from the medial epicondyle and inserting into the coronoid process. In extension the anterior fibers become tight (Fig. 30–3), and in flexion the posterior fibers become tight (Fig. 30–4). The posterior oblique ligament is more fan-shaped and inserts on the olecranon; it is tight in flexion only and lax in extension (see Chapter 3). This posterior oblique portion is absent in primates.

Anatomically and biomechanically, the anterior oblique is the major ligamentous support of the medial aspect of the elbow. In cadaveric specimens, selective transection of the posterior oblique ligament fails to create instability of the elbow in any position. With release of the stronger, thicker anterior oblique ligament, however, the elbow demonstrates gross instability to valgus stress. Additional dynamic support is probably afforded by the forearm flexor muscle mass.[43, 44]

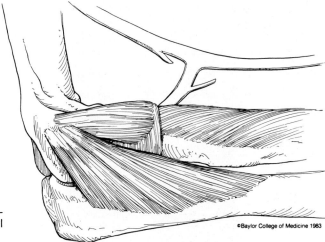

Figure 30–1. Interrelationship of the dynamic stabilizer of the elbow, the anconeus, with the radial collateral and annular ligaments.

©Baylor College of Medicine 1983

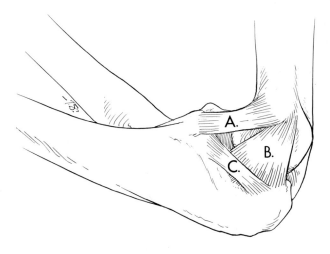

Figure 30–2. Lateral aspect of the elbow demonstrating the three components of the medial collateral ligament complex. *A*, Anterior oblique ligament. *B*, Posterior oblique ligament. *C*, Transverse ligament.

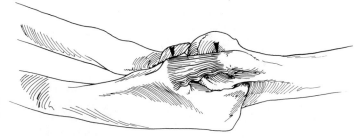

Figure 30–3. In extension, the anterior fibers of the anterior oblique ligament are taut (arrows).

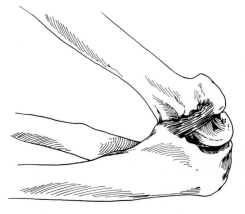

Figure 30–4. In flexion, the posterior fibers of the anterior oblique ligament become taut (arrows).

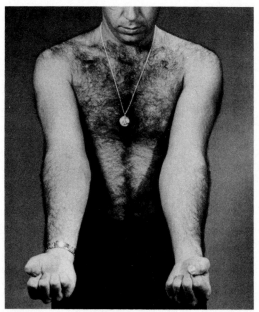

Figure 30–5. Increased valgus and hypertrophy of the left upper extremity in a professional baseball pitcher. (From King, J. W., et al.: Analysis of the pitching arm of the professional baseball pitcher. Clin. Orthop. 67:116, 1969.)

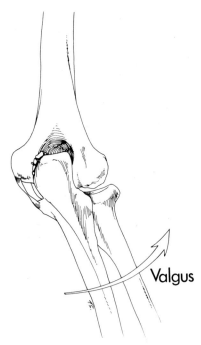

Figure 30–7. Valgus deformity of the elbow results in impingement of the medial tip of the olecranon in the olecranon fossa with loose body formation.

Response to Stress

Although the anterior oblique ligament is the primary stabilizer to valgus stress, the radiocapitellar joint also provides some secondary stability.[35] Clinically, this function is observed in throwing athletes. Repetitive valgus stress associated with the throwing act can result in microtrauma to the anterior oblique ligament. This repetitive insult results in attenuation of the ligament and compression of the lateral articulation. Two physical findings are indicative of this phenomenon: one is the presence of increased forearm valgus (Fig. 30–5), and the second is the presence of an elbow flexion contracture (Fig. 30–6). The first is caused by ligament incompetency; the second is a physiologic attempt at repair or stabilization.[27]

Progressive valgus deformity of the elbow alters the basic biomechanics of the joint. The medial tip of the olecranon may impinge on the medial wall of the olecranon fossa, and loose bodies may result (Fig. 30–7). These

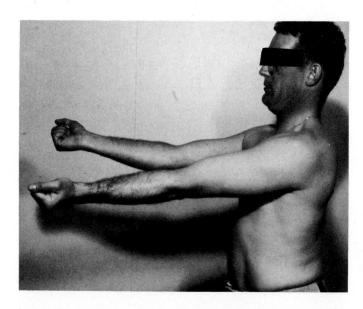

Figure 30–6. Flexion contracture of approximately 15 degrees of the right upper extremity in a professional baseball pitcher.

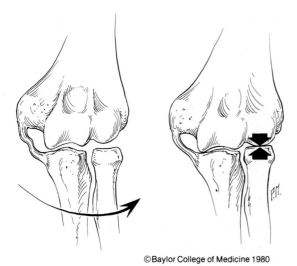

Figure 30–8. Increased valgus stress with an inadequate medial collateral ligament causes excessive compressive loads on the lateral joint, the radiohumeral articulation.

©Baylor College of Medicine 1980

have been reported in approximately 30 per cent of professional pitchers and are age-dependent.

A second change secondary to medial ligament incompetency occurs at the lateral radiocapitellar joint. In normal activity, little compressive force is transmitted to this joint. With increased valgus at the joint and an incompetent medial ligament, increased valgus stress produces abnormal compressive forces on the lateral joint (Fig. 30–8). Thus, the lateral joint acts as a secondary stabilizer to valgus stress when medial stability is lacking.[54]

Extreme examples of this phenomenon can be seen in fracture-dislocations of the elbow in which both the anterior oblique ligament is ruptured and the radial head is removed. Gross instability results, which in some cases can be improved with the use of a radial head spacer in adults.[21, 35, 55]

ACUTE VALGUS STRESS SYNDROMES IN CHILDREN

Medial Epicondylar Stress Lesions ("Little League Elbow")

In young throwing athletes, repetitive valgus stress and flexor forearm muscle pull can produce a relatively subtle stress fracture through the medial epicondyle epiphysis. Clinical manifestations include progressive pain with diminished throwing effectiveness and decreased throwing distance.

Physical findings include only point tenderness over the medial epicondyle and an elbow flexion contracture that is often greater than 15 degrees. Roentgenographic examination demonstrates fragmentation and widening of the epiphyseal lines when compared with the opposite normal elbow (Figs. 30–9 and 30–10). (This may be a normal finding in throwing athletes.) This is a benign entity and responds to rest alone for 2 to 3 weeks. Return to throwing after 6 weeks may be expected.

Medial Epicondylar Fractures

More substantial acute valgus stress from a fall or violent muscle contracture from throwing can produce a fracture through the epiphyseal plate. The result is a painful elbow with point tenderness over the medial epicondyle and an elbow flexion contracture that may be in excess of 15 degrees. The roentgenogram often shows only a minimally dis-

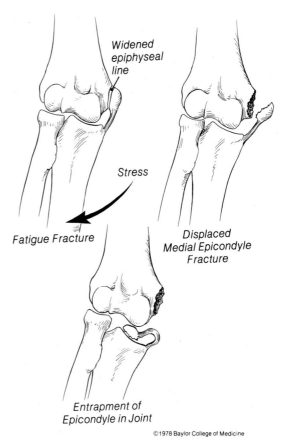

Figure 30–9. Valgus stress may cause a progressive widening of the physis in the growing individual with continued stress; the physis may separate, resulting in displacement and distal retraction. In some instances, the medial epicondyle may become entrapped in the joint. (From Schwab, G. H., et al.: Biomechanics of elbow instability: The role of the medial collateral ligament. Clin. Orthop. 146:42, 1980.)

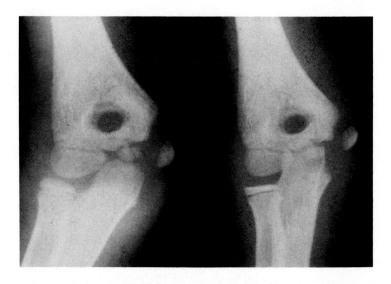

Figure 30–10. Radiograph of the elbow demonstrating normal alignment of the medial epicondyle, which displaces when valgus stress is imparted to the joint. (From Schwab, G. H., et al.: Biomechanics of elbow instabiity: The role of the medial collateral ligament. Clin. Orthop. 146:42, 1980.)

placed epicondylar fragment or marked displacement with or without entrapment of the fragment in the joint. Because the medial epicondyle is the site of origin of the flexor-pronator muscles of the forearm as well as the anterior oblique ligament, these two structures determine the extent of displacement. The weakest area of the medial epicondyle is the cartilaginous epiphyseal growth plate, and therefore separation classically occurs here. Woods has classified these lesions into two types. Type 1 occurs in younger children; the fragment is large, involving the entire epicondyle and often displaces and rotates (Fig. 30–11). The Type 2 fracture occurs in the adolescent; the medial epicondyle is fragmented, and the fracture fragment is small. Because this may be due to avulsion of the extensor tendon, the anterior oblique ligament is usually but not necessarily intact (Fig. 30–12).[62, 63]

Traditional treatment has depended on the number of millimeters of displacement of the fracture fragment. Although it is true that significant displacement (in excess of 3 to 8 mm) does reflect instability, the location of the fragment alone does not always give a true picture of the underlying pathology.

Gravity Stress Test

A simple roentgenogram using gravity to impart valgus stress can be helpful. The patient lies supine, and the shoulder is brought into maximum external rotation (Fig. 30–13). The sagittal plane of the elbow is now parallel to the floor, and the weight of the forearm is resisted only by the flexor forearm mass and

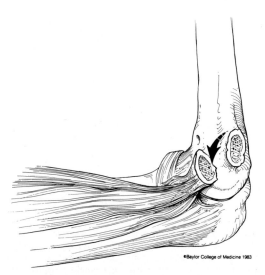

Figure 30–11. Type 1 fracture of the medial epicondyle involves a large fragment that displaces and rotates distal and anteriorly.

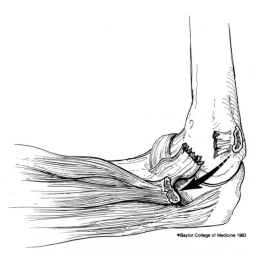

Figure 30–12. Type 2 fracture of the medial epicondyle occurs in the adolescent and involves a small fragmented portion of bone. The anterior oblique ligament does not usually tear, but it may, as demonstrated in this illustration.

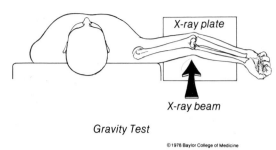

Gravity Test

©1978 Baylor College of Medicine

Figure 30–13. Method of taking a stress view of the elbow. The brachium is placed in full external rotation, allowing the forearm to deliver valgus stress to the elbow joint. (From Schwab, G. H., et al.: Biomechanics of elbow instability: The role of the medial collateral ligament. Clin. Orthop. 146:42, 1980.

the anterior oblique ligament. If the fragment moves distally, both bone and soft tissue continuity have been lost and the elbow is unstable (Fig. 30–10). Surgical reattachment should be considered.

Acute Elbow Dislocations

This topic has been discussed in Chapters 16 and 23 but should be included briefly in the context of the present discussion. Dislocation may occur with or without spontaneous reduction owing to a posteriorly directed force across the partially flexed elbow or from hyperextension. Although it is not mandatory that the medial epicondyle fracture and displace in this instance, this usually occurs in the younger child. With reduction, the displaced fractured medial epicondyle may be trapped within the joint.[43]

Examination reveals pain and tenderness medially along the joint, incomplete extension, and gross instability to valgus stress. If the fragment is incarcerated in the joint, the radiograph demonstrates an asymmetrical reduction or subluxation, absence of the medial epicondyle from its anatomic location, or the presence of the fragment in the joint (Fig. 30–14). Obviously, entrapment cannot occur unless the ligament is attached to the fractured fragment.

Inadequate reduction of unstable medial epicondyle fractures with or without dislocation can produce lifelong disability and difficult reconstructive problems. As the medial epicondyle displaces, the anterior oblique ligament is functionally lengthened. This can predispose to recurrent or late elbow dislocation, as reported by Linscheid and Wheeler.[29] More frequently, however, subtle chronic valgus instability and tardy ulnar nerve palsy may result.

A frequent and often unrecognized complication of displaced medial epicondylar fractures is entrapment of the nerve in the fracture callus. Here instability is rarely manifest; instead, a pronounced elbow flexion contracture develops, and rehabilitation efforts are unsuccessful. Insidious signs of ulnar nerve palsy develop over a period of months as the callus matures. Because reconstruction is difficult, the emphasis should be placed on early diagnosis and prompt anatomic restoration of both the nerve and the medial epicondyle. Rarely, the median nerve may become entrapped in the ulnohumeral joint following reduction of the elbow joint after apparent simple dislocation.[41]

CHRONIC VALGUS STRESS LESIONS IN CHILDREN

Osteochondritis Dissecans

Osteochondritis dissecans is one of the enigmas in orthopedic surgery. Although the condition occurs in many joints, its true etiology has never been clearly elucidated. This is particularly true of the disease in the elbow joint. Reported examples of elbow osteochon-

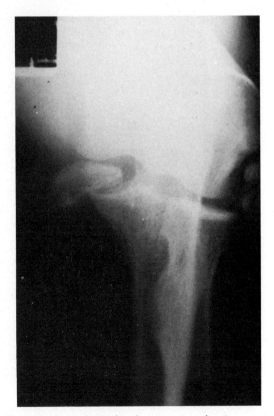

Figure 30–14. Radiographic demonstration of an incarcerating medial epicondyle fragment in the lateral joint line.

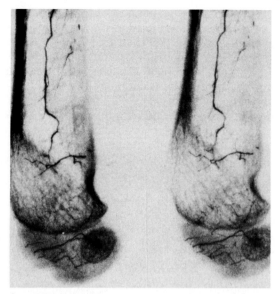

Figure 30–15. Vascular supply to the ossific nucleus of the capitellum. (From Panner, H. J.: A peculiar affection of the capitulum humeri resembling Calvé-Perthes disease of the hip. Acta Radiol. 10:234, 1928.

dritis dissecans are few—the world literature contains approximately 100 cases.

The etiology of the lesion is believed to be vascular insufficiency. Injection studies of the vascularity of the capitellum in children suggest that the blood supply is tenuous with end arterioles terminating at the subchondral plate area (Fig. 30–15). Thus compression forces at the radiocapitellar joint producing focal arterial injury and subsequent bone death is an attractive hypothesis. The implication of this theory is that repetitive stress from throwing in the teen-aged athlete may result in a significant risk of permanent injury. Although the hypothesis is attractive, there is no proof of its validity.

Several authors have emphasized the relationship between the lesion and organized throwing sports. However, a careful review of cases indicates that the lesion can and frequently does occur in the nondominant arm as well as in adolescents who have no specific history of throwing.

At the present time the process may be

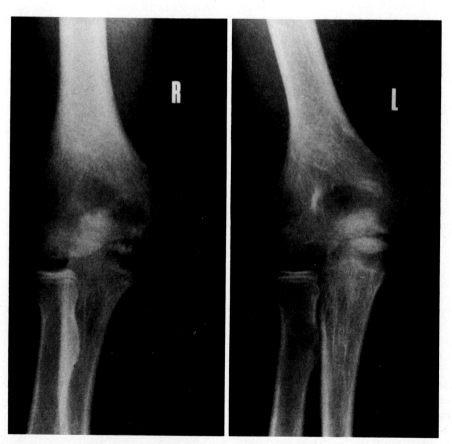

Figure 30–16. In a 13-year-old Little League pitcher with pain at the lateral aspect of the right elbow the radiograph appears reasonably normal, although a vague lucency may be detected on careful inspection. The left joint is shown for comparison.

summarized as a focal lesion that involves the capitellum, occurs in the 10- to 15-year-old age group,[18, 28] and usually, though not always, involves the dominant arm (Fig. 30–16). When present, it is a disabling process.[64] The usual presentation of osteochondritis dissecans is a young adolescent with elbow pain and a flexion contracture of 15 degrees or more. The lesion is usually focal, although in rare instances the entire capitellar fragment may be involved. The initial roentgenogram may be normal. In this instance, the antero-posterior tomogram will be helpful in defining the lesion and its extent (Figs. 30–17 and 30–18).

Because confusion periodically occurs between this entity, osteochondrosis, and Panner's disease, a brief summary of these two disease processes is shown in Table 30–1. Although some believe that osteochondritis dissecans is merely a delayed reflection of Panner's disease, the two conditions are in fact distinct processes.

The natural history of osteochondritis dissecans can be, but is not usually, benign. We

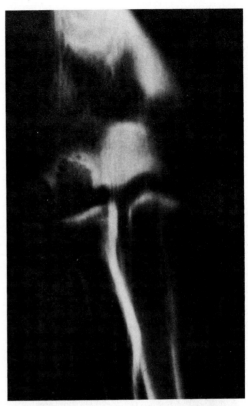

Figure 30–18. Tomogram of a 15-year-old boy showing a generalized involvement of the capitellum with osteochondritis dissecans.

have had the opportunity to follow focal capitellar lesions without exfoliation of the dead fragment for more than 10 years. Healing, although slow, can and does occur with time but residual changes can easily be seen radiographically (Fig. 30–19).[52]

Treatment

The central problem in treatment lies in determining whether the dead segment of capitellum has or has not separated. Is the over-

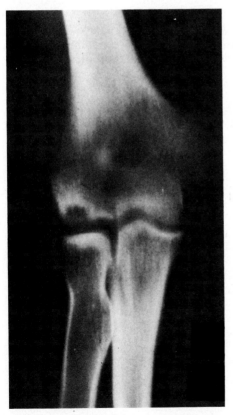

Figure 30–17. Tomogram of the same patient as seen in Figure 30–16 shows a focal but definite lucent area of the capitellum, indicating limited involvement with osteochondritis dissecans.

Table 30–1. **Characteristics of Osteochondritis Dissecans and Panner's Disease**

	Osteochondritis Dissecans	Panner's Disease
Age	Teens	~10
Onset	Insidious	Acute
X-ray	Island of subchondral bone demarcated by a rarefied zone	Fragmentation of entire capitellar ossific nucleus
Loose bodies	Present	Absent
Residual deformity of capitellum	Present	Minimal

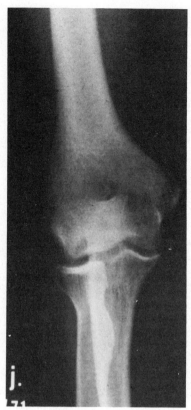

Figure 30–19. Ten-year follow-up of same patient as shown in Figure 30–16 showing a reasonably well-healed lesion of the capitellum.

the lesion with and without the use of bone graft pegs. Although results in these selected series have been good, one wonders whether it is worth the time and effort because spontaneous healing will occur if the elbow is protected.

Reinsertion of an exfoliated loose body is another matter. This is very attractive in view of the significant disability that occurs with simple excision if the lesion is large. Jobe and others[24] have attempted reattachment of large loose fragments by means of arthrotomy and fixation with multiple K wires (Fig. 30–20). In the instances presented, the results were good, and this approach seems to have merit and is worth considering.[22]

ACUTE INSTABILITY IN ADULTS

Elbow Dislocation

Elbow dislocation occurs from trauma to the extended or semiextended elbow (see Chapter 23). As the force of trauma drives the elbow into extension, the anterior capsule is stressed and subsequently ruptures, and the elbow may be forced into hyperextension. Due to the valgus tilt of the trochlea and the usual mechanism of injury, uneven stress focuses at the medial collateral ligament. Continued force levers the olecranon process in its fossa

lying cartilage intact? When a radiographic loose body is clearly seen, the problem is easy, but this is usually not the case. If the pain and contracture persist after 6 weeks of rest, the likelihood of fragmentation may be considered. On occasion, an arthrotomogram may be helpful to define either the articular fracture or the defect itself.[34] Arthroscopy, in the hands of one experienced with the technique, provides the definitive diagnosis.

Treatment is based on the existing stage of the disease process. In general, the lesion will heal if exfoliation has not occurred. In this case, simple rest alone is sufficient as the symptoms gradually disappear and the flexion contracture resolves. Because this process is slow, resumption of throwing sports is contraindicated.

Once separation has occurred, we prefer simple excision of the loose fragment regardless of size. The result will be an elbow that is functional but not able to withstand the prolonged stresses of either athletics or heavy labor activities.[47]

A variety of procedures have been utilized to promote more rapid healing of the lesion. These include drilling from above down to

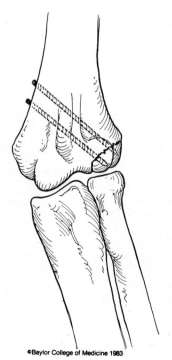

©Baylor College of Medicine 1983

Figure 30–20. Large loose fragments may be attached by arthrotomy and fixation with multiple K-wires.

and opens the joint anteriorly with attenuation or rupture of the anterior oblique ligament.

The coronoid process is levered under the trochlea, and the elbow dislocates—posteriorly because this is the direction of the dominant force and laterally because of the trochlear tilt and the mechanism of the fall.[24]

The clinical problem is, of course, not that some elbows become unstable but rather, why many more do not. We have had opportunities to study joint stability immediately after reduction and have demonstrated that the anterior oblique ligament was intact by valgus stress. How can an elbow dislocate when both medial and lateral collateral ligaments are intact? The answer must be speculative. It is possible that they are not intact at the time of dislocation. Avulsion of the anterior oblique ligament from the medial epicondyle *along with a periosteal sleeve* of soft tissue structures may occur, which would effectively lengthen the medial ligament support and allow the dislocation to occur. With reduction, the periosteum and its intact medial collateral ligament also reduce, and the elbow is stable to valgus stress (Fig. 30–21).

In about 10 per cent of cases elbow dislocation is associated with fracture of the radial head or capitellum. If the radial head is removed, stability has been compromised. In some instances, these elbows are unstable clinically and radiographically, even in 90 degrees of flexion or in plaster (Fig. 30–22). In our opinion, stabilization of this type of

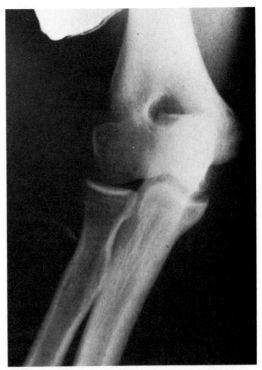

Figure 30–21. Even after dislocation the elbow may be generally stable, as shown with this stress view, due to the intact periosteal sleeve offering integrity to the medial collateral ligament.

elbow dislocation requires surgery. We feel that the simplest mechanism of providing stability in the type IV radial head fracture is the use of a radial head prosthesis or spacer (Fig. 30–23). Even though the primary stabi-

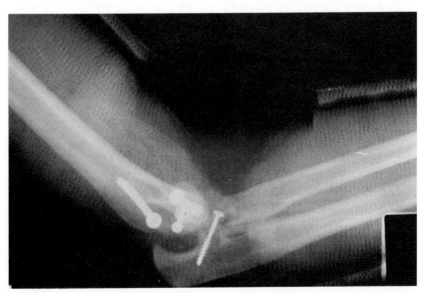

Figure 30–22. Even in a cast a posterior subluxation of the ulna was observed. This was due to the lack of integrity of the soft tissue and inadequate flexion of the elbow.

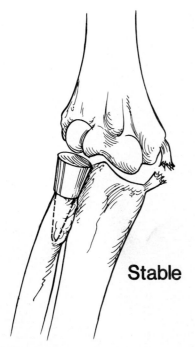

Figure 30–23. Diagram illustrating the value of some form of spacer at the radiocapitellar joint to stabilize the joint when the medial collateral ligament has been disrupted.

lizer, the ligament, has been lost, reconstructive restoration of the secondary defense mechanism may be sufficient to restore stability in the nonathlete and allow the ligament to heal without a stiff joint developing due to prolonged immobilization.[39, 40, 48]

Occasionally, a large fracture of the capitellum may occur. Anatomic restoration can at times be very difficult. If lateral stability of the joint is lost by fragment resection, then direct suture of the lacerated anterior oblique ligament is suggested.[44, 45]

Heterotopic Ossification

The topic of heterotopic ossification has been discussed in detail in Chapter 26. Some authors have correlated the development of this complication with early motion, but we cannot substantiate this position. Indeed, our impression is that heterotopic ossification in the elbow is not significantly different from the disease process in other joints. When fracture motion is present or instability is not resolved, ossification occurs.

Acute Rupture of the Medial Collateral Ligament

Isolated tears of the anterior oblique ligament of the elbow can occur, and the condition has been described in javelin throwers.[58] Although early reports suggested that this injury was rare, during the past 5 to 6 years increasing awareness has made the diagnosis much more common. To date, more than 30 patients have been diagnosed and treated.[36, 52]

The mechanism of injury in throwing athletes is almost pure valgus stress with the elbow flexed to about 60 to 90 degrees. The athlete reports acute onset of pain with or without a sensation that something "popped" in the elbow. Ecchymosis may appear about the medial joint and proximal forearm in 48 to 72 hours. Signs of ulnar nerve irritation may be present.

Differentiation between medial ligament damage and flexor forearm muscle rupture is not difficult. The precise area of local tenderness and the valgus stress test localize the injury to the ligaments (Fig. 30–24), and positive resistive flexion tests place the lesion in the flexor forearm muscle group (Fig. 30–25). Confirmation of the ligamentous injury may

Figure 30–24. Medial joint line pain due to ligamentous injury may be elicited by valgus stress and local tenderness or pain at the ulnar collateral ligament.

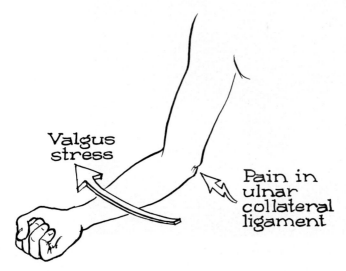

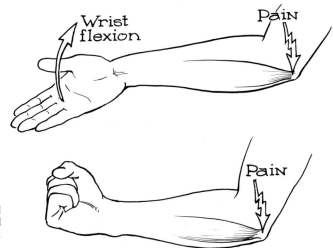

Figure 30–25. Forearm flexor muscle pain or medial tendinitis may be manifest by pain in the medial epicondyle during wrist flexion against resistance. Making a tight fist also elicits pain.

be found on the routine anteroposterior roentgenogram if a small avulsion fracture of the humeral origin of the ligament is present. Arthrograms can be helpful, particularly if they are done early, because dye extravasates from the ruptured capsule medially (Fig. 30–26).

If the diagnosis or extent of the injury is in doubt, a stress radiograph may be required (Fig. 30–27). If pain is acute or is located in a large extremity, this test should be done under anesthesia. Although this condition has not been well studied, we feel that it is not different from other acute ligament injuries with instability, and the sooner repaired, the better the results.

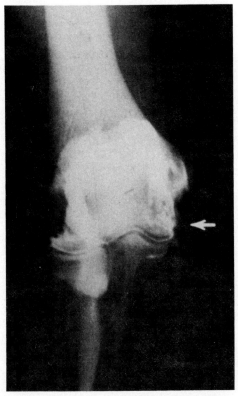

Figure 30–26. Arthrogram demonstrating poorly some extravasation of dye from the medial aspect of the capsule in a patient with a ruptured capsule (arrow).

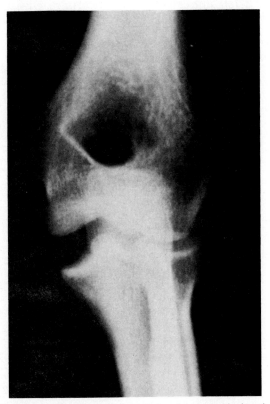

Figure 30–27. Stress roentgenogram of an individual with medial collateral ligament disruption demonstrating a wide gap at the medial aspect of the ulnohumeral joint.

Table 30–2. **32 Pitchers with X-ray Evidence of Joint Pathology**

Age	Pitchers	Pathology	Percent
26 thru 33	17	14	83
27 thru 25	21	13	62
18 thru 21	12	5	42
Total	50	32	

CHRONIC VALGUS INSUFFICIENCY IN ADULTS

Throwing Injuries

It has been shown that repetitive throwing can be detrimental to the integrity of the pitching arm.[9, 15, 20, 23] The data presented in Table 30–2 demonstrate that both periodic pain and roentgenographic findings of joint pathology are common in professional throwers. These findings become worse with advancing age.

The common site of injury is the anterior portion of the medial collateral ligament. It is speculated that repetitive valgus stress results in microtears that heal but leave functional incompetency of the medial support. Once the integrity of the medial ligament is lost, compressive injuries of the lateral joint are possible.

If left untreated, valgus deformity with or without elbow flexion contracture can result.

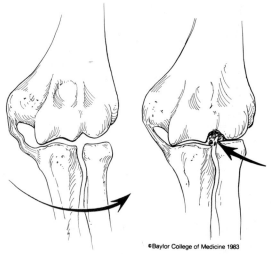

©Baylor College of Medicine 1983

Figure 30–28. Chronic instability of the elbow with resulting fragmentation and degenerative changes at the lateral aspect of the ulnohumeral joint.

Of the two, valgus deformity without elbow flexion contracture is the most disabling to a pitcher (Fig. 30–28). Incongruity develops between the olecranon process and its fossa with subsequent loose body formation (Fig. 30–29).

Nonspecific physical findings in the pitcher include muscular hypertrophy confined to those muscles dominant in the pitching act (Fig. 30–30). These include the latissimus dorsi and pectoralis major in the shoulder,

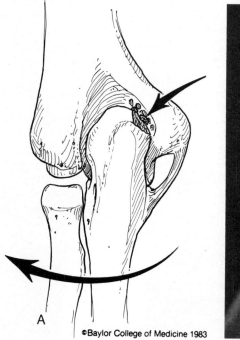

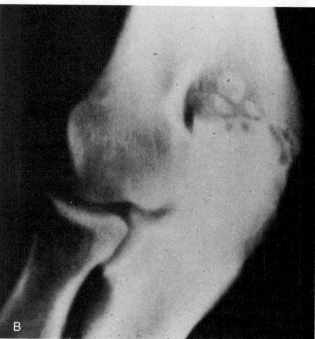

A ©Baylor College of Medicine 1983   B

Figure 30–29. A, Calcification of the medial aspect of the proximal ulna. This may be mistaken for triceps tendinitis, but it usually appears as loose bodies of the olecranon fossa (B). (B from King, J. W., et al.: Analysis of the pitching arm of the professional baseball pitcher. Clin. Orthop. 67:116, 1969.)

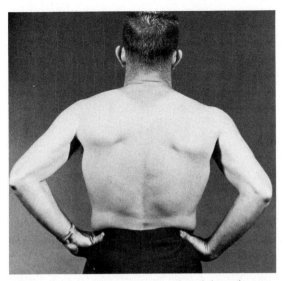

Figure 30–30. Generalized hypertrophy of the right upper extremity of a right-handed professional baseball pitcher.

which are both internal rotators of the abducted arm. In the forearm, the flexor forearm mass is noticeably hypertrophied. Roentgenographic observations include cortical hypertrophy when the pitching arm is compared with the opposite normal arm.[27]

Specific findings include increased forearm valgus and elbow flexion contractures. Medial collateral ligament tenderness may be present, but gross instability is lacking. The elbow usually does not demonstrate true locking as seen in the knee.

The roentgenographic findings can be deceptive. Fluffy calcification at the tip of the olecranon may be mistaken for triceps tendinitis (Fig. 30–29). However, because the tip of the olecranon is intra-articular, this appearance actually represents loose bodies, which can be confirmed on an anteroposterior tomogram. This study is also helpful in identifying the occasional lateral compartment loose body.

Because the disease process is due to the pitching act itself, it is apparent that no treatment will be more than palliative as long as the athlete continues to throw. This is true for surgical as well as for conservative therapy.

Barnes et al, reviewed treatment results in throwing athletes. Approximately 50 per cent were successfully returned to throwing with conservative measures such as rest, physical therapy, and anti-inflammatory measures. The other 50 per cent required surgery.[4]

Surgical procedures directed at muscle ruptures, complete or incomplete, are very diffi-

cult and probably rarely restore complete or competitive function. Resuture is tenuous, and the occasional good result may depend more on the lesion than on the surgical repair.

On the contrary, however, results with arthrotomy for loose bodies are good. With reasonable surgical discretion, accurate diagnosis, and muscle-splitting approaches, return to throwing can be anticipated. In our experience, the average professional pitcher continued to throw effectively postoperatively for 3 or more years with a range of 2 to 11 years. Thus for the professional or serious athlete this type of surgery can be easily justified.

In amateur athletes, the indications are less clear. Because surgery is directed at the result, not the cause, of the problem, it is likely that loose bodies will continue to occur if the player continues to throw. Even defining a successful result as one with improved symptoms for 3 years, an 18-year-old boy may have a very limited future regardless of his talent. For individuals of this age, particularly those of lesser talent, arthrotomy and removal of loose bodies should be followed by cessation of throwing.

Indications for reconstruction of the chronic attenuated anterior oblique ligament in throwers is less well delineated. In very experienced hands, this has been done in professional athletes. It remains to be seen whether the failure rate is acceptable and the long-term results of at least 3 years are good enough to justify the procedure. There is no question that reconstruction of the ligament is effective in nonthrowers, at least in preventing or improving gross instability.

Recurrent Elbow Dislocations

Perhaps the most interesting and one of the least common elbow lesions is that of recurrent dislocation. Few surgeons have personally seen more than one case in their lifetime. This accounts for the fact that reports discussing repair of this entity are both plentiful and inventive.[13, 25, 33, 37, 41, 43, 51] Yet in our experience many are not particularly effective.

Conceptually, the pathologic anatomy can be divided into two major categories—articular and ligamentous insufficiency.

Recurrent Dislocations Secondary to Coronoid Insufficiency.

Gartsman et al. and others discussing olecranon fractures have indicated that significant amounts of the olecranon process can be excised without essentially compromising joint stability.[2, 11, 13, 14, 16, 17, 30, 31] It is generally felt that the entire olecranon, leaving the coronoid insertion of the anterior oblique ligament, can be removed without affecting joint stability clinically.[17] The critical anterior articular surface (Fig. 30–31), which comprises approximately 20 per cent of the original joint area, includes the coronoid articulation and the anterior oblique ligament. This clinical perception has been studied in the laboratory (see Chapter 3). Small avulsion fractures of the tip of the coronoid do not cause instability and can be ignored. Large fractures may well lead to instability (Fig. 30–32). In the rare instance when significant portions of the coronoid process are absent secondary to trauma, causing elbow instability, a bone block procedure can be effective in restoring joint integrity (Figs. 30–33 and 30–34).

Recurrent Elbow Dislocations Secondary to Ligament Insufficiency

Although elbow instability due to bone loss is usually easily diagnosed, that due to ligamentous instability is more subtle. Perhaps the most common cause of recurrent elbow dislocations is the neglected medial epicondylar fracture.[29] The injury occurs in both children and adults, and the displaced fragment frequently heals with a fibrous union. When this occurs, a functionally elongated medial collateral ligament may result (Fig. 30–35). If recognized early, replacement of fragments that are displaced more than 3 mm

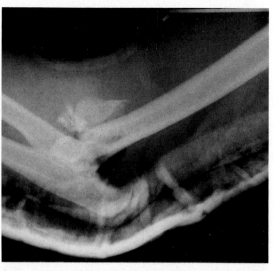

Figure 30–32. A large fracture of the coronoid causing chronic instability of the right elbow with large olecranon fragment displaced and rotated.

with pins or a screw provides predictable results (Fig. 30–36).[60] More commonly, the displaced fragment has been present many years. Yet it is usually possible to restore length and tension to the anterior oblique ligament (which is the aim of the procedure) even though anatomic restitution of the osseous anatomy is less than optimal.

More commonly, recurrent elbow dislocation is associated with a normal roentgenographic examination. The pathology lies solely in the anterior oblique ligament, which is either attenuated or absent. Initial stress views can give insight into the level of liga-

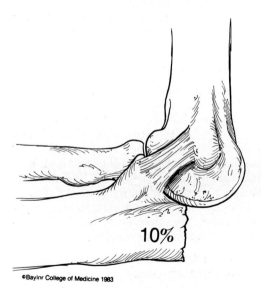

©Baylor College of Medicine 1983

Figure 30–31. A critical amount of anterior articular surface as well as the medial collateral ligament is necessary to render the elbow stable when the proximal ulna has been excised. This critical amount is probably 10 to 20 per cent of the anterior portion of the sigmoid notch.

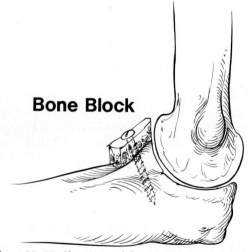

Bone Block

Figure 30–33. Chronic instability resulting from a coronoid fracture such as that shown in Figure 30–32 may be treated with a bone block to restore the coronoid of the proximal ulna.

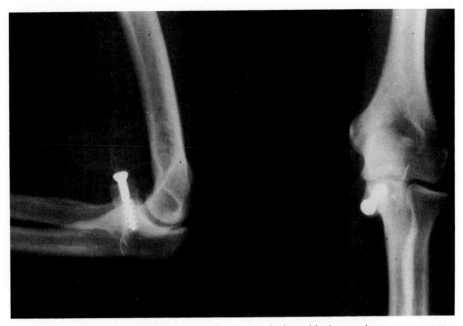

Figure 30–34. Radiographic illustration of a bone block procedure.

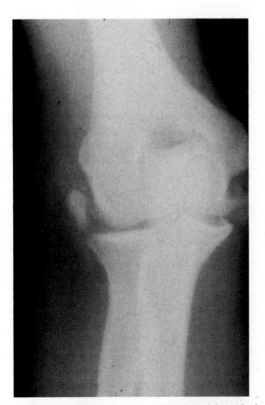

Figure 30–35. Avulsion of the lateral epicondyle with the lateral collateral ligament healed in a displaced position. Notice also the calcification of the medial collateral ligament.

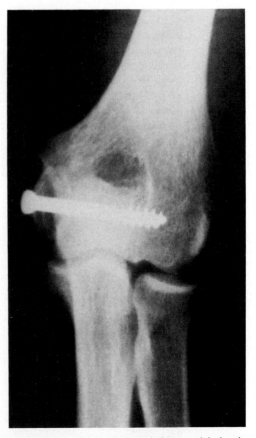

Figure 30–36. A large avulsed medial epicondyle has been replaced and repaired with a cancellous screw.

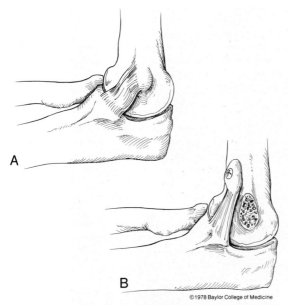

A

B

©1978 Baylor College of Medicine

Figure 30–37. For chronic elbow insufficiency, the lax anterior oblique portion of the medial collateral ligament may be stabilized by advancing the ligament superiorly and anteriorly. However, such an advancement may tend to limit elbow extension. (From Schwab, G. H., et al.: Biomechanics of elbow instability: The role of the medial collateral ligament. Clin. Orthop. 146:42, 1980.)

ment insufficiency; however, the final determination is made at surgery. If the anterior oblique is clearly present but lax, an advancement procedure using the entire medial epicondyle can be effective (Figs. 30–37, 30–38).

If the quality of the ligament is inadequate, a tendon graft reconstruction (Fig. 30–39) or reinforcement of the anterior oblique ligament is recommended. Experience with both techniques is limited; thus the final merits and liabilities of these procedures are yet to be determined.

Prior authors have advocated soft tissue reconstruction, not of the medial ligaments, but rather of the lateral side.[12, 37] There is no question that this procedure can be effective, but we agree with Spring, who proposed medial ligament reconstruction for elbow stability.[49]

AUTHOR'S PREFERRED TREATMENT METHOD

Elbow Dislocation

The patient with an elbow dislocation is taken as soon as possible to the operating room

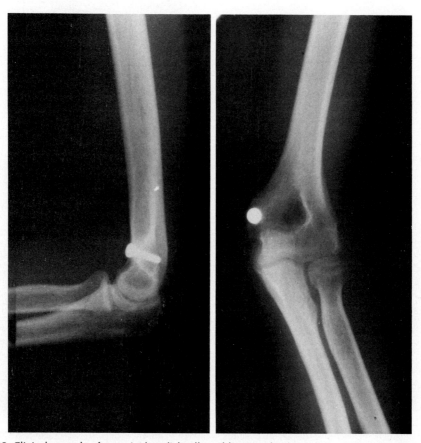

Figure 30–38. Clinical example of a repaired medial collateral ligament by the technique illustrated in Figure 30–37.

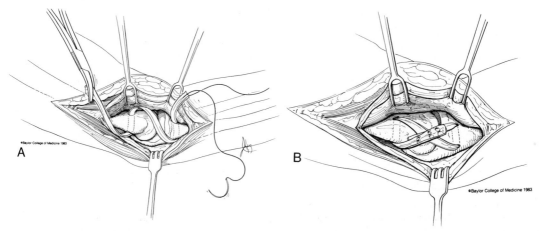

Figure 30–39. Tendon graft may be used for reconstruction of the medial collateral ligament if insufficient residual tissue is present (A). A figure-of-8 technique is used in this instance, and care is taken to attain the proper tension for both flexion and extension (B).

following adequate preoperative evaluation. Under general anesthesia, a closed reduction is performed. Only very rarely will the radial head be entrapped through the lateral extensor muscle mass, making closed reduction impossible.

Following closed reduction, the elbow is carefully taken through a range of motion to determine the presence and degree of instability. If redislocation does not occur within 20 to 30 degrees of complete extension, the elbow is probably adequately stable.

Clinical valgus stress testing is very unreliable. In most instances, the valgus force is dissipated by external rotation of the humerus, thus giving a false impression of either stability or instability.

The radiographic stress tests described above are more reliable. Careful judgment is required in the choice between surgical or conservative treatment. When the elbow is clinically stable and the medial opening minimal, the patient is placed in a posterior splint for 7 days and then given active range of motion exercises. Passive range of motion exercises are begun at 2 weeks.

If the stress examination indicates rupture of the anterior oblique ligament but the joint is still stable to motion, we prefer surgical repair, although many of these patients would do well with a posterior splint followed by a hinged cast brace for 8 weeks.

Bilateral lesions of both the radial head and the anterior oblique ligament require surgery, as discussed earlier. A cast brace is applied at 7 days followed by range of motion exercises. External support is discarded at 8 weeks.

Acute Elbow Instability with Medial Collateral Ligament Repair

In cases in which the elbow is unstable in the reduced position and can be shown to sublux posteriorly with valgus instability, exploration of the medical collateral ligament is indicated. The lateral approach may also be utilized for radial head fracture and to aid in the débridement of the elbow joint. The surgical approach to the lateral elbow is discussed in Chapter 8. Medial elbow exploration is accomplished through a curved longitudinal incision on the medial surface of the elbow just anterior to the medial epicondyle to avoid painful scarring over this prominence. The incision is carried proximally along the intermuscular septum and distally along the flexor carpi ulnaris muscle to allow adequate mobilization of the ulnar nerve. Often hemorrhage and hematoma are present in the soft tissue planes, and care must be taken to avoid damage to the ulnar nerve. The ulnar nerve is identified and carefully dissected through the groove distally to the first motor branch of the flexor carpi ulnaris. The nerve is protected and moved anteriorly. The flexor muscle mass is dissected from the medial epicondyle and reflected anteriorly to expose the medial collateral ligament. With a complete tear of the medial collateral ligament, the medial elbow joint may be inspected through the torn capsule, and débridement of the joint is carried out. If proximal disruption of the anterior oblique fibers of the medial collateral ligament has occurred, the repair consists of reinserting the ligament to the inferior anterior surface of the

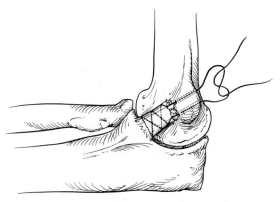

Figure 30–40. For avulsion-type injuries or when adequate substance of the anterior oblique ligament is present a Bunell-type suture may be placed through the origin of the ligament.

medial epicondyle. This is accomplished by placing drill holes through the medial epicondyle and passing a mattress suture of nonabsorbable material through the substance of the anterior oblique band of the medial collateral ligament. The suture is then passed through the drill holes and tied with the elbow at 30 degrees from full extension (Fig. 30–40). Avulsions from the ulnar attachment may be reattached with a small staple. Midportion ligament tears are repaired with nonabsorbable mattress sutures.

The posterior oblique ligament tear may be identified and can be repaired with the same techniques, but probably add little to stability. The flexor muscle mass is reattached to the medial epicondyle with nonabsorbable sutures. The ulnar nerve is transposed anterior if desired or left posterior without compression about the nerve. Soft tissue and skin closure is obtained as desired.

The elbow is initially placed in a posterior splint for 7 to 10 days until the sutures are removed. A cast brace is used to allow full flexion activities with approximately a 30 degree block to full extension. This is maintained for approximately 4 weeks at which time a cast brace to allow full flexion extension is worn for a period of 3 months.

Chronic Elbow Instability—Tendon Graft Technique

In cases of medial elbow instability that have been present for some time and constitute a chronic pattern of instability, a tendon graft procedure may be performed to allow reconstruction of the medial collateral ligament. The surgical approach is the same as that described for the acute injury. The joint is explored with a medial incision and in-

spected for loose bodies at the coronoid and olecranon articulations. A 3- to 6-mm drill hole is placed through the medial epicondyle, taking care to avoid fracture of the bone. A similar hole is placed through the medial flare of the coronoid in a volar to dorsal direction. Soft tissue dissection is required to allow adequate exposure to place the holes. At this time a tendon graft is harvested, utilizing either the palmaris longus, toe extensor, or the fascia lata. The graft is then passed through the drill holes with a carrying suture of nonabsorbable material. It may be passed in a criss-cross fashion or in a parallel fashion to reconstitute the course of the anterior oblique portion of the medial collateral ligament. The tension is adjusted with the arm approximately 30 degrees from full extension, and the tendon is sutured to itself with nonabsorbable material (Fig. 30–39). The joint is then placed through an arc of 90 degrees to full extension. The closure is accomplished in a fashion similar to that described in the acute reconstructive technique. The ulnar nerve is generally transposed anteriorly to prevent ulnar nerve symptoms due to swelling, edema, and hematoma in the area of surgery. The postoperative treatment is the same as that described for the acute reconstructive procedure.

Medial Epicondylar Transfer Technique

This procedure is utilized when the medial collateral ligament is intact but attenuated. Surgical exposure is done as in the acute reconstructive technique. The anterior oblique ligament is identified and separated from the posterior oblique fibers. At this time it is determined whether the ligament is strong enough in the attenuated position to form a suitable medial collateral support. The undersurface of the medial epicondyle is roughened and isolated, and the epicondyle predrilled with a 3.2-mm bit for attachment more proximally. An osteotome is used to remove the base of the medial epicondyle with the insertion of the anterior oblique portion of the medial collateral ligament. The epicondylar fragment is then advanced superior and anterior on the humerus to a point at which the elbow can be extended to within 30 degrees of full extension while keeping the anterior oblique portion of the medial collateral ligament taut. The site is then roughened with a rongeur or osteotome and a screw is used to secure the medial epicondylar transfer (Fig. 30–36). Closure is as described above. In the cases of medial epicondylar transfer, the arm is immobilized in a cylinder cast at approximately 30 degrees of flexion for a period of 4 weeks and then with a cast brace for a period of 2 months before return to stressful activities is allowed.

Synthetic Medial Collateral Ligament

Research in the development of a synthetic material that may replace the ligamentous structures about the elbow is ongoing. Currently, carbon fiber is being investigated to recreate or allow ingrowth of ligamentous support structures. The concept has been utilized in the reconstruction of a medial collateral ligament, but it is still too early to know if this will be successful, and thus it cannot be recommended at this time.

REHABILITATION

A rehabilitation program is established in all cases of elbow ligamentous and articular injuries. A comprehensive approach with patient, surgeon, therapist, and trainer is outlined. The use of splints, orthoses, and various strengthening modalities of rehabilitation should be integrated into the patient's activity program. Early motion is encouraged and usually begins 7 to 10 days after injury or reconstruction unless otherwise specified. A protective hinge cast brace to prevent varus, valgus, or extensor stress is utilized.

The patient is made aware of the goals of rehabilitation and knows that 6 months to 1 year will be required before the ultimate functional recovery is determined. The professional athlete realizes that the elbow is not normal and that his projected career performance may be shortened or terminated by the injury. The distinction between use and abuse is clearly explained to the athlete and to training personnel (see Chapter 31).

References

1. Adams, J. E.: Injury to the Throwing Arm: A Study of Traumatic Changes in the Elbow Joints of Boy Baseball Players. Calif. Med. 102:127, 1965.
2. Adler, S., Fay, G. F., and MacAusland, W. R.: Treatment of Olecranon Fractures, Indications For Excision of the Olecranon Fracture, Repair of the Triceps Tendon. J. Trauma 2:597, 1962.
3. Anderson, L.: Fractures. In Crenshaw, A. H. (ed.): Campbell's Operative Orthopedics, 5th Ed. St. Louis, C. V. Mosby Co., 1971.
4. Barnes, D. A., and Tullos, H. S.: An Analysis of 100 Symptomatic Baseball Players. Am. J. Sports Med. 6:62, 1978.
5. Bennett, G. E.: Shoulder and Elbow Lesions Distinctive of Baseball Players. Ann. Surg. 126:107, 1947.
6. Bennett, G. E.: Shoulder and Elbow Lesions of the Professional Baseball Pitcher. J.A.M.A. 117:510, 1941.
7. Brodgon, B. G., and Crow, N. F.: Little Leaguer's Elbow. Am. J. Roentgenol. 8:671, 1960.
8. Conn, J., and Wade, P.: Injuries of the Elbow: A Ten Year Review. J. Trauma 1:248, 1961.
9. DeHaven, K. E., and Evarts, C. M.: Throwing Injuries of the Elbow in Athletes. Orthop. Clin. North Am. 1:801, 1973.
10. DeHaven, K. E., Ferguson, A. B., Hale, C. J., Larson, R. L., and Tullos, H. S.: Symposium: Throwing Injuries to the Adolescent Elbow. Contemp. Surg. 9:65, 1976.
11. Dunn, N.: Operation for Fracture of the Olecranon. Br. Med. J. 1:214, 1939.
12. Durig, M., Mueller, W., Ruedi, T., and Gauer, E.: The Operative Treatment of Elbow Dislocations in the Adult. J. Bone Joint Surg. 61A(2):239, 1979.
13. Eppright, R. H., and Wilkins, K. E.: Fractures and Dislocations of the Elbow. In Rockwood, C. A., Jr., and Green, D. P. (eds.): Fractures. Philadelphia, J. B. Lippincott Co., 1975.
14. Eriksson, E., Sahlin, O., and Sandah, U.: Late Results of Conservative and Surgical Treatment of Fracture of the Olecranon. Acta Chir. Scand. 113:153, 1957.
15. Gainor, B. J., Piotrowski, G., Puhl, J., Allen, W. C., and Hagen, R.: The Throw: Biomechanics and Acute Injury. Am. J. Sports. Med. 8(2):114, 1980.
16. Gartsman, G. M., Sculco, T. P., and Otis, J. C.: Operative Treatment of Olecranon Fractures: Excision or Open Reduction with Internal Fixation. J. Bone Joint Surg. 63A(5):718, 1981.
17. Gartsman, G. M., and Tullos, H. S.: Unpublished data.
18. Gugenheim, J. J., Stanley, R. F., Woods, G. W., and Tullos, H. S.: Little League Survey: The Houston Study. Am. J. Sports Med. 4:189, 1976.
19. Hait, G., Boswick, J. A., and Stone, N. H.: Heterotophic Bone Formation Secondary to Trauma (Myositis Ossificans Traumatica). J. Trauma 10:405, 1970.
20. Hang, V. S., Lippert, F. G., Spolek, G. A., Frankel, V. H., and Harrington, R. M.: Biomechanical Study of the Pitching Elbow. Int. Orthop. 3:217, 1979.
21. Harrington, I. J., and Tountas, A. A.: Replacement of the Radial Head and the Treatment of Unstable Elbow Fractures. Injury 12(5):405, 1980.
22. Indelicato, P. A., Jobe, F. W., Kerlin, R. K., Carter, V. S., Shields, C. L., and Lombardo, S. J.: Correctable Elbow Lesions in Professional Baseball Players. Am. J. Sports Med. 7(1):72, 1979.
23. James, S.: Discussion of the Pitching Act. Presented at the Committee on Sports Medicine, American Academy of Orthopaedic Surgeons Post Graduate Course, San Francisco, 1971.
24. Jobe, F., and Stork, H.: Personal communication.
25. Kapel, O.: Operation for Habitual Dislocation of the Elbow. J. Bone Joint Surg. 33A:707, 1951.
26. Kerin, R.: Elbow Dislocation and its Association with Vascular Disruption. J. Bone Joint Surg. 51A(4):756, 1969.
27. King, J. W., Brelsford, H. J., and Tullos, H. S.: Analysis of the Pitching Arm of the Professional Baseball Pitcher. Clin. Orthop. 67:116, 1969.
28. Larson, R. L., and McMahan, R. O.: The Epiphysis and the Childhood Athlete. J.A.M.A. 196:607, 1966.
29. Linscheid, R. L., and Wheeler, D. K.: Elbow Dislocations. J.A.M.A. 194:1171, 1965.
30. Lou, I.: Olecranon Fractures Treated in Orthopedic Hospitals, 1936–1947. A Follow-up Examination. Acta Scand. 19:166, 1949.
31. Mains, D. B., and Freeark, R. J.: Report of Compound

Dislocation of the Elbow with Entrapment of Brachial Artery. Clin. Orthop. **106**:180, 1975.

32. McKeever, F. M., and Buck, R. M.: Fracture of the Olecranon Process of the Ulna: Treatment by Excision of Fragment and Repair of Triceps Tendon. J.A.M.A. **135**:1, 1947.

33. Milch, H.: Bilateral Recurrent Dislocation of the Ulna at the Elbow. J. Bone Joint Surg. **18**:777, 1936.

34. Mink, J. H., Eckardt, J. J., and Grant, T. T.: Arthrography in Recurrent Dislocation of the Elbow. Am. J. Radiol. **136**:1242, 1981.

35. Morrey, B. F., and An, K. N.: Stability of the Elbow Joint. A Biomechanical Assessment. (Am. J. Sports Med., submitted, 1984)

36. Morrey, B. F., Askew, L., and Chao, E. Y.: Silastic Prosthesis Replacement for the Radial Head. J. Bone Joint Surg. **63A(3)**:454, 1981.

37. Norwood, L. A., Shook, J. A., and Andrews, J. R.: Acute Medial Elbow Ruptures. Am. J. Sports Med. **9(1)**:16, 1981.

38. Osborne, G., and Cotterill, P.: Recurrent Dislocation of the Elbow. J. Bone Joint Surg. **48B**:340, 1966.

39. Panner, H. J.: A Peculiar Affection of the Capitulum Humeri Resembling Calvé-Perthes' Disease of the Hip. Acta Radiol. **10**:234, 1928.

40. Pappas, A. M.: Elbow Problems Associated with Baseball During Childhood and Adolescence. Clin. Orthop. **164**:30, 1982.

41. Pritchard, D. J., Linscheid, R. L., and Svien, H. J.: Intra-articular Median Nerve Entrapment with Dislocation of the Elbow. Clin. Orthop. **90**:100, 1973.

42. Reichenheim, P. P.: Transplantation of the Biceps Tendon as a Treatment for Recurrent Dislocation of the Elbow. Br. J. Surg. **35**:201, 1947.

43. Roberts, A. W.: Displacement of the Internal Epicondyle into the Elbow Joint. Lancet **2**:78, 1934.

44. Roberts, P. H.: Dislocation of the Elbow. Br. J. Surg. **56**:806, 1969.

45. Schwab, G. H., Bennett, J. B., Woods, G. W., and Tullos, H. S.: Biomechanics of Elbow Instability: The Role of the Medial Collateral Ligament. Clin. Orthop. **146**:42, 1980.

46. Schwab, G. H., Bennett, J. B., and Woods, G. W.: Biomechanics of Elbow Instability. Scientific Exhibit at the Annual Meeting of The American Academy of Orthopaedic Surgeons, Atlanta, February, 1980.

47. Shephard, C. W., Andrews, J. R.: Surgical Correction of Pitching Injuries of the Elbow. Submitted to Am. J. Sports Med.

48. Slocum, D. B.: Classification of Elbow Injuries from Baseball Pitching. Texas Med. **64**:48, 1968.

49. Smith, F. M.: Surgery of the Elbow, 2nd ed. Philadelphia, W. B. Saunders Co., 1972.

50. Speed, J. S., and Boyd, H. B.: Fractures about the Elbow. Am. J. Surg. **38**:727, 1937.

51. Spring, W. E.: Report of a Case of Recurrent Dislocation of the Elbow. J. Bone Joint Surg. **35B**:55, 1953.

52. Tachdijan, M. O.: Pediatric Orthopedics. Philadelphia, W. B. Saunders Co., 1972, pp. 1597-1604.

53. Trias, A., and Comeau, Y.: Recurrent Dislocations of the Elbow in Children. Clin. Orthop. **100**:74, 1974.

54. Tullos, H. S., Bennett, J. B., and Woods, G. W.: Unpublished data.

55. Tullos, H. S., Erwin, W., Woods, G. W., Wukasch, D. C., Cooley, D. A., and King, J. W.: Unusual Lesions of the Pitching Arm. Clin. Orthop. **88**:169, 1972.

56. Tullos, H. S., and King, J. W.: Lesions of the Pitching Arm in Adolescents. J.A.M.A. **220**:264, 1972.

57. Tullos, H. S., Schwab, G. H., Bennett, J. B., and Woods, G. W.: Factors Influencing Elbow Instability. **In** American Academy of Orthopaedic Surgeons, Instructional Course Lectures, Vol. 8. St. Louis, C. V. Mosby Co., 1982, pp. 185-199.

58. Wadsworth, T. G.: The Elbow. Edinborough, Churchill Livingstone, 1982.

59. Wainwright, D.: Recurrent Dislocation of the Elbow Joint. Proc. R. Soc. Med. **40**:885, 1947.

60. Waris, W.: Elbow Injuries in Javelin Throwers. Acta Chir. Scand. **93**:563, 1946.

60a. Warwick, R., and Williams, P. L. (eds.): Gray's Anatomy, 35th Brit. ed. Philadelphia, W. B. Saunders Co., 1973, pp. 324, 429.

61. Wheeler, D. K., and Linscheid, R. L.: Fracture Dislocations of the Elbow. Clin. Orthop. **50**:95, 1967.

62. Wilson, J. N.: The Treatment of Fractures of the Medial Epicondyle of the Humerus. J. Bone Joint Surg. **42B**:778, 1960.

63. Wilson, P. D.: Fractures and Dislocations in the Region of the Elbow. Surg. Gynecol. Obstet. **56**:335, 1933.

64. Woods, G. W., Elbow Instability and Medial Epicondyle Fractures. Am. J. Sports Med. **5**:23, 1977.

65. Woods, G. W., Tullos, H. S., and King, J. W.: The Throwing Arm: Elbow Injuries. Am. J. Sports Med. **1**:4, Sports Safety Supplement, 1973.

66. Woodward, A. H., and Bianco, A. J.: Osteochondritis Dissecans of the Elbow. Clin. Orthop. **110**:35, 1975.

CHAPTER 31

Rehabilitation of the Athlete's Elbow

R. NIRSCHL

Rehabilitation of the elbow begins with controlling inflammation. After the inflammatory and healing phases have been or are being treated (Chapter 9) restoration of function is attained. There are significant differences in goals and potential for rehabilitation between the athlete in competitive or high-performance sports and most other patients. A strength program is initiated first, followed by increases in flexibility, and finally, endurance is attained. For tendinitis or muscle pull injuries, limited flexibility with avoidance of tension on the injured tissue, may be combined with strength exercises. Attempts at full flexibility should not be introduced until normal strength has been attained in limited arcs of motion. Before strength exercises are undertaken, however, a period of warm-up is important.

WARM-UP

The term *warm-up*, unfortunately, is often used, and, because it is in fact a nonspecific concept, it has therefore invited a great deal of misconception and misinformation. *Warm-up* may be defined as an increase in body heat by active muscular use for the purposes of lowering soft tissue viscosity and enhancing body chemical and metabolic functions in order to protect and prepare the body for more aggressive physical activity.

Local body heat can be increased by passive means including the direct application of heat through whirlpool, heating pad, friction, ultrasound, massage, and the like. The physiologic basis of heat to the musculoskeletal system has been exhaustively studied by Lehmann and Warren.[10] This passive means of heating does not, of course, enhance the metabolic and cardiac factors that are also important in preparing the body for more rigorous activity. For elbow rehabilitation, local warming with whirlpool baths might be satisfactory, but general central muscular body activity is likely to be more productive. This can be attained by jogging in place, riding a stationary bicycle, jumping jacks, calisthenic exercise, and the like. The use of anti-inflammatory medication may also be helpful because it eliminates stiffness and soreness; buffered aspirin is usually prescribed about 15 minutes prior to rehabilitative activity. Although we do use ice to reduce postexercise soreness, the value of this modality alone has been questioned based on experimental data.[17]

STRENGTH TRAINING

Rehabilitative strength training has distinct priorities that differ from those of unrestricted strength training for physiologic enhancement or sport exercise. The potential for reinjury must be kept in mind. An exercise program pursued in the proper sequence to allow continued strengthening of uninjured tissue as well as protective exercise sequences for the injured areas is an extremely important concept. Isometric, isotonic, isoflex, and isokinetic exercises are all used (see also Chapter 5).

Isometric Exercise

Isometric exercise may be defined as strength training using the body's own resistance system with neither muscle shortening nor lengthening (i.e., without any arc of motion in the adjacent joints (Fig. 31–1). Because the patient is capable of controlling the amount of muscle tension and because there is no motion, the injured tissue is under the complete control of the patient. All adjacent muscle groups in and about the elbow including the wrist may be so exercised. It is generally recommended to hold the maximum contraction for a count of 3 to 5 seconds and progress to approximately 50 repetitions or more per day. The position of the shoulder, elbow, and

523

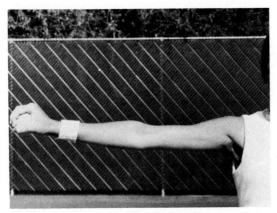

Figure 31–1. Isometric exercise. Squeezing a tennis ball or a softer racquet ball for a count of 3 to 5 seconds is an excellent form of early forearm rehabilitative exercise.

wrist can be altered in several ways to enhance strengthening of the appropriate muscle groups at different angles and lengths.

Isotonic Exercise

Isotonic exercise may be defined as a strength-training exercise utilizing a weighted resistance through the arc of motion of the selected muscle and joint (Fig. 31–2). Isotonic exercise may be performed by free weights or with a weight machine. Most machines are designed for the larger central body muscles and have less to offer the forearm and hand muscle groups. If there has been a chronic elbow problem, the entire extremity may be weak, and an additional exercise program for the shoulder including abduction, adduction, rotation, and flexion, as well as trapezius, latis-

simus dorsi, and rhomboid strengthening is important. It is our practice to have the patient selectively increase the amount of weight that can be comfortably handled until he reaches a maximum for each of the specific exercise motions outlined. Care is taken to avoid excessive weight, which causes muscle soreness[16] that can lead to loss of motion.[17] Once this maximum weight determination has been made, the recommended weight generally starts at one half of this amount, and the repetitions start at 10 and progress to 20. Three- to five-second holds at the end of each repetition are usually recommended as well. When 20 repetitions are reached an increase of approximately 10 percent in weight resistance is added, and the cycle is repeated until normal strength has been restored in each weak or injured muscle group. Return of normal strength may be determined by comparison with the uninjured arm. It should be noted that the dominant arm is usually about 10 per cent stronger in normal circumstances.

Isoflex Exercise

Physiologically, isoflex exercises produce an isotonic type of muscular contraction. Isoflex exercises consist of muscular strength training (both concentric and eccentric) through a normal arc of motion of a selected muscle and

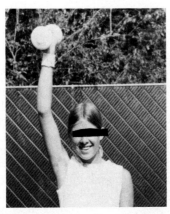

Figure 31–2. Isotonic exercise. Free weight isotonic exercise has the advantage of imposing no restrictions on arcs of motion. Because in most local injuries full arm strength is lost, a complete rehabilitation program for the upper extremity and trunk is usually indicated.

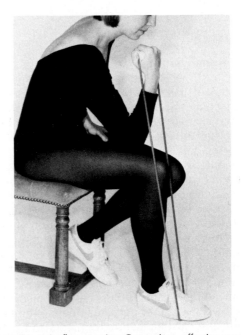

Figure 31–3. Isoflex exercise. Convenient, effective exercise system utilizing elastic tension cord resistance allows unlimited arcs of motion with both high concentric and eccentric muscle training. Favorable patient compliance has made this exercise concept extremely valuable.

adjacent joints, utilizing the resistance of an elasticized tension cord (Fig. 31–3). Like the use of free weights, this program offers the advantage of exercising in an unrestricted variety of exercise motions.

The specific exercises are similar to those described for free weights. Daily repetitions progress to 25 and are maintained for 3 to 5 seconds at the end of each exercise arc. Once the patient attains 25 repetitions, maintenance exercise is performed three times a week. After shortening the tension cord by one twist, the patient again progresses to 25 repetitions.

The major advantage of the isoflex program is that of enhanced exercise efficiency as tension resistance increases at the extremes of the exercise arc. This is contrary to the exercise efficiency of isotonic weight resistance, which usually decreases as joint motion progresses because of a shortened lever arm. By merely lengthening or shortening the cord, the resistance can be easily changed. Minimal equipment is therefore needed. Because the isoflex system is light, transportable, and convenient, patient compliance is high. One disadvantage of the isoflex system is the inability to actually calibrate the exercise resistance.

Isokinetic Exercise

Isokinetic exercise may be defined as muscular strengthening utilizing the variable resistance of a person's own individual muscular contractions through a range of motion with a fixed speed. The isokinetic devices operate with hydraulic or electrical resistance (Fig. 31–4). By presetting the speed, the power ratio and torque are controlled as well. The disadvantages of the isokinetic systems are that they are relatively expensive and, like isotonic weight machines, the arcs and angles of motion are predetermined by the machine itself. Yet the presetting of speed associated with variable resistance offers significant advantages, particularly to highly competitive athletes who, prior to returning to competition, should rehabilitate muscles to the high-speed contractile activity used in the sport. Isokinetic exercise techniques are highly individualistic but generally are continued for approximately 10 repetitions or until fatigue occurs. The ultimate resistance is the maximum the patient can generate. Most isokinetic machines accommodate wrist flexion-extension, forearm pronation and supination, and elbow flexion-extension.

FLEXIBILITY

Flexibility exercises are designed to attain as full and unrestricted an arc of joint motion as possible. As noted earlier, in the athlete premature attempts at full flexibility exercise may cause harm by placing abusive stretching force loads on the vulnerable injured tissue. It is, therefore, wise to introduce full flexibility exercise arcs at a later stage in the overall rehabilitative exercise sequence to ensure that there has been appropriate healing of injured tissue, thereby decreasing the potential of stretch overload. If there are mechanical blocks to elbow motion, these, of course, must be eliminated before a full restoration of flexibility can be anticipated. If there are soft tissue constraints that cannot be eliminated by inflammation control or mobilization, surgical release of such constraining soft tissue may be appropriate. Most soft tissue problems, however, can be resolved without surgical intervention.

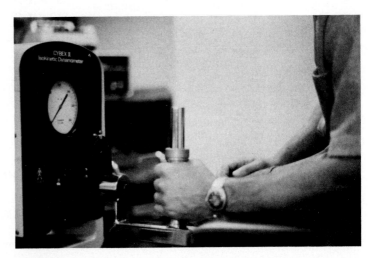

Figure 31–4. Isokinetic exercise. Fixed speed variable resistence exercise makes this system a valuable exercise tool.

The elbow responds poorly to exaggerated, premature, passive attempts at stretching to full arcs of motion. Passive manipulation can result in a further aggravation of the inflammatory response or tearing and hemorrhage of soft tissues. Passive exercise is especially difficult in long-term chronic contracture.[6] All flexibility exercises are best controlled actively by the patient through active muscle contraction and controlled joint excursion, and attempts at strength and flexibility should be carefully controlled or avoided when substantial inflammation is present. There is some clinical evidence, however, that carefully controlled passive exercise in limited arcs of motion may be beneficial in clearing tissue edema and minimizing the inflammation process.[3, 9]

Early aggressive control of the inflammatory process is therefore extremely important in the ultimate attainment of the greatest possible flexibility. In addition, because strength training itself seems to improve the overall tissue pliability and enhances the local blood supply, a proper warm-up is extremely important for the success of any flexibility program. The technical aspects of flexibility include the following:

1. Static stretch is held for 10 to 20 seconds with the patient completely relaxed and is repeated three to five times. A full warm-up, including local warmth by whirlpool and friction massage prior to stretching, is strongly recommended. All motions—flexion-extension, forearm rotation, and wrist flexion-extension— should be included.

2. Dynamic stretching may be defined as active controlled motion stretching that may be enhanced by increased momentum (e.g., holding a weight). Dynamic stretching for the elbow includes swinging a small hand dumbbell through a full arc of motion that incorporates the elbow, wrist, and shoulder into the swinging motions. The same motions discussed in Chapter 5 should be included with the dynamic exercises. The amount of weight to be used is highly individualized, but in general 2 to 5 pounds are used, and approximately 15 repetitions of each motion arc complete the exercise sequence.

3. Proprioceptive neuromuscular facilitation (PNF) exercise is defined as active muscle contraction against resistance followed by static stretching. The initial contraction facilitates flexibility. As an example, active muscular contracture of the biceps with manual resistance and subsequent relaxation is followed by a static stretch into extension. The contraction is held for 2 to 3 seconds and is followed by static stretch in the opposite direction for 5 to 10 seconds. The sequence is repeated 5 to 10 times. Clinically, the PNF technique seems to enhance the speed of progression of joint flexibility. The endpoint of any flexibility exercise is, of course, the full return and maintenance of normal motion.

ENDURANCE

Muscular endurance refers to the property of contractile strength of muscle sustained over a period of time. This topic requires consideration of the two types of muscle fibers, each of which are suited to different functions as shown in Table 31–1. We shall discuss the subject from the perspective of enhancing both aerobic and anaerobic capacity, thus, rehabilitating both muscle fibers and hence both functions.

Aerobic capacity is that property of muscle by which a physiologic steady state of nutritional and oxygen input is balanced by removal of waste products,[4] carbon dioxide, and lactic acid.[11] The muscular activity itself is evenly balanced so that there is no increase or decrease in the rhythm of muscle contracture or the generation of power.[8] This capacity of muscular activity level requires a cardiovascular system that will sustain the neurochemical and oxygen needs[2] of the body. To this end, it is important for the athlete to maintain the central cardiovascular system by general aerobic conditioning. This may include running, biking, swimming, and similar activities. A specific aerobic exercise adapted to enhance the endurance of the muscle groups in and around the elbow consists of

Table 31–1. **Types of Muscle Fibers Important in Rehabilitation**

Type I	Type II
Red	White
Slow twitch	Fast twitch
High oxidative capacity (aerobic)	Low oxidative capacity (anaerobic)
Delivery of force not a feature	Burst of forceful energy on demand
Slow contractility is expectant (irritability)	Rapid contractility (irritability)
High resistance to fatigue	Immediate fatigue

sitting behind a stationary bike and pedalling with the hands.

Anaerobic exercise utilizes the muscle chemical energy system without oxygen input on a temporary basis.[11] Anaerobic exercise is generally done at very high speeds for short periods of time with rest intervals to allow replenishment of the oxygen supply. Anaerobic exercise can occur with isoflex, isotonic, or isokinetic activity. Anaerobic fatigue is followed by a rest interval of approximately twice the time it took to develop fatigue. Four complete fatigue–rest cycles are recommended per session.

Normal aerobic and anaerobic endurance should be attained before a patient is completely rehabilitated from the injury. Rehabilitation is determined by comparison with the opposite uninjured extremity, remembering that the dominant extremity is about 10 per cent stronger than the nondominant side.[1]

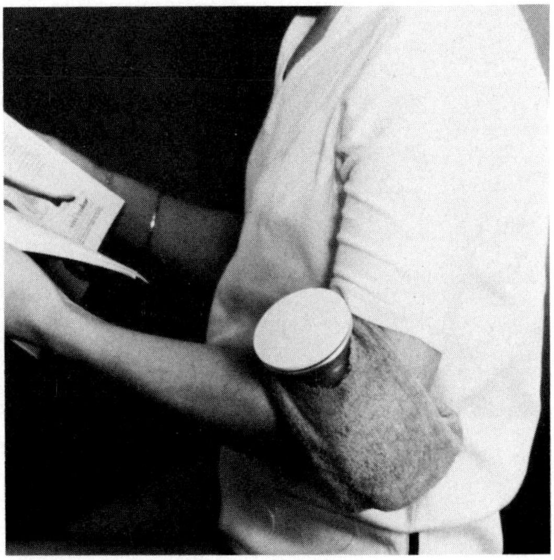

Figure 31–5. Ice strap. A convenient way to hold ice in place, increasing promptness of ice applications after activity and enhancing overall patient compliance.

AVOIDING INFLAMMATION

During progressive exercises, it is extremely important to avoid recurrence of inflammation. This is best achieved by a carefully supervised exercise program that has been initiated at the correct time and has allowed adequate healing, proper warm-up, use of ice, anti-inflammatory medication, and counterforce bracing. A word about each of these features is in order.

Careful Exercise Progression. Elbow rehabilitation cannot be left to the patient with some vague advice to "don't overdo it," but must be well supervised with specific exercises prescribed in an appropriate sequence. The patient must be informed about exactly what he is to do and how he is to do it. Recurrence of the inflammatory response is to be strictly avoided. It is our practice to have a series of printed manuals that assist the patient in all of the specifics of the exercise progression.

Warm-Up. Proper warm-up has been discussed previously. It is again emphasized that warming-up is a separate and distinct activity apart from strength or flexibility exercises.

Anti-Inflammatory Measures. Anti-inflammatory modalities and medications are used to control the potential for inflammation. The following sequence is used: (1) Buffered aspirin or an appropriate nonsteroidal anti-inflammatory medication is taken prior to exercise at the time that will ensure the proper blood level during the activity. (2) On an empirical basis, we recommend application of ice for a period of 30 minutes after the

exercise (Fig. 31–5). If soreness or swelling persists beyond the 30-minute period, we recommend intermittent application with 30 minutes on and 30 minutes off until the clinical signs of inflammation are eliminated. It is important that, if a full-scale inflammatory process has occurred, all rehabilitative exercises be discontinued until the inflammation has subsided. This may take several days or longer. If symptoms of inflammation increase during the rehabilitative exercise for that day, it is recommended that a second dose of the anti-inflammatory medication be taken at the appropriate time after exercise to sustain the blood level of the agent.

Counterforce Bracing. Counterforce bracing is a system of bracing that controls internally generated muscular forces by diminishing contractile muscle expansion or supporting the musculotendinous attachments while allowing an unimpeded arc of joint motion. The concept of Counterforce bracing, first elucidated by Ilfeld,[7] is different from rigid immobilization, joint constraint, or padding to protect from extrinsic impact forces. A similar concept was advanced by Froimson.[5] We have expanded the concept further and applied the term Counterforce.[12]

Counterforce bracing should not impede basic physiologic activity but should provide protection by gentle appropriate constraints in key pathologic areas. Recent biomechanical studies demonstrate that nonelastic, anatomically fitting counterforce bracing alters both angular velocity and the sequence of the elec-

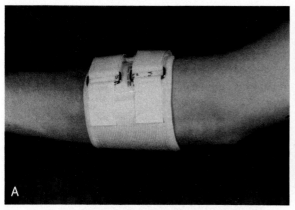 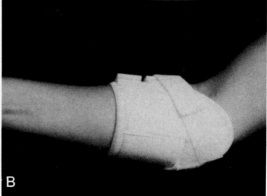

Figure 31–6. *A,* Lateral elbow counterforce brace. *B,* Medial elbow counterforce brace.

tromyographic (EMG) recording of muscular activity. This concept is utilized as a preventative measure for soft tissue problems (such as tennis elbow) as well as in a protective capacity during the initiation of rehabilitative exercises and the return of the patient to sport or occupational activities.

In the early rehabilitative phase, counterforce bracing is utilized as a protective device during the progressive exercise sequence (Fig. 31–6). The lateral brace is used as a protector of the extensor muscle groups, and the medial brace can be utilized for protection of both flexor and extensor forearm musculotendinous units as well as for pronation and supination. It is our practice to utilize counterforce braces for a period ranging from 7 to 10 days in the initial phases of the strength exercise program. Thereafter, the patient is weaned from the use of the brace for the remainder of the rehabilitative process, unless there is a recurrence of the inflammatory phase.

RETURN TO COMPETITION

The earliest safe time to return to competition is a frequent concern of the athlete and a matter of judgment for the physician. A single formula to assist in determining the appropriate timing of this decision is contained in the mneumonic SAID (Table 31–2). Return to competition may be safely recommended when the patient can Satisfactorily Adapt

Table 31–2. **When an Athlete May Return to Competition**

S–Satisfactory
A–Adaptation to
I–Imposed
D–Demands of the sport

(accomplish) to the Imposed Demands of the sport.

Following completion of the rehabilitative process (as demonstrated by objective measurements of normal flexibility, strength, and endurance), normal activity may be resumed. Flexibility is measured with a standard goniometer. Strength may be measured in several ways, including (1) a mechanical dynamometer, (2) satisfactory completion of all strength exercises equivalent to the noninjured arm, and (3) isokinetic (Cybex) testing.

For the average noncompetitive athlete, it is perfectly satisfactory to utilize the readily available spring dynamometer grip test and satisfactory completion of the prescribed exercise program. For competitive athletes, it is valuable to obtain a Cybex test result at a variety of speed settings to ensure that full power and endurance have returned at all speeds and that proper balance of protagonist-antagonist muscle groups has been attained. These determinations are critical to protect a competitive athlete while allowing participation at the highest levels of sport.

Prior to full return to sport or occupational activity, further protective measures are appropriate, including a graduated return to the desired activity. This is important because these activities may require use of the muscle tendon units at angles and speeds that are different from those of the rehabilitative program. In addition, a general check of protective arm use is appropriate as well as a review of the patient's sports equipment or workplace to eliminate undue or exaggerated force loads that may result in recurrent injury. Counterforce bracing is utilized as a final protective measure for musculotendinous injuries that may be prone to recur from intrinsic muscular overloads (e.g., medial and lateral elbow tendinitis).

MAJOR FACTORS DELAYING REHABILITATION

If the above concepts are understood and properly implemented, there should be few patients who are not rehabilitated in a predictable way. There are, however, several factors to consider that delay or even preclude a satisfactory rehabilitative process.

Type and Magnitude of Injury or Surgery. There are some injuries and diseases that permanently injure the joint or its environs. Severe fracture with permanent distortion of the normal skeletal and joint alignment will result in an altered and delayed end result. Residual ligamentous instability may not allow normal functional restoration. Progressive inflammatory disease such as rheumatoid arthritis will likewise compromise the rehabilitative effort. In these and similar circumstances, it can be appreciated that the rehabilitative process is intimately related to the initial and subsequent mechanical or inflammatory events. It is highly appropriate, therefore, to review all situations carefully when the rehabilitative process is not progressing as anticipated. It may be that removing a mechanical obstruction such as interarticular debris or some other inflammatory factor will allow resumption of a reasonable rehabilitative progression.

Lack of Inflammation Control. As has been constantly emphasized, it is critically important to control any inflammatory process prior to starting an aggressive rehabilitative exercise effort with the injured tissue. If inflammation does recur during the exercise program and does not subside when the program is decelerated, a total review of the exercise program as well as the type and character of supervision, or lack thereof, should be instituted.

Patient Motivation. A variety of motivational and emotional factors play a very important role in any rehabilitative effort, especially situations such as workman's compensation or secondary gain, which encourage a lack of progress.[15] In addition, patients who have high anxiety levels or a low pain threshold must attain emotional control in whatever manner is possible, including psychiatric counseling, biofeedback, appropriate medication, sympathetic blocks, and so on, to ensure maximum success.[13]

References

1. Askew, L. J., An., K. N., Morrey, B. F., and Chao, E. Y.: Functional Evaluation of the Elbow. Normal Motion Requirements and Strength Determinations. Orthop. Trans. 5:304, 1981.
2. Bergh, U., Thorstensson, A., Sjodin, B., Hulten, B., Piehl, K., and Karlsson, S.: Maximal Oxygen Uptake and Muscle Fiber Types in Trained and Untrained Humans. Med. Sci. Sports 10:151, 1978.
3. Coutts, R. D., Toth, C., and Kaita, J.: The Role of Continuous Passive Motion in the Rehabilitation of the Total Knee Patient. In Hungerford, D. (ed.): Total Knee Arthroplasty—A Comprehensive Approach. Baltimore, The Williams & Williams Co., 1983. (In press.)
4. Eriksson, E.: Muscle Physiology: Adaptation of the Musculoskeletal System to Exercise. Contemp. Orthop. 2:228, 1980.
5. Froimson, A. I.: Treatment of Tennis Elbow With Forearm Band Support. J. Bone Joint Surg. 53A:183, 1971.
6. Green, D. P., and McCoy, H.: Turnbuckle Orthotic Correction of Elbow-Flexion Contractures. J. Bone Joint Surg. 61A:1092, 1979.
7. Ilfeld, F. W., and Field, S. M.: Treatment of Tennis Elbow. Use of a Special Brace. J.A.M.A. 195:67, 1966.
8. Knuttgen, H. G.: Physical Conditioning and Limits to Performance. In Straus, R. H. (ed.): Sports Medicine and Physiology. Philadelphia, W. B. Saunders Co., 1979, pp. 94–110.
9. Korcok, M.: Motion, Not Immobility, Advocated for Healing Synovial Joints. J.A.M.A. 246:2005, 1981.
10. Lehmann, F., Warren, C. G., and Scham, S. M.: Therapeutic Heat and Cold. Clin. Orthop. 99:207, 1964.
11. Miller, W. E.: Kinesiology. Part V. Psychologic and Neurologic Aspects of Kinesiology. Am. J. Sports Med. 10(4):250, 1982.
12. Nirschl, R. P.: Tennis Elbow. Orthop. Clin. North Am. 4:787, 1973.
13. Sainsbury, P., and Gibson, T. G.: Symptoms in Anxiety and Tension and the Accompanying Psychological Changes in the Muscular System. J. Neurol. Neurosurg. Psychiatr. 17:216, 1954.
14. Sherman, W. M., Pearson, D. R., Plyley, M. J., Costill, D. L., Habansky, A. J., and Vogelgesang, D. A.: Isokinetic Rehabilitation After Surgery. A Review of Factors Which Are Important for Developing Physiotherapeutic Techniques After Knee Surgery. Am. J. Sports Med. 10(3):155, 1982.
15. Smith, F. M.: Surgery of the Elbow, 2nd ed. Philadelphia, W. B. Saunders Co., 1972.
16. Talag, T. S.: Residual Muscular Soreness as Influenced by Concentric, Eccentric and Static Contractions. Res. Q. 44:458, 1973.
17. Yackzan, L., Adams, C., and Francis, K. T.: The Effects of Ice Massage on Delayed Muscle Soreness. Am. J. Sports Med. 12:159, 1984.

PART V

Reconstructive Procedures of the Elbow

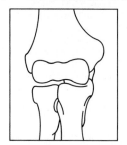

CHAPTER 32

Fascial Arthroplasty of the Elbow

PHILLIP E. WRIGHT, II, and MARCUS J. STEWARD

HISTORICAL ASPECTS

Arthroplasty, using natural or synthetic materials, has been practiced for over a century and a half. The early procedures were less refined than those used today. In 1827 Barton reported an osteotomy of an ankylosed hip, producing a pseudarthrosis. Today the term may be applied to four types of procedures: resection, functional, interposition (anatomic), or replacement arthroplasty.

Resection arthroplasty, which effectively removes the entire joint by resecting the distal humerus and proximal radius and ulna (Fig. 32–1), was first described by Verneuil in 1860 and later by Ollier in 1885. The early indication was ankylosed elbows from tuberculosis. The gross instability that resulted prompted some[14] to suggest that joint resection should not, strictly speaking, be considered an arthroplasty. Yet Buzby, as late as 1936,[6] continued to recommend this procedure as a more reliable control of pain than that realized with functional or interposition arthroplasty. Because of disabling instability (Fig.

32–2), the only real use of such a procedure today is to control a septic, usually tuberculous, process.

The so-called functional arthroplasty, described by Hass (1944),[12] is really a variety of resection arthroplasty, except that the distal humerus is fashioned in the shape of a wedge (Fig. 32–3). This is intended to provide a fulcrum about which some forearm motion is allowed. Hass has reported the long-term results of functional arthroplasty in 15 patients with an average follow-up period of 5.5 years. A satisfactory result was observed in 73 per cent, and a tendency for the bone to remodel according to its functional demands was noted. Because this is a type of resection arthroplasty, it is not surprising that 13 of the 15 procedures were in patients with previous infection.

Interposition or "anatomic" arthroplasty strives to preserve functional stability and reduce the likelihood of reankylosis by interposing a substance between the resected bone ends. In addition to the elbow, this basic technique has been used for treatment of

530

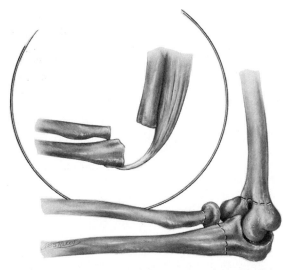

Figure 32–1. Resection arthroplasty removes the entire elbow articulation, is usually reserved for severe infection, and is rarely, if ever, indicated.

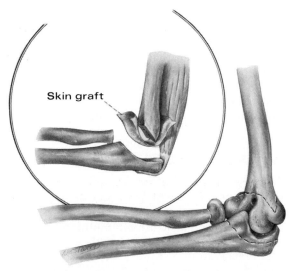

Skin graft

Figure 32–3. The so-called functional or anatomic arthroplasty resects variable amounts of distal humerus but fashions the bone as a fulcrum against which the proximal ulna pivots. Skin and other substances may be used to cover the humerus and create a new articular surface, hence the term interposition arthroplasty.

arthritis involving the temporomandibular, shoulder, wrist, knee, and hip joints. Of these, the elbow has been reported as second only to the temporomandibular as the joint most amenable to the technique.[13] In Europe arthroplasty was popularized by Putti[27] and by Payr.[25] Schüller was the first to recommend the procedure for patients with rheumatoid arthritis.[30] Various muscle flaps, animal membranes, fascia-fat transplants, skin, and other materials have been used as the interposing agent. In 1902, Murphy introduced and popularized arthroplasty in the United States.[22, 23] He advocated the use of fascia and fat as interposition surfaces. Lexer, in 1909, emphasized the value of autogenous tissue[19] and confirmed the previous impression of Murphy[23] that fat and fascia were the best substances for interposition arthroplasty. He reported that fascia remained viable and was replaced by fibrous and fibrocartilaginous tis-

sue. The mechanism of the transformation to the new articulation was also studied by Phemister and Miller.[26] Little histologic difference was noted after cartilage resection with or without interposition materials.

Baer reported early success with the so-called Baer membrane derived from pig bladder.[3] Only limited information is available about the success of the Baer membrane. Gelfoam has also been employed,[29] and the use of skin, the cutis arthroplasty, has been used by several investigators[16, 21] and was recently reported by Froimson.[11] Fascia lata has probably gained the greatest degree of popularity over the years. It is easy to harvest and conforms readily to the bony surfaces, and the donor site leaves minimal disability. Efforts to enhance its effect have been reported by

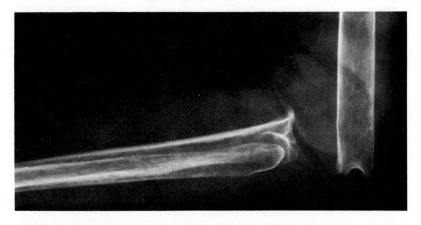

Figure 32–2. The obvious disadvantage of resection arthroplasty is incapacitating instability.

Kita using chromicized fascia lata, the so-called J-K membrane.[17] The concept has been recently reassessed after the addition of two important elements to the technique—distraction and motion. The mechanical basis[9a] and preliminary results have been encouraging.[10] This chapter will focus primarily on fascia lata interposition arthroplasty of the elbow.

GOALS OF TREATMENT

The principal goal of treating elbow arthritis or dysfunction is first the relief of pain and then the return of function to as near-normal levels as possible, while maintaining reasonable stability. Ideally, these goals are attainable. Preservation of limb length, which is so important in the lower extremity, is not essential in the upper limb.

TREATMENT OPTIONS

For the individual who has either an ankylosed or unstable elbow or is incapacitated by pain, the viable options of treatment include (1) no surgical treatment, altered activity, and continued rehabilitation activities as tolerated, (2) orthotics for controlled use of the unstable elbow, (3) arthrodesis, and (4) arthroplasty, either resection, interposition, distraction, or implant replacement.[9] Other procedures that have been used and abandoned for one reason or another include denervation of the joint[5] and so-called erasion of the joint.[32] As noted, resection arthroplasty is rarely if ever indicated at this time, the only indication being uncontrollable infection.

If the elbow is ankylosed in a functional position, no treatment may be required. If it is ankylosed in a poor position, osteotomy with correction of the position may be adequate treatment. If the patient has painful motion or an unstable elbow, an orthotic fitting may allow continuation of regular activities indefinitely or until the pain demands other treatment. The individual who is required to carry out strenuous activities such as heavy labor may not be a suitable candidate for any arthroplasty, regardless of the type of procedure.

Interposition arthroplasty is most suited for patients who require a greater arc of motion or pain relief to continue in their activities of daily living. In the young person with post-traumatic arthritis the result of replacement arthroplasty presently is unpredictable, and interposition arthroplasty is a viable option.

INDICATIONS

The basic indications for arthroplasty are either incapacitating pain or loss of motion. These conditions may, of course, co-exist. Loss of motion may follow trauma, sepsis, burns, or degenerative or inflammatory arthritis (Fig. 32–4). The cause may be bony or fibrous union across or around the joint. However, the most compelling indication for arthroplasty of the elbow is incapacitating pain. Instability is not a common indication, but satisfactory arthroplasty may be accomplished in the selected patient with limited stability. If the loss of motion and pain are postinfectious, careful evaluation must be carried out to ensure that the patient has been free of the infection for at least 6 months and preferably 1 year. The best indication, therefore, for this procedure is post-traumatic, painful loss of motion not complicated by sepsis.[32] In underdeveloped countries untreated elbow dislocation has been a common source of ankylosis and a prime indication for the procedure.[28, 31]

Selection of the proper candidate for interposition arthroplasty involves assessment of the nature of the pathology and the type of patient under consideration. Regardless of the etiology, the integrity of the soft tissue is of paramount importance for a successful outcome. Extensive scarring with adherence of skin to bone may lead to an unsatisfactory result. Of great importance is the condition of the musculature about the arm and forearm because dynamic stability is important for the success of the operation.

RELATIVE CONTRAINDICATIONS

Tuberculosis as the cause of disability and pain is considered an absolute contraindication for interposition arthroplasty.[32] If recent sepsis has occurred, no reconstruction should be considered. If epiphyseal closure has not occurred, arthroplasty should be delayed until growth is complete.

Ankylosis in a nonfunctional position is a most difficult setting in which to obtain a satisfactory result. Osteoporosis may interfere with remodeling of bone ends and may cause impairment of the final result.

PATIENT SELECTION

If the patient under consideration is a heavy laborer, fascial arthroplasty may not be as satisfactory as a painless arthrodesis of the

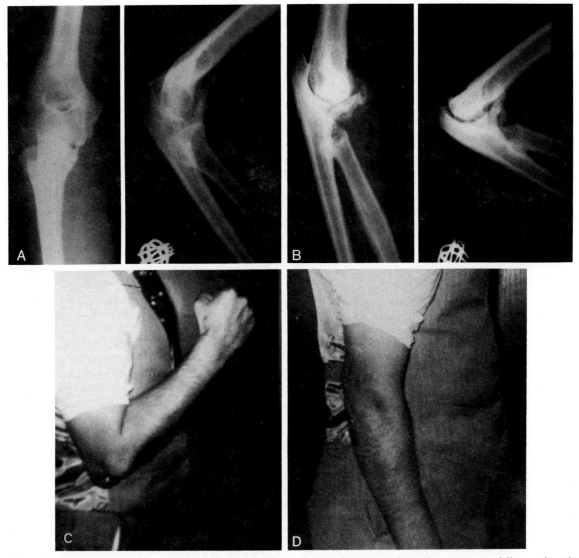

Figure 32–4. *A,* Radiographic appearance of elbow with post-traumatic arthritis. *B,* Radiographic appearance following fascial arthroplasty; left, extension; right, flexion. *C,* Flexion 5 years following surgery. *D,* Extension 5 years following surgery.

elbow in a functional position. Although fascial arthroplasty offers the patient a painless, durable joint, it cannot guarantee enough stability to allow for the activities of heavy labor.

Patients who require crutches for ambulation should be carefully evaluated prior to fascial arthroplasty. Although they may do well postoperatively, ambulation may be further impaired if they develop instability.

If multiple joints in the same extremity have become ankylosed, it will be more difficult to secure a satisfactory result.

Finally, it is of utmost importance that the patient have the motivation and fortitude to participate in a preoperative and postoperative rehabilitation program for proper devel-

opment of the musculature of the upper extremity.

RESULTS: LITERATURE REVIEW AND PERSONAL EXPERIENCE

Early reports of arthroplasty dealt with the advantages and disadvantages of resection versus interposition arthroplasty and the various type of materials used to cover the bone ends at the time of surgery. Resection arthroplasty produced a mobile, painless, but unstable joint; therefore, most surgeons developed a preference for interposition arthroplasty.

Today, the best indication for interposition

arthroplasty is probably the post-traumatic, painful, stiff joint. The procedure has been used regularly in Europe for rheumatoid arthritis.[15, 16, 34, 35] The static instability inherent to the procedure was noted to be minimized with muscle contracture during use.[16] The procedure for rheumatoid arthritis is discussed in the chapter dealing with that disease. The use of cutis arthroplasty has been recently reported by Froimson et al.,[11] Hurri et al.,[16] and Mills and Rush.[21] These investigators report consistently favorable results with this technique. The use of a chromicized fascial interposition substance was reported in 31 patients by Kita[17] in an attempt to reduce the inflammatory response initiated by fascia lata. An average of 43 to 105 degrees of motion with approximately 50 per cent excellent or good and 20 per cent poor results were observed an average of 19 years after surgery.

Campbell, in 1924, reported on 34 fascial arthroplasties of the elbow.[7] All patients obtained relief of pain and improvement of motion, and none had significant instability. In the same year, Henderson, from the Mayo Clinic, reported his experience with 30 procedures[14] after the technique of Mac-Ausland.[20] Only 63 per cent were considered excellent or good, and 20 per cent were rated as poor. This is in contrast to the 76 per cent excellent or good and only 6 per cent poor results tabulated from a collected series reported in 1918 by the same author.[13] In 1940, Speed and Smith noted that the best results could be achieved in patients between the ages of 18 and 40 years.[33] Because the elbow is not a weight-bearing joint, they felt that stability was not absolutely necessary; therefore, it was important to excise sufficient bone to permit improved motion. An arc of motion of 50 degrees (between 70 and 120 degrees of flexion) was thought to be satisfactory for most activities.

In their classic, long-term follow-up study of elbow arthroplasty, Knight and Van Zandt reviewed 45 patients.[18] Indications for the operation included fibrous or bony ankylosis, partial ankylosis with insufficient motion, and partial ankylosis with disabling pain. Causes of the ankylosis were (1) acute infectious arthritis, (2) fractures or fracture-dislocations of the elbow resulting in pain or excessive limitation of motion, and (3) "atrophic" arthritis. The best candidates were between the ages of 20 and 50 years. Their patients were followed for an average of 14 years. They reported 56 per cent good and 22 per cent fair results. Two per cent had poor results and 20 per cent were failures. On an average, these patients regained motion 6 months to 6 years after operation, and maximum strength was achieved at about 1 year.

There was little correlation between the final roentgenographic appearance of the elbow and the functional result. It is important to note that these authors found that the range of motion and stability of the arthroplasty was best in patients with good periarticular structures and good elbow flexor and extensor musculature, emphasizing the dynamic elements of joint stability.

Subsequent reports have supported the use of fascial arthroplasty of the elbow for most patients. Our experience since 1952 has been essentially the same as that reported by Knight and Van Zandt.[18] A review of our recent experience with 37 fascial arthroplasties of the elbow revealed that 26 patients (70 per cent) had excellent or good results. There was one fair result, and seven had poor results. Three patients were lost to follow-up. Most of the patients with excellent or good results had a functional range of motion and were able to return to their activities of daily living with little or no pain. The fair and poor results were due to persistent pain, loss of motion, and excessive instability. Fascial arthroplasty of the elbow has been a gratifying procedure in restoring motion to the ankylosed joint and in relieving pain in joints damaged by osteoarthritis, trauma or sepsis, or rheumatoid arthritis. The elbow in our patients has, as a rule, been reasonably stable after fascial arthroplasty, and the procedure has provided a durable joint (Fig. 32–5).

COMPLICATIONS

Complications following fascial arthroplasty of the elbow have included bone resorption, heterotopic bone formation, triceps rupture, medial and lateral subluxation with concomitant instability, infection, and seroma formation in the thigh donor site, and long-term failure. The unpredictability of the procedure for these reasons prompted the development of the total elbow arthroplasty.[9]

Bone resorption occasionally occurs at the distal humeral condyles. It may cause no difficulty, or it may contribute to instability (Fig. 32–6), especially if resorption occurs more on one side than on the other. Subluxation and instability may occur from resorption or because of technical difficulties, yet the joint may function reasonably well in spite of medial or lateral subluxation (Fig. 32–6). If the tendency to subluxate is apparent at the time the arthroplasty is performed, the

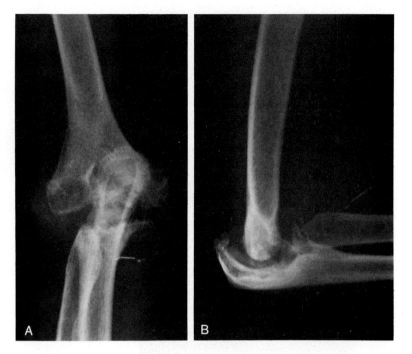

Figure 32–5. Twelve years after fascial arthroplasty this 33-year-old male developed progressive pain and loss of motion. The joint was re-explored, and a Silastic sheet was used to line the resected distal humerus *(A)*. Note lucency on AP view. One year later the motion obtained was 40 to 150 degrees flexion *(B)*, 30 degrees pronation, and 35 degrees supination. Minimal pain was present, and the patient was pleased.

elbow may be stabilized with a transarticular Steinmann pin, which is removed in about 3 weeks or prior to commencement of motion. If significant instability develops as a late sequela, ligamentous reconstruction may be beneficial.

Heterotopic bone formation rarely impairs function following elbow arthroplasty unless it is sufficiently exuberant to limit functional motion. Excision of heterotopic bone may temporarily improve motion. However, bone formation often recurs in spite of most methods used to prevent it. Triceps rupture is an uncommon complication that is related to the surgical exposure rather than to the procedure itself. If the exposure described below or the triceps is reflected in continuity, this complication should be minimized.

Infection following fascial arthroplasty should be managed promptly and aggressively. For superficial infections and cellulitis, the part should be placed at rest, elevated, and immobilized in a long arm posterior splint while appropriate antibiotics are administered. If the infection involves the deep structures, open drainage and excision of the fascial graft may be required. If bony infection occurs, removal of the involved bone may be required. Although this will leave the elbow more unstable, a useful limb can often be salvaged. Salvage with prosthetic replacement is out of the question.

If a hematoma or seroma forms in the thigh at the fascial donor site, it will usually resolve over a period of weeks. These collections rarely require drainage. If such an accumulation persists or is unusually large, drainage, if undertaken, must be done with strict aseptic technique. Needle aspiration should be attempted first.

Failure of the procedure due to pain, reankylosis, or instability may occur. As mentioned above, the result can deteriorate with time, especially in the active individual. Additional surgery may not be offered because frequently little more can be done to modify the symptoms or attain the expectations of the patient. If the precise cause of failure can be identified, revision is occasionally helpful. A Silastic membrane has been used with success in this setting (Fig. 32–6). In the older patient with reasonable expectations prosthetic replacement may become an effective salvage procedure.

AUTHOR'S PREFERRED TREATMENT METHOD

Although several techniques are available,[1, 17, 20, 35] with few modifications, the fascial arthroplasty technique we prefer is similar to that advocated by Campbell in 1939.[8] Two teams of surgeons expedite the procedure. While one team approaches the elbow, the other harvests the fascia lata graft, usually from the contralateral thigh.

With the patient supine, prepare and drape the entire arm and hand and then the contralateral thigh. Start the elbow incision about 7 or 8 cm proximal to the joint on the posterior

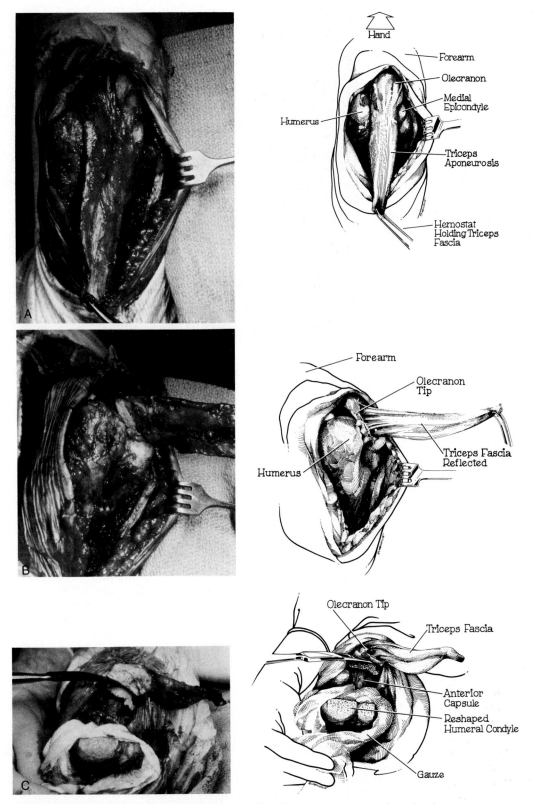

Figure 32–6. Operative technique of fascial arthroplasty. *A,* Flap of triceps aponeurosis released with incisions on each side. Humerus at bottom, ulna at top, retractor on medial side of elbow. *B,* Distal humerus has been exposed. Triceps aponeurosis at top, retractor medial to elbow. *C,* Bone is being removed from olecranon notch with curved gouge. Triceps aponeurosis at right. Distal humeral articular surface has been removed (wrapped in sponge).

Illustration continued on opposite page

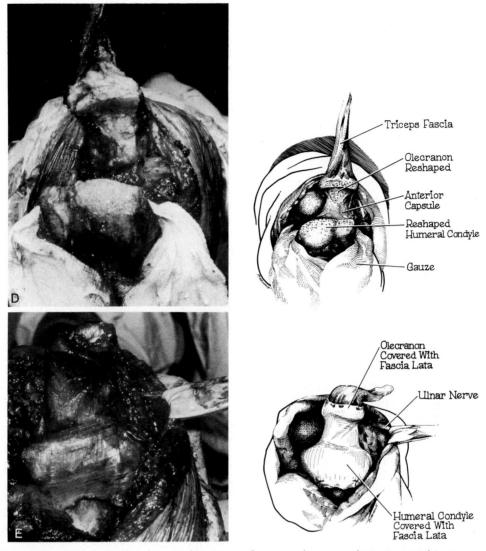

Figure 32–6 *Continued. D,* Bone removal is complete. Triceps flap at top, humerus at bottom wrapped in sponge. *E,* Fascia lata has been loosely laid over olecranon (top) and distal humerus (bottom). Retractor is medial to elbow. Penrose drain is protecting ulnar nerve.

aspect of the arm. Continue the incision distally 15 to 20 cm onto the forearm, curving lateral to the olecranon, and then back to the midline of the limb. Elevate the deep fascia laterally 2 to 3 cm to expose the triceps aponeurosis. The joint may be exposed using either of two methods. In the first of these, a transverse cut of the triceps aponeurosis is made at the proximal end of the incision and the triceps is mobilized by incising along its medial and lateral borders (Fig. 32–6A). Dissection from proximal to distal is done, and a flap of aponeurosis about 10 cm long is elevated, leaving it attached to the olecranon. Beneath the flap of the aponeurosis, the triceps muscle and periosteum are incised longitudinally in the midline over the distal

portion of the humerus (Fig. 32–6B). In the second method, also described by Campbell, the distal humerus and the elbow joint are approached by making a longitudinal incision in the midline through the aponeurosis, the triceps muscle, and the periosteum (Fig. 32–6, see also Chapter 8).

Following the exposure of the joint and distal humerus, using a periosteal elevator, strip the periosteum from the distal third of the posterior surface of the humerus. Retract the periosteum medially and laterally, exposing the radial head and olecranon. If there is osseous ankylosis of the elbow joint, use an osteotome to disrupt any fusion between the humerus and the olecranon and between the radial head and the humerus. Care should be taken at all times to isolate and protect the ulnar nerve, as well as all structures in the antecubital fossa. Anterior transplantation of the ulnar nerve is usually not required. After releasing any bony or fibrous ankylosis, flex the elbow and displace the radius and ulna medially. Using a motorized saw, osteotome, ronguer, and rasp, contour the distal end of the humerus into one condyle, convex distally from anterior to posterior (Fig. 32–6C). At times it may be helpful to fashion an inverted, shallow V-shaped notch in the humeral condyle. This should not be made into an excessively deep notch, however. Use a curved chisel or gouge to deepen and lengthen the trochlear notch of the ulna (Fig. 32–6D). Excise the head of the radius to the level of the distal portion of the trochlear notch. Smooth all bony surfaces with a rasp, and close the periosteum or a portion of fascia over the cut end of the radius.

Harvesting of the fascia lata graft can be most expeditiously done if a second surgical team proceeds with this task while the elbow is being prepared. On the lateral aspect of the thigh, make an incision in the lateral midline to expose the fascia lata. Make the skin incision long enough to allow removal of sufficient fascia lata to cover the exposed bone. A portion of fascia lata measuring about 8 to 9 cm by 20 to 25 cm is usually sufficient. Always dissect the fascia from proximal to distal. Fold the fascia in half longitudinally with the raw surface that was stripped from the muscle turned toward the bone and the smooth outer surface turned to face itself. Anchor the folded edge to the anterior capsule with three interrupted absorbable sutures, one on each side and one in the middle. Place the proximal half of the fascia over the humeral condyle and suture the fascia with interrupted sutures to the soft tissues proximal to the condyles. Use drill holes in the distal humerus to pass these sutures if the soft tissues are insufficient. Now place the distal half of the fascia over the trochlear notch and suture this portion in place. Insert a fold of fascia between the radius and ulna, cover the radial neck, and fix it with a pursestring suture (Fig. 32–6E).

Reduce the joint and hold the elbow flexed to 90 degrees. Insert suction drainage catheters as needed. Close the capsule, usually from distally to proximally. If a flap of triceps aponeurosis has been raised, suture it a bit more distally to allow elbow flexion to occur more freely. At times, after closure of the capsule, there is a tendency for the olecranon to slide from side to side. This can be avoided by placing a Steinmann pin starting in the olecranon with the elbow held at 90 degrees, passing the pin into the distal humeral medullary cavity. This pin is removed in 2 to 3 weeks.

POSTOPERATIVE CARE

A cast or posterior elbow splint is applied, holding the elbow immobilized at 90 degrees. The arm is placed on an abduction humeral splint to prevent rotation. The abduction humeral splint is worn 7 to 10 days. After wound healing is complete, in 2 to 3 weeks, the arm splint or cast is removed. A long arm posterior splint with straps and fasteners is applied. If a pin has been used for stability, it is removed at this time as well. The posterior arm splint is removed for 1 to 2 hours three or four times daily to allow active exercises to develop the elbow flexors and extensors. Three weeks after surgery, the posterior arm splint is discontinued except for night wear until a useful range of elbow motion and good muscle strength have been regained. A sling may be worn for support as needed for about 8 weeks. It is important to warn the patient that motion will be lost at this time and that there will be considerable tightening of the elbow for the next 2 or 3 months. However, if the patient will work at building up the musculature, motion will gradually return. At about 5 to 6 months after surgery motion will return and improve rapidly. Active exercises should continue for at least 12 months. About 2 years are required to regain maximum strength and motion.

References

1. Albee, F. H.: Arthroplasty of the Elbow. J. Bone Joint Surg. **15**:979, 1933.
2. Baer, W. S.: Arthroplasty With the Aid of Animal Membrane. Am. J. Orthop. Surg. **16**:1, 94, 171, 1918.
3. Baer, W. S.: Preliminary Report of Animal Membrane in Producing Mobility in Ankylosed Joint. Am. J. Orthop. Surg. **7**:3, 1909.
4. Barton, J. R.: On the Treatment of Ankylosis by the Formation of Artificial Joints. North Am. Med. Surg. J. **3**:279, 400, 1827.
5. Bateman, J. E.: Denervation of the Elbow Joint for Relief of Pain. J. Bone Joint Surg. **30B**:635, 1948.
6. Buzby, B. F.: End Results of Excision of the Elbow. Ann. Surg. **103**:625, 1936.
7. Campbell, W. C.: Mobilization of Joints with Bony Ankylosis: An Analysis of 110 Cases. J.A.M.A. **93**:976, 1924.
8. Campbell, W. C.: Operative Orthopedics. St. Louis, C. V. Mosby Co., 1939.
9. Dee, R.: Elbow Arthroplasty. Proc. R. Soc. Med. **62**:1031, 1969.
9a. Deland, J. T., Walker, P. S., Sledge, C. B., and

Farbenov, A.: Treatment of Posttraumatic Elbows With a New Hinge Destractor. Orthopedics **6**:732, 1983.

10. Ewald, F.: American Academy of Orthopedic Surgeons, Instructional Course Lecture, Atlanta, February, 1984.

11. Froimson, A. I., Silva, J. E., and Richey, D.: Cutis Arthroplasty of the Elbow. J. Bone Joint Surg. **58A**:863, 1976.

12. Hass, J.: Functional Arthroplasty. J. Bone Joint Surg. **26**:297, 1944.

13. Henderson, M. S.: What Are The Real Results of Arthroplasty? Am. J. Orthop. Surg. **16**:30, 1918.

14. Henderson, M. S.: Arthroplasty. Minn. Med. **8**:97, 1925.

15. Herbert, J. J.: Traitement des Ankyloses du Coude dans le Rheumatisme. Rev. Chir. Orthop. **44**:87, 1958.

16. Hurri, L., Pulkki, T., and Vainio, K.: Arthroplasty of the Elbow in Rheumatoid Arthritis. Acta Chir. Scand. **127**:459, 1964.

17. Kita, M.: Arthroplasty of the Elbow Using J-K Membrane. Acta Orthop. Scand. **48**:450, 1977.

18. Knight, R. A., and Van Zandt, I. L.: Arthroplasty of the Elbow: An End-Result Study. J. Bone Joint Surg. **34A**:610, 1952.

19. Lexer, E.: Über Gelenktransplantationen. Arch. Klink. Chir. **90**:263, 1909.

20. MacAusland, W. R., and MacAusland, A. R.: The Mobilization of Ankylosed Joints by Arthroplasty. Philadelphia, Lea & Febiger, 1929.

21. Mills, K., and Rush, J.: Skin Arthroplasty of the Elbow. Aust, N.Z. J. Surg. **41**:179, 1971.

22. Murphy, J. B.: Ankylosis: Arthroplasty—Clinical and Experimental. Trans. Am. Surg. Assoc. **22**:215, 1904.

23. Murphy, J. B.: Ankylosis, Clinical and Experimental. J.A.M.A. **44**:1573, 1671, 1794, 1905.

24. Ollier, L.: Traite des Resections et des Operations Conservatrices qu'on peut Practiquer sur le Systeme Osseux. Paris, G. Masson, 1885–1889.

25. Payr, E.: Über die Operative Mobilizierung Ankylosierter Gelenke. Munch, Med.Wchnschr. **37**:1921, 1910.

26. Phemister, D. B., and Miller, E. M.: The Method of New Joint Formation in Arthroplasty. Surg. Gynecol. Obstet. **26**:406, 1924.

27. Putti, V.: Arthroplasty. Am. J. Orthop. Surg. **3**:421, 1921.

28. Richard, D.: Arthroplasty of the Elbow (abstract). J. Bone Joint Surg. **49B**:594, 1967.

29. Rockwell, M.: Arthroplasty of the Elbow (abstract). J. Bone Joint Surg. **45A**:664, 1963.

30. Schüller, M.: Chirungische Mittheilungen über die Chronish Rheumatischen Gelenkentzundungen. Arch. Klin. Chir. **45**:153, 1893.

31. Silva, J. F.: Old Dislocations of the Elbow. Ann. R. Coll. Surg. Engl. **22**:363, 1958.

32. Smith, F. M.: Surgery of the Elbow, 2nd ed. Philadelphia, W. B. Saunders Co., 1972.

33. Speed, J. S., and Smith, H.: Arthroplasty: A Review of the Past Ten Years. Int. Abst. Surg. Gynecol. Obstet. **70**:224, 1940.

34. Unander-Scharin, L., and Karlholm, S.: Experience of Arthroplasty of the Elbow. Acta Orthop. Scand. **36**:54, 1965.

35. Vainio, K.: Arthroplasty of the Elbow and Hand in Rheumatoid Arthritis: A Study of 131 Operations. In Chapchal, G. (ed.) Synovectomy and Arthroplasty in Rheumatoid Arthritis. Stuttgart, Georg Thieme Verlag, 1967, pp. 66–70.

36. Verneuil, A.: De la Creation d'une Fausse Articulation par Section ou Resection Partielle de l'os Maxillaire Inferieur, Comme Moyen de Remedier L'Ankylose Orale de Fausse de la Machoire Inferieur. Arch. Gen. Med. **15**:284, 1860.

CHAPTER 33

Custom Arthroplasty and Hemiarthroplasty of the Elbow

JAMES LONDON

The profound loss of upper extremity function that occurs when there is any significant damage to the elbow joint has stimulated surgeons for many years to attempt to replace all or part of the elbow joint. The initial prostheses were custom designs that *replaced* part or all of the distal humerus or the proximal ulna. Later designs *resurfaced* the distal humerus or the proximal ulna with devices that required less bone resection. Results with these prostheses were generally but not uniformly unsatisfactory.

The modern era of joint replacement surgery was made possible by two advances made by Sir John Charnley: (1) low-friction metal on polyethylene bearings, and (2) rigid fixation of components to bone with acrylic cement. Success with the initial total hip arthroplasties led surgeons to apply the same technologic advances to elbow arthroplasty. Unfortunately, the results with the elbow have been clearly inferior to those of the hip joint. Considering the disappointing results with total elbow replacement, it is worth re-examining the early work with custom and hemiprostheses. This review is intended to help determine why most of these failed and, more important, why some demonstrated good or even excellent results.

CUSTOM REPLACEMENT ARTHROPLASTY

A search of the world literature reveals that, excluding the proximal radius, 21 custom implant arthroplasties were reported prior to 1967.[1, 8, 10, 16] The entire distal humerus was replaced in fifteen cases,[1, 7, 8, 10, 16] part of the distal humerus (capitellum) in two cases,[4] the proximal end of the ulna in one case,[5] the distal end of the humerus and the joint sur-

faces of the ulna in one case,[15] and the entire elbow joint with a hinged prosthesis in two instances.[2] Seven of those prostheses were metal (stainless steel and Vitallium),[1–5, 16] nine were acrylic,[7, 8, 12, 15] four were nylon,[7] and the first prosthesis (1925) was metal covered by dental vulcanized rubber.[10] These devices were custom designs with the configuration and dimensions being determined by radiographs of the uninvolved elbow. Fixation of the components was done by press-fitting an intramedullary stem with or without the use of additional transfixation screws.

Most of the early reports served as single or limited case reports with variable follow-up. The task of assessing the results of these early efforts accurately is difficult.

The follow-up in these 21 cases ranged from only 4 months[7] to as long as 23 years,[13] but the mean was just less than 3 years. The most impressive reported finding was the relief of pain. Although the range of motion varied, the mean arc was almost 100 degrees. Complications included wound infection, ulnar nerve palsy, joint stiffness with or without ectopic bone formation, dislocation, and loosening. When loosening occurred it tended to be slowly progressive and often caused excessive bone resorption. Pain recurred in cases when there was evidence of loosening of the prosthesis.

The largest group of custom prostheses consisted of 15 patients in whom the entire distal humerus was replaced (Figs. 33–1 and 33–2). The most complete and illustrative reports are those of MacAusland (four nylon prostheses),[7] Barr and Eaton (one Vitallium prosthesis),[1] and Street.[14] The follow-up in these cases ranged from 8 months to 23 years. Initial pain relief was satisfactory in almost all elbows, and motion was restored to a mean

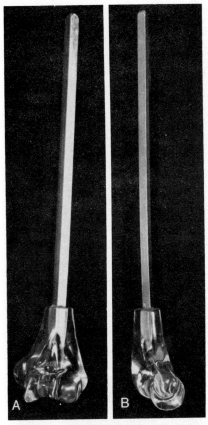

Figure 33–1. An acrylic prosthesis with an 11-mm diamond-shaped stainless steel stem designed by Dana M. Street.

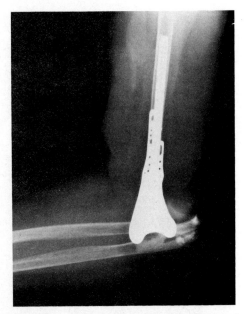

Figure 33–3. A common problem of distal humeral prosthetic replacement is instability due to the lack of collateral ligament integrity.

arc of 105 degrees. All but three arthroplasties were stable and functioned satisfactorily. Complications included dislocation, infection, loosening about the intramedullary stem, and one case of breakage of a nylon prosthesis.

The most persistent problem was instability due to loss of ligamentous support, and this is the limiting factor in the use of these devices (Fig. 33–3).

A replacement prosthesis for the proximal ulna was utilized by Johnson[5] in a case involving significant bone loss from a shotgun injury (Fig. 33–4A). The postoperative range of motion was limited to 40 degrees, but the patient had only minimal pain with strenuous, heavy work. The prosthesis lasted more than 13 years but eventually, because of instability and pain, required revision to a total elbow arthroplasty (Fig. 33–2B, C).[8]

A few custom-made ulnohumeral joint replacements were implanted prior to the modern era of total joint arthroplasty (Fig. 33–5).[2] These implants were metal or metal-hinge devices and have been used sporadically around the world[12] in cases in which there was significant bone loss or severe destruction of both sides of the elbow joint. These hinged prostheses provided stability not offered by the hemiarthroplasties, but loosening eventually occurred at the bone–prosthesis interface, and this was associated with the return of pain.

RESURFACING PROSTHESES

Because of the complications with extensive replacement surgery, resurfacing prostheses for the distal humerus or the proximal ulna were developed. These prostheses required

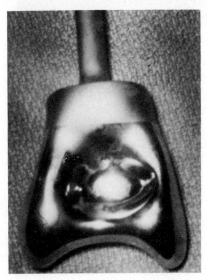

Figure 33–2. Vitallium replacement prosthesis for the distal humerus.

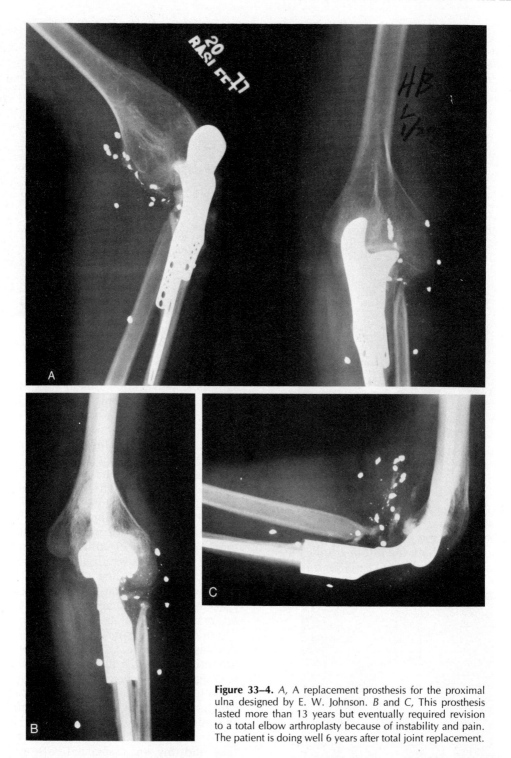

Figure 33–4. *A,* A replacement prosthesis for the proximal ulna designed by E. W. Johnson. *B* and *C,* This prosthesis lasted more than 13 years but eventually required revision to a total elbow arthroplasty because of instability and pain. The patient is doing well 6 years after total joint replacement.

less bone resection than the earlier replacement prostheses. The resurfacing prostheses demanded a variety of shapes and sizes for better accommodation of variations in anatomy, and this constraint limited their widespread use.

A Vitallium "saddle" was designed in the 1960s to resurface the proximal ulna[9] by Bic-

kle and Peterson of the Mayo Clinic (Fig. 33–6A). The prosthesis was custom-made and was draped over the articular surface of the proximal ulna, gaining considerable fixation by virtue of its geometric configuration and additional fixation by two transfixing screws. The implant was inserted in eight elbows with the primary indication of rheumatoid arthri-

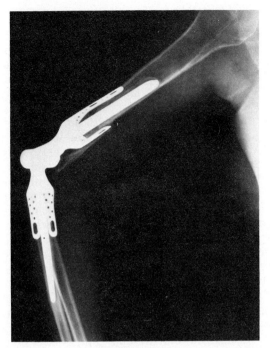

Figure 33–5. An early custom total elbow arthroplasty. Bone fixation was inadequate, and the metal-on-metal bearing was the source of considerable metal debris.

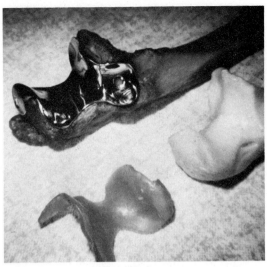

Figure 33–6. A vitallium saddle designed by Bickel and Peterson to resurface the proximal ulna. (From Peterson, L. F. A., and James, J. M.: Surgery of the rheumatoid elbow. Orthop. Clin. North Am. 2:667, 1971.)

tis. A long-term follow-up study of these cases has not been reported, but Peterson has indicated that many of these patients had satisfactory pain relief, and an acceptable range of motion.[9] An instance that was considered a moderately satisfactory long-term result 15 years after surgery is illustrated (Fig. 33–7). Loosening or joint motion limitation eventually occurred and progressed steadily.

In 1974 Street and Stevens reported on the use of a distal humerus resurfacing prosthesis made of stainless steel (Fig. 33–8).[13] This prosthesis articulated with the intact olecranon and radial head. The device was driven from the side onto the trimmed distal end of the humerus, providing for a tight fit and obviating the need for supplemental mechanical function. This represents a rather conservative approach as little bone was removed and the ligaments may be preserved. The prosthesis was provided in seven sizes with the proper size being determined preoperatively with plastic overlap from the roentgenograms.

The extent of clinical use of this prosthesis is difficult to estimate, but Street reported the results in 10 elbows: five with post-traumatic arthritis, three with rheumatoid arthritis, and two with hemophilia. Follow-up ranged from 1 to 7 years with a mean of 2 years and 4 months. Four of these elbows could be considered satisfactory at follow-up examination, with at least a 70-degree arc of motion, little or no pain, and a stable elbow joint. The follow-up period in these four elbows was a

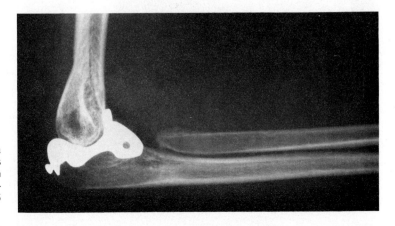

Figure 33–7. Fifteen-year follow-up of a patient with post-traumatic arthritis treated with a vitallium interposition ("saddle") arthroplasty. There was extension to 80 degrees and flexion to 135 degrees. (Courtesy of L. F. A. Peterson.)

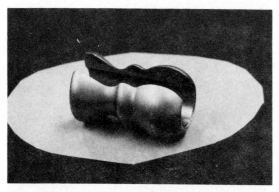

Figure 33–8. The distal humeral prosthesis designed by Dana Street and Peter Stevens.

mean of 3 years. Six elbows were graded poor at follow-up—three had ankylosed, two were unstable, and one had a markedly restricted range of motion due to ectopic bone formation. One interesting finding was evidence of new cortical bone formation inside the channel of this prosthesis (Fig. 33–9). This suggested that fixation of a resurfacing prosthesis might continue to improve if the joint reaction forces were properly transmitted to the underlying bone and stress shielding of bone was avoided. This is an observation that is pertinent today as we consider the concept of "resurfacing prostheses" or of "bone ingrowth" for prosthesis fixation.

The most frequently used partial replacement is that of the radial head. The history, indications, and results of this procedure are discussed in detail in Chapter 20.

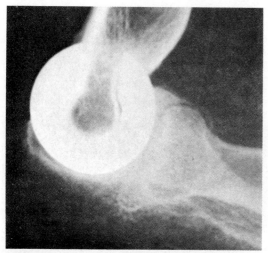

Figure 33–9. Three years following insertion of a Stevens-Street prosthesis there is new cortical bone growth inside the prosthesis. (From Street, D. M., and Stevens, P. S.: A humeral replacement prosthesis for the elbow. Results in ten elbows. J. Bone Joint Surg. 56A:1147, 1974.)

CONCLUSION

Early efforts to replace or resurface parts of the elbow joint answered some questions but raised others that persist even today. The initial concerns were whether foreign material articulating with cartilage could satisfactorily relieve pain, provide an adequate range of motion, and restore function to the extremity. The additional problem of long-term rigid fixation was also identified. These very early prostheses duplicated the size and geometric configuration of the normal elbow in only the most general way, yet tended to provide, although temporarily, a functional, relatively pain-free elbow. The primary complication with these prostheses was loosening or instability. Once loosening occurred, it tended to progress relentlessly, and the initial good results deteriorated with the passage of time. Experiences with these prostheses are not unlike our experience today with a wide variety of total elbow replacements. Loosening of the hinged, constrained components continues to be a primary problem.

As the field of joint replacement surgery advances, new materials are being developed, improved fixation of prostheses with the potential of bone ingrowth is possible* and more precise replication of excised joint parts with new modeling techniques has been reported.[11] These developments raise the question of the possible future for hemiarthroplasty of the elbow.†

New materials could provide a better surface interaction with articular cartilage. Bone ingrowth may provide adequate fixation not only of total joints but also of parts of joints. Molding techniques could quickly and exactly duplicate part or all of the articular surface of a fractured, arthritic, or neoplastic joint. These advances might again focus our attention on custom hemiarthroplasty of the elbow for selected pathologic conditions.

References

1. Barr, J. S., and Eaton, R. G.: Elbow Reconstruction with a New Prosthesis to Replace the Distal End of the Humerus. A Case Report. J. Bone Joint Surg. **47A:**1408, 1965.
2. Boerma, I., and deWaard, D. J.: Osteoplastiche Verankerung von Metallprothesen bei Pseudarthrose und bei Arthropastik. Acta Chir. Scand. **86:**511, 1942.

---

* Morrey, B. F.: Personal communication.

† Allograft replacement of all or either side of the joint is an active, ongoing, but as yet limited application of joint replacement surgery. Because of limited availability, artificial devices will continue to be used.

3. Chatzidakis, C.: Arthroplasty of the Elbow Joint Using a Vitallium Prosthesis. Int. Surg. **53**:119, 1970.

4. Jacobssom, A.: Fracture of the Capitellum of the Humerus in Adults. Treatment with Intra-Articular Chrom-Cobolt-Molybdenum Prosthesis. Acta Orthop. Scand. **26**:184, 1957.

5. Johnson, E. W., Jr., and Schlein, A. P.: Vitallium Prosthesis for the Olecranon and Proximal Part of the Ulna. Case Report with Thirteen Year Follow-Up. J. Bone Joint Surg. **52A**:721, 1970.

6. Lenggenhager, K.: Zur Frage des Kunstlichen Ellbogengelenkes. Helv. Chir. Acta **25**:338, 1958.

7. MacAusland, W. R.: Replacement of the Lower End of the Humerus with a Prosthesis. A Report of Four Cases. West. J. Surg. Gynecol. Obstet. **62**:557, 1954.

8. Mellen, R. H., and Phalen, G. S.: Arthroplasty of the Elbow by Replacement of the Distal Portion of the Humerus with an Acrylic Prosthesis. J. Bone Joint Surg. **29**:348, 1947.

9. Peterson, L. F. A., and Janes, J. M.: Surgery of the Rheumatoid Elbow. Orthop. Clin. North Am. :667, 1971.

10. Robineau, R.: Contribution of a l'Etude des Prosthesis Osseuses. Bull. Soc. Nat. Chir. **53**:886, 1927.

11. Shiba, R., Siu, D., and Sorbie, C.: Geometric Analysis of the Elbow Joint. Submitted, J. Bone Joint Surg., 1984.

12. Silva, J. F.: Arthroplasty of the Elbow. Singapore Med. J. **8**:222, 1969.

13. Street, D. M., and Stevens, P. S.: A Humeral Replacement Prosthesis for the Elbow. Results in Ten Elbows. J. Bone Joint Surg. **56A**:1147, 1974.

14. Street, D. M.: Elbow Prosthesis, A Historical View. Acta Orthop. Belg. **41**:4, 1975.

15. Tessarolo, G.: Endoprotesi Acrilica Articolare per il Gomito. Minerva Ortop. **3**:308, 1952.

16. Venable, C. S.: An Elbow and an Elbow Prosthesis: Case of Complete Loss of the Lower Third of the Humerus. Am. J. Surg. **83**:271, 1952.

CHAPTER 34

Total Joint Replacement

B. F. MORREY and R. S. BRYAN

As may be concluded from earlier chapters, total elbow arthroplasty is the logical culmination of several surgical options available for severe elbow dysfunction.

HISTORICAL PERSPECTIVES

The development of total elbow arthroplasty has been traced by Coonrad,[12] who divided elbow reconstructive surgery into four eras (Table 34–1). In the first period (1885 to 1947) resection arthroplasty for infection and interposition (anatomic) arthroplasty for post-traumatic and, less commonly, rheumatoid arthritis were predominant. The current status of this surgical philosophy is discussed in detail in Chapter 32.

In the second period (1947 to 1970) partial replacement and custom metal hinged devices were used. Reports of ulnar[35, 62] or humeral articular replacements,[4, 39, 40] usually for post-traumatic arthritis, appeared as early as 1937.[62] Resurfacing devices for the olecranon[52] and trochlea[60] were devised. Replacing both sides of the joint was reported by Boerma and deWaard in 1942[5] and by others[10] using a steel hinge articulation.[17] In general, these devices were of limited value because of the unpredictable relief of pain and the predictable instability or loosening (Chapter 33).

The third era, 1970–1975, was marked by early attempts at total elbow arthroplasty us-

ing methacrylate for component fixation. These prostheses retained a rigid metal-on-metal hinge articulation.[14, 29, 55, 59] Although follow-up was limited, the cemented prostheses were enthusiastically received because they offered more complete relief from pain and better motion and stability than did other available procedures. Unfortunately, loosening was common,[28, 59] even with the added feature of a metal on high-density polyethylene articulation.[46]

Present Era

As the inevitable failure of the constrained total elbow arthroplasty became manifest and emerging biomechanical data became available, the prostheses of the current, fourth era have evolved into two basic types—joint resurfacing and semiconstrained articulated devices. The relatively debris-free and low-friction metal and high-density polyethylene articulation is now standard with all implant designs.

RATIONALE AND DESIGN CRITERIA

More than any other peripheral joint, the elbow is unsuited to the time-honored definitive treatment for pain or dysfunction—arthrodesis. For other joints a position of usual function can be identified, but this is not

Table 34–1. **Four Eras of Total Elbow Arthroplasty**

Era	Time Period	Characteristics
First	1885 to 1947	Era of resection, interposition, and anatomic arthroplasty
Second	1947 to 1970	Era of partial and occasional total (hinge) joint arthroplasty
Third	1970 to 1975	Era of constrained metal-to-metal, hinge-joint replacement with methacrylate fixation
Fourth	1975 to present	Era of semiconstrained metal-to-polyethylene hinge of snap-fitting prostheses and unconstrained metal-to-polyethylene resurfacing arthroplasty
Fifth	The future	Biologically fixed, semiconstrained, and resurfacing devices

Table 34–2. **Design Criteria**

Kinematics
Stability
Load transmission
Materials
Friction
Wear
Fixation
Sizing and instrumentation
Can be salvaged

possible for the elbow joint (see Chapter 5). Hence, some procedure to relieve pain while preserving motion is a prerequisite for elbow function, and thus for reconstructive surgery. Historically, these basic goals have been elusive for resection as well as for anatomic or replacement arthroplasty (Table 34–2).[20]

Kinematics. All reported total elbow arthroplasties provide functional motion: 30 to 130 degrees of flexion and 50 degrees of pronation and of supination.[42] The axis of rotation is along the anterior cortex of the distal humerus[41] on the lateral projection. Not all implant designs replicate this feature even though the correct axis of rotation is important to balance the soft tissues properly.

Stability. Stability is ensured by the semiconstrained prosthesis with a captive articulation but causes increased stress at the interfaces. For resurfacing devices, stability is attained by the articular surface and the soft tissue, but the joint with this device may dislocate. For the snap-fit design, stability

may change as a function of time, with wear or cold flow of the high-density polyethylene.

Load Transmission. The joint system must withstand the peak transmitted loads as well as the routine cyclic applied forces (Fig. 34–1).[51] A force of up to three times the body weight is transmitted across the elbow joint with activities of daily living,[2, 21, 32, 49] and these are repeated as often as 1 million cycles per year.[13] Distributed forces across the radiohumeral[1, 30, 66] and ulnohumeral joints as well as rotational stresses during simple lifting (Fig. 34–2)[1] may exceed several times body weight across the radiohumeral joint alone.[3]

Theoretically, a three-component device provides more physiologic force transmission (Fig. 34–3) and increases the stability of a resurfacing device,[18] but the proper alignment of a three-piece prosthesis is difficult.

Materials. Although resistance of the present generation of metal alloys to corrosion is good,[67] the tendency and effect of ion release is uncertain.[31] It is known that metal debris does elicit harsh reactions of the soft tissue (Fig. 34–4). The convex configuration of the ultra-high molecular weight polyethylene has been shown to have a greater tendency for debris formation.[36] Further, the coefficient of friction of a polished metal and ultra-high molecular weight polyethylene is still several orders of magnitude greater than that of a normal joint.[19] Resurfacing devices imply a larger surface area of contact that may in-

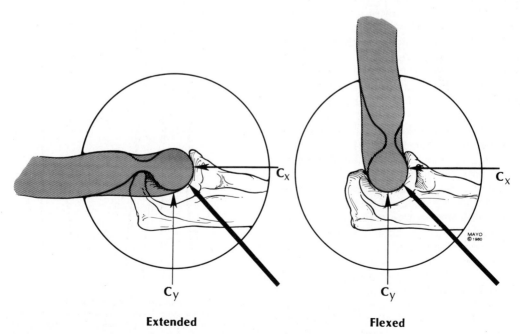

Extended   **Flexed**

Figure 34–1. The cyclic load pattern that produces first axial and then posterior displacement loads as a function of elbow position.

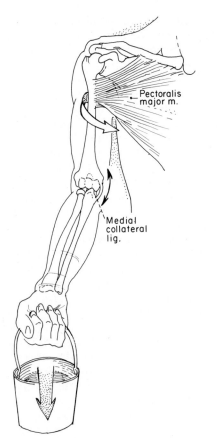

Figure 34–2. While lifting a heavy object, a rotational force is imparted to the distal humerus that stresses the collateral ligaments and tends to rotate the humeral stemmed components.

crease friction, but this is necessary for a stable joint. Further, the ultra-high molecular weight polyethylene may be deformed by cold flow,[64] unless it is sufficiently thick or reinforced by metal to prevent this.

Fixation. The elbow prosthesis should utilize as much of the distal humeral bone stock[57] as possible for fixation by cement or biologic ingrowth. Resurfacing devices that do not violate the intramedullary canal must be carefully designed so that stresses are transmitted across and not concentrated at the prosthesis–bone interface. The longer stemmed intramedullary devices tend to allow less stress transmission across the distal humerus.

Sizing and Instrumentation. Early experience with yoked humeral designs that were poorly sized caused fracture of the supracondylar bone columns.[43] Thus, several sizes should be available to fit the anatomy properly.

Salvage Potential. A failed joint replacement must allow for (1) the reimplantation of another device, (2) adequate residual function if the implant is removed, and (3) a possible arthrodesis (see Chapter 36).

These design considerations are obviously not absolute, and some concepts may conflict with others. It is clear that more than one design may be necessary for adequate treatment of the spectrum of pathology that involves the elbow joint. It is equally obvious that understanding the theoretical requirements and the clinical performance allows a more scientific approach to the difficult problem of elbow joint replacement.

INDICATIONS

As with reconstructive procedures of other joints, the indications for total elbow arthroplasty can be expected to change and broaden as improved long-term results are obtained. In general, inability to use the extremity for personal care activities or for functions of daily living because of pain, lack of motion, or instability constitutes the basis for elbow joint replacement.[6, 12, 15, 21] Gross deformity, recurrent synovitis, or significant cartilage loss are generally present before this final option is offered to the patient.

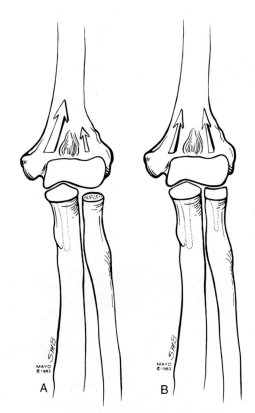

Figure 34–3. Schematic representation of elbow arthroplasty with an absent radial head. *A,* Theoretically, eccentric forces are being transmitted across the humeral prosthetic interface. *B,* With the radial head component, a more uniform distribution of forces across the distal humerus is realized.

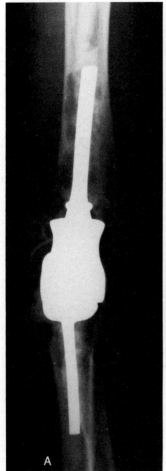

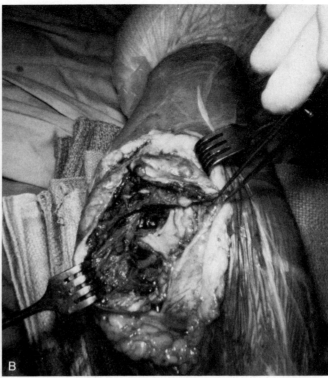

Figure 34–4. Seven years after placement of a metal-on-metal hinged prosthesis, pain and loosening are present. *A*, The scalloped border of the distal humerus suggests an active inflammatory process. *B*, At the time of revision surgery, deeply stained and discolored synovial and periarticular tissues revealed that metal debris was present in these soft tissues.

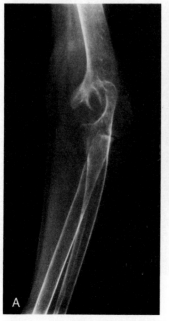

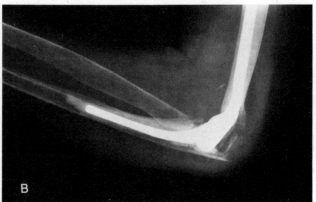

Figure 34–5. *A*, Excessive bone resorption due to chronic synovitis in a patient with rheumatoid arthritis. *B*, This degree of instability is best treated, in our opinion, by a more constrained prosthesis.

Rheumatoid Arthritis

Pain that does not respond to medical management, combined with various amounts of joint destruction, constitutes the primary indication for total elbow arthroplasty. Patients with painful synovitis but with less severe involvement of bone may be treated by syn-ovectomy and radial head excision (see Chapter 40).

Motion loss is usually considered a secondary indication for surgery. However, because ankylosis of the elbow is so disabling, this may occasionally constitute a primary indication for elbow replacement. Rheumatoid ankylosis is uncommon and is usually seen

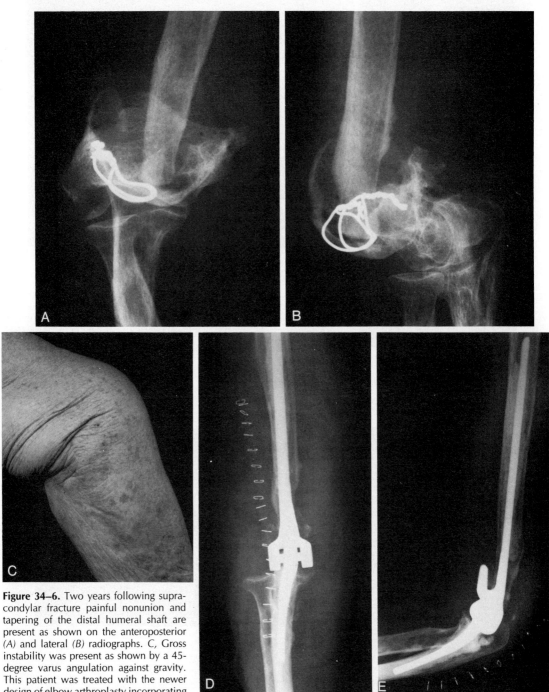

Figure 34–6. Two years following supracondylar fracture painful nonunion and tapering of the distal humeral shaft are present as shown on the anteroposterior (A) and lateral (B) radiographs. C, Gross instability was present as shown by a 45-degree varus angulation against gravity. This patient was treated with the newer design of elbow arthroplasty incorporating an anterior flange to control the rotational and posterior displacement stresses. D, The anteroposterior and (E) lateral views after replacement.

with juvenile rheumatoid arthritis; in our experience, it may recur even after replacement surgery.

Nontraumatic instability uncommonly occurs in the absence of pain. When present, however, an articulated elbow replacement effectively provides stability and relieves pain (Fig. 34–5).

In the patient with multijoint involvement, special consideration should be given to the timing of elbow surgery. To avoid stress on the elbow implant with crutch walking, elbow surgery should ideally be performed after reconstruction of the hip, knees, or ankle. Fracture of the humerus with an elbow replacement has been reported during crutch walking.[9] Shoulder surgery generally precedes elbow replacement to avoid stresses on the elbow implant during intraoperative shoulder manipulation. However, if it is perceived that elbow pain might compromise the rehabilitation program following hip, knee, or shoulder surgery, total elbow arthroplasty should be performed first. Approximation of the tips of the shoulder and elbow prostheses should be avoided to prevent stress concentration and fracture.

Post-traumatic Arthritis

As in patients with rheumatoid arthritis, the surgical indications for total elbow arthroplasty for post-traumatic arthritis are pain, loss of motion, and instability. However, because the patient may be very young, other treatment options should be considered. Interposition arthroplasty is indicated in the properly selected patient with painful post-traumatic ankylosis (see Chapter 32). Loss of bone or joint deformity with resultant instability or ankylosis is often present in these patients. Although such findings provide the basis for surgical intervention, the post-traumatic alteration of the bone architecture frequently poses difficult technical problems.

Distraction arthroplasty may prove to be an effective means of treating this type of patient.[24] Extensive bone loss may compromise the chances of a satisfactory long-term result with a prosthesis because fixation of the implant is compromised. Allograft replacement of the elbow joint has been performed in such patients on a limited basis. Supracondylar nonunion is a relatively uncommon and difficult management problem that may be successfully treated in some instances with distraction arthroplasty or with the newer generation of semiconstrained, flanged replacement devices (Fig. 34–6).

As when considering any prosthetic replacement surgery, the clinical result of a failed procedure must be weighed against the preoperative state. If the salvage procedure for a failed prosthetic replacement is judged no worse or better than the current condition, total elbow arthroplasty might be offered after a thorough discussion with the patient. Because a high failure rate has been observed to date with this group of patients, joint replacement arthroplasty is offered very cautiously for post-traumatic arthritis.

CONTRAINDICATION

The presence of an active or subacute septic process at or about the elbow is an absolute contraindication for total elbow arthroplasty. Active infection of the musculoskeletal system from any other source should delay surgery for a minimum of 3 months after treatment and after all evidence of infection has resolved.

Loss of bone stock is a contraindication for resurfacing devices. Most standardized implants do not provide adequate rotatory fixation for this type of problem. A custom design might be employed, but this increases stresses at the bone–cement interface and probably compromises the long-term result. Allograft replacement or the newer Mayo-modified Coonrad prosthesis may provide more reliable options in this difficult clinical setting.

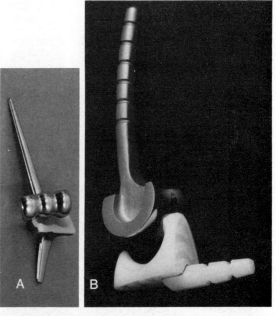

Figure 34–7. The capitellocondylar resurfacing arthroplasty (A) and the London (B) are two designs commonly used in the United States.

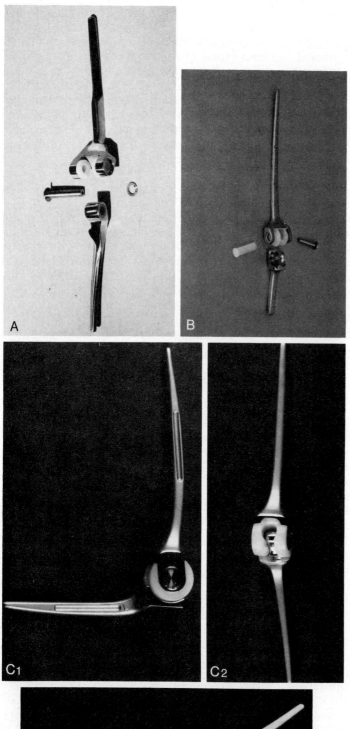

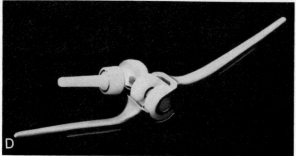

Figure 34–8. The most commonly used semi-constrained prostheses are mechanically articulated with an axis as with the Coonrad *(A)* or the Pritchard-Walker *(B)* or a snap-fit type of articulation as wih the triaxial design *(C).* The Arizona radiocapitellar device allows replacement of the radiohumeral joint as well as the snap-fit type of articulation *(D). (C* from Inglis, Allen E.: Tri-axial total elbow replacement: indications, surgical technique and results. *In* American Academy of Orthopedic Surgeons: Symposium on total joint replacement of the upper extremity. St. Louis, The C.V. Mosby Co., 1982.)

Soft tissue contracture and scarring of the flexor or extensor musculature similarly compromises the anticipated outcome. Paralysis of the extensors does not preclude this option, but absent or marked weakness of the elbow flexors is a relative contraindication for total elbow arthroplasty.

Elbow arthrodesis or painless ankylosis in a satisfactory position is considered a firm contraindication for elbow replacement at this time. If the elbow with arthrodesis is painless, stable, unilateral, and in a good position (90 degrees for unilateral involvement), a reasonably satisfactory but functionally compromised extremity results. Revision to attain motion cannot be justified because of the uncertainty of the long-term outcome of replacement surgery.

As with other joints, replacement of the elbow by a prosthetic implant in an uncooperative patient is to be avoided.

SPECIFIC REPLACEMENT OPTIONS

Two general types of joint replacement procedures are currently available—resurfacing and semiconstrained designs. The resurfacing devices tend to replicate the anatomy of the distal humerus and proximal ulna, thereby providing stability primarily by joint congruence and soft tissue constraints. Several such devices currently are commercially available, and others are under investigation in this and other countries (Fig. 34–7). A minimum amount of bone is resected. Stability is inherent in the design based on the arc of curvature of the ulnar component and varies from one design to another.[9, 59, 65]

The semiconstrained prostheses may be defined as those that possess inherent stability by a mechanical locking of the components, usually with a hinge or a snap-fit axis arrangement (Fig. 34–8).[6, 33, 56, 63] The characteristic feature of either type of device is that some rotation is allowed about all three axes—flexion, varus-valgus, and axial rotation. Slight variations in the amount of "play" exist, but generally this is about 7 to 10 degrees (see Fig. 34–9).

An additional classification may be applied according to whether the radiohumeral articulation is replaced. Theoretically, the radiohumeral joint helps distribute forces to the distal humerus.[3, 30, 63, 66] Some have stated, however, that the articulation is of no value and may be ignored.[61] It is of interest that several designs that initially ignored this joint have incorporated radiohumeral articular fea-

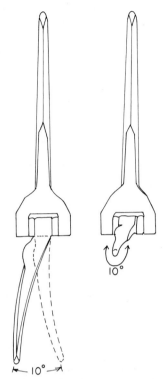

Figure 34–9. The semiconstrained devices allow some "play" at the ulnohumeral articulation. This feature is common both to the snap-fit and the axis type of articulation.

tures in subsequent modifications and others have abandoned the effort.[24] To date, however, the advantages are speculative. Alignment of the radial component has proved difficult, and no clinical data are available to support or refute the value of a prosthetic radiohumeral articulation.

Resurfacing Arthroplasty

Rationale. Replication or restoration of as near-normal anatomy as possible provides the basis for resurfacing arthroplasty. Stability is derived from the soft tissue envelope and the degree of congruence or arc of contact offered by the joint. It is generally felt that this option is "conservative" in that little bone is generally removed, thus allowing further reconstructive options in the event of failure.

Indications. In most reported series[23, 37, 38, 59, 65] the use of a resurfacing device is almost exclusively limited to and recommended for rheumatoid arthritis (Table 34–3, Fig. 34–10). Recalcitrant, painful synovitis associated with medial and lateral collateral ligament competency and adequate distal humeral and proximal ulnar bone constitutes the primary

Table 34–3. **Results of 163 Resurfacing Procedures**

Author	No. Procedures	Diagnosis	Follow-up (yr)	Extension-Flexion(°)	Pronation-Supination(°)	Pain Relief	Satisfactory Results[a]
Cavendish and Elloy (1977)	10	(?)	1.5 to 3	(?)	(?)	8/10	8
Ewald et al. (1980)	54	Rheumatoid arthritis	2 to 5	31/136	74.53	(?)	48
London (1980)	16	Rheumatoid arthritis	0.5 to 2	(?)	(?)	14/16	14
Kudo et al. (1980)	24[a]	Rheumatoid arthritis	1 to 7	42/124	29/49	22/24	21
Souter (1981)	22	Rheumatoid arthritis	0.5 to 1.5	52/143	65/66	22/22	18
Tuke et al. (1981)	27	Undefined	7 to 5	37/137	62/71	(?)	22
Wadsworth (1981)	10	Rheumatoid arthritis	0.8 to 1.2	24/133	62/74	9	9
TOTAL	163	Rheumatoid arthritis	2.7	36/131[a]	60/61	75/82 (91%)	87%

[a]Complications considered in calculation.

indication for the use of this device. The indications have been expanded somewhat by Ewald to include patients over 70 years of age with nonrheumatoid conditions.[25]

Design Options. Several devices have been designed and used around the world (Table 34–4). The common feature of all is the lack of a captive articulation, the components being readily separated with distraction. The arc of curvature of the ulnar component varies from 145 degrees in the less constrained Wadsworth device to 220 degrees in the London design.[38]* Variable amounts of gliding[61] or rotation[65] are accommodated by some designs.

Technique. Although several surgical approaches have been used, a lateral extensile Kocher approach to the joint is probably the most popular exposure (see Chapter 8). The

---

*Serboufek, J.: Personal communication.

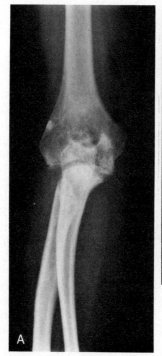

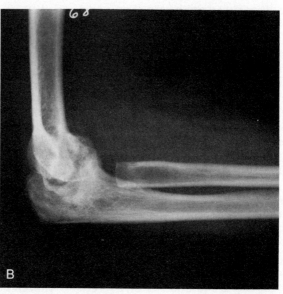

Figure 34–10. *A, B,* Severe pain and synovitis in patients with rheumatoid arthritis.

Illustration continued on opposite page

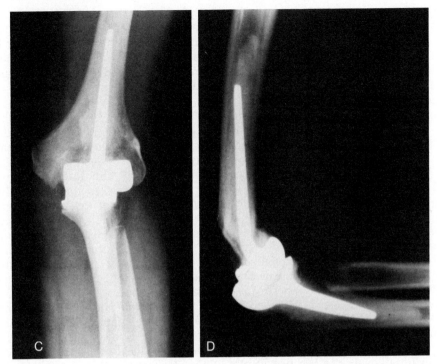

Figure 34–10. *Continued. C, D,* This amount of bone and type of presentation is felt to be particularly suitable for resurfacing arthroplasty.

radial collateral ligament is subperiosteally released from its humeral attachment and may be reattached later. The elbow is then hinged open on the medial collateral ligament, thus preserving this important structure. The ulnar nerve is not exposed. The radial head is removed routinely. The distal humerus may be prepared with the ronguer if the bone is soft. Special instrumentation is required for some of the more complex designs but often is not necessary. The contour will be a function of the specific device used. The medullary canal is identified by removing the midportion of the trochlea and achieving limited exposure in the roof of the olecranon fossa. The orientation of the humeral canal provides the complementary orientation of the humeral condyle cuts to accommodate the stemmed prosthesis.

Table 34–4. Attempts to Resurface the Elbow Joint

1. Kudo, Japan
2. Ishizuki, Japan
3. Nonblocked, West Germany
4. Liverpool, England
5. ICLH, England
6. Wadsworth, England
7. Souter, Scotland
8. London, United States
9. Capitello-condylar, United States
10. Pritchard, United States

Modified from Ewald, F. C.

A stemmed ulnar component is necessary in the rheumatoid arthritic in whom the greater sigmoid fossa is often enlarged and the bone is thinned and eroded. Because of this, careful preparation of the olecranon to avoid fracture is important. The ulnar canal is identified—it makes a valgus angle of about 5 degrees to the sigmoid notch in most individuals. Proper orientation is important to lessen the likelihood of canal perforation.

Trial reduction is extremely important when using the resurfacing devices because instability is a problem with every reported design to some extent. Thus, before the components are secured, lack of impingement and proper balance must be assessed. Lack of stability may occur because of insufficient or improper bone resection. This should be evaluated with the joint in 45 and 90 degrees of flexion. Excessive bone removal to significantly improve motion is unwise because this ignores the soft tissue contribution to elbow stability.

In our hands aftercare of the resurfacing total elbow arthroplasty consists of placing the elbow in the position of stability, usually 70 to 80 degrees of flexion, for approximately 4 or 5 days. At this time, a hinged splint is fabricated, and the patient is allowed to bend the arm as tolerated and within the arc that was demonstrated to be stable on the operating table. If subluxation appears to be a problem, a long arm cast or splint is applied for approximately 3 weeks before this program is instituted. No specific strengthening exercises are encouraged with the elbow arthroplasty, but active assisted range of motion exercises are begun as soon as comfort allows.

Results. Detailed published results of the success of resurfacing devices are limited. Brief reports of technique and design concepts are common but lack a critical analysis of the result. The published experiences of Kudo et al.,[37] Ewald et al.,[22] Souter,[59] and others,[9, 61, 65] therefore form the basis for the results summarized in Table 34–3.

Motion. The functional arc of motion is usually attained with resurfacing devices. Souter,[59] however, has noted a rather disappointing average residual flexion contracture of about 50 degrees. In general, there does appear to be a slight increase in elbow contracture with the resurfacing compared with the semiconstrained devices (see Table 34–5). This may be due to a slightly more cautious rehabilitation program due to the possibility of dislocation or because the soft tissue envelope needed to provide stability may limit extension as well.

Relief of Pain. Typically, over 90 per cent of patients attain relief of pain. This represents a significant improvement over the preoperative state and is a predictable result barring complications.

Complications. Untoward results from resurfacing arthroplasty are in many respects similar to those seen with the semiconstrained device and will be discussed below. The major difference is instability, which has been reported in 2 of 27 cases of the UCLH design,[61] in 3 of 22 procedures by Souter,[59] in

7 percent of Ewald's experience,[23] and in 10 percent by Wadsworth.[65] The vulnerability of the proximal ulna to fracture may likewise be slightly increased because of the increased preparation needed to fit the resurfaced olecranon.

Semiconstrained Devices

Rationale. This prosthesis provides inherent joint stability when loss of bone stock or instability precludes the use of a resurfacing device. Ideally, this might be considered not as an alternative to the resurfacing implant but as a means of extending the indications to individuals who are not otherwise suitable candidates for the less constrained procedures (Fig. 34–11). In practice, however, most surgeons tend to use one design or the other for most circumstances depending on their clinical experience.

Specific Indications. An unstable, painful elbow joint dictates the use of a coupled prosthesis. Some patients with advanced rheumatoid arthritis satisfy these criteria (Fig. 34–12). The post-traumatic joint in the older individual has also been considered suitable for the semiconstrained device. About one third of those treated with a semiconstrained prosthesis have post-traumatic elbow dysfunction (Table 34–5). Failed total elbow arthroplasty (Fig. 34–13) and post-traumatic loss of bone are firm indications in our opinion for the semiconstrained device if joint replacement is being considered.

Technique. The patient is placed supine, and the arm is draped free and brought across the chest. If ulnar nerve symptoms or post-traumatic arthritis are present, the joint is exposed according to the technique described by Bryan and Morrey (Chapter 8). For resur-

RHEUMATOID SURGERY OF THE ELBOW

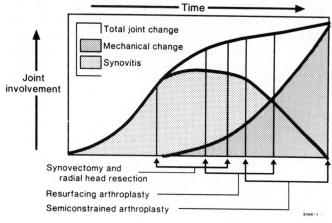

Figure 34–11. Schematic representation of the spectrum of disease pathology in rheumatoid arthritis and the general philosophy of the role of total joint replacement. The precise indications for synovectomy, resurfacing arthroplasty, and semiconstrained arthroplasty are arbitrary and to some extent based on physician preference and expertise. (Modified from Peterson, L. F. A., and Janes, J. M.: Surgery of the rheumatoid elbow. Orthop. Clin. North. Am. 2:667, 1971.)

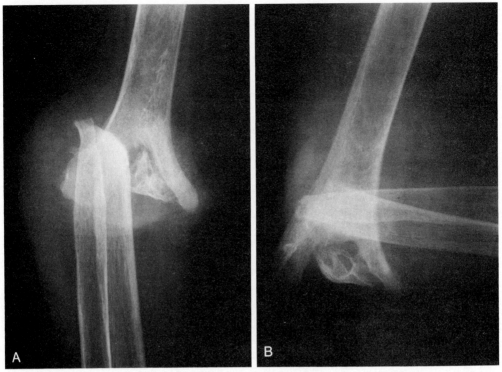

Figure 34–12. A patient with long-standing rheumatoid arthritis but without previous surgery demonstrates an apparent spontaneous fracture of the olecranon and gross instability on the anteroposterior *(A)* and lateral *(B)* radiographs. In our opinion, such instability is a contraindication to resurfacing arthroplasty.

facing devices, the extensile Kocher approach is usually employed (see Chapter 8).[23] The ulnar nerve is always identified and translocated anteriorly with the medial approach but not necessarily if the extensile Kocher approach is employed.

Particular care is also taken to preserve the soft tissue envelope about the joint for semiconstrained implants. The lateral or medial collateral ligaments are released from the humerus as necessary for adequate exposure (Fig. 34–14). The ligaments are anatomically replaced at the completion of surgery, even for semiconstrained prostheses.

The intramedullary canal is identified by resecting the midportion of the trochlea and removing the bone forming the roof of the olecranon fossa. For patients with rheumatoid disease the preparation is done with a ronguer, but an oscilating saw is required for more normal bone. The proper humeral cut is best made with an intramedullary template that shows the correct width and orientation of the cut with respect to the humeral shaft (Fig. 34–15). The capitellum is further prepared in most patients for a prosthesis that has a radial head component. The humeral intramedullary canal is prepared with rasps and burs.

The ulna is prepared by removing the tip of the olecranon, identifying the intramedullary canal, and widening the opening with a bur or rasp. Minimal bone resection is required for most of the currently employed prostheses. The 3 to 5 degrees of valgus angulation of the ulnar canal, with respect to the olecranon, must be kept in mind to avoid penetrating the ulnar cortex during preparation of soft rheumatoid bone.

The radial head is removed by a transverse cut made by rotating the forearm during the resection. If replacement is desired, difficulty may be encountered in obtaining an adequate radiohumeral articulation through the full range of elbow motion. If this occurs, the ulnohumeral relationship should be reassessed. Radial head prostheses in variable thicknesses are available, but if the radial head cannot be made to articulate accurately with the humeral component, it should not be used. Again, its value is theoretical.

Trial reduction of all components is essential. The exact order of cementing the prosthesis depends on the mechanism of the articulation. The snap-fit type of joint allows insertion of either component alone or at the same time, and the joint is assembled after the cement has hardened. If an axis is re-

Table 34–5. Clinical Results of Semiconstrained Elbow Prosthesis

Author	Prosthesis	No.	With Rheumatoid Arthritis	Mean Follow-up (Range-yr)	Extension Flexion	Pronation-Supination	Pain Relief	Compli-cations %	Revised for Loosening	Satisfactory Results
Morrey[a] (1983)	Coonrad[b]	17	9	2.9 (2–5)	26/130	70/57	16	3	0	16
Morrey (1983)	Pritchard (II)	26	19	3.0 (2–5)	29/126	64/62	23	10	1	22
Pritchard (1981)	Pritchard (II)	92	55	2.5 (—3)	—	—	90	14	2	85
Volz (1978)	Arizona	15	13	2.0 (5–3)	39/135	73/65	14	1	0	14
Inglis (1978)	Triaxial	44	28	3.5 (—)	—	—	39	16	1	?
		194	124 (64%)	2.7	30/131	68/61	94%	23%	2%	91%

[a]Unpublished data
[b]Loose hinge, since 1978

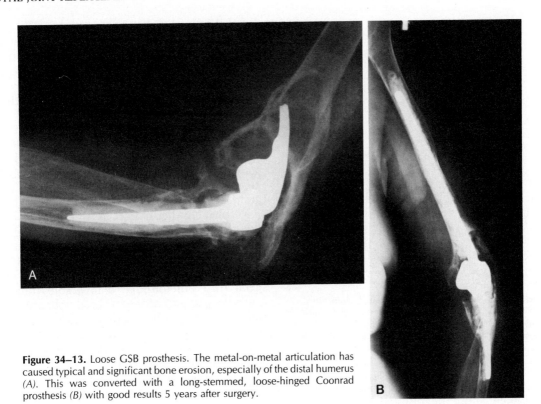

Figure 34–13. Loose GSB prosthesis. The metal-on-metal articulation has caused typical and significant bone erosion, especially of the distal humerus (A). This was converted with a long-stemmed, loose-hinged Coonrad prosthesis (B) with good results 5 years after surgery.

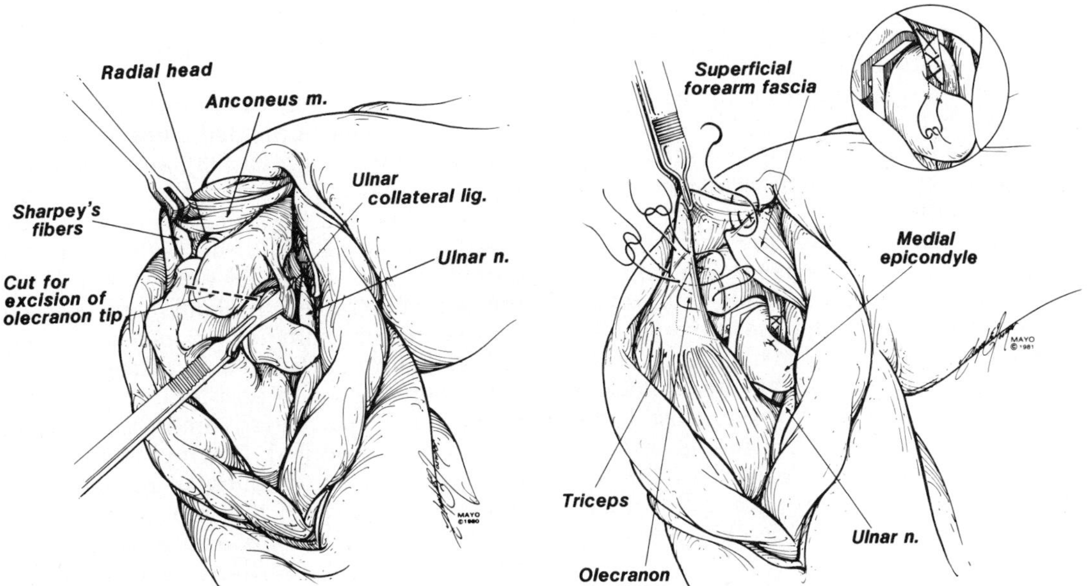

Figure 34–14. The triceps reflection technique exposes the distal humerus. A, Proper access to the joint may be facilitated by subperiosteal release of the medial collateral ligament from the undersurface of the medial epicondyle. B, If this is done, the ligament must be replaced anatomically to its original position through holes placed in the medial epicondyle. See insert (B).

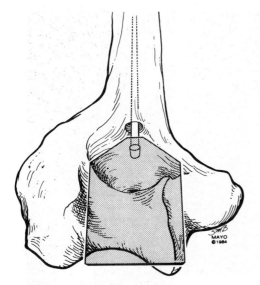

Figure 34–15. The intramedullary canal is sufficiently exposed through the trochlea to allow insertion of an intramedullary stemmed template that permits the surgeon to estimate the proper width and orientation of the distal humeral cut.

quired, it should be inserted last. The joint is articulated before the humeral portion is completely seated.

Cement is placed in the ulnar canal with a 60-ml nasogastric type of syringe, and a 5-cm length of suction tubing is applied to the tip. For the humerus, a femoral injecting system is used with a piece of suction tubing placed from inside the cartridge. The injector gun inserts the cement as distally as necessary. The proximal medullary canal is considerably larger than the opening made in the roof of the olecranon through which the prosthesis is inserted, so bone chips may be used to plug the canal and provide some resistance to the injected cement.

Hemostasis is obtained, and two or three drains are used. The triceps tendon complex is reattached with nonabsorbable sutures that have been placed through the proximal olecranon before cementing the ulnar prosthesis. Again, the collateral ligaments are reattached to their anatomic origin with a nonabsorbable suture. A compressive dressing is applied with the elbow in extension with an anterior splint. Flexion with a posterior splint might exert undue pressure on the skin overlying the olecranon.

Postoperative Management. The surgical dressing is removed on the third to fifth postoperative day, and a light dressing is applied. If the skin is of concern, motion is delayed with a protective splint. Swelling is controlled with an Ace bandage and elevation.

Rehabilitation after elbow replacement generally is not difficult. The major goal during this period is to begin active assisted motion. Active flexion is limited to 90 degrees, and strengthening exercises are avoided to decrease excessive forces at the joint. Functions of daily living are begun at once, and the patient is dismissed from the hospital at the end of 10 to 14 days. If the joint was stiff or ankylosed preoperatively, we have used the continuous passive motion machine for about 10 days and then instituted the above program.

Results. No distinction in function between the snap-fit and hinge-axis semiconstrained device is apparent at this time. Results of both devices are thus summarized in Table 34–5. Given the shortcomings of compiling data from different authors, a favorable trend is definitely apparent when these data are compared with similar results previously compiled with the more constrained prostheses.[44]

Follow-up with these devices remains limited, averaging less than 3 years. However, the loosening rate is less than 3 percent compared with approximately 25 percent observed with the constrained prostheses. Patient satisfaction exceeds 90 percent. The arc of motion remains at about 30 to 130 degrees of flexion, 60 degrees of pronation, and 60 degrees of supination. This is well within the amount of motion shown to be required for daily living.[42] Insufficient data are available for a critical comparison of the snap-fit with the loose-hinge or the three-part with the two-part prosthesis.

At our institution, 102 semiconstrained devices have been implanted since 1976 of the Pritchard (39), Coonrad (33), and Mayo-modified Coonrad (30) designs. Of those 42 cases with a minimum 2-year follow-up (see Table 34–5), loosening requiring revision has occurred in only one.[47] Of further note is that the semiconstrained implants have been employed in approximately 35 percent of individuals with nonrheumatoid disease.

Among those with post-traumatic arthritis, we have been particularly impressed with the use of the modified Coonrad device as a treatment for supracondylar humeral nonunion. The flange of this prosthesis controls posterior displacement and rotation of the prosthesis. This prosthesis has a humeral component length of 6 inches. Coonrad[12] feels strongly that the longer stem is a definite advantage in decreasing the incidence of loosening of this semiconstrained prosthesis (see Fig. 34–13). Our data, while preliminary, tend to substantiate this impression.

Table 34–6. **Some of the More Common Complications and the Relative Frequency of Each**

Complication	Frequency (%)
Loosening (semiconstrained)	3
Instability	5–10
Mechanical failure	
Humeral component fracture[a]	12
Articular uncoupling	5
Infection	5–10
Nerve injury	7
Triceps deficiency	7
Wound healing	4
Fracture	
Cortex penetration	50[b]
Humerus	5

[a]High density polyethylene humeral component
[b]For revision surgery

However, elimination of early loosening and other complications is still only the first step in a truly successful, reliable surgical option. Loosening from biologic rather than mechanical failure is certainly possible with any implant. The wear features of the bearing surfaces remain untested. Long-term tissue reaction to the implant is still unknown. The uncertainties must be constantly considered before offering total elbow arthroplasty as an option, particularly to the younger individual.

COMPLICATIONS

Complications after total elbow arthroplasty have been reported in 23[53, 63] to 59 percent[54] of patients. The most frequently recognized problems, to date, have been the inordinately high incidence of loosening of the constrained prostheses, dislocation of the resurfacing designs, and infection (Table 34–6).[44] In general, an explanation of the high incidence of complications rests on the fact that the elbow is a complex joint that is subcutaneous in location and is intimately associated with a major nerve. Further, most patients who are candidates for the procedure have rheumatoid arthritis or post-traumatic arthritis that has been previously operated on. Both groups of patients are at increased risk for complications from other joint replacements.[26, 68]

Complications Causing Revision

Loosening

Loosening of the components of total elbow arthroplasty was first recognized with noncemented constrained implants. The use of polymethyl methacrylate only delayed the appearance of this complication. About 25 percent of patients will show loosening by 3 years after total elbow arthroplasty with a constrained hinge-type device.[44] The humeral side loosens about twice as often as does the ulnar component. Several factors account for the nonseptic loosening of these implants: prosthetic design, surgical technique, and patient selection.

Prosthetic Design. Built-in motion of approximately 7 degrees of rotation and 7 degrees of varus-valgus[11] at the coupling of the semiconstrained devices appears to have markedly altered the early loosening of this device. Improved distal humeral flexion is considered essential for proper absorption of the considerable translation and rotatory forces that occur at this joint. The flanged device meets this requirement.

Technique. As was true of hip joint replacement,[50] inadequate cementing technique is directly associated with a higher incidence of radiolucent lines and loosening (Fig. 34–16).[44] Experimental and clinical data have shown

CEMENTING TECHNIQUE AND LOOSENING

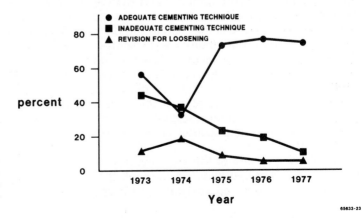

● ADEQUATE CEMENTING TECHNIQUE
■ INADEQUATE CEMENTING TECHNIQUE
▲ REVISION FOR LOOSENING

Figure 34–16. A 5-year period showed decreased early mechanical failure with improvement of cementing technique. (From Morrey, B. F., and Bryan, R. S.: Complications of total elbow arthroplasty. Clin. Orthop. 170:204, 1982.)

65633-23

the need to obtain a more secure bone–cement interface at the time of the initial procedure.

Patient Selection. The limitation of activity imposed upon the rheumatoid patient by the disease appears to act, to some extent, as a protection or safeguard against loosening. The individual with post-traumatic arthritis demonstrates loosening more often and earlier than the patient with rheumatoid arthritis.[48] If these high-risk patients are avoided, the results will obviously improve.

Treatment. When the loose prosthesis becomes symptomatic, five options are available: (1) arthrodesis, which may be nearly impossible to accomplish and functionally unacceptable; (2) removal of the prosthesis, leaving a resection arthroplasty; (3) modification of the existing residual bone stalk to provide a normal interposition or resection arthroplasty;[16] (4) allograft replacement; or (5) revision, usually with a different type of prosthetic design. Revision is discussed in detail in Chapter 35.

Component Failure

Mechanical failure of an elbow replacement is uncommon and occurs in one of three ways: (1) fracture of a component, (2) uncoupling of the articulating device, and (3) dislocation of the articulating components.

Humeral component fracture has been observed in 12 to 16 percent if the component is made of high-density polyethylene. We have seen one instance of a polyethylene ulnar component fracture. Fracture of a metal component has not been reported.

The articulating mechanism may become uncoupled in about 4 percent of the Pritchard-Walker prostheses (Fig. 34–17).[53, 54] This has not been reported after other pin-axis semiconstrained designs.

Of more concern, however, is prosthesis instability that develops in 5 to 10 percent of cases as a result of wear of the snap-fit polyethylene and metal articulation.[34, 63] Although loose-fitting, semicaptive designs tend to cause less stress at the bone–cement interface and thus decrease the chances of loosening, the relatively small tolerances imposed by the elbow geometry can result in a rather small polyethylene component that is subject to wear and renders the joint unstable. With longer follow-up, evidence suggests that the incidence of this complication may increase significantly.[64]

Treatment. Revision of the coupling device is obviously required when failure of this mechanism has occurred. Instability may also

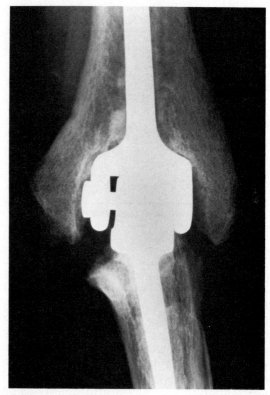

Figure 34–17. The hinged coupling device has become loose and appears to be backing out while being blocked by bone approximately 1 year after implantation of the Pritchard-Walker device.

be treated by replacement of the high-density polyethylene bushing. However, since the potential problem still exists, revision to another prosthetic design or to a resection arthroplasty should be considered in a younger or more active person.

Infection

Deep infection is more frequent after elbow than after hip or knee replacement surgery. The incidence has been reported as 3[33] to 11 per cent.[61] Recently, we analyzed our experience with 156 total elbow replacements and found that 14 (9 per cent) had deep sepsis.[45] Several explanations might be offered. The subcutaneous joint provides poor soft tissue coverage and hence compromised vascularity. Arthroplasty is performed in patients with rheumatoid arthritis and post-traumatic arthritis; both of these groups are known to be at greater risk of deep sepsis.[26] Finally, 4 of the 14 patients in our series developed a deep infection more than 3 years after the prosthesis had been implanted. Two of these four had outside-in type infections with skin lesions developing first, followed by deep sepsis. Two patients had spontaneous and apparently hematogenous infections 3 years after implantation.

Treatment. The most important first step in treatment is prevention. Any history of sepsis of the joint is a relative contraindication to elbow implant surgery. If the posterior skin condition is poor, consideration should be given to attaining better soft tissue by using a muscle pedicle before or concurrent with the arthroplasty. Early motion should be avoided if the skin is tenuous and splinting should be in extension.

The usual treatment for infected arthroplasty is removal of the foreign body.[23, 45] This was performed in two of three cases reported by Ewald[23] and in 12 of 14 reported in our series.[45] Only one of the initial 14 patients was successfully treated by debridément. We have since salvaged two individuals with deep sepsis with serial debridément. Reimplantation after negative cultures has also been performed in two patients who are asymptomatic 12 and 13 months following revision. Of the 10 individuals with resection arthroplasty, 8 considered the joint more functional and less painful than it was before the initial procedure (Fig. 34–18). Others have also observed the surprisingly good functional result after component removal for sepsis.[23, 34, 61] If the resection is painful and if significant function is lost, there is no evidence of infection at 1 year, the organism is not a resistant pathogen, and the soft tissues are of good quality, then reimplantation can be considered in some instances. Generally, however, reimplantation is not recommended.

Complications Causing Nonrevision Surgery

Neurapraxia

The frequency of ulnar nerve dysfunction, although temporary, has been a major problem with elbow joint replacement, averaging about 7 percent among several reports.[12, 22, 34, 43, 54] Excessive traction, trauma from exposure, intraneural hematoma, mechanical pressure, thermal damage from polymethylmethacrylate, and translocation causing constriction must all be considered and carefully avoided. A pre-existing subclinical neuropathy, which occasionally occurs in a patient with rheumatoid arthritis or tardy ulnar nerve palsy from old, untreated condylar fractures, should also be noted. If motor weakness exists for more than 12 hours after operation, the nerve should probably be explored and decompressed. Unless neurolysis is performed early, motor function may not return to normal. Sensory changes are a less compelling reason to re-explore the nerve. In our early experiences at the Mayo Clinic, the ulnar nerve was re-explored in 2 instances out of 125 procedures.

Triceps Insufficiency

The poor quality of the triceps tendon in patients with rheumatoid arthritis is well recognized. Triceps rupture or insufficiency has

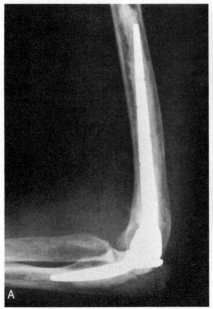
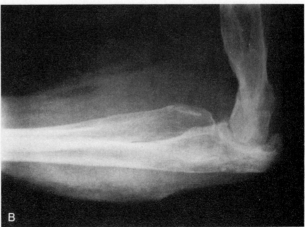

Figure 34–18. *A,* The Pritchard-Walker prosthesis was mechanically sound, but deep infection caused its removal. *B,* Two years later the patient has a functional resection arthroplasty. Although the distal humerus was fractured in order to remove the prosthesis, this patient rated 95 on a scale of 100, and had no pain and surprisingly good stability. (From Morrey, B. F., and Bryan, R. S.: Infection after total elbow arthroplasty. J. Bone Surg. 65A(3):330, 1983.)

been reported in 7 percent in the early experience.[22, 33, 43] At our institution, release of the triceps at its insertion was associated with a 29 percent incidence of triceps weakness, and the Van Gorder approach was followed by triceps insufficiency in 10 percent. Two of these patients required reattachment of the triceps because of avulsion, an experience observed by others.[8, 33] Triceps problems cause revision surgery in about 1 percent of patients. This complication has not been observed if the extensor mechanism is reflected in continuity either from medial to lateral as reported by Bryan and Morrey or from lateral to medial as in the modified extensile Kocher exposure (see Chapter 8).

Motion Loss

As in the experience with other replacement procedures, postoperative motion is related to the motion that was present preoperatively. Two early attempts at our institution to increase joint motion that was lost by soft tissue contracture in the postoperative period have proved unsuccessful. Further, we have not observed, nor have we seen reported, significant problems with heterotopic bone causing limitation of motion after a total elbow arthroplasty.

Wound Healing

Wound healing problems occur in 3 to 5 percent of patients reported from several series.[22, 33, 43] Less than 25 percent will require additional surgical procedures. Inglis and Pellicci[33] observed four wound hematomas and two instances of skin slough after 36 procedures, and Ewald et al.[22] reported that 3 of 64 patients had wound hematomas after capitellocondylar arthroplasties with a Campbell posterior triceps-splitting approach. We experienced 10 of 125 instances of poor wound healing or hematoma formation, but only one required additional surgery. Wound care during and after surgery cannot be overemphasized, because hematoma and tissue necrosis may further dispose this already too vulnerable joint to the development of deep sepsis. The patient with extensive soft tissue scarring after trauma or surgery is at particular risk.

Treatment. Most wound complications can be avoided. A straight incision placed medially or laterally away from the tip of the olecranon is recommended. The tourniquet should be deflated, securing meticulous hemostasis. Two drains are used, and the elbow is placed in as much extension as possible with an anteriorly placed splint. If a skin slough does occur, extensive plastic surgical procedures may be required to close the deficit. A rotational flap or the more difficult latissimus dorsi musculocutaneous pedicle flap or brachioradialis pedicle flap may be necessary to obtain soft tissue coverage.

Intraoperative Fractures

Supracondylar Bony Column. Fracture of the lateral or, more commonly, medial supracondylar bone was observed in as many as 10 percent of the cases in our early experience[44] and appeared to compromise fixation.[43] This complication should now occur rarely, if ever, because different sizes of prostheses are available and because greater awareness of the possibility exists. No specific treatment is necessary for the undisplaced fracture. In the postoperative course, if it appears that this complication has compromised fixation, a period of splinting or casting of 3 to 4 weeks is appropriate.

Cortex Penetration. Little is documented about the frequency of this complication. It is most commonly seen after revision surgery[48] (see Chapter 35), but it can occur during the initial procedure if the bone is very thin, as in a patient with rheumatoid arthritis. Evidence of extramedullary extravasation of cement confirms the occurrence of this event, and this may increase the chance of fracture at this site or cause local symptoms. No specific treatment is usually necessary for simple penetration of the medullary canal; soft tissue or nerve irritation is an indication for resection of the irritating focus. A bone graft taken from the resected bone might be helpful to avoid cement extravasation, and incorporation of the graft may eliminate the stress riser effect.

Postoperative Fractures

Following Trauma. Post-traumatic fracture of the humerus was identified in 2 of 36 patients with triaxial semiconstrained prostheses and in 1 of 69 after resurfacing procedures. Four of 35 patients with a Pritchard implant were noted to have post-traumatic fractures of the humerus occurring above the stem.[27, 54] These fractures occur because of the compromised quality of the bone or from the stress concentration caused by perforation of the cortex during preparation (Fig. 34–19). The rapid change in the elastic modulus between the composite acrylic cement-prosthesis-bone distally and normal bone proximally are additional features that predispose to fracture.

Treatment. If possible, patients with fracture of the humeral or ulnar shafts are treated by

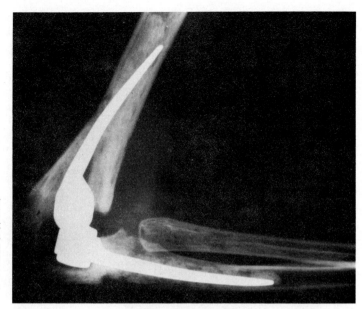

Figure 34–19. Humeral fracture occurred after a fall on the outstretched hand. The distal humeral bone may have been devitalized at the time of surgery, but this patient (who was referred from another hospital) had no record of cortical penetration at the time of the initial procedure. (From Morrey, B. F., and Bryan, R. S.: Complications of total elbow arthroplasty. Clin. Orthop. 170:204, 1982.)

simple immobilization.[22, 33, 44, 54] If the fracture is severely comminuted or the prosthesis is loose, treatment may be best performed in stages. The prosthesis might have to be removed and the fracture allowed to heal. If the resulting resection arthroplasty is painless, no further treatment is offered. If it is painful and if adequate bone stock is available, reimplantation surgery may be considered at a later date. If a fracture has occurred at the tip of a prosthesis and if no loosening has occurred, the fracture should heal, and revision will not be necessary.

Fractures Caused by Loosening

A loose humeral prosthesis may cause cortical resorption or penetration and sufficient weakening of the bone to predispose to fracture along the length of the stem or at the tip (Fig. 34–20). Ewald has also reported two instances of loose ulnar components that apparently predisposed to olecranon fracture.[22]

   Treatment. Probably the most important consideration with this fracture is to avoid its occurrence. If a prosthesis has become loose and is causing bone resorption, it should be removed or revised, even if the patient is having minimal pain (see Chapter 35). To ignore such a situation is only to invite a clinical circumstance that is much more difficult to manage. If a fracture has occurred in the presence of a loose prosthesis, the implant should be removed. This results in resection arthroplasty, or in some circumstances a longer intramedullary stem may be inserted. Additional exposure and bone graft of the fracture may or may not be necessary.

Instability

Elbow instability is a unique complication of the resurfacing devices or the snap-fit implants. With the resurfacing options, 5 to 10 per cent of instability persists (see Table 34–6).[25, 38, 59, 61, 65] In most instances, the instability may be treated nonoperatively (Fig. 34–21). Occasionally, revision is necessary in order to control the problem. The uncoupling of a snap-fit semiconstrained device occurs in 5 to 10 percent of cases according to current

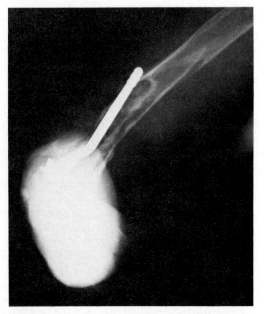

Figure 34–20. A loose Mayo prosthesis eroded through the humeral cortex, thus predisposing the patient to a spiral fracture.

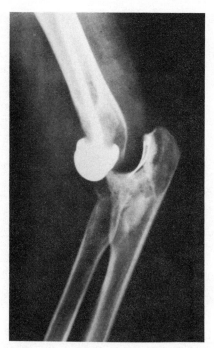

Figure 34–21. A specific complication with the resurfacing device has been a tendency toward instability in a small percentage of cases. This complication does not necessarily require revision. (From Morrey, B. F., and Bryan, R. S.: Prosthetic arthroplasty for the elbow. In Surgery of the Musculoskeletal System. New York, Churchill Livingstone, 1983.)

reports.[33, 64] However, the incidence of this complication may increase in a nonlinear fashion if a certain critical amount of high-density polyethylene is worn away, as suggested by the experience of Volz.[64]

Treatment. The dislocated elbow, if it occurs early, may be treated by immobilization for 3 to 6 weeks followed by use of a hinged splint. If recurrent dislocation occurs in spite of this treatment, then revision should be considered. If the dislocation occurs early and is not rendered stable with closed reduction, the joint should be re-explored and the cause of the instability corrected. This is usually due to the tensions that have been developed in the static (collateral ligaments) or dynamic (triceps, soft tissues) elements related to the amount of bone removed.

In the snap-fit prosthesis, a high-density polyethylene bushing might be replaceable, which would render the joint stable. However, unless there is a significant alteration in design that would indicate that the modification or revision surgery would preclude a recurrence of the complication, the entire joint should be replaced, either with a resection-type arthroplasty or with insertion of another design of implant.

AUTHOR'S PREFERRED TREATMENT METHOD

Rheumatoid Arthritis

This disease is usually managed with non-operative measures. The generalized process should be controlled and the joint rested and exercised under the careful supervision of a rheumatologist (see Chapter 40). Recurrent or recalcitant painful synovitis is the primary indication for surgical intervention, and the first procedure of choice is radial head resection and synovectomy. This is performed when the patient has (1) a functional arc of motion, (2) no significant instability, and (3) reasonable preservation of the joint. We do not require the presence of a normal articular surface. Severe destruction of the radiohumeral joint is still amenable to this procedure because the radial head is routinely removed at surgery.

As the spectrum of pathology increases so that the patient begins to notice increased limitation of motion, grating or instability with motion or activity, persistent pain, and radiographic evidence of some degree of bone loss, resurfacing arthroplasty is considered. If the patient is 60 years or older, and has instability as well as painful limitation of motion, and if the radiograph shows more extensive destruction of the joint and subchondral bone, semiconstrained total elbow arthroplasty is considered.

Post-traumatic Arthritis

A painless ankylosis or spontaneous arthrodesis in an acceptable position between 80 and 100 degrees is left alone unless the specific position markedly affects the patient's daily activity. If the position of ankylosis is unacceptable, usually due to excessive extension or occasionally forearm rotation, and if the joint is reasonably well preserved so that the pathology is largely periarticular or extra-articular, then we prefer soft tissue releases and removal of heterotopic bone as necessary to attain motion. If ankylosis is associated with intra-articular pathology and if the patient is under 55 years of age, we consider interposition arthroplasty an acceptable treatment option. When a painful ankylosis is present and it is felt that resection arthroplasty will not provide adequate motion or predictable relief of pain, the semiconstrained total elbow arthroplasty is our treatment of choice. Distraction arthroplasty is also considered a viable option in such cases.[24]

In the individual with instability because

of loss of bone, we proceed to semiconstrained total elbow arthroplasty. The special case of a supracondylar nonunion is difficult to treat, and no single treatment modality is considered optimum (see Chapter 19). Our experience has indicated that the flanged humeral component makes total elbow arthroplasty a viable option in this type of patient (see Fig. 34–6). A custom device is not felt to be necessary for bone loss up to 5 to 10 mm above the roof of the olecranon fossa, since the axis of rotation is not appreciably altered by inserting a prosthesis at this level. Further loss of length is not very noticeable cosmetically, and in fact function may be improved owing to the increased motion that occurs

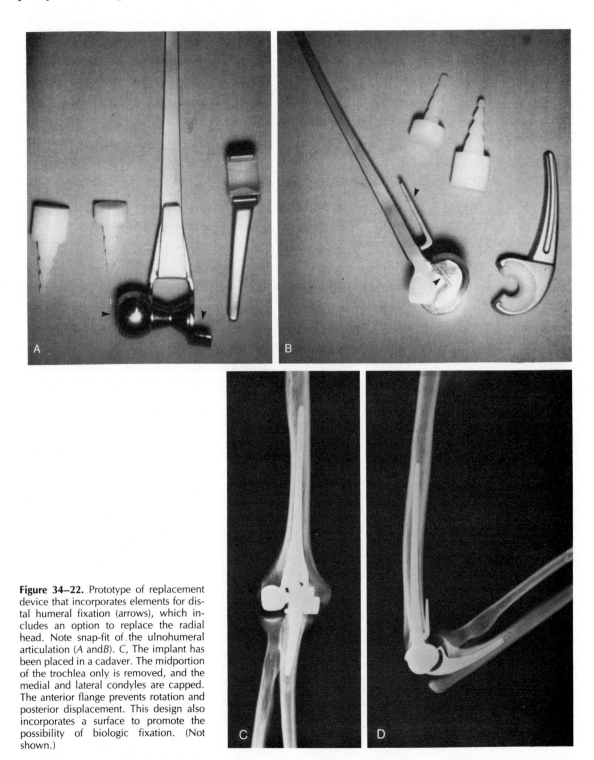

Figure 34–22. Prototype of replacement device that incorporates elements for distal humeral fixation (arrows), which includes an option to replace the radial head. Note snap-fit of the ulnohumeral articulation (*A* and *B*). *C,* The implant has been placed in a cadaver. The midportion of the trochlea only is removed, and the medial and lateral condyles are capped. The anterior flange prevents rotation and posterior displacement. This design also incorporates a surface to promote the possibility of biologic fixation. (Not shown.)

when slightly greater resection has been performed. When the distal humeral bone has been lost, we feel that some type of flanged prosthesis is absolutely essential to help control rotation stresses that contribute to loosening.

THE FUTURE

The three-component prosthesis will continue to be assessed in the future. Its theoretical advantage will motivate attempts to employ the radiohumeral articulation for both resurfacing and the semiconstrained prosthesis. The difficulty of obtaining proper alignment and tracking of this third component will remain a problem and will probably limit its use. Clinical results with and without such a component will be required to resolve this issue. A thicker, high-density polyethylene component may well be required for the snap-fit type of joint replacement to avoid progressive instability with time. These designs will seek to attain as much distal humeral fixation as possible (Fig. 34–22).

Biologic Fixation

In our opinion, this is the field of greatest potential in the future. In fact, several workers have performed preliminary design modifications, and some prototype humeral and ulnar implants of both the resurfacing and semiconstrained designs have been inserted without cement.

The progress made in total elbow arthroplasty has been encouraging but not rapid. However, because total elbow arthroplasty still provides the most predictable relief of pain and a functional arc of motion, we can recommend the procedure with cautious optimism. The avoidance of complications and successful long-term results are achieved with considerable experience and meticulous surgical technique.

References

1. Amis, A. A., Dowson, D., and Wright, V.: Muscle Strengths and Musculoskeletal Geometry of the Upper Limb. Eng. Med. **8**:41, 1979.
2. Amis, A. A., Dowson, D., and Wright, V.: Elbow Joint Force Predictions for Some Strenuous Isometric Actions. J. Biomechan. **13**:765, 1980.
3. Amis, A. A., Miller, J. H., Dowson, D., and Wright, V.: Biomechanical Aspects of the Elbow. Joint Forces Related to Prosthesis Design. Engin. Med. **10**:2:65, 1981.
4. Barr, J. S., and Eaton, R. G.: Elbow Reconstruction With a New Prosthesis to Replace the Distal End of the Humerus. J. Bone Joint Surg. **47A**:1408, 1965.
5. Boerma, I., and deWaard, D. J.: Osteoplastic Verankerung von Mettal Prosthesis bei Pseudarthrose und bei Arthroplastic. Acta Chir Scand. **86**:511, 1942.
6. Bryan, R. S.: Total Replacement of the Elbow Joint. Arch. Surg. **112**:1092, 1977.
7. Bryan, R. S., and Morrey, B. F.: Extensive Posterior Exposure of the Elbow: A Triceps-Sparing Approach. Clin. Orthop. **166**:188, 1982.
8. Brumfield, R. H., Jr., and Volz, R. G.: Total Elbow Arthroplasty: A Clinical Review of 30 Cases Employing the Mayo and AHSC Prostheses. American Academy of Orthopedic Surgeons Presentation, Atlanta, 1980.
9. Cavendish, M. E., and Elloy, M. A.: A Simple Method of Total Elbow Replacement. In Joint Replacement in the Upper Limb. London, Mechanical Engineering Publications, 1977, p. 93.
10. Chatzidakis, C.: Arthroplasty of the Elbow Joint Using a Vitalium Prosthesis. Int. Surg. **53**:119, 1970.
11. Coonrad, R. W.: History of Total Elbow Arthroplasty. In Inglis, A. E. (ed.), Upper Extremity Joint Replacement (Symposium on Total Joint Replacement of the Upper Extremity, 1979). St. Louis, C. V. Mosby Co., 1982.
12. Coonrad, R. W.: Seven-Year Follow-Up of Coonrad Total Elbow Replacement. In Inglis, A. E. (ed.): Upper Extremity Joint Replacement (Symposium on Total Joint Replacement of the Upper Extremity, 1979). St. Louis, C. V. Mosby Co., 1982.
13. Davis, P. R.: Some Significant Aspects of Normal Upper Limb Functions. Conference on Joint Replacement of the Upper Extremity. London, Institute of Mechanical Engineers, 1977.
14. Dee, R.: Total Replacement Arthroplasty of the Elbow for Rheumatoid Arthritis. J. Bone Joint Surg. **54B**:88, 1972.
15. Dee, R.: Total Replacement of the Elbow Joint. Orthop. Clin. North Am. **4**:415, 1973.
16. Dee, R.: Revision Surgery After Failed Elbow Endoprosthesis. In Inglis, A. E. (ed.): Upper Extremity Joint Relacement (Symposium on Total Joint Replacement of the Upper Extremity, 1979). St. Louis, C. V. Mosby Co., 1982.
17. Driessen, A. P. P. M.: Thirty Years With a Complete Elbow Prosthesis. Arch. Chir. Neerl. **24–II**:87, 1972.
18. Dubrow, E., Gurtowski, J., Manley, M. T., Stern, L., and Dee, R.: Biomechanical Comparison of Non-Constrained Total Elbow Prostheses. Orthop. Trans. **701**:284, 1983.
19. Duff-Barclay, I., and Spillman, D. T.: Total Human Hip Joint Prostheses—A Laboratory Study of Friction and Wear. Proc. Inst. Mech. Enginrs. **181(3J)**:90, 1966.
20. Elloy, M. A., Wright, J. T. M., and Cavendish, M. E.: The Basic Requirements and Design Criteria for Total Joint Prostheses. Acta Orthop. Scand. **47**:193, 1976.
21. Ewald, F. C.: Total Elbow Replacement. Orthop. Clin. North Am **6**:685, 1975.
22. Ewald, F. C., Scheinberg, R. D., Poss, R., Thomas, W. H., Scott, R. D., and Sledge, C. B.: Capitellocondylar Total Elbow Arthroplasty: Two- to Five-Year Follow-Up in Rheumatoid Arthritis. J. Bone Joint Surg. **62A**:1259, 1980.
23. Ewald, F. C.: Nonconstrained Metal-to-Plastic Total Elbow Replacement. In Inglis, A. E. (ed.): Upper Extremity Joint Replacement (Symposium on Total Joint Replacement of the Upper Extremity, 1979). St. Louis, C. V. Mosby Co., 1982.
24. Ewald, F. C.: Presentation to Meeting of Shoulder and Elbow Surgeons, Rochester, November, 1983.
25. Ewald, F. C.: American Academy of Orthopedic Sur-

geons Instructional Course Lecture, Atlanta, February, 1984.

26. Fitzgerald, R. H., Jr., Nolan, D. R., Ilstrup, D. M., Van Scoy, R. E., Washington, J. A., II, and Coventry, M. B.: Deep Wound Sepsis Following Total Hip Arthroplasty. J. Bone Joint Surg. 59A:847, 1977.

27. Frykman, G. K., Wood, V. E., and Rogers, F. R.: Elbow Replacement Arthroplasty. Orthop. Trans. 6:105, 1982.

28. Garrett, J. C., Ewald, F. C., Thomas, W. H., and Sledge, C. B.: Loosening Associated with GSB Hinge Total Elbow Replacement in Patients With Rheumatoid Arthritis. Clin. Orthop. 127:170, 1977.

29. Gschwend, N., Scheier, H., and Bahler, A.: GSB Elbow-, Wrist-, and PIP-Joints. In Joint Replacement in the Upper Limb. London, Institution of Mechanical Engineers, 1977, p. 107–116.

30. Halls, A. A., and Travill, A.: Transmission of Pressures Across the Elbow Joint. Anat. Rec. 150:243, 1964.

31. Heath, J. C., Freeman, M. A. R., and Swenson, S. A. V.: Carcinogenic Properties of Wear Particles from Prostheses Made From Cobalt-Chromium Alloys. Lancet 1:564, 1971.

32. Hui, F. C., Chao, E. Y., and An, K. N.: Muscle and Joint Forces at the Elbow Joint During Isometric Lifting (abstract). Orthop. Trans. 2:169, 1978.

33. Inglis, A. E., and Pellicci, P. M.: Total Elbow Replacement. J. Bone Joint Surg. 62A:1252, 1980.

34. Inglis, A. E.: Tri-Axial Total Elbow Replacement: Indications, Surgical Technique, and Results. In Inglis, A. E. (ed.): Upper Extremity Joint Replacement (Symposium on Total Joint Replacement of the Upper Extremity, 1979). St. Louis, C. V. Mosby Co., 1982.

35. Johnson, E. W., Jr., and Schlein, A. P.: Vitallium Prosthesis for the Olecranon and Proximal Part of the Ulna. Case Report with Thirteen-Year Follow-Up. J. Bone Joint Surg. 52A:721, 1970.

36. Kempson, G. E., and Tuke, M. A.: As quoted by Tuke: The ICLH Elbow. Engin. Med. 10:75, 1981.

37. Kudo, H., Iwano, K., and Watanabe, S.: Total Replacement of the Rheumatoid Elbow with a Hingeless Prosthesis. J. Bone Joint Surg. 62A:277, 1980.

38. London, J. T.: Resurfacing Total Elbow Arthroplasty. Presentation to the American Academy of Orthopedic Surgeons Annual Meeting, Atlanta, February, 1980.

39. MacAusland, A. R.: Replacement of the Lower End of the Humerus With a Prosthesis: A Report of Four Cases. West. J. Surg. Obstet. Gynecol. 62:557, 1954.

40. Mellen, R. H., and Phalen, G. S.: Arthroplasty of the Elbow by Replacement of the Distal Portion of the Humerus with an Acrylic Prosthesis. J. Bone Joint Surg. 29:348, 1947.

41. Morrey, B. F., and Chao, E. Y.: Passive Motion of the Elbow Joint: A Biomechanical Analysis. J. Bone Joint Surg. 58A:501, 1976.

42. Morrey, B. F., Askew, L. J., An, K. N., and Chao, E. Y.: A Biomechanical Study of Normal Functional Elbow Motion. J. Bone Joint Surg. 63A:87, 1981.

43. Morrey, B. F., Bryan, R. S., Dobyns, J. H., and Linscheid, R. L.: Total Elbow Arthroplasty: A Five-Year Experience at the Mayo Clinic. J. Bone Joint Surg. 63A:1050, 1981.

44. Morrey, B. F., and Bryan, R. S.: Complications of Total Elbow Arthroplasty. Clin. Orthop. 170:204, 1982.

45. Morrey, B. F., and Bryan, R. S.: Infection After Total Elbow Arthroplasty. J. Bone Joint Surg. 65A:3:330, 1983.

46. Morrey, B. F., and Bryan, R. S.: Prosthetic Arthroplasty for The Elbow. In Surgery of the Musculo-

47. Morrey, B. F.: Unpublished data, 1984.

48. Morrey, B. F., and Bryan, R. S.: Revision for Failed Total Elbow Arthroplasty. Presented at the American Academy of Orthopaedic Surgeons Annual Meeting, Atlanta, February, 1984.

49. Nicol, A. C., Berme, N., and Paul, J. P.: A Biomechanical Analysis of Elbow Joint Function. In Joint Replacement in the Upper Limb. London, Institution of Mechanical Engineers, 1977.

50. Oh, I., Carlson, C. E., Tomford, W. W., and Harris, W. H.: Improved Fixation of the Femoral Component After Total Hip Replacement Using a Methacrylate Intramedullary Plug. J. Bone Joint Surg. 60A:608, 1978.

51. Pearson, J. R., McGinley, D. R., and Butzel, L. M.: A Dynamic Analysis of the Upper Extremity. Planar Motions. Hum. Factors 5:59, 1963.

52. Peterson, L. F. A., and Janes, J. M.: Surgery of the Rheumatoid Elbow. Orthop. Clin. North Am. 2:667, 1971.

53. Pritchard, R. W.: Long-Term Follow-Up Study: Semi-Constrained Elbow Prosthesis. Orthopedics 4:151, 1981.

54. Rosenfeld, S. R., and Anzel, S. H.: Evaluation of the Pritchard Total Elbow Arthroplasty. Orthopedics, 5:713, 1982.

55. Scales, J. T., Lettin, A. W. F., and Bayley, I.: The Evolution of the Stanmore Hinged Total Elbow Replacement 1967–1976. In Joint Replacement in the Upper Limb. London, Mechanical Engineering Publications, 1977, p. 53.

56. Schlein, A. P.: Semiconstrained Total Elbow Arthroplasty. Clin. Orthop. 121:222, 1976.

57. Seireg, A., and Arvikar, R. J.: The Prediction of Muscular Load Sharing Joint Forces in the Lower Extremities During Walking. J. Biomechan. 8:89, 1975.

58. Souter, W. A.: Arthroplasty of the Elbow: With Particular Reference to Metallic Hinge Arthroplasty in Rheumatoid Patients. Orthop. Clin. North Am. 4:395, 1973.

59. Souter, W. A.: A New Approach to Elbow Arthroplasty. Engin. Med. 10:2:59, 1981.

60. Street, D. M., and Stevens, P. S.: A Humeral Replacement Prosthesis for the Elbow. J. Bone Joint Surg. 56:1147, 1974.

61. Tuke, M. A.: The ICLH Elbow. Engin. Med. 10(2):75, 1981.

62. Virgen (1937): Cited in Schlein, A. P.: Semiconstrained Total Elbow Arthroplasty. Clin. Orthop. 121:223, 1976.

63. Volz, R. G.: Development and Clinical Analysis of a New Semiconstrained Total Elbow Prosthesis. In Inglis, A. E. (ed.): Upper Extremity Joint Replacement (Symposium on Total Joint Replacement of the Upper Extremity, 1979). St. Louis, C. V. Mosby Co., 1982.

64. Volz, R. G.: Total Elbow Arthroplasty. American Academy of Orthopedic Surgeons, Instructional Course Lecture. The Upper Extremity. Tuscon, February, 1983.

65. Wadsworth, T. G.: A New Technique of Total Elbow Replacement. Engin. Med. 10:2:69, 1981.

66. Walker, P. S.: Human Joints and Their Artificial Replacement. Springfield, Ill., Charles C Thomas, 1977.

67. Williams, D. F., and Roaf, R.: Implants in Surgery. P. 173, London, W. B. Saunders Co., 1973, p. 173.

68. Woo, R. Y. G., and Morrey, B. F.: Dislocations After Total Hip Arthroplasty. J. Bone Joint Surg. 64A:1255, 1982.

skeletal System. New York, Churchill Livingstone, 1983, p. 273.

CHAPTER 35

Revision Joint Replacement

B. F. MORREY

Obviously, the best treatment for a failed elbow prosthesis is to avoid its occurrence, but the need to treat this condition is an unfortunate reality. The unsuccessful elbow implant may necessitate revision in one of five clinical settings: (1) infection, (2) fracture, (3) material failure, (4) unstable resurfacing or snap-fit device, or (5) loosening of a stemmed prosthesis. The characteristic features of each should be considered when reviewing the treatment options.

CLINICAL PRESENTATION

In general, a septic joint may be diagnosed early in the perioperative period by the char-

acteristic features of a febrile clinical course, erythema, swelling, and drainage. Late infections from direct spread or hematogenous inoculations may be more difficult to diagnose accurately. The sedimentation rate is not always elevated and is even less helpful in the patient with rheumatoid arthritis. Radiolucency at the bone-cement interface may be due to mechanical or septic factors, but the lucent line is not universally present with the septic joint (Fig. 35–1). This factor complicates the treatment because removal of the prosthesis may result in fracture of the bone.

Material failure may involve the fixation or articular aspects of the device. Only the high-density polyethylene components have

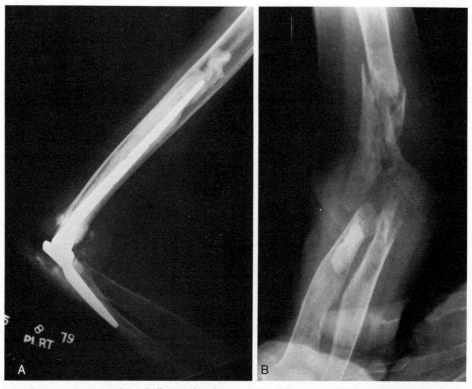

Figure 35–1. *A,* Sepsis can occur with total elbow arthroplasty, causing soft tissue manifestations without radiolucency of the bone–cement interface. *B,* This presentation may pose difficulties for teatment because the distal humerus may often be fractured at the time of revision. Fortunately, these fractures tend to consolidate and may provide acceptable results after salvage procedures. (*B* from Morrey, B. F., and Bryan, R. S.: Complications of total elbow arthroplasty. Clin. Orthop. 170:204, 1982.)

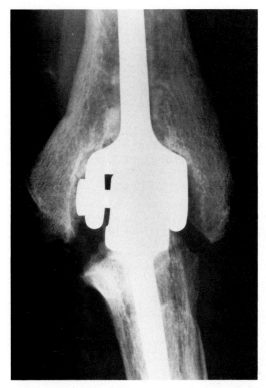

Figure 35–2. Mechanical failure of the articulation, such as occurred in this instance with axis failure of a Pritchard-Walker prosthesis, is usually managed by reinserting the failed articular component. The structural components are left intact.

shown any tendency to fracture, and these are no longer in use, so this mode of failure should no longer be seen. The articulation has dislocated in the snap-fit designs,[7, 13] and the axis has backed out in several of the Pritchard-Walker devices (Fig. 35–2). This type of failure does not usually necessitate the removal of the entire prosthesis, but only the coupling mechanism.

With resurfacing prostheses, early instability is not unusual. Chronic subluxation is noted in some patients with certain activities or sometimes even with simply flexing and extending the elbow. In the questionable case, examination under fluoroscopy may demonstrate the pathologic cause. Frank dislocation is usually posterior and is considerably more disabling, allowing the diagnosis to be made with ease (Fig. 35–3). Dislocation is painful, often occurs early in the postoperative or perioperative period, and may require a general anesthetic for reduction.

Mechanical loosening of the stem and prosthesis occurs about twice as often with the humeral as with the ulnar component.[10] Pain is a constant feature. If a prosthesis has become loose, it is important to recognize that careful follow-up is very important to ensure that excessive bone resorption does not occur (Fig. 35–4). When cortical thinning or "bal-

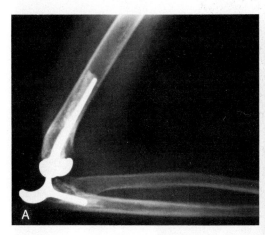

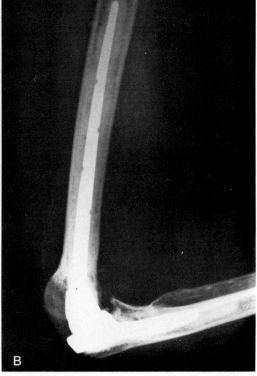

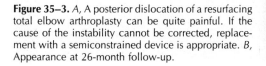

Figure 35–3. *A*, A posterior dislocation of a resurfacing total elbow arthroplasty can be quite painful. If the cause of the instability cannot be corrected, replacement with a semiconstrained device is appropriate. *B*, Appearance at 26-month follow-up.

looning" of the humerus or ulna is present, the prosthesis should be removed. If the condition is allowed to progress, fracture may result (Fig. 35–4B). Resorption of a significant amount of bone can pose major problems to the reconstructive plan, especially when it is complicated by fracture. Fracture of the humerus has been seen in some instances without a loose prosthesis, usually at the level of the proximal aspect of the humeral stem.[12] Fractures that are not caused by loosening are

commonly, but not always, successfully treated by simple cast immobilization (Fig. 35–5).

TREATMENT OPTIONS

Prosthesis Retained

In the patient with an early postoperative subluxation or dislocation stability may often be achieved by casting with or without subsequent brace protection. Nonrevision salvage

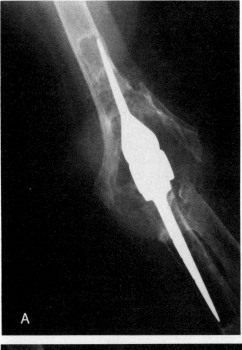

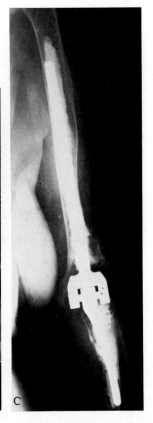

Figure 35–4. A, B, Marked bone resorption along the shaft of the humeral and ulnar prostheses. The distal humerus has fractured posteriorly. In this instance a long-stemmed semiconstrained prosthesis was used (C) with a satisfactory result 5 years later.

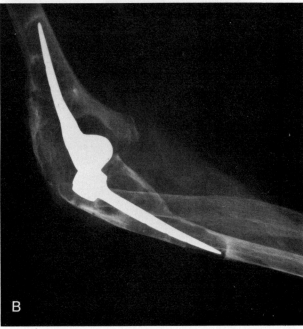

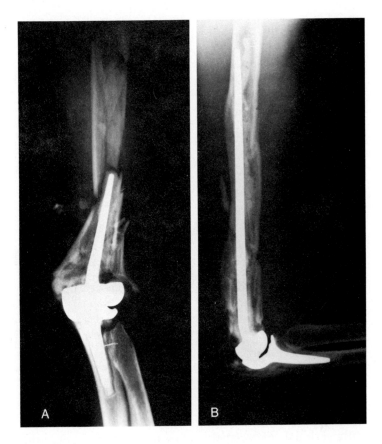

Figure 35–5. A, Resurfacing prosthesis with fracture of the humerus after a serious traumatic event 1 year after surgery. B, Because nonunion developed with casting, a custom, long-stemmed humeral prosthesis was inserted. The patient is doing well 1 year later.

of an infected total elbow has been successfully performed but only occasionally, and such treatment can be expected to be successful only when infection is diagnosed in the early postoperative period.[9] Mechanical failure of the articulation may also require additional surgery, but the cemented components need not be revised—only the articular mechanism that has failed.

Prosthesis Removal

If the implant has failed in such a way that it requires removal of the components, treatment options will depend on the factors that resulted in the failure. These aspects are specifically reflected in the amount of bone and quality of soft tissue remaining after implant removal (Fig. 35–6), both of which directly influence the revision option (Table 35–1). As suggested in Table 35–1, several variables must be considered when choosing the treatment for a failed elbow prosthesis. We shall discuss the subject with respect to the salvage options available.

Arthrodesis

In our judgment, arthrodesis is rarely indicated for the elbow. First, there is no predom-

inant position of function in the elbow to allow an optimum position for arthrodesis. Second, if adequate bone stock is present to allow arthrodesis, such a joint would probably do well with a simple resection arthroplasty. If an infected prosthesis is removed, the resection arthroplasty often provides a very functional result.[7, 9] Rarely, persistent infection with poor soft tissues may require an arthrodesis, but we have not yet encountered such a patient.

Interposition Arthroplasty

The indications for this procedure are preserved distal humeral condyles, ideally in the younger patient with post-traumatic arthritis. If the olecranon and condyles are preserved, some have recommended the interposition of skin over the distal humerus to provide a formal interposition arthroplasty.[2] Removal of a resurfacing arthroplasty will tend to preserve the distal humeral bone because little is initially removed (Fig. 35–6). Because stability of resurfacing prostheses requires a rather formal ulnar component, the olecranon may be jeopardized at the time of implant removal. This event precludes the ability to perform an interposition arthroplasty.

From a practical standpoint, because too

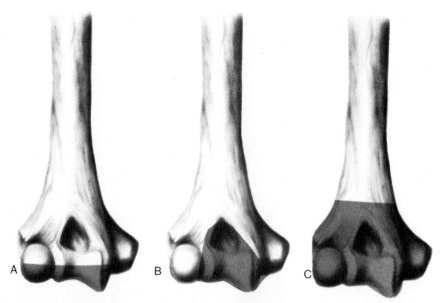

Figure 35–6. Condition of the distal humerus after removal of various types of prostheses. *A*, For failed resurfacing devices, no additional treatment other than closure and motion may be required. If a yolked device has been removed and the supracondylar bone preserved, nothing more need be done in some instances. *B*, However, reimplantation of a prosthesis of a different design that avoids the cause of the initial failure is a viable option. *C*, When the entire distal humerus has been resected, this joint is felt to be too flail simply to leave alone. In this instance, an allograft or reimplantation with a device that allows potential for bone grafting and biologic fixation is our choice of treatment.

little residual bone remains after removal of a yolked prosthesis, resurfacing arthroplasty is not an option when this type of prosthesis fails. There are no data to indicate the success of interposition arthroplasty, and we question whether or not resurfacing or interposing tissue over the distal humerus enhances the likelihood of a good result to such an extent that the additional surgery required is justified. Distraction arthroplasty may be an alternative to a formal interposition arthroplasty. With this method, the healing scar tissue

provides the interposed tissue. Motion is maintained with favorable early results.[5]

Resection Arthroplasty

Resection arthroplasty is indicated in the presence of septic stemmed prostheses, loose, unstable or fractured resurfacing constrained prostheses. Resection arthroplasty might be subcategorized into two types—those with and those without supracondylar bone. The determining feature for this type of result resides in the design of the initial prosthesis. In joints in which the supracondylar bone has been preserved, the salvage procedure although technically classed as a resection will function quite well owing to the stability offered by the supracondylar columns (Fig. 35–7).

If a significant amount of humeral bone is resected of if ulnar bone is lost and no bone graft is performed owing to a septic process or poor soft tissues, an extensive bone resection will be necessary (Fig. 35–8). The anatomic and functional differences and implications between this and the previous type of resection are dramatic. These joints are grossly unstable, and although there will be virtually no pain, the extremity is almost completely without function due to the weakness and complete instability that result.

Table 35–1. Factors That Influence Salvage of Failed Elbow Prosthesis

Cause of Revision	Possible Status of Bone	Salvage Procedures Available
Infection	Condyles present	Arthrodesis
Resurfacing— unstable	Condyles removed— supracondylar bone present	Interposition arthroplasty (resurfacing failure)
Loose-stemmed prosthesis		
Loose-stemmed prosthesis with fracture	Entire distal humerus absent	Allograft replacement (supracondylar bone absent)
	Olecranon absent—fracture	Reimplantation arthroplasty (supracondylar bone present or absent)

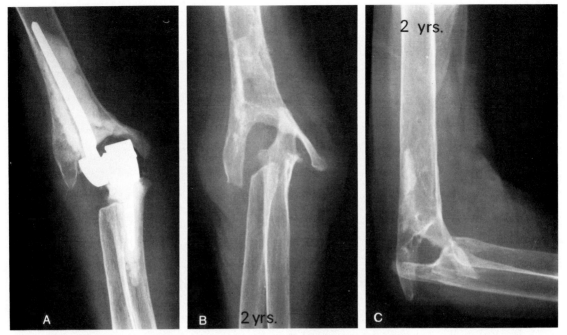

Figure 35–7. *A,* A loose Mayo prosthesis was removed, leaving the supracondylar bone *(B)* and proximal ulna *(C)* intact. This patient had a satisfactory functional result after 2 years.

Allograft Replacement

If loss of bone is so extensive that it renders the extremity functionless (Fig. 35–8B), an allograft replacement is a viable option, particularly in the younger patient (Fig. 35–9). Theoretically, stability, infection, incorporation of the graft, and chondrolysis could all be problems, yet this remains an attractive option in selected patients. However, the difficulty of obtaining an appropriate sized specimen presents a major limitation to the widespread use of this reconstructive option.

Prosthetic Reinsertion

This option is indicated for nonseptic removal of the resurfacing or semiconstrained prosthesis, ideally in an older individual with good bone stock.

If the bone and soft tissue are of good quality, reimplantation may be considered. The new device must overcome the shortcomings of the first prosthesis. This usually implies a stem that bypasses any cortical weakness or fracture, provision for adequate distal humeral or ulnar fixation, and a stable articulation. Bone grafting of any cortical defect and biologic fixation are also considered desirable aspects of a revision design (Fig. 35–10). Unless these criteria are met, reimplantation will not be successful. It must be reemphasized that for reimplantation to be considered a viable option, the mechanical or biologic causes of the initial failure must be overcome with the new design.

TECHNIQUE

Several factors should be considered prior to revising a failed total elbow arthroplasty. Successful intervention requires careful planning to anticipate potential complications and to make available all the options that may be required at the time of surgery to attain a successful result. Preoperative planning includes

1. Assessment of the bone stock and the potential for injury to the bone at the time of revision.
2. Ensuring availability of the appropriate array of tools necessary to remove both the components and the cement, especially if the device was inserted elsewhere.
3. Preparation of the iliac crest or availability of bone-bank bone if bone supplementation is required.
4. Ensuring that external fixation or distraction devices are available if needed.
5. Ensuring the availability of several sizes of the prosthesis if reimplantation is considered. A long-stemmed device is desirable for revision operations.[1, 11]

In addition, several aspects of the surgical procedure should likewise be considered:

Skin. Skin coverage in this group of patients is often compromised even at the time of the initial procedure. Thus, there should be serious concern about the quality of the skin at the time of the revision procedure, particularly in patients with post-traumatic or rheumatoid arthritis when reinsertion is considered. A local or remote pedicle flap may be necessary to ensure adequate wound healing. The importance of providing soft tissue coverage over the posterior aspect of the elbow cannot be overemphasized.

Ulnar Nerve. The ulnar nerve, in our opinion, must routinely be identified in the revi-

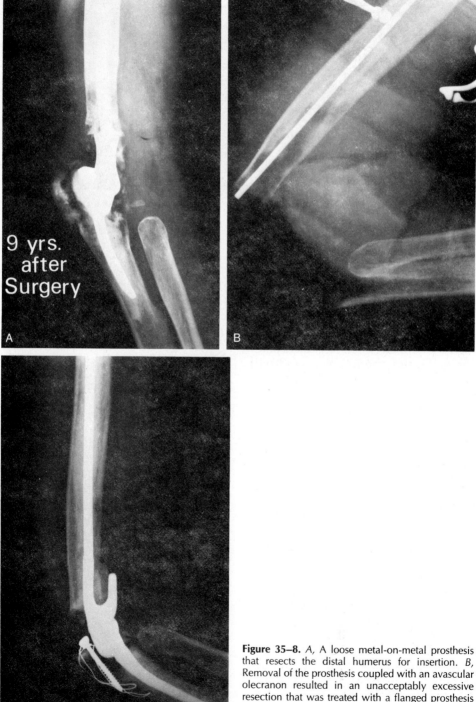

9 yrs. after Surgery

Figure 35–8. *A,* A loose metal-on-metal prosthesis that resects the distal humerus for insertion. *B,* Removal of the prosthesis coupled with an avascular olecranon resulted in an unacceptably excessive resection that was treated with a flanged prosthesis *(C).* The olecranon has been reconstructed with a bone graft.

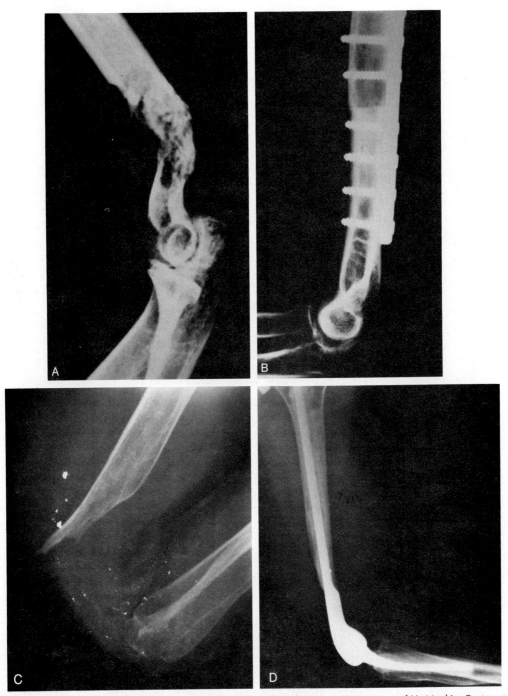

Figure 35–9. *A,* Distal humeral bone tumor was treated by allograft replacement *(B)* (courtesy of H. Mankin, Boston, Mass.). Although we have no experience with this treatment, we have treated extensive bone loss *(C)* with a custom-made prosthesis with satisfactory results after 7 years *(D).*

sion procedure. In many instances it will have already been transferred anteriorly, but regardless, it must be sufficiently identified and protected during the course of the procedure. Depending on the cause of previous failure and the type of prosthesis, more or less dissection may be necessary, and this will dictate the extent to which the ulnar nerve is exposed and protected.

Triceps. In our experience, the triceps, if adequately attached or managed during the first procedure, can be reflected in continuity from the tip of the olecranon during the revision procedure. Scarring and loss of compliance are minimized with either medial or lateral triceps reflection approaches. We have not used the triceps mechanism as an interposition substance as recommended by some[3]

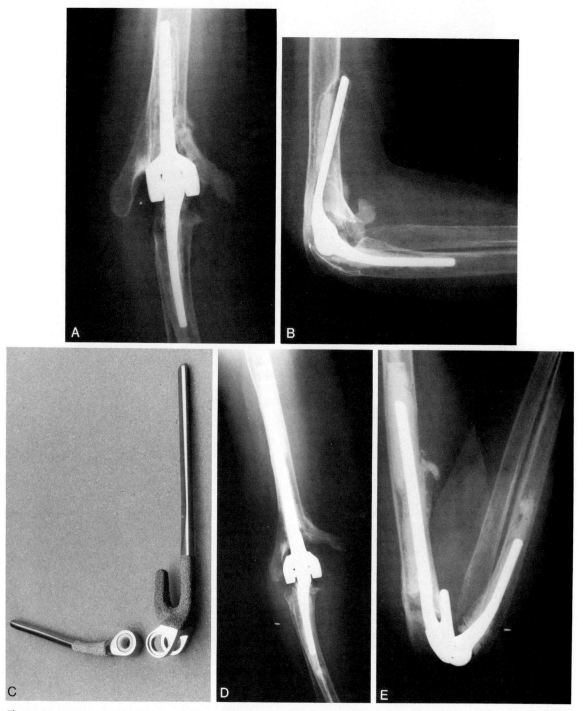

Figure 35–10. *A, B,* A common mode of failure is anterior proximal migration of the proximal aspect of the humeral component. The cortical defect was bone-grafted. *C,* The 6-inch humeral stem, which has an anterior flange just proximal to the articulation and a loose hinge, has been an acceptable type of revision prosthesis in our experience. The spray coating of the distal humerus and proximal ulna provide the potential for biological fixation, but these implants are usually cemented in place, except for the area with the spray coating, which is bone-grafted. At two years, the patient shows no symptoms. *D, E,* Incorporation of the bone graft appears to have taken place. (All but Part C from Morrey, B. F., Bryan, R. S.: Complications of total elbow arthroplasty. Clin. Orthop. 170:204, 1982.)

and if there is any consideration of further surgery, this obviously should be avoided.

Ligaments and Soft Tissue. The soft tissue envelope about the joint is no less important at the time of the revision than during the initial procedure. The periosteum and collateral ligament should be reflected subperiosteally whenever possible. In addition, the medial or lateral collateral ligament complex should be left intact depending on the nature of the exposure and the type of problem. If there has been significant bone resected at the time of the initial procedure, the ligaments are, of course, absent. We do not feel obliged to reattach the flexor or extensor muscle groups to the distal humeral shaft when there has been marked bone loss. With respect to strength, elbow instability is a more significant factor than is an unstable origin of these muscles, particularly since the scar tissue does provide some stability of the flexor and extensor muscle masses.

Distal Humerus. The preservation of bone must be a foremost priority at the time of revision.

Loose Prostheses. If the prosthesis is loose, it is easily removed, but all or some cement may be left. If the option of interposition or resection arthroplasty has been selected, all the cement from the medullary canal need not be removed. If implantation is considered, removal of the cement must be done very carefully because cortical penetration or fracture may occur (Fig. 35–11). In the presence of infection all cement must be removed, and this does frequently result in fracture of the distal humerus (Fig. 35–11). In this setting, generous exposure of this bone should minimize the chance of fracture.

Prosthesis Is Not Loose. If the prosthesis has not become loose, its removal may result in some bone loss, particularly in the patient with rheumatoid arthritis. To minimize damage to the bone, adequate exposure of the distal humerus should be achieved at the time of the prosthetic removal. Infection requires all foreign material to be removed, again requiring exposure of the distal humerus.

Ulna. Regardless of the bone–cement–prosthesis bond, one must be constantly vigilant to avoid fracture or penetration of the ulnar cortex. This bone presents a very small medullary canal distal to the coracoid process. The valgus angulation of the shaft likewise makes removal of the cement with straight instruments difficult and hazardous. Resurfacing prostheses may involve a fair amount of dissection or fashioning of the proximal ulna, and this may predispose to fracture

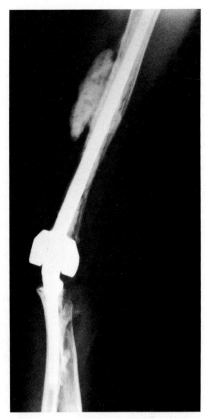

Figure 35–11. Cortical penetration of the humerus is not uncommon and must be avoided if it is necessary to remove the medullary cement.

when the component is removed. This is particularly the case in the rheumatoid patient who has olecranon involvement. The subcutaneous exposure of the proximal ulna may be necessary to remove cement without penetration of the cortex.

Closure. Depending on the particular revision option selected, the triceps should be reattached to bone. Two drains are left in the depths of the wound, and the tourniquet is deflated to develop meticulous hemostasis. The skin is carefully inspected. If there is any question about the status of the cutaneous circulation, the elbow is casted in extension for 10 to 21 days.

Postoperative Management. For resection arthroplasty, the joint is protected in a cast for 3 weeks. This allows optimum opportunity for the skin and soft tissue to heal as well as for scarring to occur about the joint, thereby rendering it stable. With interposition arthroplasty, if ankylosis is a concern, early motion with the distractor device might be considered, but we have had no experience with this. If a reimplantation has taken place, careful inspection of the skin in 5 days with initiation of motion is recommended. The elbow is rested in an orthoplast splint for most of the time when the elbow is not being formally exercised by the patient.

Again, if questions exist with regard to the healing of the soft tissue, the arm is simply rested in a splint or cast for 2 to 3 weeks.

RESULTS

Comments have appeared in the literature about various techniques of revision.[2, 3, 7] There are, however, no data about the results of any of the techniques discussed above. We have previously reported our experience with resection arthroplasty for the septic joint,[9] and this is discussed in Chapter 34. After sepsis, 8 of 10 patients with resection arthroplasty achieved a satisfactory rating on the elbow rating scale and considered their condition improved compared with their initial condition prior to joint replacement.

Analysis of our experience with revision reimplantation of total elbow arthroplasty for nonseptic loosening over a 10-year period has recently been reported.[11] Of 24 procedures, 9 (37 per cent) were in individuals with post-traumatic arthritis. The average time to revision was 43 months in those with rheumatoid and 17 months in those with post-traumatic disease. This difference is statistically significant ($p<.01$). In this group the humeral component was loose in 11, the ulnar component was loose in 2, and both components were loose in 7. In four implants, material failure caused revision. Of note is that six patients had fracture of the humerus before or during revision due to bone resorption caused by the loose prosthesis.

With a mean follow-up of 3.5 years (range, 2 to 5 years), 17 (71 per cent) have a satisfactory outcome from the surgery. The motion averages 27 to 130 degrees of flexion, 72 degrees of pronation, and 67 degrees of supination. This is approximately the same as the motion attained after the first procedure. The mean time of surgery was approximately 20 minutes more than the time required for the first implant. Seven have required another operation, five because of loosening. Each of those that reloosened was initially revised with a prosthesis similar to the first device. Thus, in this limited series with short follow-up, reimplantation has been an acceptable alternative, especially when a 6-inch stem, loose-hinge, anterior flanged prosthesis is bone grafted at the time of surgery (see Fig. 35–10).

COMPLICATIONS

All the complications presented in the previous chapter and previously discussed[8] can occur with revision surgery. In our series of 24 revision procedures, material failure of the implant, infection, and postoperative humeral fracture occurred in two instances each. One case of ulnar neuropathy and one of ulnar fracture was likewise documented. Excluding the patients with loosening discussed above, the complication rate was 11 in 24 (46 per cent). One specific complication was noted. Cortical penetration, as evidenced by extravasation of polymethylmethacrylate on the roentgenographic film, had occurred in eight humeral and five ulnar bones (Fig. 35–11). One patient developed an ulnar fracture through the stress riser effect of the penetrated ulnar cortex (Fig. 35–12).

AUTHOR'S PREFERRED TREATMENT METHOD

Revision for Sepsis

Because removal of components leaving a resection arthroplasty provides good results

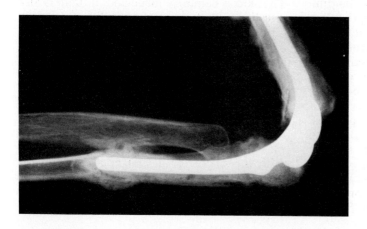

Figure 35–12. Undisplaced fracture at the tip of the revised ulnar component occurred because the cortex was penetrated. This fracture healed uneventfully by casting. (From Morrey, B. F., and Bryan, R. S.: Complications of total elbow arthroplasty. Clin. Orthop. 170:204, 1982.)

in most individuals, simple removal is the recommended treatment.[4, 6, 9] The extremity is casted for about 3 to 4 weeks; stability is surprisingly good if not too much bone has been removed. If fracture of the distal humerus occurs, it will heal with 8 to 12 weeks of casting.

Revision for Resurfacing Devices

In an early postoperative course, a subluxing resurfacing device is treated by casting for 3 to 6 weeks. A hinged splint is used as needed. In most instances this will result in enhanced stability. If symptomatic chronic instability, subluxation, or dislocation develops, revision is considered. If the cause of the instability is clearly identified and is amenable to nonrevision treatment, the resurfacing device is preserved. If the present implant must be removed and the quality of bone stock and soft tissues is good, reinsertion of a 6-inch stemmed, anterior flanged device with a loose hinge is employed. The plasma spray coat of the distal humerus and proximal ulna allows supplementary bone grafting for the possibility of enhancing biologic fixation. If the bone has been fractured or if an inadequate shell of bone is present, and particularly if the soft tissues are scarred and of poor quality, the prosthesis is simply removed and the wound closed. A hinged brace is used to provide stability while still allowing early motion.

Loosening of a Semiconstrained Prosthesis

Because loosening usually occurs at the bone–cement interface, the component and the cement can be removed without too much difficulty in many instances. Treatment at this point is similar to removal of a resurfacing device. If a significant amount of bone has been removed or was destroyed due to disease or the initial procedure, a 6- or, rarely, an 8-inch humeral component is employed for reimplantation. Once again, bone grafting around the distal humerus or in the presence of fracture or cortical penetration is employed. If the supracondylar bone has been resected, we employ the flanged revision prosthesis with bone grafting of the distal humerus. If extensive bone is lost, an allograft would be considered an acceptable option. We have not performed this procedure.

A most important element that must be carefully discussed with all patients initially and especially with patients undergoing revision is the absolute necessity of limiting activity. The goal of the surgery is to allow the elbow to place the hand in space but not to provide a stable fulcrum for lifting, twisting, or carrying. It must be understood that at this time total elbow arthroplasty has not developed enough to allow normal stresses to be carried across the joint and to be absorbed by the bone–cement or biologic interface. This limitation of revision arthroplasty should be kept in mind before the initial surgical procedure is offered.

References

1. Coonrad, R. W.: Seven-Year Follow-Up of Coonrad Total Elbow Replacement. In Inglis, A. E. (ed.): Upper Extremity Joint Replacement (Symposium on Total Joint Replacement of the Upper Extremity, 1979). St. Louis, C. V. Mosby Co., 1982.
2. Dee, R.: Revision Surgery After Failed Elbow Endoprosthesis. In Inglis, A. E. (ed.): Upper Extremity Joint Replacement (Symposium on Total Joint Replacement of the Upper Extremity, 1979). St. Louis, C. V. Mosby Co., 1982.
3. Dee, R.: Reconstructive Surgery Following Total Elbow Endoprosthesis. Clin. Orthop. 170:196, 1982.
4. Ewald, F. C., Scheinberg, R. D., Poss, R., Thomas, W. H., Scott, R. D., and Sledge, C. B.: Capitellocondylar Total Elbow Arthroplasty: Two to Five-Year Follow-Up in Rheumatoid Arthritis. J. Bone Joint Surg. 62A:1259, 1980.
5. Ewald, F. C.: Distraction Arthroplasty. Presented at the Annual Meeting of the Society of Shoulder and Elbow Surgeons. Rochester, NY November, 1983.
6. Inglis, A. E., and Pellicci, P. M.: Total Elbow Replacement. J. Bone Joint Surg. 62A:1252, 1980.
7. Inglis, A. E.: Revision Surgery Following a Failed Total Elbow Arthroplasty. Clin. Orthop. 170:213, 1982.
8. Morrey, B. F., and Bryan, R. S.: Complications of Total Elbow Arthroplasty. Clin. Orthop. 170:204, 1982.
9. Morrey, B. F., and Bryan, R. S.: Infection After Total Elbow Arthroplasty. J. Bone Joint Surg. 65A:3:330, 1983.
10. Morrey, B. F., and Bryan, R. S.: Prosthetic Arthroplasty of the Elbow. In Surgery of the Musculoskeletal System, Vol. 3, no. 2. New York, Churchill Livingstone, 1983, p. 273.
11. Morrey, B. F., and Bryan, R. S.: Reimplantation Revision for Failed Total Elbow Arthroplasty. American Academy of Orthopedic Surgeons Annual Meeting, Atlanta, February, 1984.
12. Rosenfeld, S. R., and Anzel, S. H.: Evaluation of the Pritchard Total Elbow Arthroplasty. Orthopedics 5:713, 1982.
13. Volz, R. G.: Total Elbow Arthroplasty. In American Academy of Orthopedic Surgeons Continuing Education Course. The Upper Extremity. Tuscon, February, 1983.

CHAPTER 36

Arthrodesis

ROBERT D. BECKENBAUGH

Arthrodesis of the elbow is a procedure designed to achieve pain relief and stability (power) in afflictions of the elbow without the associated hazards and long-term complications of joint replacement. Historically, most experience with fusion of the elbow has come from spontaneously occurring arthrodesis following tuberculosis or rheumatic disease of the elbow. The elbow functions with the shoulder to place the hand in space. Because of this, one of the prerequisites for elbow fusion is satisfactory function of the shoulder. In the absence of abduction and internal rotation of the shoulder, adaptive positioning of the hand is impossible if the elbow is fused. In disease states involving both the elbow and the shoulder, arthroplasty must, therefore, be selected. In addition, arthrodesis is not indicated in bilateral elbow disease because functional limitations are too great. Functionally, a limited range of 100 degrees in midposition is enough for most daily activities, but removing all elbow motion restricts the majority of activities either away from the body or at the mouth.[8]

The optimum position for fusion depends on associated joint involvement, occupation of the patient, or specific patient functional requirements. Little objective information about the position of fusion has been set forth.

Ninety degrees of flexion is probably the best position of arthrodesis in a dominant arm with good shoulder and wrist motion. At this position the hand may reach the mouth with adaptive neck, shoulder, and wrist motion, and writing may be performed comfortably. Special needs may occur in the nondominant arm that prompt fusion in 30 degrees or 60 degrees of flexion if, for example, bench work or assistive activities are required.[11]

INDICATIONS

Because of the above-mentioned limitations, arthrodesis of the elbow is not commonly indicated. If this reconstructive procedure has a place in the surgeon's armamentarium, it would be in patients with post-traumatic unilateral arthrosis of the elbow requiring strength and stability. In patients with bilateral disease and limited shoulder or wrist motion, arthroplasty with or without joint replacement is preferred. In unilateral postinfectious arthrosis, arthrodesis may be indicated but generally occurs spontaneously with adequate immobilization.

TECHNIQUE

Most of the limited reports concerning arthrodesis deal with various fusion techniques. These may be broadly classified according to the intra-articular procedure and the technique of fixation.

The elbow is one of the most difficult joints to fuse surgically. The hand and forearm act as a long lever arm, producing strong bending forces across the potential fusion site.

Joint Preparation

Depending on the underlying diagnosis, the amount and quality of existing bone, and the degree of joint destruction, the articulation may be entered and cancellous bone surfaces fashioned (see Figs. 36–4, 36–12, 36–13, and 36–14). In some instances the joint may be fixed after minimal removal or fashioning of the joint surfaces (see Figs. 36–1 and 36–7).

Stabilization

In general, both autogenous grafts and mechanical fixation are now utilized, although in the past fixation was achieved with grafts alone. In the presence of active infection, external skeletal fixation is preferred. In the presence of ancient sepsis or arthrosis with limited motion and minimal deformity, arthrodesis may be achieved with limited internal fixation (screws) without bone grafts. If significant instability or deformity is present preoperatively, internal fixation with screws supplemented with external skeletal fixation may be utilized, or occasionally plates may be used.

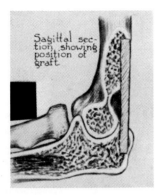

Figure 36–1. Steindler technique of elbow fusion. Cortical screws may be placed through graft, humerus, and olecranon. (From Steindler, A.: Reconstructive Surgery of the Upper Extremity. New York, Appleton-Century-Croft, 1923.)

Early Surgical Techniques

Steindler

Steindler uses a single posterior tibial cortical graft keyed into the olecranon for fusion (Fig. 36–1).[14] A posterior lateral incision is made over the olecranon and distal part of the humerus. The triceps tendon is detached from the olecranon, and the joint is flexed to allow removal of cartilage and subchondral bone from the semilunar notch and trochlea. A cortical graft, 1.5 by 8 cm, is removed from the superior surface of the tibia. A groove is prepared in the tip of the olecranon, and a matching bed is made on the posterior surface of the humerus. The graft is impacted in place with the elbow in 90 degrees of flexion and is fixed with cortical screws to the humerus and olecranon. Postoperatively, a cast is worn for 8 weeks, and then the elbow is braced until union has occurred.

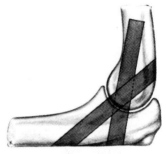

Figure 36–2. Crossed tibial graft technique of Brittain. (From Brittain, H.A.: Architectural Principles in Arthrodesis, 2nd ed. Edinburgh, E. & S. Livingstone Ltd., 1952.)

Brittain

Brittain developed a technique of crossed grafts through the elbow joint.[3, 5] Noting that gravitational forces tended to compress the ends of the graft, he believed that the crossing of the grafts was important (Fig. 36–2).

Two corticocancellous grafts, 1 by 6 cm each, are removed from the anterior medial surface of the tibia. A straight longitudinal incision is made over the back of the elbow and is deepened directly to bone. Two holes are drilled into the olecranon at its middle portion, and a 1-cm osteotome is driven from the olecranon across the elbow into the humerus nearly parallel to the medullary canal of the humerus. The osteotome is gently worked to and fro to accommodate the thickness of the graft. Two holes are drilled into the humerus just above the olecranon fossa, and a second osteotome is driven across the joint distally to the olecranon so that the two osteotomes form an X. The first osteotome is left in place, and the second is driven across to prevent impingement of the grafts against each other (Fig. 36–3). The grafts are driven

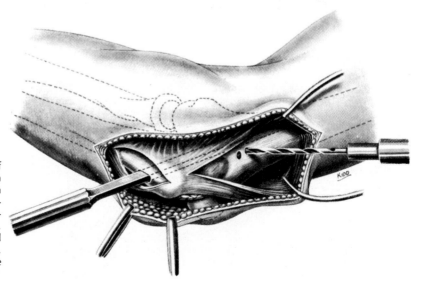

Figure 36–3. Brittain method of arthrodesis. Osteotomes are driven across the elbow in crossed fashion after predrilling of cortex. Two osteotomes are used to prevent interference of grafts with each other. (From Brittain, H.A.: Architectural Principles in Arthrodesis, 2nd ed. Edinburgh, E. & S. Livingstone Ltd., 1952.)

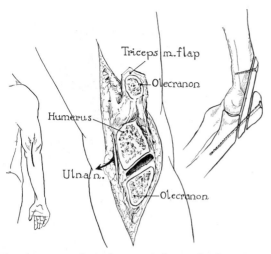

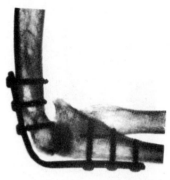

Figure 36–5. Spier technique of compression plate arthrodesis of elbow. (From Spier, W.: Beitrag zur Technik der Druckarthrodese des Ellenbogengelenks. Monatsschr. Unfallheilkd. 76:274, 1973.

Figure 36–4. Staples technique of elbow arthrodesis. (From Staples, O.S.: Arthrodesis of the elbow joint. J. Bone Joint Surg. 34A:207, 1952.)

across the elbow in the slots prepared by the osteotomes. Postoperatively, the elbow is immobilized in a cast for 4 months or until union appears evident. Koch and Lipscomb have described a modification of this technique consisting of a tibial graft placed through a large drill hole in the humerus and ulna and additional cancellous grafts to the joint.[7]

Staples

Staples uses a corticocancellous iliac graft through the posterior portion of the elbow and oblique humeral and olecranon intra-articular resection (Fig. 36–4).[13] A posterior incision is made over the elbow. The ulnar nerve is freed and retracted medially. An oblique osteotomy is made through the middle of the olecranon at the desired degree of fusion. The triceps is split medially and laterally, and the olecranon triceps flap is re-

tracted proximally. The posterior part of the humerus is then resected obliquely in line with the olecranon osteotomy to produce a broad, cancellous flat surface at the angle of desired fusion. A flat, corticocancellous graft is removed from the anterior iliac crest and fixed to the elbow posteriorly with one screw through the humerus. A second screw is placed from the olecranon across the graft and into the ulna. Postoperatively, a plaster cast is worn for 3 months or until fusion is evident.

Recent Surgical Techniques

With the advent of improved internal and external skeletal fixation devices, several alternatives exist in attempts to achieve arthrodesis of the elbow.[6] Spier[12] and Plank[10] have described a compression arthrodesis that makes use of a bent plate and external compression device (Fig. 36–5). Bonnel has reported a successful case of elbow arthrodesis (for arthroplasty that failed) in which external skeletal fixation was combined with bone grafting (Fig. 36–6).[2]

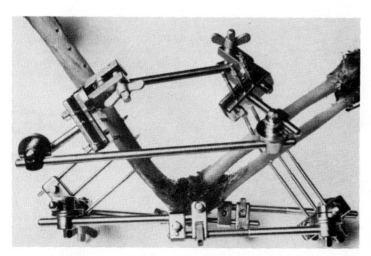

Figure 36–6. Fixation of humerus, radius, and ulna with Hoffman device for arthrodesis of elbow. (From Bonnel, F.: Technique d'arthrodese du coude par fixateur externe. J Chir. (Paris) 107:79, 1974.)

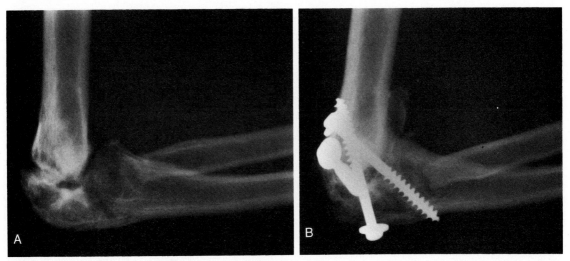

Figure 36–7. *A,* Post-traumatic elbow arthrosis. Patient has 10 degrees of painful motion. *B,* After compression screw application across elbow without bone graft.

For post-traumatic arthrosis of the elbow with minimal motion but significant pain, I have used compression fixation of the elbow with screws. The procedure involves partial débridement of remaining articular surfaces and compression screw fixation without grafts (Fig. 36–7).

External Skeletal Fixation

In the presence of active sepsis, synovectomy and débridement of the radial head and articular surfaces followed by external skeletal fixation will allow spontaneous arthrodesis to occur in the desired position. Fixation is best achieved through a bilateral trapezoidal frame.

Two transfixing pins are placed in the midhumerus and proximal ulna. Care must be taken to avoid the radial and ulnar nerves. Three nontransfixing pins are placed in the midradius and midulna, and the trapezoidal configuration is completed (Fig. 36–8).[4]

In tuberculous arthrosis, in which fusion is easy to achieve, a single external frame may be utilized as follows: three nontransfixing pins are placed in the lateral humerus, proximal ulna, and midulna, and a triangular compression (Fig. 36–9) or quadrangular frame is applied (Fig. 36–10).

Limited Internal Fixation With Screws

In patients with active draining sinuses with tuberculosis of the elbow, Arafiles has described a technique that locks the olecranon in the humeral fossa and is stabilized by screw fixation.[1] In 13 patients with tuberculosis he

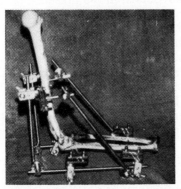

Figure 36–8. Skeletal representation of trapezoidal configuration for external fixation of the elbow. (From Connes, H.: Hoffman's External Anchorage: Techniques, Indications and Results. Paris, Editions GEAD, 1977.)

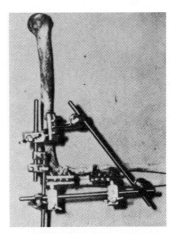

Figure 36–9. Skeletal representation of single lateral frame complex for fusion of tuberculous arthrosis. (From Connes, H.: Hoffman's External Anchorage: Techniques, Indications and Results. Paris, Editions GEAD, 1977.)

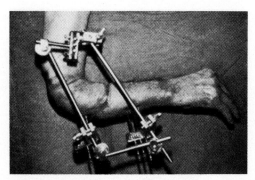

Figure 36–10. Lateral skeletal fixation frame for fusion in tuberculous arthrosis. (From Connes, H.: Hoffmann's External Anchorage: Techniques, Indications and Results. Paris, Editions GEAD, 1977.)

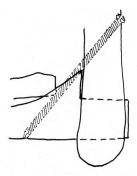

Figure 36–12. Screw fixation following resection and impaction of bone surfaces. (From Arafiles, R. P.: A new technique of fusion for tuberculous arthritis of the elbow. J. Bone Joint Surg. 63A:1397, 1981.)

achieved healing of the arthrodesis within 3 months.

A straight longitudinal incision is made over the posterior elbow. The triceps tendon is split longitudinally and detached distally for 5 cm with medial and lateral periosteal sleeves. The ulnar nerve is freed and retracted, and the distal humerus is freed subperiosteally, elevating the soft tissues off the condyles, including the flexor and extensor origins. The radial head and both humeral condyles are resected. Complete synovectomy and removal of the articular cartilage is performed. The proximal ulna and the olecranon fossa are shaped into matching triangular sets (Fig. 36–11). After insertion of the olecranon into the trochlea, a single cortical screw is placed from the posterior olecranon and humerus obliquely into the ulna (Fig. 36–12). The triceps is repaired anatomically, the ulnar nerve is transposed anteriorly, and the flexor and extensor origins are sutured to the triceps fascia.

Postoperatively, a long arm cast is worn for 3 months, and then mobilization is allowed. Appropriate chemical therapy is initiated preoperatively and continued as necessary through 18 months.

AO Compression

The AO group incorporates axial compression with external fixation with a cancellous lag screw into the humeral shaft (Fig. 36–13).[9] Through a posterior approach, the surfaces of the distal humerus and olecranon are resected to provide a wedge fit. The radial head is excised, and a Kirschner wire is passed from the olecranon up the humeral shaft. Transverse pins are inserted through the olecranon and humerus, the Kirschner wire is removed, and a long cancellous screw is inserted with a washer up the shaft of the humerus. External compression clamps are then applied.

Author's Preferred Method of Treatment

The Unstable Elbow

Without Sepsis. In the presence of an unstable elbow without sepsis, the application of internal fixation with screws will achieve immediate stability and allow application of additional bone grafts if necessary. This, in conjunction with cast fixation, should produce simplified and more rapid union.

With Infection. In the presence of infection, however, I prefer, in an unstable elbow, to use simple external skeletal fixation with cancellous graft if necessary. There is often a hypertrophic bony response in the presence of infection. Hence, external skeletal fixation with the bilateral or unilateral triangular configuration can achieve compression and good immobilization and allow the wounds to be left open for gradual closing in anticipation

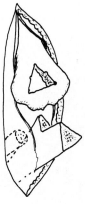

Figure 36–11. Triangular resection of olecranon and enlargement of trochlear fossa. (From Arafiles, R.P.: A new technique of fusion for tuberculous arthritis of the elbow. J. Bone Joint Surg. 63A:1397, 1981.)

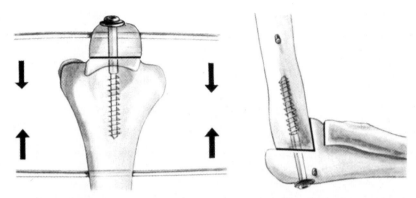

Figure 36–13. AO technique of axial fixation and external skeletal fixation for arthrodesis of the elbow. (From Muller, M.E., et al.: Manual of Internal Fixation: Techniques Recommended by the AO-Group, 2nd ed. New York, Springer-Verlag, 1979.)

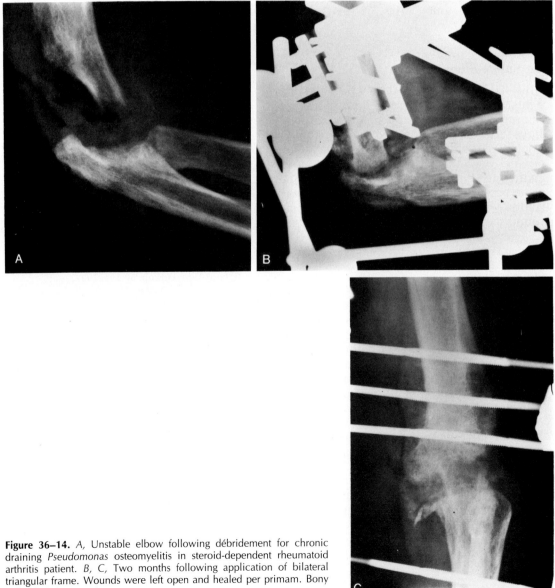

Figure 36–14. *A*, Unstable elbow following débridement for chronic draining *Pseudomonas* osteomyelitis in steroid-dependent rheumatoid arthritis patient. *B, C,* Two months following application of bilateral triangular frame. Wounds were left open and healed per primam. Bony arthrodesis is occurring.

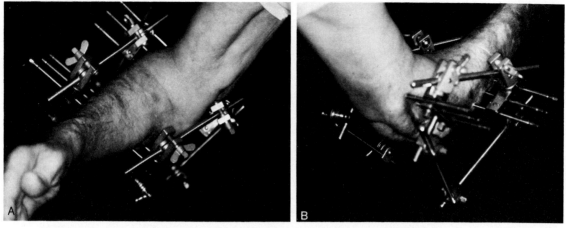

Figure 36–15. *A, B,* Bilateral triangular frame of the type used in Figure 36–14 for unstable infected elbow.

of spontaneous union (Figs. 36–14 and 36–15).

The Stable Elbow

In the stable elbow without infection, the use of internal fixation with cancellous compression screws is a very simple method that will allow more rapid union and earlier mobilization. Grafts are generally not necessary, and minimal débridement of cortical surfaces is required to allow the fusion to mature. Again, in the presence of infection external skeletal fixation with articular débridement and open wound packing will promote union.

COMPLICATIONS

Nonunion. Few data are available about the incidence of successful primary arthrodesis. Koch and Lipscomb reported that primary arthrodesis failed in 9 of 17 patients treated at the Mayo Clinic.[7] Six of 11 elbows treated for tuberculosis failed to unite. Extensive joint destruction and unavailability of chemotherapy were cited as contributory factors to account for this poor rate of fusion. With better chemotherapy, control of infection, and improved fixation techniques, the success rate of primary fusion should improve.

Fracture. The long lever arm created by elbow fusion causes increased stress along the entire extremity. Fracture through or proximal to the fused or ankylosed joint is not uncommon and was observed in 4 of 17 patients reported by Koch and Lipscomb.[7]

References

1. Arafiles, R. P.: A New Technique of Fusion for Tuberculosis Arthritis of the Elbow. J. Bone Joint Surg. **63A**:1396, 1981.
2. Bonnel, F.: Technique d'Arthrodese du Coude par Fixateur Externe. J. Chir. (Paris) **107**:79, 1974.
3. Brittain, H. A.: Architectural Principles in Arthrodesis, 2nd ed. Edinburgh, E. & S. Livingstone, 1952, p. 161.
4. Connes, H.: Hoffmann's External Anchorage: Techniques, Indications and Results. Paris, Editions GEAD, 1977, p. 118.
5. Crenshaw, A. H.: Campbell's Operative Orthopaedics, 5th ed. St. Louis, C. V. Mosby Co., 1971, p. 1191.
6. Dahl, H. K.: A-O-Metoden ved Osteotomi og Arthrodese. Nord. Med. **85**:599, 1971.
7. Koch, M., and Lipscomb, P. R.: Arthrodesis of the Elbow. Clin. Orthop. **50**:151, 1967.
8. Morrey, B. F., Askew, L. J., An, K. N., and Chao, E. Y.: A Biomechanical Study of Normal Functional Elbow Motion. J. Bone Joint Surg. **63A**:872, 1981.
9. Muller, M. E., Allgower, M., Schneider, R., and Willenegger, H.: Manual of Internal Fixation: Techniques Recommended by the AO-Group, 2nd ed. Berlin, Springer-Verlag, 1979, p. 387.
10. Plank, E., and Spier, W.: Die Arthrodese des Ellenbogens. Aktuel Probl. Chir. Orthop. **2**:41, 1977.
11. Snider, W. J., and De Witt, H. J.: Functional Study for Optimum Position for Elbow Arthrodesis or Ankylosis. *In* Proceedings of the American Academy of Orthopedic Surgeons. J. Bone Joint Surg. **55A**:1305, 1973.
12. Spier, W.: Beitraz zur Technik der Druckarthrodese des Ellenbogengelenks. Montasschr. Unfallheilkd. **76**:274, 1973.
13. Staples, O. S.: Arthrodesis of the Elbow Joint. J. Bone Joint Surg. **34A**:207, 1952.
14. Steindler, A.: Reconstructive Surgery of the Upper Extremity. New York, D. Appleton & Co., 1923.

CHAPTER 37

Flaccid Dysfunction of the Elbow

EUGENE T. O'BRIEN

Flaccid paralysis of the elbow severely limits the ability of the patient to position and stabilize the hand so that it can function. The patient with paralysis of the elbow flexors (biceps, brachialis, and brachioradialis) is unable to reach his face for eating, shaving, washing, and combing his hair. Most jobs require that the hand be held at frequently changing levels for lifting and carrying, and this is impossible when the elbow flexors are paralyzed. Paralysis of the elbow extensors results in loss of ability to work with the extremity held above the horizontal position, as when reaching to obtain an object off a high shelf. Stabilizing an object in space or on a surface, such as holding a loaf of bread while it is being sliced, is also impossible. The patient who needs to transfer or use crutches is unable to do so without active elbow extension. Supination of the forearm is necessary in lifting and carrying and in using the hand around the face. Pronation is important for positioning the hand for most activities such as writing, working at a bench, and driving a car.

Most of the operations developed to restore elbow flexion were developed for patients paralyzed from poliomyelitis. Currently, the majority of tendon transfers to restore elbow function are performed in patients who have had an injury of the brachial plexus. Most commonly, the injury results from a fall from a motorcycle or being thrown out of an automobile at the time of impact. A permanent lesion of the C5 and C6 root or upper trunk results in a flaccid paralysis of the elbow flexors with preservation of nearly normal hand function. Birth palsy involving the upper portion of the brachial plexus (Erb's palsy) results in paralysis or weakness of elbow flexion that may require reconstructive surgery. Irreparable damage to the musculocutaneous and radial nerves proximal to the muscles innervated by them results in a flaccid paralysis of the elbow. Extensive direct muscle injury may occasionally necessitate a tendon and muscle transfer to replace lost function. Radical excision of the entire flexor or extensor muscle compartment to eradicate a malignant soft tissue tumor may require a muscle transfer or transplant. In the tetraplegic patient, tendon transfers are sometimes performed to restore elbow extension, making transfer activities easier. The severely compromised function of the upper extremity in a child with arthrogryposis can be improved by a tendon transfer to restore some elbow flexion. Patients with progressive neurologic or muscular diseases involving the entire upper extremity and resulting in flaccid paralysis of the elbow are rarely, if ever, candidates for elbow tendon transfers.

GENERAL PRINCIPLES

Timing. Because there is often a reasonable expectation of some spontaneous recovery of elbow flexion following stretching injuries of the brachial plexus, especially those involving the upper trunk, reconstructive surgery to replace elbow function should not be undertaken until 12 to 18 months after the injury. If the patient shows any sign of recovery of elbow motor function at 1 year, reconstructive surgery should be postponed another 6 months or so to be certain that it is really necessary. In the tetraplegic patient, likewise, reconstructive surgery to replace triceps function should not be undertaken less than a year after injury. In the child with arthrogryposis, transfers to gain elbow flexion can be done after 5 years of age. Usually reconstruction should be done on only one side so that one extremity can be used for activities requiring flexion while the unoperated elbow is used for actions requiring extension. After the traumatic loss of a flexor or extensor muscle compartment, it is advisable to wait until the tissues about the elbow joint are supple before proceeding with tendon transfer.

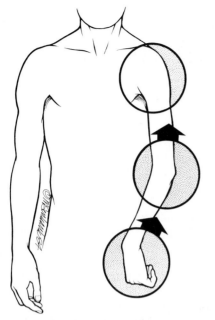

Figure 37–1. Order of reconstruction of paralyzed upper extremity.

Order of Reconstructive Procedures for Adjacent Joint Paralysis. Reconstructive surgery to restore active flexion or extension of the elbow is indicated only if the patient has useful or restorable hand function.

In general, most authors have advised proceeding in a distal to proximal direction—that is, doing the hand first, followed by the elbow and, finally, the shoulder (Fig. 37–1). Carroll, however, advised performing flexorplasty before hand surgery because the results of tendon transfer in the hand were better if the origin of the transferred muscle was transferred in advance.[16] Zancolli advised that in the tetraplegic patient surgery on the elbow should precede that on the hand.[76] Moberg also felt that it may be desirable to operate on the elbow first because this surgery prevents the patient from using the hand to eat with for about 4 months, a boring situation once he has already learned to use his reconstructed hand.[50]

Stabilization of the shoulder is usually carried out after performance of hand and elbow surgery. Seddon and Nyholm, however, both advised performing arthrodesis of the shoulder before carrying out the transfer to restore elbow flexion.[51,59] Seddon believed that the prolonged immobilization of the extremity required for the shoulder to fuse might be harmful to the elbow that had been operated on already.

Except when performing a Steindler flexorplasty, I believe that reconstructive hand surgery should precede elbow surgery. However, when the same muscles that are transferred proximally on the humerus are used for transfers to restore hand function, it seems more reasonable to perform the hand transfers after the origin has already been shifted proximally. The elbow transfer should always be done before the shoulder arthrodesis for several reasons. As noted by Clark, it is best to wait and see if the restored elbow flexion really needs assistance by stabilization of the shoulder, and one is then capable of choosing the best fusion position to supplement the new elbow flexion. The elbow transfer surgery, especially if it is a Steindler flexorplasty, is also technically easier to perform if it is done prior to shoulder stabilization.

Correction of Pre-existing Joint Contracture. Acceptable passive motion of the elbow must be obtained prior to transfer. This often requires physical therapy in which the joint and muscle contractures are gently stretched out and the functioning muscles are strengthened by progressive resistance exercises. At least 120 degrees of passive flexion is desirable before tendon transfer is carried out. The principle of the turnbuckle splint is very useful in regaining passive extension.[32] Occasionally, surgery is required to release a severely damaged elbow flexor, extensor muscle, or joint capsule before the joint can be mobilized. Soft tissue cover may have to be added to a severely scarred flexor or extensor surface of the arm before tendon transfer can be carried out.

Choosing an Appropriate Muscle for Transfer. The most common cause of failure in tendon transfers about the elbow, as elsewhere, is underestimating the strength of the transferred muscle. The muscle to be transferred should contract against gravity and some resistance (grade 4) if significant function is to be anticipated (Table 37–1).

Table 37–1. **Muscle Strength Grading System**

Grade	Definition	Explanation
0	Absent	No function
1	Trace	Slight contraction No motion
2	Poor	Complete motion Gravity eliminated
3	Fair	Complete motion against gravity
4	Good	Complete motion against gravity and some resistance
5	Normal	Apparently normal strength

In addition to muscle strength, which is determined by clinical examination, it is also important to know something about the comparative work capacities of the various muscles available for transfer.[72] The work capacity is determined by multiplying the power of the muscle (3.65 kg × cm^2 of physiologic cross section) by its amplitude (the distance through which the tendon moves when its muscle contracts). The work capacity of the biceps for elbow flexion is 4.8 kg-m (kilogram-meters), and for forearm supination it is 1.1 kg-m. The sternocostal head of the pectoralis major muscle has nearly three times as much work capacity at 10.4 kg-m. By contrast, the total forearm flexor (pronator teres, flexor carpi radialis and ulnaris, and palmaris longus) work capacity is 3.8 kg-m.[37]

The mechanical advantages of the different elbow flexor transfers have been calculated by Holtmann et al.[37] They found that the transferred triceps or sternocostal portion of the pectoralis major required less force to support a given load than did the transferred forearm flexors but more force than the normal biceps. The mechanical advantage of the sternocleidomastoid approximated that of the normal biceps because of its similarity in angle of approach to the bicipital tuberosity of the radius.

The expendability of the transferred muscle must be considered in choosing a muscle for transfer around the elbow. Triceps transfer for elbow flexion is not often indicated because the triceps is not really expendable. The latissimus dorsi is not expendable in the polio patient, who relies on it to elevate the pelvis when the other pelvic elevators are paralyzed.

Cosmesis is sometimes a consideration in the choice of a muscle transfer. The bowstringing of the sternocleidomastoid transfer across the side of the neck makes it an undesirable transfer even though, theoretically, it is one of the most mechanically efficient transfers. Restoration of near-normal bulk of the arm in a patient with loss of flexor or extensor muscle mass is a nice cosmetic by-product of the bipolar latissimus or pectoralis muscle transplant.

RESTORATION OF ELBOW FLEXION

Elbow flexion has been restored by a variety of methods. The insertion of a muscle can be transferred: triceps,[14] pectoralis major,[9] and sternocleidomastoid.[12] All or part of the origin of a muscle or muscle group can be trans-ferred: forearm flexor-pronator,[64] sternocostal portion of pectoralis major,[21] latissimus dorsi,[38] and pectoralis minor.[61] The entire muscle can be transplanted on its neurovascular pedicle: latissimus dorsi,[56] pectoralis major.[19] And, finally, a muscle can be transplanted using a microneurovascular anastomosis, as with the gracilis.[31]

Steindler Flexorplasty

In 1918, Steindler first described his simple but ingenious concept of proximally shifting the origin of the flexor-pronator muscle group to increase its lever arm and markedly improve its mechanical efficiency in flexing the elbow.[62, 63] His technique consisted in the subperiosteal dissection of the origin of the flexor-pronator muscles of the forearm from the medial epicondyle. The muscle flap was then transposed proximally between the brachialis and the triceps and sutured to the medial epicondylar ridge through two drill holes 2 inches above the epicondyle. Steindler recommended the procedure only if the wrist flexors were normal or only slightly weakened.

Subsequent authors differed on the prerequisites for a Steindler flexorplasty. Mayer and Green believed that the epicondylar muscle group strength should be at least grade 3 or better and re-emphasized the need for strong wrist flexors for the operation to succeed.[47] They described a simple test in which the arm is abducted to 90 degrees to eliminate gravity. If the patient can flex his elbow in this position (using the epicondylar muscle group), he is a candidate for the operation. Nyholm believed that the criteria for forearm muscle strength should be liberalized because all his patients achieved 90 degrees of elbow flexion even though a relatively large number had forearm muscles that were "primarily paretic."[51] Dutton and Dawson performed the operation if the strength of the forearm flexor-pronator group was rated fair or better.[28] It would seem that there is considerable leeway in the preoperative muscle strength needed for active flexion, and in this operation the axiom that the muscle loses a grade in transferring it does not seem to apply.

Subsequent authors have modified and refined Steindler's original operation. These modifications have been directed at increasing flexor strength and decreasing the tendency toward development of a pronation deformity. Bunnell described prolonging the common tendon of origin with a fascia lata graft that would reach 2 inches up the lateral border of the humerus.[12] According to the author, this resulted in a moderate but not complete correction of the pronation tendency. Mayer and Green detached the flexor-pronator origin with a portion of the medial epicondyle and attached it through a window cut in the anterior cortex of the humerus 5 to 7.5 cm proximal to the joint.[47] Their description of the technical details of the Steindler flexorplasty, which includes a careful dissection of the ulnar and median motor branches, is the best in the literature. Lindholm and Einola used a screw to fix the epicondylar fragment to the humerus in two cases.[44] Eyler advocated omitting the flexor carpi ulnaris because this would allow the surgeon to work in the "internervous plane" between the flexor sublimis anteriorly and the flexor profundus and flexor carpi ulnaris dorsally.[29]

Attempts have been made to augment the strength of elbow flexion, especially in patients who have weakness of the flexor-pronator muscle group. In one of his earlier communications,[64] Steindler recommended proximal transfer of the radial wrist extensor muscle origins off the lateral epicondyle in conjunction with the medial transfer but did not comment on it in his later communications. Mayer and Green noted difficulty in mobilizing the lateral epicondylar muscle group without damaging the nerve supply[47] and gave up the procedure[47] after two unsatisfactory results. Lindholm and Einola were unable to detect any increase in flexion strength in the six patients who had the additional lateral transfer.[44]

Anatomy. The pronator teres arises by two heads: the humeral head originates from the medial supracondylar ridge and medial intermuscular septum and from the common flexor tendon, whereas the smaller ulnar head arises from the coronoid process of the ulna. The median nerve enters the forearm between the two heads of the pronator teres. The flexor carpi radialis, palmaris longus, and humeral head of the flexor superficialis all originate from the common flexor tendon. The flexor carpi ulnaris arises by two heads: the humeral head originates from the common flexor tendon, and the ulnar head originates along the medial border of the olecranon and posterior border of the upper three fifths of the ulna. Branches originating from the medial surface of the median nerve supply the pronator teres (C6 and C7), flexor carpi radialis (C6 and C7), palmaris longus (C7 and C8), and humeral head of flexor superficialis (C8 and T1). The flexor carpi ulnaris (C8 and T1) is innervated by two or three branches of the ulnar nerve,

the first of which usually leaves the nerve just as it passes between the two heads of the muscle.

Technique (Modified from Mayer and Green). See Figure 37–2. A sandbag is placed under the opposite hip. A tourniquet is usually not employed. The incision begins on the anterior aspect of the arm about 7.5 cm above the elbow and swings gently in a medial direction; at the elbow it runs just posterior to the epicondyle. It then curves anteriorly, following the direction of the pronator teres, ending about 10 cm below the elbow. The ulnar nerve is isolated, gently lifted from its bed with a vessel loop, and freed distally until the branches to the flexor carpi ulnaris are seen. Preserving these motor branches, the dissection is continued distally for 5 cm. The lacertus fibrosus is divided, and the median nerve is exposed above the elbow and dissected distally, exposing the motor branches (all of which leave the medial aspect of the nerve) to the common flexor-pronator muscle group. The common flexor-pronator muscle origin is then detached with a flake of epicondyle (cartilage in children and bone in adults). The flake of bone or cartilage is then grasped with a clamp, and, while traction is made in a distal and anterior direction, the muscles are stripped from the anterior surface of the joint and from the coronoid process of the ulna. As the ulnar head of the flexor carpi ulnaris is detached from the ulna with an elevator, the assistant puts gentle traction on the median and ulnar nerves, thus demonstrating the motor twigs that must be carefully avoided. Dissection is continued distally as far as permitted by the anatomic distribution of the nerves. The common tendon is then transfixed with a modified pull-out suture of #1 Prolene. The elbow is then flexed to 120 degrees, and traction is exerted on the transfer to determine how far above the elbow it will reach. This is usually between 5 and 7.5 cm. The ulnar nerve often seems to have less tension on it if it is transferred anterior to the epicondyle. The atrophied fibers of the brachialis are slit longitudinally, the periosteum is incised, and the anterior humerus is exposed subperiosteally. An air drill is then used to make an opening in the anterior cortex of the humerus nearer to the lateral border than the medial at the point to which the transplant reaches when the elbow is flexed. Two small drill holes are made from anterior to posterior through this cortical window. The Prolene suture ends are then threaded through the holes and out through the triceps muscle and skin. The nerves are inspected as the

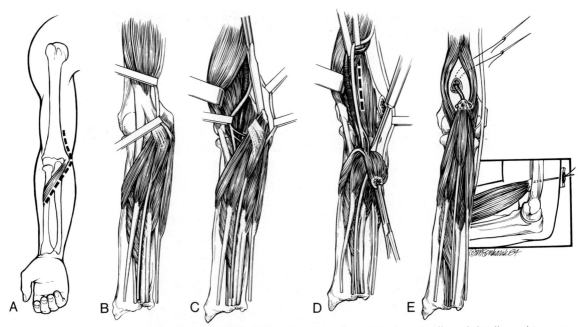

Figure 37–2. Steindler flexorplasty. *A,* The incision. *B,* The ulnar nerve is mobilized proximally and distally, and its motor branches to the flexor carpi ulnaris are identified and protected. *C,* The common flexor-pronator origin is detached with a flake of medial epicondyle. The motor branches of the median nerve to the flexor-pronator group are identified and protected. *D,* The detached flexor-pronator group is mobilized distally as far as the motor branches of the median and ulnar nerves will permit. The brachialis muscle is divided. *E,* The distal humerus is prepared, and a Prolene pull-out suture is used to anchor the transferred muscles to the anterolateral surface of the humerus 5 to 7.5 cm above the elbow. (After Mayer and Green.)

transfer is pulled into the cortical window to be sure that they are not subjected to undue tension on twisting. The distal portion of the wound is closed up to the bend in the elbow. The sutured ends are drawn tight with the elbow in maximum flexion and tied over a button under which a thick piece of felt has been placed. Several auxiliary sutures between the periosteum and the transplanted epicondylar tissues are taken, and the remainder of the wound is closed with a drain.

A posterior splint is then applied with the elbow in about 120 degrees of flexion and the forearm in full supination. Four weeks after surgery, the pull-out suture is removed by cutting one end and pulling out the other end. A removable orthoplast splint is applied, and active flexion and supination and extension exercises are begun. No special retraining is required because the muscles transferred functioned as an accessory elbow flexor prior to transfer.[23] The splint is discontinued 6 to 8 weeks after surgery, the longer time being utilized in patients with normal triceps function. A dynamic extension splint is often useful if the patient has no triceps function (Fig. 37–3).

Results. The results in the literature for Steindler flexorplasty reflect a high degree of success in achieving a functional range of elbow flexion against gravity. The majority of transfers reported have been performed for poliomyelitis. Steindler achieved 79.48 per cent good results (flexion against gravity of not less than 90 degrees) in 39 cases.[66] Fifteen good results (useful range of flexion with good to fair power) in 27 flexorplasties were reported by Carroll and Gartland.[15] Using strict criteria for success, including subtracting from the total score for flexion contracture over 15 degrees and for supination of less than 45 degrees, Mayer and Green recorded 11 excellent, 5 good, 4 fair, and 2 poor results in the 22 flexorplasties they followed.[47] Segal et al. compared the results of 13 Steindler flexorplasties (transplantation of both flexor and extensor origins) and 17 Clark pectoralis major transfers.[60] The flexorplasty results were better than the pectoralis transfers, but the average flexion contracture in the flexorplasty group was 60 degrees, whereas in the Clark transfer group, it rarely exceeded 15 degrees. Kettelcamp and Larson, evaluating 15 flexorplasties using Mayer and Green's scoring system, noted eight excellent or good results, six fair results, and one poor result.[39] They also measured the carry-lift strength (flexion against gravity, plus weight at 1-

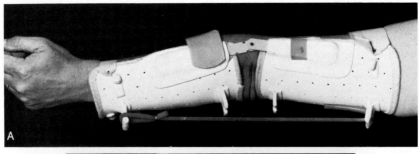

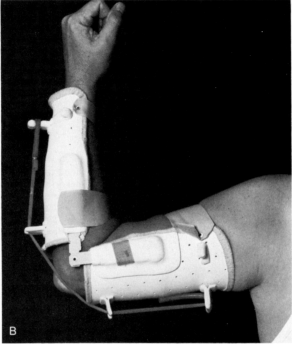

Figure 37–3. *A, B,* A dynamic flexion and extension elbow splint. The dynamic extension is particularly useful in the patient who has a Steindler flexorplasty but lacks triceps function.

pound increments), and found that 9 of the 14 patients who were able to flex the elbow 110 degrees or more against gravity were able to flex through this range with 1 pound or more. The maximum weight lifted was 6 pounds by one patient.

Nyholm reported 24 patients, one fourth of whom achieved a normal degree of elbow flexion following flexorplasty.[51] Five patients (three with brachial plexus trauma and two with polio) achieved some recovery of biceps function, which did not seem to be compromised by the previous flexorplasty. Nyholm noted that all of the patients except two preferred to flex the elbow with the forearm pronated and hand clenched.

The largest series of flexorplasties was reported by Lindholm and Einola,[44] who found that 50 of their 61 cases achieved a range of flexion of at least 90 degrees. Eleven patients were able to lift a weight of over 1 kg at right angles. Dutton and Dawson, using Mayer and Green's criteria in evaluating 25 flexorplasty patients, noted that 20 patients had excellent or good function of the transferred muscles.[28] Eighteen of the patients could lift 1 to 2 kg through an arc of full elbow motion.

Many authors have noted the beneficial effect of arthrodesis of the flail shoulder in the patient who has had a flexorplasty.[28, 39, 44, 65] Shoulder arthrodesis permits abduction at the scapulothoracic joint that decreases the gravitational forces that have to be overcome by the transferred flexor-pronator muscle group. Stabilizing the humerus also maximizes the power of the transfer in preventing backward movement of the elbow, which diminishes the advantage of the flexion contracture by increasing the length of the arc through which the flexorplasty must move the weight against gravity.[39]

Complications. The main complications of

the Steindler transfer are development of a pronation contracture of the forearm and a flexion contracture of the elbow. The development of a pronation contracture is related to two things: the preoperative absence of active supination in most of these patients and the tightening of the pronator teres that results from its proximal shift. Inserting the transfer more anteriorly and laterally on the humerus diminishes this tendency, but if no active supination is present, pronation deformity may still be a problem. Segal et al.[60] and Nyholm[51] did not notice any great change in passive supination after Steindler flexorplasty in their patients. Carroll and Gartland noted that half of the 23 patients who were improved by the flexorplasty had a pronation defect.[15] Lindhol and Einola encountered a pronation contracture in 17 of 61 patients who had a flexorplasty, but 14 of these patients had had no active supination preoperatively.[44] Dutton and Dawson noted an average loss of supination of 39 degrees in the 25 patients they reported.[28]

The degree of fixed flexion contracture of the elbow that is considered acceptable varies a good deal among the different authors. The strength of the transferred muscles, the duration of immobilization, and the strength of the opposing triceps muscle all affect the extent of the flexion contracture. A flexion contracture of the elbow does increase the mechanical advantage of the transferred muscle, and this is especially important in the patient who has significant weakness of the transferred muscle group. Steindler felt that a 60-degree flexion contracture was acceptable,[65] and Carroll and Gartland accepted 40 degrees.[15] Kettelcamp and Larsen observed that when strength rather than appearance was important (men and patients with severe paralysis of the opposite extremity), flexorplasties are more satisfactory with a flexion contracture of between 30 and 60 degrees.[39] Mayer and Green were not satisfied if the flexion contracture exceeded 15 degrees, and they used turnbuckle splints postoperatively to minimize the flexion deformity.[47] Dutton and Dawson preferred a flexion contracture of 15 to 30 degrees, which allows the arm to hang at the side more normally, in a patient concerned with appearance, and a 30- to 45-degree contracture in the patient more concerned with function.[28]

Transient ulnar nerve paresthesias were reported in two patients by Dutton and Dawson.[28] Lindholm and Einola also reported two patients with postoperative ulnar nerve paresthesias; one of them was still having symptoms at follow-up.[44] Pulling-out of the trans-

ferred muscle is the other complication that has been reported. Steindler reported one patient who achieved an excellent result after the pulled-out transfer was reinserted.[65] Lindholm and Einola noted that on x-ray follow-up four epicondylar attachments had pulled loose, but they did not comment on the clinical significance of this finding.[44] Kettelcamp and Larson recorded one poor result in a patient whose transfer pulled loose 4 months after operation.[39]

Latissimus Dorsi Transfer-Transplantation

History

Schottstaedt et al. were the first to report the successful restoration of elbow flexion in two patients by rotating the entire latissimus dorsi muscle on its neurovascular pedicle, reattaching its insertion to the coracoid and its origin to the distal biceps muscle and tendon.[56] One patient could lift 4 pounds, and in the other patient elbow stability was increased and supination had been regained, but the follow-up was only 6 weeks. They noted that the procedure was contraindicated if the latissimus dorsi was the only muscle capable of elevating the pelvis for a forward step. Zancolli and Mitre refined the technique described by Schottstaedt and associates and coined the term "bipolar transfer" for the procedure.[76] Brones et al. reported the use of a bipolar myocutaneous latissimus dorsi flap to restore contour and function in a patient who had sustained a severe soft tissue crush and avulsion injury of his arm.[8]

Restoration of elbow flexion by transferring only the origin of the latissimus dorsi to the biceps insertion (unipolar transfer) was reported by Hovnanian in 1956.[38] He noted that the cross-sectional area, fiber length, and excursion of the latissimus dorsi muscle compared favorably with that of the biceps and brachialis. Axer et al. modified the unipolar technique by using only the upper third of the latissimus dorsi, transferring its origin off several spinous processes to the biceps tendon.[2] An excursion of 7 cm was obtained by stimulating this part of the muscle. According to these authors, transferring only a portion of the muscle avoids the sometimes bulky enlargement of the arm that results when the whole muscle is used. Preservation of some function in the undisturbed portion of the latissimus dorsi was noted in one of the patients.

Free latissimus dorsi muscle or myocutaneous flaps have become very popular for reconstruction of defects in the lower extremity. The latissimus dorsi can be easily rotated on its neurovascular pedicle to replace the elbow flexors or extensors, so free transplantation of this muscle for replacing elbow motors is not indicated.

Anatomy

The latissimus dorsi is a broad, thin muscle (Fig. 37–4) with a wide origin from the lower six thoracic vertebrae, from the spinous processes of the lumbar and sacral vertebrae by an aponeurosis, by an aponeurosis from the iliac crest, and by muscular slips from the lower four ribs. It inserts into the medial wall and floor of the intertubercular groove of the humerus. The major vascular pedicle of the muscle is the thoracodorsal artery, a terminal branch of the subscapular artery. Tobin et al.'s study of 114 latissimus dorsi muscles showed that in 94 per cent of the specimens there was a bifurcation of the common neurovascular trunk into lateral (parallel to the lateral border of the muscle) and medial (parallel to the upper border) branches.[68] Bartlett et al. studied 50 latissimus dorsi muscles and noted the same bifurcation in 56 per cent of the dissections.[3] These studies provide the anatomic basis for the clinical findings noted by Axer et al.[2] The thoracodorsal nerve (C6–C8) is derived from the posterior cord and enters the muscle with the artery and its vein on its deep surface approximately 10 cm from its insertion. There are from one to three branches from the thoracodorsal artery to the serratus muscle that have to be ligated to allow the complete mobilization of the latissimus during a bipolar transfer. In the study by Bartlett et al., the vascular pedicle to the latissimus dorsi had a mean length of 11 cm, and the thoracodorsal nerve had a mean length of 12.3 cm.[3]

Technique

The bipolar transplantation is preferable to the unipolar transfer for several reasons: The mechanical efficiency of the transplant is increased by the more anterior placement of the origin into the coracoid process, the proper length is easier to determine when the distal insertion is completed first, and there is less chance for kinking the neurovascular pedicle.

Bipolar Transplantation. This description follows that of Zancolli and Mitre (Fig. 37–5).[76] The operation is carried out in four steps.

1. The latissimus dorsi muscle origin and insertion are divided while preserving its neurovascular pedicle.
2. Both ends of the biceps muscle are exposed through separate incisions.
3. Transplantation of the latissimus dorsi muscle under a cutaneous bridge in the axilla to the bed of the paralyzed biceps and brachialis, resecting the biceps muscle if need be to provide room for the latissimus dorsi.
4. Fixation of the transposed muscle to the coracoid process and biceps tendon.

The operation is carried out with the patient turned onto his side on a beanbag with the upper extremity draped free. A longitudinal incision is made parallel to the lateral border of the latissimus dorsi muscle, extending from the posterior border of the axilla to the iliac

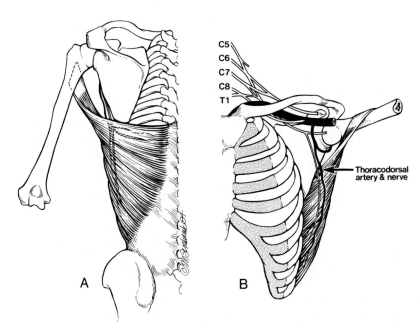

Figure 37–4. A, B, The anatomy of the latissimus dorsi. Shortly after entering the muscle the single neurovascular pedicle (thoracodorsal nerve and artery) divides into lateral and medial branches.

Thoracodorsal artery & nerve

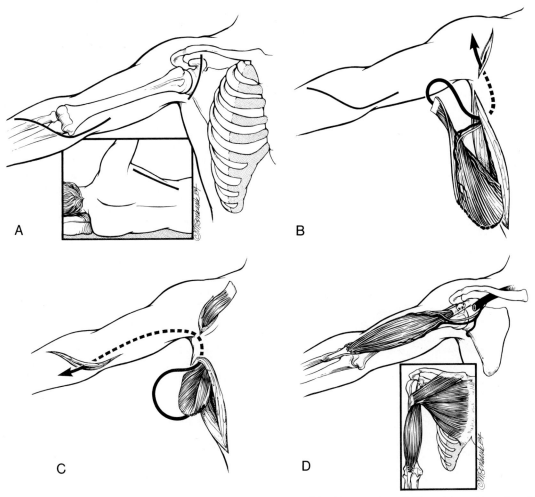

Figure 37–5. Bipolar transplantation of latissimus dorsi. *A*, Incisions used for this procedure. *B*, The origin and insertion of the latissimus dorsi are divided, and the muscle is mobilized on its neurovascular pedicle. *C*, Transplantation of the muscle under a cutaneous bridge in the axilla; the origin is redirected through a subcutaneous tunnel in the arm to the biceps tendon. *D*, The distal anastomosis is completed first, and the proximal attachment to the coracoid process and its conjoined tendon is used to set the tension. (After Zancolli, E., and Mitre, H.: Latissimus dorsi transfer to restore elbow flexion. J. Bone Joint Surg. 55A:1265, 1973.)

crest. The dissection of the muscle is begun along its lateral border from distal to proximal. The neurovascular pedicle must be freed up to its origin in the axilla, and this requires the ligation of any branches of the thoracodorsal artery that enter the serratus anterior. Once the neurovascular pedicle is freed, the origin and insertion of the latissimus dorsi are sectioned. When the muscle is small, it is transplanted completely, but when it is completely normal, it may be necessary to transplant only its lateral half. It is also possible to fold over the vertebral border of the muscle to make it more tubular in shape.

A deltopectoral incision is used to expose the coracoid process and free the tendon of the pectoralis major, behind which the transposed latissimus dorsi will be routed. The insertion of the biceps is then exposed through a bayonet incision over the anterior aspect of the elbow. If the paralyzed biceps is to be resected it is carried out through these two incisions, taking care to protect the neurovascular bundle of the arm and preserving a long segment of distal biceps tendon. The latissimus dorsi muscle is then passed under the skin bridge of the axilla, protecting its neurovascular pedicle from any kinking or tension. The insertion of the transposed muscle is passed deep to the pectoralis major tendon and up to the coracoid process while its distal end is passed downward toward the elbow beneath the skin of the arm. It is convenient at this time to close the thoracic incision over several drains. The distal biceps aponeurosis is opened up and spread out so

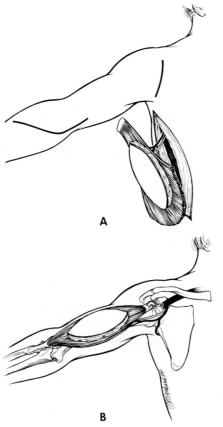

Figure 37–6. Technique used for a myocutaneous latissimus dorsi transplantation.

that it can be wrapped around the distal end of the latissimus dorsi. A significant amount of distal latissimus muscle usually has to be excised because it is too long. After the distal anastomosis is completed, the distal skin incision is closed. Fixation of the proximal end is then carried out at the junction of the conjoined tendon with the coracoid process, adjusting the length of the transplant so that the elbow remains spontaneously at 90 to 100 degrees of flexion with some trial sutures in place. After the proper length has been determined, the final suturing of the proximal end is carried out, and the shoulder wound is closed. A plaster Velpeau bandage is then applied with the elbow flexed and the forearm supinated.

The drains are removed at 48 hours. Postoperative immobilization is maintained for 6 weeks. Flexion exercises are then permitted (with gravity eliminated) with gradually decreasing extension block splinting over the next 2 weeks. At 8 weeks, flexion against gravity is begun. Four to 6 months are required before maximum strength of the transplant is attained.

A myocutaneous transplantation of the latissimus dorsi is performed using the same technique except that an appropriate sized segment of skin is left attached to the muscle (Fig. 37–6).

Unipolar Transfer. This description is based on that of Hovnanian (Fig. 37–7). Placement

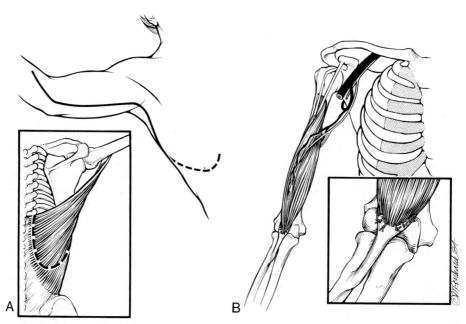

Figure 37–7. Unipolar transfer of the latissimus dorsi for elbow flexion. *A,* Incisions employed. *B,* The detached origin, rotated on its neurovascular pedicle, is attached to the biceps tendon and aponeurosis.

of the patient is the same as that used for the bipolar transfer. The incision begins in the loin, extends along the lateral margin of the latissimus to the posterior axillary fold, and continues across the axilla and downward along the medial arm to the elbow. The muscle is detached from its origin, preserving part of the aponeurosis with it, and freed up proximally. Branches from the thoracodorsal artery to the serratus anterior muscle are ligated. The muscle is then transferred to the anterior arm, where it is attached to the biceps tendon and periosteal tissues of the bicipital tuberosity. The arm is bandaged to the thorax for 3 to 4 weeks, at which time active and passive exercises are started.

Results

Hovnanian reported one patient who achieved satisfactory elbow flexion following a unipolar transfer. Zancolli and Mitre followed eight patients who had a bipolar transplantation of the latissimus dorsi for more than 4 years.[76] Active flexion ranging from 105 to 140 degrees was achieved, and flexion strength varied from 0.7 to 5 kg. Flexion contractures of the elbow of 10 degrees and 15 degrees occurred in two patients, and active supination from 20 to 50 degrees was achieved in six of the patients. Axer et al. reported one patient with a unipolar partial transfer of the latissimus dorsi who achieved 125 degrees of elbow flexion against gravity and moderate resistance.[2] Bostwick et al. reported one patient who had full flexion and could lift 60 kg 18 months after a unipolar transfer.[5] Stern et al. reported two patients who had a bipolar latissimus dorsi myocutaneous transposition to restore soft tissue coverage in the arm and elbow flexion at the same time.[67] One patient had 125 degrees of flexion and a 20-degree flexion contracture 4 months after surgery. The other patient achieved 140 degrees of flexion, lacked 15 degrees of extension, and could flex his elbow to 100 degrees holding an 8-pound weight 5 months later. Brones et al. also reported a good result (15 pounds of elbow flexion and return to work as a laborer 14 months postoperatively) in a patient who had a bipolar myocutaneous latissimus dorsi flap.[8] No complications were reported by any author.

Pectoralis Muscle Transfer

History

The first use of the pectoralis major muscle to restore elbow flexion was reported in the European literature in 1917 by Schulze-Berge, who transferred its tendon of insertion directly into the belly of the biceps.[58] Subsequent modifications of the method of insertion of the pectoralis major included the use of fascia lata or strands of silk to form tendons of insertion, either into the biceps tendon or directly into the ulna.[36, 42, 43, 55] Clark reported the first really successful physiologic transfer of the pectoralis major in 1946.[21] In his procedure, the sternocostal origin of the muscle with its separate nerve (medial pectoral) and blood supply was mobilized, passed subcutaneously down the upper arm, and attached to the biceps tendon. Seddon modified Clark's operation by elevating a segment of rectus abdominis sheath in continuity with the distal end of the transplant to act as a tendon.[59]

Brooks and Seddon described a unipolar transfer of the entire pectoralis major muscle, employing the devascularized long head of the biceps muscle as its tendon of insertion.[9] They recommended this operation instead of a Clark transfer in patients in whom either the lower part of the pectoralis major was paralyzed, the clavicular head being strong, or the whole muscle was weak.[60]

In 1955 Schottstaedt et al. first reported the bipolar transplantation of the chondrosternal portion (lower two thirds) of the pectoralis major on its neurovascular pedicle to restore elbow flexion.[56] The humeral insertion was detached and shifted to the coracoid process, and the origin was transplanted to the biceps tendon. Carroll and Kleinmann transplanted the entire pectoralis major muscle on both of its neurovascular pedicles.[19] The muscle origin with its attached anterior rectus abdominis sheath was attached to the biceps tendon, and its tendon of insertion was secured to the anterior aspect of the acromion. They reasoned that using the entire available muscle mass was more desirable than using only part of it, especially when the muscle is weaker than normal. With bipolar transplant of the entire muscle, they noted increased shoulder stability, negating the need for shoulder arthrodesis, and improved mechanical efficiency for elbow flexion compared with the unipolar transfer.

Tsai et al. added a unipolar transfer of the pectoralis minor muscle to a bipolar pectoralis major transplant, noting excellent strength of elbow flexion without endangering the two muscles' common neurovascular bundles.[70] The lateral half of the clavicular origin of the pectoralis major was left intact to preserve shoulder adduction.

Bradford first described the transfer of the

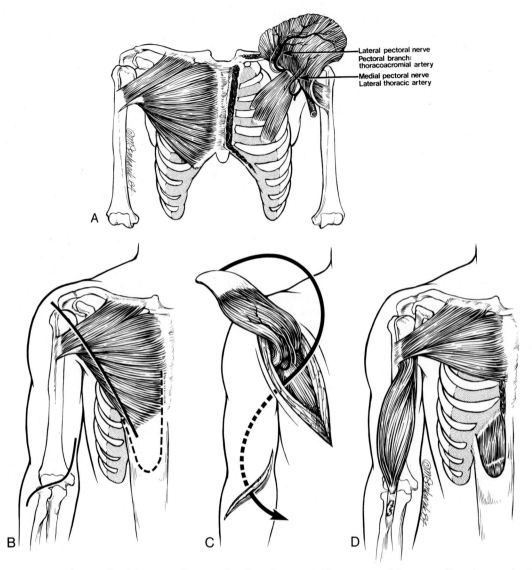

Figure 37–8. Unipolar transfer of the pectoralis major for elbow flexion. *A,* The anatomy of the pectoralis major muscle. The lateral pectoral nerve and pectoral branch of the thoracoacromial artery supply the clavicular portion and the upper part of the sternocostal portion of the muscle. The medial pectoral nerve and branches from the lateral thoracic artery supply the lower part of the sternocostal portion and the abdominal portion (when present) of the pectoralis major. *B,* Incisions employed in performing a unipolar transfer of the lower sternocostal portion of the pectoralis major (Clark's transfer). *C,* The lower third of the pectoralis major, detached with a 6-cm segment of anterior rectus abdominis sheath, is mobilized proximally on its neurovascular pedicle. *D,* The detached origin with the attached rectus abdominis sheath is passed through a subcutaneous tunnel and attached to the biceps tendon.

pectoralis minor to the paralyzed biceps to restore elbow flexion in 1910.[6] Spira reported one patient who had complete paralysis of the pectoralis major secondary to poliomyelitis who obtained excellent function following the transfer of the origin of the pectoralis minor into the distal biceps. [61]

Anatomy

Phylogenetically, the pectoralis major muscle evolved from three separate muscles, and it retains a segmental morphology with an independent neurovascular supply (Fig. 37–8A). The pectoralis major muscle has two constant (clavicular and sternocostal) and one inconstant (abdominal) subunits. The clavicular portion of the muscle originates from the medial third of the clavicle. The sternocostal portion arises from the anterior surface of the manubrium and the body of the sternum and cartilage of the first six ribs. The abdominal portion, when present, arises from the aponeurosis of the external oblique muscle and is found posterior to the axillary border of the sternocostal portion. A morphologically distinct abdominal subunit was found by Tobin et al. in 44 per cent of the 88 cadaver muscles they examined.[69] The lateral pectoral nerve, derived from the lateral cord and containing fibers from C5, C6, and C7, supplies the clavicular and upper portion of the sternocostal parts of the muscle. The medial pectoral nerve, derived from the medial cord and containing fibers from C8 and T1, innervates the lower sternocostal and abdominal parts of the pectoralis major after piercing the pectoralis minor or passing around its lateral edge as it also innervates this muscle. The clavicular and upper sternocostal portions of the pectoralis major are supplied by the pectoral branch of the thoracoacromial artery. The lower sternocostal portion (and the abdominal portion when present) receives its blood supply from the lateral thoracic artery.

Technique

Unipolar Transfer. This approach is based on that of Clark[21] and Holtmann et al.[37] (Fig. 37–8B-D). The patient is supine with a sandbag behind the shoulder. The arm is draped free and supported on a hand table or Mayo stand. An incision is made parallel to the lateral border of the pectoralis major muscle from the axilla to the seventh rib. The origin of the lower third of the muscle is detached from the sternum and fifth and sixth costal cartilages in continuity with a 6-cm segment of anterior rectus abdominis sheath. The sternocostal segment is freed from the rest of the pectoralis major muscle, taking care to protect its nerve (medial pectoral) and vascular (lateral thoracic branches) supply.

The biceps tendon is exposed through an oblique incision over the anterior aspect of the distal arm and elbow. A large forceps is then thrust upward from this distal incision to create a subcutaneous tunnel continuous with the upper end of the other incision. The muscle is then pulled through the tunnel, and its rectus sheath segment is woven through the biceps tendon with the elbow at 125 degrees flexion and the forearm fully supinated. With the shoulder in adduction and internally rotated, the elbow and forearm are immobilized in acute flexion and supination for 6 weeks. Isometric contractions are begun at 3 weeks, followed by active elbow flexion from an initial position of 90 degrees elbow flexion.

Partial Bipolar Transplantation of Pectoralis Major. This description follows that of Schottstaedt et al.[56] The muscle is exposed through an incision extending from 2.5 cm distal to the margin of the axilla along the lateral border of the pectoralis major muscle to within 5 cm of the midline. The lower half of the pectoralis major muscle is detached from its sternocostal origin and separated from the underlying pectoralis minor, taking care to protect its nerve (medial pectoral) and vascular supply (lateral thoracic arterial branches). As the muscle is freed from its origin, several large perforating vessels, which are not of any importance in preserving the viability of the muscle, are sectioned.

Through a separate 10-cm deltopectoral incision, the pectoralis major tendon of insertion is detached. The clavicular fibers of insertion should be detached from the freed tendon. At this point, the lower portion of the muscle is detached from the upper portion of the muscle in line with its fibers; it is now completely free on its neurovascular pedicle. The biceps tendon is exposed in the distal arm and antecubital space through an oblique 12-cm incision extending from proximal medial to distal lateral. A subcutaneous tunnel is created upward to the deltopectoral incision, and the sternocostal origin of the muscle is drawn through the tunnel so that it overlies the paralyzed biceps. The pectoralis muscle is then sewed to the biceps tendon and opened-up aponeurosis with heavy, nonabsorbable sutures. The distal wound is then closed, and the pectoralis major insertion is attached to the conjoined tendon at the coracoid by weaving it through several times. The muscle tension should be such that the muscle is under maximum tension with the elbow in approximately 125 degrees of flexion while the proximal suturing is performed. At this point, it can be noticed that the pedicle is made more lax by relieving some of the downward pull placed upon it initially when the muscle was sutured to the distal biceps. According to Schottstaedt et al., an extension of length using rectus abdominis sheath is usually unnecessary.

The postoperative position of immobilization and the exercise program are similar to those used with the unipolar transfer.

Complete Bipolar Transplantation of Pectoralis Major. This procedure is based on that of Carroll and Kleinman[19] (Fig. 37–9). The patient is placed in the supine position with a flat bolster under the blade of the scapula and the upper extremity draped free. A long, curvilinear incision is made from the seventh sternocostal joint proximally to two fingerbreadths inferior to the clavicle. The incision

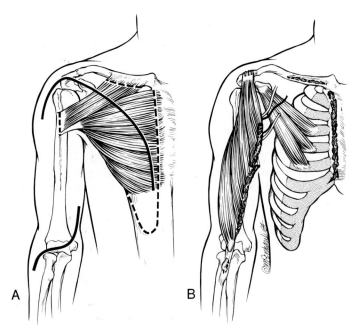

Figure 37–9. Bipolar transplantation of the pectoralis major muscle for elbow flexion. *A,* Incisions employed. Solid lines indicate skin incisions and dotted lines indicate the extent of detachment of the pectoralis major and rectus abdominis sheath. *B,* The completely detached pectoralis major is rotated on its two neurovascular pedicles. Its origin is attached to the biceps tendon, and its insertion is attached to the acromion through drill holes.

continues laterally to the coracoid process, then distally along the anteromedial aspect of the arm to the level of the axilla.

With the acromion and the entire pectoralis major muscle exposed, a second curvilinear incision is made over the antecubital fossa with its transverse limb across the fossa and the longitudinal limb extending medially and distally 6 cm. The entire pectoralis major muscle is then detached from its origin along the medial half of the clavicle and its sternocostal border with a 10- by 4-cm strip of attached rectus abdominis fascia. In the process of freeing the pectoralis major from the chest wall and the underlying pectoralis minor, meticulous care is given to preservation of its two neurovascular pedicles. The entire muscle mass is then rotated 90 degrees on its two neurovascular pedicles. The clavicular and sternocostal origins with the attached rectus sheath are rolled into a tube and directed through the subcutaneous tunnel, exiting through the second incision. With the elbow flexed 135 degrees, the fascial tube is enclosed under maximal tension to the biceps tendon with nonabsorbable sutures, including a transcutaneous stay suture tied over a bolster. The tendon of insertion is then detached, directed proximally, and anchored securely to the anterior acromion by nonabsorbable sutures through drill holes.

The elbow is immobilized for 6 weeks with the joint flexed 135 degrees using a collar and cuff with a swathe before exercises are commenced.

Results

Clark's original report included one patient who had flexion limited by only 15 degrees, extension limited by 5 degrees, and flexion power 40 per cent of normal 16 weeks after a partial bipolar transfer of the pectoralis major.[21] Seddon noted excellent results (powerful flexion against gravity and resistance) in 7 of 16 Clark transfer patients he reported.[59] In the remainder, the elbow could be flexed against gravity and slight resistance. Seven patients regained supination against resistance (from 10 to 90 degrees). In four cases in which the pectoralis major power was subnormal, the pectoralis minor was used in addition. D'Aubigne reported excellent active flexion, independent of shoulder adduction, in two patients who had a Clark transfer.[24] Using the unipolar transfer of the pectoralis major into the devascularized long head of the biceps, Brooks and Seddon achieved three excellent, three good, and two fair results (active flexion less than passive or flexion against gravity but not resistance), and two complete failures.[9] Two of the good results, however, required a second operation (triceps to biceps) because of simultaneous action of the pectoralis major and the triceps, a phenomenon they ascribed to axonal confusion during regeneration after brachial plexus lesions.

Segal, Seddon, and Brooks, using a combined objective and subjective evaluation, compared the results of 13 flexorplasties, 3 triceps transfers, 17 Clark transfers, and 8 Brooks-Seddon transfers.[60] Fifty-three per cent of the Clark transfers and 75 per cent of the Brooks-Seddon transfers were either fair or failed, whereas only 31 per cent of the flexorplasties had a fair result and there were no failures. The decreased flexion contracture of the elbow, simultaneous contraction of the triceps when the pectoralis transfer flexed the elbow, and undesirable shoulder adduction and internal rotation movements accompanying elbow flexion all contributed to less satisfactory results in the pectoralis transfer group. These authors, as well as Clark himself, advised against using the pectoralis transfer if some biceps activity was present or could be anticipated.[22] Holtmann et al. noted useful active elbow flexion through a mean range of 96 degrees, accompanied by supination of the forearm, in all seven Clark transfers they reported.[37] Four of the patients had arthrogryposis, and in all cases the transfer was extended with a 6-cm-long segment of anterior rectus sheath.

Discussing the use of Clark's pectoralis major transfer in the arthrogrypotic child, Lloyd-Roberts and Lettin observed that a preliminary posterior release and triceps lengthening may be necessary to secure passive flexion.[45] They modified Clark's transfer by obtaining a longer anterior rectus abdominis sheath and inserting the transfer into the ulna because the biceps tendon is frequently absent. All seven patients who had the modified transfer could get their hands to their mouth against gravity and some resistance, although two patients required secondary repair with fascia lata when the bony attachment pulled loose.

The first reports of a bipolar pectoralis major transplantation were by Schottstaedt et al., who noted active elbow flexion in all seven cases, although two of the operations had to be revised in order to tighten the transfer.[56] Doyle et al. reported seven cases of arthrogryposis in which a bipolar transfer of the entire sternal head of the pectoralis major with a generous tongue of anterior rectus abdominis sheath was performed.[26] All seven cases achieved improved elbow motion, and six achieved single-hand feeding. Three of the four patients reported by Carroll and Kleinman who had a bipolar transfer of the entire pectoralis major muscle achieved an excellent result.[19] Because of the increased shoulder stability achieved with this operation, shoulder arthrodesis was not required. Tsai et al. employed a modified bipolar transplantation of the pectoralis major (leaving the lateral half of the clavicular origin intact), supplemented with a unipolar transfer of the pectoralis minor, in four patients.[70] Three of the four achieved excellent results (full extension with at least 60 degrees of flexion), and the other patient required a secondary Steindler flexorplasty.

Spira achieved strong flexion through a range of 135 degrees with virtually full extension in a patient with total paralysis of the pectoralis major and elbow flexors secondary to poliomyelitis in whom he transferred the pectoralis minor origin to the biceps tendon.[61]

Complications

Doyle et al. reported two patients who developed transient nerve palsies, one median and one radial, following pectoralis major transfer.[26] Both resolved completely after several weeks. Simultaneous contraction of the triceps when the elbow is flexed by the transfixed pectoralis major was noted in three cases by Segal et al.[60] All three had brachial plexus injuries and initially had had paralysis of the triceps and elbow flexors. Axon confusion following regeneration seems to be the likely explanation, but the complication cannot be predicted because in six other cases in which the triceps was paralyzed initially and recovered later, no simultaneous flexor-extensor action developed.

Triceps Transfer

History

Transfer of the triceps muscle to restore elbow flexion was mentioned by Steindler in 1939 only to condemn it because "loss of the normal function of the triceps is too great a sacrifice."[65] Bunnell described the pull-out wire technique for inserting the triceps tendon, which had been elongated with a 1½-inch graft of fascia lata, into the tuberosity of the radius, and stated that he had used the method with success.[11] In his opinion, "it is more important to flex than to extend the elbow, and the loss of the triceps as an extensor robs the patient only of the ability to push the arm up or away from the body."[12] In 1952, Carroll described the technical details of triceps transfer,[14] and in 1970 Carroll and Hill reported the results in 15 patients.[18] They advised against performing triceps transfer bilaterally or in the patient who used crutches.

Anatomy

The triceps muscle arises by three heads—one from the scapula (long head) and two from the posterior humerus (lateral and medial heads). The medial head has an extensive origin from the posterior shaft of the humerus, extending from the insertion of the teres major to within 2.5 cm of the trochlea of the humerus. The muscle is supplied by the radial nerve (C7 and C8, with a smaller contribution from C6) through branches that all arise above the spiral groove, except the posterior branch to the medial head, which leaves the radial nerve just as it enters the groove.[7]

Technique

This description is based on that of Carroll (Fig. 37–10). The patient is placed on his side with the affected extremity draped free. A posterior midline incision is made, extending over the distal two thirds of the arm and then curving lateral to the olecranon and extending distally over the subcutaneous border of the ulna for 5 cm. The skin flaps are widely undermined so that the ulnar nerve can be exposed medially and the lateral intermuscular septum laterally. As long a tail of periosteum as possible is raised from the ulna in continuity with the triceps insertion, and the medial head is mobilized from the distal third of the shaft of the humerus. The radial motor nerves enter the muscle in the interval between the lateral and medial heads as the radial nerve enters the spiral groove. The raw surface of the stripped medial head is then covered by suturing its two edges together into a tube.

The biceps tendon is then exposed through a curvilinear incision in the antecubital fossa, and the tendon is dissected free to its insertion onto the radius. The biceps tendon is split longitudinally. The triceps tendon is

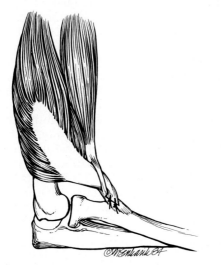

Figure 37–10. Transfer of triceps insertion around the lateral side of the elbow to the biceps tendon.

passed through a laterally placed subcutaneous tunnel between the two incisions, superficial to the radial nerve. The triceps tendon is then passed through the split biceps tendon and sutured in place under maximum tension with the elbow at 90 degrees of flexion and the forearm in full supination. As an alternative method, the triceps tendon can be attached to the radial tuberosity using a pullout wire technique as described by Bunnell.[12] The elbow is immobilized in a posterior splint at 90 degrees of flexion and full supination for 4 weeks, at which time active exercises are begun.

Results

Carroll and Hill recorded the results of 15 triceps transfers.[18] Five successes (flexion against gravity with ability to bring the hand to the mouth), one limited result, and one failure were noted in the seven post-traumatic and paralytic patients. In the eight patients with arthrogryposis, there were five successes, one limited result, and two failures. The average range of motion was 116 degrees, with an average flexion contracture of 24 degrees in the first group, but motion averaged only 43 degrees with an average fixed flexion deformity of 59 degrees in the arthrogrypotic group. Seven of the eight arthrogrypotic patients required adjunctive procedures such as excision of a dislocated radial head or a modified elbow arthroplasty to achieve an acceptable passive range of motion prior to triceps transfer. Williams reported improvement in all 19 arthrogrypotic elbows submitted to triceps transfer, and he did not hesitate to perform the procedure bilaterally.[73] A successful case achieved elbow flexion against gravity and resistance; however, in his series, extension was usually restricted to approximately a right angle because of the tenodesis effect of the triceps. Four of seven arthrogrypotic patients reported by Doyle et al. achieved improved motion and single-hand feeding ability following triceps transfer.[26] Other authors have noted little or no improvement following triceps transfer in the arthrogrypotic patient.[33, 48]

No complications were reported by any of the authors.

Miscellaneous Transfers for Elbow Flexion

Sternocleidomastoid Transfer

In 1951 Bunnell reported a single patient with a paralyzed upper extremity secondary to poliomyelitis in whom elbow flexion was obtained by transferring the insertion of the sternocleidomastoid muscle, prolonged with a strip of fascia lata, into the bicipital tuberosity.[12] The patient could flex his elbow freely and with moderate strength. Carroll reported 80 per cent satisfactory results in 15 cases of almost total paralysis of the entire upper extremity.[17] The sternocleidomastoid was extended with a tube of fascia lata to restore elbow flexion.

Flexor Carpi Ulnaris Transfer

In 1975 Ahmad published a single case report of a patient with a brachial plexus palsy who achieved 130 degrees of elbow flexion following the transfer of the insertion of the flexor carpi ulnaris, turned back on itself, into the distal humerus.[1] No subsequent reports of this transfer have appeared in the literature.

Free Muscle Transplants

Gilbert reported an excellent result in a 5-year-old child who had a free transplantation of the gracilis, using the musculocutaneous nerve as the recipient nerve, after a traumatic destruction of the biceps muscle.[31] Five other patients (two with poliomyelitis and three with brachial plexus palsies), however, achieved no useful flexion following a gracilis transplantation that was innervated through a long nerve graft connected to the sternocleidomastoid nerve. O'Brien et al. also recorded a failure in one patient 8 years after a free gracilis transplantation that was innervated by the second and third intercostal nerves.

RESTORATION OF ELBOW EXTENSION

Latissimus Dorsi Transfer or Transplant

History

Hohmann,[36] Lange,[42] and Harmon[34] each proposed the unipolar transfer of the latissimus dorsi insertion into the extensor mechanism at the back of the arm to restore elbow extension. Harmon also added the teres major to the latissimus dorsi transfer in the single case report he published. Hovnanian devised a unipolar transfer of the latissimus dorsi in which its origin was transferred to the triceps tendon.[38] A myocutaneous unipolar transfer of the latissimus dorsi was reported by Landra to provide skin cover and elbow extension at the same time.[41] Tobin et al. performed a similar procedure but used only the lateral

segment of the latissimus dorsi with an attached island of skin.[68]

Bipolar transplantation of the latissimus dorsi was first reported by Schottstaedt et al. in 1955.[56] The origin was sutured to the triceps tendon, and the insertion was moved to the acromion. DuToit and Levy emphasized the necessity for discarding the distal 3 inches of the latissimus dorsi to get the transplant tight enough.[27]

Technique

Unipolar Transfer. This description is based on that of Hovnanian (Fig. 37–11). The patient is placed on his side with the arm completely draped free. The technique of exposing, detaching, and mobilizing the latissimus dorsi on its neurovascular pedicle is the same as that described above for flexor replacement. The incision on the arm, however, is carried over from the posterior axillary fold onto the posteromedial aspect of the arm without

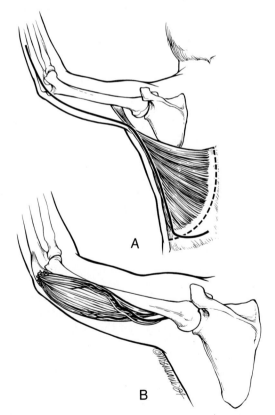

Figure 37–11. Unipolar transfer of the latissimus dorsi for elbow extension. *A,* Incisions employed. The solid line indicates skin incisions, and the dotted line indicates the muscle incision. *B,* The insertion is undisturbed, and the muscle is rotated on its long neurovascular pedicle. Its origin (after appropriate shortening) is attached to the triceps tendon and olecranon periosteum under maximum tension with the elbow fully extended.

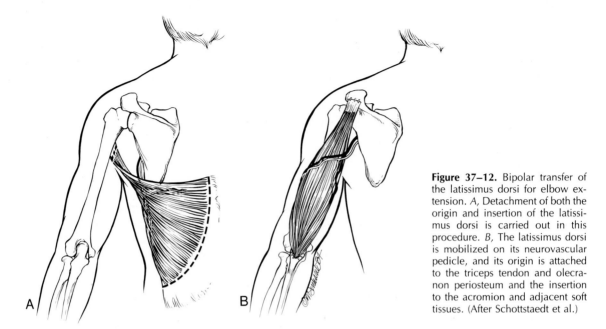

Figure 37–12. Bipolar transfer of the latissimus dorsi for elbow extension. *A,* Detachment of both the origin and insertion of the latissimus dorsi is carried out in this procedure. *B,* The latissimus dorsi is mobilized on its neurovascular pedicle, and its origin is attached to the triceps tendon and olecranon periosteum and the insertion to the acromion and adjacent soft tissues. (After Schottstaedt et al.)

crossing the neurovascular bundle. Distally, the incision is carried over the medial epicondyle onto the posterior aspect of the proximal ulna. The aponeurotic fascia at the free end of the latissimus dorsi muscle is then sutured under tension to the triceps tendon, the periosteum over the olecranon, and the connective tissue and muscle septa on the extensor surface of the forearm, keeping the elbow in full extension. Considerable muscle usually has to be excised in order to make the transfer maximally tight.

The elbow is immobilized in extension and bandaged to the side of the body. Passive and active elbow movements are begun after 3 to 4 weeks.

Bipolar Transplantation. This description is based on the technique of Schottstaedt et al. (Fig. 37–12). The latissimus dorsi muscle is exposed, freed, and completely detached on its neurovascular pedicle through an incision extending from the posterior axillary fold along the muscle's lateral margin to within 5 to 7.5 cm of the iliac crest. The lower triceps and olecranon is exposed through a posterior incision. A subcutaneous tunnel is then created between this incision and the dorsolateral incision and the origin of the latissimus dorsi is drawn through it. This portion of the muscle is then attached to the triceps tendon and adjacent soft tissue around the olecranon. The acromion is exposed through a 5-cm transverse incision over its posterior edge. The insertion of the latissimus dorsi is then drawn up over the deltoid and sutured securely through drill holes to the acromion and the adjacent soft tissues under maximum

tension with the elbow fully extended. The elbow is maintained in full extension for 3 to 4 weeks before flexion is allowed.

Results

Hovnanian reported satisfactory results in two patients who had a unipolar latissimus transfer.[38] Schottstaedt et al. achieved full extension of the elbow against gravity after a bipolar transplantation of the latissimus dorsi in a 5-year-old child with poliomyelitis.[56] DuToit and Levy reported a 44-year-old man who was able to do push-ups after a bipolar transplantation of the latissimus dorsi.[27] They noted that the distal 3 inches of muscle had to be discarded to secure the proper tension in the transplant, and they made the proximal acromial attachment before the distal attachment. Tobin et al. used a unipolar transfer of the lateral portion of the latissimus dorsi with a large island of attached skin to restore extension and cover a large ulcer involving the elbow joint in a 58-year-old man with syringomyelia.[68] Active elbow extension was achieved. The wound was covered, and latissimus dorsi muscle function in the donor site was said to be preserved by the innervated medial muscle branch retained in situ.

No complications were reported by any author.

Posterior Deltoid Transfer

History

In 1949, d'Aubigne mentioned transferring the posterior part of the deltoid into the triceps as a good method of restoring active extension of the elbow.[24] The technique, however, was not described, and no cases were reported. In 1975 Moberg described mobilizing the separately innervated posterior part of the deltoid, extending it with multiple toe extensor tendon grafts inserted into the triceps aponeurosis, to restore elbow extension in 16 tetraplegic patients.[49] Converting the transferred deltoid from a one-joint to a two-joint muscle achieved elbow extension without any detectable shoulder dysfunction. Following Moberg's initial communication, there have been five subsequent reports by other authors, all dealing with tetraplegic patients in which posterior deltoid transfer with several modifications has been successfully used to achieve elbow extension. Bryan performed bilateral posterior deltoid transfers at the same sitting and inserted the tendon grafts through drill holes in the olecranon.[10] Hentz et al. used fascia rather than tendon grafts to extend the transfer to the olecranon.[35] They also employed a polycentric adjustable splint postoperatively, which blocks flexion at any chosen angle. Castro-Sierra and Lopez-Pita used two opposing periosteal flaps, one from the deltoid insertion and one turned backward from the triceps insertion into the olecranon, to join the deltoid and triceps.[20]

Anatomy

The deltoid muscle is supplied by two terminal branches of the circumflex nerve, which divides approximately 6 cm below the level of the acromion. The posterior branch is short and runs almost horizontally to supply the portion of the deltoid arising from the spine of the scapula. The anterior branch is longer and runs horizontally to supply the acromial and clavicular portions of the deltoid.[7]

Technique

This procedure is based on that of Moberg (Fig. 37-13). Through a slightly curved incision along the posterior border of the deltoid, the posterior half of the muscle is exposed to its insertion. There is usually a natural cleavage between the two parts of the deltoid where the separation can be accomplished mostly by blunt dissection. Because the deltoid muscle lacks a large tendon of insertion, both the tendon of insertion and the surrounding periosteum, as well as a rectangular strip of fascia from the adjacent brachialis muscle, should be maintained attached to the deltoid muscle. The posterior deltoid is mobilized proximally until 3 cm of amplitude (the amplitude necessary for elbow extension) are obtained, tak-

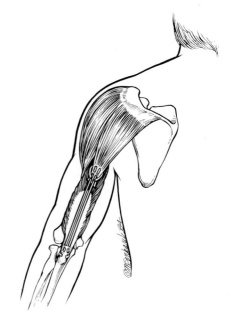

Figure 37–13. Transplantation of the posterior third of the deltoid, extended with toe extensor grafts, to the triceps tendon. This transfer is used to retore extension in the tetraplegic patient.

ing care to avoid injury to the axillary nerve branches. Careful hemostasis is important.

The triceps aponeurosis is exposed through separate, slightly curved, longitudinal incisions proximal to the olecranon. The conjoined extensor tendons to the second, third, and fourth toes (functionless in the tetraplegic patient) are removed with the aid of a Brand tendon stripper. Attaching the graft to the deltoid muscle is accomplished by looping the end of the graft through the deltoid tendon and adjacent fascia and periosteum at least twice and suturing the graft to the adjacent structures. The graft is then passed distally through a subcutaneous tunnel created between the two incisions. The tendon graft is then looped twice through and sutured to the triceps aponeurosis, passed again subcutaneously in a proximal direction, and again attached to the deltoid muscle. Suturing of the graft should be done with the elbow extended fully and the shoulder abducted 30 degrees. The posterior deltoid muscle is infiltrated with 20 ml of 1 per cent Xylocaine with epinephrine 1:200,000 to prevent a disruption of the anastomosis during recovery from anesthesia.

Aftercare

A long arm cast, applied from the upper humerus to just proximal to the wrist with the elbow in 10 degrees of flexion, is worn for 6 weeks. At that time, the patient begins active extension exercises; however, in order to prevent stretching of the newly transferred muscle tendon unit, elbow flexion is restricted to increments of only 10 degrees per week. A polycentric adjustable elbow splint that allows full extension but blocks flexion at whatever position desired is very useful.[35] During the rehabilitation period, elbow extension power must be closely monitored. If a decrease in extension power occurs temporarily, reimmobilization in the extended position is carried out until active full extension is regained. Bryan believes that late stretching is due to stretching in the central portion of the grafts during their revascularization and advised protection from flexion past 90 degrees for 3 months after surgery.[10]

Results

Moberg's cumulative experience with the posterior deltoid transfer includes 38 procedures,[50] and he reports only one failure in the entire group. In general, elbow extension power was noted to be several times stronger with the extremity at the side in the position for lifting the body than with the limb extended over the head. Bryan reported satisfactory results in 10 of 14 deltoid transfers performed in seven tetraplegic patients.[10] In all but one of the patients, bilateral deltoid to triceps transfers were performed at the same operation. De Benediti evaluated 13 tetraplegic patients with 14 deltoid to triceps transfers.[25] Using a 0 to 5 muscle grading system, he noted a postoperative average of 3.6 compared with a preoperative average of 0.5. Castro-Sierra and Lopez-Pita noted satisfactory results in 13 tetraplegic patients using Moberg's technique, but were able to shorten the postoperative immobilization period to 35 days and to obtain satisfactory results with ten transfers in seven patients using a new technique of anastomosis.[20] A proximally based flap of triceps tendon with an attached flap of olecranon periosteum is turned back on itself and sutured to the deltoid insertion with its attached flap of periosteum. Lamb and Chan reported satisfactory results after 16 Moberg transfers in 10 tetraplegic patients.[40] Hentz et al. used a tubed fascia lata strip inserted through drill holes in the olecranon and allowed up to 30 degrees of immediate flexion postoperatively.[35] Splinting was continued for only 4½ weeks, but no follow-up was given for this modified procedure.

Complications

Stretching out and disruption of the proximal or distal anastomosis may result and require reoperation. Spasticity of the elbow flexors may prejudice the result.

Miscellaneous Transfers for Elbow Extension

Brachioradialis Transfer

In 1938, Ober and Barr described the posterior transfer of the freed anterior margin of the brachioradialis into the proximal ulna, olecranon, and triceps tendon to restore active elbow extension. Addition of the extensor carpi radialis to strengthen the brachioradialis was advised if its power was insufficient. Immobilization of the elbow in full extension and supination was advised, and exercises were started at 10 days. Six cases were operated on, and in each case extension of the elbow against gravity was possible. No subsequent reports of the procedure have appeared in the literature.

Biceps to Triceps Transfer

Friedenberg, in 1954, reported a patient with poliomyelitis who had difficulty arising from a chair and walking with crutches because of bilateral absent triceps function.[30] Lateral subcutaneous transfer of the biceps tendon into the triceps aponeurosis was performed on both elbows 8 months apart. Following surgery, the patient was able to support 7.5 pounds in extension on the right and 8.5 pounds on the left and was able to transfer independently and to use crutches without difficulty. He reported another patient, a tetraplegic, who also underwent bilateral biceps to triceps transfer but did not become independent. Hentz et al.[35] and Lamb and Chan[40] both recorded tetraplegic patients in whom biceps to triceps transfer had failed to achieve the desired result.

TRANSFERS FOR RESTORATION OF FOREARM ROTATION

Transfers for Pronation

History

Paralytic supination deformity of the forearm, most commonly the result of obstetric palsy, is secondary to a partial or complete paralysis of the flexor-pronator muscles in the presence of unopposed biceps and supinator muscles. The deformity is not only cosmetically displeasing but seriously limits the function of the hand for grasping and two-handed activities. Nondynamic correction of the supination deformity by closed osteoclasis[4] or open osteotomy of the forearm bones[13, 77] was advised by earlier authors.

Schottstaedt et al. suggested changing the biceps from a supinator to a pronator by transferring its tendon to the side of the radial tuberosity opposite its normal insertion but did not report their results.[57] Zancolli modified the technique by performing a long Z-lengthening of the tendon, rerouting the distal strip of the tendon around the neck of the radius.[74] All 14 of his patients also required a release of the contracted soft tissues, particularly the interosseous membrane, in order to obtain passive correction of the supination deformity prior to the biceps rerouting. Manske et al. believed that soft tissue releases could be avoided by performing the biceps rerouting earlier; if correction was not satisfactory, a secondary percutaneous osteoclasis of the radius and ulna was recommended.[46]

Technique

This description is based on those of Zancolli[74] and Manske et al.[46] (Fig. 37–14). A high tourniquet is employed, and the biceps tendon is exposed through an incision starting on the medial aspect of the distal arm, extending across the flexion crease of the elbow and distally on the lateral aspect of the forearm. The lacertus fibrosus is incised, and the median nerve and brachial artery are retracted medially. The biceps tendon is exposed to its insertion into the bicipital tuberosity, and the

radial recurrent leash of vessels is divided. The tendon is divided by a long Z-plasty to its insertion, and the distal segment is passed posteriorly around the radial neck at the level of the tuberosity using a ligature carrier. The tendons are reattached by side-to-side suture, effectively lengthening the tendon by about 1.5 cm. A long arm cast is applied with the forearm in the neutral position and the elbow at a right angle for 4 to 6 weeks. If the deformity is longstanding and the patient is older, soft tissue releases are often required to obtain passive forearm rotation. The interosseous membrane and supinator muscle can be released through a long dorsal incision overlying the ulna. The extensor muscles are retracted radialward, and this protects the interosseous nerve. Owings et al. suggested releasing the supinator from the volar lateral surfaces of the radius through the anterior incision.[54]

Results

Zancolli performed soft tissue releases and biceps tendon rerouting in 14 patients with paralytic supination contracture of the forearm (four poliomyelitis, eight birth palsies, and two tetraplegia).[74] Correction to the neutral position or some pronation was maintained in all patients, and eight had 10 to 60 degrees of active pronation. Owings et al. reported 9 good, 11 satisfactory, and 2 poor results in 26 patients who had biceps tendon

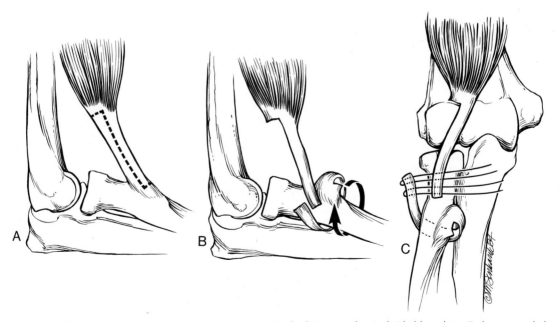

Figure 37–14. Biceps tendon rerouting to restore pronation. *A,* The biceps tendon is divided by a long Z-plasty extended to its insertion. *B, C,* The distal end of the divided tendon is passed around the neck of the radius using a ligature passer. The two layers of the tendon are reattached side to side, effectively lengthening the tendon by about 1.5 cm. (After Zancolli.)

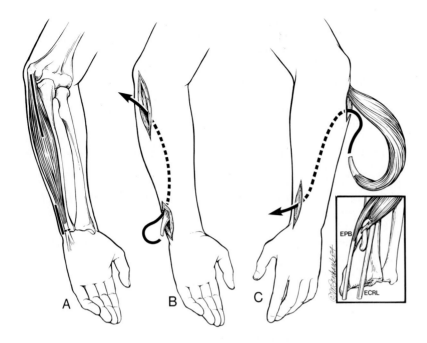

Figure 37–15. Transfer of flexor carpi ulnaris to restore supination. *A,* The flexor carpi ulnaris tendon is detached distally, mobilized proximally, and brought out through the proximal incision. *B, C,* The dorsoradial aspect of the distal radius is exposed. The flexor carpi ulnaris is redirected through a subcutaneous tunnel and attached to the radius through a drill hole. (After Steindler.)

rerouting using the Z-plasty technique.[54] The two poor results were related to problems with stability of the proximal radius. Manske et al. reported the results of Zancolli's biceps tendon rerouting in 11 patients with supination deformity secondary to obstetric paralysis.[46] The neutral position was obtained in nine of the patients, and six of the patients had active supination-pronation movement averaging 42 degrees (15 to 65 degrees). Two patients, neither of whom had preoperative passive pronation to neutral, obtained satisfactory results after a secondary percutaneous osteoclasis of the radius and ulna. These authors recommended that surgical correction of paralytic supination deformity of the forearm be done between 3 and 6 years of age.

Complications

Zancolli reported two patients who had overcorrection, presumably because the biceps tendon suture was under excessive tension.[74] Owings et al. reported one patient who had persistent weakness of thumb extension, two patients with proximal radial instability, and one patient who developed excessive pronation.[54]

Transfers for Supination

History

Because it is infrequently indicated, muscle transfer to regain supination in the paralyzed upper extremity has received scant attention

in the literature. Steindler described transferring the flexor carpi ulnaris tendon into the dorsal aspect of the distal radius.[65] Tubby described transferring the flexor carpi radialis and pronator teres through the interosseous space to the back of the radius to achieve supination in the spastic upper extremity.[71] Schottstaedt et al. noted that providing active supination, using the flexor carpi ulnaris or palmaris longus redirected dorsally into the radial shaft, was often necessary after Steindler flexorplasty.[57]

Technique of Transferring Flexor Carpi Ulnaris to Radius

This technique is based on that of Steindler[65] (Fig. 37–15). The flexor carpi ulnaris tendon is detached, and its distal half is mobilized through a 12-cm incision along the volar-ulnar aspect of the forearm. The dorsolateral surface of the distal radius is exposed between the extensor pollicis brevis and the extensor carpi radialis longus tendons using a 5-cm longitudinal incision. A subcutaneous tunnel is created between this incision and the proximal end of the first incision, and the flexor carpi ulnaris tendon is pulled through. A hole is drilled through the distal radius and the tendon is fed through the hole from dorsal to volar. Its end is reflected back and sutured to itself under tension with the forearm supinated and the elbow flexed. A long arm cast with the wrist slightly dorsiflexed, the forearm in full supination, and the elbow at a right angle is worn for 3 weeks. Part-time splinting is continued for 2 months.

Results

Steindler reported 11 good and 5 poor results in 16 flexor carpi ulnaris transfers to the radius.[66] A good transfer functioned actively through a useful arc with at least 40 degrees of pronation-supination movement.

CHOOSING A TRANSFER: AUTHOR'S PREFERRED METHOD

A Steindler flexorplasty, the transfer that has been around the longest, is relatively simple to perform and works well, even when the wrist flexor muscle strength is not normal. The large number of satisfactory cases that have been published attests to its dependability. Using Mayer and Green's simple clinical test, it is easy to predict which patient is a candidate for the procedure.[47] Post-traumatic brachial plexus palsy is now the most common cause of loss of elbow flexion power, and flexorplasty works well in restoring function, especially in the irreparable C5–C6 lesion (Fig. 37–16). I have also been pleasantly surprised to see functional elbow flexion re-

stored in some patients with C5, C6, and C7 involvement. The transfer functions best if there is some triceps function present, although the absence of active elbow extension does not preclude its use. If triceps function is absent, the use of a dynamic extension elbow splint helps to prevent excessive fixed flexion contracture (Fig. 37–3). Late recovery of some motor function in the biceps is not affected by a flexorplasty, unlike other transfers that tie into the biceps.

Steindler flexorplasty does have some drawbacks. It is not as strong as some of the other transfers (latissimus dorsi and pectoralis major), and active supination is not achieved with the procedure. The development of a pronation deformity after flexorplasty was a problem with the original proximal medial shift of the flexor pronator origin. Pronation deformity has not been as great a problem with the more anterolateral insertion currently employed. Fascial extension to permit a more lateral shift of the origin is usually unnecessary.

Bipolar transplantation of the latissimus dorsi to restore either elbow flexion or extension is an excellent procedure. Its long single neurovascular pedicle allows greater mobility

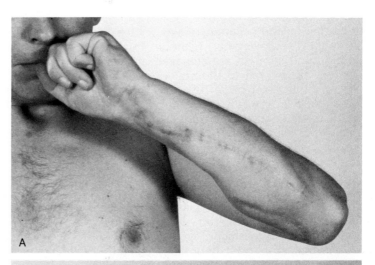

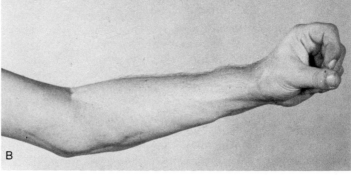

Figure 37–16. *A,* This 21-year-old man sustained a brachial plexus injury in a motorcycle accident. A Steindler flexorplasty performed 16 months after injury restored excellent elbow flexion. Subsequent transfer of the flexor carpi ulnaris into the extensor carpi radialis brevis restored wrist extension, and finger and thumb extension was restored using the superficialis muscle of the middle and ring fingers. A shoulder arthrodesis was also performed. *B,* Fixed flexion deformity of 35 degrees was present after the Steindler flexorplasty.

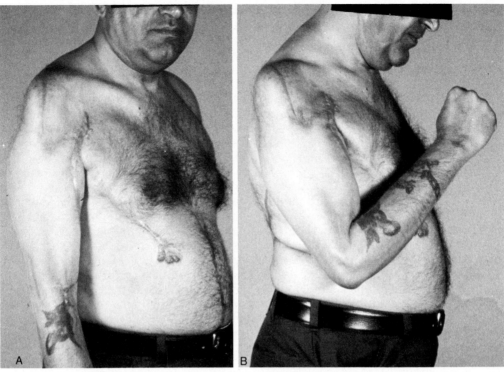

Figure 37–17. *A, B,* This 36-year-old man who had C5–6 paralysis following a closed brachial plexus injury underwent a bipolar transfer of the latissimus dorsi 3 years after injury. Good elbow flexion was restored *(A)*, and nearly full extension of the elbow was maintained *(B)*. A shoulder arthrodesis was also performed.

than that for the pectoralis major, which has a double neurovascular pedicle. Excellent motion and strength are achieved and good contour is restored to the arm (Fig. 37–17). Preoperative evaluation of the latissimus dorsi muscle strength is often difficult. Its main innervation comes from C7 (with contributions from C6 and C8), so it is a useful transplant for restoring flexion in the irreparable C5–C6 brachial plexus lesion. It is a more formidable procedure than the Steindler flexorplasty, and hematoma formation and delayed wound healing sometimes occur following the large posterior dissection. It is more technically demanding, and achieving proper tension is most important. Enough of the muscle toward the origin must be excised so that the transplant will be under maximum tension with the elbow flexed to 120 degrees. It seems that it is almost impossible to get it too tight. Shoulder stabilization by arthrodesis significantly improves the function of both the flexor-pronator and latissimus dorsi transfers for elbow function.

Bipolar transplantation of part or all of the pectoralis major muscle is becoming a popular method of restoring elbow flexion. Brooks and Seddons' unipolar transfer of the pecto-

ralis major into the devascularized long head of the biceps muscle should no longer be performed because there are better and more predictable ways to transfer the muscle. The results reported for Clark's unipolar transfer of the inferior sternocostal portion of the pectoralis major have been quite good except for the occasional patient who develops simultaneous contraction of the transfer and the triceps when elbow flexion is attempted. This is presumably due to axonal confusion during regeneration and cannot be predicted preoperatively.

The lower (C8–T1) segmental innervation of the inferior pectoralis major makes it available for transfer in brachial plexus palsies extending to and involving C7. My experience with the pectoralis major transfers is limited; however, I would favor a bipolar transfer of the pectoralis on both of its neurovascular pedicles (as described by Carroll and Kleinman) over the bipolar transplantation of only a portion of the muscle. The superior vascular pedicle (pectoral branch of the thoracoacromial artery) is much larger and more dominant than the inferior pedicle (branch of lateral thoracic artery). If one is careful in the dissection, the muscle can be adequately mobi-

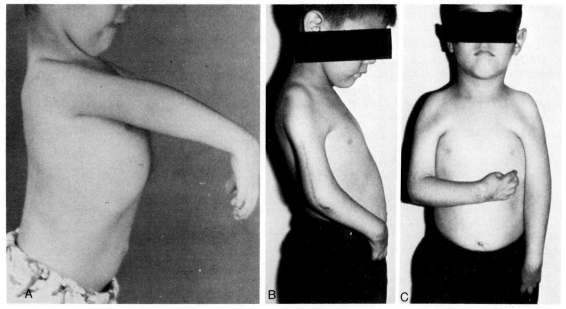

Figure 37–18. *A,* This 5-year-old boy with arthrogryposis multiplex congenita underwent triceps transfer on the right. *B,* Six months after surgery he was able to flex the elbow to 95 degrees, and gravity extension was possible to 50 degrees. *C,* The opposite elbow was left in extension.

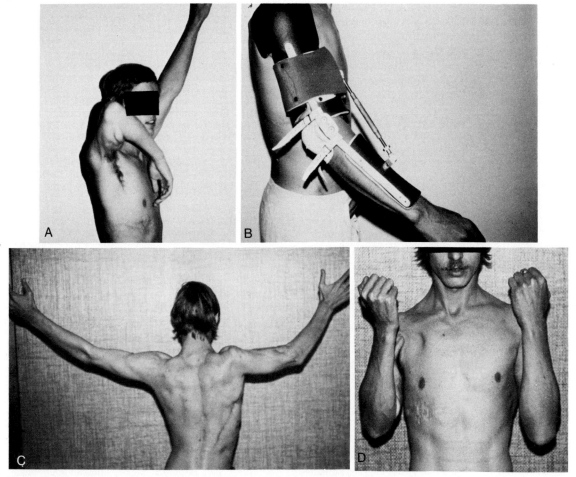

Figure 37–19. *A,* This 19-year-old airman sustained a severe posterior compartment soft tissue injury and an open comminuted fracture of the humerus in a half-track accident. There was complex loss of elbow extension. *(B),* The humeral fracture united after two bone grafting procedures, and passive extension of the elbow was obtained with a turnbuckle splint. *C,* Bipolar transplantation of the latissimus dorsi restored satisfactory elbow extension, and full flexion of the elbow was maintained *(D).*

613

lized and transplanted without undue tension or kinking of the pedicles. The bipolar transplantation, according to its proponents, may preclude the need for a shoulder fusion.

Triceps to biceps transfer is rarely indicated because the loss of active elbow extension is usually too great a price to pay for elbow flexion. Almost always, other procedures are available that allow preservation of elbow extension. I have only used the transfer with the arthrogrypotic elbow and have been pleased with the hand-to-mouth function that is restored (Fig. 37–18). In my opinion, bilateral elbow transfers to regain flexion should not be performed in the child with arthrogryposis.

Restoration of active elbow extension can be achieved very nicely using the bipolar transplantation of the latissimus dorsi when it is available (Fig. 37–19). In the tetraplegic patient, transfer of the posterior third of the deltoid into the triceps aponeurosis using multiple toe extensor tendon grafts is the procedure of choice for restoring elbow extension. Careful attention to postoperative detail, including the prolonged use of an adjustable flexion-blocking splint, is necessary to prevent late stretching of the transfer.

References

1. Ahmad, I.: Restoration of Elbow Flexion by a New Operative Method. Clin. Orthop. **106**:186, 1975.
2. Axer, A., Segal, D., and Elkon, A.: Partial Transposition of the Latissimus Dorsi. J. Bone Joint Surg. **55A**:1259, 1973.
3. Bartlett, S. P., May, J. W., and Yaremchuk, M. J.: The Latissimus Dorsi Muscle: A Fresh Cadaver Study of the Primary Neurovascular Pedicle. Plast. Reconstr. Surg. **67**:631, 1981.
4. Blount, W. P.: Osteoclasis for Supination Deformities in Children. J. Bone Joint Surg. **22**:300, 1940.
5. Bostwick, J., Nahai, F., Wallace, J. G., and Vasconez, L. O.: Sixty Latissimus Dorsi Flaps. Plast. Reconstr. Surg. **63**:31, 1979.
6. Bradford, E. H.: The Operative Treatment of Paralysis of the Shoulder Following Anterior Poliomyelitis. Am. J. Orthop. Surg. **8**:21, 1910.
7. Brash, J. C.: Neuro-vascular Hila of Limb Muscles. Edinburgh, E. & S. Livingstone Ltd., 1955.
8. Brones, M. F., Wheeler, E. S., and Lesavoy, M. A.: Restoration of Elbow Flexion and Arm Contour with the Latissimus Dorsi Myocutaneous Flap. Plast. Reconstr. Surg. **69**:329, 1982.
9. Brooks, D. M., and Seddon, H. J.: Pectoral Transplantation for Paralysis of the Flexors of the Elbow: A New Technique. J. Bone Joint Surg. **41B**:36, 1959.
10. Bryan, R. S.: The Moberg Deltoid-Triceps Replacement and Key Pinch Operations in Quadriplegia: Preliminary Experiences. Hand **9**:207, 1977.
11. Bunnell, S.: Surgery of the Hand, 2nd ed. Philadelphia, J. B. Lippincott Co., 1948, p. 584.
12. Bunnell, S.: Restoring Flexion to the Paralytic Elbow. J. Bone Joint Surg. **33A**:566, 1951.
13. Burman, M.: Paralytic Supination Contracture of the Forearm. J. Bone Joint Surg. **38A**:303, 1956.
14. Carroll, R. E.: Restoration of Flexor Power to the Flail Elbow by Transplantation of the Triceps Tendon. Surg. Gynecol. Obstet. **95**:685, 1955.
15. Carroll, R. E., and Gartland, J. J.: Flexorplasty of the Elbow. J. Bone Joint Surg. **35A**:706, 1953.
16. Carroll, R. E.: Discussion Paper by Mayer, L., and Green, W.: Experiences with the Steindler Flexorplasty at the Elbow. J. Bone Joint Surg. **36A**:858, 1954.
17. Carroll, R. E.: Restoration of Elbow Flexion by Transplantation of Sternocleidomastoid Muscle. J. Bone Joint Surg. **44A**:1039, 1962.
18. Carroll, R. E., and Hill, N. A.: Triceps Transfer to Restore Elbow Flexion. J. Bone Joint Surg. **52A**:23, 1970.
19. Carroll, R. E., and Kleinman, W. B.: Pectoralis Major Transplantation to Restore Elbow Flexion to the Paralytic Limb. J. Hand Surg. **4**:501, 1979.
20. Castro-Sierra, A., and Lopez-Pita, A.: A New Surgical Technique to Correct Triceps Paralysis. Hand **15**:42, 1983.
21. Clark, J. M. P.: Reconstruction of the Biceps Brachii by Pectoral Muscle Transplantation. Br. J. Surg. **34**:180, 1946.
22. Clark, J. M. P.: Reconstructive Surgery in Paralysis of the Elbow. Physiotherapy **56**:295, 1970.
23. Colson, J. H. C.: Physical Treatment of Pectoral Transfer and Flexorplasty. Physiotherapy **56**:300, 1970.
24. D'Aubigne, R. M.: Treatment of Residual Paralysis After Injuries of the Main Nerves (Superior Extremity). Proc. Roy. Soc. Med. **42**:831, 1949.
25. De Bendetti, M.: Restoration of Elbow Extension Power in the Tetraplegic Patient Using the Moberg Technique. J. Hand Surg. **4**:86, 1979.
26. Doyle, J. R., James, P. M., Larson, L. J., and Ashley, R. K.: Restoration of Elbow Flexion in Arthrogryposis Multiplex Congenita. J. Hand Surg. **5**:149, 1980.
27. Du Toit, G. T., and Levy, S. J.: Transposition of Latissimus Dorsi for Paralysis of Triceps Brachii. Report of a Case. J. Bone Joint Surg. **49B**:135, 1967.
28. Dutton, R. O., and Dawson, E. G.: Elbow Flexorplasty. An Analysis of Long-Term Results. J. Bone Joint Surg. **63A**:G064, 1981.
29. Eyler, D. L.: Modification of Steindler Flexorplasty. Georgia Warm Springs Foundation, Warm Springs, Georgia, Unpublished circular letter, Oct. 19, 1950.
30. Friedenberg, Z. B.: Transposition of the Biceps Brachii for Triceps Weakness. J. Bone Joint Surg. **36A**:656, 1954.
31. Gilbert, A.: Free Muscle Transfer. Int. Surg. **66**:33, 1981.
32. Green, D. P., and McCoy, H.: Turnbuckle Orthotic Correction of Elbow-Flexion Contractures After Acute Injuries. J. Bone Joint Surg. **61A**:1092, 1979.
33. Greene, M. H.: Cryptic Problems of Arthrogryposis Multiplex Congenita. J. Bone Joint Surg. **45A**:885, 1963.
34. Harmon, P. H.: Muscle Transplantation for Triceps Palsy. The Technique of Utilizing the Latissimus Dorsi. J. Bone Joint Surg. **31A**:409, 1949.
35. Hentz, V. R., Brown, M., and Keoshrian, L. A.: Upper Limb Reconstruction in Quadriplegia: Functional Assessment and Proposed Treatment Modifications. J. Hand Surg. **8**:119, 1983.
36. Hohmann, G.: Ersatz des Gelähmten Bizeps Brachii Durch den Pectoralis Major. Munch. Med. Wochenschr. **65**:1240, 1918.
37. Holtmann, B., Wray, R. C., Lowrey, R., and Weeks, P.: Restoration of Elbow Flexion. Hand **7**:256, 1975.

38. Hovnanian, A. P.: Latissimus Dorsi Transplantation of the Elbow. Ann. Surg. **143**:493, 1956.

39. Kettelkamp, D. B., and Larson, C. B.: Evaluation of the Steindler Flexorplasty. J. Bone Joint Surg. **45A**:513, 1963.

40. Lamb, D. W., and Chan, K. M.: Surgical Reconstruction of the Upper Limb in Traumatic Tetraplegia. J. Bone Joint Surg. **65B**:291, 1983.

41. Landra, A. P.: The Latissimus Dorsi Musculocutaneous Flap Used to Resurface Defect on the Upper Arm and Restore Extension to the Elbow. Br. J. Plast. Surg. **32**:275, 1979.

42. Lange, F.: Die Epidemische Kinderlahmung. Munich, J. F. Lehmann, 1930, p. 298.

43. Lange, M.: Orthopaedisch-Chirurgische Operationslehre. Munich, J. F. Bergmann, 1951, p. 301.

44. Lindholm, T. S., and Einola, S.: Flexorplasty of Paralytic Elbows. Analysis of Late Functional Results. Acta Orthop. Scand. **44**:1, 1973.

45. Lloyd-Roberts, G. C., and Lettin, A. W. F.: Arthrogryposis Multiplex Congenita. J. Bone Joint Surg. **52B**:494, 1970.

46. Manske, P. R., McCarroll, H. R., and Hale, R.: Biceps Tendon Rerouting and Percutaneous Osteoclasis in the Treatment of Supination Deformity in Obstetrical Palsy. J. Hand Surg. **5**:153, 1980.

47. Mayer, L., and Green, W.: Experiences with Steindler Flexorplasty of the Elbow. J. Bone Joint Surg. **36A**:775, 1954.

48. Meade, N. G., Lithgow, W. C., and Sweeney, H. J.: Arthrogryposis Multiplex Congenita. J. Bone Joint Surg. **40A**:1285, 1958.

49. Moberg, E.: Surgical Treatment for Absent Single-Hand Grip and Elbow Extension in Quadriplegia. Principles and Preliminary Experience. J. Bone Joint Surg. **57A**:196, 1975.

50. Moberg, E.: The Upper Limits in Tetraplegia: A New Approach to Surgical Rehabilitation. Stuttgart, Thieme, 1978.

51. Nyholm, K.: Elbow Flexor Plasty in Tendon Transposition (an Analysis of the Functional Results in 26 Patients). Acta Orthop. Scand. **33**:32, 1963.

52. Ober, F. R., and Barr, J. S.: Brachioradialis Muscle Transposition for Triceps Weakness. Surg. Gynecol. Obstet. **67**:105, 1938.

53. O'Brien, B., Morrison, W. A., MacLeod, A. M., and Weinglein, O.: Free Microneurovascular Muscle Transfer in Limbs to Provide Motor Power. Ann. Plast. Surg. **9**:381, 1982.

54. Owings, R., Wickstrom, J., Perry, J., and Nickel, V. L.: Biceps Brachii Rerouting in Treatment of Paralytic Supination Contracture of the Forearm. J. Bone Joint Surg. **53A**:137, 1971.

55. Rivarola, R. A.: Tratamiento de las Paralisis Definitivas del Miembro Superior. Bul. Trabajos Soc. Cirug. Buenos Aires **12**:688, 1928 (reported in Sernana Med. Buenos Aires **2**:1294, 1928).

56. Schottstaedt, E. R., Larsen, L. J., and Bost, F. C.: Complete Muscle Transportation. J. Bone Joint Surg. **37A**:897, 1955.

57. Schottstaedt, E. R., Larsen, L. J., and Bost, F. C.: The Surgical Reconstruction of the Upper Extremity Paralyzed by Poliomyelitis. J. Bone Joint Surg. **40A**:633, 1958.

58. Schulze-Berge: Ersatz der Benger des Voderarmes (Bizeps und Brachialis) durch den Pectoralis Major. Deutsche Med. Wochenschrift **43**:433, 1917.

59. Seddon, H. J.: Transplantation of Pectoralis Major for Paralysis of the Flexors of the Elbow. Proc. R. Soc. Med. **43**:837, 1949.

60. Segal, A., Seddon, H. J., and Brooks, D. M.: Treatment of Paralysis of the Flexors of the Elbow. J. Bone Joint Surg. **41B**:44, 1959.

61. Spira, E.: Replacement of Biceps Brachii by Pectoralis Minor Transplant. J. Bone Joint Surg. **39B**:126, 1957.

62. Steindler, A.: Orthopaedic Reconstruction Work on Hand and Forearm. N. Y. Med. J. **108**:1117, 1918.

63. Steindler, A.: A Muscle Plasty for the Relief of Flail Elbow in Infantile Paralysis. Interstate Med. J. **25**:235, 1918.

64. Steindler, A.: Operative Treatment of Paralytic Conditions of the Upper Extremity. J. Orthop. Surg. **1**:608, 1919.

65. Steindler, A.: Tendon Transplantation in the Upper Extremity. Am. J. Surg. **44**:260, 1939.

66. Steindler, A.: Muscle and Tendon Transplantation at the Elbow. In American Academy of Orthopaedic Surgeons, Instructional Course Lectures on Reconstruction Surgery. Ann Arbor, J. W. Edwards, 1944, pp. 276–283.

67. Stern, P. J., Neale, H. W., Gregory, R. O., and Kreilein, J. G.: Latissimus Dorsi Musculocutaneous Flap for Elbow Flexion. J. Hand Surg. **7**:25, 1982.

68. Tobin, G. R., Shusterman, B. A., Peterson, G. H., Nichols, G., and Bland, K. I.: The Intramuscular Neurovascular Anatomy of the Latissimus Dorsi Muscle: The Basis for Splitting the Flap. Plast. Reconstr. Surg. **67**:637, 1981.

69. Tobin, G. R., Bland, K. I., and Adcock, R.: Surgical Anatomy of the Musculus Pectoralis Major and Neurovascular Supply. American College of Surgeons, 1981. Surg. Forum **32**:574, 1981.

70. Tsai, T., Kalisman, M., Burns, J., and Kleinert, H. E.: Restoration of Elbow Flexion by Pectoralis Major and Pectoralis Minor Transfer. J. Hand Surg. **8**:186, 1983.

71. Tubby, A. H.: Deformities Including Diseases of the Bones and Joints. London, MacMillan, 1912, pp. 730–734.

72. VonLanz, T., and Wachsmuth, W.: Praktische Anatomie, 2nd ed. Berlin, Springer-Verlag, 1959, pp. 93–96, 166.

73. Williams, P. F.: The Elbow in Arthrogryposis. J. Bone Joint Surg. **55B**:834, 1973.

74. Zancolli, E. A.: Paralytic Supination Contracture of the Forearm. J. Bone Joint Surg. **49A**:1275, 1967.

75. Zancolli, E. A.: Structural and Dynamic Bases of Hand Surgery, 2nd ed. Philadelphia, J. B. Lippincott Co., 1979.

76. Zancolli, E. A., and Mitre, H.: Latissimus Dorsi Transfer to Restore Elbow Flexion. J. Bone Joint Surg. **55A**:1265, 1973.

77. Zaoussis, A. L.: Osteotomy of the Proximal End of the Radius for Paralytic Supination Deformity in Children. J. Bone Joint Surg. **45B**:523, 1963.

CHAPTER 38

Spastic Dysfunction of the Elbow

M. M. HOFFER, R. L. WATERS, and D. E. GARLAND

THE CEREBRAL PALSIED CHILD

Cerebral palsy is a perinatal disorder that is nonhereditary and is not progressive. This disorder is characterized by developmental, cognitive, and sensory problems.[16] Although any of these features may predominate in the clinical presentation, the disability is usually classified by its motor manifestations (Table 38–1). The spastic disorder involves fluctuations in muscle tone, which are demonstrated by stretch reflexes and even by clonus. The result is often postural changes that make function of the extremity difficult or impossible. These are the patients that are most often helped by surgical or orthotic devices. Patients with motion disorders (ataxia, dyskinesia, athetosis, and tremors) are characterized by variable changes in muscle tone that are markedly affected by position and activity. The motion disorders are currently treated by experimental attempts at drug therapy and brain surgery. Many disorders have both motor and spastic components. Unpredictable results occur in the surgery of the spastic limb when there is an admixture of these motion disorders.[9]

Diagnosis

Clinical Features

The diagnosis is frequently delayed in the first year of life. The key factor in evaluating

Table 38–1. **Simple Classification of Cerebral Palsy**

Geographic Distribution
Hemiplegia, primarily one-sided
Diplegia, primarily upper extremity involvement
Total involvement, all four extremities plus speech

Type
Spastic, increased stretch reaction
Motion disorders, ataxias, athetosis, chorea
Mixed

Most elbow problems occur in spastic hemiplegia, although occasionally those with total involvement develop fixed contracture.

the infant is achievement of developmental milestones. Normal infants become free of perinatal tonic neck reflexes and develop sitting balance, for example, by 6 months of age. A dominant extremity is not developed until the child is 18 to 24 months of age. The normal child develops two-handed activity and bilateral grasp and progresses from a two-handed approach to objects to a unilateral approach using the ulnar and then the radial portion of the hands in grasping at about the age of 18 to 24 months.

The cerebral palsied child generally is slow to develop balance and remains dominated by perinatal tonic neck reflexes. Early hand preference is usually a sign of poor function in the minor limb. The normal sequence of grasp may not occur, but primitive grasplike reflexes may be elicited.

The typical elbow deformity in cerebral palsy is one of elbow flexion and forearm pronation (Fig. 38–1). Rarely is a supinated and flexed posture observed. We have not seen extension deformities in the spastic elbow of children. Posterior dislocation of the radial head occurs occasionally in spastic children.[12] No treatment is usually advised.

Testing

The most important elements in testing the cerebral palsied child for function of the upper extremity are cognition, hand placement, and sensibility.[9]

Cognition is the complex of processes that indicates intelligence. This includes perception, abstract reasoning, and communication. The testing of cognition is difficult in patients with communication problems. Children graded in the first standard deviation of normal are termed normal. Those between the first and second standard deviations are considered educable, and those between the second and third standard deviations are considered trainable. Children below this level are thought to be profoundly retarded. Only those individuals with cognitive abilities that are

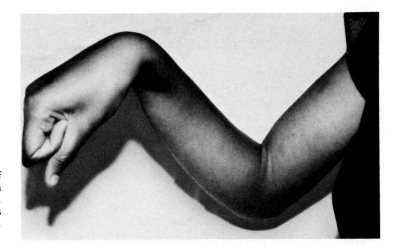

Figure 38–1. Typical flexion-pronation of the dysfunctional upper extremity in a patient with cerebral palsy. (From Mital, M. A.: Lengthening of the elbow flexors in cerebral palsy. J. Bone Joint Surg. 61A:515, 1979.)

educable or higher can expect to have functional results from upper extremity surgery.

Hand placement is simply assessed by requiring an individual to place a hand on the opposite knee and the top of head in 10 seconds.

Sensibility is best tested by texture discriminations in a 2- to 3-year-old, object identification in a 4- to 5-year-old, graphesthesia in the 6- to 9-year old, and two-point discrimination in the older child. Only those children with three of five correct object identifications, number perception in the palm, or two-point discrimination of less than 10 mm can be expected to have functional results after upper extremity surgery.

Definition of Goals

Functional tasks that should be tested in each patient are dressing, toileting, feeding, two-handed assisted work, grasp and release, and side pinch. After cognition, placement, and sensibility are tested, the functional goals for the hand should be established. One can then determine if the anticipated function is being accomplished by the patient.

The goal should be developed according to the expected function of the hand. The elbows in these cerebral palsied children merely place and position the hand. If there is no expected function in the hand, then surgery about the elbow may also be directed toward achieving self-care (hygiene) or cosmesis. Thus, a thorough hand evaluation in a cerebral palsied child prior to instituting an elbow procedure is mandatory.

Functional Test

In developing surgical goals for the upper extremity affected by cerebral palsy, children with cognition below the educable level, pre-

cise hand placement from head to knee of longer than 5 seconds, and sensibility test results of less than three of five objects or poor graphesthesia and two-point discrimination should be considered to be capable of achieving self-care (hygiene) as a result of elbow surgery.

If the child does have cognition in the educable range or higher but still has poor placement and sensibility test results, hygiene remains the goal, but cosmesis of the upper extremities may also be important to such a patient.

In those individuals with educable or better cognition, hand to knee placement of less than 5 seconds, and good sensibility results as described above, a good functional upper extremity should be the surgical goal. This group of patients should be considered for the more complex procedures.

Treatment

Several types of intervention may be offered for the spastic, contracted elbow, generally with variable and unpredictable results.[2, 3, 9, 10, 11, 14, 15]

Neurectomy

Musculocutaneous neurectomy is an effective procedure for the flexed elbow with contractures of less than 30 degrees in a patient whose main problem is that of excessive flexor tone. Neurectomy is contraindicated when elbow function in flexion depends on the biceps and brachialis alone. A Xylocaine block of the musculocutaneous nerve along the medial proximal border of the biceps is helpful in separating the results of flexor tone from those of contracture. It should be suspected that contracture will ensue if the spastic posture has been present for years. This block will also predict brachioradialis elbow flexion capability after the neurectomy.

Technique

We use an axillary approach to the musculocutaneous nerve (Fig. 38–2). The biceps and lateral cord of the brachial plexus are located. The nerve is identified prior to its penetration in the biceps and is further identified by nerve stimulation. It is severed in patients with cerebral palsy. We have injected the nerve sheath with 5 per cent phenol in glycerin to give temporary relief of flexor tone that is required in patients with head injury or stroke (see below, Acquired Spasticity).

Biceps-Brachialis Lengthening

This procedure is used to achieve the goals of cosmesis and hygiene. It is indicated when there are fixed contractures that interfere with

hygiene and should not be performed when flexion function may be lost. The results are variable and unpredictable[2,15] and occasionally excessive weakness may result.

Technique

Mital performs biceps-brachialis lengthenings through a curved antecubital approach.[11] The lacertus fibrosus is excised, and a Z-plasty of the biceps tendon and release of the brachialis aponeurosis are performed (Fig. 38–3). Occasionally the anterior elbow capsule must be released. Three weeks of postoperative immobilization are followed by bivalved elbow positioning splints in both of these operative procedures.

Flexor-Pronator Release

The flexor slide may be performed to achieve the goals of hygiene and cosmetic lengthening of the elbow, wrist, and finger flexors. We and

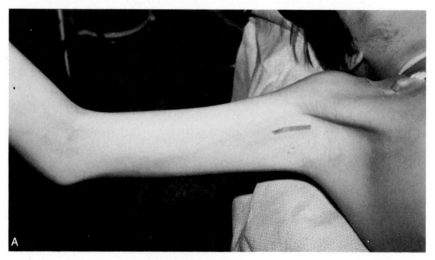

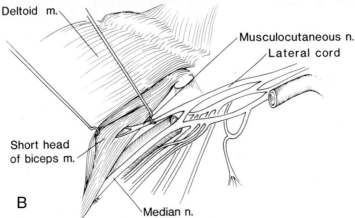

Figure 38–2. *A,* Axillary exposure provides access to the musculocutaneous nerve, which usually branches from the brachial plexus high in the axilla and is isolated between the biceps and the coracobrachialis *(B).* The nerve may be injected with phenol or severed as desired. (From Garland, et al.: Current uses of open phenol nerve block for adult acquired spasticity. Clin. Orthop. 165:217, 1982.)

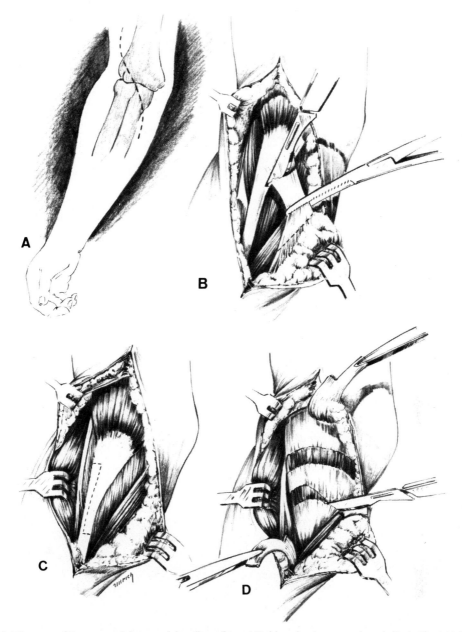

Figure 38–3. Diagrams of the sequential steps of the elbow-flexor Mital lengthening procedure *A–D*. *A,* The initial incision of the operation. *B,* The exposure of the tendon of the biceps and the excision of the lacertus fibrosus. *C,* Third step of the elbow-flexor lengthening procedure: the Z-lengthening of the biceps tendon. *D,* The incision of the aponeurotic fibers covering the brachialis. (From Mital, M. A.: Lengthening of the elbow flexors in cerebral palsy. J. Bone Joint Surg. 61A:515, 1979.)

others[10] have found that this procedure may also cause excessive weakness in finger flexors and thus, because it is sometimes unpredictable, it may not be a good surgical option in cerebral palsy.

If surgery is offered, we prefer a careful fractional lengthening of the forearm and hand muscles at their musculotendinous junctions (Fig. 38–4). This is an easier, more precise procedure than the slide procedure. However, when pronation, elbow flexion, and forearm, wrist, and hand flexion all interfere with hygiene, this flexor-pronator release may be helpful. Many surgeons find that this procedure improves function in the spastic, contracted hand and elbow.

Technique

The origin of the pronator-flexor group is released through a volar incision from the medial epicondyle to the distal forearm. The ulnar and median nerves are identified and protected while all the structures between

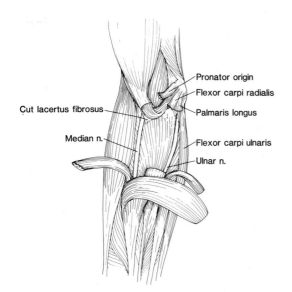

Figure 38–4. Modified flexor-pronator release. The muscles from the medial epicondyle and occasionally the flexor carpi ulnaris are released, exposing the ulnar nerve.

them, including the pronator teres, flexor carpi radialis and ulnaris, the flexor digitorum superficialis and profundus, and flexor pollicus, are allowed to slide distally from the medial epicondyle, ulna, and radius. This slide should permit adequate wrist and finger extension. A positioning plaster is utilized for 4 weeks, and then intermittent braces are used as necessary.

Acquired Spasticity

Acquired brain damage in childhood occurs most commonly from trauma. Anoxia, cerebrovascular anomalies, slow-growing or arrested cerebral neoplasms, and progressive cerebrosclerosing syndromes are rarer causes of acquired brain damage. The spasticity resulting from acquired brain damage usually does not reach its maximum point until 1 to 2 months after the incident. Then muscle tone may gradually decrease during the next 2 years.

We do not perform definitive procedures in children with acquired brain damage in the first 2 years after the insult. However, we advise positioning drop-out plasters for elbows with great flexor tone during this period (Fig. 38–5). A solid long arm plaster is placed with the arm in maximum comfortable extension. Then either the humeral extensor half of the plaster or the forearm extensor half is removed. This allows elbow extension while blocking flexion. If this fails, phenol injection of the musculocutaneous nerve (previously mentioned) is carried out.

Another problem in the child with acquired brain injury is heterotopic bone formation, usually about the anterior elbow.[13] Most children will eventually resorb the heterotopic bone. Thus, we advise gentle motion and re-evaluation at least 6 months prior to any attempt at excision.

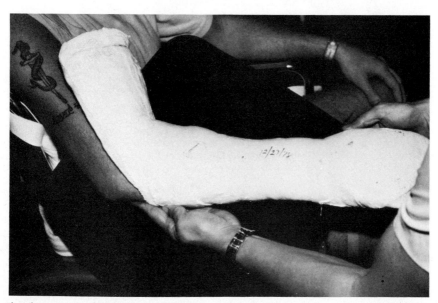

Figure 38–5. The drop-out cast has been used effectively as a nonoperative means of controlling excessive flexion or maintaining the correction that has been obtained in surgery. (From Garland, D. E., et al.: Musculocutaneous neurectomy for spastic elbow flexion in nonfunctional upper extremities in adults. J. Bone Joint Surg. 62A:108, 1980.)

STROKE AND HEAD TRAUMA IN THE ADULT

Adult stroke and head trauma produce permanent impairment in a total of approximately 3 million individuals in the United States. Abnormal elbow function due to spasticity and loss of motor control is a common disability. The surgeon treating these conditions must be fully cognizant of the complex rehabilitation process that ensues following central nervous system illness, particularly hand function, as noted above for the patient with cerebral palsy. Surgery is undertaken only after careful assessment of many of the factors (including cognition, motor control, spasticity at other joints, and sensory perception) that determine the patient's potential to use the limb.[1]

Cerebral vascular accident most commonly involves the middle cerebral artery or one of its branches in the region of the cerebral cortex supplying the upper extremity. Consequently, the upper extremity is usually more severely and frequently affected than the lower extremity. Elbow flexion contractures are nearly always preventable in the stroke population if range of motion therapy, splinting, and other standard preventative measures are instituted early. In contrast, head-injured individuals often have excessive elbow flexor tone due to decerebrate or decorticate rigidity. The degree of tone may be so severe that nonoperative measures alone may not prevent or correct elbow flexion deformity.

Elbow flexion contracture due to spasticity is the most common problem that requires surgical attention and usually occurs in patients with nonfunctional hands. Surgery is indicated to correct contractual deformities interfering with hygiene or causing pain; rarely, it is used to improve cosmesis (Fig. 38–6). Operative intervention is usually performed after neurologic recovery is completed, which usually occurs from 6 to 18 months afterward depending on the nature of the insult. If progressive elbow flexion deformity occurs in a patient with severe flexor spasticity prior to the time of neurologic recovery, despite a trial of nonoperative therapy that includes passive range of motion exercise, splints, and serial casts, phenol injection of the musculocutaneous nerve is performed.[8] Rarely is surgery indicated to improve active elbow extension in a functional arm.[17]

Potential for Functional Recovery

Substantial neurologic recovery generally occurs following the onset of stroke or head injury. In the stroke patient, most neurologic recovery is completed in the first 6 months; however, substantial recovery occurs in head trauma patients during the first year and a half.[4] Definitive surgical procedures to improve function are delayed until after these time periods so that the patient's neurologic

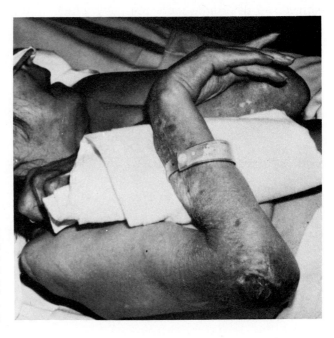

Figure 38–6. Flexion deformity in a nonfunctional hand is frequently seen in the decerebrate posturing after a motor vehicle accident. Note the poor condition of the skin that is common in such patients. An operation is indicated to improve hygienic care. (From Garland, D. E., et al.: Musculocutaneous neurectomy for spastic elbow flexion in nonfunctional upper extremities in adults. J. Bone Joint Surg. 62A:108, 1980.)

condition has become stabilized, he has learned to cope with his disability, and he has had sufficient time to receive appropriate nonoperative therapy. When elbow flexion spasticity is excessive in the acute recovery phase, either open phenol injection of the motor branches of the musculocutaneous nerve or percutaneous motor point phenol block is utilized to reduce elbow flexion tone.[8] The effects of phenol are transient, and spasticity is temporarily decreased until the completion of the recovery phase, when definitive procedures can be performed if necessary.

Preoperative Evaluation

Vestibular reflexes potentiate flexor responses in the upper extremity. So that the influence of spasticity on performance can be accurately assessed, the patient is examined in the sitting position. Range of motion of the elbow is determined by quickly and slowly extending the elbow. Quick stretch excites the velocity-sensitive components of the muscle spindle and may elicit clonus if spasticity is severe. Consequently, a greater range of extension can often be obtained by slow extension (often lasting 1 or 2 minutes) in the supine position. Even when the elbow is slowly stretched and maintained in the furthest extended position possible, tonus may persist. Consequently, spasticity can be differentiated from fixed contracture only by preoperative nerve block or examination under general anesthesia.

Dynamic electromyography is becoming increasingly useful as a tool that enables the surgeon to determine more precisely which flexor muscles are responsible for deformity (Fig. 38–7) or whether surgical ablation of function of a given muscle will be effective.

This information is particularly valuable in a patient with functional elbow motion because it enables the surgeon to release or lengthen only the most involved muscles and preserve those that are less involved. Volitionary elbow flexion and extension are assessed at slow and fast speeds. Attempts to move the elbow rapidly enhance an abnormal flexor response (Fig. 38–8).

Anterior and posterior radiographs of the elbow are taken prior to any surgical procedure. Arthritis or other conditions commonly present in the adult patient may be responsible for intrinsic joint restriction and decrease the probability of a successful surgical outcome.

Lastly, preoperative evaluation always includes a detailed assessment by a therapist. This assessment includes a detailed evaluation of motor and perceptual function not only of the elbow but also of the hand and shoulder. In addition, cognitive, vocational, and social factors that are important determinants of arm function are also assessed.

Surgical Techniques

Nonfunctional Elbows

When elbow flexion contracture is present, lengthening of the biceps tendon alone will not significantly improve elbow flexion deformity, and attention must be directed to the brachialis muscle as well. Myostatic contracture is differentiated from spasticity by anesthetic block of the musculocutaneous nerve (axillary nerve block) or by examining the patient under anesthesia. If there is less than 90 degrees of fixed deformity, musculocuta-

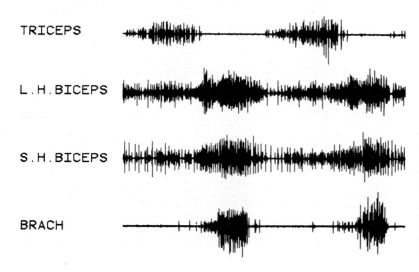

TRICEPS

L.H.BICEPS

S.H.BICEPS

BRACH

Figure 38–7. Dynamic electromyogram of head-injured patient with spasticity during slow extension-flexion–extension-flexion cycle of elbow. Triceps displays normal bursts of activity during extension phase. The brachialis is also normally active in flexion. Note that both the long and the short head of the biceps is inappropriately active during attempted elbow extension indicating obstructive tone.

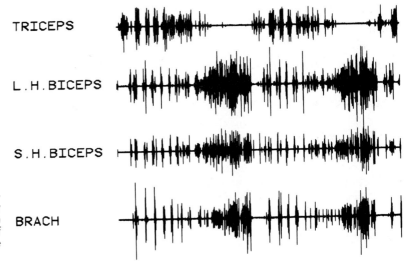

TRICEPS

L.H.BICEPS

S.H.BICEPS

Figure 38–8. Dynamic electromyogram during attempted fast elbow motion. Note clonic firing pattern in all muscles, which is indicative of severe spasticity in all muscle groups.

BRACH

neous neurectomy is performed.[5] Residual deformity is corrected after surgery by dropout or serial casts (Fig. 38–5).

Even when minimal or no fixed myostatic or joint contracture is present, spasticity may cause the elbow to assume a flexed posture that interferes with function. Among hemiplegics it is common for the elbow to assume a flexed posture while walking, and it may bounce up and down owing to clonus. The patient may purposely walk slowly to decrease clonus. Musculocutaneous neurectomy will improve cosmesis and eliminate clonus.[5] Following musculocutaneous neurectomy, the loss of elbow flexion strength is not important because most stroke patients with excessive elbow flexion have nonfunctional hands. Because the brachioradialis is innervated by the radial nerve, which is left intact, some elbow flexion will persist following surgery if this muscle was active preoperatively, and the loss of musculocutaneous sensation is not bothersome. In the patient without volitional brachioradialis control or spasticity, this procedure should not be performed because musculocutaneous neurectomy will leave a completely flail elbow.

Musculocutaneous neurectomy is performed through a longitudinal incision extending distally from the tendon of the pectoralis major in the interval between the short head of the biceps and the coracobrachialis.[5] This incision can be extended proximally or distally if further exploration to locate the nerve is required. A 1-cm segment of the nerve is excised (Fig. 38–2).

When deformity is longstanding and considerable myostatic contracture has occurred,

flexor release is performed. Using a lateral incision, the origin of the brachioradialis is released, providing access to the biceps tendon, which is lengthened or tenotomized, and the brachialis, which is myotomized. Thirty to 40 degrees of correction (Fig. 38–9) are usually obtained, and further elbow extension is blocked by the contracture of the neurovascular structures and skin. Excessive tension on the neurovascular elements is unnecessary and may lead to vascular compromise. It is not usually necessary to release the anterior capsule. Further correction is easily obtained postoperatively by a program of serial casting. Because this procedure is usually performed on nonfunctional limbs, full extension is not necessary, and surgery in combination with postoperative serial casting will provide adequate correction.

Functional Elbow

Patients who have intact hand function and lack adequate elbow extension occasionally benefit by selective release of contracted or spastic elbow flexor muscles. Operative procedures that rely on releasing or lengthening the elbow flexors may reduce elbow flexion strength and range. Preoperative dynamic electromyography may enable determination of a specific flexor that is more severely spastic, and surgery can be restricted to this muscle. Preoperative motor point block with Xylocaine enables the surgeon to evaluate the effects of deletion of tone in a specific flexor muscle prior to surgery.

Some voluntary extension strength must be available preoperatively to move the elbow through the full range of available extension after obstructive flexor spasticity or contracture is reduced.

Essential to surgical success is a postoperative therapy program to teach the patient to incorporate the increased elbow extension into routine daily living activities.

Heterotopic Ossification

Heterotopic ossification of the elbow is a severe complication that occurs in approximately 3 per cent of head-injured patients. It most commonly occurs when severe hypertonus is present at the elbow owing to rigidity from decorticate or decerebrate posturing or spastic hemiplegia (Fig. 38–10). Heterotopic ossification generally is apparent within the first 6 months following head trauma with the peak occurrence at 2 months. The typical stroke patient infrequently develops heterotopic ossification. In the head-injured patient, the complication occurs more often posteriorly than anteriorly.[6a]

The incidence of traumatic heterotopic ossification in combined head and elbow injuries is 90 per cent.[6a] Heterotopic ossification most commonly occurs in the collateral ligaments but may form in all planes about the elbow. Formation in the ulnar collateral ligament may contribute to an acute ulnar palsy

from the localized swelling or a tardy ulnar palsy resulting from chronic pressure.

Heterotopic ossification is heralded by swelling, pain, and limited motion at the elbow. Evidence of heterotopic ossification on bone scans is apparent 2 to 3 weeks before radiographic evidence of calcification appears. Muscular hypertonus exerts continuous forces across the inflamed joint, intensifying the pain. Pain consequently increases spasticity, thus completing the vicious cycle. If the patient's neurologic condition rapidly improves, the amount of heterotopic ossification is lessened, and no significant impairment may result if an adequate range of elbow motion is maintained. On the other hand, if elbow range becomes severely restricted or the elbow becomes ankylosed, extremity function may be difficult even if neurologic recovery has occurred. Even in the nonfunctional arm, hygiene of the elbow flexor crease and limb positioning are difficult in the patient with severe limb flexion deformity and ankylosis.

Treatment of heterotopic ossification begins with prompt recognition. Joint motion is preserved by range of motion exercises. Movement should be slowed to minimize pain. Elbow splints are useful to enable the elbow

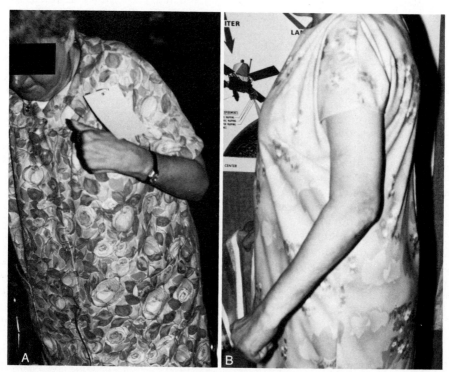

Figure 38–9. *A,* A severe flexion contracture was present in this individual following a cerebral vascular accident. *B,* Approximately 40 degrees of correction was obtained after a flexor release. (From Garland, D. E., et al.: Musculocutaneous neurectomy for spastic elbow flexion in nonfunctional upper extremities in adults. J. Bone Joint Surg. 62A:108, 1980.)

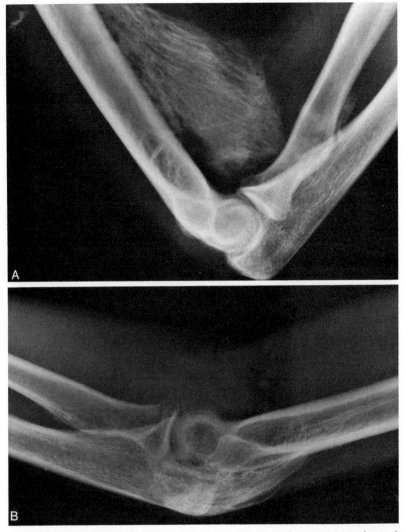

Figure 38–10. Decerebrate rigidity may be associated with myositis ossificans in the anterior muscles *(A)* but even more often in the posterior aspect of the elbow *(B)*. (From Garland, D. E., et al.: Periarticular heterotopic ossification in head-injured adults. J. Bone Joint Surg. 62A:143, 1980.)

to be positioned in maximum extension. Diphosphonate therapy is initiated if diagnosis was prompt, and treatment is continued for 3 to 6 months. Phenol injection of the musculocutaneous nerve may be helpful to reduce muscle tone in the biceps and brachialis muscles. The temporary reduction of elbow flexor tone permits the therapist to perform range of motion exercises more easily to maintain elbow extension. Forceful manipulation of the elbow under anesthesia may also be helpful to maintain or increase elbow range.[7]

Because the incidence of heterotopic ossification is so high, prophylactic or early diphosphonate treatment may be indicated. This type of heterotopic ossification is not related to the severity of the head injury, and spasticity about the joint may not be present.

Resection of heterotopic ossification is performed after the bone is skeletally mature.[6,13] In our experience, volitional flexion and extension enabling active motion are essential to maintain joint range following surgery. Diphosphonates are given preoperatively for 2 weeks and postoperatively for 3 to 6 months.

References

1. Caldwell, C., and Braun, R. M.: Spasticity in the Upper Extremity. Clin. Orthop. **104**:80, 1974.
2. Carroll, R. E., and Craig, F. S.: The Surgical Treatment of Cerebral Palsy—The Upper Extremity. Surg. Clin. North Am. **31**:385, 1951.
3. Colton, C. L., Ransford, A. O., and Lloyd-Roberts, G. C.: Transposition of the Tendon of the Pronator Teres in Cerebral Palsy. J. Bone Joint Surg. **58B**:220, 1976.

4. Garland, D. E., and Waters, R. L.: Orthopedic Evaluation in Hemiplegic Stroke. Orthop. Clin. North Am. **9**:291, 1978.

5. Garland, D. E., Thompson, R., and Waters, R. L.: Musculocutaneous Neurectomy for Spastic Elbow Flexion in Non-functional Upper Extremities in Adults. J. Bone Joint Surg. **62A**:108, 1980.

6. Garland, D. E., Blum, C. E., and Waters, R. L.: Periarticular Heterotopic Ossification in Head-Injured Adults. J. Bone Joint Surg. **62A**:1143, 1980.

6a. Garland, D. E., and O'Hallaren, R. M.: Fractures and Dislocations About the Elbow in Head Injured Adults. Clin. Orthop. **168**:38, 1982.

7. Garland, D. E., Razza, B., and Waters, R. L.: Forceful Joint Manipulation in Head Injured Adults With Heterotopic Ossification. Clin. Orthop. **169**:133, 1982.

8. Garland, D. E., Lucie, R. S., and Waters, R. L.: Current Uses of Open Phenol Nerve Block for Adult Acquired Spasticity. Clin. Orthop. **165**:217, 1982.

9. Hoffer, M. M.: Cerebral Palsy: Operative Hand Surgery. *In* Green, D. (ed.): Operative Hand Surgery. New York, Churchill Livingstone, 1982, pp. 185–194.

10. McCue, F. C., and Honner, R.: Deformities of the Upper Limb in Cerebral Palsy. South. Med. J. **63**:355, 1970.

11. Mital, M. A.: Lengthening of the Elbow Flexors in Cerebral Palsy. J. Bone Joint Surg. **61A**:515, 1979.

12. Pletcher, D., Hoffer, M. M., and Kohman, N.: Non-traumatic Dislocation of Radial Head in Cerebral Palsy. J. Bone Joint Surg. **58**:104, 1976.

13. Roberts, J. B., and Pankratz, D. G.: The Surgical Treatment of Heterotopic Ossification at the Elbow Following Long-Term Coma. J. Bone Joint Surg. **61A**:760, 1979.

14. Sakellarides, H. T., and Mital, M.: Treatment of the Pronator Contracture of the Forearm in Cerebral Palsy. J. Hand Surg. **1**:79, 1976.

15. Samilson, R. L., and Morris, V. M.: Surgical Improvement of the Cerebral Palsied Upper Limb. J. Bone Joint Surg. **46A**:1203, 1964.

16. Samilson, R. L.: Principles of Assessment of the Upper Limb in Cerebral Palsy. Clin. Orthop. **47**:105, 1966.

17. Waters, R. L., Wilson, D. J., and Savinelli, R.: Rehabilitation of the Upper Extremity Following Stroke. *In* Hunter, J. M., et al. (ed.): Rehabilitation of the Hand. St. Louis, C. V. Mosby Co., 1978, p. 505.

CHAPTER 39

Amputation*

ERNEST M. BURGESS and MORRIS A. DODGE

Amputations through and about the elbow joint are infrequent. Little has been written to describe this subject, and this discussion is followed therefore by a list of general rather than specific references. Amputations about the elbow result primarily from trauma and neoplasm. By far the most frequent cause of all major elective amputations in the western world is ischemia due to peripheral vascular disease. Because less than 5 per cent of these amputations occur in the upper limb, the elbow is a relatively rare site for ischemic limb loss. In contrast, congenital limb deficiency is seen with some frequency near the elbow joint. The very short below-elbow transverse hemimelia is the congenital upper limb amputation most often encountered. Although the number of these patients is also small, they do present a challenge in amputation management and in prosthetic substitution.

Elbow disarticulation has not been viewed kindly by prosthetists. If normal, segmental, bilateral arm length is to be achieved, it is necessary to use external hinges at the prosthetic elbow joint. Because the elbow must be positioned and stabilized before useful control of the terminal prosthetic device (hand or hook) can be achieved, an elbow-locking mechanism is essential. This requirement calls for a somewhat complicated mechanical modification of the single-axis or the polycentric elbow hinge in order to allow voluntary positioning and locking. The more refined, intrinsic, body-controlled elbow mechanisms used for above-elbow prostheses require so much additional upper arm prosthetic length that undesirable problems with the fitting of clothing to the arm and with appearance result when the device is incorporated at elbow disarticulation level. For these reasons many surgeons and prosthetists discourage amputation through the elbow joint and favor a

somewhat higher level through the lower humerus. In this way, modern intrinsic elbow mechanisms can be spatially accommodated in the prosthesis yet the normal elbow level is maintained.

In terms of successful prosthetic function, however, elbow disarticulation is a most satisfactory level of amputation (Fig. 39–1). It should not be converted to a higher level simply for the purpose of less complicated prosthetic design. The distal condyles of the humerus with their irregular contours provide a good source of rotary stability and suspension of the prosthesis. Effective muscle stabilization is surgically feasible without technical difficulty, thereby allowing retainment of a more physiologic residual limb. It is hoped that continued research in engineering design, especially of myoelectric prostheses, will enhance the usefulness of elbow disarticulation as a preferred amputation level.

PRINCIPLES AND TECHNIQUE

Amputation surgery is reconstructive surgery. The surgeon is reconstructing a terminal end-organ for contact with the environment, specifically the prosthesis. In this respect, the surgery is technically comparable to similar procedures performed on the intact hand.

The basic principle of all upper limb amputations is preservation of maximum length consistent with satisfactory surgical wound management. Equally important is the conservation of functional tissue in the remaining portion of the limb. This includes muscles, nerves, blood supply, and, whenever possible, healthy skin. Retained functional muscle is useful not only to provide contour and strength. The voluntary myoelectric currents arising in the muscles of the stump initiate the signals that control almost all externally powered prostheses that are presently available. Retention of voluntary stump muscle activity is, then, a fundamental requirement for a physiologic amputation. The severed muscles or tendons need a fixed distal end point for effective use. This requirement im-

*ACKNOWLEDGMENTS. This work is supported with Veterans Administration Rehabilitation Research and Development funds, Contract No. V663P-1323.

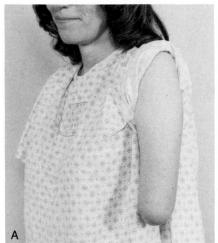

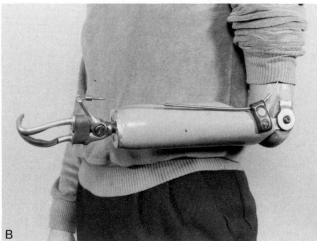

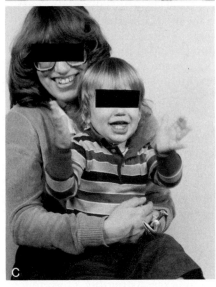

Figure 39–1. *A,* Healed amputation at elbow disarticulation level. *B,* Same patient wearing conventional body-powered prosthesis. *C,* Functional support using prosthesis.

plies distal muscle stabilization at a length that avoids proximal joint restriction yet permits effective, forceful, voluntary contraction. Muscle stabilization, then, when surgically feasible, is very important for elbow disarticulation.

As with all amputations and, in fact, with all areas of surgery, the principles of appropriate wound healing apply. Well-nourished and sensible skin is needed to cover the amputation site. Skin flaps are developed and placed with plastic surgical technique and with knowledge and consideration of the replacement device. The prosthetic contact with the limb, the interface, is the vital functional bridge. Almost all prostheses today totally contact the stump. Scar placement is elective and depends primarily on the surgical circumstances. The scar should be nontender, not adherent to bone or other deeper, rigid structures, and sufficiently healthy to withstand interface contact and force transfer. Un-

derlying bone must be well contoured and smooth. Major nerves should be subjected to moderate traction, ligated, and sharply sectioned. In this manner they are allowed to retract back into the soft tissues where neuroma formation will not be a source of irritation.

The final need is early, progressive rehabilitation. Upper limb amputations are particularly responsive to immediate or early functional prosthetic use. Whether body-powered or externally powered, the rapid use of provisional functional prostheses, the immediate fit technique, has been a revolutionary advance in successful rehabilitation.

ELBOW DISARTICULATION

Skin

The skin flaps are ordinarily anteroposterior and equal in length (Fig. 39–2). They are fashioned short, and closure should be suffi-

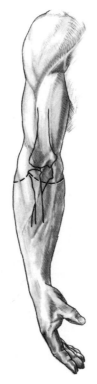

Figure 39–2. Skin incision for elbow disarticulation and very long above-elbow amputation.

lage surfaces, or folded and redundant will compromise limb fit. Skin grafts are not a contraindication to prosthetic fit. Their use may be indicated, particularly in burn amputations. Skin on upper limb amputations is far less subject to pressure, shear, and stretching than it is in the weight-bearing lower limb. Skin of somewhat poorer than normal quality and well-nourished skin grafts will improve in socket tolerance with time provided socket contact is permitted to adjust slowly to tolerance. It is important to maintain skin sensation and good skin nutrition to the maximum degree possible.

Nerves and Blood Vessels

Major nerves about the elbow are ligated under moderate tension. A fine, nonabsorbent suture is used. The ligated nerve end is then allowed to retract into the adjacent soft tissues away from the amputation site and away from areas where it could become adherent and a source of pressure irritation from the socket wall.

Adequate hemostasis by ligature is necessary. Cautery is used only for very small vessels. Wounds are drained for 48 hours. Postoperative hematomas must be avoided.

Bone

Through-elbow amputation is carried out as a true disarticulation (Fig. 39–3). Minor contouring of the margins of the distal humerus is needed to eliminate sharp condylar prominences. It is necessary to plan the soft tissue coverage carefully to ensure that it is adequate to avoid pressure-sensitive areas. Not infrequently, the trauma leading to the amputation has distorted and damaged the distal humeral

ciently loose to allow free mobility of the skin. The position of the skin closure scar will vary depending on the surgical circumstances. The nature of the trauma, including burns, may require extensive modification of the classic equal flap closure. Because the prosthetic socket will totally contact the amputation site, scar placement can be adjusted to the available skin provided the closure is appropriate. Skin that is adherent, of poor viability, stretched tight over bone and carti-

Figure 39–3. Cross section of elbow disarticulation preparatory to myoplasty closure. The myoplastic flaps must be sectioned with sufficient length to permit closure with tension.

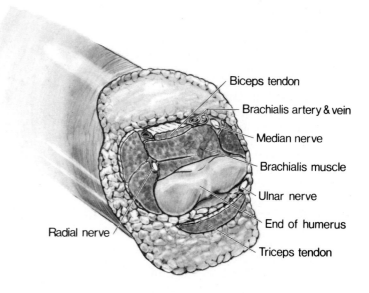

Biceps tendon

Brachialis artery & vein

Median nerve

Brachialis muscle

Ulnar nerve

End of humerus

Triceps tendon

Radial nerve

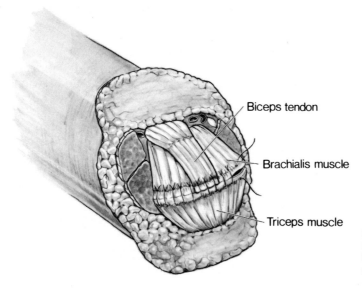

Figure 39–4. Muscle stabilization using anteroposterior myofascial flaps over contoured distal humerus at elbow level. The flaps must be stabilized directly to the periosteum or bone.

surfaces. When the distal humerus has been so injured, the remaining bone and joint surface is carefully modified and rounded to avoid sharp prominences and rough bone edges.

Muscle Stabilization

Whenever possible, the sectioned proximal muscles and tendons are stabilized at or near the end of the humerus at the amputation site (Fig. 39–4). The triceps tendon with aponeurosis is retained and brought forward through and over the trochlea to be sewn under *moderate* tension to the brachialis muscle. The biceps tendon can also be interwoven into the brachialis muscle near the amputation site, thus giving excellent stump muscle control. Should the biceps tendon be damaged and of inadequate length to sew down at the amputation site, the more proximal tendon or the musculotendinous junction may be carefully stabilized into the brachialis muscle.

Muscle stabilization requires firm fixation to the distal bone. When opposing muscles are sewn to each other over the bone or joint end without firm distal fixation, a slinglike effect can develop that causes bursa formation, reduces effectiveness of the muscles, and is not infrequently painful. A myodesis with two or four small drill holes through the distal humerus may be necessary to accomplish good muscle tie-down. Individual circumstances resulting from trauma will require innovation. The principle of muscle stabilization, however, is employed as effectively as the surgical circumstances permit.

A properly performed elbow disarticulation provides an excellent well-contoured stump with freely moveable, sensible, nontender skin and good muscle control, giving strength to the remaining arm and for myoelectric signaling when electric-powered prostheses are used.

The closed wound is drained. Suction drainage, a soft rubber through-and-through drain, or a combination of both can be used (Fig. 39–5). When rigid dressings are applied postoperatively, the suction drain can be brought out through the dressing or above it. Drains are ordinarily removed on the second postoperative day.

POSTOPERATIVE MANAGEMENT

Worldwide experience during the last 15 years has established the immediate postsurg-

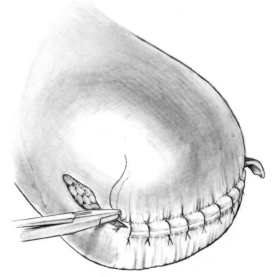

Figure 39–5. Skin closure with drainage.

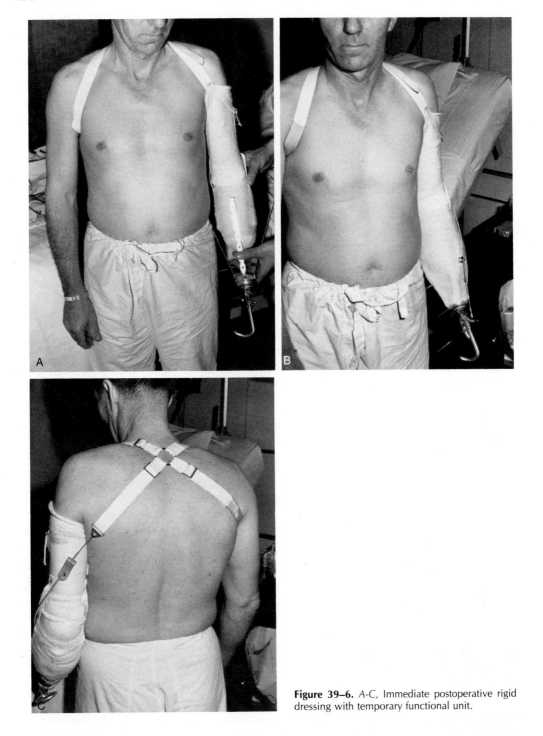

Figure 39–6. *A-C,* Immediate postoperative rigid dressing with temporary functional unit.

ical rigid dressing technique as the most effective management for supporting uncomplicated wound healing and early rehabilitation (Fig. 39–6). At completion of surgery, dry, gently compressive dressings are applied with distal wound support. A contoured sterile polyurethane compression pad is used over the distal end of the stump, and the entire remaining limb up to shoulder level is immobilized in a supportive cast. Suspension is

accomplished by dressing adherence to the skin and a light Dacron suspension-strap harness.

A terminal device can often be fitted the day following surgery. Body-powered prosthetic use with a conventional shoulder-girdle harness permits rapid accommodation to limb loss and a progressively increasing ability to resume bimanual activities (Figs. 39–7 and 39–8).

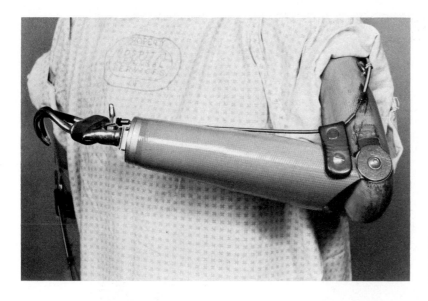

Figure 39–7. Conventional body-powered elbow disarticulation prosthesis using external locking hinged joints with terminal hook.

If electrical external power is planned, surface electrodes are placed on appropriate muscle signal areas in the inner wall of the cast. Instrumentation is then fitted to the rigid dressing, and training in myoelectrical control begins. In uncomplicated circumstances the terminal device quickly becomes functional either by body power or by electrical control. Functional loss is minimized under this rapid rehabilitation technique (Figs. 39–9 and 39–10).

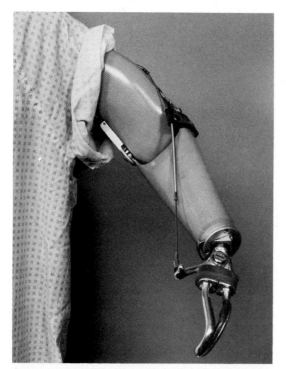

Figure 39–8. Same prosthesis as shown in Figure 39–7. Incorporated wrist flexion unit improves range of function of terminal device.

As noted earlier, the drain is normally removed 48 hours after surgery. Serial cast changes are carried out when indicated either by loosening the cast or at appropriate intervals when removing sutures and inspecting the wound. Shoulder and shoulder-girdle exercises are started immediately following amputation. Disability is minimized by early temporary limb fit and active physical therapy. Young, active patients are frequently able to achieve effective control of the temporary prosthesis and terminal device a few days after limb loss.

Conventional soft dressings with elastic wrap can be used when the rigid dressing technique is unavailable or when it is appropriate to inspect the wound at frequent intervals. Even in the presence of open wounds and tissues of marginal viability, the rigid dressing technique is still effective. When the amputation site is infected, the nature of the pathology will dictate the postoperative management (i.e., soft dressings or closed cast treatment), and as healing progresses, the temporary prosthetic device will be used first followed by the definitive prosthesis. At elbow disarticulation level the uncomplicated amputation will generally be healed and ready for a permanent prosthesis 5 to 6 weeks following the date of surgery.

AMPUTATIONS IMMEDIATELY ADJACENT TO THE ELBOW

Severe trauma through the elbow joint may require a low transcondylar amputation. In the adult with closed distal humeral epiphyses, the surgical and immediate postoperative treatment is essentially the same as

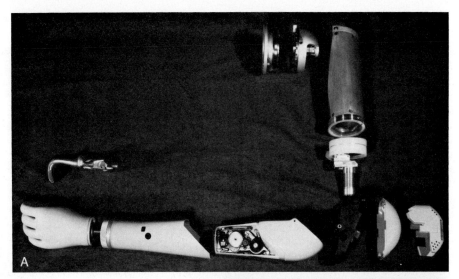

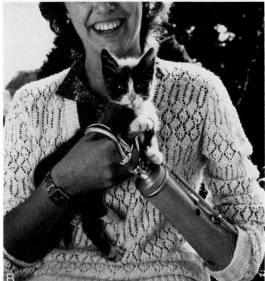

Figure 39–9. *A, B,* Myoelectric "Utah" arm available for amputations through and about the elbow joint. This is the most effective external electrically powered prosthesis available in the world today. (Courtesy of Motion Control Inc., 1005 South 300 West, Salt Lake City, Utah 84101.)

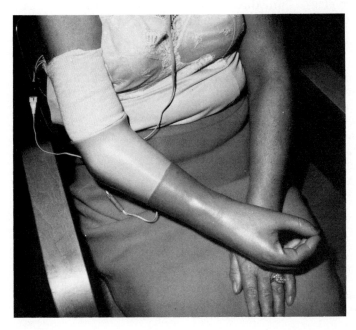

Figure 39–10. U.S. Veterans Administration externally powered prosthesis.

that outlined for elbow disarticulation. It is important to contour the distal humerus adequately and to provide good soft tissue and skin coverage, disregarding, if necessary, classic equal flap closure. Muscle stabilization is accomplished by appropriate myoplasty or myodesis. Angulation osteotomy of the distal humerus is in general reserved for the occasional distal humerus amputation in children. The indications and techniques for this bone contour augmentation have been well outlined by Marquardt.[14, 15]

Amputation through the forearm just distal to the elbow joint presents certain characteristics that require surgical modifications other than those outlined for elbow disarticulation. If the elbow joint itself is badly damaged, with pain and marked restriction of motion, it may be necessary to proceed with a formal elbow disarticulation. The elbow, however, should not be saved at all costs. In general, even very short below-elbow amputation should be preserved, leaving the integrity of the elbow joint. The muscles providing elbow control retain their attachments when ablation has occurred at this level. The advantages of elbow retention for the very short below-elbow level are related to improved suspension of the prosthesis and the simplicity of the elbow joint mechanism.

Section of the biceps tendon at its distal insertion increases the depth of the cubital fossa, making socket fit more stable. Some surgeons prefer to transfer the biceps tendon to the underlying brachialis muscle just proximal to the elbow joint. Such a transfer does not significantly disturb function of the biceps but does permit a modern and effective electrical signal when an external powered prosthesis is used.

If surgically appropriate, it is desirable to leave the ulna slightly longer than the radius in the very high forearm amputation. The bone ends must be carefully tailored to avoid rough and prominent surfaces. The loss of elbow flexion strength by distal biceps tendon transfer has not been a troublesome source of weakened prosthesis control. The brachialis muscle is sufficiently strong as an effective flexor to accomplish elbow flexion with the prosthesis in place.

ELBOW DISARTICULATION IN CHILDREN

Surgery is rarely needed in congenital limb deficiencies at or approximately at elbow level. Transverse hemimelia just distal to the elbow joint rarely needs surgical intervention

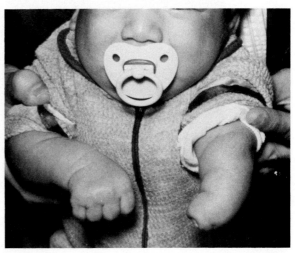

Figure 39–11. Congenital, very short below-elbow transverse hemimelia.

(Fig. 39–11). The prosthetic management is well standardized and effective. These children generally present with a short below-elbow residual limb that is painless, freely moveable, and generally permits full flexion and 10 to 25 degrees of hyperextension. Such children routinely become efficient users of prostheses. In acquired amputations in the immature skeleton the epiphyses should be preserved wherever possible. Elbow disarticulation is the *level of choice* for neoplasms requiring ablation of the forearm.

PROSTHETIC MANAGEMENT

The success of an artificial organ, that is, a prosthesis designed to replace limb loss, can be measured by the degree of function, appearance, and comfort it provides. The development of an artificial arm to replace limb loss at the elbow disarticulation level is a monumental task. In contrast to the loss of certain vital internal organs, limb loss does not pose a threat to life. Nonetheless, an artificial limb is in fact an artificial organ. Understanding the physical characteristics of the lost part and the psychological impact will be the first step in an intelligent approach to inert replacement.

The complexity and integration of function and grace in the hands and arms of a concert violinist or pianist, a professional magician, a world-class gymnast, a calligrapher, or a weight-lifter overwhelm the engineer involved in biomedical design. Coordinated musculoskeletal behavior is highly complex and not fully understood even by those most knowledgeable in anatomy, biology, and engineering. A constant flow of many thousands of nerve signals is continually transmitted to the central nervous system, then synchronized, processed, and directed to initiate appropriate motor response.

This afferentation arises from nerve-tendon organs that monitor muscle tensions, from a variety of proprioceptive sources that determine the configuration of the limb in space, from thousands of muscle spindle receptors that continually monitor the contraction speed and length of muscles, and from a wide variety of skin receptors that respond to pressure, temperature, tension, vibration, motion speed, and many other factors.

This huge, continuous source of information is further augmented by vision, by the vestibular organs, and by electrical, chemical, and mechanical changes in the external environment itself. Functional adaptation, learning as well as information accrual and storage, add to the complexity of limb substitute design.

The muscles themselves are remarkable energy-conversion machines. The transfer of chemical energy into mechanical force in a highly efficient, quiet, and coordinated manner depends on rapid self-adaption to numerous physical circumstances including the nature of bone and joints, physical loading, and large numbers of other performance characteristics. Factors of general body metabolism, nutrition, and tissue perfusion are a few of the additional performance variables influencing function.

Last, the psychological impact of limb loss must be considered. Self-image and social relevance as with peer response all place additional demands on the cosmesis, for example, of the replacement device.

The prosthetic engineer, in surveying the physiologic mechanisms he must replace, immediately realizes that a system of priorities is the first need. Certain principles and priorities surface at once in fabricating and servicing an elbow disarticulation prosthesis.

A surgically adequate elbow disarticulation in a properly contoured, total-contact socket gives the amputee excellent opportunities for prosthetic control. The arm muscles assist in retaining the limb with a minimum of harnessing. The patient can mechanically flex the hinged or prosthetic elbow and rotate the prosthesis by shoulder positioning. With proper training and reasonable coordination, an elbow disarticulation amputee with currently available prostheses can quickly learn to remove a card, comb, or other small item from his shirt or pants pocket as well as to

assist in and skillfully perform many bimanual living needs.

PROSTHETIC ELBOW JOINT

Currently, there are several outside-locking hinge arrangements designed for the elbow disarticulation or the very short below-elbow amputee. The stump-activated locking hinge for the short below-elbow amputee allows the individual to flex the forearm with the elbow unlocked. This is accomplished by a dual control, above-elbow cable with the stump in the extended position. When forearm flexion is desired, the stump is flexed, engaging a lock on the elbow hinge. Holding tension on the stump keeps the elbow locked and increases the ability to retain the prosthesis while lifting or pulling. A problem that is often encountered with this type of prosthesis occurs when the prosthetic frame is severely twisted or pulled. The stump-activated lock bar occasionally becomes twisted, inhibiting the free forearm flexion and extension needed for operation.

With the advent of the Muenster prosthesis (Fig. 39–12), interest in the "locking lever" short below-elbow prosthesis diminished. Prosthetists and patients alike generally accept a modest limitation in flexion and exten-

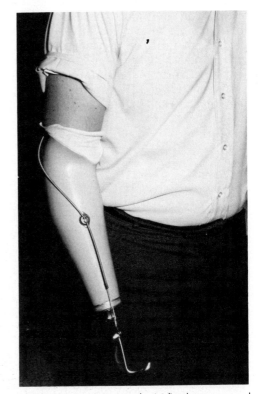

Figure 39–12. Muenster prosthesis fitted to a very short below-elbow amputation.

sion coupled with a more simple and trimmer prosthesis in preference to the alignment and fitting problems related to the stump-activated lock.

The standard of acceptance in the elbow disarticulation prosthesis is usually the outside-locking hinge. This unit comes in several sizes from the small child unit to the extra large, heavy-duty adult hinge. Care must be taken in application as the prosthesis tends to become bulky or wide at the elbow owing to necessary relief for the humeral condyles and the need to keep the hinges exactly parallel.

Normally, the locking half of the hinge is located on the medial side with from five to seven locking positions; the more "slim" free hinge is located laterally. Harnessing is accomplished by a normal figure-of-eight harness and elbow lock control in the normal deltopectoral triangle area and by a firm elastic under the lock cable to assist in returning the locking mechanism to neutral. Occasionally, with a well-contoured stump and good retaining musculature, the prosthetist can abbreviate the suspension to a simple figure-of-eight loop for terminal control and a heavy elastic for some socket retention and elbow lock cycle ability. This type of socket can often be worn mainly as a suction suspension with a sheath-type sock to facilitate donning and removing the limb. This arrangement is quite adaptable to the use of a hand—cosmetic, mechanical, or myoelectric terminal device. With a battery-operated hand, the elbow can be fabricated with a free swing and the hand activated with a myosensor in the socket or a switch control where the lock

normally attaches. Although this type of elbow system limits the lift ability of the amputee, it does give a lighter and more functionally cosmetic appliance for the "non–heavy duty" user.

Sometimes the elbow disarticulation is fitted with the standard type elbow using a turntable, outside-cable lock exit and a conventional above-elbow type of forearm. This adds the ability to rotate the forearm easily at the elbow turntable for various activities and gives a smaller elbow width through the condyle area. The disadvantage, of course, is the extended humeral section and shortened forearm, making approximation of the face, neck, and hair with terminal devices rather difficult.

TERMINAL DEVICES

A great many terminal devices are available for both the externally powered and body-powered upper limb prostheses. These include special purpose units, cosmetic hands that provide function, and the nonfunctional cosmetic "dress" hand. There is no specific terminal device most suited for the elbow disarticulation level. Patient preference will prevail (Fig. 39–13).

Most standard mechanical elbow units have eleven lock positions and are relatively strong. By comparison, the outside-lock internal mechanism units must necessarily be small and more delicate in engineering design, even in the strongest example of its type.

Much engineering research and development has been deployed on the elbow disarticulation and long above-elbow prosthesis since World War II. The older wood and

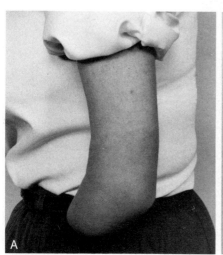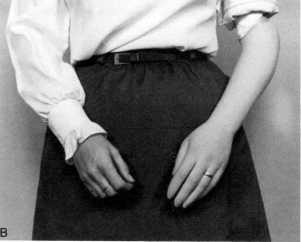

Figure 39–13. *A,* Very short below-elbow amputation retaining active elbow flexion and extension. *B,* Cosmetic replacement prosthesis.

rawhide limbs with manually locking elbows gradually gave way to fiber, metal, plastic, and composite materials; the Carnes arm with stump-controlled elbow flexion, supinating wrist flexion unit, and integral hand; the Fitch arm with its cleverly activated, nonlocking elbow controlled by flexion and extension of the humerus; and the Northrop-Sierra plastic laminated arm with the revolutionary inside-locking elbow controlled without manual operation by the sound hand. All are still available. More currently, various endoskeletal designs with soft, tissuelike contoured exteriors enhance the cosmesis and "touch" of the prosthesis. Unfortunately, all were somewhat inconsistent with elbow disarticulation amputation until the 1950s, when a real breakthrough in design occurred to help this particular amputee with his relatively trouble-free amputation. Prosthetists welcomed this new outside-locking hinge, located rather inconspicuously on the medial side of the arm. Most prosthetists enjoy the challenge of fitting one of these amputations. After trauma, this amputation is usually well designed surgically, strong, mobile, and not hypersensitive to prosthetic activity. Some 30 years later, prosthetists now look forward equally to more research with the current development using small electric motors, sensors, and batteries.

The surgeon, prosthetist, and engineer can coordinate their efforts to effect a technology transfer that will provide an effective, comfortable, and functional prosthesis that is suitable for the training and acquisition of numerous skills and affords the amputee an enhanced quality of life.

References

1. American Academy of Orthopedic Surgeons: Atlas of Limb Prosthetics: Surgical and Prosthetic Principles. St. Louis, C. V. Mosby Co., 1981.

2. Banerjee, S. N. (ed.): Rehabilitation Management of Amputees. Baltimore, Williams & Wilkins Co., 1982.

3. Burgess, E. M.: General Principles of Amputation Surgery. In American Academy of Orthopedic Surgeons: Atlas of Limb Prosthetics: Surgical and Prosthetic Principles. St. Louis, C. V. Mosby Co., 1981, pp. 14–18.

4. Burgess, E. M.: Postoperative Management. In American Academy of Orthopedic Surgeons: Atlas of Limb Prosthetics: Surgical and Prosthetic Principles. St. Louis, C. V. Mosby Co., 1981, pp. 19–23.

5. Burgess, E. M.: Wound Healing after Amputation: Effect of Controlled Environment Treatment. J. Bone Joint Surg. 60A:245, 1978.

6. Burkhalter, W. E., Mayfield, G., and Carmona, L. S.: The Upper Extremity Amputee. Early and Immediate Postsurgical Prosthetic Fitting. J. Bone Joint Surg. 58A:46, 1976.

7. Friedman, L. W. (ed.): The Surgical Rehabilitation of the Amputee. Springfield, Ill., Charles C Thomas, 1978.

8. Gerhardt, J. J., King, P. S., and Zettl, J. H.: Amputations: Immediate and Early Prosthetic Management. Bern, Hans Huber, 1982.

9. Hierton, T. (ed.): Amputations Kirurgi och Proteser. Uppsala, Tiden/Folksam, 1980.

10. Herndon, J. H. (ed.): Symposium on Orthopedic Surgery. Surg. Clin. North Am., 63:1, 1983.

11. Herndon, J. H., and LaNone, A. M.: Salvage of a Short Below-Knee Amputation with Pedicle Flap Coverage. Inter-Clin. Info. Bull. 12(7):5, 1973.

12. Kostuik, J. P. (ed.): Amputation Surgery and Rehabilitation. The Toronto Experience. New York, Churchill Livingstone, 1981.

13. Marquardt, E.: Amputationen im Bereich der Oberen Extremitaten. Vortrag auf der Unfallmedizinschen Arbeitstagung, Baden Baden, October, 1975.

14. Marquardt, E., and Neff, G.: The Angulation Osteotomy of Above-Elbow Stumps. Clin. Orthop. 104:232, 1974.

15. Marquardt, E., and Roesler, H.: Prothesen und Prothesenversorgungen der Oberen Extremitat. In Witt, A. N., Retig, H., Schlegel, F. K., Hackenbrock, M., and Hupfauer, W. (eds.): Orthopadie in Praxis und Klinik, Vol. 2. Stuttgart, Georg Thieme Verlag, 1981.

16. Nickel, V. L. (ed.): Orthopedic Rehabilitation. New York, Churchill Livingstone, 1982.

17. Schmidl, H.: The INAIL Experience Fitting Upper-Limb Dysmelia Patients with Myoelectric Control. Bull. Prosth. Res. 10(27):17, Spring, 1977.

18. Slocum, D. B. (ed.): An Atlas of Amputations. St. Louis, C. V. Mosby Co., 1949.

PART VI

Septic and Nontraumatic Conditions of the Elbow

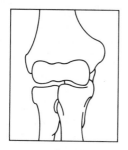

CHAPTER 40

Rheumatoid Arthritis

ALLAN E. INGLIS*

Rheumatoid arthritis of the elbow may seriously limit the overall function of the patient afflicted with this disease, and the process usually involves this joint within the first 5 years of onset.[13] Rheumatoid involvement of the elbow joint actually includes a variety of disease entities including systemic lupus erythematosus, psoriatic arthritis and enteropathic arthropathy, the variants of ankylosing spondylitis, or a combination of these diseases. These entities are discussed in Chapter 41. Early in the disease it may be only painful synovitis that limits flexion and extension of the elbow, thereby limiting the patient's capacity to bring the hand to the face or to extend the hand in space for useful work. A nonfunctional elbow, whether due to pain, weakness, or gross instability, is like attempting to answer the telephone by lifting the cord. In patients afflicted with rheumatoid arthritis, 20 to 50 per cent will ultimately show elbow involvement,[11, 34] and there is frequently involvement of the adjacent shoulder, wrist, and hand as well. A therapeutic program designed for the elbow must always include the needs of these articulations as well.

PATHOLOGY

Rheumatoid arthritis may disrupt elbow function in a variety of ways. The extent of involvement follows a rather characteristic pattern, thus allowing a reasonably reliable classification of the gross pathology (see below). Initially, the patient may have only an intense synovitis with painful distention of the joint capsule. This inflamed joint may be so involved that flexion and extension are restricted as well as rotation of the forearm. In about 10 per cent of patients, spontaneous resolution will occur (Fig. 40–1).[1] In an effort to relieve the pain and distention the patient frequently prefers to keep the elbow in a flexed position, resulting in a fixed flexion contracture. If the synovitis remains uncontrolled, the hyaline cartilage on the joint surfaces may be eroded in time, first at the edges and then eventually over the entire articular surface. As the hyaline cartilage is lost, cyst formation and small, bony excrescences or osteophytes appear along the margins of the joint (Fig. 40–2). These small bony excres-

*Appreciation is extended to Richard Tompkins, Rheumatology Department, Mayo Clinic, for the recommendations on medical management.

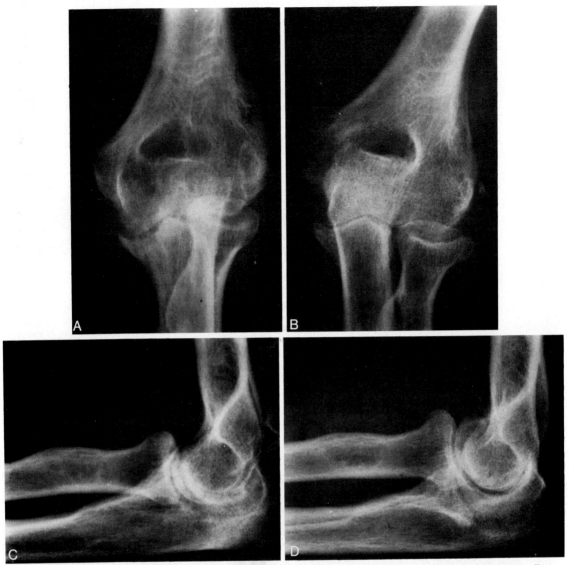

Figure 40–1. Elbow of a 49-year-old man with rheumatoid arthritis. *A,* Anteroposterior view showing osteopenia, effusion, erosion of bone, and cystic changes. *B,* Same elbow 7 years later. Bony surfaces are regular, and osteopenia is gone. *C,* Lateral view shows cystic changes in olecranon. *D,* Seven years later, cystic changes are gone. (From Bryan, R. S., and Morrey, B. F.: Rheumatoid arthritis of the elbow. *In* Evarts, C. M. (ed.): Surgery of the Musculoskeletal System, Vol. 2, no. 3. New York, Churchill Livingstone, 1983.)

cences interfere with the normal functioning of the joint capsule and ligamentous supports. As the destruction of the cartilaginous surface progresses, there is additional damage to the subchondral bone with loss of joint space and increasing degrees of elbow instability (Fig. 40–3). The joint gradually self-destructs and dissolves, resulting in a weak, unstable articulation (Fig. 40–4).

The rheumatoid synovitis may also directly affect the ligamentous support about the elbow.[2] Destruction of the annular ligament surrounding the radial neck may permit the radial head to become unstable and to be displaced anteriorly toward the antecubital fossa by the powerful unopposed biceps brachii muscle. This is particularly troublesome when the radial head has been eroded by the synovitis surrounding the radiocapitellar articulation. The anterior medial ligament is the major supporting, stabilizing ligament of the elbow joint.[31, 35] This ligament passes between the sublime tubercle of the ulna and the medial epicondyle of the humerus[25] and may be damaged or weakened by rheumatoid synovitis. Destruction or attenuation of this ligament, when combined with cartilaginous and bony loss, will result in gross medial-lateral instability of the elbow joint.

At times, the synovitis may be so intense

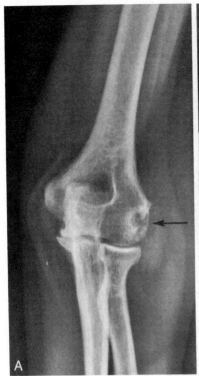

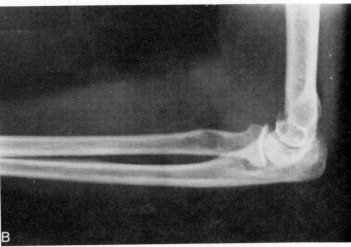

Figure 40–2. *A,* Radiograph of grade II rheumatoid disease of the elbow. Note the marginal osteophytes along the medial edges of the ulna and trochlea of the humerus. Also, there are early joint changes at the radiocapitellar joint. There is a large cyst in the capitellum beneath the humeral attachment of the lateral collateral ligament (arrow). *B,* Lateral radiograph of grade II rheumatoid disease showing good preservation of the articular surfaces of the trochlea of the humerus and of the semilunar notch of the ulna.

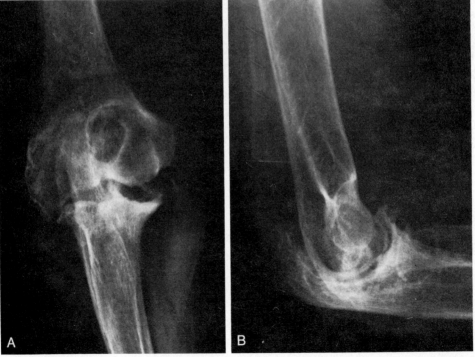

Figure 40–3. *A,* Anterior view of dominant joint in a 77-year-old female showing severe medial erosion and joint widening. *B,* Lateral view of the same joint shows severe erosion and thinning of the olecranon coronoid and radial head. (From Bryan, R. S., and Morrey, B. F.: Rheumatoid arthritis of the elbow. *In* Evarts, C. M. (ed.): Surgery of the Musculoskeletal System, Vol. 2, no. 3. New York, Churchill Livingstone, 1983.)

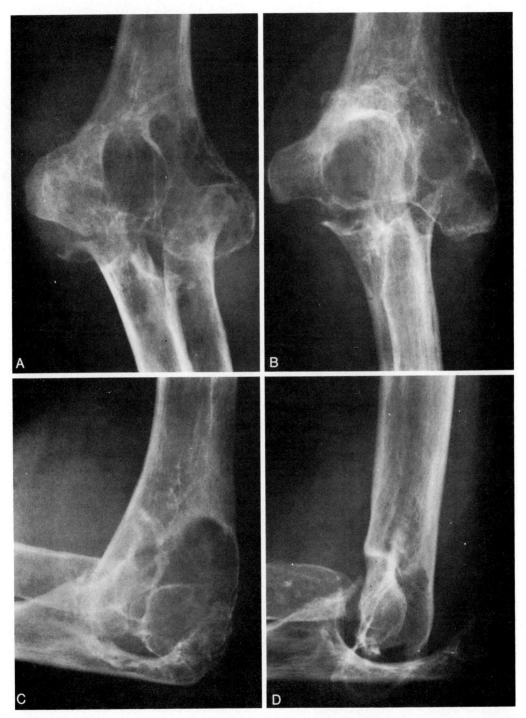

Figure 40–4. Elbow of a 51-year-old man with rheumatoid arthritis. *A, B,* Anteroposterior views taken 3 years apart show severe cystic involvement with progressive joint collapse. *C, D,* Lateral views of same patient taken 3 years apart, showing extreme bone resorption. (From Bryan, R. S., and Morrey, B. F.: Rheumatoid arthritis of the elbow. *In* Evarts, C. M. (ed.): Surgery of the Musculoskeletal System, Vol. 2, no. 3. New York, Churchill Livingstone, 1983.)

that large evaginations of synovium and capsule may extend distally into the forearm (Fig. 40–5), giving rise to forearm vascular, neural,[28] and muscular dysfunction. Additionally, the synovitis may be of sufficient severity that it will produce a small synovial and capsular herniation medially into the cubital tunnel, causing direct compression on the ulnar nerve with concomitant ulnar nerve signs and symptoms (Fig. 40–6). The rheumatoid synovitis may also produce intraosseous synovial cysts within the intra-articular portion of the humerus and the coronoid (Fig. 40–5) or the olecranon processes (Fig. 40–4) of the ulna. These cysts may also be seen in the trochlea (Fig. 40–4A) and in the capitellum (Fig. 40–2). The process may become so extensive that the overlying bone may give way, resulting in a state in which the elbow joint actually caves in on itself (Fig. 40–4B).

Rheumatoid disease may also involve the olecranon bursa. This bursa may become so distended that not only is it cosmetically

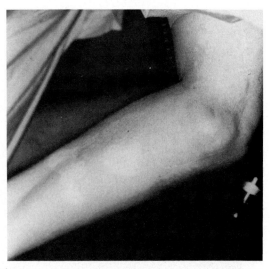

Figure 40–6. Recurrent mass behind the medial epicondyle. Two prior local excisions had failed to relieve symptoms of ulnar neuropathy. Following elbow synovectomy and debridément, patient has had no further joint or nerve symptoms.

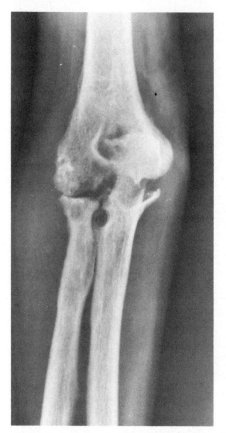

Figure 40–5. Radiograph of grade III-A rheumatoid disease of the elbow. Note the cysts beneath the thin subchondral bone. As these cysts enlarge, the subchondral bone weakens and collapses. This results in loss of joint surface integrity and support, which in turn results in instability. Note cystic changes distal to the radioulnar joint and of the coronoid.

unpleasing but also it reduces the function of the upper extremity, particularly in patients who must write or rest their arms on flat surfaces at work. At times, in addition to bursitis, the patient may develop rheumatoid nodules on the extensor surface of the ulna. These nodules may be large and multiple. Because of their location, these bursae and nodules are both prone to local irritation and secondary infections.

CLASSIFICATION

Several classifications of rheumatoid arthritis have been suggested. Some are based on clinical presentation and functional implications.[37] The Hospital for Special Surgery classification of rheumatoid arthritis defines the degree or level of joint involvement as determined by clinical and radiographic criteria. Grade I disease indicates only a mild to moderate degree of synovitis and no radiographic changes and is managed with aspirin or nonsteroidal, anti-inflammatory drugs. Grade II synovitis indicates a recalcitrant synovitis that cannot be managed with aspirin and requires intermittent arthrocentesis and steroid injection for control. The roentgenogram shows minimal architectural changes (Fig. 40–2). Grade III-A disease indicates unremitting, active synovitis and variable signs of joint articular damage with or without cyst formation (Figs. 40–5 and 40–7). Grade III-B disease occurs when there is extensive articular damage as well as loss of nearby sub-

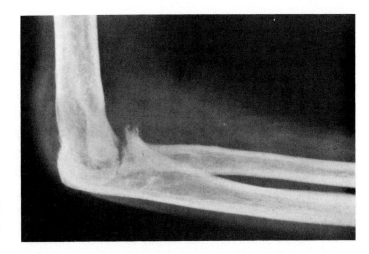

Figure 40–7. Lateral radiograph of grade III-A rheumatoid disease of the elbow. Note the loss of the normal contour of the semilunar notch of the ulna and of the radial head. The trochlea of the humerus is eroded.

chondral bone and gross ligamentous instability (Fig. 40–4) or ankylosis of the joint (Fig. 40–8). These classifications are useful to the treating physician as an aid in designing a therapeutic program. Further, this classification may be applied not only to rheumatoid arthritis but also to any of the other varieties of rheumatoid conditions.

EVALUATION

It should always be kept in mind that rheumatoid disease of the elbow is only part of a systemic disorder in which other joints or organ systems may be involved. Therefore, a complete evaluation of the patient and his disease is required. Surgical assessment of the disease should always be conducted in concert with a rheumatologist or other physician who is fully acquainted with the complexities of rheumatoid arthritis. A careful historical study must be made of the patient's problems, including the duration, severity, and extent of the disease. Additionally, an assessment of the patient's life needs, both vocational and avocational, must be determined.

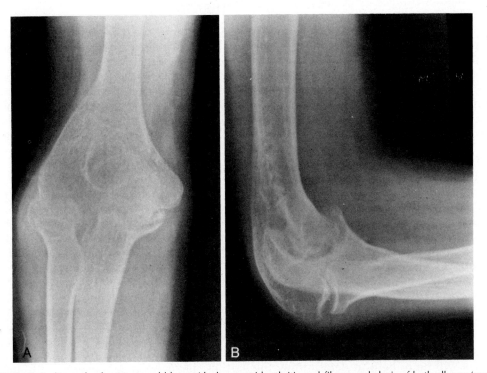

Figure 40–8. A, Radiograph of a 15-year-old boy with rheumatoid arthritis and fibrous ankylosis of both elbows (grade III-B). Both elbows underwent replacement arthroplasty. Patient is now a third-year student in medical school and is asymptomatic. B, Preoperative bony overgrowth of capitellum, trochlea, and semilunar notch of ulna.

Besides routine laboratory studies, special laboratory determinations including sedimentation rate, latex fixation, HLA titers, and complement level should be obtained to assess the type and severity of the disease. *All joints should be studied for synovitis, stability, range of motion, and pain.* Radiographs of the involved joints should be obtained.

Physical Examination. Examination of the elbow joint with symptomatic rheumatoid synovitis may be difficult (see Chapter 4). Inspection of the joint may reveal the presence of an involved olecranon bursa or rheumatoid nodules. The patient is asked to demonstrate an active range of flexion, extension, and rotation of the forearm, which should be carefully noted and recorded. Additional passive motion, particularly of flexion, should also be recorded. A fixed internal block to motion is suggested when passive and active motion are equal. However, if the passive range of motion exceeds the active motion range, then the problem may be due to guarding from painful synovitis or a fluid-filled, distended joint.

Careful evaluation of ulnar nerve function will provide data about possible compression of the ulnar nerve by synovitis bulging out between the trochlea of the humerus and the semilunar notch of the olecranon process. Inability to extend the fingers may be due to extensor tendon rupture or posterior interosseous nerve dysfunction from synovitis at the elbow.[28] Normally, the articular margins in the elbow are difficult to locate and palpate. The only articular margin that can be uniformly palpated is the radiocapitellar articulation, just distal to the lateral epicondyle of the elbow. Even this joint cannot be identified with any degree of accuracy when the elbow is in flexion. However, in extension, the joint can be accurately located by palpation and studied by rotating the forearm. With the elbow in extension, the radial head can be felt to rotate against the capitellum. Frequently, in this same area there will be palpable bulging of the synovium. Only two standard radiographs are of value in the radiographic assessment of the elbow joint. True lateral and anteroposterior views are sufficient. Frequently, however, the requested true lateral is in fact somewhat oblique (Fig. 40–8B), and this may lead to a distorted lateral study of the joint. Oblique radiographs are confusing and unnecessary. If an implant arthroplasty is anticipated, radiographs taken at 60 inches will be of help in determining the true medullary geometry of the ulna and the humerus. If indicated, a more detailed geometric evaluation of the humerus and ulna can be obtained by calibrated computed tomography (CT) scans.

Arthrocentesis of the elbow joint for diagnosis or therapeutic purposes is always accomplished from the lateral side of the joint. Attempted aspiration of the elbow joint medially risks the possibility of injuring the ulnar nerve, which lies directly over the ulnohumeral joint. The forearm can be rotated enough so that the exact interval between the radius and the capitellum can be determined. Arthrocentesis performed with a large diameter needle is somewhat difficult owing to the curved shape of the radial head and the capitellum and the narrow interval between these two structures.

After the completion of the history and physical and radiographic examinations, the diagnosis and overall plan of treatment can be designed and discussed with the patient based on the extent or classification of the disease process. The natural history of the disease and the therapeutic priorities should be discussed in detail. Although 10 per cent will enjoy a remission,[1] an equal or greater number develop a progressive and relentless course. Most (80 per cent) will be confronted by chronic, slow progression of the synovitis.[13]

TREATMENT

Rheumatoid synovitis of the elbow can usually be managed by nonsurgical conservative measures. Rheumatoid arthritis is a chronic disease, and its management requires a long-term commitment from the treating physician. Education of the patient about the nature of the disease is most important. Modification of lifestyle and work habits may be necessary.

Nonoperative Treatment

Medical therapy is usually initiated with a salicylate, most commonly aspirin. The ideal serum salicylate level is 20 mg per 100 ml. In some patients tinnitus or upper gastrointestinal tract intolerance limits the use of salicylates. In these instances, one of the nonsteroidal anti-inflammatory drugs (NSAID) can be used (Table 40–1).[35a] These medications are therapeutically equivalent, but they have different doses and schedules of administration. Although the nonsteroidal drugs have more gastrointestinal tolerance than aspirin, they have been associated with headache, tinnitus, gastric intolerance, peptic ulcer disease, abnormal liver function tests, diarrhea,

Table 40–1. **Nonsteroidal Anti-inflammatory Drugs**

Drug	Dose
Anthranilic acids	
Meclofenamate (Meclumen)	50–100 mg 3 or 4 times a day
Arylalkanoic acids	
Fenoprofen (Nalfon)	300–600 mg 3 times a day
Ibuprofen (Brufen, Motrin)	400–600 3 or 4 times a day
Naproxen (Naprosyn)	250–500 mg 2 times a day
Indoleacetic acids	
Indomethacin (Indocin)	25–50 mg 3 or 4 times a day
Sulindac (Clinoil)	150–200 mg 2 times a day
Tolmetin (Tolectin)	400 mg 3 times a day
Oxicams	
Piroxicam (Feldene)	10–20 mg once a day
Pyrazolones	
Phenylbutazone (Azolid, Butazolidin)	100 mg 3 or 4 times a day— no longer than 7 days
Oxyphenbutazone (Tandearil)	100 mg 3 or 4 times a day— no longer than 7 days
Salicylates	
Acetylsalicylic acid (aspirin)	600–900 mg 4 times a day
Choline magnesium trisalicylate (Trilisate)	500 mg 2 times a day
Diflunisal (Dolobid)	500 mg immediately, then 250–500 mg 2 times a day
Salicylosalicylic acid (Disalcid)	1000 mg 2 or 3 times a day
Sodium salicylate	600–900 mg 4 times a day

cross sensitivity with aspirin, and renal failure.[3a]

Neither salicylates nor NSAIDs influence the eventual outcome of rheumatoid arthritis. Patients who develop the chronic form of the disease deserve a trial of a disease-remitting agent (Table 40–2).[34a] In mild disease, an antimalarial can be tried, but if the disease is progressive, either a gold salt or D-penicillamine is tried. Usually, gold is employed first and D-penicillamine is reserved for patients who do not respond to gold therapy. D-Penicillamine can, however, be used before gold therapy. Both drugs can have serious side effects such as leukopenia, thrombocytopenia, and progenuria. Further, D-penicillamine can be associated with fever, myopathy, pulmonary reactions, serositis, and glomerulonephritis. It is precisely because of these additional potential side effects that gold is tried first, although gold must be administered parenterally whereas D-penicillamine is given orally.

Table 40–2. **Disease-Remitting Agents**

Aurothioglucose (Solganal)
Gold sodium thiomalate (Myochrysine)
Hydroxychloroquine (Plaquenil)
D-Penicillamine (Cuprimine, D-Pen)

Table 40–3. **Immunosuppressive Agents**

Alkylating agents
  Chlorambucil
  Cyclophosphamide
Folic acid antagonists
  Methotrexate
Purine analogues
  Azathioprine

Both require careful monitoring through periodic complete blood counts and urinalysis.

Immunosuppressive agents (Table 40–3) are reserved for relentlessly progressive disease that is unresponsive to less toxic therapy.[34b] The administration must be carefully monitored, and the patient should be fully informed about the potential risks and benefits.

Corticosteroids are frequently used in the management of rheumatoid arthritis. These drugs function as nonspecific anti-inflammatory agents, but although they provide symptomatic relief, they do not influence the ultimate course of the disease. Hypercortisonism can be more devastating than the disease and should be avoided, but most patients tolerate doses of less than 7.5 mg predisone daily reasonably well.

Basic physical medicine principles of rest, range of motion, and muscle conditioning are important. Rest may require the use of simple,

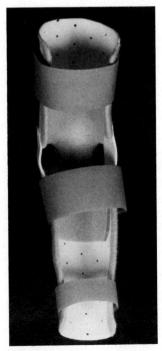

Figure 40–9. Well-padded resting splint secured with Velcro straps. Patient usually wears a loose-fitting stockinette to prevent any local skin irritation.

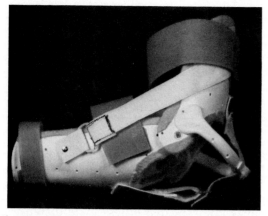

Figure 40–10. The adjustable flexion-extension splint. The side and posterior straps are adjustable. Usually the patient alternates nightly between flexion and extension depending on the motion deficiencies.

static splints (Fig. 40–9). These can be fabricated in an occupational therapy department or can be made in the physician's office with plaster and secured with a loose-fitting Ace bandage. The device can be worn at night or when the patient expects to be carrying out activities that usually cause pain. This treatment modality is extremely useful in reducing synovitis and pain, and the splints are not costly. When instability is the major symptom, a dynamic splint that permits flexion and extension but limits lateral and medial movements may be employed (Fig. 40–10). When the dynamic splints are fabricated, they should be as lightweight as possible and carefully padded to avoid local irritation over the epicondyles, olecranon process, and long diaphysis of the ulna. In general, however, the simple resting splints are sufficient for the relief of painful synovitis.

In our experience, corticosteroid injections into the elbow joint are of considerable value in controlling painful synovitis. Therapeutic, intra-articular injections are performed with a small-diameter, short needle inserted directly between the radial head and the capitellum, usually all the way to the hilt. If the needle cannot be completely inserted, it is incorrectly placed and should be redirected into the center of the joint. Long-acting corticosteroids are recommended because of their prolonged effect. Many physicians also inject a small amount of long-lasting local anesthetic, thereby affording the patient some degree of immediate pain relief. Although this is a temporary measure, it may provide a helpful level of relief during the period when other systemic medications are gradually beginning to become effective.

The goal of initial treatment of painful syn-ovitis of the elbow joint is, therefore, to provide adequate systemic medications, rest the joint with splints, and, if necessary, administer local steroid injections within the joint itself. If these measures fail to bring the problem under control, then other therapeutic modalities must be considered.

Operative Treatment

Extra-articular Procedures

Rheumatoid involvement of the olecranon bursa may be treated locally with aspiration and steroid injections. Usually, however, the local steroid injections are of short-term benefit because the synovitis is of the proliferating type and is combined with an inflamed, thickened bursal capsule. Communication with the joint is occasionally seen. If surgical removal of rheumatoid nodules or the olecranon bursa is needed, the patient must be advised that these nodules or bursa may recur or new nodules may appear. Removal of nodules or bursa should *not* be combined with other surgery on the upper extremity because, first, the surgery can be very time-consuming, thereby compromising the primary surgical procedure, and second, these wounds will occasionally heal by secondary intention, thus complicating a postoperative rehabilitation program. This "minor" surgery may therefore place other surgical sites at risk due to postoperative infection.

Intra-articular Procedures

Surgical therapy for uncontrolled rheumatoid disease within the elbow should be considered when conservative measures have failed to bring the problem under control. Frequently, these patients may have severe disabling arthritis of multiple joints, all of which require surgical treatment. In general, surgical therapy should be directed to those joints that are most painful and disabling to the patient, whether they are the weight-bearing or the upper extremity joints. At times, the surgeon should consider the use of two teams so that one can, for example, carry out corrective foot surgery while the other is performing corrective elbow surgery. This has the obvious advantage of reducing the total number of anesthetics and rehabilitation periods. These patients frequently do not have the emotional strength to undergo multiple hospitalizations for corrective surgery, and these procedures might thus be optimally combined to minimize hospitalization, surgical stresses, and the physical dependency that this treatment entails.

If there are multiple major disabilities in the upper extremity, a decision must be made about whether the hand, wrist, elbow, or shoulder has precedence. The most painful articulation must be corrected first. However, if all factors are equal, the treatment plan should proceed centripetally, that is, the hand and wrist should be corrected first, followed by the elbow and shoulder. The hand should receive prime consideration because if this function is limited, the ultimate result of elbow surgery will be commensurably decreased. Therefore, when the hand has been successfully treated, surgical therapy for the elbow can be recommended. When the elbow is functioning satisfactorily, attention can then be directed to the shoulder. If the reverse plan is instituted, that is, correction is done first of the shoulder, then of the elbow, and finally of the hand, but a poor surgical result occurs with the hand, the other two operations will have been for nothing. Additionally, a poor result following hand surgery, such as a wound infection or wound slough, places the prior arthroplasties at risk of infection. Again, it is highly desirable to have a well-functioning hand before elbow surgery is undertaken.

Arthrodesis

The most definitive surgical procedure for a painful, unstable elbow joint is arthrodesis. This produces a painless, functionless joint, but there are rarely, if ever, any indications for this treatment in rheumatoid disease of the elbow (see Chapter 36). Loss of ulnar and humeral bone stock makes it difficult to achieve the necessary apposition of the bone ends to produce a solid arthrodesis. More important, however, there is nearly always rheumatoid disease in the adjacent shoulder and hand joints. An arthrodesed rigid elbow places an increased functional burden on these nearby joints. Therefore, with the exception of the cervical spine and the foot, and at times the wrist and hand, there is little role for joint fusion in patients with rheumatoid arthritis. These patients need flexibility with stability and motion, particularly when considering the generalized nature of their disease and the high possibility of disease involvement with the contiguous articulations.

Interposition Arthroplasty

Fascial arthroplasty has been used in patients with severe rheumatoid arthritis of the elbow where there is either ankylosis or gross instability. Certain patients with painful synovitis in which there has been gross destruction of the elbow joint have successfully undergone this procedure. The joint is débrided and the remaining bony surfaces sculptured and covered with a layer of fascia lata or other interposition substance such as fat, skin, or Gelfoam.[15, 19, 42] Although this operation was initially designed for post-traumatic ankylosis, gratifying results have been reported in patients with rheumatoid arthritis.[19, 42] Our experience with this procedure has also been satisfactory. Even when the patient has a rather alarming degree of medial-lateral instability, sufficient flexion and extension are usually obtained to carry out most activities of daily living. The result of this procedure is considered satisfactory if about 90 degrees of near-painless motion with mild instability is attained. Using this standard, about 75 to 80 per cent of results have been satisfactory.[19, 42]

Fascial arthroplasty has been used less in patients with rheumatoid arthritis in most major centers since the early 1970s, when implant replacement arthroplasty became available. Since that time, joint replacement has been the procedure of choice in patients with grades III-A and III-B disease who have unstable elbows due to loss of joint surfaces and in patients with ankylosis in whom motion with stability and power is required.[7, 10, 14, 21]

Synovectomy

First described at the turn of the century for the knee by Mignon,[16] this procedure was soon adapted to the elbow.[39] Elbow synovectomy and débridement has proved to be an effective method of managing patients with grade II involvement.[8, 12, 20] In these patients, there is uncontrolled, painful synovitis of the elbow joint with pain and limitation of function. At the same time, there is no extensive joint or ligamentous destruction. Although some have suggested chemical synovectomy,[9] such as with osmic acid,[32] the potential for cartilage damage with such agents[18, 29] has limited this approach in this country.[6]

Hence, surgery is preferred and should be performed early before there is gross joint destruction rather than later when the more destructive grade III levels of disease have occurred. Yet, according to some, even rather extensive involvement is not a contraindication to synovectomy.[8, 34, 40]

There are only two major contraindications to synovectomy and débridement. The first, already alluded to, is the presence of gross joint destruction and instability. The second is the presence of severe stiffness resulting from inflammatory fibroarthrosis. In this situation, there is capsular and ligamentous scarring and thickening that will not respond postoperatively to even the best designed rehabilitation program. Yet when the painful synovial lining of a stiff joint has been completely excised, pain relief may be observed.[43] However, some patients may go on to complete fibrous or bony ankylosis.[20]

There are several versions of this operation depending on whether the radial head is excised and the extent to which the synovectomy is carried out. Simple synovectomy without removal of the radial head has been reported with adequate results.[8, 44] Excision of the radial head has, however, become the accepted practice.[4, 5, 24, 34]

A limited, subtotal synovectomy with removal of the radial head performed through a lateral approach to the elbow joint is the common procedure.[3, 4, 24, 27, 34, 40, 41, 44] This allows for removal of the bulk of the synovium within the elbow joint, but it is not possible to remove all the synovium along the medial joint recesses or posteriorly within the olecranon fossa. This limited synovectomy has, however, proved extremely useful in many surgeons' hands[8, 27, 40] because the short du-

ration of the surgical procedure makes it compatible with a wrist or hand operation. In fact, repeat synovectomy has even been reported as successful in some instances.[34]

Synovectomy and débridement, using a transolecranon approach, has been frequently used with excellent results.[20] With this approach, an osteotomy is performed through the midportion of the olecranon process, allowing reflection of the proximal olecranon with the triceps muscle. This approach allows an extensive exposure of the elbow joint (Fig. 40–11A, B). A radial head resection is then carried out, and a complete anterior synovectomy, including removal of the synovium from the anterior aspect of the joint along the medial joint recesses, and a complete synovectomy of the posterior aspect of the joint can then be accomplished. The removal of the damaged radial head improves rotation of the forearm, but it also reduces impingement problems between the radial head and the capitellum. Although suggested by some,[26, 38] we have not found that silicone radial head replacement is useful or strictly necessary in a patient with rheumatoid disease of the elbow. The olecranon fragment is replaced with

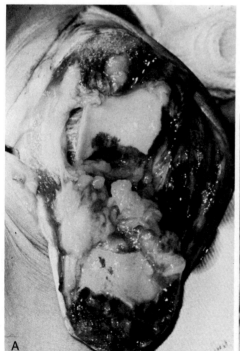
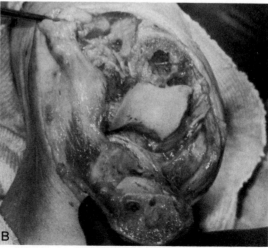

Figure 40–11. *A,* Exposure of the posterior aspect of the elbow joint through the transolecranon approach. In the center is the well-preserved trochlea with a small area of pannus. Note proliferative synovitis and the rheumatoid cyst in the osteotomized olecranon process. *B,* Appearance of the elbow after synovectomy and débridement. The radial head has been removed and an anterior synovectomy completed. Note the pitting and penetration of the cartilage and subchondral bone beneath the area where the pannus has been excised.

an olecranon screw, and then the osteotomy site is further secured with a figure-of-eight wire. The fragment is made secure enough that early motion can be initiated.

More recently, synovectomy and débridement has been performed through a medial triceps flap approach as described by Bryan and Morrey.[5] With this surgical approach, the triceps muscle, along with the portion of the epimysium of the flexor carpi ulnaris, is elevated as a laterally based flap (see Chapter 8). The radial head is easily exposed and excised. The entire elbow articulation can then be viewed and a complete synovectomy performed. The triceps flap is repositioned and secured well enough to allow early motion. This approach eliminates the possible complications of failure of the olecranon fixation that can occur with the transolecranon approach, especially when the sigmoid fossa has expanded, leaving little bone (Fig. 40–4D).

Rehabilitation following synovectomy and débridement is of great importance. All patients should be advised that it may be necessary for them to remain in the hospital under active treatment for 10 days to 2 weeks following their surgery. Indeed, the major portion of their hospitalization will be spent in the rehabilitation programs. Whether the limited or complete synovectomy, the transolecranon, or the triceps flap approach has been used, all patients should begin active flexion and extension within 3 to 4 days following surgery or when the wound is sealed. Protective splints are used when the patient is not actively participating in the exercise program (Fig. 40–9). Active and active resistive exercises are emphasized. Occasionally, active assistive flexion exercises may also be required. This assistive exercise program must be carefully monitored to be certain that excessive force is not applied to the olecranon osteotomy or to the triceps repair. Rarely, in certain patients with very low pain thresholds, a gentle examination under general anesthesia may prove useful early to lyse adhesions.

Results. The results reported in the literature are surprisingly consistent (Table 40–4). Most patients will experience a functional range of motion.[30] Motion is usually unchanged (45 per cent) but improves in about 40 per cent and decreases slightly in another 15 per cent. Instability has not been a major problem. Most important, relief of pain is regularly seen in about 90 per cent of patients for about 3 years (Fig. 40–12). The 5-year overall success rate is therefore about 75 to 80 per cent.[6] Recurrence of the synovitis is, however, common after about 5 years. Of interest is that similar results are reported even if rather significant joint destruction is present preoperatively.[8, 40] Finally, failure of the procedure does not preclude further reconstructive measures including replacement arthroplasty.

Complications. The major complications with synovectomy and débridement are usually technical and thus are avoidable. Ankylosis may occur if the operation is performed in an individual with a stiffening form of arthritis or in whom there are major psychological barriers to a rehabilitation program. Breakage of the olecranon fixation devices occurred in 8 per cent of our patients who underwent synovectomy and débridement through a transolecranon approach. If the olecranon fossa is moderately eroded, the osteotomy is done through a thin portion of bone (Fig. 40–4D), thus causing potential problems of union, and thus should be avoided in this patient. This complication usually did not require reoperation or affect the long-term result, and the patients did not have weakness in triceps or elbow extensor function. This complication is now avoided with the triceps-sparing approach.

As noted above, the condition of a number of patients undergoing synovectomy who initially did well was found to have deteriorated with the passage of time. In our experience, these patients had grade III disease initially, and their elbows were already architecturally damaged. Contrary to the opinion of others,[8, 34] these patients would be candidates for replacement arthroplasty in our judgment today.

Joint Replacement Arthroplasty

This topic has been discussed in detail in Chapters 34 and 35. However, because rheumatoid arthritis is currently the best indication for this operation, we shall briefly outline our philosophy and technique of joint replacement arthroplasty.

Patients with grades III-A and III-B levels of disease in whom there has already been destruction of the articular surfaces or of ligamentous support have in the past posed a difficult problem for the reconstructive surgeon.[33] Early in the 1970s joint replacement arthroplasty first became available. Arthritis surgeons in the United States, aware of the disappointing results from replacement arthroplasty achieved in Britain owing to implant loosening,[10, 36] designed devices to reduce the torque forces across the bone-cement

Table 40–4. **Result of Elbow Synovectomy for Rheumatoid Arthritis**

Author	Year	No. of Procedures	No. of Radial Heads Removed	Recommended Approach	Result							Follow-Up (mo)	
					Pain Relief		Motion (%)			Satisfac-tory		Mean	Range
					No.	%	Gained	No Change	Lost				
Laine and Vainio[24]	1969	92	92	Lateral and medial	71	77	39	48	13	80		12	?
Torgerson and Leach[41]	1970	5	5	Lateral	5	100	5	0	0	100		29	24–60
Inglis et al.[20]	1971	28	28(9)[a]	Transolecranon	28	100	54	18	28	89		42	12–72
Marmor[27]	1972	19	19(10)[a]	Posterior lateral	13	68	36	32	32	92		42	8–89
Wilson et al.[44]	1973	55	28	Lateral and medial	51	92	54	32	14	78		19	6–48
Porter et al.[34]	1974	154	154	Lateral and medial	—	—	16	68	16	71		29	12–72
Brattstrom[4]	1975	118	118	Lateral	91	87	38	52	10	83		45	15–72
Taylor et al.[40]	1976	44	44	Lateral	38	86	0	0	11	91		60	6–96
Copeland and Taylor[8]	1979	30	16	Lateral and medial	22	88	73	23	3	80		51	12–120
Eichenblat et al.[12]	1982	25	25	Lateral	22	88	80	0	20	100		60	24–132
Total		560	529		341	83	38	46	16	80		34	6–96

[a]Darrah procedure.

Modified from Bryan, R. S., and Morrey, B. F.: Rheumatoid Arthritis of the Elbow. In Evarts, C. M. (ed.): Surgery of the Musculoskeletal System. London, Churchill Livingstone, 1983.

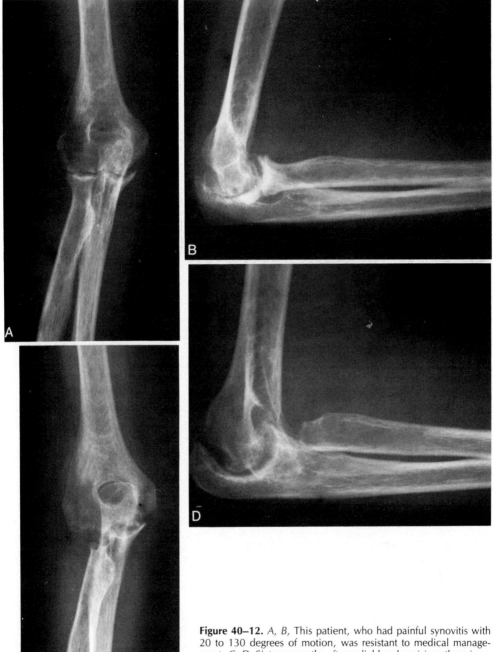

Figure 40–12. *A, B,* This patient, who had painful synovitis with 20 to 130 degrees of motion, was resistant to medical management. *C, D,* Sixteen months after radial head excision, there is no pain, motion has not changed, and she has returned to an active job.

bond by preventing loosening of the implant, and replacement arthroplasty then became a viable surgical procedure.[7, 14, 21]

Two approaches have been followed. In one, a cemented resurfacing type of replacement retains the ligamentous structures and the surrounding muscles for joint stability.[14] The other uses a bearing system that has sufficient laxity to prevent high torsional impact loading on the prosthetic bone–cement interface but provides stability independent of ligamentous integrity. At this time, we recommend implant arthroplasty for patients with grades III-A and III-B rheumatoid disease of the elbow, including even active, youthful patients with grade III disease. Patients with disabling ankylosis, in a poorly functioning position, may also be considered for elbow replacement arthroplasty if hand and shoulder function is adequate.

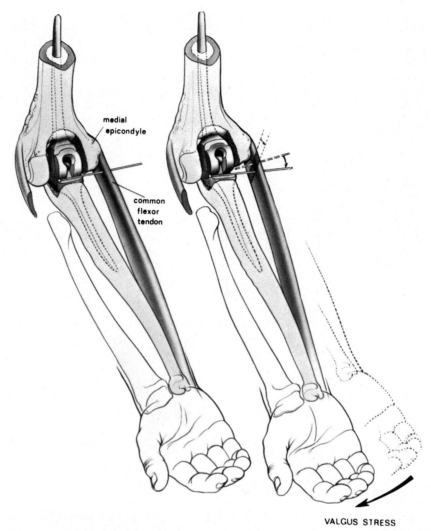

medial
epicondyle

common
flexor
tendon

VALGUS STRESS

Figure 40–13. Diagrammatic illustration of the muscular protection of the implant. The effect of the epicondyle is the muscle space times the distance from the muscle to the inner edge of the prosthesis *squared*. Hence, the wider the epicondyles, the greater the reduction of torque force at the cement-bone interface.

Contraindications for implant arthroplasty in rheumatoid arthritis are, first, severe prior septic arthritis. The surgeon must be aware that patients with rheumatoid arthritis are prone to sepsis.[17] Destruction of the medial and lateral epicondyles is also a contraindication. Our bioengineering studies have pointed out the need for the medial and lateral epicondyles and their muscular attachments. These attachments, through their normal viscoelastic tension and stretch reflexes, tend to minimize the torque forces across the bone-cement bond in the humerus (Fig. 40–13). In our series of more than 90 elbow implants, we have only one loose humeral component and no loose ulnar components. The only loose humeral component occurred in an elderly patient with an old supracondylar frac-

ture who had no medial or lateral epicondyles.

Preferred Technique. Within the last 4 years, the surgical technology for elbow implant surgery has improved immensely[22] (see Chapter 34). Earlier surgical techniques resulted in high levels of soft tissue complications.[23] The triceps insertion was incised to gain access to the joint and closed at the end of the procedure as a flap. We now employ the medial triceps reflection exposure (discussed above and in Chapter 8).

A trial reduction with the implant in place must be performed after preparation of the ulna and humerus to ensure that the elbow joint can be fully extended. If not, more bone may have to be removed, usually from the distal humerus or occasionally from the proximal ulna. Physical therapy will not achieve more motion than that attained in the operating room. The triceps muscle must be accurately reattached to the olecranon process, but must not be excessively advanced because this may increase triceps muscle tension and prevent flexion of the elbow. This attachment should be tested at the time of reattachment to be certain that the correct triceps tension has been achieved.

The elbow is placed in 45 degrees of extension, thereby reducing local tissue tension surrounding the implant. The dressings are changed on the third postoperative day. If the wound is dry and sealed, the rehabilitation program is initiated. The main purpose is to encourage active and active resistive flexion exercises of the elbow. Pronation and supination exercises are also started at this time. Assistive flexion and extension are cautiously administered if the elbow is slow to achieve the desired daily goals in the rehabilitation program. On rare occasions, in patients with low pain thresholds, we have used an examination under general anesthesia and gentle manipulation.

The patient should achieve the preoperative functional goals before discharge from the hospital. These goals consist of the capacity to reach the back of the head and to extend the elbow to 30 degrees. When the patient has achieved this level of movement, he can be discharged and followed closely on a home rehabilitation program. Patients are provided with a flexion extension splint secured with Velcro straps (Fig. 40–10). This splint has a hinge that allows placement in flexion one night and extension the next, for emphasis of whatever mode of motion is needed. This splint also has a rubber band–loaded device that can be used to increase extension when needed. The device is fabricated individually, thereby maximizing comfort and use by the patient.

Initially, the complications of total elbow arthroplasty were related to surgical technique. When using the triceps attachment and repair technique we have had no triceps dehiscence, wound slough, or hematomas, all of which were related to the soft tissue aspects of the surgery. In our group of 90 cases, we have had three patients in which an epicondyle has been fractured either during the operation or during the rehabilitation period. All of these have healed promptly and have not compromised the final result. Two patients, neither of whom had rheumatoid arthritis, had persistent ulnar neuropathy consisting of dysesthesias and hypalgesia. Neither of these patients noted any ulnar nerve motor loss. Two patients in our series have had persistent dislocation of the snap-fit bushing system.[21] Both of these patients have required reoperation and replacement of the high-density polyethylene bushing system. Preoperative assessment should have suggested that these patients were vulnerable to this complication because they had poor quality tissues and extremely weak upper extremities. This problem could have been avoided if an implant with a fixed axle, still retaining the laxity design, had been recommended and used.

Another complication worth emphasizing occurred when a patient sustained a nondisplaced fracture between the tip of the humeral component and the tip of a total shoulder humeral component (Fig. 40–14). This small isthmus of bone between the stems of the implant did not possess sufficient strength to sustain the load requirements of this patient.

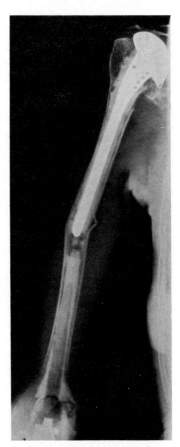

Figure 40–14. Radiograph of a fracture between two cemented implants. Better operative planning could have avoided this complication by shortening the stems of these implants or reinforcing the diaphyseal interspace.

Preoperative planning should be performed to prevent this complication by either shortening both humeral stems, thereby lengthening the area for more uniform dispersal of force, or reinforcing the area between the stems with cement and fine wires.

The results achieved in elbow implant arthroplasty in patients with rheumatoid arthritis have been excellent. Patients should expect 120 degrees of flexion and extension to 35 degrees. Many patients will gain nearly full extension. Pronation and supination should exceed 40 degrees in each quadrant. Freedom from pain is uniform.

Finally, these patients are cautioned to avoid all activities that involve high-impact loading. This includes hammering, tennis, golf, and so on. We have many patients who are able to use canes and crutches within 3 weeks of elbow replacement arthroplasty. The possible need for ambulatory assists is an obvious and important consideration in patients with rheumatoid arthritis, who always face the possibility of lower extremity involvement requiring the use of canes and crutches. Postoperatively, both vocational and avocational caveats about the implant frequently go unheeded by these patients once there is relief of pain and restoration of strength and motion. However, implant material failure remains uncommon.

In summary, the successful overall management of a patient with rheumatoid arthritis of the elbow is complex. The managing physician must first assess the general condition of the patient and then determine the activity of the disease within the elbow articulation. A specialist in rheumatoid arthritis should seek an early orthopedic consultation, both for elbow assessment and for an overall musculoskeletal evaluation, and then recommend a comprehensive treatment program. Similarly, the orthopedic surgeon should seek the assistance of a rheumatologist or someone experienced in the field of rheumatology for his or her assessment and recommendations for the medical management of the patient's multisystem disease. These two physicians should devise an overall program that should include the assistance of social workers, physical therapists, occupational therapists, and psychological counselors.

The initial thrust of treatment is to assure the patient that the problem will be brought under control with the simplest and most uncomplicated treatment program possible. The initial treatment should consist of resting splints and medication. If this fails to achieve the desired response, then arthrocentesis and intra-articular steroid injection should be tried. A careful range of motion exercise program should be initiated to reduce stiffness and prevent a flexion contracture. The responsible surgeon should consider early surgery and not allow the patient to "get behind," so that he later needs three to four major surgical procedures. Similarly, the rheumatologist must not wait too long before altering the medical program to bring the disease under control. If this synovitis is uncontrolled and the patient remains in grade II, elbow synovectomy can be recommended with confidence. If the patient is in grade IIIA, it may already be too late for elbow synovectomy, and an implant arthroplasty may be required. The technical problems of this operation have been reduced sufficiently to allow it to be recommended in patients with severe rheumatoid arthritis of the elbow.

At present, there are a wide variety of therapeutic modalities that can be tried in the patient with disabling rheumatoid arthritis of the elbow. The rheumatologist and the reconstructive surgeon must be prepared to manage these problems in concert. If the programs are comprehensive and well designed, there will be excellent patient compliance, thereby enhancing a good therapeutic result.

References

1. Allison, N., and Coonse, G. K.: Synovectomy in Chronic Arthritis. Arch. Surg. **18**:824, 1929.
2. Amis, A. A., Hughes, S. J., Miller, J. H., and Wright, V.: A Functional Study of the Rheumatoid Elbow. Rheum. Rehab. **21**:151, 1982.
3. Anderson, L. D., and Heppenstall, M.: Synovectomy of the Elbow and Excision of the Radial Head in Rheumatoid Arthritis. In Cruess, R. L., and Mitchell, N. S. (eds.): Surgery of Rheumatoid Arthritis. Philadelphia, J. B. Lippincott Co., 1971.
3a. Blackshear, J. L., Napier, J. S., Davidman, M., and Stillman, M. T.: NSAID-Induced Nephrotoxicity. Drug Therapy Hospital Edition 8:47–51, 55, 56, 65, 68, November, 1983.
4. Brattstrom, H., and Khudairy, H. A.: Synovectomy of the Elbow in Rheumatoid Arthritis. Acta Orthop. Scand. **46**:744, 1975.
5. Bryan, R. S., and Morrey, B. F.: Extensive Posterior Exposure of the Elbow: A Triceps-Sparing Approach. Clin. Orthop. **166**:188, 1982.
6. Bryan, R. S., and Morrey, B. F.: Rheumatoid Arthritis of the Elbow. In Evarts, C. M. (ed.): Surgery of the Musculoskeletal System. London, Churchill Livingstone, 1983.
7. Coonrad, R. W.: Seven Year Follow-Up of Coonrad Total Elbow Replacement. In Inglis, A. E. (ed.): Symposium on Total Joint Replacement of the Upper Extremity. St. Louis, C. V. Mosby Co., 1982.
8. Copeland, S. A., and Taylor, J. G.: Synovectomy of the Elbow in Rheumatoid Arthritis. The Place of Excision of the Head of the Radius. J. Bone Joint Surg. **61B**:69, 1979.

9. d'Aubigne, R. M., and Delbarre, F.: Synovectomy of the Elbow in Rheumatoid Arthritis. In Hijmans, W., Paul, W. D., and Herschel, H. (eds.): Early Synovectomy in Rheumatoid Arthritis. Amsterdam, Excerpta Medica Foundation, 1969, p. 119.

10. Dee, R.: Total Replacement of the Elbow Joint. Orthop. Clin. North Am. 4:415, 1973.

11. DeSeze, S., Debeyre, N., and Djian, A., et al.: The Elbow Joint. International Congress Series No. 61. Amsterdam, Excerpta Medica, 1963.

12. Eichenblat, M., Hass, A., and Kessler, I.: Synovectomy of the Elbow in Rheumatoid Arthritis. J. Bone Joint Surg. 64A:1074, 1982.

13. Ellison, M. R., Kelly, K. J., and Flatt, A. E.: The Results of Surgical Synovectomy of the Digital Joints in Rheumatoid Disease. J. Bone Joint Surg. [Am.] 53:1041, 1971.

14. Ewald, F. C., Scheinberg, R. D., Poss, R., Thomas, W. H., Scott, R. D., and Sledge, C. B.: Capitellocondylar Total Elbow Arthroplasty. J. Bone Joint Surg. 62A:1259, 1980.

15. Froimson, A. I., Silva, J. E., and Richey, D. G.: Curtis Arthroplasty of the Elbow Joint. J. Bone Joint Surg. 58A:863, 1976.

16. Geens, S.: Synovectomy and Debridement of the Knee in Rheumatoid Arthritis. Part I. Historical Review. J. Bone Joint Surg. [Am.] 51:617, 1969.

17. Gelman, M. I., and Ward, J. R.: Septic Arthritis: A Complication of Rheumatoid Arthritis. Radiology 122:17, 1977.

18. Goldberg, V. M., Rashbaum, R., and Zika, J.: The Role of Osmic Acid in the Treatment of Immune Synovitis. Arth. Rheum. 19:737, 1976.

19. Hurri, L., Pulkki, T., and Vainio, K.: Arthroplasty of the Elbow in Rheumatoid Arthritis. Acta Chir. Scand. 127:459, 1964.

20. Inglis, A. E., Ranawat, C. S., and Straub, L. R.: Synovectomy and Debridement of the Elbow in Rheumatoid Arthritis. J. Bone Joint Surg. [Am.] 53:652, 1971.

21. Inglis, A. E., and Pellicci, P. M.: Total Elbow Replacement. J. Bone Joint Surg. 62A:1252, 1980.

22. Inglis, A. E.: Triaxial Total Elbow Replacement: Indications, Surgical Technique, and Results. In Inglis, A. E. (ed.): Symposium on Total Joint Replacement of the Upper Extremity. St. Louis, C. V. Mosby Co., 1982.

23. Inglis, A. E.: Revision Surgery Following a Total Elbow Arthroplasty. Clin. Orthop. 170:213, 1982.

24. Laine, V., and Vainio, K.: Synovectomy of the Elbow. In Hijmans, W., Paul, W. D., and Herschel, H. (eds.): Early Synovectomy in Rheumatoid Arthritis. Amsterdam, Excerpta Medica Foundation, 1969, p. 117.

25. Last, R. J.: Anatomy, Regional and Applied, 6th ed. Boston, Little, Brown & Co., 1966, p. 111.

26. MacKay, I., Fitzgerald, B., and Miller, J. H.: Silastic Radial Head Prosthesis in Rheumatoid Arthritis. Acta Orthop. Scand. 53:63, 1982.

27. Marmor, L.: Surgery of the Rheumatoid Elbow: Follow-up Study on Synovectomy Combined with Radial Head Excision. J. Bone Joint Surg. [Am.] 54:573, 1972.

28. Millender, L. H., Nalebuff, E. A., and Holdsworth, D. E.: Posterior Interosseous Nerve Syndrome Secondary to Rheumatoid Synovitis. J. Bone Joint Surg. 55A:753, 1973.

29. Mitchell, N., Laurin, C., and Shepard, N.: The Effect of Osmium Tetroxide and Nitrogen Mustard on Normal Articular Cartilage. J. Bone Joint Surg. [Br.] 55:814, 1973.

30. Morrey, B. F., Askew, L., and An, K. N., et al.: A Biomechanical Study of Normal Functional Elbow Motion. J. Bone Joint Surg. 63A:872, 1981.

31. Morrey, B. F., and An, K. N.: Articular Ligamentous Contributions to the Stability of the Elbow Joint. Am. J. Sports Med. 11:315, 1983.

32. Oka, M., Rekonen, A., and Ruotsi, A.: The Fate and Distribution of Intra-articularly Injected Osmium Tetroxide (Os-191). Acta Rheum. Scand. 15:35, 1969.

33. Peterson, L. F. A., and Janes, J. M.: Surgery of the Rheumatoid Elbow. Orthop. Clin. North Am. 2:667, 1971.

34. Porter, B. B., Park, N., Richardson, C., et al.: Rheumatoid Arthritis of the Elbow. The Results of Synovectomy. J. Bone Joint Surg. [Br.] 56:427, 1974.

34a. Rodnan G. P., and Schumacher H. R.: Clinical Pharmacology of the Antirheumatic Drugs. In Primer on Rheumatic Diseases, 8th ed. Atlanta, Arthritis Foundation, 1983.

34b. Rodnan and Schumacher: Principles in the Use of Immunosuppressive Agents. In Primer on Rheumatic Diseases, 8th ed. Atlanta, Arthritis Foundation, 1983.

35. Schwab, G. H., Bennett, J. B., Woods, G. W., and Tullos, H. S.: Biomechanics of Elbow Instability: The Role of the Medial Collateral Ligament. Clin. Orthop. 146:42, 1980.

35a. Simon, L. S., and Mills, J. A.: Nonsteroidal Antiinflammatory Drugs. N. Engl. J. Med. 302:1179, 1237, 1980.

36. Souter, W. A.: Arthroplasty of the Elbow with Particular Reference to Metallic Hinge Arthroplasty in Rheumatoid Patients. Orthop. Clin. North Am. 4:395, 1973.

37. Steinbrocker, O., Traeger, C. H., and Batterman, R. C.: Therapeutic Criteria in Rheumatoid Arthritis. J.A.M.A. 140:659, 1949.

38. Swanson, A. B.: Flexible Implant Resection Arthroplasty in the Hand and Extremities. St. Louis, C. V. Mosby Co., 1973.

39. Swett, P. P.: The Present Status of Synovectomy. Am. J. Surg. 6:807, 1929.

40. Taylor, A. R., Mukerjea, S. K., and Rana, N. A.: Excision of the Head of the Radius in Rheumatoid Arthritis. J. Bone Joint Surg. [Br.] 58:485, 1976.

41. Torgerson, W. R., and Leach, R. E.: Synovectomy of the Elbow in Rheumatoid Arthritis. Report of Five Cases. J. Bone Joint Surg. [Am.] 52:371, 1970.

42. Vainio, K.: Arthroplasty of the Elbow and Hand in Rheumatoid Arthritis: A Study of 131 Operations. In Chapehal, G. (ed.): Synovectomy and Arthroplasty in Rheumatoid Arthritis. Stuttgart, George Thieme, Verlag, 1967, p. 66.

43. Wilkinson, M. C., and Lowry, J. H.: Synovectomy for Rheumatoid Arthritis. J. Bone Joint Surg. [Br.] 47:482, 1965.

44. Wilson, D. W., Arden, G. P., and Ansell, B. M.: Synovectomy of the Elbow in Rheumatoid Arthritis. J. Bone Joint Surg. [Br.] 55:106, 1973.

CHAPTER 41

Nonrheumatoid Inflammatory Arthritis

RICHARD B. TOMPKINS

Accurate diagnosis of any condition involving the elbow is necessary for successful treatment. To achieve this, emphasis needs to be placed on an appropriate history and physical examination. Evaluation of other joints, especially those above and below the elbow, may be helpful. Radiographs, appropriate laboratory investigations, and synovial fluid analysis help in arriving at a diagnosis.

A precise diagnosis of the cause of the painful elbow should be possible in most instances. A short but complete history and physical examination will enable the examiner to tell if the elbow problem is an isolated one or part of a systemic disease. Systemic inflammatory rheumatic diseases may begin as monarticular arthritis, and olecranon bursitis may be the primary manifestation of gout. Tenderness of the epicondyles, swelling of the olecranon bursa, and swelling of the elbow joint should be distinguished from each other, although in some patients all three findings will be present. Rheumatoid nodules and gouty tophi may be found in the olecranon bursa or along the proximal ulna. Limitation of extension of the elbow is usually indicative of intra-articular disease.

In systemic diseases, one may find a mild normochromic normocytic anemia, an elevation of the Westergren sedimentation rate, a decrease in the serum albumin, and an increase in the serum alpha-2 globulins. Eighty per cent of rheumatoid arthritis patients have a positive rheumatoid factor, and almost all systemic lupus erythematosus patients have positive antinuclear antibody tests. Gout is usually but not always associated with elevated uric acid levels. In hemorrhagic disorders, clotting studies, including those evaluating platelet function as well as the clotting cascade, can lead to a specific diagnosis.

Radiography can help determine the presence of trauma, tumor, and chronic inflammatory or degenerative arthritis. Synovial fluid analysis can lead to a specific diagnosis of crystalline-induced synovitis and infection. It can help in establishing a diagnosis but is not diagnostic of other rheumatic diseases. A partial list of the conditions that can cause pain and swelling in and around the elbow is shown in Table 41–1. Rheumatoid arthritis, infections, bleeding disorders, neuropathic arthropathies, and tumors are discussed elsewhere (see Chapters 40, 42, 43, 44, and 46).

Crystalline-Induced Arthropathies

Sodium urate, calcium pyrophosphate, and hydroxyapatite crystals can involve the joints and periarticular structures including the olecranon bursa. Sodium urate crystals almost always cause acute symptoms, calcium pyrophosphate crystals cause acute and chronic symptoms, and hydroxyapatite crystals cause chronic symptoms.

Table 41–1. **Conditions Associated with Swelling In and Around the Elbow**

Bleeding disorders (Chapter 43)

Crystalline arthritis
   Calcium pyrophosphate dihydrate
   Hydroxyapatite
   Sodium urate

Degenerative joint disease

Infectious arthritis (Chapter 42)

Inflammatory arthritis of unknown cause
   Rheumatoid arthritis (Chapter 40)
   Spondyloarthropathies
   Systemic lupus erythematosus

Neurotrophic arthritis (Chapter 44)

Osteochondritis dissecans (Chapters 15 and 30)

Traumatic arthritis

Tumors (Chapter 46)
   Osteochondromatosis
   Pigmented villonodular synovitis
   Synovioma

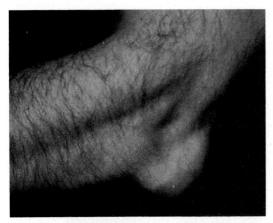

Figure 41–1. Acute olecranon bursitis is a very common clinical manifestation of gout. Often this presentation is rather dramatic and may be a common location for tophi as well.

Gout

Gout[9] is characterized by precipitation of monosodium urate crystals within synovial spaces, leading to acute inflammatory reactions by development of nodular collections of sodium urate in and around the joints (tophi) or by deposits of uric acid in the parenchyma or tubules of the kidneys. Monosodium urate is not very soluble in body fluids and will precipitate on the surface and within the substance of the articular cartilage and synovium as well as in adjacent struc-

tures such as bursae. Acute gouty arthritis is the inflammatory response that results from phagocytosis of the precipitated sodium urate crystals. The presence of these crystals within the cytoplasm of phagocytic cells aspirated from the synovial space is pathognomonic for the disease. A diagnosis of gout should be considered in any patient with an acutely inflamed joint or bursal cavity. Although much more commonly involving the metatarsophalangeal joints, it may begin as acute olecranon bursitis (Fig. 41–1)[3] or occasionally acute elbow synovitis. When it involves the elbow, the classic erosion with the overhanging margin is not usually seen (Fig. 41–2), but rarely bone resorption may occur (Fig. 41–3) in the presence of long-standing synovitis. The olecranon bursa is also a common location for tophi.

Calcium Pyrophosphate Dihydrate Deposition Disease (CPDD)

Calcium pyrophosphate dihydrate crystals[7] can precipitate attacks of acute synovitis that are indistinguishable from gout, and therefore this condition is commonly referred to as pseudogout. The synovitis most commonly affects the knees and the wrists. The elbows, hands, ankles, shoulders, and hips are involved with approximately equal frequency.[12] Unlike many other joints, the elbow is often symptomatic when roentgenographic evi-

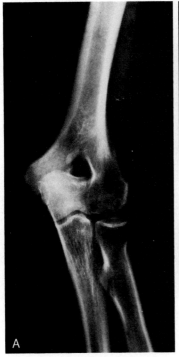
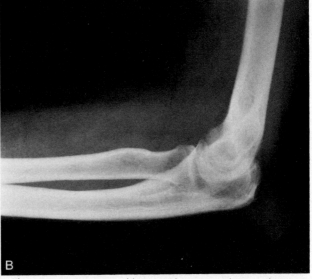

Figure 41–2. A 45-year-old man with a 12-year history of intermittent acute burning pain in the region of the right big toe and ankle. Gout was diagnosed. *A,* Cystic erosion of the capitellum joint is noted, particularly on the anteroposterior view. *B,* On the lateral projection, a small erosion is noted at the tip of the olecranon, and an enlarged olecranon bursa can be seen.

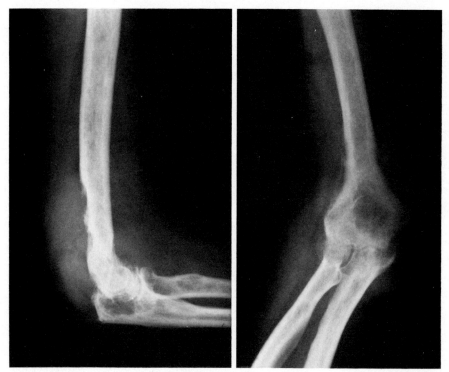

Figure 41–3. This 50-year-old woman had a long history of joint pains and swelling with a uric acid level of over 9 mg per 100 ml. A large, soft tissue mass is present in the posterior aspect of the elbow as well as erosive changes along the posterior distal humerus. Cystic changes of the olecranon fossa and proximal radius are best seen on the lateral projection. An elbow flexion contracture was present.

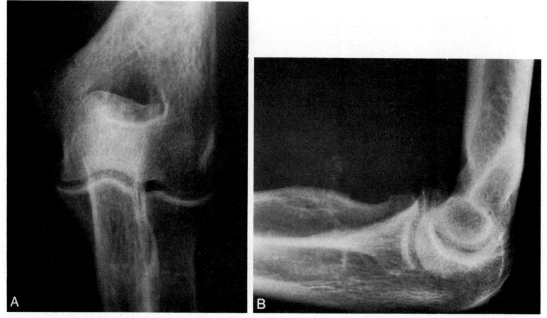

Figure 41–4. A 57-year-old man was given a diagnosis of chondrocalcinosis at age 41 when he developed knee pain. Minimal symptoms were referable to the elbow, but the radiograph does show calcification about the capsule of the medial aspect of the joint on the anteroposterior view *(A)* as well as articular calcification of the radiohumeral joint. On the lateral view *(B)*, calcification in the region of the biceps tuberosity as well as the insertion of the triceps is observed.

dence of the disease is present.[12] The most common clinical presentation is elbow flexion contraction.[5, 12] The presentation may be rather acute and difficult to distinguish from a septic joint. Precipitation of an attack is sometimes seen after a surgical procedure.[4] The finding of typically positive birefringent crystals within phagocytic cells is the hallmark of the disease. The deposition of these crystals in the capsule and within the articular cartilage leads to linear calcification, which can be detected by roentgenologic examination of the involved joints (Fig. 41–4).[5] In its chronic form, this disease is indistinguishable from degenerative joint disease.

Hydroxyapatite Arthropathy

Hydroxyapatite crystals[13] have been found in association with bursitis, periarthritis, inflammatory reactions in subcutaneous sites, and chronic arthritis. These crystals are quite small individually and can be detected only by electron microscopy. However, they can aggregate into masses that are not birefringent and have a pasty-white appearance. Definitive identification of the crystals is possible only by x-ray diffraction techniques. Although acute and chronic forms of periarthritis are the most common forms of apatite disease, attacks may occur in such joints as the elbows, shoulders, wrists, digits, and knees. Usually only one site is involved at a time, and the disease may be associated with a chronic erosive process. Radiographic examinations may demonstrate calcification in and around the joints. These calcifications are usually found in soft tissues and are distinguishable from linear calcification of cartilage typically seen in calcium pyrophosphate deposition disease.

Spondyloarthropathies

The spondyloarthropathies[1] have in the past been referred to as rheumatoid variants or rheumatoidlike arthritides. They consist of ankylosing spondylitis, the arthritis associated with inflammatory bowel disease, psoriatic arthritis, and the arthritis of Reiter's disease. These diseases share the common features of inflammatory peripheral arthritis, clinical or radiologic evidence of sacroiliitis with or without spondylitis, and mucocutaneous, ocular, genital, or gastrointestinal manifestations. The flocculation test for rheumatoid factor is negative, and rheumatoid nodules are absent. There tends to be familial clustering, and there is a frequent association

with HLA-B27 antigen, particularly when sacroiliitis or spondylitis is present. The concept of spondyloarthropathies developed after the discovery of the association between each of these diseases and the HLA-B27 antigen. This antigen is one of the transplantation antigens found on the surface of cells; in the laboratory it is detected serologically on the surface of lymphocytes. The transplantation antigens are coded for by genes contained in the major histocompatibility complex that is located on the short arm of the sixth chromosome. This complex also contains the genetic determinant for a number of characteristics that regulate the immune response. These genes exert their action through cell surface components that appear to be involved in the cell-cell interactions. HLA-B27 is normally found in 4 per cent of North American black and 8 per cent of North American white males. It is detected in 90 to 100 per cent of patients with ankylosing spondylitis, 70 to 90 per cent of patients with endemic Reiter's syndrome, 50 to 60 per cent of patients with psoriatic arthropathy with sacroiliitis, 50 to 70 per cent of patients with inflammatory bowel disease with sacroiliitis, and 40 to 60 per cent of patients with juvenile polyarthropathy with sacroiliitis. The relationship between the presence of this antigen and the development of the disease manifestations is unclear. Because the antigen is found in a large number of healthy individuals and because some patients who have spondyloarthropathy clinically do not have the antigen, its presence alone cannot be used for diagnosis. In suspicious clinical situations, however, detection of the antigen can heighten awareness of the possibility of a spondyloarthropathy. The peripheral arthritis of these diseases may be very similar to that of rheumatoid arthritis. It may also be oligoarticular and asymmetrical and may have a predilection for larger joints such as elbows, shoulders, ankles, and knees.

Primary Degenerative Arthritis

Degenerative arthritis of the elbow is conspicuously rare as a primary form of involvement. Primary degenerative arthritis was the underlying diagnosis in less than 5 per cent of those undergoing total elbow arthroplasty at the Mayo Clinic.[10] Ortner has studied the incidence of hypertrophic arthritis of two populations based on cadaver studies.[11] In this curious effort, which included post-traumatic changes, an 18 per cent incidence was found in the Alaska Eskimo population, compared

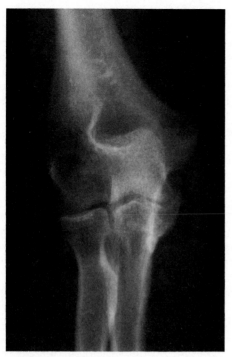

Figure 41–5. Ten years after elbow dislocation, medial ulnohumeral joint narrowing and ulnar osteophyte formation are present. The patient has minimal pain.

with 5 per cent among Peruvian Indians. When degenerative changes are observed, osteophyte formation of the medial ulnohumeral joint is the most common radiographic finding (Fig. 41–5). Degenerative changes of the cartilage of the radiohumeral joint have been studied by Goodfellow and Bullock,[6] but the process appears to be largely asymptomatic. From a practical standpoint, degenerative arthritis of the elbow usually presents as a mild to moderate flexion contracture, and is treated symptomatically.

Miscellaneous Diseases

A wide variety of infectious agents including viruses, bacteria, mycobacteria, fungi, and spirochetes can cause joint inflammation. Viruses,[8] which have been implicated in arthritis, include hepatitis B, rubella, mumps, varicella, Epstein-Barr virus, echovirus, adenovirus, and group A arboviruses. Lyme arthritis[14] has been shown to be due to a spirochete. For the most part, the viral arthritides do not become chronic and resolve without permanent damage to the involved joints. Bacterial, mycobacterial, and fungal infections can cause severe joint damage if they are not treated promptly and appropriately.

LABORATORY EXAMINATIONS USED FOR DIAGNOSIS

General

General laboratory tests such as hemoglobin, white blood cell count, differential white blood cell count, and Westergren sedimentation rate may give clues to underlying systemic diseases. In conditions localized primarily to the elbow, these tests are often normal. In systemic diseases a mild normocytic normochromic anemia (usually not less than 10 g) as well as an elevated Westergren sedimentation rate can be seen. General chemistry testing is most often not helpful in arriving at a diagnosis. Gouty arthritis is usually but not always associated with hyperuricemia.

Serologic tests for rheumatoid factor, antinuclear antibodies, and HLA-B27 antigen may, if positive, raise suspicion of the presence of rheumatoid arthritis, systemic lupus erythematosus, and spondyloarthropathy, respectively, but are not diagnostic for these diseases.

In infectious arthritis, distant sources should be looked for. Local cultures as well as blood cultures for common pathogens, mycobacteria, and fungi should be performed. Acute and convalescent antibody titers to viruses are sometimes helpful in arriving at a diagnosis.

Synovial Fluid Analysis

All synovial joints contain clear, pale yellow, viscous, nonclotting fluid.[2] This fluid is an ultrafiltrate of plasma and usually contains less than 200 white blood cells per cubic millimeter, most of which are mononuclear cells. It serves as a source of nutrition for cartilage and helps in joint lubrication. Type B synovial lining cells synthesize hyaluronic acid, a high molecular-weight glycosaminoglycan that imparts viscosity to synovial fluid. Synovial fluid glucose level is similar to or slightly lower than that of serum. Uric acid, electrolyte, and nonprotein nitrogen levels are about the same as those in plasma. All the proteins of the complement cascade are present, but fibrinogen and many clotting factors are absent from synovial fluid. In inflammatory synovial fluid increased vascular permeability allows the clotting factors to be present, and an anticoagulant such as ethylenediamine tetra-acetate (EDTA) should be used to keep synovial fluid from clotting.

Table 41–2. **Conditions Associated with Types of Synovial Fluids**

Group 1	Group 2	Group 3	Hemorrhagic
Acromegaly	Acute rheumatic fever	Acute tuberculosis	Anticoagulant therapy
Acute rheumatic fever	Ankylosing spondylitis	Bacterial infections	Hemophilia and other bleeding disorders
Aseptic necrosis	Arthritis of inflammatory bowel disease		Neuropathic joint disorders
Degenerative joint disease	Chronic infectious tuberculosis		Pigmented villonodular synovitis
Hypertrophic osteoarthropathy	Crystal-induced synovitis		Synovioma
Neuropathic arthropathy	Fungus arthritis		Thrombocytopenia
Osteochondritis dissecans	Psoriatic arthritis		Thrombocytosis
Osteochondromatosis	Reiter's disease		Trauma
Systemic lupus erythematosus	Rheumatoid arthritis		
Trauma	Systemic lupus erythematosus		
	Viral arthritis		

Through the use of simple laboratory tests and direct observation, synovial fluid can be divided into four groups (Table 41–3). These are noninflammatory or group 1 effusions, inflammatory or group 2 effusions, septic or group 3 effusions, and hemorrhagic effusions. Conditions associated with the various types of synovial fluid are listed in Table 41–2. If synovial fluid is classified as either group 2 or group 3 crystalline and infectious etiologies should be sought. Gram stain can be performed, but a negative result does not exclude the presence of infection. Cultures for bacteria, mycobacteria, and fungi should be performed.

Crystals can be detected by using a polarizing microscope with a first-order red compensator.[15] The needle-shaped, negatively birefringent crystals of sodium urate can be distinguished from the rhomboid, positively birefringent crystals of calcium pyrophosphate dihydrate (Fig. 41–6). Corticosteroid crystals are birefringent and may be confused with the crystals of sodium urate and calcium pyrophosphatase dihydrate. The steroid may remain in a joint for several weeks following therapeutic instillation and may be phagocytosed by polymorphonuclear leukocytes. The use of crystalline substances such as oxalate should be avoided as anticoagulants for synovial fluid.

If crystalline-induced synovitis and infections are ruled out as the cause of inflammatory synovial fluid, further testing can be performed to help distinguish between other causes of the inflammation. However, it is rarely possible to make a specific diagnosis based on synovial fluid analysis alone. Total hemolytic complement can be measured in the synovial fluid and is almost always low in rheumatoid arthritis. It can be either low or normal in systemic lupus erythematosus and has been reported to be high in Reiter's disease. Rheumatoid factor is positive in the

Table 41–3. **Classification of Synovial Effusions**

	Normal	Noninflammatory (Group 1)	Inflammatory (Group 2)	Septic (Group 3)	Hemorrhagic
Viscosity	High	High	Low	Variable	Variable
Color	Pale yellow	Pale to dark yellow	Yellow to green	Variable	Bloody
Clarity	Transparent	Transparent	Translucent	Opaque	Opaque
WBC (mm³)	200	200–100	2000–75,000	Often 100,000	Same as blood
PMNs (%)	25	25	50 (often)	75	Same as blood
Culture	Negative	Negative	Negative	Often positive	Negative
Mucin clot	Firm	Firm	Friable	Friable	Friable
Glucose	Nearly equal to blood	Nearly equal to blood	25 mg per 100 ml lower than blood	25 mg per 100 ml lower than blood	Same as blood

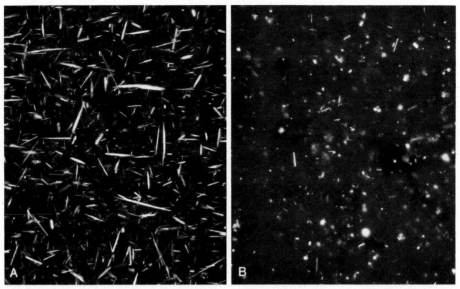

Figure 41–6. *A,* Classic sodium urate and *(B)* calcium pyrophosphate dihydrate crystals. The needle shape of the urate crystal is distinguishable from the rhomboid shape of the calcium pyrophosphate crystal. The positive birefringent nature of the pyrophosphate crystals *(B)* contrasts with that of the crystals of gout, which have a negative birefringent property *(A).* Both fields were taken in polarized light with ×400 magnification.

synovial fluid of some rheumatoid arthritis patients, and occasionally lupus erythematosus cells can be seen in synovial fluid. Polymorphonuclear leukocytes containing inclusion bodies in their cytoplasm are very common in rheumatoid arthritis but can be seen in other inflammatory conditions as well. The Reiter's cell, a phagocytic cell containing intact polymorphonuclear leukocytes, was felt to be diagnostic of Reiter's disease but is now known to occur in a variety of inflammatory conditions.

THERAPY

Treatment of elbow synovitis depends primarily on the proper diagnosis. Prompt treatment of trauma, tumors, and infections is most important. If blood is present in the joint and a bleeding disorder is excluded, trauma is the most likely diagnosis, and appropriate treatment should be instituted. Crystals should be looked for, and if found, treatment with one of the nonsteroidal anti-inflammatory drugs is appropriate. Butazolidin in a dose of 100 mg four times a day for 5 days and Indocin in a dose of 25 to 50 mg four times a day for 5 days are the most commonly used nonsteroidal anti-inflammatory drugs for these situations. Intra-articular or intrabursal instillation of corticosteroids also can be helpful in the management of these patients, but

this treatment should be followed by use of an oral nonsteroidal anti-inflammatory drug for 3 to 4 days to prevent a recrudescence of the inflammatory reaction. In a postoperative period if a patient cannot take medications orally, intravenous colchicine can be used in a dose of 2 mg given intravenously for a minute or two followed by 1 mg in 12 hours. Subsequent 1-mg doses can be repeated no more frequently than every 12 hours and for not longer than 4 days to prevent recrudescence.

In chronic inflammatory arthritis, it is important to treat the primary associated diseases such as inflammatory bowel disease, Reiter's disease, and psoriasis. If a coagulopathy, such as hemophilia, is present, prompt treatment of the bleeding episode is necessary through replacement of the missing clotting factor (see Chapter 43). The peripheral arthritis of inflammatory bowel disease and psoriasis usually parallels the manifestations of the underlying disease. The spondylitis conditions, however, run a course independent of that of the underlying disease. Treatment of rheumatoid arthritis is discussed in Chapter 40.

Physical therapy, which can be very important in the management of acute and chronic arthritis of the elbow, employs the principles of rest, splinting, and progressive range of motion. Salicylates and nonsteroidal anti-inflammatory drugs are used in the management of chronic elbow synovitis. Intra-articular instillation of corticosteroids should not be the primary form of treatment for chronic synovitis because if they are given too often, they can lead to a neurotrophic type of arthritis. Synovectomy is rarely indicated except in rheumatoid arthritis.

References

1. Arthritis Foundation: Ankylosing Spondylitis. Primer on the Rheumatic Diseases, 8th ed. 1983, p. 85.
2. Blau, S. P.: The Synovial Fluid. Orthop. Clin. North Am. **10**:21, 1979.
3. Canoso, J. J., and Yood, R. A.: Reaction of Superficial Bursae in Response to Specific Disease Stimuli. Arth. Rheum. **22**:1361, 1979.
4. Duffy, J. D.: Pseudogout Syndrome in Hospital Patients. J.A.M.A. **226**:42, 1973.
5. Genant, H. K.: Roentgenographic Aspects of Calcium Pyrophosphate Dehydrate Crystal Deposition Disease (Pseudogout). Arth. Rheum. **19**:307, 1976.
6. Goodfellow, J. W., and Bullough, P. G.: The Pattern of Aging of the Articular Cartilage of the Elbow Joint. J. Bone Joint Surg. **49B**:175, 1967.
7. Howell, D. S.: Disease Due to the Deposition of Calcium Pyrophosphate and Hydroxyapatite. In Kelley, W. N., Harris, E. D., Jr., Ruddy, S., and Sledge, C. B. (eds.): Textbook of Rheumatology. Philadelphia, W. B. Saunders Co., 1981.
8. Hyer, F. H., and Gottlieb, N. L.: Rheumatic Disorders Associated with Viral Infection. Sem. Arth. Rheum. **8**:17, 1978.
9. Kelley, W. N.: Gout and Disorders of Purine Metabolism. In Kelley, W. N., Harris, E. D., Jr., Ruddy, S., and Sledge, C. B. (eds.): Textbook of Rheumatology. Philadelphia, W. B. Saunders Co., 1981.
10. Morrey, B. F., Bryan, R. S., Dobyns, J. D., and Linscheid, R. L.: Total Elbow Arthroplasty: A Five Year Experience at the Mayo Clinic. J. Bone Joint Surg. **63A**:1050, 1981.
11. Ortner, D. J.: Description and Classification of Degenerative Bone Changes in the Distal Joint Surfaces of the Humerus. Am. J. Phys. Anthrop. **28**:139, 1968.
12. Resnick, D., Niwagama, G., Goergen, T. G., Utsinger, D., Shapiro, R. F., Haselwood, D. H., and Wiesner, K. B.: Clinical, Radiographic, and Pathological Abnormalities in Calcium Pyrophosphate Dehydrate Deposition Disease (CPPD): Pseudogout. Radiology **122**:1, 1971.
13. Schumacher, H. R., Miller, J. L., Ludivico, C., and Jessar, R. A.: Erosive Arthritis Associated with Apatite Crystal Deposition. Arth. Rheum. **24**:31, 1981.
14. Steere, A. C., Grodzicki, R. L., Kornblatt, A. N., Craft, J. E., Barbour, A. G., Burgdorfer, W., Schmid, G. P., Johnson, E., and Malawista, S. E.: The Spirochetal Etiology of Lyme Disease. N. Engl. J. Med. **308**:733, 1983.
15. Zaharopoulos, P., and Wong, J. Y.: Identification of Crystals in Joint Fluids. Acta Cytol. **24**:197, 1980.

CHAPTER 42

Septic Arthritis

K. P. BUTTERS and B. F. MORREY

General Considerations

An infection may be defined as the clinical manifestation of a host response to a given inoculum. Aspects of the inoculum include the amount of bacteria, the type of entry, and the nature or virulence of the pathogen. The host factors that influence the nature and course of the infection may be classified as congenital or acquired. Congenital immunoincompetence syndromes are associated with deficiencies of the humeral or bursal immunologic systems and have been well described in standard medical text books. Acquired failures or alteration of immunocompetence may be either generalized or localized. Generalized processes include diabetes mellitus, steroid therapy, cancer with or without immunosuppressive therapy, and alcohol or other chemical addiction or abuse. Local processes that alter normal host resistance include scar formation from previous surgery, burns, radiation, or prior infection. In applying these observations specifically to the elbow, it should be noted that this is a subcutaneous joint. Hence, soft tissue coverage is poor, making the elbow vulnerable to direct inoculation of a pathogen, particularly after local host resistance is altered.

Three types of infection occur about the elbow: osteomyelitis, septic arthritis, and septic bursitis.

OSTEOMYELITIS

Infection of the bone has been classified according to the source of the inoculum: (1) hematogenous, (2) direct inoculation after surgery or open fracture, and (3) contiguous spread from a local process.[44]

Hematogenous Infection

Hematogenous infection is the most common type of osteomyelitis and has been reported to occur at the elbow in about 4 per cent of such cases.[44] In the growing child, the end-arterial loop of the metaphyseal bone causes

sluggish bone blood flow. The lack of phagocytic activity in these loops allows maturation of a septic thrombus at the arterial site.[23] The abscess spreads through the haversian system into the subperiosteal space. If the metaphysis is intra-articular, as at the hip or shoulder, a septic joint will then result,[42] but this is not the case at the elbow. As with other sites, acute hematogenous osteomyelitis is most common in children under 3 and over 7 years of age. The first group is vulnerable owing to the lack of acquired host immunity; the second corresponds to the growth spurt.[31]

Presentation and Diagnosis. The clinical presentation is typical and includes local pain, warmth, and swelling. The patient may be afebrile but is not necessarily systemically ill. A predisposing, traumatic event is common,[30] and a remote focus is sometimes definable. The elbow is held in flexion and pseudoparalysis or reflex inhibition may be present. Because the elbow is a subcutaneous joint, the physical examination is rewarding.

Two important features should be carefully elicited:

1. The specific point of maximal tenderness should be determined by gentle palpation. The focus of the septic process can often be accurately localized in this way, even before radiographic changes are apparent.
2. Gentle passive motion of the joint should be done to rule out septic arthritis. With joint infections, all motion is resisted; with metaphyseal osteomyelitis, gentle, supported passive motion is possible.

Except in the very acute stages, an elevated white cell count has not been reliable in our experience,[31] but the differential count tends to demonstrate a shift to the left in two thirds of the cases. The erythrocyte sedimentation rate has been the most sensitive blood test; it is elevated in the early stages of infection in about 80 per cent of individuals. Interestingly, the rate is statistically higher in joint than in bone infections and is a valuable means of following the treatment and resolution of the infection.[30] Radiographs are not helpful early. After 7 to 14 days, osteoporosis may be present, followed by periosteal elevation or erosions.

Radioactive bone scanning with the technetium (^{99m}Tc) isotopes measures the blood flow in the early phase and bone formation in later stages. More specifically, gallium (^{67}Ga) isotope is taken up by acute chronic inflammatory cells and is felt to offer the earliest confirmation of osteomyelitis. However, Sullivan found that half of children with acute hematogenous osteomyelitis had scans that were subtle or nondiagnostic.[40] The initial phase of ^{99m}Tc uptake measures the "blood pool" and thus may be used to distinguish cellulitis from bone infection; osteomyelitis shows the increased uptake in the later images. Hence, some feel that early views are unnecessary.[40] The classic appearance of osteomyelitis by bone scan is a well-defined focal area of increased uptake at the site of active infection (Fig. 42–1). The ^{99m}Tc scan may be positive as early as 24 hours after the onset of symptoms in a patient with osteomyelitis.[13] The increased activity of equal intensity on both sides of the joint indicates joint disease, arthritis, or synovitis but is not reliable in the neonate. The ^{67}Ga scan shows increased uptake in areas of infection even when the ^{99m}Tc scan is negative. However, nonspecific inflammatory arthritides of rheumatoid arthritis or gout as well as soft tissue infections may demonstrate a positive ^{67}Ga scan.[20] At the present time, we recommend first a ^{99m}Tc scan as a low-cost screening test to provide immediate results and localization and then a ^{67}Ga scan if the ^{99m}Tc scan is inconclusive. Finally, the indium white blood cell scan may emerge as the most specific test to date to demonstrate active infection but its role is still evolving.

Direct Inoculation

Direct inoculation is probably the most common cause of infection about the elbow joint. The poor soft tissue coverage predisposes to compound fractures that may become secondarily infected. Elective surgery of the elbow region has been associated with an infection rate of about 5 per cent, significantly greater than the commonly quoted 1 per cent for elective orthopedic procedures.

The diagnosis in this setting is made by applying standard diagnostic judgment to the clinical setting: pain, warmth, and erythema, often with a febrile course or frank drainage.

Spread from a Contiguous Focus

This type of infection occurs at the elbow from a septic joint or from an infected olecranon bursa. These circumstances are most commonly seen in a patient with rheumatoid arthritis, and the management is the same as that for a septic joint. Because a sympathetic sterile effusion may occur with metaphyseal osteomyelitis, even though the metaphysis is extra-articular, the joint should be aspirated to exclude septic arthritis if an effusion is present.

Microorganisms

The most common pathogen causing acute hematogenous osteomyelitis is *Staphylococcus aureus*. Opportunistic organisms are isolated in the debilitated patient, and *Pseudomonas aeruginosa* is most commonly associated with drug addiction or chronic,

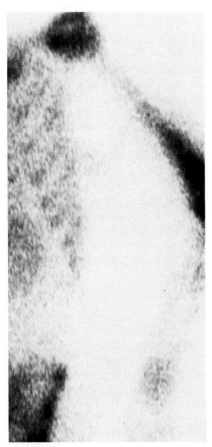

Figure 42–1. Technetium bone scan of a rheumatoid patient (note uptake of shoulder) with an infected total elbow arthroplasty. Notice the increased uptake on the humeral side of the joint.

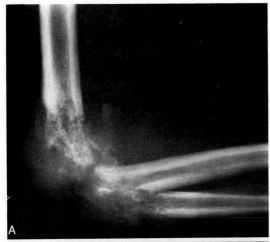

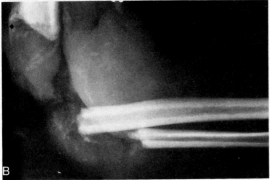

Figure 42–2. This 70-year-old man sustained a severe burn of the upper extremity 56 years previously. He developed chronic osteomyelitis by direct spread from skin breakdown. *A,* Sclerosis and loss of bone has occurred at the distal humerus as well as at the proximal ulna. *B,* Because of the chronic nature of the process and the poor soft tissue coverage, an extensive débridement was carried out. Although this procedure did control the infection, such extensive resection of bone is undesirable because it renders the joint unstable, leaving the upper extremity with significantly impaired function. (From Morrey, B.F., et al.: Diphtheroid osteomyelitis. J. Bone Joint Surg. 59A:529, 1977.)

draining wounds. Organisms not generally considered pathogenic must be viewed as such when isolated on several occasions, particularly in patients with compromised resistance. In one report, two of the three cases with diphtheroid osteomyelitis involved the elbow, and both patients had altered local immunocompetency (Fig. 42–2).[32] *Serratia* infection of open fractures has also been reported in the humerus and forearm in about one third of such cases.[25] After joint replacement, *Staphylococcus aureus* remains the most common organism, but less virulent microbes are also isolated.[33] This particular problem is addressed in more detail in Chapter 34.

Treatment

There are no unique features of management of acute hematogenous osteomyelitis of the distal humerus or proximal ulna or radius except that prolonged immobilization is to be strictly avoided. In cases diagnosed early, antibiotics alone may be adequate.[6, 31] Surgery is indicated when there is no response to parenteral antibiotic therapy after 36 to 48 hours. It has been our experience that acute hematogenous osteomyelitis in which symptoms have been present less than 10 days may be treated with specific intravenous antibiotics for approximately 2 to 3 weeks. If symptoms have been present for more than 10 days, a discrete soft tissue or bone abscess has often developed and must be surgically decompressed. Needle aspiration is sometimes helpful in accurately defining this localization.

Intravenous antibiotics should be continued for about 3 weeks. Oral agents for an additional 4 weeks may be used, but bacteriocidal levels should be attained and monitored.[27] The precise antibiotic dosage and duration of treatment will, of course, vary according to the organism, host response, and other variables discussed above. Infection involving bone may become subacute or chronic, and in this instance, incision and drainage with limited bone débridement and secondary soft tissue healing may be necessary. An extensive débridement of bone severely impairs function because the joint becomes disfunctionally unstable and is almost impossible to fuse (see Fig. 42–2); thus, this should be avoided if possible.

In the acute phase of treatment, the joint should be splinted, elevated, and put to rest. As the process resolves, gentle active motion is encouraged as soon as possible. Devices that provide passive motion may prove to be beneficial in some patients to avoid ankylosis or adhesions.

Results

In the preantibiotic area, Welinsky reported that 3 of 18 patients developed spontaneous ankylosed elbows owing to immobilization for osteomyelitis of the elbow region.[45] Other long-term residual effects include sinus tract formation, recurrent infection, pathologic fracture, growth disturbances, and development of chronic osteomyelitis. West et al. observed that chronic osteomyelitis of the humerus appears to have a better prognosis than chronic infection of the tibia or femur.[46] The most important aspect of a satisfactory result is clearly the duration of the septic process.[31, 35] Hence, a thorough evaluation to make the diagnosis is most important.

Summary

In summary, aggressive, specific antibiotic therapy for a minimum of 3 weeks with judicious early splinting followed by active and passive motion and surgical intervention for that individual who does not respond to the initial treatment is the recommended program for osteomyelitis about the elbow. Early diagnosis remains the most prominent factor in prognosis. Subperiosteal needle aspiration and bone scan can aid in rapid diagnosis and isolation of the organism, thus allowing early treatment of the condition. Specifically, prolonged immobilization and extensive resection of the elbow is to be avoided if possible.

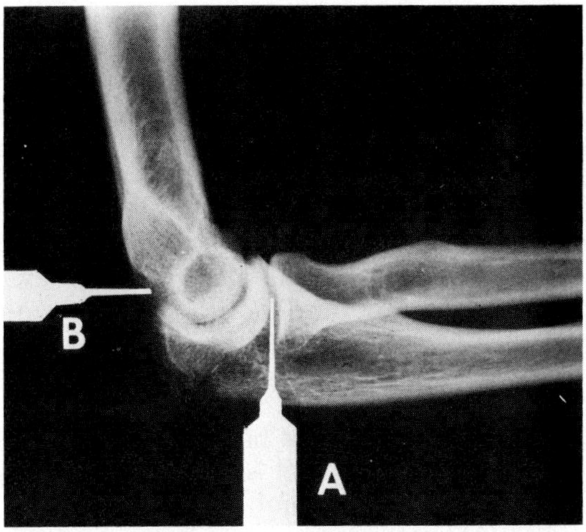

Figure 42–3. Aspiration of the elbow is carried out through the lateral portal between (A) the radial head, lateral epicondyle, and tip of the olecranon. B, Alternatively, with significant joint distention, a posterolateral approach into the olecranon fossa may be used.

SEPTIC ARTHRITIS OF THE ELBOW

In the adult, suppurative arthritis of the elbow is relatively more frequent than is osteomyelitis of this region. Yet joint infection is more common in children than in adults. In the experience of the Mayo Clinic, elbow involvement occurred in 6 per cent of adults with septic arthritis[24] and 3 per cent of children with this complaint.[30] Goldenberg places the incidence of elbow involvement at about 9 per cent, and Argen reported an incidence of 13 per cent, indicating that the ages at risk were those "at the extremes of life." The frequent association of septic arthritis with rheumatoid arthritis has been described.[17, 26, 36] Kellgren et al. reported that septic joints in 4 of 12 rheumatoid arthritis patients (33 per cent) involved the elbow.[26] Also noted was the high incidence of *Staphylococcus aureus* organisms (83 per cent) and multiple sites of involvement in all 12.

Diagnosis

An incorrect initial diagnosis is common.[24] The clinical examination and an index of suspicion are crucial to a prompt and correct diagnosis. The maximum capacity of the joint is at about 60 degrees of flexion, so the patient will present with the joint held in this position. Pain and swelling about the elbow are invariably present, and gentle, passive motion is quite painful.

Differential diagnosis of an infected elbow in the child includes juvenile rheumatoid arthritis, unrecognized trauma, acute rheu-

matic fever (which affects the elbow in about 15 per cent of cases), and transient synovitis. In the adult, 5 per cent of patients with gout or pseudogout will have involvement of the elbow. Differentiation from osteoarthritis or post-traumatic arthritis should not be a difficult problem. Rheumatoid arthritis with a secondary infection is, of course, a difficult clinical diagnosis that is usually resolved only with aspiration.

Systemic symptoms are variably present and distinction from an underlying disease is difficult. A leukocytosis is often present early, but the shift to the left of the differential cell count is more reliable. The sedimentation rate is invariably increased, but this does not distinguish the patient with active rheumatoid arthritis. As with any joint infection, the key to the diagnosis is joint aspiration. The distended joint is easy to enter either from the lateral "triangle" or at the posterior olecranon fossa (Fig. 42–3). In addition to joint aspiration for culture and cell count, gas-liquid chromatography may be helpful in differentiating a bacterial from a nonseptic inflammatory process.[7]

The radiographic assessment is not helpful in the early diagnosis of elbow infection, but an increased amount of synovial fluid may show an anterior or posterior fat pad sign. Later, osteopenia and subtle bone erosion at the synovial attachment occur, progressing to uniform thinning of the articular cartilage and then more extensive erosions and subchondral disruption. Joint aspiration must be done under sterile conditions, because inoculation of the sterile joint is possible with aspiration and has been reported.[3]

Additional laboratory investigations include blood cultures, which are positive in about 40 to 70 per cent of patients[3, 16, 31] and in up to 90 per cent if multiple joints are involved. We have observed that the limited use of antibiotics will tend to result in a negative blood culture, but the joint aspirate will still reveal the organism.[31]

Staphylococcus aureus is isolated in about two thirds of cases of bacterial arthritis in adults[24] and in at least half of those in children.[30] In the neonatal age group, coliform and gram-positive organisms are not uncommon.[34] At ages 3 months to 3 years, the child is at risk for *Hemophilus influenzae*, but in children older than 3 years, *Staphylococcus aureus* is the predominant organism.[30]

Treatment

Initial specific antibiotic treatment is first based on the Gram stain. If infection is suspected and no organism is isolated, initial antibiotic treatment should be based on age and presentation. This should include penicillin in the young healthy patient, *Staphylococcus* and gram-negative coverage in the older patient with underlying disease, and drugs for *Hemophilus influenzae* in the young child. Mayo Clinic treatment consists of 3 to 4 weeks of intravenous antibiotics, but this may be somewhat conservative, and the duration should be tailored to the clinical setting. Others have begun an appropriate oral antibiotic approximately 1 week after serum bacteriocidal levels have been obtained.[27] Serial monitoring of the serum antibiotic levels is continued on an outpatient basis.

In addition to systemic antibiotics, the treatment of septic arthritis of the elbow, as in any diarthrodial joint, requires removal of accumulated cellular debris and pus. Cartilage is destroyed by digestion from enzymes elaborated from neutrophils, synovium, and bacteria.[10] Aspiration is easily done in this superficial joint. When there is capsular distention, entry through the soft tissue triangle between the olecranon, lateral epicondyle, and radial head or posterior lateral aspect of the olecranon fossa provides ready access to the joint (Fig. 42–3). Rather than simple aspiration for diagnosis, we strongly recommend that the joint be lavaged with sterile saline at the time of aspiration. This has been clearly shown to be effective in preventing collagen loss in the rabbit.[10] Suc-

cessive decreasing cell counts from the joint aspirate may also be used as an indicator of recovery.[14, 15] Intermittent joint distention-suction through percutaneous catheters may prevent synovial adhesions and improve drainage.[21] To avoid secondary infection the tube should be removed in 3 or 4 days.[30]

Intra-articular antibiotics are controversial in the treatment of septic arthritis. Adequate levels of antibiotics do occur in the synovial fluid from parenteral treatment, and post-infection synovitis lasting up to 8 weeks in as many as 40 per cent of the cases has been related to the intra-articular use of penicillin.[3] Yet, experimental evidence indicates that the joint can be sterilized more rapidly by intra-articular injection of antibiotic.[5] Lacking evidence that the chemical synovitis is harmful to the joint, if there has been a delay in diagnosis of 4 to 5 days, we inject a half gram of cefazolin sodium diluted in 10 ml of sterile water, particularly if a gram-positive organism is suspected.

In contrast to the preantibiotic era,[14, 30, 45] aspiration and lavage rather than surgical drainage are now favored as initial treatment for elbow sepsis. For infections that are subacute, postoperative, or due to direct inoculation, adequate clearance by aspiration is not reliable, and open drainage may be necessary. If a significant amount of soft tissue involvement is present, the joint may be left open, but in any event, early motion is begun. Although recently popularized for the knee,[4] early motion with the joint exposed was recommended 65 years ago by Willems, who reported good results with both knee and elbow infections.[47] The basis of the beneficial effect of early motion has been carefully studied by Salter et al.,[38] who concluded that this technique (1) prevents adhesions, (2) improves nutrition of cartilage, (3) enhances clearance of lysosomal enzymes, and (4) stimulates the living chondrocytes.

Arthroscopy of the elbow allows inspection, clearance of loculations and adhesions, thorough irrigation, and synovial tissue culture as well as insertion of drainage catheters. Hence, this appears to be a valuable potential alternative to open drainage if repeated aspiration proves to be inadequate. Posterior lateral and anterior lateral puncture sites are preferred (see Chapter 7).

Results

Unsatisfactory results occur from the degeneration of articular cartilage and the development of fibrous adhesions.[30] Delay in diagnosis and treatment is probably more important than the exact type of treatment, and is the most important factor affecting prognosis.[15, 26, 30] A normal joint is unlikely if treatment is delayed for more than 1 week after the onset of symptoms.[30, 35] Other variables have been studied in relation to the influence of prognosis.[14] Virulence of the organism is an important variable. In one series, complete recovery occurred in 90 per cent of those infected with *Streptococcus*, 60 per cent of those with *Staphylococcus*, and less than one third of patients infected with a gram-negative organism.[15] Gram-negative in-

fection has a poor prognosis and is often associated with compromised host resistance. Gonococcal arthritis also involves the elbow in about 10 per cent of cases,[29] and treatment offers predictably good results. Nongonococcal *Neisseria* infections have also been reported to involve the elbow, again often with compromised host resistance or in association with a crystalline-induced arthritis.[11] The prognosis for this type of infection depends on the premorbid condition of the joint.[11]

Loss of function, not recurrence, is the most common sequela of this infection (Fig. 42–4). In the Mayo series of 103 septic joints, acute

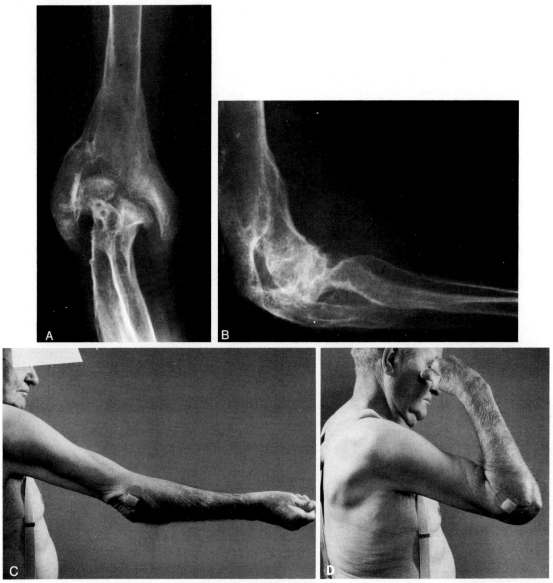

Figure 42–4. This 60-year-old patient with rheumatoid arthritis was treated with joint resection for an infected elbow and did well for 2½ years. He had significant loss of bone but the resection-type arthroplasty functioned reasonably well, as shown in the AP *(A)* and lateral *(B)* projections. The arc of motion of the elbow was between 15 and 135 degrees *(C and D)* with no significant discomfort.

infection was eradicated in all but one, with only four recurrences. Argen found no evidence of reinfection or chronic osteomyelitis in any of the elbow infections, and we found no secondary procedures necessary in elbow infections in children.[30] As stated above, the ultimate functional outcome greatly depends on the state of the joint before the infectious process.

Nonbacterial Infections

The elbow joint is involved in approximately 10 per cent of all skeletal infections from tuberculosis.[28] Unlike suppurative arthritis, the adjacent bone may also be involved. A tuberculous infection of the elbow is diagnosed by aspiration in 25 to 75 per cent of instances, but most consistently (95 per cent), it results from biopsy of the synovial tissue. Pulmonary tuberculosis is present in only about half of the cases.[49] Atypical *Mycobacterium* infection, for example, *M. kansasaii*,[50] may also occur, both from direct inoculation and from lung involvement.

The articular cartilage is preserved in the elbow well into the course of the disease. The radiographic stages are well exemplified in the elbow: soft tissue involvement (Fig. 42–5), localized cystic lesions in the bone (Fig. 42–6), or resorption with cystic subchondral changes (Fig. 42–7).

In a study of 29 joints involved with tuberculosis, 28 attained a useful joint after 12 months of treatment with chemotherapy alone.[28] Currently, chemotherapy with early motion is the treatment of choice, surgery being used only to make the diagnosis. For residual dysfunction, a synovectomy and radial head resection might be considered as well as excisional arthroplasty. Arthrodesis

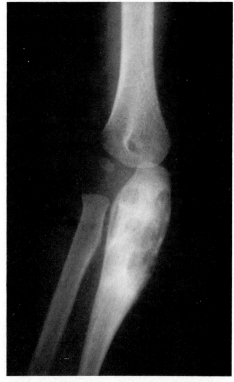

Figure 42–6. Tuberculosis of the elbow may present as a cystic and sclerotic type of osteomyelitis. In this instance extensive involvement of the proximal ulna is present. (Courtesy of Dr. Richard Marks, Cape Town, South Africa.)

may be difficult[2] and is recognized as a poor salvage procedure that should be used only if the infection cannot be controlled.

Coccidioidomycosis caused by *Coccidioides immitis* has been reported in the elbow in 3 of 25 joint infections.[48] The treatment recommended is synovectomy with intravenous amphotericin-B for the disseminated disease.

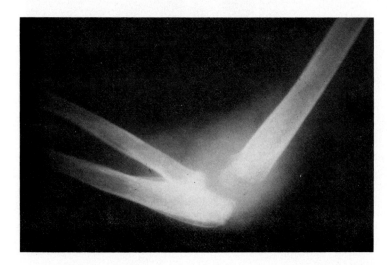

Figure 42–5. Typical radiographic appearance of tuberculosis of the elbow joint demonstrating severe soft tissue reaction about the joint without dramatic changes of the bone itself at this stage. (Courtesy of Dr. Richard Marks, Cape Town, South Africa.)

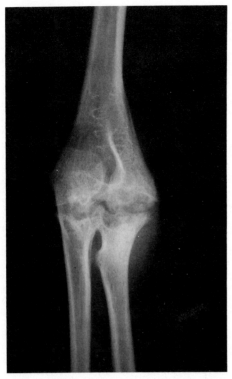

Figure 42–7. Classic radiographic picture of tuberculosis involving both sides of the elbow joiint with subchondral cyst formation. Subchondral sclerosis is variably present.

SEPTIC OLECRANON BURSITIS

The superficial location of the extensor surface of the elbow places the olecranon bursa at increased risk of trauma,[37] especially in certain occupations.[8] A pre-existing local infection or associated conditions such as diabetes mellitus or alcoholism have also been noted. Infection of the olecranon bursa does not imply elbow joint infection because normally the two structures do not communicate. However, the bursa may communicate with the elbow in rheumatoid arthritis,[43] and elbow joint aspiration and sinogram may be necessary for an accurate diagnosis. Of those who do develop a septic olecranon bursa, about one third give a history of a previous noninfected olecranon bursitis.[1]

The presentation varies widely from acute onset of cellulitis (Fig. 42–8) to a low-grade subacute process of two or more weeks' duration. Fluid aspirate yields S. aureus in 90 per cent of cases.[9, 18] Other less common organisms include group A streptococcus,[18] anaerobic,[41] tuberculosis,[39] and even paracytic organisms.[1]

Sterile hemodialysis olecranon bursitis is a well-known entity, and probably occurs from the sustained pressure that occurs in the arm with the vascular access.[22] If the bursa becomes secondarily infected, usually with S. aureus, the condition may appear indistinguishable from noninfected bursitis, and the diagnosis must be confirmed by aspiration.

Examination for crystals should be done, because gout may co-exist with or even predispose to bursal sepsis (see Chapter 41).[12] A key point is that aspiration with cell count, crystal determination, and Gram stain probably should be done prior to steroid injection into the bursa in all cases. Cell counts below 1000 are not worrisome, but those above are at least suspicious. Clinical findings include bursal swelling with or without fever. Importantly, pain and erythema are suspicious of a septic rather than a mechanical process. The range of motion is restricted at the extremes only, aiding the differentiation of bursal from elbow joint sepsis. The differential diagnosis includes septic, traumatic, or inflammatory bursitis, and, in patients with rheumatoid arthritis, septic elbow.[8, 12, 19, 37]

The relationship with septic arthritis in the patient with rheumatoid arthritis is particularly important. The co-existence of the two is well established, and septic arthritis may occasionally present as an infected olecranon bursitis.[43]

Prior to choosing treatment, the underlying disease, extent of infection (local and systemic), and any roentgenographic pathology

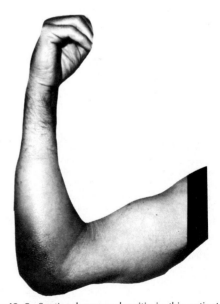

Figure 42–8. Septic olecranon bursitis in this patient presented with marked cellulitis, swelling, and pain over the entire posterior aspect of the elbow region. *Staphylococcus aureus* was isolated at the time of aspiration. The process resolved with 5 days of intravenous antibiotics and 10 days of oral antibiotics.

should be considered. Initial treatment should include adequate drainage and antibiotics. Initially, a single aspiration and oral antibiotic treatment may suffice in the mild case. Intravenous antibiotics and a second aspiration may be required if erythema or systemic symptoms are present. Surgical drainage is performed for (1) failed aspiration and antibiotic treatment, (2) long-standing resistant infections, (3) chronic, recurrent infection, (4) an infected bursa that has been altered by a prior inflammatory process or surgery, and (5) infection with a resistant organism not responding to treatment[18] (see Chapter 48).

The length of treatment with antibiotics is based on the clinical response and the duration of symptoms. A sterile aspiration serves as an appropriate end-point, but usually the clinical course is an adequate indicator. Other factors that may influence the duration of treatment include the underlying disease, the completeness of bursal drainage, the appropriateness of antibiotic treatment, and, most important, the duration of infection prior to the initiation of treatment. Ho recommends continued treatment for 5 days after a sterile aspirate has been obtained.[19]

Indications for excision of the olecranon bursa include prolonged drainage after surgical incision or rupture, recurrent septic bursitis, and chronic bursitis with contiguous osteomyelitis. Ablation is difficult, especially in the patient with rheumatoid arthritis. We have found that meticulous dissection under magnification with preliminary staining of the bursal wall using methylene blue and hydrogen peroxide is helpful. The incision should be lateral to the midline, not over the center of the bursa.

References

1. Ahbel, D. E., et al.: Protothecal Olecranon Bursitis. J. Bone Joint Surg. 62A:835, 1980.
2. Arafiles, R.: A New Technique of Fusion for TB Arthritis of the Elbow. J. Bone Joint Surg. 63A:1396, 1981.
3. Argen, R. J., Wilson, C. H., and Wood, P.: Suppurative Arthritis. Arch. Intern. Med. 117:661, 1966.
4. Ballard, A., et al.: The Functional Treatment of Pyogenic Arthritis of the Adult Knee. J. Bone Joint Surg. 57A:1119, 1975.
5. Bardenheier, J. A., Morgan, H. C., and Stamp, W. G.: Treatment and Sequelae of Experimentally Produced Septic Arthritis. Surg. Gynecol. Obstet. 122:249, 1966.
6. Blockey, N. J., and McAllister, T. H.: Antibiotics in Acute Osteomyelitis in Children. J. Bone Joint Surg. 54B:299, 1972.
7. Brook, I., Reza, M., Bricknell, K. S., Bluestone, R., and Finegold, S. M.: Abnormalities in Synovial Fluid of Patients With Septic Arthritis Detected by Gas-

8. Canoso, J. J.: Idiopathic or Traumatic Olecranon Bursitis. Arth. Rheum. 20:1213, 1977.
9. Canoso, J. J., and Sheckman, P. R.: Septic Subcutaneous Bursitis. Report of Sixteen Cases. J. Rheum. 6:1, 1979.
10. Daniel, D., Akeson, W., Amiel, D., Ryder, M., and Boyer, J.: Lavage of Septic Joints in Rabbits: Effects of Chondrolysis. J. Bone Joint Surg. 58A:393, 1976.
11. Degan, T. J., Rand, J. A., and Morrey, B. F.: Musculoskeletal Infection with Nongonococcal Neisseria Species Not Associated With Meningitis. Clin. Orthop. 176:206, 1983.
12. Gerster, J. C., et al.: Olecranon Bursitis Related to Calcium Pyrophosphate Dihydrate Crystal Deposition Disease. Arth. Rheum. 25:989, 1982.
13. Gilday, D. L., et al.: Diagnosis of Osteomyelitis in Children by Combined Blood Pool and Bone Imaging. Radiology 117:331, 1975.
14. Goldenberg, D. L., et al.: Treatment of Septic Arthritis. Arth. Rheum. 18:83, 1975.
15. Goldenberg, D. L., and Cohen, A. S.: Acute Infectious Arthritis. Am. J. Med. 60:369, 1976.
16. Goldenberg, D. L., and Cohen, A. S.: Synovial Membrane Histopathology in Differential Diagnosis of Arthritis. Medicine 57:239, 1978.
17. Gristina, H.: Spontaneous Septic Arthritis in Rheumatoid Arthritics. J. Bone Joint Surg. 56A:1180, 1974.
18. Ho, G., et al.: Septic Bursitis in the Prepatellar and Olecranon Bursae. Ann. Int. Med. 89:21, 1978.
19. Ho, G., and Su, E. Y.: Antibiotic Therapy of Septic Bursitis. Arth. Rheum. 24:905, 1981.
20. Hughes, S.: Radionuclides in Orthopedic Surgery. J. Bone Joint Surg. 62B:141, 1980.
21. Jackson, R. W., and Parsons, C. J.: Distension-Irrigation Treatment of Major Joint Sepsis. Clin. Orthop. 96:160, 1973.
22. Jain, V. K., et al.: Septic and Aseptic Olecranon Bursitis in Patients on Maintenance Dialysis. Clin. Exp. Dialysis Apheresis 5:4, 1981.
23. Kahn, D. S., and Pritzker, K.: The Pathophysiology of Bone Infection. Clin. Orthop. 96:12, 1973.
24. Kelley, P. J., et al.: Bacterial (Suppurative) Arthritis in the Adult. J. Bone Joint Surg. 52A:1595, 1970.
25. Kelley, P. J.: Musculoskeletal Infections Due to Serratia. Clin. Orthop. 96:76, 1973.
26. Kellgren, J. H., Ball, J., Fairbrother, R. W., and Barns, K. L.: Suppurative Arthritis Complicating Rheumatoid Arthritis. Br. Med. J. 1:1193, 1958.
27. Kolyvas, E., et al.: Oral Antibiotic Therapy of Skeletal Infections in Children. Pediatrics 65:867, 1980.
28. Martini, M., and Gottesman, H.: Results of Conservative Treatment of TB of the Elbow. Int. Orthop. 4:83, 1980.
29. Masi, A. T., and Eisenstein, B. I.: Disseminated Gonococcal Infection and Gonococcal Arthritis. Sem. Arth. Rheum. 10:173, 1981.
30. Morrey, B. F., and Bianco, A. J.: Septic Arthritis in Children. Orthop. Clin. North Am. 6:923, 1975.
31. Morrey, B. F., and Peterson, H. A.: Hemotogenous Pyogenic Osteomyelitis in Children. Orthop. Clin. North Am. 6:935, 1975.
32. Morrey, B. F., Fitzgerald, R. H., Kelly, P. J., Dobyns, J. H., and Washington, J. A., III: Diphtheroid Osteomyelitis. J. Bone Joint Surg. 59A:527, 1977.
33. Morrey, B. F., and Bryan, R. S.: Infection After Total Elbow Arthroplasty. J. Bone Joint Surg. 65A:330, 1983.
34. Nelson, J. D.: The Bacterial Etiology and Antibiotic Management of Septic Arthritis in Infants and Children. Pediatrics 50:437, 1972.

Liquid Chromatography. Ann. Rheum. Dis. 39:168, 1980.

35. Peterson, S., Knudsen, F. U., Andersen, E. A., and Egebald, M.: Acute Hematogenous Osteomyelitis and Septic Arthritis in Children. Acta Orthop. Scand. **51**:451, 1980.
36. Rimoin, D. L., and Wennberg, J. F.: Acute Septic Arthritis Complicating Chronic Rheumatoid Arthritis. J.A.M.A. **196**:109, 1966.
37. Saini, M., and Canoso, J. J.: Traumatic Olecranon Bursitis. Acta Radiol. Diag. **23**:255, 1982.
38. Salter, R. B., Bell, R. S., and Kelley, F. W.: The Protective Effect of Continuous Passive Motion on Living Articular Cartilage in Acute Septic Arthritis. Clin. Orthop. **159**:223, 1981.
39. Sharma, S. V., et al.: Dystrophic Calcification in Tubercular Lesions of Bursae. Acta Orthop. Scand. **49**:445, 1978.
40. Sullivan, D. C., et al.: Problems in the Scintigraphic Detection of Osteomyelitis in Children. Radiology **135**:731, 1980.
41. Tollerud, A.: Anaerobic Septic Bursitis (Letter). Ann. Int. Med. **91**:494, 1979.
42. Trueta, J.: Three Types of Acute Hematogenous Osteomyelitis. J. Bone Joint Surg. **41B**:671, 1959.
43. Viggiano, D. A.: Septic Arthritis Presenting as Olecranon Bursitis in Patients with Rheumatoid Arthritis. J. Bone Joint Surg. **62A**:1011, 1980.
44. Waldvogel, F. A., Medoff, G., and Swartz, M. D.: Osteomyelitis: A Review of Clinical Features, Therapeutic Considerations and Unusual Aspects. N. Engl. J. Med. Part I: **282**:316, 1970; Part 2: **282**:260, 1970; and Part 3: **282**:198, 1970.
45. Wilensky, A. O.: Osteomyelitis. Its Pathogenesis, Symptomatology, and Treatment. New York, Macmillan & Co., 1934.
46. West, W. F., Kelley, P. J., and Martin, W. J.: Chronic Osteomyelitis. J.A.M.A. **213**:1837, 1970.
47. Willems, C.: Treatment of Purulent Arthritis by Wide Arthrotomy Followed by Immediate Active Mobilization. Surg. Gynecol. Obstet. **28**:546, 1919.
48. Winter, W. G., et al.: Coccidioidal Arthritis and Its Treatment. J. Bone Joint Surg. **57A**:1152, 1975.
49. Wolfgang, G. L.: Tuberculous Joint Infection. Clin. Orthop. **136**:257, 1978.
50. Zretina, J. R., et al.: *Mycobacterium kansasii* Infection of the Elbow Joint. J. Bone Joint Surg. **61A**:1099, 1979.

CHAPTER 43

Hematologic Arthritis

GERALD S. GILCHRIST

This chapter will focus on the effects on the elbow of some of the inherited diseases of blood coagulation and diseases characterized by the presence of sickle hemoglobin. Although joint involvement is not infrequent at the time of presentation or relapse of acute leukemia, involvement of the elbow is rare and virtually never occurs without simultaneous involvement of other joints.[16, 18] Arthropathy is also a feature of hereditary hemosiderosis and resembles rheumatoid arthritis in many respects.[7, 11] Only hemophilia and sickle cell arthropathy will be discussed in detail because the elbow is vulnerable in both of these conditions.

HEMOPHILIA

The term *hemophilia* applies to a group of clinical conditions characterized by an inherited functional deficiency of one or another of the plasma coagulation factors. In general, only hemophilia A (classic hemophilia, Factor VIII deficiency) and hemophilia B (Christmas disease, Factor IX deficiency) are associated with hemarthrosis and then only if the coagulation deficiency is moderately severe (a plasma Factor VIII or IX level of 1 to 5 per cent of normal) or severe (less than 1 per cent of normal clotting activity). Occasionally, patients with von Willebrand's disease, an autosomally inherited disorder characterized by reduced levels of components of the Factor VIII molecule necessary for normal blood coagulation and normal platelet function, may have problems with joint bleeding, and this is usually associated with very low levels of Factor VIII coagulant activity.[22]

Incidence

In many series, including our own, the elbow is one of the more frequently involved joints. A study in Sweden that surveyed 114 patients with hemophilia A and 43 with hemophilia B documented involvement of the elbow in 145 joints.[1] Sixty-six of the 95 severely affected and 20 of the 38 moderately severely affected patients had elbow involvement.

Fifty-nine had bilateral involvement. The severity of the arthropathy increased with age. In a group of children 9 years of age or younger, only six involved joints were documented in 26 patients, and all of these were classified as grade 2 or 3. In contrast, of 22 patients with severe disease aged between 20 and 29 years, 40 involved joints were documented, 9 of which were classified as grade 4 and 23 as grade 3. Grade 4 arthropathy was not seen in any patient with moderately severe hemophilia before the age of 40 years. A review of the experience over a 3-year period at the Nuffeld Orthopedic Center in Oxford, England, identified 366 acute hemarthroses in 113 patients.[6] One hundred and fifty-one bleeds had involved the knees, 109 had affected the elbows, 73 had occurred in the ankles, 9 involved the wrists, 8 the shoulders, and 5 the hips. In order of frequency, therefore, elbow joint involvement ranks second only to involvement of the knee in our experience and in most large reported series.

Anatomy

Radiologic Aspects

A number of classifications of hemophilic arthropathy have been developed based on the roentgenographic findings.[1, 16] The system used by Arnold and Hilgartner[2] at New York Hospital–Hospital for Special Surgery provides for five stages according to the following definitions (Figs. 43–1 to 43–4):

Stage I. No skeletal abnormalities. Soft tissue swelling present.

Stage II. Osteoporosis, particularly in the epiphyses with overgrowth of the epiphyses. Joint integrity maintained without narrowing of cartilage space. No bone cysts.

Stage III. Disorganization of the joint but no significant narrowing of cartilage space. Subchondral cysts are visible. The synovium may be opacified, and the trochlear notch of the ulna is usually widened.

Stage IV. Joint space narrowing and destruction of the cartilage with progression of changes noted in stage III.

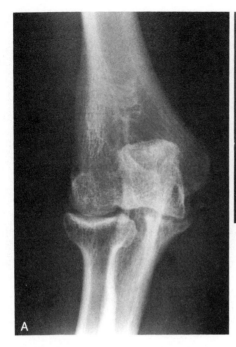

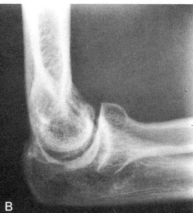

Figure 43–1. *A, B,* Stage II arthropathy with overgrowth of the ends of the bones, particularly the radial head. The joint space is maintained.

Stage V. Fibrous joint contracture, loss of joint space, extensive enlargement of the epiphyses, and substantial disorganization of joint structures.

Clinical Aspects

Acute Hemarthrosis. Most acute hemarthroses are not preceded by identifiable trauma but are characterized by a prodromal phase of pain and stiffness. As the intraarticular hemorrhage progresses, the joint be-

comes more painful, swollen, tender, and warm. Characteristically, the elbow is held in a flexed position with restricted range of motion due to a combination of pain and muscle spasm as well as the actual hemarthrosis. With continued bleeding, the joint may become excruciatingly tender, and the overlying skin may even become tense, shiny, and erythematous.

Subacute Hemarthrosis. Subacute hemarthroses usually develop after a series of acute

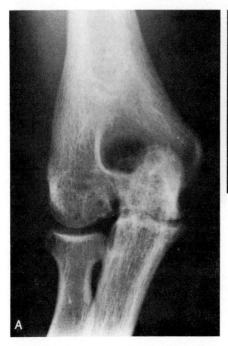

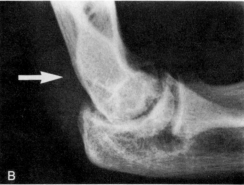

Figure 43–2. *A,* An example of stage III arthropathy demonstrating subchondral cysts in the distal humerus, the capitellum, and the trochlea. *B,* The joint spaces are fairly well preserved in the lateral view; however, there is some narrowing of the ulnohumeral joint space and opacification of the synovium (arrow).

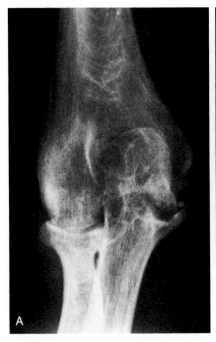

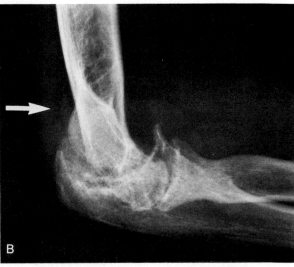

Figure 43–3. *A,* X-ray films of the same patient shown in Figure 43–2 taken 5 years later show progressive changes with loss of the joint space narrowing and loss of cartilage (stage IV). *B,* Again the arrow shows opacification of the synovium.

hemarthroses, and this phase usually coincides with the early x-ray changes defined as stage II above. There is some loss of motion, and the synovium is felt to be thickened and boggy.

Chronic Hemarthrosis. Chronic arthropathy develops after months or years of subacute joint involvement complicated by superimposed acute hemorrhages. The end-stage of hemophilic arthropathy consists of fibrotic, contracted, periarticular structures and destruction of the articular cartilage and results in a totally destroyed elbow.

Pathology

The earlier structural changes in the process of hemophilic arthropathy are the appearance

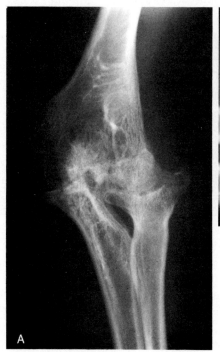

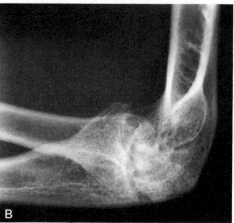

Figure 43–4. *A, B,* Stage V arthropathy showing marked loss of joint space with extensive enlargement of the epiphysis. Some degree of contracture is evident by the incomplete extension visible on the AP film.

of an abnormally thickened synovium with varying degrees of fibrovascular proliferation and pannus and villus formation together with hemosiderin staining. The increased vascularity may set the stage for further bleeding. Chronic hyperemia leads to epiphyseal overgrowth, and the synovium becomes friable and hypertrophic. Fibrillation of cartilage follows severe repeated hemarthroses, ultimately leading to cartilaginous degeneration.[2] In this report, the advanced changes are similar to those seen in osteoarthritis, although in hemophilia, the destructive changes are more conspicuous, subchondral pseudocysts are common, and the productive changes—eburnation and osteophytes—are less prominent.

Pathophysiology

The biologic basis for the predisposition to bleeding in the hemophilic joint has not been clarified. The phenomenon occurs most characteristically with deficiencies of coagulant Factors VIII and IX; it also occurs in various animal species with inherited deficiencies of these clotting factors.

Once bleeding into a joint has occurred, the subsequent series of events are reasonably well established in experimental animals and in studies in humans. In response to bleeding into the joint, the inflamed synovium plays a role in the liberation of proteolytic enzymes such as cathepsin-D, acid phosphatase, and various collagenases that produce digestion of ground substance of cartilage, and degeneration of collagen. White cells that enter the joint during an episode of hemarthrosis may also contribute to the release of proteolytic enzymes. The high levels of fibrinolytic activity in the neovascularized synovium may also contribute to rebleeding and reactivation of the process.

Increases in intra-articular pressure may also play a role in producing the degenerative changes.[19] Although it has been postulated that iron deposition may affect the development of hemophilic arthropathy, conventional histologic examination has failed to identify siderotic pigmentation of fibrous replacement cartilage as a consistent feature of hemophilic joint disease.[19]

In addition to pathologic changes in the joint as a direct result of bleeding, the reflex inhibition induced by pain and swelling and the immobilization provided by well-meaning physicians and surgeons produces muscle atrophy. In the weight-bearing joints this con-

tributes to instability of the joint and can result in inability to ambulate. The function of the upper extremity can be markedly impaired when the elbow joint is significantly involved.

Treatment and Results

The management of patients with hemophilia requires a multidisciplinary team approach. The orthopedic surgeon should be closely involved in the periodic evaluation of such patients and should be available for consultation if unusual or unexpected joint problems occur. Major surgical procedures should be undertaken only in centers with facilities for defining the coagulation abnormality, screening inhibitors, and monitoring factor levels.

Acute Hemarthrosis. Here the primary goal is to prevent or control bleeding into the joint and maintain function. It is impractical to limit activities to protect joints, and for most people, routine prophylactic administration of the missing clotting factor is neither practical nor economically feasible. Thus early, prompt intravenous replacement therapy is advised at the *earliest* sign of bleeding into the joint. Patients and families are carefully instructed in the early signs and symptoms of hemarthrosis, and many patients are now being trained in home infusion of factor concentrates. The material is either administered by a family member or a friend or is self-infused. Patients not trained for home infusion are directed to the nearest treatment facility, where it is desirable to keep an ongoing prescription for replacement therapy on file. Unless the patient or family identifies something unusual about the hemorrhagic episode, routine examination by a physician is not necessary and could in many instances delay treatment unnecessarily.[10]

All replacement concentrates for routine use are derived from normal human plasma, and various clotting factors are concentrated to varying degrees. For treatment of acute elbow hemarthrosis, we advise infusion of enough material to produce a 20 to 50 per cent rise in the plasma level of the missing factor.

Joint aspiration is reserved for situations in which immediate relief of pain from extreme swelling is needed or when the possibility of pyarthrosis is being considered.

Splint immobilization is not necessary and is probably contraindicated unless padding is needed to protect a particularly painful joint from trauma. Early mobilization and restoration of joint function must be encouraged as soon as symptoms have resolved sufficiently even if the joint is still swollen.

Ulnar nerve palsies have been reported in association with elbow hemarthrosis and in one patient who had severe arthropathy and a large medial synovial cyst.[14]

Recurrent Hemarthroses

Recurrent bleeding into a single joint with clinical and radiologic evidence of synovitis requires evaluation to ensure that the patient is responding with appropriate rises in blood levels of coagulation factors. Specific inhibitors to the administered factors, which are gamma globulins, develop in up to 10 per cent of patients with severe hemophilia A, and specialized laboratory tests are necessary to identify them.

If it is established that the patient does not have an inhibitor and that in vivo increments of Factor VIII or Factor IX are appropriate, consideration should be given to a 3- to 6-month trial of prophylactic replacement therapy aimed at maintaining levels above 3 to 5 per cent of normal.[10] Alternatively, a course of oral prednisone therapy has been found to be useful in reducing the inflammatory process in the joint.[13] These procedures are aimed at reducing the vascularity and friability of the synovium and the tendency to rebleed. If neither of these programs succeeds in eliminating the recurrent hemarthroses, surgical synovectomy should be considered. Synovectomy often produces a decrease in joint function but can effectively reduce or even eliminate bleeding into the joint and provide relief from pain. In a series of 12 elbow synovectomies, Kaye et al. noted a reduction in the average number of bleeding episodes from 24 per year (range, 8 to 52) before surgery to 3 per year (range, 1 to 18) following the procedure.[12] During a follow-up period of 12 to 58 months (average, 29.5 months) after synovectomy, 8 of 12 elbow joints lost an average of 19 degrees of flexion-extension mobility, and the other 4 joints gained 5 to 35 degrees. With respect to supination-pronation, three patients were improved (10 to 95 degrees), three remained unchanged, and six lost between 5 and 45 degrees of range of motion.[12] Ideally, synovectomy should be undertaken before significant changes have occurred on radiography. Medical synovectomy using osmic or radioactive gold has been used in knee joints, but the elbow has been the subject of only a few reports on this procedure.[15, 20]

Joint contractures can be prevented or min-imized during early phases of arthropathy by prompt, effective replacement therapy, early mobilization, and an active physical therapy program aimed at maintaining muscle strength and range of motion. This aspect of management tends to be overlooked in the elbow because patients are usually able to maintain reasonably normal function in spite of significant restrictions of motion at this joint. Long-term corrective rigid bracing is rarely indicated in the elbow or other joints, but adjustable elbow splints can be useful for temporary protection of a tender joint following acute hemorrhage. These splints are also useful at night to prevent recurrent hemorrhage.[3]

Pain control can become a problem in this phase. Aspirin and aspirin-containing drugs should be avoided because of their adverse effect on platelet function. Some of the nonsteroidal anti-inflammatory drugs have a more transient effect on platelet function and could be tried with cautious observation in selected patients. We have been impressed by the anti-inflammatory effects of nonacetylated salicylates such as Trilisate (choline magnesium trisalicylate) and Disalcid (salicylasalicylic acid) in relieving arthritic symptoms. Particularly in patients with established hemophilic arthropathy, drug abuse and addiction can be serious problems and must be guarded against.

Chronic Arthropathy

Chronic arthropathy is associated with pain, motion restrictions, stiffness, discomfort, and muscle atrophy. A well-designed exercise program can maintain the elbow in a functional range.[3] In children, premature closure of the epiphyseal centers can occur. Forearm rotation is restricted by involvement of the radial head and capitellum, and this loss of rotatory function is more disabling than loss of flexion or extension. Periodic use of the adjustable elbow splint may provide some relief from pain and discomfort.

Radial head excision and partial synovectomy can provide pain relief, reduce the incidence of hemarthrosis, and improve forearm rotation in selected patients.[9] Total elbow arthroplasty may be indicated when there is severe functional limitation (Fig. 43–5).

In the patient with chronic arthropathy, adequate analgesia must be provided, particularly in drug-dependent patients undergoing major surgical procedures. The involvement of a chemical abuse team can be very helpful in handling this aspect of hemophilia management.

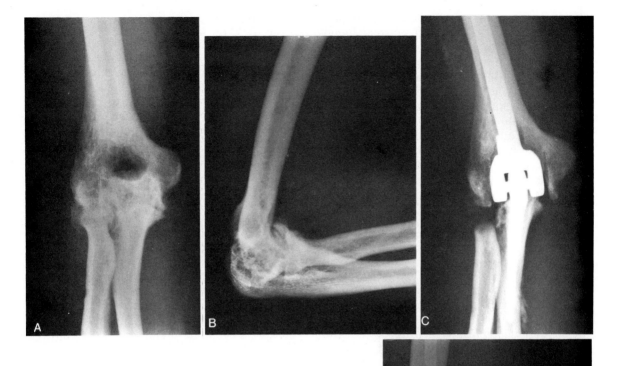

Figure 43–5. *A, B,* Extensive changes of hemophilic arthropathy, showing overgrowth, subchondral cysts, and marked narrowing of the joint space with evidence of contracture. Also, observe the narrowing of the medullary canal. *C, D,* Same patient following insertion of an elbow prosthesis. Note absence of the use of cement in this press fit technique.

SICKLE CELL DISEASE

The term *sickle cell disease* is used to include various inherited diseases characterized by the presence of hemoglobin S (sickle hemoglobin, Hbs). Hbs imparts a sickle shape to deoxygenated red cells. Most of the clinical features of sickle cell disease result from an increase in blood viscosity produced by the abnormal rheologic properties of sickle cells. Perfusion of organs and tissue is impaired, and the resulting stagnation leads to reductions in oxygen tension and further sickling, producing a "vicious cycle of erythrostasis." These vasocclusive crises can affect the blood supply to various organs or tissues including bone, bone marrow, periosteum, and periarticular tissues.[21]

Approximately 8 per cent of blacks in the United States carry the gene for Hbs, with an incidence of homozygous sickle cell anemia (SS disease) at birth of 1 in 625. Hemoglobin SC disease affects about 1 in 833 blacks in the United States, and hemoglobin S-thalassemia affects 1 in 1667. Double heterozygote states for Hbs and a second disorder of hemoglobin synthesis are less common.[21]

Incidence

Patients with sickle cell trait (hemoglobin AS) and aseptic necrosis of bone have been reported, but joint involvement is exceedingly rare. A study of 94 individuals with sickle cell trait found no significant difference in the frequency of joint symptoms or objectively demonstrable joint disease when compared with 114 black patients with normal hemoglobin electrophoretic patterns.[5]

In contrast, most if not all of those with homozygous sickle cell anemia experience bone or joint crises, with the first episode usually occurring before the age of 6 years and rarely under the age of 2. In a prospective study of 56 adults with SS disease, Espinoza et al. documented 61 separate episodes of joint involvement in 31 individuals during a 6- to 18-month observation period.[8] The elbow was affected at one time or another in 13 patients (42 per cent), usually in association with involvement of other large joints.[8]

Anatomy

Radiologic Aspects

Soft tissue swelling is the most common x-ray manifestation. Evidence of prior bone infarction and periostitis may be seen in the adjacent long bones. Widening of the joint space due to effusion is infrequent. Degenerative and hypertrophic changes are rarely seen in the elbow unless there is superimposed infection.[4]

Clinical Aspects

Acute onset of pain, swelling, warmth, and limitation of joint function is characteristic. Erythema is often present. Polyarticular symptoms are observed in more than 80 per cent of cases and are usually symmetrical. Fever is a prominent feature.[8]

Because of the increased susceptibility of these patients to develop infection, the possibility of septic arthritis or osteomyelitis must be considered, particularly in those with monarticular presentations. Osteomyelitis may involve multiple sites, and in more than half the cases this involvement is due to Salmonella.[3] Polyarticular involvement is sometimes migratory and may mimic rheumatic fever. The clinical picture may be further complicated by the presence of cardiomegaly and heart murmurs related to the chronic anemia and involvement of the heart by hemosiderosis. Acute gouty arthritis has been described in sickle cell disease, and serum uric acid levels are often elevated. Uric acid crystals were not identified in joint fluid in any of the 13 cases studied by Espinoza et al. in spite of an elevated serum uric acid level in about one fourth of their patients.[8] Hypertrophic pulmonary osteoarthropathy might be suggested by the periosteal elevation adjacent to the joint in association with pulmonary infiltrates.[17]

Pathology

Clinical and microscopic observations clearly indicate that vascular occlusion is responsible for the bone and joint manifestations of sickle cell disease. It is speculated that the joints are affected by avascular necrosis of adjacent bone. The sinusoidal circulation of the bone marrow provides an ideal bed for the sickling phenomenon.

Studies on synovial fluid have produced variable results. The fluid varies in color from yellow and clear to a cloudy brown. It is sometimes hemorrhagic. Synovial fluid viscosity is normal to decreased with good mucin clot formation. White blood cells, predominantly polymorphonuclear leukocytes, are always present with counts of up to 270,000 per mm^3 without evidence of infection. Sickled erythrocytes are present in about half the cases.[8] Glucose levels are usually normal, but total protein may be elevated, often in association with high levels of total hemolytic complement.[8]

Synovial biopsies generally reveal microvascular thrombosis with occasional intraluminal sickled cells and perivascular fibrosis. Mononuclear inflammatory cell infiltration is variable.[17] Electron microscopy confirms the vascular occlusion with a thickened, sometimes multilaminated vascular basement membrane.[8] The synovial surface may be covered in some areas by fibrin deposits.[8, 17]

Pathophysiology

The fundamental defect in sickle cell disease is an inherited substitution of valine for glutamic acid in position 6 of the beta chain of hemoglobin.[3] This minor change in structure produces profound alterations in the stability and solubility of the hemoglobin molecule. Deoxygenation produces polymerization of Hbs molecules leading to the formation of a semisolid gel and the sickle-shape deformity. Sickling is further aggravated by slight drops in pH and is often irreversible.

The vasocclusive episodes are often preceded by an infectious episode, particularly in children. They can also occur with sudden changes in altitude or during periods of hypoxia, for example, during or after general anesthesia. Fever, dehydration, acidosis, and impaired pulmonary and tissue perfusion contribute to further sickling. Microvascular occlusion produces avascular necrosis, particularly in areas without collateral circulation.

Treatment and Results

There is no specific therapy for vasocclusive crises. A wide variety of therapeutic modalities have been proved ineffective. The prevention or treatment of infection, dehydration, hypoxemia, and acidosis can prevent or modify intravascular sickling. The major goal of treatment is to correct factors that might precipitate or aggravate the intravascular occlusive process.

Fluid replacement is essential and must compensate for the hyposthenuria that is inevitably present and is not reversible by transfusion beyond the age of 4 to 5 years.[3] In addition, fluid and electrolyte losses related to fever, vomiting, and diarrhea must be replaced. Acidosis should be corrected. Underlying infection must be sought and treated as appropriate. Conventional oxygen therapy is of doubtful benefit, and blood transfusions do not modify the course of an established crisis. Pain control is important; acetaminophen is preferable to aspirin, which tends to impose an additional acid load.

Narcotic addiction must be guarded against, particularly in adults who have frequent crises. Since virtually all patients with joint involvement present with fever and leukocytosis with neutrophilia, these features cannot be used as evidence for or against osteomyelitis or suppurative arthritis. One third of patients with uncomplicated sickle cell arthropathy have an elevated erythrocyte sedimentation rate. If clinical evaluation suggests the possibility of septic arthritis, particularly in the patient presenting with monarticular involvement, synovial fluid should be examined *and* cultured. It is important for the clinician to recognize that large numbers of neutrophils are seen in uncomplicated cases of sickle cell arthropathy, and the fluid is sometimes frankly purulent in spite of negative cultures.[8]

Arthritic manifestations clear in 3 to 10 days, and the clinical presentation, pattern of joint involvement, and disease course tend to repeat themselves from crisis to crisis in individual patients. Atypical clinical or laboratory features should alert one to the possibility of other complications. Until a reliable treatment is developed for vasocclusive events, treatment remains supportive, and the outcome is largely determined by the individual's pattern of response.

References

1. Ahlberg, A.: Haemophilia in Sweden. VII. Incidence, Treatment, and Prophylaxis of Arthropathy and Other Musculoskeletal Manifestations of Haemophilia A and B. Acta Orthop. Scand. Suppl. **77**:20, 1965.
2. Arnold, W. D. and Hilgartner, M. W.: Hemophilic Arthropathy. J. Bone Joint Surg. **59A**:287, 1977.
3. Boone, D. C.: Common Musculoskeletal Problems and Their Management. *In* Boone, D. C. (ed.): Comprehensive Management of Hemophilia. Philadelphia, F. A. Davis Co., 1976, pp. 52–85.
4. Diggs, L. W.: Bone and Joint Lesions in Sickle-Cell Disease. Clin. Orthop. **52**:119, 1967.
5. Dorwart, B. B., Goldberg, M. A., Schumacher, H. R., et al.: Absence of Increased Frequency of Bone and Joint Disease with Hemoglobin AS and AC. Ann. Int. Med. **86**:66, 1977.
6. Duthie, R. B., Matthews, J. M., Rizza, C. R., Steel, W. M., and Woods, C. G.: The Management of Musculoskeletal Problems in the Hemophiliac. Oxford, Blackwell, 1972, pp. 29-127.
7. Dymock, I. W., Hamilton, E. B. D., Laws, J. W., and Williams, R.: Arthropathy of Haemochromatosis: Clinical and Radiologic Analysis of 63 Patients With Iron Overload. Ann. Rheum. Dis. **29**:469, 1970.
8. Espinoza, L. R., Spilberg, I., and Osterland, C. K.: Joint Manifestations of Sickle Cell Disease. Medicine **53**:295, 1974.
9. Gilbert, M. S., and Glass, K. S.: Hemophilic Arthropathy in the Elbow. Mt. Sinai J. Med. **44**:389, 1977.
10. Gilchrist, G. S.: Hemorrhagic Disorders. *In* Gellis, S. S., and Kagen, B. M. (eds.): Current Pediatric Therapy, 11th ed. Philadelphia, W. B. Saunders Co., 1984.
11. Hamilton, E., Williams, R., Barlow, K. A., and Smith, P. M.: The Arthropathy of Idiopathic Haemochromatosis. Q. J. Med. **37**:171, 1968.
12. Kaye, L., Stainsby, D., Buzzard, B., Fearns, M., Hamilton, P. J., Owen, P., and Jones, P.: The Role of Synovectomy in the Management of Recurrent Hemarthroses in Hemophilia. Br. J. Haemat. **49**:53, 1981.
13. Kisker, C. T., and Burke, C.: Double-Blind Studies on the Use of Steroids in the Treatment of Acute Hemarthrosis in Patients With Hemophilia. N. Engl. J. Med. **282**:639, 1970.
14. Lancourt, J. E., Gilbert, M. S., and Posner, M. A.: Management of Bleeding and Associated Complications of Hemophilia in the Hand and Forearm. J. Bone Joint Surg. **59A**:451, 1977.
15. Rivard, G. E., Girard, M., Cliche, C. L., Guay, J. P., Belanger, R., and Besner, R.: Synoviorthesis in Patients With Hemophilia and Inhibitors. Can. Med. Assoc. J. **127**:41, 1982.
16. Schaller, J.: Arthritis as a Presenting Manifestation of Malignancy in Children. J. Pediatr. **81**:793, 1972.
17. Schumacher, H. R., Andrews, R., and McLaughlin, G.: Arthropathy in Sickle-Cell Disease. Ann. Int. Med. **78**:203, 1973.
18. Silverstein, M. N., and Kelly, P. J.: Leukemia With Osteoarticular Symptoms and Signs. Ann Int. Med. **59**:637, 1963.
19. Sokoloff, L.: Biomechanical and Physiological Aspects of Degenerative Joint Diseases With Special Reference to Hemophilic Arthropathy. Ann. N. Y. Acad. Sci. **240**:285, 1975.
20. Storti, E., and Ascari, E.: Surgical and Chemical Synovectomy. Ann. N. Y. Acad. Sci. **240**:316, 1975.
21. Wintrobe, M. M., Lee, S. R., Boggs, D. R., Bithell, T. C., Foerster, J., Athens, J. W., and Leukens, J. N.: Clinical Hematology, 8th ed. Philadelphia, Lea & Febiger, 1981, pp. 1158–1205.
22. Wintrobe, M. M., Lee, G. R., Boggs, D. R., Bithell, T. C., Foerster, J., Athens, J. W., and Lukens, J. N.: Clinical Hematology, 8th ed. Philadelphia, Lea & Febiger, 1981, pp. 835–859.

CHAPTER 44

Neurotrophic Arthritis

J. C. STEVENS

The occurrence of a neurotrophic arthritis of the elbow is distinctly unusual. Although a large number of causes of neurotrophic arthritis are recognized (Table 44–1), diagnosis is made simpler by the fact that only five or six of these affect the upper extremity joints and only three with any frequency at all. In this section the causes and pathogenesis of neurogenic arthropathy of the elbow are discussed, along with laboratory investigations and differential diagnosis. Arthropathy of lower limb joints and the spine will not be

considered, but references cited in Table 44–1 are provided to direct the interested reader to other sources of information. Excellent reviews of the subject have been written by Bruckner and Howell[9] and by Rodnan.[51]

PATHOGENESIS

Debate about the pathogenesis of neurotrophic arthritis began with Charcot's paper in 1886, and today our understanding of the pathophysiology remains incomplete. Charcot, observing the posterior column demyelination of tabes dorsalis, suggested loss of a trophic function protecting joints. This view was soon challenged by those who felt that the disorder resulted from trauma. A major advance in our understanding followed the often-quoted work of Eloesser,[27] who sectioned the posterior roots of the hind limb of cats. Deafferentation combined with thermocautery of the joint cartilage led to the rapid development of neurogenic arthropathy, bone fractures and dislocations emphasizing the role of insensitivity and trauma. Chemical analysis and tests of bone strength and elasticity were normal—evidence against Charcot's view that the joints and bones wasted from an abnormality of trophic nerves. The roles of insensitivity, activity, and trauma were further emphasized by Corbin and Hinsey, who found that cats with loss of sensation developed a Charcot joint only if they were allowed to roam freely in the cage while those kept in restricted space did not.[19] They were impressed by the importance of proprioceptive loss, which allowed an abnormal range of joint movement. It is also recognized that limbs splinted by spasticity rarely develop an arthropathy. Knowledge about the importance of activity and trauma in the development of a neurotrophic arthropathy is now being appreciated clinically. Harris and Brand reported that joint breakdown in the neuropathy of leprosy can be minimized or prevented by proper protection.[37] Johnson emphasized the importance of unrecognized and untreated

Table 44–1. Etiology of Neurogenic Arthropathy

I. Brain
  A. Congenital indifference (asymbolia) to pain[31, 49, 57]
  B. "Stoic" individual[38]
  C. Functional abnormality of enkephalins, endorphins or opiate receptors?[25]
II. Spinal cord
  A. Tabes dorsalis[16, 41, 54, 62, 67, 68]
  B. Syringomyelia[33]
  C. Paraplegia[65]
  D. Radiation myelopathy[68]
  E. Myelomeningocele[13]
  F. Subacute combined degeneration[36]
  G. Arachnoiditis—Tbc[46] spinal anesthetic[69]
  H. Multiple sclerosis[57]
  I. Idiopathic?[5, 43]
  J. Spinal cord tumor
III. Peripheral Nerve
  A. Metabolic neuropathy
    1. Diabetes mellitus[6, 12, 17, 29, 45, 50, 58]
    2. Amyloidosis[48, 55]
    3. Gigantism[21]
  B. Inherited Neuropathies
    1. Hereditary motor and sensory neuropathy[22]
      (a) Type I—Charcot-Marie-Tooth[8, 10]
      (b) Type II—Dejerine-Sottas[53]
    2. Hereditary sensory and autonomic neuropathy[22, 23, 24]
      (a) Type I
      (b) Type II
      (c) Type III[11, 35]
      (d) Type IV
      (e) Type V
    3. Subclinical neuropathy with neurogenic arthropathy and recurring fractures[25]
  C. Infection—leprosy[28]
  D. Nutritional—alcoholism[54]
  E. Traumatic—sciatic and other peripheral nerves[40, 56]
IV. Corticosteroids—Charcotlike neuropathy[2, 14, 26, 63]

fractures, especially stress fractures in the development of neurogenic arthropathy.[38]

The most widely held view on the pathogenesis of Charcot's joints, then, involves a loss of protective joint nociception and position sense that subjects the joint to repeated trauma that is not recognized by the affected individual. The injured joint in a neurologically normal patient quickly announces its presence by the development of pain and loss of function leading to immobilization and a search for appropriate medical treatment. In the neurologically impaired person, on the other hand, unrecognized injury is untreated and leads to a vicious circle of compounding injuries. This explanation is intuitively reasonable, particularly in the presence of severe superficial and deep loss of pain perception. It is more difficult to invoke when joint destruction evolves but sensory loss is minimal or difficult to demonstrate. For example, we recently studied patients with subclinical inherited neuropathy with severe neurotrophic arthropathy of various joints and recurring fractures who had no sensory symptoms or findings on clinical examination.[25] Even with sophisticated tests, including computer-assisted sensory examination, periosteal nociception, and morphometric and graded teased fiber evaluation of cutaneous nerves, only a mild neuropathic abnormality was found. Methods of measuring joint capsule and articular bone pain perception are not available; however, cortical bone is known to contain both unmyelinated and myelinated fibers, and presumably some of these subserve nociception.[18] Joint capsules, particularly in their external layers, contain several types of formed corpuscles and naked nerve endings. Synovia have not been observed to contain nerve endings. Although pain sense is carried by both small myelinated and unmyelinated fibers, the relative importance of these two systems in normal protective joint sensation is unknown. In those puzzling patients in whom sensation appears to be normal, a new method of measuring joint pain perception or afferent nerve fiber activity is needed.

There are a number of situations in which the neurotraumatic hypothesis seems inadequate to explain joint destruction entirely, even in the neurologically impaired person, and the additional factor of a trophic vascular mechanism becomes attractive. This theory has been most recently articulated by Brower and Alman.[7] The neurovascular theory suggests that neurologic disease triggers increased bone blood flow and active bone resorption by osteoclasts and that fractures and joint damage follow. The arguments in favor of the hypothesis are enumerated below.

First, a proportion of patients with Charcot joints are said to have no neurologic disease when joint destruction develops, making it difficult to blame joint insensitivity. It may be, however, that many of these patients would be found to harbor neurologic disease following intensive neurologic investigation. Second, there are instances in which neurotrophic joints develop in bedridden patients in whom weight bearing is impossible and repeated severe joint trauma unlikely. Third, a few patients suffer joint destruction and resorption of articular structures in a matter of weeks to a few months, making pure mechanical destruction hard to accept as the sole mechanism.[47] Last, many neurotrophic arthropathies are associated with long bone fractures that seemingly occur spontaneously or without unusual trauma. This implies a metabolic abnormality of bone, possibly related to abnormal blood flow; however, no abnormality of bone chemical analysis or stress tests have been found in experimental animals or human subjects. Although histologic examination is said to show pathologically increased vascularity, it is also a fact that acutely damaged joints become hot and swollen from increased blood flow and exudation as part of the body's normal repair process, making pathologic vascularity difficult to prove. Hind limb sympathectomy might be expected to increase blood flow; however, in experimental animals, at least, it does not lead to joint damage or abnormalities in the chemical composition of bone.[19] It is still possible, however, that local hyperemia is exaggerated in some patients, leading to rapid bony softening and resorption, and it is not possible to discard this hypothesis out of hand (Fig. 44–1).

Joint infection has been suggested in the past as a cause of neurogenic arthropathy, and although sepsis undoubtedly occurs in some cases, it is clearly not present in the majority. Trophic ulceration, lymphangitis, and cellulitis, however, can result in osteomyelitis, which accelerates joint destruction and leads to digit resorption. Tuberculosis of the elbow can cause resorptive and destructive changes similar to those in a neurotrophic joint (Fig. 44–2).

Environmental factors can adversely add to the effect of nociceptive loss in a number of ways. Neurotrophic arthropathy is more common in weight-bearing joints and in men,

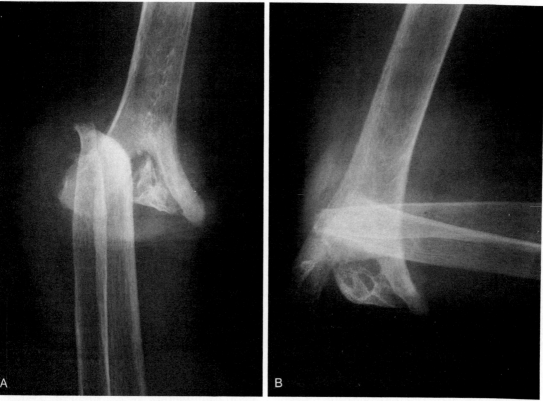

Figure 44–1. This figure shows the gross resorption destruction of the elbow joint due to rheumatoid arthritis (A, B), although no hypertrophic changes are present as in the typical neurotrophic joint. This illustration does, however, seem to represent an example of hyperemic arthropathy, one of the etiologic considerations of neurotrophic joints.

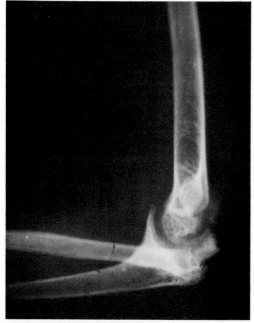

Figure 44–2. Gross destruction of an elbow joint involved with tuberculous arthritis. Note that both sides of the joint are involved. A distinction between this entity and a neurotrophic arthropathy in the early stages is complicated by the possibility that the two conditions co-exist.[46] (Courtesy of Dr. Richard Marks, Cape Town, South Africa.)

perhaps because of occupations involving manual labor and physical activity. Additional factors include the presence of mental retardation, psychosis, the metabolic effect of diabetes, and rheumatoid arthritis or metabolic bone disease. The so-called stoic personality, while admitting pain, seems to be able to ignore it and continue to walk and work unimpeded. There are also those who, although experiencing considerable pain, may out of economic necessity cling to a job in spite of deforming arthritis.

The administration of steroids particularly by the intra-articular route, in the treatment of patients with degenerative joint disease occasionally is followed by rapid joint disintegration. Patients reported with this complication have not had any neurologic disease, and therefore the joint destruction cannot be called a neurotrophic arthropathy. The administration of steroids, however, relieves joint pain and allows a level of increased activity that leads to further joint damage. The interplay of multiple factors in the genesis of bone and joint complications is emphasized in Figure 44–3.

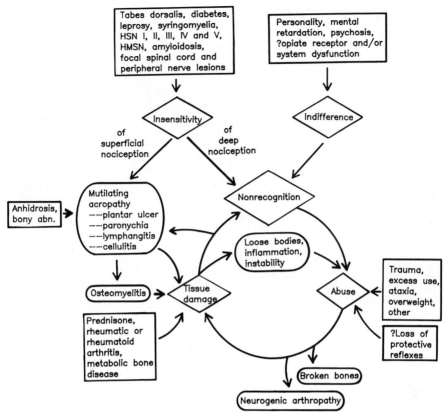

Figure 44–3. Schematic representation of the inter-relationship between the etiology and pathophysiology of neurotrophic arthropathy.

CONDITIONS CAUSING NEUROARTHROPATHY OF THE ELBOW

Tabes Dorsalis

Although syphilis used to be responsible for up to 90 percent of neurotrophic joints, antibiotic treatment of the condition during the last 30 years has resulted in a steadily declining incidence. New cases of tabes dorsalis are rarely seen, and locomotor ataxia is now an uncommon cause of neuroarthropathy. Approximately 10 percent of all tabetics will develop a Charcot joint, the majority occurring between the ages of 40 and 60 years, some 20 years or more after the primary infection. In approximately 78 percent of cases, the lower limbs are affected,[32] with the knee most frequently involved, followed by the hip, ankle, and tarsus. Spinal arthropathy affects the lumbar and lower thoracic segments. In the upper limbs, the shoulder, elbow, hands, and wrists are affected.[3, 20, 32, 61, 64, 66] Polyarticular involvement is seen in up to 40 percent. Clinical features include the presence of lightening pains, neurogenic bladder disturbances, optic neuritis, and visceral crises. Most patients have pupillary abnormalities, and loss of pupillary reflexes to light (Argyll-Robertson pupils) are seen in up to 62 percent. Vibration and position sense are reduced, and deep pain sensation may be absent. Pain perception may be delayed. Muscular hypotonia and sensory ataxia are frequent. Lower limb reflexes are usually reduced or absent. Although the VDRL may be negative, newer and more specific tests such as the FTA-ABS are usually positive. Elbow movement may be restricted, or the elbow may be subluxed and hypermobile with marked instability (Fig. 44–4).[3] Spontaneous fractures can occur. Roentgen examination may show extensive destruction of the bone ends, disintegration of the joint, abundant periosteal callus formation, valgus deformity, and free bodies in the articulation.[64]

Syringomyelia

In contrast to tabes dorsalis, 80 percent of the joints involved in syringomyelia are in the upper extremities.[32] It is estimated that approximately 25 percent of those affected will develop joint breakdown. Neuropathic dis-

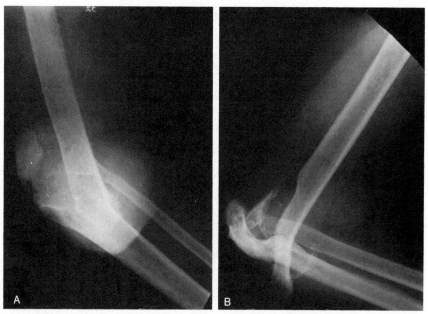

Figure 44–4. The deformity associated with this Charcot joint is obvious by inspection, and the joint is grossly unstable (A, B). (From Beetham, W. P. et al: Charcot's joints. Ann. Int. Med. 58:1002, 1963.)

ease involves the shoulder most commonly, followed by the elbow and wrist. Degenerative changes in the cervical spine are not uncommon. The process evolves gradually with paresthesias of the hands, followed by progressive weakness and wasting of the small hand muscles, and then atrophy of arm and shoulder muscles.[30] Loss of pain and temperature sense affects the arms and upper thoracic segments. As the syrinx enlarges long tract signs appear, and a Horner's syndrome is seen. The Arnold-Chiari malformation is commonly associated and is related to the development of syringomyelia.

Roentgenographic examination of the cervical spine may show widening of the spinal canal, but the major diagnostic procedure is myelography including films taken in the supine position to demonstrate tonsillar herniation. Computed tomography with metrizamide contrast enhancement of the cerebrospinal fluid may demonstrate spinal cord enlargement and cavitations in some instances.

Elbow arthropathy may follow neurologic symptoms, but is sometimes a presenting complaint.[4] A history of trauma is usually lacking. Joint swelling due to effusion may be marked, and pain is experienced in some cases. Atrophic changes in the bone, particularly of the shoulder, are more common than in tabes dorsalis.[67] Although extremely rapid destruction of the shoulder may occur with resorption of the humeral head,[42, 59] the elbow seems less likely to be affected in this fashion.

The roentgenogram of the elbow shows resorption of bone ends and often of the entire joint (Fig. 44–5). Reparative callus is evident along with gross deformity and instability.

Diabetes Mellitus

The importance and diagnosis of diabetes mellitus as an increasing cause of neurotrophic arthropathy is being recognized. Indeed it has probably surpassed tabes dorsalis as the leading cause of neurotrophic arthropathy. The arthropathy usually develops in diabetics who have had the disease for some time and who have suffered the additional complication of a symmetrical sensorimotor polyneuropathy. In diabetic "pseudotabes" severe sensory and autonomic impairment leads to an ataxic gait, pupillary abnormalities, neurogenic bladder, and lightening pains reminiscent of tabes dorsalis. Diabetic arthropathy primarily affects the joints of the feet, with less frequent involvement of the ankles and knees.[6, 17, 45, 50, 58] The distal predominance of the arthropathy is in keeping with the stocking pattern of sensory loss, which is maximal in the feet. Bony abnormalities in the upper extremities of diabetics are quite uncommon, but involvement of the shoulder, elbow,[12] and wrist[29] has been recorded. Campbell[12] and Feldman[29] illustrate a

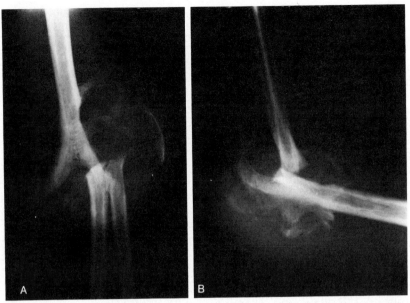

Figure 44–5. Gross destruction of an elbow joint in a 34-year-old woman with syringomyelia. *A,* Anteroposterior view. *B,* Lateral view. The classic features of joint obliteration and resorption followed by an abortive effort of callus formation resulting in instability are obvious.

radiograph of the elbow in a 59-year-old patient showing marked disorganization of the joint with destruction of the articular surfaces, numerous bone fragments, and periosteal new bone formation typical of a Charcot joint.

Congenital Indifference and Insensitivity to Pain

The concept of indifference to pain implies that these patients perceive pain stimuli in a normal fashion but fail to react in the usual defensive manner, a kind of asymbolia for pain, whereas insensitivity denotes an inability to receive a painful stimulus because of a neurologic deficit. Most patients with the former disorder have not had detailed electrophysiologic, biomechanical, and pathologic examinations, and it is likely that previously reported cases have had a congenital sensory and autonomic neuropathy of type IV or V.[24] Nevertheless, occasional patients in this group may develop a neurotrophic arthropathy or fracture that may affect the elbow.[31, 44, 57] Involvement of the elbow in Charcot-Marie-Tooth disease has also been recorded.[9]

Miscellaneous

A case of idiopathic arthropathy of the elbow was reported by Meyn and Yablon in 1973;[43] however, syringomyelia was not excluded be-cause the patient refused myelography. A second example of "idiopathic" arthropathy of the elbow may also have been syringomyelia.[5] In a poorly studied patient reported by Karten[39] with the CRST variant of systemic sclerosis and multiple neuropathic joints including the elbows, it was suggested that hysterical indifference to pain was a major factor. This seems an unlikely explanation, however, because muscle weakness and atrophy and absence of deep pain were present. Another unusual patient, described by Alajouanine and Boudin,[1] had elbow arthropathy associated with distal muscular atrophy, subcutaneous and vascular calcification, and abnormal calcium and phosphorus metabolism. There were no sensory changes, and the cause of the arthropathy is obscure.

INVESTIGATION

The examination of a patient with a neurotrophic arthropathy of the elbow should focus on a search for evidence of syringomyelia, tabes dorsalis, and diabetes because almost all patients will be found to harbor one of these disorders. When physical signs of these diseases are lacking, the patient should be examined carefully for evidence of pes cavus, hammer toes, enlargement of peripheral nerves, and distal sensory loss, which may suggest the presence of a peripheral neuropathy. A dissociated sensory loss is found in syringomyelia but may also be present in amyloid neuropathy, familial dysautonomia, hereditary sensory and autonomic neuropathy type II, and Tangier disease. Evidence of an autonomic neuropathy is important because small myelinated and unmyelinated pain afferents that provide joint nociception are often involved as well. Loss of sweating, orthostatic hypotension, urinary incontinence, and impotence are the most important symptoms of autonomic dysfunction seen in a variety of small fiber neuropathies. Other neuropathies may have a more generalized sensory disturbance that affects both large and small fibers. A profound loss of pain sense, however, is not a necessary prerequisite for the development of neurogenic arthropathy, and the patient's complaint of pain and the presence of normal or nearly normal nociception should not deter further investigation. It is often helpful to interview and examine family members even when no apparent disease is known to kin. This is particularly necessary in patients with a peripheral neuropathy or only slight neurologic abnormalities in whom the hereditary nature of the disorder may become evident only after intensive investigation of relatives. The clinician should also look for wasting of small hand muscles and ulnar sensory loss because the nerve may be compromised behind the medial epicondyle by the deformity associated with the Charcot joint.

Laboratory investigations that we have found useful in the investigation of neurogenic arthropathy, in addition to "routine tests," are listed in Table 44–2. Some of these studies require special expertise and equipment not readily available at smaller centers. We have found the computer-assisted sensory examination, and electromyography and nerve conduction studies helpful in detecting disease in minimally affected patients and family members. In a few patients nerve biopsy, including teased fiber preparations,

Table 44–2. Laboratory Investigations

1. Serologic tests for syphilis (blood and CSF)
2. Fasting blood glucose
3. Serum vitamin B_{12}
4. Serum protein electrophoresis and special serum and urine protein studies
5. MMPI, psychometric evaluation
6. Thermoregulatory sweat test
7. Computer-assisted sensory examination
8. Periosteal bone nociception
9. Computed tomography
10. Myelography
11. Sural nerve biopsy

Table 44–3. Differential Diagnosis of Neurogenic Arthropathy

1. Osteoarthritis
2. Traumatic arthritis
3. Acute infective arthritis
4. Tuberculosis arthritis
5. Rheumatoid arthritis
6. Gout
7. Malignant disease
8. Thrombophlebitis, cellulitis
9. Osteoblastic metastases and Paget's disease (spine)

quantitative morphometry, electron microscopy, histochemistry, analysis of myelin lipids, the in vitro nerve action potential, and studies of axonal transport may be needed for complete evaluation of the specimen. The differential diagnosis of neurogenic arthropathy is listed in Table 44–3.

TREATMENT

Two stages of the disease process should be identified for treatment. During the early stages of development, the neurotrophic joint should be protected with a long arm cast or molded splint. The appropriate diagnosis is obviously important during this stage. Thus, some knowledge of the existence of this entity as well as the etiologic factors is important (see Table 44–1). As the active process resolves, the residual dysfunction should be assessed. Pain is rare. Hence, stability is the primary consideration in most clinical settings. This residual is usually treated with an orthoplast splint with hinges to retain function. Surgical fusion is extremely difficult and should be considered rarely only as a procedure of last resort.[60]

References

1. Alajouanine, T., and Boudin, G.: Sur un Complexus Clinique Caracterise par une Atrophie Musculaire, Myelopathique de Type Distal avec Grosses Deformations des Pieds, Arthropathies du Caude et de la Colome Vertebrale Nodosites Calcaires Sous-Cutanees et Arterite Calcaire avec Perturbation du Metabolisme Phosphocalcique. Rev. Neurol. **77**:193, 1945.
2. Alarcon-Segovia, D., and Ward, L. E.: Carcot-like Arthropathy in Rheumatoid Arthritis. Consequences of Overuse of a Joint Repeatedly Injected with Hydrocortisone. J.A.M.A. **193**:1052, 1965.
3. Beetham, W. P., Kaye, R. L., and Polley, H. F.: Charcot's Joints. A Case of Extensive Polyarticular Involvement, and Discussion of Certain Clinical and Pathologic Features. Ann. Int. Med. **58**:1002, 1963.
4. Bhaskaran, R. K., Suresh, K., and Iyer, G. V.: Charcot's Elbow. J. Postgrad. Med. **27**:194, 1981.
5. Blanford, A. T., Keane, S. P., McCarty, D. J., and Albers, J. W.: Idiopathic Charcot Joint of the Elbow. Arth. Rheum. **21**:923, 1978.

6. Boehm, H. J.: Diabetic Charcot Joint. Report of a Case and Review of the Literature. N. Engl. J. Med. **267**:185, 1962.
7. Brower, A. C., and Alman, R. M.: Pathogenesis of the Neurotrophic Joint: Neurotraumatic vs. Neurovascular. Radiology **139**:349, 1981.
8. Bruckner, F. E.: Double Charcot's Disease. Br. Med. J. **2**:603, 1968.
9. Bruckner, F. E., and Howell, A.: Neuropathic Joints. Sem. Arth. Rheum. **2**:47, 1972.
10. Bruckner, F. E., and Kendall, B. E.: Neuroarthropathy in Charcot-Marie-Tooth Disease. Ann. Rheum. Dis. **28**:577, 1969.
11. Brunt, P. W.: Unusual Cause of Charcot Joints in Early Adolescence (Riley-Day Syndrome). Br. Med. J. **4**:277, 1967.
12. Campbell, W. L., and Feldman, F.: Bone and Soft Tissue Abnormalities of the Upper Extremity in Diabetes Mellitus. Am. J. Roentgenol. **124**:7, 1975.
13. Carr, T. L.: The Orthopaedic Aspects of One Hundred Cases of Spina Bifida. Postgrad. Med. J. **32**:201, 1956.
14. Chandler, G. N., Jones, D. T., Wright, V., and Hartfall, S. J.: Charcot's Arthropathy Following Intra-articular Hydrocortisone. Br. Med. J. **1**:952, 1959.
15. Charcot, J. M.: Sur Quelques Arthropathies qui Paraissent Dependre d'une Lesion Cerveau ou de la Moelle Epiniere. Arch. Physiol. Normale Pathol. **1**:161, 1868.
16. Cleveland, M., Smith, A., and De, F.: Fusion of the Knee in Cases of Charcot's Disease. Report of Four Cases. J. Bone Joint Surg. **13**:849, 1931.
17. Clouse, M. E., Gramm, H. F., Legg, M., and Floyd, T.: Diabetic Osteoarthropathy. Clinical and Roentgenographic Observations in 90 Cases. Am. J. Roentgenol. **121**:22, 1974.
18. Cooper, R. R.: Nerves in Cortical Bone. Science **160**:327, 1968.
19. Corbin, K. B., and Hinsey, J. C.: Influence of the Nervous System on Bone and Joints. Anat. Rec. **75**:307, 1939.
20. Das, P. C., Banerji, A., Roy, A., and Basu, S.: Neurogenic Arthropathies (Charcot's Joints). J. Indian Med. Assoc. **54**:368, 1970.
21. Daughaday, W. H.: Extreme Gigantism. N. Engl. J. Med. **297**:1267, 1977.
22. Dyck, P. J.: Inherited Neuronal Degeneration and Atrophy Affecting Peripheral Motor Sensory and Autonomic Neurons. In Dyck, P. J., Thomas, P. K., Lambert, E. H., and Bunge, R. G. (eds.): Peripheral Neuropathy. Philadelphia, W. B. Saunders Co., 1984.
23. Dyck, P. J.: Neuronal Atrophy and Degeneration Predominantly Affecting Peripheral Sensory Neurons. In Dyck, P. J., Thomas, P. K., Lambert, E. H., and Bunge, R. G. (eds.): Peripheral Neuropathy. Philadelphia, W. B. Saunders Co., 1984.
24. Dyck, P. J., Mellinger, J. F., Reagan, T. J., Horowitz, S., McDonald, J. W., Litchy, W. J., Daube, J. R., Fealey, R. D., Go, V. L., Kao, P. C., Brimijoin, W. S., and Lambert, E. H.: Not "Indifference to Pain," but Varieties of Hereditary Sensory and Autonomic Neuropathy. Brain **106**:373, 1983.
25. Dyck, P. J., Stevens, J. C., O'Brien, P. C., Oviatt, K. F., Lais, A. C., Coventry, M. B., and Beabout, J. W.: Neurogenic Arthropathy and Recurring Fractures with Subclinical Inherited Neuropathy. Neurology **33**:357, 1983.
26. Eibel, P.: Painless Arthropathy Complicated by Massive Hemorrhagic Effusion. Clin. Orthop. **60**:149, 1968.
27. Eloesser, L.: On the Nature of Neuropathic Affections of the Joints. Ann. Surg. **66**:201, 1917.
28. Faget, G. H., and Mayoral, A.: Bone Changes in Leprosy: A Clinical and Roentgenologic Study of 505 Cases. Radiology **42**:1, 1944.
29. Feldman, M. J., Becker, K. L., Reefe, W. E., and Longo, A.: Multiple Neuropathic Joints Including the Wrist, in a Patient with Diabetes Mellitus. J.A.M.A. **209**:1690, 1969.
30. Finlayson, A. E.: Syringomyelia and Related Conditions. In Baker, A. B., and Baker, A. L. (eds.): Clinical Neurology. Philadelphia, Harper & Row, 1982.
31. Fitzgerald, J. A. W.: Neuropathic Arthropathy Secondary to Atypical Congenital Indifference to Pain. Proc. R. Soc. Med. **61**:663, 1968.
32. Floyd, W., Lowell, W., and King, R. E.: The Neuropathic Joint. South. Med. J. **52**:563, 1959.
33. Foster, J. B., and Hudgson, P.: Traditional Concepts of Syringomyelia. In Barnett, H. J. M., Foster, J. B., and Hudgson, P. (eds.): Syringomyelia. Philadelphia, W. B. Saunders Co., 1973.
34. Frewin, D. B., Downey, J. A., Feldman, F., and Myers, S. J.: Neuropathic Arthropathy: A Report of Two Cases. Aust. N.Z. J. Med. **3**:587, 1973.
35. Goldberg, M. F., Payne, J. W., and Brunt, P. W.: Ophthalmologic Studies of Familial Dysautonomia. The Riley-Day Syndrome. Arch. Ophthal. **80**:732, 1968.
36. Halonen, P. I., and Jarvinen, A. J.: On the Occurrence of Neuropathic Arthropathies in Pernicious Anemia. Ann. Rheum. Dis. **7**:152, 1948.
37. Harris, J. R., and Brand, P. W.: Patterns of Disintegration of the Tarsus in the Anaesthetic Foot. J. Bone Joint Surg. **48B**:4, 1966.
38. Johnson, J. T. H.: Neuropathic Fractures and Joint Injuries. J. Bone Joint Surg. **49A**:1, 1967.
39. Karten, I.: CRST Syndrome and "Neuropathic" Arthropathy. Arth. Rheum. **12**:636, 1969.
40. Kernwein, G., and Lyon, W. F.: Neuropathic Arthropathy of the Ankle Joint Resulting from Complete Severence of the Sciatic Nerve. Ann. Surg. **115**:261, 1942.
41. Key, J. A.: The Treatment of Tabetic Arthropathies. Urol. Cutan. Rev. **49**:161, 1945.
42. Meyer, G. A., Stein, J., and Poppel, M. H.: Rapid Osseous Changes in Syringomyelia. Radiology **69**:415, 1957.
43. Meyn, M., and Yablon, I. G.: Idiopathic Arthropathy of the Elbow. Clin. Orthop. **97**:90, 1973.
44. Mooney, V., and Mankin, H. J.: A Case of Congenital Insensitivity to Pain with Neuropathic Arthropathy. Arch. Rheum. **9**:820, 1966.
45. Muggia, F. M.: Neuropathic Fracture. Unusual Complication in a Patient with Advanced Diabetic Neuropathy. J.A.M.A. **191**:336, 1965.
46. Nissenbaum, M.: Neurotrophic Arthropathy of the Shoulder Secondary to Tuberculous Arachnoiditis. Clin. Orthop. **118**:169, 1976.
47. Norman, A., Robbins, H., and Milgram, J. E.: The Acute Neuropathic Arthropathy—A Rapid, Severely Disorganizing Form of Arthritis. Radiology **90**:1159, 1968.
48. Peitzman, S. J., Miller, J. L., Ortega, L., Schumacher, H. P., and Fernandez, P. C.: Charcot Arthropathy Secondary to Amyloid Neuropathy. J.A.M.A. **235**:1345, 1976.
49. Petrie, J. G.: A Case of Progressive Joint Disorders Caused by Insentivity to Pain. J. Bone Joint Surg. **35B**:399, 1953.
50. Robillard, R., and Gagnon, P. A.: Diabetic Neuroarthropathy: Report of Four Cases. Can. Med. Assoc. J. **91**:795, 1964.
51. Rodnan, G. P.: Neuropathic Joint Disease. In McCarty,

D. J. (ed.): Arthritis and Allied Conditions. Philadelphia, Lea & Febiger, 1979.

52. Rosenthal, H. S.: Neurotrophic Arthropathy in Multiple Sclerosis. Bull. Hosp. Joint Dis. **26:**109, 1965.

53. Russell, W. R., and Garland, H. G.: Progressive Hypertrophic Polyneuritis with Case Reports. Brain **53:**376, 1930.

54. Samilson, R. L., Sankaran, B., Bersani, F. A., Smith, A., and De, F.: Orthopedic Management of Neuropathic Joints. Arch. Surg. **78:**115, 1959.

55. Scott, R. B., Elmore, S., Brackett, N. C., Harris, W. O., and Still, W. J. S.: Neuropathic Joint Disease (Charcot Joints) in Waldenströms Macroglobulinemia with Amyloidosis. Am. J. Med. **54:**535, 1973.

56. Shands, A. R.: Neuropathies of the Bones and Joints. Report of a Case of an Arthropathy of the Ankle Due to a Peripheral Nerve Lesion. Arch. Surg. **20:**615, 1930.

57. Silverman, F. N., and Gilden, J. J.: Congenital Insensitivity to Pain: A Neurologic Syndrome with Bizarre Skeletal Lesions. Radiology **72:**176, 1959.

58. Sinha, S., Munichoodappa, C. S., and Kozak, G. P.: Neuro-Arthropathy (Charcot Joints) in Diabetes Mellitus. Medicine **51:**191, 1972.

59. Skall-Jensen, J.: Osteoarthropathy in Syringomyelia. Acta Radiol. **38:**382, 1952.

60. Smith, F. M.: Surgery of the Elbow, 2nd ed. Philadelphia, W. B. Saunders Co., 1972.

61. Soto-Hall, R., and Haldeman, K. O.: The Diagnosis of Neuropathic Joint Disease (Charcot Joint). J.A.M.A. **114:**2076, 1940.

62. Sprenger, H. R., and Foley, C. J.: Hip Replacement in a Charcot Joint. Clin. Orthop. **82:**191, 1982.

63. Steinberg, C., Duthie, R. B., and Piva, A. E.: Charcot-like Arthropathy Following Intra-Articular Hydrocortisone. J.A.M.A. **181:**851, 1962.

64. Steindler, A.: The Tabetic Arthropathies. J.A.M.A. **29:**250, 1931.

65. Stepanek, V., and Stepanek, P.: Changes in the Bones and Joints of Paraplegics. Radiol. Clin. North Am. **29:**28, 1960.

66. Storey, G.: Charcot Joints. Br. J. Vener. Dis. **40:**109, 1964.

67. Storey, G.: Charcot Joints. Ann. Rheum. Phys. Med. **10:**312, 1970.

68. Wirth, C. R., Jacobs, R. L., and Rolander, S. D.: Neuropathic Spinal Arthropathy. A Review of the Charcot Spine. Spine **5:**558, 1980.

69. Wolfgang, G. L.: Neurotrophic Arthropathy of the Shoulder—A Complication of Progressive Adhesive Arachnoiditis. Clin. Orthop. **87:**217, 1972.

CHAPTER 45

Nerve Entrapment Syndromes

M. SPINNER and R. L. LINSCHIED

Overview

The diagnosis of a nerve entrapment lesion arising at the elbow can be relatively easy to make if the history, physical examination, and electromyographic studies all confirm the diagnosis and the localization of the lesion.[6, 38, 66] However, if the history and physical examination do not dovetail, then problems can arise. It is not uncommon for an elderly patient to say that her fingers are "stiff," when in reality the fingers are numb. Stiffness suggests an arthritic process, whereas numbness suggests involvement of the peripheral neurologic system in the pathologic process. Similarly, persistent pain about the lateral aspect of the elbow that is resistant to all forms of conservative treatment as well as operative treatment directed to the lateral epicondyle may suggest entrapment of the posterior interosseous nerve. However, it can be difficult to establish the diagnosis of resistant "tennis elbow" due to posterior interosseous nerve compression if the electromyographic studies do not confirm the diagnosis and localization of the pathologic process. The persistence of pain anteriorly over the course of the posterior interosseous nerve should make this structure suspect as the cause of the patient's symptomatology. Unfortunately, patients may have pain due to both lateral epicondylar involvement and posterior interosseous nerve compression. Knowledge that lateral epicondylitis and posterior interosseous nerve compression can coexist is essential. Only management of both lesions simultaneously can relieve the patient's resistant tennis elbow symptoms. A nerve can be compressed at more than one level, that is, it may be a "double crush" lesion. Unfortunately, more than one nerve can be involved at one time.[14] It is necessary to direct one's conservative or surgical attention on occasion to two nerves or two sites on one nerve to relieve all the patient's symptoms and neurologic findings. One must be certain that when more than one nerve is suspect in the neural compression process the brachial plexus is not the site of pathology. Careful serial examinations and electromyographic studies can usually localize the lesion or lesions. Furthermore, some patients are prone or predisposed to multiple sequential neural compression lesions. The care of one neural compression lesion may be completed successfully, only to be followed by another neural compression problem in another peripheral nerve a few months or years later.[67] Obviously, a detailed understanding of the complex normal anatomy of this region is essential for proper diagnosis and treatment of these conditions (Fig. 45–1).

Neurophysiology of Nerve Compression Lesions

Nerve compression may be categorized as first-, second-, third-, or fourth-degree neural lesions. This method was first described by Sir Sidney Sunderland.[93] The earlier classification of Sir Herbert Seddon (1943)[77] utilizes the terms of neurapraxia, axonotmesis, and neurotomesis and can be correlated with Sir Sunderland's in the following manner.

A first-degree lesion is a neurapractic lesion. A second- or mild third-degree lesion is an axonotmetic lesion. The neurotmetic lesion comprises all the fourth-degree lesions (the neuroma in continuity) and the advanced third-degree lesions. We prefer utilizing Sunderland's classification when correlating our clinical problems with the underlying nerve fiber pathology present (Table 45–1).[67]

With neural compression lesions it is rare to have a pure first-, second-, or third-degree lesion. Most often, these lesions are mixed. One of the degrees of injury usually predominates in a particular case.[66] The lesion mix can be determined by serial physical examinations, pre- and postoperative serial electro-

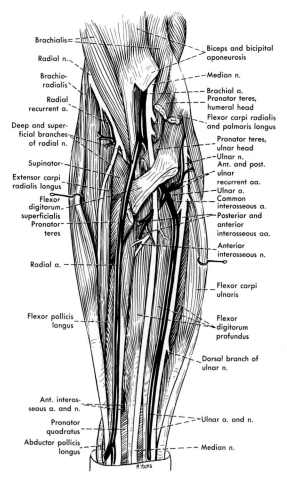

Figure 45–1. Major neurovascular and muscular relationships of the elbow region. (From Hollinshead, W.H.: Anatomy for Surgeons, Vol. 3, 3rd ed. New York, Harper & Row, 1982.)

myographic studies, and knowledge of the duration of the partial or complete nerve compression lesions. A fourth-degree nerve compression lesion is found most often when motor and sensory complete paralysis of a particular nerve has existed for more than 18 months.

Table 45–1. **Correlation of Seddon and Sunderland Classification of Nerve Injuries**

Seddon	Sunderland (degree)				
	First	*Second*	*Third*	*Fourth*	*Fifth*
Neurapraxia	▨				
Axonotmesis		▨	▨		
Neurotmesis				▨	▨

Shaded areas indicate equivalent terms.

The factors that affect return of nerve function following entrapment lesions are (1) the nerve fiber pathology, (2) the duration of the lesion and whether it is complete or partial, (3) the status of the end organs, motor and sensory, and (4) the level of the lesion.

When a nerve is entrapped, it is the peripheral fibers that are the most vulnerable to the pathologic process. Similarly, the heavy myelinated fibers are more susceptible to compressive forces. There appear to be several types of first-degree injury. These lesions are correlated best when both the nerve fiber pathology and the clinical recovery following neurolysis are analyzed temporally. There are ionic[42] and vascular[19, 49, 92] lesions of nerve fibers that respond to release by prompt recovery within, at times, hours of surgery. These are the nonstructural, first-degree lesions of nerves. There is a structural first-degree lesion, described by Gilliatt[30] and Ochoa,[65] in which there is segmental injury to the nerve fiber consisting of segmental demyelinization and remyelinization of just a few nodal segments of the fibers. In this instance, the entire recovery process takes 30 to 60 days. The clinical implications of this particular lesion are as follows: whether the lesion is high or low in the nerve, it takes 30 to 60 days for neural function to be restored. In contrast, in the second-degree lesion of nerve compression there is degeneration from the point of injury distally. Regeneration of the nerve fibers occurs within the intact basement membrane. This usually progresses at the rate of 1 mm or more a day from the site of the lesion. A low second-degree lesion recovers much more rapidly than a high lesion with second-degree compression. A second-degree brachial plexus injury often takes 14 months before the intrinsic muscles in the hand recover. The more proximal extrinsic muscles of the forearm recover function at about the ninth to the twelfth month following a second-degree entrapment lesion of the brachial plexus.

Third-degree injury due to neural entrapment occur most frequently when other mechanical factors affecting nerves, such as traction and friction, are superimposed on the compression neuropathologic process. In the third-degree lesion there is increased fibrosis in and about the nerve fibers that causes further structural change and neural dysfunction. Nerves move with motion of the limb. If their mobility is restricted by adherence of the nerve about a joint, as for example at the site of a supracondylar fracture in which the ulnar nerve adheres to the posterior aspect of the distal humerus, movement of the joint without movement of the nerve can cause traction neuritis of the ulnar nerve, which in turn can produce a stove-pipe appearance of the nerve. A markedly thickened ulnar nerve can be the source of chronic pain even when it is intact and functioning.

RADIAL NERVE

The radial nerve and its major branches, the posterior interosseous nerve and the superficial radial nerve, are vulnerable to compression forces from the level of the lateral head of the triceps through the region of the elbow, proximal forearm, and even into the distal forearm.[25, 63] Between these areas, the arcade of Frohse,[26] adhesions at the anterior aspect of the distal humerus, muscular anomalies, vascular aberrations,[20] bursae,[1] ganglionic[5] fibrotic bands proximally within the midportion or at the distal end of the supinator muscle,[79] inflammatory thickening and adherence of the extensor carpi radialis brevis[58] tendinous origin to the proximal edge of the supinator on its radial side,[10, 11] thrombotic recurrent radial vessels, thickened proliferating rheumatoid synovium from the radiocapitellar joint,[9] tumors,[3, 72, 102] fractures,[87] and fracture-dislocations[59, 84] can all produce symptomatology of radial nerve compression (Fig. 45–2). Depending on which branch of the nerve is involved, predominantly motor posterior interosseous nerve paralysis without superficial nerve involvement is observed with compression of the radial nerve at the elbow. On occasion, the superficial radial nerve is involved as well.[97] Isolated superficial radial nerve entrapment can occur owing to a proximal forearm or elbow lesion.

Relevant Anatomy

The radial nerve in the distal third of the arm passes anteriorly 10 cm proximal to the lateral epicondyle (Fig. 45–3).[35] At the level of the radiocapitellar joint it divides into its major branches, the posterior interosseous and the superficial radial nerves. In this passage, the radial nerve passes just deep to the fascia of the brachioradialis. Above the elbow it innervates the brachioradialis and the extensor carpi radialis longus. The motor branch to the extensor carpi radialis brevis arises from the superficial radial nerve in 58 per cent of the population.[76] It frequently arises as a separate terminal branch of the radial nerve with the posterior interosseous and superficial radial nerves.

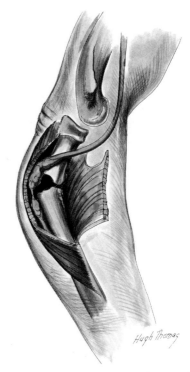

Figure 45–2. Fractures of the proximal radius often demonstrate posterior angulation, which places the posterior interosseous nerve in jeopardy. (From Omer, G., and Spinner, M.: Peripheral Nerve Problems. Philadelphia, W.B. Saunders Co., 1980.)

At the elbow, the posterior interosseous nerve passes between the two heads of the supinator muscle.[18] The proximal edge of the supinator forms an arch for the posterior interosseous nerve, the arcade of Frohse. The superficial radial nerve passes superficial to the supinator muscle. It is covered anteriorly by the brachioradialis. Recurrent vessels of the radial artery cross superficial and deep to these radial nerve branches.

Posterior Interosseous Nerve Syndrome

The posterior interosseous nerve can be compressed at the level of the proximal edge of the supinator (arcade of Frohse), in its midportion,[15] and as it passes through the supinator muscle at its distal end. The most common site is at the proximal edge in the region of the arcade of Frohse.[57, 64, 73, 80, 83]

Classically, the clinical presentation of this nerve paralysis is thought to be typically motor because the posterior interosseous nerve basically carries motor fibers destined to innervate the extensor digitorum communis, extensor digiti minimi, extensor carpi ulnaris, abductor pollicis longus, extensor pollicis longus and brevis, and extensor in-

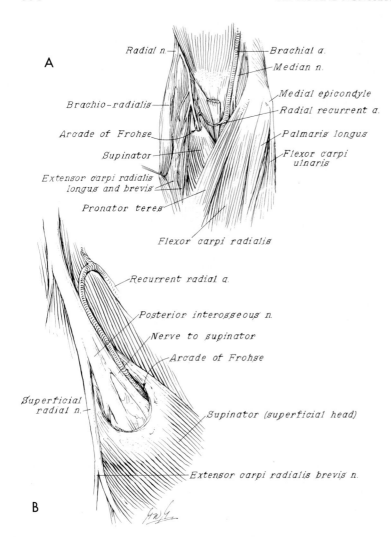

Figure 45–3. *A,* Dissection of the anterior aspect of the elbow demonstrating the anatomic relationship with the radial nerve. *B,* An enlarged view of the antecubital fossa shows the relationship of the posterior interosseous nerve to the supinator muscle and the arcade of Frohse. Note how the proximal superficial radial nerve is spared from compression by the arcade. (From Spinner, M.: Injuries to the Major Branches of the Forearm, 2nd ed. Philadelphia, W. B. Saunders Co., 1978.)

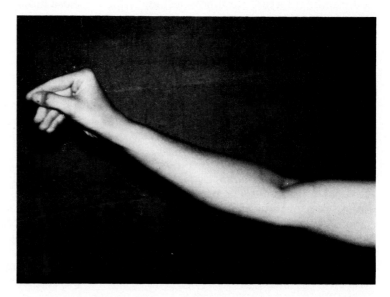

Figure 45–4. Patient with a posterior interosseous nerve paralysis showing inability to extend the fingers at the metacarpophalangeal joints as well as an inability to extend the thumb. (From Spinner, M.: Injuries to the Major Branches of the Forearm, 2nd ed. Philadelphia, W. B. Saunders Co., 1978.)

dicis. However, pain simulating lateral epicondylitis is now recognized as a common early presentation (see below).[11, 74] As the posterior interosseous nerve passes through the supinator, it innervates this muscle with multiple branches. The proximal or distal location of the compression of this nerve in the supinator can be determined by evaluating the electromyogram. Fibrillations in the supinator muscle suggest that the compression is proximal, at the arcade of Frohse. The pattern of involvement of this nerve varies depending on whether the entire nerve is compressed or whether there is a partial paralysis. When the entire nerve is compressed, the fingers and thumb cannot extend at the metacarpophalangeal level and the wrist deviates in a radial direction with wrist extension (Fig. 45–4).[7, 100] With partial paralysis, some of the digits, for example, the fourth and fifth fingers at the metacarpophalangeal joints, do not extend but the others do.[20, 31, 34, 62] The hand looks like a pseudoulnar claw hand. In reality there is no clawing but only a drop at the metacarpophalangeal joint and no true hyperextension of the metacarpophalangeal joints of the fourth and fifth fingers as seen in low ulnar nerve palsy.

The posterior interosseous nerve courses in a dorsoradial direction in the proximal forearm. As it passes through the supinator it innervates this muscle by multiple branches. Approximately 8 cm below the elbow joint this nerve emerges from the supinator muscle where it divides into its terminal motor branches to the extensor digitorum communis, extensor digiti minimi, extensor carpi ulnaris, abductor pollicis longus, extensor pollicis longus and brevis, and extensor indicis. Another clinical presentation of partial posterior interosseous nerve paralysis is an inability to extend metacarpophalangeal joints of the long and ring fingers while the thumb, index, and little fingers extend. In both partial and complete posterior interosseous nerve paralysis, sensation in the autonomous region on the dorsum of the first web space of the hand is uninvolved.

Resistant Tennis Elbow

For the most part, resistant tennis elbow is caused by lateral epicondylitis and its associated fascial tears or calcifications or by bursitis in close vicinity to the lateral epicondyle. On occasion, persistent complaints may be due to either compression of the posterior interosseous nerve or to a combination of nerve compression and persistent localized epicondylitis.[11, 74, 81] Resistant pain about the lateral epicondyle should suggest that entrapment of the adjacent interosseous nerve may be an underlying, unrecognized factor. Physical findings not infrequently reveal tenderness both over the lateral epicondyle and anteriorly over the course of the posterior interosseous nerve as it passes through both heads of the supinator. On occasion, pain can be localized to the distal end of the supinator where the nerve regresses between both heads of the supinator posteriorly at the junction of the middle and upper thirds of the proximal third of the forearm. Pain in the elbow on resistance to extension of the long finger with the elbow extended is also a common finding. There are no sensory abnormalities in the hand. Electromyographic studies in cases of resistant tennis elbow due to entrapment of the posterior interosseous nerve may be positive, especially if the condition has been present for 7 to 9 months. Conduction delays are observed occasionally. Stress testing, as described by Werner,[98] has sometimes been helpful in confirming the diagnosis. Fibrillations in some of the muscles innervated by this nerve, most frequently the extensor indicis, are observed. Individual muscles innervated by the posterior interosseous nerve should be studied for electromyographic abnormalities. In partial lesions, only a few of the muscles may show changes, whereas in the full-blown posterior interosseous nerve paralysis all of them do. The supinator muscle, if it does not reveal any neuroelectromyographic abnormalities, should lead to suspicion that the compression lesion is at the distal end of this muscle rather than at its usual proximal end. It should be remembered that the motor supply to the supinator muscle is given segmentally to this muscle after the nerve passes through the arcade of Frohse, which is located at the proximal end of the muscle. The brachioradialis and the extensor carpi radialis longus and brevis should not reveal any abnormalities in the typical posterior interosseous nerve syndrome because these muscles are innervated by the radial nerve proximal to the arcade of Frohse.

Author's Preferred Operative Exposure for the Entire Course of the Posterior Interosseous Nerve

When exposure of the entire posterior interosseous nerve is needed, the plane between the extensor carpi radialis brevis and the extensor digitorum communis (Fig. 45–5) is developed. The incision commences 5 cm

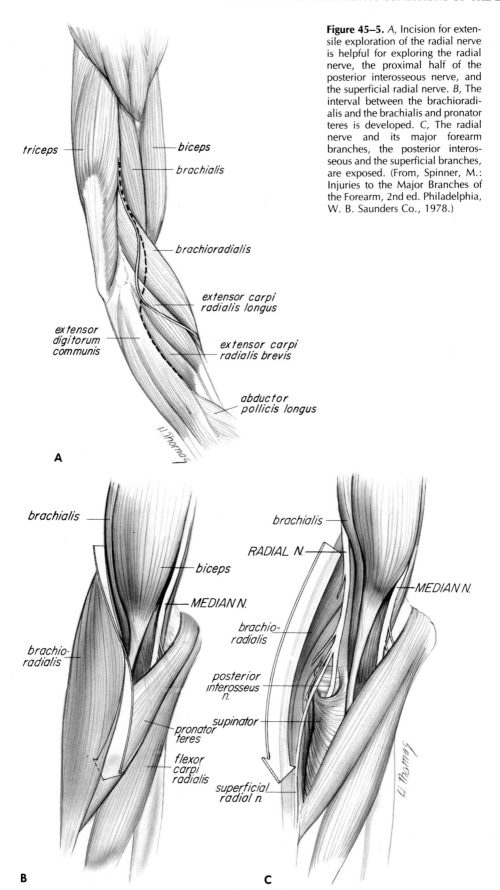

Figure 45–5. *A,* Incision for extensile exploration of the radial nerve is helpful for exploring the radial nerve, the proximal half of the posterior interosseous nerve, and the superficial radial nerve. *B,* The interval between the brachioradialis and the brachialis and pronator teres is developed. *C,* The radial nerve and its major forearm branches, the posterior interosseous and the superficial branches, are exposed. (From, Spinner, M.: Injuries to the Major Branches of the Forearm, 2nd ed. Philadelphia, W. B. Saunders Co., 1978.)

proximal to the lateral epicondyle and passes over the lateral epicondyle down to the region of the origin of the outcropping muscles (abductor pollicis longus, extensor pollicis longus and brevis). The aponeurotic plane between the extensor carpi radialis brevis and the extensor digitorum communis is developed from distal to proximal (Fig. 45–6). The supinator muscle is seen in the depth of the wound as these muscles are liberated. To gain complete exposure to the proximal end of the supinator, the extensor carpi radialis brevis tendon is detached from its origin at the pit of the lateral epicondyle of the humerus. Adherence of the tendinous origin of this muscle to the lateral portion of the supinator muscle is frequently found and is freed to give exposure to the proximal end of the

supinator. By flexing the elbow and by palpating the course of the posterior interosseous nerve as it passes obliquely through the supinator in a dorsoradial direction, one can identify the posterior interosseous nerve. By gently spreading longitudinally on both sides of the nerve with a right radial-angled hemostat, the nerve can be isolated. Because there are recurrent vessels in the vicinity, dissection must be gentle. Any vessels crossing the nerve should be clamped and tied individually. When the posterior interosseous nerve is identified proximal to the arcade of Frohse, a rubber band is passed about it so that its identity and continuity are maintained. Often the arcade of Frohse is found to be thickened. A hemostat is placed deep to the arcade but superficial to the nerve, and the arcade is

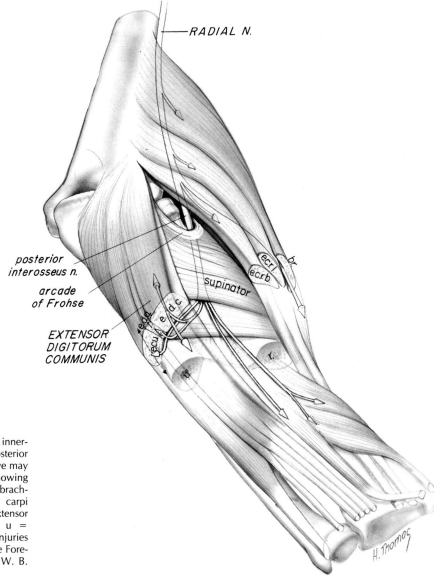

Figure 45–6. Details of the innervation provided by the posterior interosseous nerve. The nerve may be traced to the supinator showing the terminal branches (br = brachioradialis; ecrl = extensor carpi radialis longus; ecu = extensor carpi ulnaris; r = radius; u = ulna). (From Spinner, M.: Injuries to the Major Branches of the Forearm, 2nd ed. Philadelphia, W. B. Saunders Co., 1978.)

incised, liberating the most proximal portion
of the nerve. If further surgery is necessary to
identify the full course of the nerve, this can
be accomplished by tracing the entire posterior interosseous nerve and bringing it into
direct view. Compression of the proximal and
distal region has been described as well as
compression of the nerve in its midportion.
Epineurotomy of the interosseous nerve at the
site of its compression may be necessary.
Microsurgical technique should be utilized
when this is indicated.

The detailed anatomy of the nerve supply
to the extensor digitorum communis is important because this muscle obtains its innervation from branches of the terminal portion
of the posterior interosseous nerve that run at
right angles to the plane of the forearm in the
distal portion of the proximal third of the
forearm (Fig. 45–6). The operating surgeon
should not sweep the planes between the
extensor digitorum communis and the supinator because these branches are vulnerable.
Furthermore, strong retraction medially of the
extensor digitorum communis in this area
could damage the nerve supply to this important muscle.

The tendinous origin of the extensor carpi
radialis brevis tendon is not reattached.
Rather, a 3- to 4-cm portion of its most proximal tendinous origin is excised. The tourniquet is released, and hemostasis is obtained.
If the patient had lateral epicondylar pain and
tenderness preoperatively, then at this time
the lateral epicondyle can be drilled or a small
portion excised. The skin is closed, and the
arm is immobilized in long arm plaster splints
with the elbow at 90 degrees, the forearm in
midposition, and the wrist in a functional
position. The immobilization is continued for
3 weeks, and then the arm is gradually mobilized.

If a limited anterior exposure of the posterior interosseous nerve is needed, we prefer
the approach to the arcade of Frohse by developing the plane proximal to the elbow
between the brachialis and brachioradialis.
Distal to the elbow, the anatomic dissection
is continued, and the plane between the brachioradialis and the pronator teres is developed. If the dissection is difficult because of
muscle anomalies, the superficial radial nerve
can be identified and traced distally through
the proximal supinator. Any obstructing collateral vessels are ligated. The proximal third
of the posterior interosseous nerve can be
visualized with this exposure. If necessary,
the rest of the nerve can be followed by a
separate posterior approach.

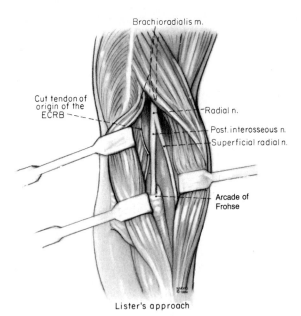

Figure 45–7. An extensile exposure of the forearm to demonstrate the radial nerve may be accomplished by the surgical
excisions shown here. The data outlined by Lister may be
used to aid in performing an extensile exposure to the carpal
tunnel.

A longitudinal transbrachioradialis approach as popularized by Lister[48] provides
direct access to the nerve from the radiohumeral level to the midsupinator (Fig. 45–7).

THE ULNAR NERVE

Relevant Anatomy

At the elbow, the ulnar nerve passes posterior
to the medial epicondyle. In the proximal
arm, the nerve descends in the anterior compartment to the wrist. In the majority of upper
extremities, the ulnar nerve crosses from the
anterior to the posterior compartment of the
arm through the arcade of Struthers,[89, 90] 8 cm
proximal to the medial epicondyle (Fig. 45–
8). The ulnar nerve, similarly, passes from the
posterior to the medial epicondyle to the
anterior compartment of the forearm a few
centimeters distal to the medial epicondyle;
it does so a few centimeters distal to the
cubital tunnel. In the arm there usually are
no branches of the ulnar nerve of significance.
Occasionally there is a variant high takeoff of
a motor branch to the flexor carpi ulnaris in
the distal arm. The sensory branch to the
dorsoulnar aspect of the hand has, rarely,
been observed to arise in the proximal forearm
rather than in the distal forearm. At the elbow
level, there is an expendable articular branch
just distal to the medial epicondyle; there are
numerous varying branches of the flexor carpi

ulnaris and the motor branch to the fourth and fifth flexor digitorum profundus muscles.

Etiology

Ulnar nerve compression lesions may be due to many factors.[32, 50, 68, 69, 95, 97] At the elbow level, spontaneous compression neuritis is well known as the cubital syndrome.[23] Flexion of the elbow may cause tightening and narrowing of the cubital tunnel as the posterior fascial aponeurosis and the epicondylar olecranon ligament become taut. The tendinous origin of the flexor carpi ulnaris can compress this nerve between its ulnar and humeral heads with elbow flexion.[2] A hypermobile ulnar nerve and at times a snapping nerve can produce symptomatology.[12] This usually occurs during elbow flexion, and the nerve rides ulnarly along the undersurface of the epicondyle. The anconeus epitrochlearis,[45a] an anomalous muscle crossing the ulnar nerve in the region of the medial epicondyle, may also be a causative factor.[71] Ganglia,[6a] tumors, cubitus valgus deformities,

and tethering adhesions may also produce late ulnar nerve symptomatology at the elbow. Fractures and dislocations, old medial epicondylar fractures, arthritic changes, rheumatoid arthritis,[20a, 46] or osteoarthritis may also be implicated.

Iatrogenic causes of secondary ulnar nerve compression are numerous and technical in nature. Compression may occur when the ulnar nerve is translocated subcutaneously and is insufficiently mobilized, proximally and distally.[85] Iatrogenic compression can be established proximally at the level of the arcade of Struthers or distally where the ulnar nerve passes from a posterior location at the elbow to the anterior compartment of the proximal forearm in the region of the common aponeurosis for the humeral head of the flexor carpi ulnaris and the origin of the flexor digitorum superficialis (Fig. 45–8).[37] If these two aponeurotic arches are not released proximally and distally, potential secondary sites of entrapment can produce symptomatology.[86] Whether translocated subcutaneously or deep, the ulnar nerve should be transposed

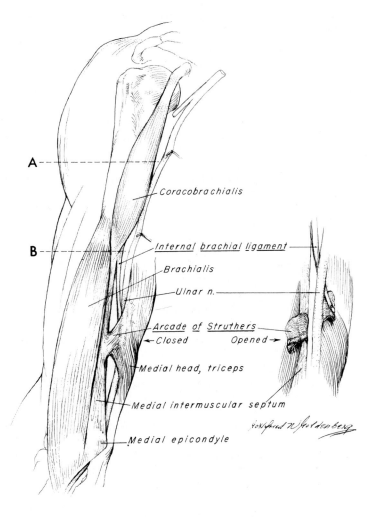

Figure 45–8. Anatomic distribution of the ulnar nerve crossing the intermuscular septum and passing under the arcade of Struthers. Impingement in the midbrachium from the internal brachial ligament should be recognized. Insert: the arcade of Struthers has been released, demonstrating the internal brachial ligament within the arcade. (From Spinner, M., and Kaplan, E. B.: The relationship of the ulnar nerve to the medial intermuscular septum in the arm and its clinical significance. Hand 8:239, 1976.)

Coracobrachialis

Internal brachial ligament

Brachialis

Ulnar n.

Arcade of Struthers

←Closed   Opened→

Medial head, triceps

Medial intermuscular septum

Medial epicondyle

anteriorly without kinking. Furthermore, the nerve should not be transposed into a groove in the flexor-pronator group of muscles because traction neuritis is commonly produced. When the nerve heals in the muscular groove, the longitudinal fibrotic aponeuroses of flexor muscles of the medial aspect of the elbow produce a secondary traction neuritis. The medial intermuscular septum should be removed because it too is a common cause for secondary ulnar nerve entrapment.

Clinical Presentation

An ulnar nerve lesion at the elbow usually begins with intermittent paresthesias in the ring and little fingers that are aggravated by elbow flexion and frequently awaken the patient. Sensory loss in the fourth and fifth fingers of the hand usually occurs later, but sensory loss in the dorsoulnar aspect of the hand is a classic localizing sign. Usually, there are no sensory abnormalities in the forearm. In the motor area weakness may be progressive in both extrinsics and intrinsics and at times occurs with minimal sensory symptoms. With paralysis of the flexor digitorum profundus to the fourth and fifth fingers, there is usually minimal clawing or no clawing of the fourth and fifth fingers. With partial lesions, clawing may be more pronounced if the flexor digitorum profundus muscles are intact and the intrinsic muscles are atrophic.[53, 92] There are numerous variations in fibers carried within the ulnar nerve at the elbow level.[85] In 15 per cent of upper extremities, the median nerve will carry many of the intrinsic motor fibers to pass from the median nerve or the anterior interosseous nerve branch of the median nerve to the ulnar nerve in the midforearm. Hence, a mechanical lesion of the ulnar nerve, at the elbow, in different patients, may present with different clinical patterns because of the presence or absence of neural anomalies and the extent of involvement of the nerve. Similarly, if the metacarpophalangeal joints of the ring and little fingers cannot hyperextend because of innate tightness of the volar plates, then clawing will also not be observed.

Similarly, the sensory pattern typical of an ulnar nerve lesion at the elbow with diminished or absent sensation on the dorsoulnar aspect of the hand[44] may not be observed. This occurs when other sensory nerves take over the area usually supplied by the ulnar dorsal cutaneous branch of the hand. One variant sensory pattern is observed when the superficial radial nerve innervates not only the dorsal radial aspect of the hand but also extends to supply the dorsoulnar aspect. Furthermore, all of the ring and long fingers can be anesthetic in some complete ulnar nerve lesions.

Differential Diagnosis

In the differential diagnosis, a nerve lesion, which involves the cervical foramina as in cervical arthritis, can present with ulnar nerve symptoms. There usually is restriction and pain on movement of the neck. Positive foraminal compression maneuvers, arthritic changes seen roentgenologically, and cervical paravertebral muscle electrical abnormalities are usually seen. Short segment stimulation may be effective in isolating the level of the compression.[21]

Another frequent site for exclusion is the thoracic outlet. The medial components of the plexus are most frequently involved. Radiation of paresthesia along the inner aspect of the arm with symptomatology referable to the fourth and fifth fingers is a common neural presentation. Clinical signs localizing the pathology to the outlet, a positive Tinel sign, a positive Adson sign, and an arterial bruit with abduction extension should all be considered. Confirmatory localizing electromyographic studies, specifically conduction delays across the thoracic outlet, help in differentiating the level of nerve entrapment.[21] Absence of ulnar f-wave abnormalities, cervical paravertebral fibrillations, and an ulnar nerve conduction delay distally are strong confirmatory findings.

Entrapment in the forearm and hand rarely occurs. Depending on the level of nerve involvement, varying clinical signs and symptoms become manifest. A full-blown lesion in Guyon's canal is accompanied by sensory loss in the fourth and fifth fingers of the hand. There is usually clawing of these digits because the flexor digitorum profundus is functioning. The sensation on the dorsoulnar aspect of the hand is intact, and the palmar aspect of the hand can also be free of symptomatology, although some hypesthesia on the ulnar aspect of the palm may be observed. Lesions of the ulnar nerve in the proximal forearm are similar to the findings at the elbow, whereas in the mid and distal forearm, symptomatology depends on the relationship of the lesion to the motor branch of the flexor digitorum profundus and the branch of the dorsal sensory cutaneous nerve of the hand. A lesion proximal to this clinically presents with numbness in the dorsoulnar aspect of the hand. A lesion distal to the takeoff of the motor branch of the flexor digitorum profundus usually is seen in patients with no clawing. On rare occasions, clawing of the ring and little fingers may be observed even with a neural compression proximal to the motor branch. This occurs when the flexor digitorum profundus to the fourth and fifth fingers is anomalously innervated by the median nerve or the anterior interosseous nerve.

Operative Procedure

When there is evidence of nerve fiber pathology, as demonstrated by electromyographic studies for a lesion in the cubital tunnel, our preferred operative procedure is the Learmonth technique. In contrast, in symptomatic patients when there is no evidence of electromyographic nerve fiber pathology, either release of the cubital tunnel[13] or anterior subcutaneous translocation[24] is recommended (Fig. 45–9). If the patient has no fat in the subcutaneous tissue, I also prefer to perform the Learmonth procedure, the submuscular anterior translocation of the ulnar nerve.[45]

The Learmonth Procedure

The incision we utilize extends 8 to 10 cm proximal to the medial epicondyle and 8 to 10 cm distal to the medial epicondyle on the medial side of the arm and forearm. At the level of the medial epicondyle, the incision darts anteriorly for 5 cm, and then below the medial epicondyle it extends to the medial aspect of the forearm (Fig. 45–10A). The V-shaped flap formed at the elbow level is undermined subcutaneously and is retracted medially. The medial cutaneous nerves of the forearm and arm are identified and preserved by placing a rubber band about them. The vulnerable branch of the medial cutaneous nerve of the forearm, which innervates the skin over the olecranon, is identified and preserved. There are other variable branches that cross medially that are preserved if possible. Avoidance of injury to the medial cutaneous nerve of the forearm and its branches is important because patients afflicted with ulnar entrapment lesions are vulnerable to symptomatic postoperative skin neuromas. The plane between the subcutaneous fat and the brachial and antibrachial fascia in the distal arm is delineated and undermined. The medial intermuscular septum is seen, and the ulnar nerve is identified just posterior to the medial intermuscular septum in the distal third of the arm. In approximately 70 per cent of limbs, muscular fibers of the medial head of the triceps will be found to cross the ulnar nerve and attach to the arcade of Struthers, 8 cm proximal to the medial epicondyle. If these muscular fibers of the medial head of

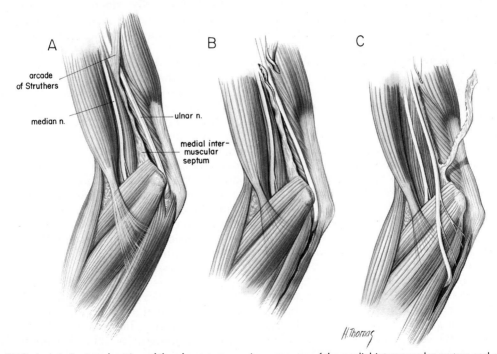

Figure 45–9. *A,* Anterior translocation of the ulnar nerve requires exposure of the medial intermuscular septum and arcade of Struthers. *B,* The arcade has been released. *C,* Intermuscular septum is then removed and the ulnar nerve is brought forward anterior to the flexion axis of the elbow. (From Spinner, M.: Injuries to the Major Branches of the Forearm. 2nd ed. Philadelphia, W. B. Saunders Co., 1978.)

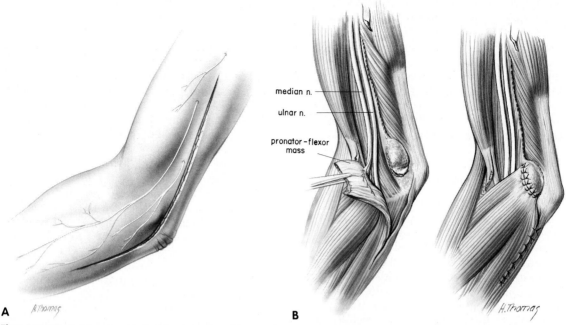

Figure 45–10. *A,* Extensive skin incision is employed for translocation of the ulnar nerve. This allows exposure of the proximal aspect of the intermuscular septum and the arcade of Struthers. *B,* Submuscular translocation (Learmonth) technique requires proximal dissection of the ulnar nerve and release of the intermuscular septum approximately 8 cm proximal to the flexor pronator muscle group, which is elevated from the medial epicondyle, and the ulnar nerve is brought forward to lie next to the median nerve. The flexor pronator group is then reattached to the medial epicondyle *(B).* Particular care is taken not to injure the interosseous branch of the median nerve, which arises in this region. (From Spinner, M.: Injuries to the Major Branches of the Forearm, 2nd ed. Philadelphia, W. B. Saunders Co., 1978.)

the triceps are noted, it is a clear indication that the ulnar nerve must be liberated from the arcade in this area. The medial intermuscular septum is identified and cleared posteriorly of muscular fibers to the level of the humerus (Fig. 45–10*B*). Anteriorly, the medial intermuscular septum is separated with care from the neural vascular bundle. The inferior ulnar collateral vessels, which penetrate the intermuscular septum, can be preserved, and the medial intermuscular septum is excised. The ulner nerve is mobilized. Its external longitudinal vessels are kept in continuity with the nerve. The transverse components of the vascular supply can be cauterized, keeping the external and internal vascular supply intact. At the level of the posterior aspect of the medial epicondyle, the ulnar nerve is liberated, and an articular branch to the adjoined surface is sacrificed. One or two rubber bands are placed about the ulnar nerve to aid in the dissection. Distal to the medial epicondyle, the ulnar nerve is identified as it passes through the cubital tunnel. The tendinous arch for the origin of the flexor carpi ulnaris of the humerus and ulna in the proximal region is identified. The humeral attachment is detached, and the interval between the common aponeurosis of the flexor carpi ul-

naris humeral head and the flexor digitorum superficialis is defined. The ulnar nerve is identified distally, deep to the flexor carpi ulnaris. Its common fibrous aponeurosis is liberated to free the ulnar nerve in the proximal forearm. The multiple branches of the flexor carpi ulnaris are preserved. The motor branch to the flexor digitorum profundus of the ring and little fingers is also identified and preserved. The ulnar nerve is mobilized in the proximal third of the forearm to allow for anterior translocation. Utilizing loupe magnification, the motor branches are mobilized using microsurgical technique to permit nontethered anterior translocation of the ulnar nerve. If the nerve is to be placed in the subcutaneous plane, the dissection in the mobilization of the nerve stops at this point.

To proceed with the Learmonth procedure, the median nerve is identified proximal to the lacertus fibrosus in the distal arm, and a rubber band is placed about it (Fig. 45–10*B*). The median nerve is found deep to the brachial fascia at the elbow level medial to the brachial artery. The lacertus fibrosus in the proximal forearm is incised longitudinally. The next step in the dissection is to detach the muscles of the flexor-pronator group 1 cm distal to the medial epicondyle. To accomplish this, after the median nerve has been identified and the ulnar nerve has been mobilized, a tonsillar clamp is placed from the radial side of the flexor-pronator group of muscles, 1 cm distal to the medial epicondyle, and passed medially deep to the flexor-pronator group of muscles to the exit in the region of the cubital tunnel. The tonsillar clamp is passed superficial to the ulnar collateral vessels on the anterior aspect of the medial side of the forearm. By sharp dissection, 1 cm distal to the medial epicondyle, the flexor-pronator group of muscles is incised. The brachial fascia is identified. By a combination of sharp dissection and periosteal stripping, the flexor-pronator group of muscles is stripped distally. The tourniquet is released. Any additional bleeding is brought under control either by ties or with hyfrecator. The ulnar nerve is translocated radially adjacent to the median nerve, and the flexor-pronator group of muscles is resutured, using 0 chromic sutures (Fig. 45–10C). The subcutaneous tissues and skin are closed with either interrupted or subcuticular sutures. The elbow is dressed well, and the wrist and elbow are immobilized at 90 degrees of flexion and with the forearm in midposition. The fingers and thumb are free. The immobilization is continued for 3 weeks followed by progressive active mobilization.

I have had no experience with medial epicondylectomy for ulnar nerve neuritis. It has been reported to be successful in relieving the symptomatology of ulnar nerve neuritis by other surgeons.[17, 27, 36] Unfortunately, it may adversely affect the moment arm of the flexor-pronator group. I believe that the choice of operative procedure should be fitted to the patient's symptoms and the electromyographic findings.

Simple fascial release over the common flexor tendon and forearm fascia is recommended by some.[13] We have had no experience with this but do not feel that this technique is routinely indicated or predictably effective.

THE MEDIAN NERVE

The median nerve at the level of the elbow is susceptible to a compressive neuropathy from the level of the supracondyloid process superiorly to the flexor superficialis arch distally. Between these the ligament of Struthers, the lacertus fibrosus, the deep head of the pronator teres, muscles, distended bursae, or vascular malformations may produce symptomatic median nerve compression.

Relevant Anatomy

The median nerve lies beneath the brachial fascia on the medial aspect of the arm resting on the brachialis muscle (Fig. 45–11A).[35] The brachial artery and veins lie laterally in close proximity and adjacent to the biceps tendon. The medial intermuscular septum lies posteriorly and attaches to the medial epicondylar flare. The median nerve passes first alongside the humeral origin of the pronator teres and then beneath it to lie on the deep surface. It most often passes between the humeral head and the ulnar head of the pronator muscle but may pass deep to both heads, or the ulnar head may be absent. The motor branches of the pronator teres usually arise from the medial aspect of the nerve beneath the upper margin of the muscle but variably arise above the antecubital area. The branch to the ulnar head may arise from the main branch or as a separate branch from the median nerve. The anterior interosseous branch arises deep and usually laterally at the level of the deep head of the pronator teres and in close approximation to the bifurcation of the radial and ulnar arteries from the brachial artery. The main branch of the median nerve next passes beneath the tendinous arch of origin of the flexor superficialis and lies in close approximation to the deep surface of this muscle (Fig. 45–11B). The anterior interosseous nerve runs onto the index profundus muscle and the flexor pollicis longus.

The pronator teres usually arises from the common origin of the medial epicondyle but may extend proximally along the medial epicondylar flare. The lacertus fibrosus passes from the biceps tendon to the antebrachial fascia obliquely over the flexor-pronator group of muscles.

Anatomic variations sometimes play an important part in nerve compression syndromes. The most important of these are the supracondyloid process and ligament of Struthers,[90] Gantzer's muscle,[28] the palmar profundus,[85] the flexor carpi radialis brevis,[85] a three-headed biceps with reduplicated lacertus fibrosus, and vascular perforation or tether involving the nerve. Distal humeral fracture or dislocation is well known to cause median nerve injury.[47, 70]

Supracondyloid Process

Compression of the median nerve at the level of the distal humerus may occur when the nerve passes beneath the osseous process, which extends obliquely medioanteriorly and continues to the medial epicondyle as the

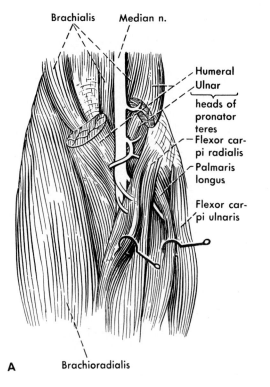

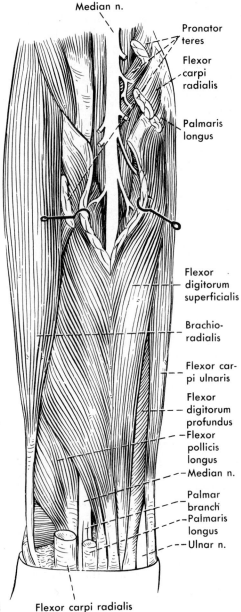

Figure 45–11. *A,* As the median nerve enters the forearm it gives off branches to the humeral and ulnar heads of the pronator teres, which originate from the medial aspect of the nerve. (From Hollinshed, W. H.: Anatomy for Surgeons, Vol. 3, 2nd ed. New York, Harper & Row, 1969.)

B, The median nerve is followed deeper into the forearm. The anterior interosseous nerve is shown entering the forearm under the flexor digitorum superficialis and innervating this structure. The nerves to the flexor pronator group are demonstrated. (From Hollinshed, W. H.: Anatomy for Surgeons, Vol. 3, 2nd ed. New York, Harper & Row, 1969.)

ligament of Struthers.[29] Muscle hypertrophy or strenuous use may facilitate the irritant effect of this structure.[35]

Pronator Syndromes

The pronator syndrome has been recognized comparatively recently as a neural compression syndrome within the proximal forearm.[40, 60, 78] The symptoms are often vague, consisting of discomfort in the forearm with occasional proximal radiation into the arm. A fatigue-like pain description may be elicited. Numbness of the hand in the median distribution is often secondary. Repetitive stren-

uous motions, such as industrial activities, weight training or driving, often provoke the symptoms. Nocturnal symptoms are infrequent. Numbness may affect all or part of the median distribution. Occasionally, patients may insist on emphasizing numbness of the little finger or the "whole hand."

Women seem to be at greater risk than men of developing these symptoms, especially if they are exposed to highly repetitive, moderately strenuous industrial occupations in which alternating pronosupinatory motions are required. The symptoms usually develop insidiously, but occasionally a specific event or sudden onset of pain in the forearm is

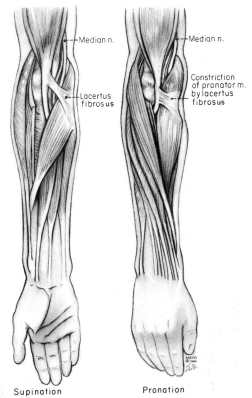

Figure 45–12. When the arm pronates, contraction of the pronator muscle may result in indentation of this structure by the lacertus fibrosus. Such a process may give rise to entrapment of the median nerve and the so-called pronator syndrome.

associated with heightened susceptibility to muscular stress. Renal dialysis patients with arteriovenous fistulae have been reported to develop pronator symptoms suddenly. The syndrome may also occur following crushing or contusion of the proximal forearm, or stretching of the spastic flexor musculature by casting in patients with cerebral palsy.

Diagnosis is often delayed because of the vague, poorly related history, lack of easily observed findings, and association with workers compensation evaluation. At times, the patient seems more interested in recriminatory association with his job than with resolution of the problem.

Examination

Physical findings are often subtle, and several suggestive observations help to make the diagnosis: (1) An indentation of the pronator flexor muscle mass below the medial epicondyle suggests that the lacertus fibrosus exerts a constrictive effect at that level. The indentation may be increased by active or passive pronation of the forearm. This should be compared with the opposite arm (Fig. 45–12). (2) The flexor pronator musculature feels indurated or tense in comparison with the opposite arm or with resisted pronation. (3) Resisted pronation for a period of 60 seconds may initiate the symptoms by contracting the flexor pronator muscle (Fig. 45–13). (4) Re-

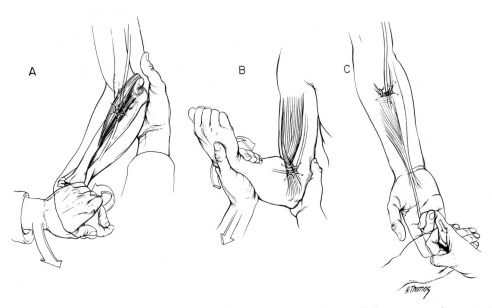

Figure 45–13. Features of the physical examination that help to demonstrate the so-called pronator syndrome. *A,* Proximal forearm pain is increased by resistance to pronation and elbow flexion as well as to flexion of the wrist. *B,* Pain in the proximal forearm that is increased by resistance to supination is also suggestive of compression by the lacertus fibrosus. *C,* Resistance of the long finger flexor produces pain in the proximal forearm when compression of the median nerve occurs at the flexor digitorum superficialis arch. (From Spinner, M.: Injuries to the Major Branches of the Forearm, 2nd ed. Philadelphia, W. B. Saunders Co., 1978.)

sisted elbow flexion and forearm supination may elicit similar symptoms, also presumably by tensing the lacertus fibrosus. (5) Resisted flexion of the long finger PIP joint by tightening the fibrous arch of origin of the superficialis muscle may also induce symptoms, although this test is positive far less frequently than the previous two. (6) Direct pressure over the proximal portion of the pronator teres by the examiner's thumb approximately 4 cm distal to the antebrachial crease while exerting moderate resistance to pronation has been the most reliable test in my experience. It should be compared with results of a similar test on the asymptomatic forearm. (7) The median nerve is sensitive to direct pressure, tapping, or rolling beneath the finger in the antecubital space. (8) Occasionally, passive stretching of the finger and wrist flexors will accentuate the symptoms, but this is unlikely to be positive before the preceding tests. (9) Weakness of the median innervated muscles is infrequent, but careful comparison of strength between the two hands is indicated. The flexor pollicis longus and index profundus are the most likely to show weakness. It is important to verify whether these tests mimic or reproduce exactly the symptoms that brought the patient to the physician (see below, Anterior Interosseous Syndrome).

This syndrome is most likely to be confused with carpal tunnel syndrome, and unfortunately the two conditions may occur simultaneously, or one may antedate the other, suggesting a susceptibility factor (see below, Double Crush Syndrome).

Some factors that help to differentiate between the two syndromes are indicated in Table 45–2. Obviously, careful clinical judgment is required to ensure the correct diagnosis.

Indications for surgery depend largely on the severity of the patient's symptoms. Aside

from avoidance of the activities associated with aggravation of the symptoms there is little available treatment for conservative care. On occasion we have carefully injected a mixture of lidocaine and hydrocortisone paraneurally with temporary beneficial effect. This may provide an additional diagnostic aid if effective.

Electromyography

Electromyographic findings as an aid in the diagnosis of the pronator syndromes have been disappointing.[8] In only 10 per cent of patients with the diagnosis of pronator syndrome were there findings that adequately supported the diagnosis. Slowed conduction velocity across the median nerve below the elbow is seldom detected. The best explanation for this is the size and complexity of the nerve, which is insufficiently compressed to prevent a stimulus progressing at normal velocities down a significant number of fascicles of the nerve. The slowed impulses in affected fascicles are blurred and dampened in the recording. Muscle studies are seldom specific. Isolated fibrillations, particularly in the pronator teres, have been observed. Insertional changes are often nonspecific, and fasciculations are infrequent.

Intraoperative studies of conduction velocities and voltages were carried out before and after median nerve release in 10 forearms in the early part of our series.[23] Significant increases in recorded velocities or voltages at the distal electrodes were noted in only five instances. Newer techniques may improve the diagnostic acuity of electromyography, but at this time the history and physical examination must be relied upon for the diagnosis.

Operative Findings

The median nerve seldom shows the flattening, indentation, or pseudoneuroma formation so common at the carpal tunnel. The lacertus fibrosus is usually quite apparent in its course from the biceps tendon to its interdigitations with the longitudinally directed fibers of the antebrachial fascia over the proximal third of the flexor-pronator muscle group. An indentation of the pronator teres is apparent with passive pronation (Fig. 45–14). At times this finding may be quite dramatic. After release of the lacertus and antebrachial fascia, the median nerve is apparent lying adjacent to the humeral head of the pronator teres (Fig. 45–15). The median nerve is followed under the humeral head of the pronator, where it encounters the ulnar head of the

Table 45–2. **Comparison of Findings Between the Pronator Syndrome and the Carpal Tunnel Syndrome**

	Carpal Tunnel Syndrome	Pronator Syndrome
Nocturnal symptoms	+	−
Muscular fatigue	−	+
Proximal radiation	±	+
Medial hypohidrosis	+	−
Thumb paresthesias	±	+
Thenar atrophy	+	−
Phelan's sign	+	−
Pronator signs	−	+
EMG	+	−

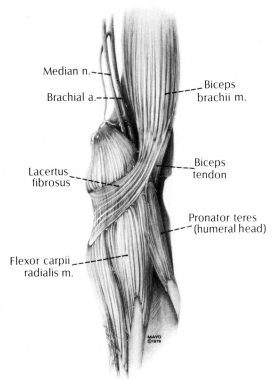

Figure 45–14. Course of the lacertus fibrosus in the antecubital fossa. The median nerve may be trapped under this structure as it compresses the origin of the pronator teres.

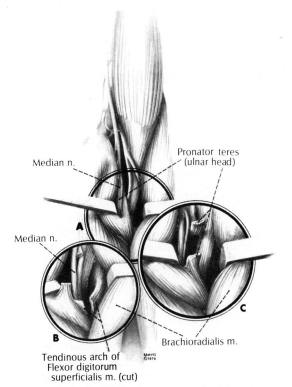

Figure 45–15. *A,* Release of the lacertus fibrosus reveals the median nerve as it enters the pronator teres muscle. *B,* Release of the ulnar head sometimes reveals a tight arch of the flexor digitorum superficialis muscle. *C,* If the ulnar head of the pronator teres is the offending part, it is released.

muscle, which varies considerably in size. It may be primarily a fleshy head, but usually the tendon of origin of the muscle arises laterally and crosses the nerve. It may vary from a structure measuring 1 or 2 mm in diameter to a band of 1 or 2 cm in width. This structure lies just distal to the overlying lacertus fibrosus. Occasionally the tendon arises medially, thus allowing the nerve to pass under rather than through the pronator teres. Sometimes no ulnar head is discernible, and forearms with this arrangement are probably far less susceptible to the condition. In the majority of patients with the pronator syndrome the combination of a tight tendinous band of the ulnar head associated with hypertrophy of the flexor-pronator musculature, which is constricted by the enveloping antebrachial fascia and lacertus fibrosus, produce the combination of pressure and tension on the nerve that induces symptoms.

The fibrous arch of origin of the superficialis lies 1 to 2 cm distal to the deep head of the pronator (Fig. 45–15B). This too may be constricting, especially when there is a large sharp edge to the band and hypertrophy of both the deep flexors and overlying muscle groups is present.

In a similar fashion aberrant or vestigial muscles such as Gantzer's muscle, palmaris profundus, or flexor carpi radialis brevis may act to produce constriction. Less common factors that act to compress the median nerve are vascular malformations or distention of the bicipital bursa. The nerve may be perforated by a branch of the radial artery and accompanying veins or overlain by a taut vascular bridge.

The Anterior Interosseous Syndrome

Isolated paresis or paralysis of the anterior interosseous nerve gained modern acceptance from the report of Kiloh and Nevin in 1952 and is often referred to as the Kiloh-Nevin syndrome.[39] Perhaps originally described by Tinel in 1918,[94] a number of authors have cited case reports or small series.[22, 43, 51, 75, 79, 82] In our experience this syndrome is seen as an isolated entity in a ratio of 1 to 40 with the pronator syndrome. There is an occasional overlap between the two conditions, especially with minor weakness in the motor distribution of the anterior interosseous nerve in the pronator syndrome. It is surprising that there is not a greater correlation between the two conditions, given the similarity of etiologic conditions within the same anatomic area and the close association of the nerves.

Symptoms

Commonly, a deep unremitting pain in the proximal forearm initiates the symptoms, which subside within 8 to 12 hours. The patient may then note a lack of dexterity or weakness of pinch that fails to resolve. If the patient was seen previously diagnoses from tendinous rupture to multiple sclerosis may have been entertained, particularly if the onset has been insidiously painless.

Physical Findings

The findings are those associated with denervation of the classic distribution of the anterior interosseous nerve to the flexor pollicis longus, the index and long finger profundus, and the pronator quadratus. The stance of the thumb and index finger when attempting to pinch is characteristic (Fig. 45–16). Because of inability to flex the distal joints, they are approximated in hyperextension along their distal phalanges. Pinch is weak, and manipulative facility is impaired. Isolated testing shows marked weakness or paralysis of the flexor pollicis longus or index profundus. The long finger is usually less affected depending on the relative contributions of the ulnar and median nerves to the profundi.

Weakness in pronation is seldom a recognizable complaint of the patient because it is submerged in the general discomforts of weakness and clumsiness of the extremity. The pronator quadratus is tested by placing both elbows against the side and resisting pronation with the elbows flexed to a right angle. This effectively reduces the strength contribution of the pronator teres humeral head, allowing comparison of the pronator quadratus.

Tenderness over the proximal forearm is usually absent, and sensory disturbance is not apparent.

Electromyographic findings of fibrillations are present in the affected muscles.[4]

Anastomotic nerve variations such as the Martin Gruber anastomosis may occur between the anterior interosseous nerve and the ulnar nerve as well as between the median and ulnar nerves. The former fibers are likely to innervate intrinsic muscles on the radial aspect of the hand. It is therefore necessary to differentiate partial apparent ulnar paralysis from the anterior interosseous syndrome.

Operative Findings

The operative findings are similar to those described above for the pronator syndrome. The usual finding is a constriction due to the tendon or origin of the ulnar head of the pronator teres across the posterolateral aspect of the anterior interosseous nerve as its separation from the median nerve becomes obvious. There may be a fibrous reaction in the area that is probably associated with the acute episode of pain, suggesting a localized vascular reaction such as thrombosis or ischemia (Fig. 45–17).

Author's Preferred Treatment

The spectrum of median nerve problems at the elbow suggests that the initial incision should be adaptable to unsuspected findings. We therefore prefer a longitudinally oriented incision curved at the antecubital crease or zigzagged to increase exposure and decrease tension on the scar line during healing (see Fig. 45–7). The medial antebrachial cutaneous nerve should be sought and protected. Major veins are retracted after ligating communicating veins. The plane over the brachial and antebrachial fascia is cleared to observe the effect of the lacertus fibrosus on passive pronation. A deep indentation of the flexor pronator group is significant. The origin of the pronator is inspected. If it is prolonged proximally, the muscle often covers the median nerve above the elbow. The medial intermuscular septum and brachial fascia tend to envelop the nerve in this situation. A true ligament of Struthers may be present if there is a supracondyloid process. Although such a diagnosis is usually made roentgenographically, palpation of the lower humerus through this

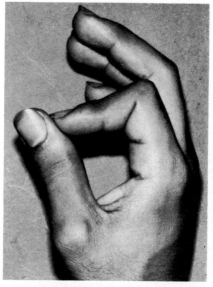

Figure 45–16. Anterior osseous nerve paralysis, demonstrating the characteristic pinch of this paralysis. (From Spinner, M.: Injuries to the Major Branches of the Forearm, 2nd ed. Philadelphia, W. B. Saunders Co., 1978.)

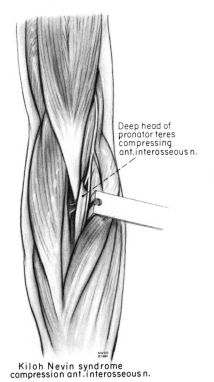

Deep head of
pronator teres
compressing
ant.interosseous n.

Kiloh Nevin syndrome
compression ant.interosseous n.

Figure 45–17. Compression of the anterior interosseous nerve can occur at its entrance to the pronator muscle near its origin. This constriction was first described by Kiloh and Nevin, and the syndrome thus bears this name.

wound may indicate an unsuspected supra-condyloid process. It may be important to extend the incision proximally in these instances—hence, draping to the edge of a tourniquet placed as high in the axilla as possible is a wise precaution. A sterile tourniquet is preferred for this reason. Reflection of the brachial fascia to expose the nerve is followed by release of the lacertus fibrosus. Pronation and retraction of the humeral head of the pronator allows the nerve to be exposed distally (Fig. 45–15). Motor branches usually exit from the nerve medially, thus allowing safe dissection along the lateral margin. Small vessels crossing the interval over the nerve are ligated. Electrocoagulation close to the nerve must be used cautiously, and bipolar coagulation is preferable. The ulnar head of the pronator teres usually crosses the nerve; it may appear as either a fleshy muscle, a tendinous band, or a combination of the two. Frequently a tendinous portion of the muscle is seen lying on the nerve if the fleshy portion is reflected. Resection of the tendon allows exposure of the nerve distally to beneath the tendinous origin of the superficialis muscle. The tautness of this band may be assessed by lifting it up with a dental probe. Scissor sectioning presents little problem.

Anomalous structures may be obvious, but anticipation is desirable. Extension of the incision is always indicated if identification of the neurovascular structures is difficult.

The reduplicated lacertus fibrosus, Gantzer's muscle, palmaris profundus, or flexor carpi radialis brevis, vascular perforations, or tethers at times pose problems. Rarely, the nerve itself will appear to be unusually taut and to bowstring on elbow extension. One of us (MS) has released the radial insertion of the pronator teres to allow the nerve to be positioned subcutaneously, after which the tendon is repaired.

When the anterior interosseous nerve is of primary concern, this branch should be identified and followed distally past the superficialis origin. Epineurolysis with magnification and microsurgical instruments may be helpful if the nerve feels scarred and indurated. Fascicular neurolysis is not indicated at this level.

The tourniquet is released before closure and hemostasis obtained. A suction drain may be used, although a passive drain is usually adequate. Subcuticular closure and adhesive strips to reduce skin tension improve the late appearance. Unfortunately, scars in this area are often hypertrophic. Active motion is commenced as tolerated after 4 to 5 days.

MUSCULOCUTANEOUS NERVE

Compression neuropathy of the lateral antebrachial cutaneous nerve is a recently recognized syndrome.[4]

Relevant Anatomy

The musculocutaneous nerve, after supplying the coracobrachialis, biceps, and brachialis, continues in the interval between the latter two muscles as a sensory nerve to supply the skin over the anterolateral aspect of the forearm, often as far as the thenar eminence. It emerges from beneath the biceps tendon laterally and penetrates the brachial fascia just above the elbow crease to course down the forearm (Fig. 45–18).

Clinical Findings

Bassett and Nunley described both acute and chronic problems.[4] A distinct mechanism of injury consisting of elbow hyperextension and pronation was elicited from their patients; presumably the nerve was compressed between the biceps tendon and the brachialis fascia because both the nerve and the tendon

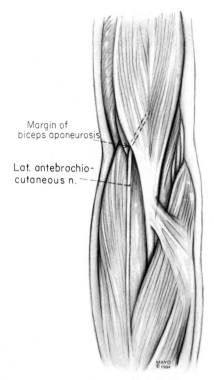

Margin of
biceps aponeurosis

Lat. antebrachio-
cutaneous n.

Figure 45–18. The lateral antebrachial cutaneous nerve has been reported to be compressed at the lateral margin of the biceps aponeurosis at the level of the lateral epicondyle.

were rendered taut by the forearm position. Burning dysthesia in the distribution of the nerve is seen acutely. In chronic phases the patient complains of a vague discomfort in the forearm with some dysthetic qualities that are sometimes made worse by supinopronatory activities with the elbow extended.

On physical examination a dysesthetic area on the anterolateral aspect of the forearm may be elicited by gently stroking across the skin transversely with a blunt point. Tenderness to direct pressure on the lateral aspect of the bicipital tendon just proximal to the elbow crease is characteristic; loss of extension and pronation is often exhibited with this maneuver.

Treatment

For the acute injury rest, splinting, avoidance of extension-pronation, and anti-inflammatory medication are indicated. Steroidal injections at the area of tenderness may help if exacerbation occurs. In chronic syndromes or those failing to respond to conservative care surgical decompression is effective. Under tourniquet control a zigzag incision across the lateral aspect of the elbow crease allows exposure of the lateral antebrachial nerve. The

site of compression usually occurs where the nerve emerges beneath the bicipital tendon. A tight band of antebrachial fascia at the elbow crease has been noted to alter the course of the nerve to an acute angle in one of our patients. Release of the brachial fascia and excision of a triangular portion of the bicipital tendon at the point of impingement is recommended. Obliteration of the vascular marking at the site of compression may be noted.

Results

Symptoms may subside after an acute episode, but the nerve thereafter is apparently more susceptible to further irritation. Surgical decompression can be expected to produce relief of pain, improvement in sensibility, and restoration of motion.

References

1. Agnew, D. H.: Bursal Tumor Producing Loss of Power of Forearm. Am. J. Med. Sci. **46:**404, 1863.
2. Apfelberg, D. B., and Larson, S. J.: Dynamic Anatomy of the Ulnar Nerve at the Elbow. Plast. Reconstr. Surg. **51:**76, 1973.
3. Barber, K. W., Jr., Bianco, A. J., Jr., Soule, E. H., and MacCarty, C. S.: Benign Extramural Soft Tissue Tumors of the Extremities Causing Compression of Nerves. J. Bone Joint Surg. **44A:**98, 1962.
4. Bassett, F. H., and Nunley, H. A.: Compression of the Musculotendon Nerve at the Elbow. J. Bone Joint Surg. **64A:**1050, 1982.
5. Bowen, T. L., and Stone, K. H.: Posterior Interosseous Nerve Paralysis Caused by a Ganglion at the Elbow. J. Bone Joint Surg. **48B:**774, 1966.
6. Boyes, J. H.: Bunnell's Surgery of the Hand, 5th ed. Philadelphia, J. B. Lippincott Co., 1970, pp. 418–419.
6a. Brooks, D. M.: Nerve Compression by Simple Ganglia. J. Bone Joint Surg. **34B:**391, 1952.
7. Bryan, F. S., Miller, L. S., and Panijaganond, P.: Spontaneous Paralysis of the Posterior Interosseous Nerve: A Case Report and Review of the Literature. Clin. Orthop. **80:**9, 1971.
8. Buchthal, F., Rosenflack, A., and Trojaborg, W.: Electrophysiological Findings in Entrapment of the Median Nerve at Wrist and Elbow. J. Neurol. Neurosurg. Psychiat. **37:**340, 1974.
9. Campbell, C. S., and Wulf, R. F.: Lipoma Producing a Lesion of the Deep Branch of the Radial Nerve. J. Neurosurg. **11:**310, 1954.
10. Capener, N.: Posterior Interosseous Nerve Lesions. Proceedings of the Second Hand Club. J. Bone Joint Surg. **46B:**361, 1964.
11. Capener, N.: The Vulnerability of the Posterior Interosseous Nerve of the Forearm. J. Bone Joint Surg. **48B:**770, 1966.
12. Childress, H. M.: Recurrent Ulnar-Nerve Dislocation at the Elbow. Clin. Orthop. **108:**168, 1975.
13. Clark, C. B.: Cubital Tunnel Syndrome. J.A.M.A. **241:**801, 1979.
14. Cohen, B. E.: Simultaneous Posterior and Anterior Interosseous Nerve Syndromes. J. Hand Surg. **7:**398, 1982.

15. Comtet, J. J., and Chambaud, D.: Paralysie "Spontanee" du Nerf Inter-osseox Posterieur par Lesion Inhabituelle. Deux Observations. Rev. Chir. Orthop. 61:533, 1975.

16. Comtet, J. J., Chambaud, D., and Genety, J.: La Compression de la Branche Posterieur du Nerf Radial. Une Etiologie Meconnue de Certaines Paralysies et de Certaines Spicondylalgies Rebelles. Nouv. Presse Med. 5:1111, 1976.

17. Craven, P. R., Jr., and Green, D. P.: Cubital Tunnel Syndrome. J. Bone Joint Surg., 62A:986, 1980.

18. Davies, F., and Laird, M.: The Supinator Muscle and the Deep Radial (Posterior Interosseous) Nerve. Anat. Rec. 101:243; 1948.

19. Denny-Brown, D., and Brenner, C.: Paralysis of Nerve Induced by Direct Pressure and by Tourniquet. Arch. Neurol. Psychiat. 51:1, 1944.

20. Dharapak, C., and Nimberg, G. A.: Posterior Interosseous Nerve Compression. Report of a Case Caused by Traumatic Aneurysm. Clin. Orthop. 101:225, 1974.

20a. Erhlich, G. E.: Antecubital Cysts in Rheumatoid Arthritis—A Corollary to Popliteal (Baker's) Cysts. J. Bone Joint Surg. 54A:165, 1972.

21. Escobar, P. L.: Short Segment Stimulations in Ulnar Nerve Lesions Around Elbow. Orthop. Rev. 12(10):65, 1983.

22. Farber, J. S., and Bryan, R. S.: The Anterior Interosseous Nerve Syndrome. J. Bone Joint Surg. 50A:521, 1968.

23. Feindel, W., and Stratford, J.: The Role of the Cubital Tunnel in Tardy Ulnar Palsy. Can. J. Surg. 1:296, 1958.

24. Foster, R. J., and Edshage, S.: Factors Related to Outcome of Surgically Managed Compressive Ulnar Neuropathy at the Elbow Level. J. Hand Surg. 6:181, 1981.

25. Freundlich, B. D., and Spinner, M.: Nerve Compression Syndrome in Derangements of the Proximal and Distal Radioulnar Joints. Bull. Hosp. Joint Dis. 19:38, 1968.

26. Frohse, F., and Frankel, M.: Die Muskeln des Menschlichen Armes. Bardelenben's Handbuch der Anatomie das Menschlichen. Jena, Fisher, 1908.

27. Froimson, A. I., and Zahrawi, F.: Treatment of Compression Neuropathy of the Ulnar Nerve at the Elbow by Epicondylectomy and Neurolysis. J. Hand Surg. 5(4):391, 1980.

28. Gantzers, C. F. L.: De Musculorum Varietates. Thesis, Berlioni, J. F. Starckie, 1813.

29. Gessini, L., Jandolo, B., and Pietrangeli, A.: Entrapment Neuropathies of the Median Nerve at and Above the Elbow. Surg. Neurol. 19:112, 1983.

30. Gilliatt, B. W., Ochoa, J., Rudge, P., and Neary, D.: The Cause of Nerve Damage in Acute Compression. Trans. Am. Neurol. Assoc. 99:71, 1974.

31. Goldman, S., Honet, J. C., Sobel, R., and Goldstein, A. S.: Posterior Interosseous Nerve Palsy in the Absence of Trauma. Arch. Neurol. 21:435, 1969.

32. Harrelson, J. M., and Newman, M.: Hypertrophy of the Flexor Carpi Ulnaris as a Cause of Ulnar-Nerve Compression in the Distal Part of the Forearm. Case Report. J. Bone Joint Surg. 57A:554, 1975.

33. Hartz, C. R., Linscheid, R. L., Gramse, R. R., and Daube, J. R.: Pronator Teres Syndrome: Compressive Neuropathy of the Median Nerve. J. Bone Joint Surg. (Am.) 63A:885, 1981.

34. Hobhouse, N., and Heald, C. B.: A Case of Posterior Interosseous Paralysis. Br. Med. J. 1:841, 1936.

35. Hollinshead, W. H.: Anatomy for Surgeons, Vol. 3. The Back and Limbs, 3rd ed. New York, Harper & Row, 1982.

36. Jones, R. E.: Medial Epicondylectomy for Ulnar Nerve Compression Syndrome at the Elbow. Clin. Orthop. 139:174, 1979.

37. Kane, E., Kaplan, E. B., and Spinner, M.: Observations of the Course of the Ulnar Nerve in the Arm. Ann. Chir. 27:487, 1973.

38. Kaplan, E. B.: Functional and Surgical Anatomy of the Hand, 2nd ed. Philadelphia, J. B. Lippincott Co., 1965.

39. Kiloh, L. G., and Nevin, S.: Isolated Neuritis of the Anterior Interosseous Nerve. Br. Med. J. 1:850, 1952.

40. Kopell, H. P., and Thompson, W. A. L.: Pronator Syndrome. N. Engl. J. Med. 259:713, 1958.

41. Kopell, H. P., and Thompson, W. A.: Peripheral Entrapment Neuropathies. Baltimore, Williams & Wilkins, 1963.

42. Kuszynski, K.: Functional Micro-Anatomy of the Peripheral Nerve Trunks. Hand 6:1, 1974.

43. Lake, P. A.: Anterior Interosseous Nerve Syndrome. J. Neurosurg. 41:306, 1974.

44. Learmonth, J. R.: A Variation of the Radial Branch of the Musculo-Spinal Nerve. J. Anat. 53:371, 1919.

45. Learmonth, J. R.: Technique for Transplanting the Ulnar Nerve. Surg. Gynecol. Obstet. 75:792, 1942.

45a. LeDouble, A. F.: Traite des Variations du Systeme Musculaire de l'Homme. Paris, Schleicher, 1897.

46. Leffert, R. D., and Dorfman, H. D.: Antecubital Cyst in Rheumatoid Arthritis. Surgical Findings. J. Bone Joint Surg. 54A:1555, 1972.

47. Lipscomb, P. R., and Burelson, R. J.: Vascular and Neural Complications in Supracondylar Fractures in Children. J. Bone Joint Surg. 37A:487, 1955.

48. Lister, G. D., Belsole, R. B., and Kleinert, H. E.: The Radial Tunnel Syndrome. J. Hand Surg. 4:52, 1979.

49. Lundborg, G.: Ischemic Nerve Injury. Experimental Studies on Intraneural Microvascular Pathophysiology and Nerve Function in a Limb Subjected to Temporary Circulatory Arrest. Scand. J. Plast. Reconstr. Surg. [Suppl.] 6:1, 1970.

50. MacNicol, M. F.: Extraneural Pressures Affecting the Ulnar Nerve at the Elbow. Hand 14(4):5, 1982.

51. Maeda, K., Miura, T., Komada, T., and Chiba, A.: Anterior Interosseous Nerve Paralysis. Report of 13 Cases and Review of Japanese Literatures. Hand 9:165, 1977.

52. Mangini, U.: Flexor Pollicis Longus Muscle. Its Morphology and Clinical Significance. J. Bone Joint Surg. 42A:467, 1960.

53. Mannerfelt, L.: Studies on the Hand in Ulnar Nerve Paralysis. A Clinical-Experimental Investigation in Normal and Anomalous Innervation. Acta Orthop. Scand. Suppl. 87, 1966.

54. Marmor, L., Lawrence, J. F., and Dubois, E.: Posterior Interosseous Nerve Paralysis Due to Rheumatoid Arthritis. J. Bone Joint Surg. 49A:381, 1967.

55. Marquis, J. W., Bruwer, A. J., and Keith, H. M.: Supracondyloid Process of the Humerus. Proc. Staff Mayo Clin. 37:691, 1957.

56. Marshall, S. C., and Murray, W. R.: Deep Radial Nerve Palsy Associated With Rheumatoid Arthritis. Clin. Orthop. 103:157, 1974.

57. Mayer, J. H., and Mayfield, P. H.: Surgery of the Posterior Interosseous Branch of the Radial Nerve. Surg. Gynecol. Obstet. 84:979, 1947.

58. Millender, L. H., Nalebuff, E. A., and Holdsworth, D. E.: Posterior Interosseous Nerve Syndrome Secondary to Rheumatoid Synovitis. J. Bone Joint Surg. 55A:753, 1973.

59. Morris, A. H.: Irreducible Monteggia Lesion With Radial-Nerve Entrapment. J. Bone Joint Surg. 46A:608, 1964.

60. Morris, H. H., and Peters, B. H.: Pronator Syndrome:

Clinical and Electrophysiological Features in Seven Cases. J. Neurol. Neurosurg. Psychiat. **39:**461, 1976.

61. Mowell, J. W.: Posterior Interosseous Nerve Injury. Int. Clin. **2:**188, 1921.

62. Mulholland, R. C.: Non-Traumatic Progressive Paralysis of the Posterior Interosseous Nerve. J. Bone Joint Surg. **48B:**781, 1966.

63. Nicolle, F. V., and Woolhouse, F. M.: Nerve Compression Syndromes of the Upper Limb. J. Trauma **5:**313, 1965.

64. Nielsen, H. O.: Posterior Interosseous Nerve Paralysis Caused by Fibrous Band Compression at the Supinator Muscle. A Report of Four Cases. Acta Orthop. Scand. **47:**304, 1976.

65. Ochoa, J.: Schwann Cell and Myelia Changes Caused by Some Toxic Agents and Trauma. Proc. Soc. Med. **67:**3, 1974.

66. Omer, G., and Spinner, M.: Peripheral Nerve Problems. Philadelphia, W. B. Saunders Co., 1980.

67. Omer, G., and Spinner, M.: Peripheral Nerve Testing and Suture Techniques. In American Academy of Orthopaedic Surgeons, Vol. 24. Instructional Course Lectures. St. Louis, C. V. Mosby Co., 1975, p. 122.

68. Osborne, G.: Compression Neuritis of the Ulnar Nerve at the Elbow. Hand **2:**10, 1970.

69. Osborne, G.: The Surgical Treatment of Tardy Ulnar Neuritis. J. Bone Joint Surg. **39B:**782, 1957.

70. Pritchard, D. J., Linscheid, R. L., and Svien, H. J.: Intra-articular Median Nerve Entrapment With Dislocation of the Elbow. Clin. Orthop. **90:**100, 1973.

71. Reis, N. D.: Anomalous Triceps Tendon as a Cause for Snapping Elbow and Ulnar Neuritis: A Case Report. J. Hand Surg. **5:**361, 1980.

72. Richmond, D. A.: Lipoma Causing a Posterior Interosseous Nerve Lesion. J. Bone Joint Surg. **35B:**83, 1953.

73. Riordan, D. C.: Radial Nerve Paralysis. Orthop. Clin. North Am. **5:**283, 1974.

74. Roles, N. C., and Maudsley, R. H.: Radial Tunnel Syndrome. Resistant Tennis Elbow as a Nerve Entrapment. J. Bone Joint Surg. **54B:**499, 1972.

75. Rosk, M. R.: Anterior Interosseous Nerve Entrapment: Report of Seven Cases. Clin. Orthop. **142:**176, 1979.

76. Salsbury, C. R.: The Nerve to the Extensor Carpi Radialis Brevis. J. Surg. **26:**95, 1938.

77. Seddon, H. J.: Three Types of Nerve Injury. Brain **66:**237, 1943.

78. Seyffarth, H.: Primary Myoses in the M. Pronator Teres as Cause of Lesion of the N. Medianus (The Pronator Syndrome). Acta Psychiat. Neurol. Suppl. **74,** 1951.

79. Sharrard, W. J. W.: Anterior Interosseous Neuritis. Report of a Case. J. Bone Joint Surg. **50B:**804, 1968.

80. Sharrard, W. J. W.: Posterior Interosseous Neuritis. J. Bone Joint Surg. **48B:**777, 1966.

81. Somerville, E. W.: Pain in the Upper Limb. Proceedings of the British Orthopaedic Association. J. Bone Joint Surg. **45B:**621, 1963.

82. Spinner, M.: The Anterior Interosseous Nerve Syn-

drome. With Special Attention to Its Variations. J. Bone Joint Surg. **52A:**84, 1970.

83. Spinner, M.: The Arcade of Frohse and Its Relationship to Posterior Interosseous Nerve Paralysis. J. Bone Joint Surg. **50B:**809, 1968.

84. Spinner, M., Freundlich, B. D., and Teicher, J.: Posterior Interosseous Nerve Palsy as a Complication of Monteggia Fracture in Children. Clin. Orthop. **58:**141, 1968.

85. Spinner, M.: Injuries to the Major Branches of the Forearm, 2nd ed. Philadelphia, W. B. Saunders Co., 1978.

86. Spinner, M., and Kaplan, E. B.: The Relationship of the Ulnar Nerve to the Medial Intermuscular Septum in the Arm and Its Clinical Significance. Hand **8:**239, 1976.

87. Strachan, J. C. H., and Ellis, B. W.: Vulnerability of the Posterior Interosseous Nerve During Radial Head Resection. J. Bone Joint Surg. **53B:**320, 1971.

88. Struthers, J.: Anatomical and Physiological Observations, Part I. Edinburgh, Sutherland and Knox, 1854.

89. Struthers, H.: On a Peculiarity of the Humerus and Humeral Artery. Monthly J. Med. Sci. **8:**264, 1848.

90. Struthers, J.: On Some Points in the Abnormal Anatomy of the Arm. Br. For. Med. Chir. Rev. **14:**170, 1854.

91. Sunderland, S.: The Innervation of the Flexor Digitorum Profundus and Lumbrical Muscles. Anat. Rec. **83:**317, 1945.

92. Sunderland, S.: Nerve Lesions in the Carpal Tunnel Syndrome. J. Neurol. Neurosurg. Psychiat. **39:**615, 1976.

93. Sunderland, S.: Nerves and Nerve Injuries. Baltimore, Williams & Wilkins Co., 1968, p. 749.

94. Tinel, J.: Nerve Wounds. New York, William Wood, 1918, pp. 183–185.

95. Vanderpool, D. W., Chalmers, J., Lamb, D. W., and Whiston, T. B.: Peripheral Compression Lesions of the Ulnar Nerve. J. Bone Joint Surg. **50B:**792, 1968.

96. Wadsworth, T. G.: The External Compression Syndrome of the Ulner Nerve at the Cubital Tunnel. Clin. Orthop. **124:**189, 1977.

97. Wartenberg, R.: Cheiralgia Paresthetica (Isolierte Neuritis des Ramus Superficialis Nervi Radialis). Z. Neurol. Psychiat. **141:**145, 1932.

98. Werner, C. O.: Lateral Elbow Pain and Posterior Interosseous Nerve Entrapment. Acta Orthop. Scand. [Suppl.] **174:**1, 1979.

99. Whitely, W. H., and Alpers, B. J.: Posterior Interosseous Palsy With Spontaneous Neuroma Formation. Arch. Neurol. **1:**226, 1959.

100. Woltman, H. W., and Learmonth, J. R.: Progressive Paralysis of the Nervus Interosseus Dorsalis. Brain **57:**25, 1934.

101. Wu, K. T., Jordan, F. R., and Eckert, C.: Lipoma. A Cause of Paralysis of Deep Radial (Posterior Interosseous) Nerve. Report of a Case and Review of the Literature. Surgery **75:**790, 1974.

CHAPTER 46

Neoplasms of the Elbow

D. J. PRITCHARD and D. C. DAHLIN

Most benign and malignant tumors of bone and soft tissue are relatively rare, and their occurrence in the region of the elbow is even more unusual. Although there are no valid statistics on soft tissue tumors, a simple compilation of lesions from Dahlin's textbook, *Bone Tumors: General Aspects and Data on 6221 Cases*, shows that only 1 per cent, 62 tumors, occurred in the bones at the elbow joint (Table 46–1).[12] Hence, no single entity is apt to be encountered very often at this site.

Unfortunately, comparable figures are not available for benign and malignant soft tissue tumors, although our impression is that the most common benign soft tissue tumor in the elbow region is the lipoma. Ganglia and myxomas are also occasionally seen in this region. Of the malignant soft tissue tumors, epithelioid sarcoma and synovial sarcoma are probably the most frequently encountered at this joint. The locally aggressive desmoid tumor may also occur at or near the elbow.

Tumors that occur in the region of the elbow are unique in that, because there are a relatively large number of important structures in a relatively small and confined area, there is little normal tissue that can be spared, and it may be difficult or impossible to remove a tumor with a margin of normal tissue

on all sides without severely compromising the function of the forearm and hand. In this respect, tumors that occur at the elbow, particularly those in the antecubital fossa, are comparable with tumors that occur in the region of the knee. However, the upper extremity is probably considered more important by most patients and their doctors; hence, amputation surgery is probably less apt to be carried out for these tumors than for those of the lower extremity. In addition, it is generally considered difficult to fit a patient with an upper limb prosthesis, and even if upper limb prosthetic devices are prescribed, patients are often reluctant to use them. In contrast, most patients readily accept the use of a lower limb prosthesis. An amputation may be required for aggressive or malignant tumors to achieve adequate surgical margins, and yet both the patient and the physician may be reluctant to accept this radical treatment.

Clinical Presentation

As with mesenchymal tumors arising in other locations, patients usually complain of either a lump or pain or perhaps both. Lesions in the region of the elbow may cause some limitation of motion, and this may be the first symptom the patient notices. In addition, swelling or increased warmth may be noted by either the patient or the physician. Dilated veins may be the first indication that there is an underlying tumefaction. Symptoms may occur because of localized compression of one or more of the nerves that cross the elbow joint, causing either local or referred pain, numbness, or paresthesia. Symptoms are not very helpful in terms of distinguishing among the diagnostic possibilities but merely serve to call the problem to the attention of the patient and ultimately to the attention of the physician. A long history suggests that the lesion is benign. If the patient describes a mass that seems to fluctuate in size, a ganglion or hemangioma may be considered.

Table 46–1. **Bone Tumors**

	Number at Elbow	Total Number
Benign		
Osteoid osteoma	12	158
Osteochondroma	9	579
Giant cell tumor	6	264
Chondromyxoid fibroma	1	30
Osteoblastoma	1	43
Malignant		
Lymphoma	11	327
Ewing's sarcoma	8	299
Osteosarcoma	7	962
Fibrosarcoma	3	158
Hemangioendothelioma	2	25
Chondrosarcoma	1	470
Malignant giant cell tumor	1	20

Preoperative Evaluation

In addition to the usual history and physical examination, the physician should pay particular attention to the palpation of any tumor mass that may be encountered. The consistency of the mass may give a clue to its nature. Is it firm, or does it feel cystic? Is it freely movable, or does it appear to be attached to some underlying structure? Is there a palpable thrill? As with soft tissue masses in other locations, a stethescope should be utilized to listen for the presence of a bruit. Transillumination of the mass with a pen light in a darkened room may suggest the presence of a cystic mass. Pain or paresthesias referred to the forearm or the hand at the time of palpation of the tumorous mass may suggest the presence of a neurogenic tumor such as a neurofibroma.

Following the clinical examination, x-ray films in at least two planes should be obtained.[20] In addition to plain x-rays, several additional studies may occasionally be useful. Xeroradiography is particularly helpful in finding and outlining soft tissue masses. Computerized tomography with a comparison of the opposite elbow joint may also yield useful information, particularly in terms of planning for the surgical procedure. We have not found the performance of routine arteriography to be particularly helpful in this or any other site; however, if one needs to know the relationship of the tumor to the adjacent major vessels, contrast material can be utilized when computerized tomography is performed, thereby supplying this information more simply and safely than by performing routine arteriography. The role of the nuclear magnetic resonator in the examination of bone and soft tissue tumors is not yet defined but appears to be a promising new modality for the preoperative evaluation of mesenchymal tumors.

Radioisotopic bone scans may also be useful not only in defining the extent of the lesion in the elbow but also by ruling out additional disease in other sites. Although it is unusual for tumors of any type to metastasize to the elbow, it is possible and should be considered whenever a primary mesenchymal neoplasm is being considered. In addition, all other modalities utilized in the evaluation of mesenchymal tumors in other locations should be employed as well. Routine blood chemistries and hematologic studies should be obtained. The relevance of these tests to certain specific entities will be discussed later as these entities are considered in more detail.

Certainly a routine chest x-ray should be obtained in every patient. If there is any possibility that a sarcoma may be found, one should consider obtaining a computerized tomographic evaluation of the lung fields before any surgical procedure is carried out. If biopsy is done first and the computerized tomographic examination is obtained later, the findings might be confusing, particularly if a general anesthetic is utilized; atelectasis or other changes may occur in the lungs because of the anesthetic. Again, it should be stressed that as much information as possible should be obtained about the patient and the tumor before any surgical procedure is carried out.

Biopsy

As with musculoskeletal tumors in other locations, the biopsy procedure should be considered at least as important as the definitive surgical procedure. The biopsy procedure should be planned with the definitive surgery in mind and should probably not be undertaken unless one is willing and prepared to proceed with whatever surgery may be indicated, depending on the results of the histologic examination and whether the pathologist can render a judgment on the basis of the frozen section. If one is approaching a lipoma or a ganglion cyst, for example, this usually becomes readily apparent to the surgeon so that he can perform a simple excisional biopsy as a one-stage procedure. If subsequent histologic examination of the permanent section should reveal something unexpected, definitive surgery can be carried out later. The frozen section can and should be utilized to determine at least whether a representative specimen of tumor tissue is obtained. The pathologist should be prepared to tell the surgeon whether the tissue sampled is reactive or whether it is tumorous, i.e., neoplastic.

The biopsy procedure itself should be performed meticulously. Very careful hemostasis should be obtained to prevent the dissemination of tumor cells in the hematoma. If the tumor lies under a muscle belly, it is usually better to go straight through the muscle rather than to dissect around the muscle, which may contaminate additional tissue planes. The general principle that incisions on extremities should be made vertically rather than transversely holds for the region of the elbow, although for lesions in the region of the antecubital fossa, it may be desirable to make an S-shaped incision with the transverse portion crossing the crease of the elbow. The biopsy wound should be closed with sutures placed close to the wound edges; if a drain is utilized it should be brought out either through the wound or very close to the wound edge so that if a surgical resection is subsequently required the biopsy site can be included in the resected specimen.

Staging

The staging system of Enneking and Spanier, which includes both soft tissue and bone sarcomas, seems to be useful.[22] This system has two main factors, the first of which is the biologic potential of the lesion. If the lesion is benign it is labeled G_0. If malignant, it is judged to be either a low-grade (G_1) or a high-grade (G_2) lesion, the high-grade lesions having greater potential for metastatic spread. The second factor is the anatomic site of the lesion—that is, whether it is entirely within a surgical compartment (T_1) or whether it extends outside the compartment (T_2). For purposes of definition, a tumor located entirely within a bone without evidence of soft tissue extension is considered to be within a single compartment. Alternatively, a lesion that has broken through the cortex into the surrounding soft tissues is considered to be extracompartmental. Similarly, a soft tissue lesion that is confined to a single fascial compartment is considered to be intracompartmental; one that extends beyond the confines of a single fascial plane is extracompartmental. With these classifications, a low-grade malignant tumor that is entirely within a single compartment is a 1A lesion; a low-grade lesion that extends into a second compartment is a 1B lesion; a high-grade malignant tumor that is confined to a single compartment is a 2A lesion; and a high-grade tumor that extends into a second compartment is a 2B lesion. Any tumor that shows evidence of metastatic spread is considered a grade 3 lesion.

In the past there has been no consensus about the nomenclature describing surgical procedures. The terminology suggested by Enneking is now generally accepted.[21] Thus, if a lesion is entered at surgery, the procedure should be considered an intralesional resection; if a tumor is "shelled out," the procedure should be considered a marginal resection; and if there is a margin of normal tissue on all aspects of the resected specimen, the operation should be considered a wide excision. For the procedure to be judged a radical resection, all the structures within the involved compartment must be resected. When the lesion involves bone, the entire bone must be removed if the procedure is to be considered a radical resection.

The same terminology is applicable to amputation surgery. Thus, if the amputation cuts through the tumor, even though the procedure may be considered radical by the patient and the surgeon, the procedure is called an intralesional amputation. For the procedure to be considered radical, the entire compartment must be amputated. For a lesion of bone, this means that disarticulation is necessary to achieve a radical amputation. Acceptance of this concept will make comparisons of results from different institutions possible. At present, there is no general consensus about what surgical procedure constitutes an adequate resection for each surgical stage of disease. Although some surgeons believe that any stage 2B lesion requires a radical resection, others feel that a wide resection is acceptable. It must be emphasized that although the adequacy of resection remains controversial, the terminology of the procedures involved and the staging utilized are not.

With these general principles in mind, we will now discuss some of the entities that are likely to be encountered in the region of the elbow.

BONE TUMORS

Benign Bone Tumors

Osteoid Osteoma

Osteoid osteoma arising in an intra-articular location is relatively uncommon; however, it may occur in the region of the elbow. This small benign bone tumor occurs in patients of any age, most commonly children and young adults. As with most bone tumors, males are more commonly affected than females. Unremitting pain is the usual symptom for which the patient seeks medical attention. Night pain is particularly prominent. Aspirin may afford very dramatic relief of pain; in fact, this dramatic relief of pain with aspirin may suggest the diagnosis of osteoid osteoma. Occasionally, the pain may be experienced at a site remote from the lesion. Another peculiar feature of this tumor is its occasional association with atrophy of the adjacent soft tissues.

When osteoid osteoma occurs at or near the elbow joint, there is characteristically loss of some flexion or extension, but pronation and supination are preserved. In addition, there may be a synovial reaction that may further confuse the diagnosis.

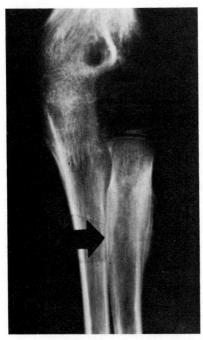

Figure 46–1. Osteoid osteoma in a 10-year-old boy, upper radial shaft. Rarefied nidus with central sclerotic area and surrounding bone formation.

The osteoid osteoma is by definition quite small, usually no more than 1.5 cm in diameter. Lesions that are clinically and histologically similar but are 2 cm or more in diameter are referred to as osteoblastomas; these lesions have clinical features somewhat different from those of osteoid osteoma.[39] Osteoblastoma, like osteoid osteoma, consists principally of irregularly arranged trabeculae of osteoid bone. It may grow to several centimeters in diameter and often lacks the classic pain of osteoid osteoma. Osteoid osteoma is small when first encountered and remains small.[27]

An extensive diagnostic evaluation is usually required to determine the precise location of the osteoid osteoma.[10, 30] When the patient complains of unremitting pain in the elbow, plain roentgenograms are usually obtained (Fig. 46–1). These may or may not reveal the presence of the tumor. The lesion typically appears as a central small nidus, which is a radiolucent area usually surrounded by an area of sclerosis. It is this sclerosis that is usually seen[33]; the central area of the nidus is more difficult to identify. When the lesion is located on the surface of the bone, there may be periosteal new bone formation that further obscures the nidus. Cronemeyer et al. described an unusual roentgenographic feature of osteoid osteoma in the elbow joint—subperiosteal new bone formation in adjacent

bones, for example, an osteoid osteoma in the distal end of the humerus that exhibits periosteal new bone formation in the proximal radius and ulna.[11] These authors concluded that "awareness of this association will prevent misdiagnosis of the benign neoplasm as an inflammatory arthritis."

Recently, the use of technetium-99m scintigraphy has been shown to be helpful in locating these lesions. If scintigraphy reveals no abnormality, an osteoid osteoma is unlikely to be found. If, however, the bone scan is positive, further diagnostic studies of the involved area should be undertaken. If there is any significant synovial reaction, there may be increased uptake due to the synovitis as well as to the lesion itself.[42] Further diagnostic studies of the involved area are frequently required. Tomograms in two planes often reveal the suspected lesion. Sometimes multiple roentgenograms must be taken before the lesion can be identified. Computerized tomography may be helpful; however, the tumor is so small that it can be easily missed on this examination.[44]

Grossly, there is usually some sclerotic bone surrounding a central nidus. This nidus may be somewhat redder than the surrounding cortical bone and has been described as having the appearance of a small cherry. The pathologist may have trouble identifying this nidus unless the lesion is very well localized preoperatively and the entire block of tissue is submitted for examination. It is sometimes helpful to obtain roentgenograms of the excised block of tissue before the pathologist cuts into the block. Microscopic examination of the surrounding bone shows no unusual features; the nidus itself consists of a network of osteoid trabeculae. These trabeculae have no pattern to their arrangement except that there is usually more mineralization in the center of the lesion and less on the surface. The cells mantling the osteoid trabeculae are benign, and the background consists of benign fibroblastic tissue usually containing thin-walled blood vessels. The lesion is circumscribed.

The treatment of osteoid osteoma is surgical excision of the nidus. It is not necessary to remove all of the sclerotic bone. The main problem with this type of surgery is identification of the lesion and confirmation of its removal by the pathologist, which may be difficult. Ghelman et al. described a method for localizing an osteoid osteoma intraoperatively using a scintillation probe.[24] This technique may simplify the localization of the lesion at the time of surgery. Patients whose lesions are not completely excised will probably continue to have the same pain and will probably require a second operation.[41]

Osteochondroma

Osteochondroma is probably the most common benign bone tumor, but it is not very commonly encountered in the elbow. The incidence may be somewhat higher than that reflected in our surgical experience, however, because many osteochondromas in other locations are asymptomatic and presumably may also be in the region of the elbow. The osteochondroma is not inherently painful but causes symptoms by pressure on adjacent structures. In addition, the tumor may produce a deformity that is either structurally or cosmetically undesirable. Occasionally, an osteochondroma may fracture at its base, and this may cause symptoms. The tumor may be found in a patient of any age, but it usually stops growing when skeletal maturity is reached. An osteochondroma may arise from the surface of any bone but most commonly does so in the metaphyseal region of long bones (Fig. 46–2). The tumor tends to project away from the joint along the direction of attached muscles. The tumor may be pedunculated on a stalk or may be sessile and have a broad base (Fig. 46–3). The cortical surface of the underlying normal bone extends up into the stalk. The tumor is covered by a

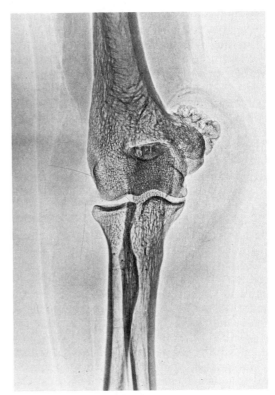

Figure 46–3. Osteochondroma of distal humerus in a 41-year-old man. Note soft tissue reaction.

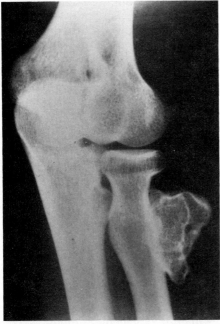

Figure 46–2. Osteochondroma in a 23-year-old woman. Radial shaft with cortical and medullary bone extending into tumor.

cartilage cap, which contributes to the bone formation by enchondral ossification. This cartilage cap may not be visible on roentgenographic examination; thus, the tumor may appear larger by clinical examination than by roentgenographic examination. If the cartilage cap becomes markedly thickened, the possibility of sarcomatous transformation must be considered; if it is more than 1 cm thick the risk of secondary chondrosarcoma is relatively high. The age of the patient must be taken into consideration, however, because in children the cartilage cap is normally thicker than in adults. Probably less than 1 per cent of osteochondromas ever become malignant.[26]

Multiple osteochondromas sometimes occur, a condition that tends to be familial. When multiple bones are involved there may be some element of dysplasia in the deformity. Patients with multiple osteochondromas are much more likely to develop sarcomatous transformation of one or more of these lesions. Although the true incidence of sarcomatous change is not known, it is probably near 10 per cent. Thus, patients with multiple osteochondromas need to be carefully observed by periodic follow-up examinations. When and if there is evidence of change or any new symptoms, excision must be considered.

Osteochondromas in the region of the elbow may cause mechanical difficulties, specifically, interference with the motion of the elbow joint. In addition, the cartilage cap may impinge on important neurovascular structures, causing symptoms in this way. If there are symptoms or mechanical or cosmetic difficulties, excision of the osteochondroma should be considered. The osteochondroma should be excised completely, together with the overlying cartilage cap. Excision usually involves using an osteotome to shave the lesion level with the underlying cortical bone. Such simple excision generally results in cure, although local recurrence may occasionally be noted, indicating that part of the cartilaginous cap was left behind.

The pathologist should examine the cartilage cap carefully by making sections at right angles to the surface of the lesion so that the exact thickness can be measured. If the cap is thicker than 1 cm in an adult, the lesion must be carefully studied histologically to exclude the possibility of a sarcoma. Histologic criteria of malignancy include relatively numerous multinucleated cells, enlargement of nuclei, and invasion into surrounding tissues.

Giant Cell Tumor

Benign giant cell tumors are occasionally encountered in the region of the elbow. In general, giant cell tumors more commonly affect females than males, contrary to the situation with most benign and malignant bone tumors. About 80 per cent of giant cell tumors occur in persons who are more than 20 years of age. This point may be helpful in differentiating a giant cell tumor from an aneurysmal bone cyst, which may be radiographically similar but tends to occur in persons who are less than 20 years of age.

Giant cell tumors nearly always occur in the epiphyseal region and may extend to the articular surface of the bone (Fig. 46–4). Campanacci and colleagues have attempted to grade giant cell tumors according to radiographic criteria; thus grade 1 lesions are radiographically indolent and grade 3 tumors are radiographically aggressive. Unfortunately, the majority of giant cell tumors are probably what Campanacci and colleagues refer to as grade 2, in which the roentgenographic appearance is aggressive, but the tumor has not yet broken through cortical bone. Radiographic grading may be important in helping the surgeon decide on the appropriate treatment.[8]

Grossly, the tumor consists of a red, soft tissue that typically extends up the subchon-

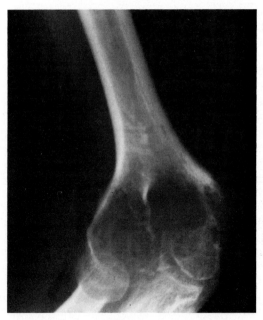

Figure 46–4. Giant cell tumor of the distal end of the humerus of a 75-year-old woman. The zone of rarefaction is associated with "expansion of the bone."

dral bone at the articular surface. There may be thinning and erosion of the cortical bone with extension of the tumor into the surrounding soft structures. Histologically, it is the appearance of the stromal cells that is important. These cells are histologically benign and usually contain a round or oval-shaped nucleus that has an appearance similar to the nuclei of the giant cell. Mitotic figures are not uncommon, and bone formation may be seen. These findings may lead to the erroneous diagnosis of osteosarcoma. Attempts have been made to grade giant cell tumors by histologic criteria, but this has not proved to be useful because the histologic appearance of any one giant cell tumor is apt to be similar to all others. Those giant cell tumors that appear to be more aggressive histologically do not necessarily behave more aggressively clinically.[15]

The extent of surgery required to eradicate giant cell tumors is somewhat controversial. In the region of the elbow particularly difficult problems may be encountered. The distal end of the humerus does not lend itself well to surgical excision by curettage unless the lesion is radiographically a grade 1 lesion. Total excision of the distal end of the humerus, although it would probably cure the patient and prevent local recurrence, creates a very serious problem for the reconstructive surgeon. Allograft replacement might be considered in this setting, but the decision about the method of treatment is often exceedingly difficult. Excision by curettage in other locations results in a local recurrence rate of approximately 25 per cent. It is probably reasonable to accept this risk and to try curettage for the first treatment because the alternative of resection of the distal end of the humerus is so drastic. However, if the tumor has already broken through the cortex into the surrounding soft structures, curettage is unlikely to be effective. For tumors of the proximal end of the ulna, curettage might be more reasonable because there is more bone to work with—hence, a larger margin of normal bone can be included in the resected specimen, whether resection is done by curettage or actual excision. If the proximal radial head is involved with a reasonably small tumor, it is probably best treated by simple excision.[25, 29]

Radiation therapy for benign giant cell tumors should be avoided if possible. In our previous experience, radiation of benign giant cell tumors was accompanied by significant risk of subsequent malignant transformation.

Aneurysmal Bone Cyst

This benign lesion typically contains abundant benign giant cells in scattered zones and formerly was included among the giant cell tumors. It is different, however, because it nearly always contains blood-filled spaces, is somewhat fibrogenic, and usually has zones with osteoid formation and trabeculae of bone. The proliferating cells of this lesion are benign, although mitoses may be numerous in some areas. This introduces the risk of mistaking the process for sarcoma. The tumor is considered to be a non-neoplastic reactive process that sometimes does not recur even after subtotal removal. Rare pertinent examples are predominantly solid and resemble

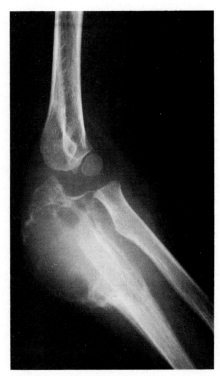

Figure 46–5. Aneurysmal bone cyst of the ulna in a 5-year-old boy. Note circumscription of the mass, which is associated with destruction of the shaft and end of the bone.

florid heterotopic ossification of the soft tissues.

An aneurysmal bone cyst may arise de novo, or a similar reactive change may be seen in various benign and even in malignant tumors of bone. It is necessary to rule out any causative underlying process because this will dictate the capability of the lesion.

In the Mayo Clinic experience with 134 aneurysmal bone cysts unrelated to pre-exist-

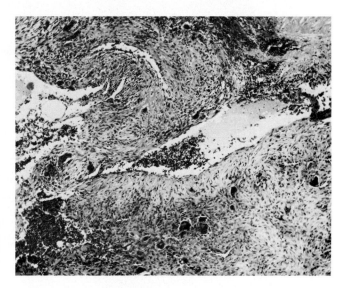

Figure 46–6. Aneurysmal bone cyst showing space from which the blood has partially escaped. Septa contain fibrogenic cells, which show maturation and some osteoid production. The cells are benign (hematoxylin and eosin, ×100).

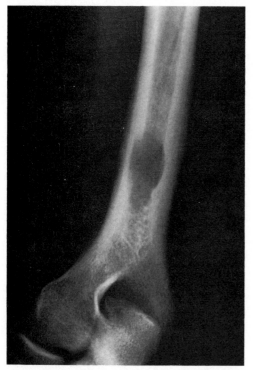

Figure 46–7. Histiocytosis X producing a well-defined rare-faction of the humeral shaft. This completely benign lesion is associated with a good prognosis, especially if it is solitary.

ing disease, 43 per cent occurred in males. In contrast to the age of predilection for giant cell tumors, 78 per cent of the patients were less than 20 years old. Pain and swelling are the most common features. A minority of the lesions are near the elbow.[12]

Roentgenologically, the diseased area is sometimes confusingly like that of a malignant tumor, but the zone of rarefaction is usually well circumscribed, eccentric, and associated with an obvious soft tissue extension of the process (Fig. 46–5). Classically, the soft tissue extension is produced by bulging of the periosteum and a resultant layer of roentgenologically visible new bone that delimits the periphery of the tumor. Fusiform expansion may be produced, especially when small bones such as a fibula or a rib are affected. The lesion is usually metaphyseal in location.[5, 16]

Pathologically, an aneurysmal bone cyst contains anastomosing cavernomatous spaces that usually comprise the bulk of the lesion (Fig. 46–6). The spaces are usually filled with unclotted blood, which may well up into, but does not spurt from, the tumor when it is unroofed. The eggshell-thick layer of subperiosteal new bone that delimits the lesion peripherally is ordinarily readily discernible. Reconstruction of the cavernomatous spaces from the curetted fragments may be difficult. The most important thing to recognize histologically is the benign quality of the constituent cells.[14, 37] Telangiectatic osteosarcoma may simulate aneurysmal bone cyst when viewed at low magnification.

Treatment is essentially the same as that for benign giant cell tumors. Curettage and bone grafting are usually required, and the majority of lesions treated in this way will be cured. Perhaps 25 per cent of these cases will recur and require additional surgery.

Other Benign Bone Tumors and Tumor Simulators

Benign tumors of bone at the elbow other than those previously discussed may rarely be encountered (Fig. 46–7). In addition, there

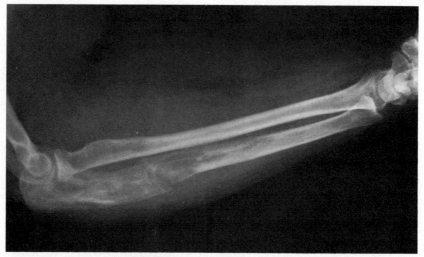

Figure 46–8. Paget's disease of proximal two-thirds of ulna. This classic lesion is associated with pathologic fracture and extends to the end of the bone. Paget's disease of bone is very rare in patients less than 40 years old.

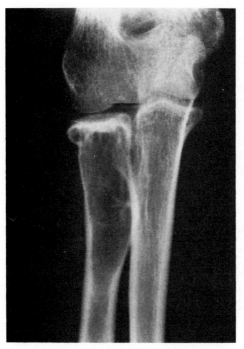

Figure 46–9. Fibrous dysplasia producing rarefaction and slight expansion of the proximal part of the radius of a 20-year-old woman. Symptoms produced by a lesion of fibrous dysplasia may require surgical management.

are a number of lesions that may occur in any bone and that may simulate or mimic a primary bone tumor (Figs. 46–8 to 46–10). Benign cartilage tumors are very rare at the elbow; nevertheless, they do occasionally occur (Figs. 46–11 to 46–13).

Malignant Bone Tumors

Lymphoma of Bone

Currently the term *malignant lymphoma* is used for those small round cell tumors of bone that previously were referred to as reticulum cell sarcoma.[34] Lymphoma tends to occur in middle-aged or elderly adults; young people are uncommonly affected. Patients with lymphoma generally present with pain and perhaps swelling in the region of the lesion. The tumor may arise primarily in any bone including bones in the region of the elbow. When a destructive lesion is encountered in the region of the elbow and when biopsy confirms the diagnosis of lymphoma, staging must be carefully done to rule out the presence of other disease. Staging usually includes technetium-99m bone scans, chest

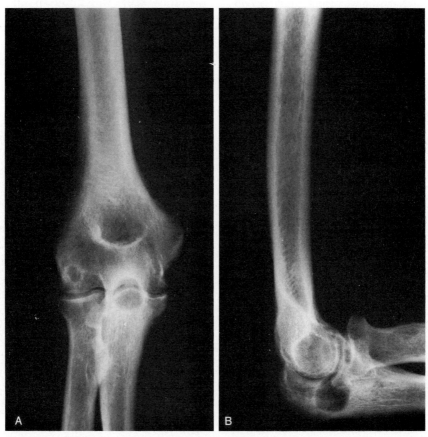

Figure 46–10. *A, B,* Cyst of upper part of the ulna secondary to degenerative joint disease at the elbow.

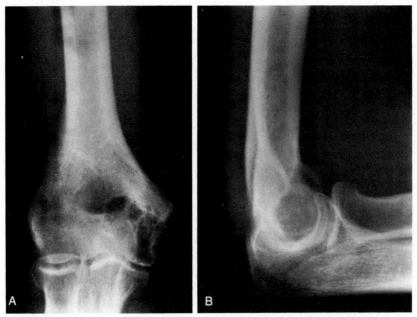

Figure 46–11. *A, B,* Benign chondroblastoma of distal end of the humerus in a 25-year-old man. Note discrete zone of rarefaction. Such lesions are more innocuous than giant cell tumors.

x-rays, and computerized tomographic examination of the lungs, pelvis, and abdomen. In addition, bone marrow aspirates and special smears of peripheral blood must be obtained. Lymphangiography is no longer routinely obtained when these other modalities are utilized.

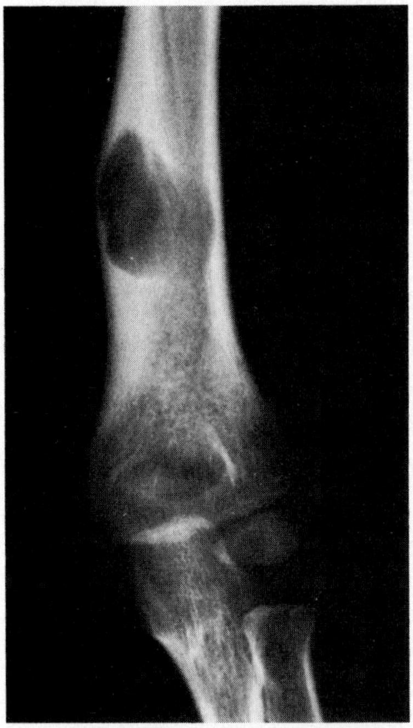

The roentgenographic features of lymphoma are nonspecific (Fig. 46–14). There is usually a diffuse, destructive, mottled appearance with indistinct margins. Variable degrees of sclerosis may be present in the lesion; the cortical bone is usually eroded, and the tumor may extend into the adjacent soft tissues. Periosteal new bone formation is not usually a prominent feature.

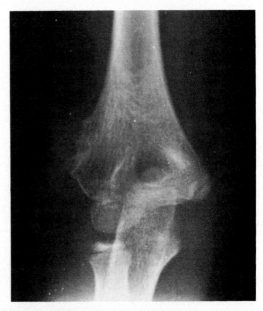

Figure 46–12. Chondromyxoid fibroma of the humerus in a 6-year-old boy. This rare benign lesion has almost no capability of becoming a malignant tumor.

Figure 46–13. Periosteal chondroma on the medial distal humerus. The benign lesion lies in a concavity of the bone.

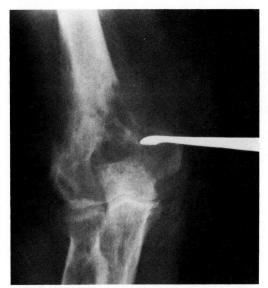

Figure 46–14. Malignant lymphoma producing malignant-appearing destruction of the distal part of the humerus in a 60-year-old woman.

Grossly, lymphoma tissue is usually gray or white and very soft. The area of involved bone may be extensively destroyed with areas of necrosis. Microscopically, lymphoma is usually composed of a mixture of cell types that cannot be reliably subclassed in the same way that is characteristic of lymphomas of lymph nodes. Reticulum cells are frequently encountered. These cells tend to be larger than those seen in Ewing's sarcoma and tend to have grooving or infolding of the nuclei. Lymphocytes and lymphoblasts are also usually present. These cells tend to form an alveolar pattern with cells surrounded by a reticular network. Reticulum stains are helpful in delineating this network. If lymphocytes are prominent, this may lead to an erroneous diagnosis of osteomyelitis. Histiocytosis X can also be confused with lymphoma of bone, although the cells of histiocytosis X lack the features suggestive of malignancy.

Lymphoma is generally treated with radiation therapy if there is only a solitary lesion of bone. For lymphoma in the region of the elbow joint, some morbidity can probably be expected from the radiation therapy. Radiation therapists generally try to avoid circumferential treatment of an extremity in order to allow some normal lymphatic channels to remain open. Failure to do so may result in significant swelling distal to the treatment area. It may be difficult or impossible to avoid treating the entire circumference of the extremity in the region of the elbow. In addition, when radiation exceeds approximately 4000 rads, radiation therapists generally try to direct treatment away from the articular surface. Again, this may be difficult or impossible to achieve in the region of the elbow.

There is no clear-cut or obvious advantage to the use of adjunctive chemotherapy at the time of initial treatment if only a solitary lesion is present. Obviously, patients with lymphoma need to be followed closely with frequent examinations and repeat studies with the expectation that chemotherapy will be utilized if systemic or metastatic disease develops.[40]

In general, lymphoma presenting primarily in bone has a long-term survival of about 60 per cent.[6] However, no figures are available for the occurrence of lymphoma of bone specifically at the elbow.

Ewing's Sarcoma

Ewing's sarcoma may arise in any bone, including those in the region of the elbow. Ewing's sarcoma is more frequently found in children than adults; very young infants, however, very rarely have this tumor. Most patients with Ewing's sarcoma complain of pain that seems to become worse with time, and many complain of swelling or intermittent low-grade fever.

The usual roentgenographic appearance of Ewing's sarcoma is that of a mottled or moth-eaten destructive lesion that may contain both lytic and blastic areas (Fig. 46–15). There is frequently periosteal reactive new bone, which may form layers, forming the "onion skin" appearance that is said to be typical of this disease. We have noted, however, that this feature is not pathognomonic for Ewing's sarcoma because it may be found with other bone lesions, both benign and malignant. Any portion of any bone may be involved. It should be emphasized that the radiographic and occasionally the clinical appearance of Ewing's sarcoma is similar to that of osteomyelitis. The roentgenographic appearance combined with the presence of fever and an elevated erythrocyte sedimentation rate may lead to the erroneous diagnosis of osteomyelitis.

Grossly, Ewing's sarcoma may be very soft or even semiliquid; indeed, the appearance may simulate the purulence of infection. The tumor may be solid, but it is not encapsulated. There frequently is more involvement of the bone than can be appreciated on the roentgenogram. Microscopically, Ewing's sarcoma is very cellular, and the cells are remarkably similar to each other. There is usually very little stromal tissue; the lack of stromal tissue

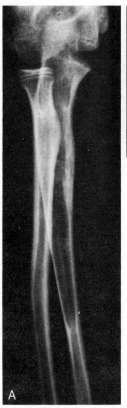
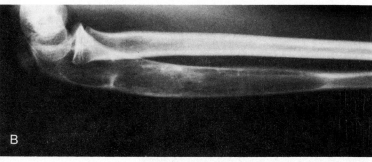

Figure 46–15. A, B, Recurrent Ewing's sarcoma with cystlike lesion of upper half of the ulna in a 21-year-old woman. The original tumor had been treated 10 years previously.

can be demonstrated with a reticulum stain. Individual cells are small and round and have round or oval nuclei. Areas of extensive necrosis may be identified. Periosteal new bone formation, if present, may complicate the histologic interpretation.[38]

Treatment of Ewing's sarcoma of bone in the region of the elbow is similar to that for other sites. That is, the local lesion is generally treated with radiation therapy, and systemic combination chemotherapy is generally utilized in an attempt to prevent micrometastases. Although there is a growing trend toward considering a larger role for surgery in the treatment of the primary lesion, there is little enthusiasm for resecting malignant tumors in the region of the elbow because it is difficult to achieve adequate margins in this region without damaging important normal structures.[35] Even if an adequate resection could be achieved, satisfactory reconstruction would be difficult or impossible. This is particularly true when dealing with children with open physes. In general, then, Ewing's sarcoma of the elbow is probably best treated by radiation therapy plus chemotherapy. This treatment is the same for Ewing's sarcoma as for lymphoma in the region of the elbow.[4, 28] A major side effect is soft tissue fibrosis causing a stiff joint.

An identical small round cell tumor may occur outside of bone in the somatic soft tissue,[2] and once again, the treatment principles that apply for Ewing's tumor of bone are used for Ewing's tumor of soft tissue.

Osteosarcoma

Osteosarcoma is the most common primary malignant bone tumor but in our experience is not the most common primary malignant bone tumor in the region of the elbow. Nevertheless, it does occasionally occur. Osteosarcoma generally affects persons in the second decade of life. Males are more commonly affected than females. This tumor usually causes pain and swelling.

Roentgenographically, osteosarcoma usually appears to be aggressive with evidence of cortical destruction. There may be reactive periosteal new bone formation, which in the distal humerus may be abundant and give a "sunburst" appearance. Some osteosarcomas present as almost entirely lytic lesions, whereas others may appear entirely sclerotic. The precise extent of the lesion may not be apparent on plain radiographs (Fig. 46–16). The tumor can usually be more accurately assessed with a technetium or gallium bone scan. Other studies, such as computerized tomography, may be utilized to help deter-

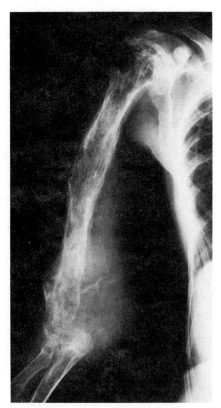

Figure 46–16. Grade 4 osteosarcoma of the distal end of the humerus in a patient with Paget's disease of the entire bone.

mine the extent of soft tissue involvement if it is present. Grossly, the tumor may vary from being almost entirely sclerotic to being almost entirely soft. Almost always, however, there are areas of soft tumorous tissue that may be obtained for biopsy. The reactive new bone formation at the periphery of the lesion should not be sampled for biopsy because this will simply lead to confusion in the interpretation of the histologic findings. If there is a soft tissue extension of the tumor, this is the area that is best to biopsy because it is usually the most malignant and the easiest to process in the pathology laboratory. Frozen sections should be utilized to assess whether an adequate sample has been removed for examination by the pathologist.

By definition, to be considered an osteosarcoma the lesion must contain areas of malignant cells that are producing osteoid (Fig. 46–17). There are no procedures or stains that are specific for osteoid; hence, considerable judgment and experience on the part of the pathologist is necessary for the proper interpretation of this lesion. About one half of these tumors are predominantly fibrous or cartilaginous and the remainder are predominantly bone-forming. Because any one of these three types of differentiation may predominate, the

lesions may be subtyped into fibroblastic, chondroblastic, or osteoblastic osteosarcoma. Sometimes the lesion contains a more or less equal mixture of these three elements, and the histologic diagnosis cannot be subclassified. This subclassification may be important because the osteoblastic subtype appears to have a worse prognosis than the other two subtypes.[13, 17, 46–48]

Malignant fibrous histiocytoma of bone is a recently recognized variant of osteosarcoma.[18] From a practical standpoint, the clinical management of this malignancy is essentially identical with that of osteosarcoma (Figs. 46–18 and 46–19).

The initial evaluation and staging of a patient with osteosarcoma includes careful examination of the lung fields. In addition to plain roentgenography, computed tomography has proved to be particularly useful in detection of occult metastatic disease. In our own experience, 8 to 10 per cent of patients with newly diagnosed osteosarcoma are found to have metastatic disease, either by plain roentgenography or computed tomography.

The usual treatment for osteosarcoma, as for other radioresistant malignant bone tumors, is surgical ablation. For many years amputation was required. However, today there is considerable interest in various limb salvage procedures as an alternative to amputation. There is very little experience with

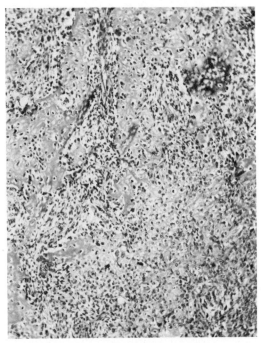

Figure 46–17. Grade 3 osteosarcoma. The malignant cells are producing osteoid, which is slightly mineralized in the darker staining areas (×100).

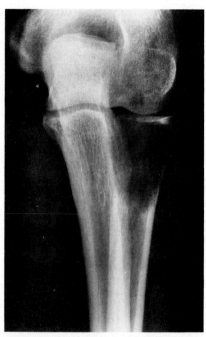

Figure 46–18. Grade 4 malignant fibrous histiocytoma producing malignant-appearing destruction of the upper part of the ulna in a 45-year-old man.

this approach, however, for tumors in the region of the elbow. Unless such a tumor is unusually small, amputation is probably preferable to attempts at resection in this area.[7, 43, 45]

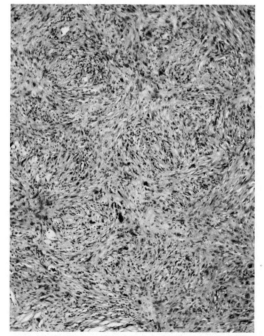

Figure 46–19. Grade 3 malignant fibrous histiocytoma with fibrogenic cells showing a storiform pattern. Scattered, highly malignant cells and a pathologic mitosis are present (hematoxylin and eosin, ×100).

SOFT TISSUE TUMORS

Mesenchymal soft tissue tumors, especially the malignant types, are probably the least understood of all tumors. There are numerous varieties of mesenchymal tumors, and yet most of these entities are rarely encountered. A full discussion of all of these tumors is well beyond the scope of this chapter.

Many benign soft tissue tumors are commonly encountered; however, because some soft tissue sarcomas may grow very slowly, both the patient and the physician may be misled into thinking that a soft tissue mass is benign. When this happens, a definitive diagnosis may be delayed, sometimes for years. When the patient does seek medical attention, it is not uncommon for the physician to perform a biopsy procedure that may jeopardize subsequent surgical care. As with bone tumors, proper placement of the biopsy incision is critical, and any subsequent resection surgery for malignant tumors demands that the biopsy site be included in the resected specimen. If the biopsy incision is not well placed, inclusion of the site at surgery may be difficult or impossible to achieve. Again, because the vast majority of lumps and bumps are benign, the initial treating physician may not suspect an emergency, and therefore may be misled into performing an improper biopsy procedure. If the mass is small and is situated in a favorable location, it is far preferable to perform an excisional biopsy, leaving a margin of normal tissue on all aspects of the suspected lesion. If an incisional biopsy is done, sufficient tissue must be removed to allow adequate representative sampling of the tumor so that the pathologist can arrive at the correct diagnosis. Perhaps no other factor is as important in the management of patients with soft tissue tumors as the proper performance of the biopsy procedure.

The management of soft tissue tumors is made even more difficult by the problems encountered by the surgical pathologist. Soft tissue sarcomas not only are relatively rare but also are notoriously difficult to diagnose accurately. Relatively few surgical pathologists claim considerable experience and expertise in dealing with these lesions. As a result, the initial histologic diagnosis may be in error and the patient may receive inappropriate treatment. Often the original pathologist seeks additional consultation from other surgical pathologists. Occasionally in this situation more than one histologic diagnosis may be suggested, leading to further confusion and delay. It is not unusual in such instances for definitive surgery to be delayed for several months from the time the patient initially seeks medical attention.

If a soft tissue mass is encountered or suspected, some information may be obtained from the history and physical examination. Patients may complain of a lump or pain or both. Small painful lumps may represent benign tumors—neurilemmoma, neurofibroma, schwannoma, vascular myoma, glomus tumor, and fat necrosis should all be considered in this situation. Sometimes these lesions may be occult, particularly when they are small and buried in the deep soft tissues. When the patient complains of well-localized persistent pain, these entities should be considered.

The presence of a slowly growing mass that has been present perhaps for several years should lead to a suspicion of such sarcomas as synovial sarcoma, clear-cell sarcoma, or even a well-differentiated sarcoma of a more common histologic type, such as a liposarcoma, rhabdomyosarcoma, or malignant fibrous histiocytoma. When the lesion is located in the upper extremity, epithelioid sarcoma should be considered.

Some of the commonly encountered soft tissue lumps may be reasonably diagnosed on the basis of the history and physical examination alone. This is particularly true for lipomas, which are commonly encountered by all physicians. When the lesion is asymptomatic and has characteristic features on the clinical examination, biopsy is probably not necessary. Certainly, biopsy is unnecessary for most lipomas. However, caution is needed because even the most benign-appearing soft tissue tumor may be malignant. When a decision is made not to perform an excisional biopsy on the basis of the physician's clinical judgment, the patient should be followed up closely and should understand that any change in the situation warrants further medical attention.

Laboratory and radiographic evaluations of the patient will depend largely on the clinical situation. If a sarcoma is suspected, then a full battery of routine laboratory tests should be obtained. In addition, various radiographic techniques may be helpful. Again, depending on the situation encountered, plain roentgenograms may be helpful, particularly if the radiologist uses special soft tissue techniques. Calcium or even ossification may be present within the lesion. In addition, the relationship of the lesion to the surrounding structures may be ascertained. This is particularly true if there is erosion of the underlying skeleton.

Xeroradiographs in general give more precise information about soft tissue tumors than do plain roentgenograms. If the lesion is totally lucent and has very sharply circumscribed margins, it may be a lipoma. If, however, the lesion has irregular margins and a nonhomogeneous density, sarcomatous change must be suspected.

In summary, the clinical evaluation of the patient with a suspected soft tissue tumor depends largely on the experience and judgment of the treating physician. However, when in doubt as much information as possible should be obtained before the performance of the biopsy procedure.

Benign Soft Tissue Tumors

Lipomas

Lipoma is probably the most frequently encountered benign soft tissue neoplasm. This tumor is usually solitary, but multiple lipomas have occurred in virtually all locations in the body. In some instances of multiple lipomas, there is probably some disturbance in adipose metabolism. The tumor is simply a localized collection of adipose tissue that is histologically and chemically similar to ordinary fat.

Most lipomas are small, asymptomatic, and relatively dormant in that they seem to remain approximately the same size. In other instances, however, the tumor may continue to grow and become symptomatic. If there is trauma to the area, necrosis may develop within the lipoma, and this is usually symptomatic. Deep-seated lipomas, especially those that arise in the belly of a muscle, seem to have a particular tendency to increase in size. Indeed, these tumors may be difficult to eradicate. Most lipomas consist almost entirely of adipose tissue; however, there may be increased vascularity, in which case the lesion is referred to as angiolipoma.[19]

The majority of lipomas require no treatment other than simple observation. The patient should be made aware that if the lesion continues to increase in size or if it becomes symptomatic, medical consultation should be sought. Most of these lesions can be easily and confidently diagnosed on the basis of the clinical examination alone; however, some lipomas may not have the clinical characteristics of the usual subcutaneous lipoma and may require further diagnostic modalities. Radiographs will usually reveal a homogeneous lucency. Xeroradiography is particularly helpful in the assessment of such tumors; a uniform fat density is seen. For very large tumors, computed tomography is helpful. If there are areas within the lesion that are not homogeneous, the possibility of liposarcoma or some other soft tissue sarcoma must be considered.

Surgical excision should be considered for lipomas that increase in size, are symptomatic or cosmetically undesirable, or interfere with function and in situations when the diagnosis is not certain. For most such tumors, a simple marginal excision is all that is indicated. However, when a lipoma is located within the belly of a muscle, it may be necessary to sacrifice some normal muscle tissue on all aspects in order to minimize the risk of local recurrence.

Ganglion

A ganglion is a cystic lesion generally found in the hands, wrists, and feet, but it may be found less commonly in the region of the elbow. A true ganglion has no or only a poorly defined synovial lining. The cyst is filled with a mucoid, colorless, semiliquid substance that has been reported to have the appearance of apple jelly. Although the ganglion may connect with the joint, it does not always do so; indeed, the lesion may occur within a tendon, in a muscle, or even on occasion in bone. Characteristically, the size of these lesions varies, as do the patient's symptoms. Many such lesions are probably ignored by patients who do not seek medical attention unless the lesion appears to be increasing in size or is symptomatic. Treatment is simple excision, ensuring that the entire lesion has been removed. Not all ganglia require excision, however, and most patients may be treated symptomatically by splinting, injections, and other conservative measures.

Myxoma

Myxomas occasionally occur in the soft tissues at the elbow. This tumor is a very soft, almost mucoid, lesion that consists of cells in a loose matrix of reticulin and collagen fibers. Histologically, the tissue may be similar to that seen in the lining of a ganglion; however, myxomas do not contain cysts. A myxoma is relatively small and is usually encountered in the superficial soft tissues. It is not uncommon for this tumor to arise within the substance of a major muscle.

The treatment for myxoma is excision; however, a wide excision rather than a marginal resection is probably indicated because this tumor tends to recur if it is marginally excised.

Pigmented Villonodular Synovitis

Jaffe and associates described this lesion and suggested the name *villonodular synovitis*. In the past, the disease had various names including xanthoma, xanthogranuloma, giant cell tumor of the tendon sheath, and myeloplaxoma. Pigmented villonodular synovitis probably belongs in the middle of the spectrum of diseases, within the general category of fibrous histiocytoma. Pigmented villonodular synovitis involves the synovium, bursae, or tendon sheaths. The knee is the most common site of involvement; however, involvement of the fingers, hip, ankle, and foot and even the iliopectineal bursa has been reported. Rare lesions of this type occur in the elbow. The lesion tends to occur in young adults, but it may be found in teenagers and older adults. Men and women are about equally affected.

Clinically, there are two forms of the disease—nodular and diffuse. The nodular or localized form is probably most frequently encountered in the small joints of the fingers, whereas the diffuse form is most commonly found in the knee joint. The usual presenting symptom is swelling, although some patients complain of mild to moderate pain. On physical examination, the only finding may be swelling, with a suggestion of increased thickening of the synovium. Roentgenograms may reveal cystic erosions on either side of the joint (Fig. 46–20). When erosions are found and there is no loss of joint space and no demineralization of the surrounding bone, the diagnosis should be suspected. In most cases of pigmented villonodular synovitis, however, there is no bony erosion, but there is evidence of lobular swelling of the soft tissues.[3]

Pathologically, the diffuse form is predominantly villous, and the nodular form may show a localized focus of synovial enlargement. The hypertrophic synovial tissue may show numerous villi that vary in color from yellow to dark brown. The pigmentation is due to hemosiderin and lipid. Sometimes the tissue may be seen eroding into the surrounding bone, and the question of malignancy may be considered. However, the lesion is not malignant and should not be confused with a synovial sarcoma.

Microscopic study shows a stromal background of reticulin and collagen fibers in which various different cells may be found. The firm nodular lesions have more collagenous stroma, whereas the soft villous lesions have less stroma. There may be numerous

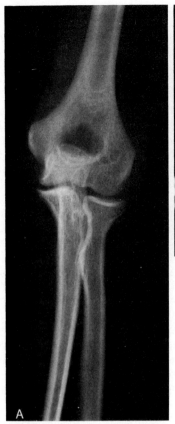
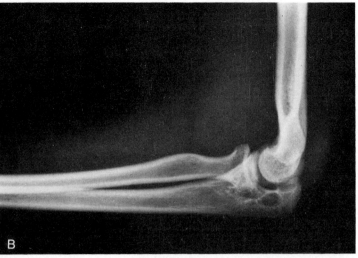

Figure 46–20. Pigmented villonodular synovitis in a 17-year-old girl, with a 3-year history of pain and swelling. Note cystic erosions.

small vessels, which have normal structures. The cells are usually mononuclear, but benign multinucleated giant cells in variable numbers are present. Histiocytic cells containing hemosiderin or lipid are usually present. Some lesions may be highly cellular, and occasional mitotic activity is noted. However, the cytologic features of malignancy are not present.

In the nodular form, the nodule may be simply excised with the expectation that a cure will be achieved in most cases. However, the results of treatment of the diffuse form are discouraging. Even aggressive surgery is likely to be followed by local recurrence, which is more frequent when there is evidence of bony erosion. Even multiple synovectomies have not always been curative; because of this, various alternative treatments have been attempted. Radiation therapy has been utilized and has resulted in regression. However, there is no documented evidence that such treatment will actually eliminate the disease and prevent local recurrences. In addition, if high doses of radiation are used in the region of a joint, the complications of the treatment may be worse than the original disease. Thus, one or more synovectomies probably should be

done, but if this treatment leads to symptomatic local recurrence, then arthrodesis must be considered in most joints. In the elbow, however, since this joint does poorly with an arthrodesis, resection or replacement arthroplasty may allow successful management of the patient's pain, even though the disease is not totally eradicated.

Chondromatosis of the Synovium

Chondromatosis includes "osteochondromatosis" of the synovium, but occasionally there is no actual bone present in the discrete cartilaginous tumors. It is the same process as chondromatosis, and the same treatment is used. Chondromatosis is a benign, tumorous, multifocal, chondromatous or chondro-osseous metaplastic proliferation involving the subsynovial connective tissue of joints, tendon sheaths, or bursae. The process can involve any joint. The average age of the patients is about 40 years; males are affected more often than females. Symptoms include pain and limited motion. The duration of symptoms may be long or relatively short before diagnosis is made. In the Mayo Clinic series, only two thirds of the roentgenograms showed radiopaque masses (Fig. 46–21).[32] Di-

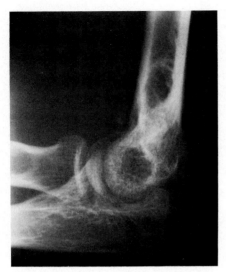

Figure 46–21. Synovial chondromatosis of the elbow. Note that a small mineralized focus is evident in the antecubital fossa.

agnosis is difficult because the roentgenogram may not reveal ossific bodies even when they are present.

Longstanding pain localized to one joint may be associated roentgenographically with only mild osteoporosis or with multiple, diffuse, calcified, osteocartilaginous bodies. If they are only slightly calcified, osteochondromatous bodies may be seen with special roentgenographic techniques that blur out soft tissue shadows.

When the roentgenologic diagnosis is indefinite and symptoms persist without any other obvious cause, diagnostic arthrotomy is indicated. Because osteochondromatosis may be sharply localized and may not be a diffuse condition of the entire synovium, careful inspection of the whole synovial lining is important. Generally, diagnosis can be made by the gross appearance and confirmed by immediate histologic examination using frozen section techniques.

The treatment of osteochondromatosis consists of removing any loose osteochondromatous bodies and the involved synovium from which they arise. In general, complete synovectomy is necessary, and complete exposure of the elbow joint from an extensile posterior approach is required. The condition may recur because nests of synovium may be left behind. If this happens, a second arthrotomy is necessary. Frequently, the longstanding synovial osteochondromatosis creates secondary osteoarthritis. General principles of treatment of chondromatosis at other sites apply to chondromatosis at the elbow (see Chapter 47).

Radiation therapy is to be condemned. Although irradiation may have some inhibiting effects on synovial growth, its potential for causing later malignant change is notorious.

Myositis Ossificans (Heterotopic or Ectopic Ossification)

Heterotopic ossification, often erroneously called myositis ossificans, may occur near the elbow, either in muscle or other soft tissue. In its early or "florid" stage, there may be such pronounced cellular activity that it may be mistaken for sarcoma. The relative rarity of this disease has delayed understanding of the peculiar tissue reaction associated with it. For this reason, a brief discussion is appropriate here, although the topic has been thoroughly reviewed in Chapter 26.

The patient sometimes has experienced significant recent trauma to the area in which the lesion develops. A mass commonly occurs in as short a time as a week or two; rarely, it may recur just as rapidly after surgical removal. This rapid rate of development affords a diagnostic clue because most sarcomas grow much more slowly.

Roentgenologic study, in the earliest stages, may show no evidence of mineralization in the lesion. Shortly, however, an extraosseous mass develops, and the mineralization that develops in it tends to be peripherally located. There may be some associated periosteal reaction. As the soft tissue process matures, it becomes increasingly ossified (Fig. 46–22).

Pathologically, the tumor is well circumscribed except in the very early stages. It is usually in the belly of a muscle but may occur in soft tissues apart from a muscle. It is generally obvious that the lesion did not arise from bone, but a similar reactive change may be related to periosteum or even deeper osseous structures. Ossification is found to be more mature at the periphery of the mass, the central part usually being the most cellular; often, numerous mitoses are formed in this central zone (Fig. 46–23). This central portion is fibroblastic, and its tissue differentiates and exhibits osseous metaplasia as the periphery is approached. The trabeculae of bone that are formed are disposed in a parallel fashion that simulates the appearance of callus. This "functional" arrangement of the osteoid and osseous trabeculae, combined with the lack of true anaplasia in the proliferating cells, provides the histopathologist with the necessary clues to exclude sarcoma.[1] Sometimes a chondroid phase is interposed between that of the proliferating fibroblasts and that of the osseous trabeculae.

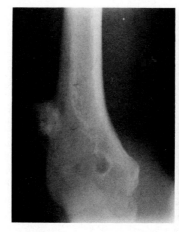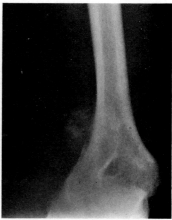

Figure 46–22. Heterotopic ossification (myositis ossificans) mainly in the soft tissues adjacent to the humerus. Note some rarefaction of the central portion.

Treatment is often unnecessary, and certainly any surgical removal should be conservative.

A similar non-neoplastic benign, reactive process may occur in the deeper portions of the skin. the poorly defined small mass that is found may also show prominent mitotic activity. The lesion is called proliferative fasciitis and has been mistaken for such entities as liposarcoma or fibrosarcoma.[9] The rapidly proliferating cells again do not show true anaplasia. Another related entity is proliferative myositis.[23] In this condition, there is a tumefactive, intramuscular proliferation of benign fibroblastic cells but no discernible osseous metaplasia. Mitotic activity may be pronounced, making it possible to mistake this lesion for a malignant tumor.

Malignant Soft Tissue Tumors

Synovial Sarcoma

Synovial sarcoma, or synovioma, is a malignant soft tissue tumor that usually arises in the extremities or limb girdles; about 70 per cent of lesions involve the lower extremity, most commonly the thigh. This tumor occasionally arises in the region of the elbow. Although the name of this tumor suggests a relationship with synovial tissue, actually the tumor is believed to develop de novo from ubiquitous mesenchyme of the somatic soft tissue rather than from pre-existent synovial tissue. In the Mayo Clinic experience, only the tumors of about 20 per cent of patients had suggestive evidence of origin from anatomic synovium. This tumor can be found in patients of any age, but young or middle-aged adults seem to be most commonly affected.

Symptoms may be present for many years before diagnosis. In the Mayo Clinic experience, the average duration of symptoms before

diagnosis was 2½ years. In addition to physical examination, roentgenographic examination may be helpful because about a third of patients with synovial sarcoma show evidence of calcification. When calcification is found in a soft tissue tumor, synovial sarcoma should be included in the differential diagnosis.

The tumor is lobular, circumscribed, gray, and contains areas of calcification, hemorrhage, necrosis, or cyst formation, Microscopic study reveals a bimorphic pattern with

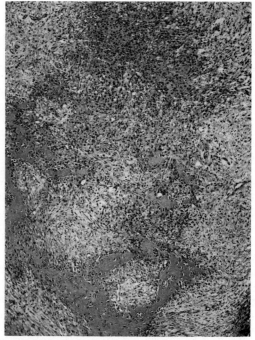

Figure 46–23. Florid heterotopic ossification. There are foci of marked cellularity, but there is maturation to osseous trabeculae. The cellular zones, often containing numerous mitotic figures, introduce the possibility of misinterpretation as an osteosarcoma. The cells lack the anaplasia of sarcoma (hematoxylin and eosin, ×64).

fascicles of spindle cells and aggregates ranging from plump spindle cells to epithelial elements that line glandlike spaces or clefts.

Close cooperation between the pathologist and the surgeon is essential if the diagnosis is to be made at operation. Local excision of the tumor generally results in a local recurrence; with local recurrence, the prognosis for survival is lessened. In the Mayo Clinic experience, the overall 5-year survival rate was 38 per cent, and the 10-year rate was 23 per cent, with a median survival of 39 months.[49] However, for patients treated after 1960, the 5-year survival rate has been 55 per cent, and the 10-year rate has been 38 per cent. Patients who had the best prognosis were those treated by wide excision or radical surgery.

Liposarcoma

The pathologic diagnosis of liposarcoma may be difficult, especially when the lesion is histologically low-grade. A lipoma that shows evidence of growth should be suspected of being malignant. Furthermore, on palpation, a liposarcoma is frequently firmer than a lipoma. Most liposarcomas do not have enough normal fat to be radiolucent compared with the surrounding muscle. However, both radiolucency and radiopacity may be noted within the substance of a liposarcoma. Thus, roentgenograms are not as diagnostic for liposarcoma as they are for lipoma, but the combination of more dense and less dense tissues may be characteristic of liposarcoma. Computed tomography is very helpful not only in defining the extent of the lesion but also in showing relative densities. Most soft tissue sarcomas are not homogeneous; thus, if the entire lesion is of one density, it is less likely to be malignant. Liposarcomas are recognized because of their component of malignant lipoblasts.

Liposarcomas may arise in any part of the body and are occasionally found at the elbow. Older adults are more commonly affected than younger people.

The extent of treatment depends at least in part on both the size and the grade of the tumor. Lesions that are grade 1 or grade 2 probably can be safely excised with a margin of normal tissue on all aspects. Even if the lesion does recur, it can probably be excised without the need for radical surgery. However, the higher grade lesion probably should be treated by wide resection and perhaps by radical resection unless the tumor can be totally and widely removed without sacrifice of limb function. This is difficult to do with

tumors in the region of the elbow, and amputation may be necessary. In the Mayo Clinic experience, about 50 per cent of all patients currently treated for liposarcoma may expect to survive for 5 years and be free of evidence of disease progression.[36]

Malignant Fibrous Histiocytoma

Malignant fibrous histiocytoma is now the most commonly encountered malignant soft tissue tumor of the extremities. The upper extremity and, more specifically, the region of the elbow are not uncommonly affected by this tumor. This tumor can arise in any age group. As with other malignant soft tissue tumors, there are no unique clinical or radiographic features characteristic of this lesion. Plain roentgenograms and xeroradiographs may be useful in defining its extent. More recently, computed tomography has been utilized to define the extent and relationship of the tumor with surrounding structures.

Grossly, this tumor is usually soft, white or gray. It may vary in consistency and color from patient to patient, and indeed, even in different areas of the same tumor. There also may be an area of firm, white tumor adjacent to a yellow mucoid necrotic area. Tumors arising in the upper extremity in general tend to be smaller than those arising in the buttock or lower extremity, probably because they are noticed by the patient earlier in their evolution. Hence, there is usually less necrosis in the smaller tumors than there is in the larger lower extremity tumors. Microscopically, the lesion may vary from the most benign-appearing spindle cells with small nuclei and relatively few mitotic figures, such as those seen in a grade 1 lesion, to the wildly anaplastic, bizarre histiocytic cells found in grade 4 lesions. Generally, there is a mixture of fibroblastic cells that may exhibit a storiform pattern and malignant cells with the quality of histiocytes. Considerable variation exists in the spectrum of what is called malignant fibrous histiocytoma. Myxoid, fibrous, inflammatory angiomatoid, giant cell, and histiocyte subtypes are recognized. There is growing evidence, however, that the grade of the lesion as manifested by anaplasia is a more important predictor of behavior than are these histologic subtypes. It is recognized that various of these subtypes may be represented in different parts of a given tumor.

There is no one universally acceptable treatment for this lesion. Relatively small tumors may be excised with a margin of normal tissue on all aspects. Larger lesions or those

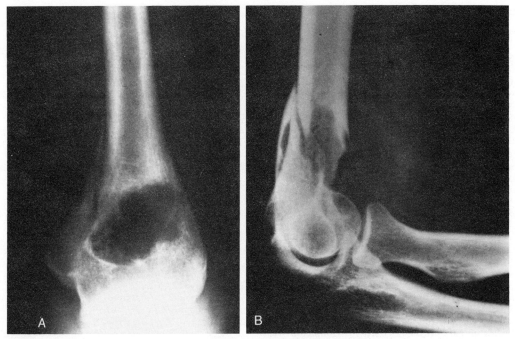

Figure 46–24. *A, B,* Epithelioid sarcoma that has eroded into and destroyed much of the distal part of the humerus in a 27-year-old woman.

that are histologically higher grade require a more aggressive approach. In this situation, we now favor a course of preoperative radiation therapy using approximately 5000 rads, followed after several weeks by excision of the lesion with a margin of normal tissue on all aspects. Additional external beam radiation may be given following the surgery if the tumor is found to be still viable or if the margins are questionable. Adjunctive chemotherapy has not been helpful in our experience, either for management of the primary lesion or as a means of controlling or preventing systemic metastatic disease.

Malignant fibrous histiocytoma, as described above, may occur as a lesion primary in bone.

Epithelioid Sarcoma

This rare, slowly growing malignant tumor usually begins in the superficial tissues of the hand or forearm and may occur at the elbow. Small, poorly defined tumor nodules composed of epithelioid cells or histiocytic aggregates comprise the tumor. Sometimes central necrosis in these aggregates of cells suggests that the disease is a granulomatous infection. There is often a delay in recognition of the malignant nature of the disease, and the long-term prognosis for life is poor. Rarely, the tumor erodes into underlying bone (Figs. 46–

24 and 46–25). Lymphatic or hematogenous metastasis is common, especially in the later stages of this disease.

Treatment for cure requires wide excision. Marginal or intralesional excision almost always results in tumor recurrence and subsequent disease progression. The relatively slow growth of the tumor and the unusual nature of the histology may tend to dissuade the surgeon from performing adequate surgery.

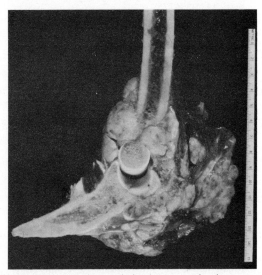

Figure 46–25. Another epithelioid sarcoma that has caused osseous destruction at the elbow.

References

1. Ackerman, L. N.: Extra-Osseous Localized Non-Neoplastic Bone and Cartilage Formation (So-Called Myositis Ossificans). Clinical and Pathologic Confusion with Malignant Neoplasms. J. Bone Joint Surg. **40A**:279, 1958.
2. Angervall, L., and Enzinger, F. M.: Extraskeletal Neoplasm Resembling Ewing's Sarcoma. Cancer **36**:240, 1975.
3. Atmore, W. G., Dahlin, D. C., and Ghormley, R. K.: Pigmented Villonodular Synovitis. A Clinical and Pathologic Study. Minn. Med. **39**:196, 1956.
4. Bacci, G., Picci, P., Gitelis, S., Borghi, A., and Campanacci, M.: The Treatment of Localized Ewing's Sarcoma. The Experience at the Istituto Rizzoli in 163 Cases Treated With and Without Adjuvant Chemotherapy. Cancer **49**:1561, 1982.
5. Bonaledarpeun, A., Levy, W. M., and Aegerter, E.: Primary and Secondary Aneurysmal Bone Cyst: A Radiologic Study of 75 Cases. Radiology **126**:75, 1978.
6. Boston, H. C., Jr., Dahlin, D. C., Ivins, J. C., and Cupps, R. E.: Malignant Lymphomas (So-Called Reticulum Cell Sarcoma) of Bone. Cancer **34**:1131, 1974.
7. Campanacci, M., and Cervellati, G.: Osteosarcoma: A Review of 345 Cases. Ital. J. Orthop. Traumatol. **1**:5, 1975.
8. Campanacci, M., Giunti, A., and Olmi, R.: Giant Cell Tumors of Bone: A Study of 209 Cases With Long-Term Follow-Up in 130. Ital. J. Orthop. Traumatol. **1**:249, 1975.
9. Chung, E. B., and Enzinger, F. M.: Proliferative Fasciitis. Cancer **36**:1450, 1975.
10. Corbett, J. M., Wilde, A. H., McCormick, L. J., and Evarts, C. M.: Intra-articular Osteoid Osteoma, A Diagnostic Problem. Clin. Orthop. **98**:225, 1974.
11. Cronemeyer, R., Kirchmer, N. A., Desmet, A. A., and Neff, J. R.: Intra-articular Osteoid Osteoma of the Humerus Simulating Synovitis of the Elbow: A Case Report. J. Bone Joint Surg. **63A**:1172, 1981.
12. Dahlin, D. C.: Bone Tumors. General Aspects and Data on 6221 Cases. Springfield, Ill., Charles C Thomas, 1978, p. 445.
13. Dahlin, D. C.: Pathology of Osteosarcoma. Clin. Orthop. **111**:23, 1975.
14. Dahlin, D. C., Besse, B. E., Jr., Pugh, D. G., and Ghormley, R. K.: Aneurysmal Bone Cysts. Radiology **64**:56, 1955.
15. Dahlin, D. C., Cupps, R. E., and Johnson, E. W., Jr.: Giant Cell Tumor: A Study of 195 Cases. Cancer **25**:1061, 1970.
16. Dahlin, D. C., and McLeod, R. A.: Aneurysmal Bone Cyst and Other Non-Neoplastic Conditions. Skel. Radiol. **8**:243, 1982.
17. Dahlin, D. C., and Unni, K. K.: Osteosarcoma of Bone and Its Important Recognizable Varieties. Am. J. Surg. Pathol. **1**:61, 1977.
18. Dahlin, D. C., Unni, K. K., and Matsuno, T.: Malignant (Fibrous) Histiocytoma of Bone—Fact or Fancy? Cancer **39**:1508, 1977.
19. Dionne, G. P., and Seemayer, T. A.: Infiltrating Lipomas and Angiolypomas Revisited. Cancer **33**:732, 1974.
20. Edeiken, J., and Hodes, P. J.: Roentgen Diagnosis of Diseases of Bone, 2nd ed., Vols. 1 and 2. Baltimore, Williams & Wilkins, 1973.
21. Enneking, W. F.: Musculoskeletal Tumor Surgery, Vol. 1. New York, Churchill Livingstone, 1983.
22. Enneking, W. F., Spanier, S. S., and Goodman, M. A.: A System for the Surgical Staging of Musculoskeletal Sarcoma. Clin. Orthop. **153**:106, 1980.
23. Enzinger, F. M., and Dulcey, F.: Proliferative Myositis. Report of Thirty-Three Cases. Cancer **20**:2213, 1967.
24. Ghelman, B., Francesca, M., Thompson, F. M., William, D., and Arnold, W. D.: Intra-operative Radioactive Localization of an Osteoid Osteoma: Case Report. J. Bone Joint Surg. **63A**:826, 1981.
25. Goldenberg, R. R., Campbell, C. J., and Bonfiglio, M.: Giant Cell Tumor of Bone. An Analysis of 218 Cases. J. Bone Joint Surg. **52A**:621, 1970.
26. Harsha, W. N.: The Natural History of Osteocartilaginous Exostoses (Osteochondroma). Am. Surg. **20**:65, 1954.
27. Jaffe, H. L., and Lichtenstein, L.: Osteoid-osteoma: Further Experience with This Benign Tumor of Bone; With Special Reference to Cases Showing the Lesion in Relation to Shaft Cortices and Commonly Misclassified as Instances of Sclerosing Non-Suppurative Osteomyelitis or Cortical-Bone Abscess. J. Bone Joint Surg. **22**:645, 1940.
28. Johnson, R. E., and Pomeroy, T. C.: Evaluation of Therapeutic Results in Ewing's Sarcoma. Am. J. Roentgenol. **123**:583, 1975.
29. Larsson, S. E., Lorentzon, R., and Boquist, L.: Giant-Cell Tumor of Bone: A Demographic, Clinical, and Histopathological Study of All Cases Recorded in the Swedish Cancer Registry for the Years 1958 Through 1968. J. Bone Joint Surg. **57A**:167, 1975.
30. Marcove, R. C., and Freiberger, R. H.: Osteoid Osteoma of the Elbow: A Diagnostic Problem. Report of Four Cases. J. Bone Joint Surg. **48A**:1185, 1966.
31. Matsuno, T., Unni, K. K., McLeod, R. A., and Dahlin, D. C.: Telangiectatic Osteogenic Sarcoma. Cancer **38**:2538, 1976.
32. Murphy, F. P., Dahlin, D. C., and Sullivan, C. R.: Articular Synovial Chondromatosis. J. Bone Joint Surg. **44A**:77, 1962.
33. Norman, A., and Dorfman, H. D.: Osteoid Osteoma Inducing Pronounced Overgrowth and Deformity of Bone. Clin. Orthop. **110**:223, 1975.
34. Parker, F., Jr., and Jackson, H., Jr.: Primary Reticulum Cell Sarcoma of Bone. Surg. Gynecol. Obstet. **68**:45, 1939.
35. Pritchard, D. J., Dahlin, D. C., Dauphine, R. T., Taylor, W. E., and Beabout, J. W.: Ewing's Sarcoma: A Clinicopathological and Statistical Analysis of Patients Surviving Five Years or Longer. J. Bone Joint Surg. **57A**:10, 1975.
36. Reszel, P. A., Soule, E. H., and Coventry, M. B.: Liposarcoma of the Extremities and Limb Girdles. A Study of Two Hundred Twenty-Two Cases. J. Bone Joint Surg. **48A**:229, 1966.
37. Sanekin, N. G., Mott, M. G., and Roylance, J.: An Unusual Intraosseous Lesion With Fibroblastic, Osteoclastic, Osteoblastic, Aneurysmal, and Fibromyxoid Elements. "Solid" Variant of Aneurysmal Bone Cyst. Cancer **51**:2278, 1983.
38. Schajowicz, F.: Tumors and Tumor-like Lesions of Bones and Joints. New York, Springer-Verlag, 1981, p. 581.
39. Schajowicz, F., and Lemos, C.: Osteoid Osteoma and Osteoblastoma. Closely Related Entities of Osteoblastic Derivation. Acta Orthop. Scand. **41**:272, 1970.
40. Shoji, H., and Miller, T. R.: Primary Reticulum Cell Sarcoma of Bone: Significance of Clinical Features Upon the Prognosis. Cancer **28**:1234, 1971.
41. Sim, F. H., Dahlin, D. C., and Beabout, J. W.: Osteoid

Osteoma: Diagnostic Problems. J. Bone Joint Surg. **57A**:154, 1975.

42. Snarr, J. W., Abell, M. R., and Martel, W.: Lympho-fallicular Synovitis with Osteoid Osteoma. Radiology **106**:557, 1973.

43. Spanos, P. K., Payne, W. S., Ivins, J. C., and Pritchard, D. J.: Pulmonary Resection for Metastatic Osteogenic Sarcoma. J. Bone Joint Surg. [Am]. **58**:624, 1976.

44. Swee, R. G., McLeod, R. A., and Beabout, J. W.: Osteoid Osteoma—Detection, Diagnosis, and Localization. Radiology **130**:117, 1979.

45. Taylor, W. F., Ivins, D. C., Edmonson, J. H., and Pritchard, D. J.: Trends and Variability in Survival from Osteosarcoma. Mayo Clin. Proc. **53**:695, 1978.

46. Unni, K. K., Dahlin, D. C., and Beabout, J. W.: Periosteal Osteogenic Sarcoma. Cancer **37**:2476, 1976.

47. Unni, K. K., Dahlin, D. C., Beabout, J. W., and Ivins, J. C.: Parosteal Osteogenic Sarcoma. Cancer **37**:2466, 1976.

48. Weatherby, R. P., Dahlin, D. C., and Ivins, J. C.: Postradiation Sarcoma of Bone. Review of 78 Mayo Clinic Cases. Mayo Clin. Proc. **56**:294, 1981.

49. Wright, P. H., Sim, F. H., Soule, E. H., and Taylor, W. F.: Synovial Sarcoma. J. Bone Joint Surg. **64A**:112, 1982.

CHAPTER 47

Loose Bodies

B. F. MORREY

Loose bodies, first described in the knee by Anbrose Paré[18] in 1558, occur in the elbow with a frequency second only to that in the knee.[19] As with other joints, a distinction between congenital or developmental variants and acquired lesions is sometimes difficult to determine with certainty. A useful classification of elbow loose bodies is shown in Table 47–1.

ACCESSORY OSSIFICATION

Three accessory ossicles about the elbow have been described as congenital variations of normal. These occur distal to the medial epicondyle; proximal to the tip of the olecranon, the patella cubiti; and in the olecranon fossa, the os supratrochlea dorsale.

Medial Epicondyle Accessory Ossicle

A smooth, rounded ossicle is sometimes seen just distal to the medial epicondyle and is considered an accessory ossification of the medial epicondyle.[10] Probably more than in any other site, confusion exists about whether or not this radiographic appearance represents a traumatic or a congenital event. The distinction is further blurred by assuming trama as an etiology common to all accessory ossicles.[22] Instances of a discrete, rounded, smooth ossicle that is radiographically consistent with the appearance of an accessory

Table 47–1. **Classification of Loose Bodies**

Congenital (developmental)	Medial epicondyle—accessory ossification
	Olecranon—os patella cubiti
	Olecranon fossa—os supratrochlea dorsale
Acquired	Articular fracture— osteochondritis dissecans
	Degenerative
	Synovial proliferation— synovial chondromatosis

ossicle have been observed in the region of the medial epicondyle (Fig. 47–1) in patients who have had no history of injury to this region. An irregular or malshaped medial epicondyle is suggestive of a traumatic origin. However, the formation of a fully developed medial epicondyle does not necessarily prove the diagnosis because in a child the medial epicondyle can remodel and appear normal in later years (Fig. 47–1).

Patella Cubiti

The so-called patella cubiti is rare but has been well described in the older literature.[8, 11, 20] A thorough review of the topic has been presented by Habbe.[8] This ossicle occurs in the triceps tendon near its insertion and is considered a true sesamoid bone.[11a] The proximal position is so characteristic in appearance that little doubt should exist about its origin (Fig. 47–2). This structure should be distinguished from avulsion of the olecranon apophysis, which appears more distally, and calcification of the olecranon bursa. Because of its superficial location, this ossicle may be subject to direct trauma and even fracture[4] but will generally respond to symptomatic treatment.

Os Supratrochlea Dorsale

The radiographic density observed within the olecranon fossa has been the source of recent controversy. Characteristically the ossicle consists of a round, smooth, oval shape that is often best seen in the lateral projection but is also demonstrated in the anteriorposterior view (Fig. 47–3). In early descriptions of this entity its etiology was considered to be a form of osteochondritis dissecans of the trochlea.[16] The precise origin of this osseous structure is still the subject of some discussion, and trauma is often considered its cause.[2] This opinion is supported by the mechanism of injury. With hyperextension, impaction of the

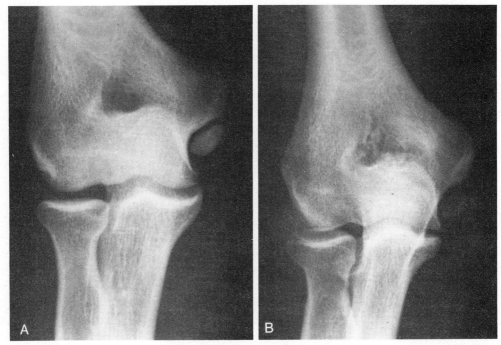

Figure 47–1. *A,* The occurrence of a smooth ossicle at the inferior aspect of the medial epicondyle without a history of injury represents an accessory ossicle. *B,* A prior medial epicondyle fracture may have the same appearance, but the epicondyle may remodel in the young patient (see Chapter 13). Notice loose bodies in olecranon fossa *(B)*.

tip of the olecranon into the olecranon fossa may cause development of a spur at the tip of the olecranon. This can conceivably dislodge, form a nidus, and grow into the characteristic appearance of the os supratrochlea.

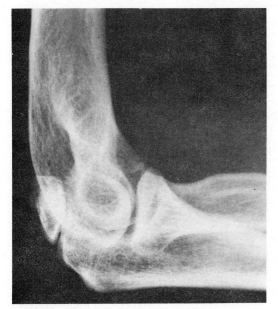

Figure 47–2. The os patella cubiti is present in the triceps tendon; the proximal location helps distinguish this from a variation of the olecranon ossification center.

Certainly this mechanism has been implicated in the formation of loose bodies in the olecranon fossa (Fig. 47–4).[21] The problem has been recently discussed in detail and clarified by Obermann and Loose, who concluded that the os supratrochlea dorsale is most likely a congenital accessory bone.[17] Rather than being caused by trauma, it is subject to trauma with secondary chondrometaplasia and resulting symptomatology. When this occurs, the ossicle may demonstrate a post-traumatic appearance with an irregular margin.

Thus, the distinction between an ossicle caused by or subjected to trauma remains obscure (Fig. 47–4). Regardless of the source, the treatment is obvious. The mere radiographic presence of the osseous density does not imply that it needs to be removed. If it is painful due to an injury caused by hyperextension or a direct blow, symptomatic treatment should allow resolution of pain. If catching, locking, or persistent pain is present, the ossicle is easily excised through a limited posterior lateral incision.

ACQUIRED LOOSE BODIES

Loose or pedunculated cartilaginous or osseocartilaginous bodies are thought to originate from a small nidus.[19] The sequence of mor-

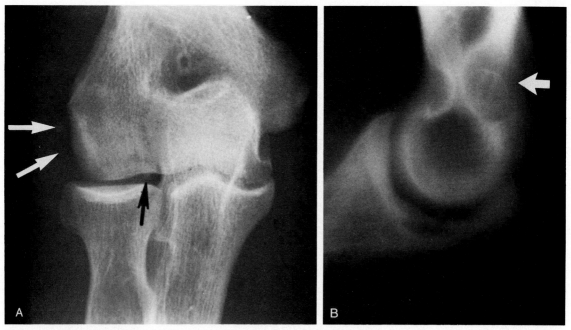

Figure 47–3. A smooth, rounded ossicle in the olecranon fossa, observed on the anteroposterior *(A)* and sometimes more obvious on the lateral radiograph *(B)*, is consistent with the diagnosis of os supratrochlea. Other small densities are present on the anteroposterior view (arrows).

phologic alterations that subsequently occur is common to all free bodies regardless of their origin.[13] Surface proliferation of chondroblasts and osteoblasts nourished by the synovial fluid creates a laminar or layered effect that is seen in about 87 per cent of those with a predominantly cartilaginous component and in 80 per cent of those with a predominantly osseous composition (Fig. 47–5).[13] The growth process continues as long

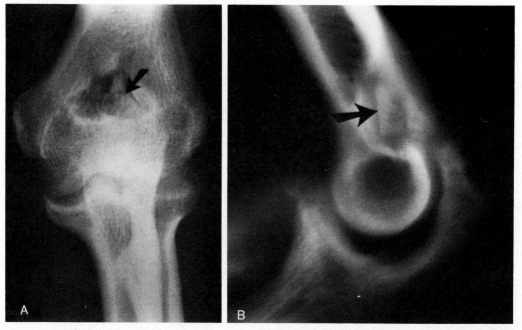

Figure 47–4. *A, B,* Subject to trauma, the appearance of this ossicle may sometimes take on an irregular shape, leading some to suspect that the etiology is a traumatic event or even osteochondritis dissecans of the trochlea. Hyperextension of the elbow may cause spur formation of the tip of the olecranon and multiple loose bodies in the olecranon fossa, a condition that should be distinguished from the os supratrochlea.

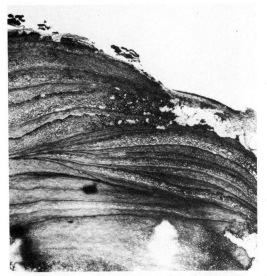

Figure 47–5. Classic demonstration of the laminar effect of a cartilaginous loose body, which is responsible for the growth of these structures. (From Milgram, J. W.: The development of loose bodies in human joints. Clin. Orthop. 124:295, 1977.)

as the free or pedunculated body is present and is exposed to the synovial fluid.

Etiology

Our understanding of intra-articular loose bodies has been greatly enhanced by the work of Milgram.[12–14] The clinical findings and presentation allow classification of acquired free or pedunculated bodies into three groups: osteochondral fractures, degenerative disease of the articular surface, and a proliferative disorder of the synovium, synovial chondromatosis. Milgram[13] defines three types of cartilage associated with loose bodies consistent with their supposed site of origin: articular cartilage cells, osteophytic cells from a proliferating osteophyte in a degenerative joint, and lobular cartilage from the synovial lining cell. Pathologically, these loose bodies may originate from a joint fracture, degenerative osteophytes or de novo as a proliferative disease of the synovium.

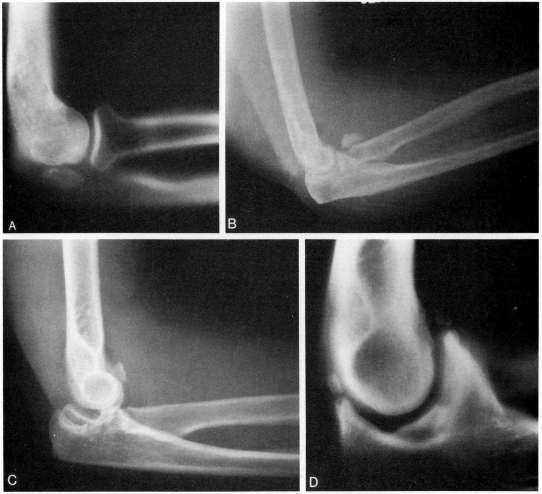

Figure 47–6. Post-traumatic loose body originating from fracture of the capitellum *(A)*, radial head *(B)*, and coronoid process *(C)* after dislocation. The potential for osteophytic loose bodies exists even without frank fracture *(D)*.

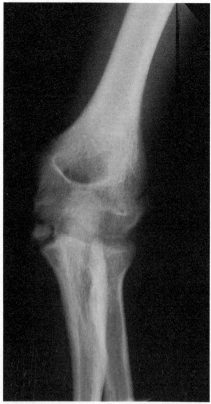

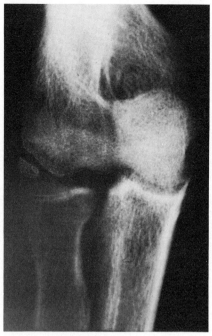

Figure 47–8. Osteochondritis dissecans of the capitellum has caused an osteocartilaginous loose body in the joint.

Figure 47–7. Entrapment of the medial epicondyle in the ulnohumeral joint after fracture-dislocation of the elbow.

Osteochondral Fracture

Fracture of the joint surface may be acute or chronic as is the case with osteochondritis dissecans. A shear fracture of the capitellum may involve little osseous substance, as in

the type II lesion (see Chapter 18). In the acute stage, localization and diagnosis of this fracture may be missed, leading to development of an intra-articular loose body (Fig. 47–6). Elbow dislocation often leads to fractures of the coronoid, capitellum, or radial head and subsequent development of loose or attached intra-articular osseous bodies (Fig. 47–6). Postreduction ossification is common even without fracture, but the clinical behav-

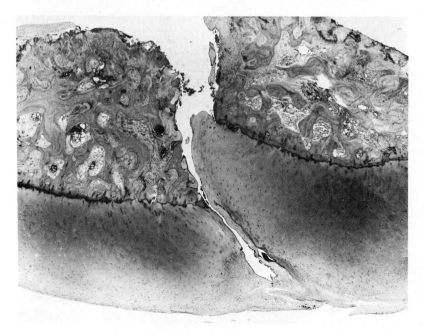

Figure 47–9. A fragment of capitellum from a 24-year-old male with a 7-year history of intermittent restricted range of motion. No viable blood supply is present even though the surgeon had to cut through the articular cartilage to excise the underlying osseous defect. It can be seen that there is no reactive change in the articular cartilage chondrocytes even though this fragment has fractured. However, the bone does show reactive changes although the articular cartilage does not (Courtesy of J. W. Milgram).

ior is of a painful arc of motion rather than limited motion with locking or catching. An avulsed medial epicondyle at the time of dislocation can also cause entrapment in the joint with reduction, but this process is obvious (Fig. 47–7) and should cause no problems with diagnosis or treatment.

The development of osteochondritis dissecans of the capitellum has been thoroughly discussed in Chapters 15 and 30. This condition can progress to fragment detachment, forming a loose body in the joint (Fig. 47–8). The subtle occurrence of pain, loss of extension, grating, snapping, or frank locking of the joint may occur owing to separation of a loose osteocartilaginous fragment of osteochondritis dissecans or a lesion of the capitellum or other portions of the articular surface or margin (Fig. 47–9). In fact, trauma as the accepted etiology for loose bodies in the elbow joint has prompted some to attribute all extranuous ossific densities, even accessory ossicles, to trauma,[1, 15, 16, 22] Although the clinical features and precise etiology vary, the presence of a bony nidus is the common pathologic finding with each of these traumatic lesions.[12]

Loose Bodies of Degenerative Origin

Theoretically, degenerative joint disease can elicit loose body formation by creating a nidus from a fragmented joint surface, from a degenerative osteophyte, or from the synovium of the joint with degenerative cartilaginous

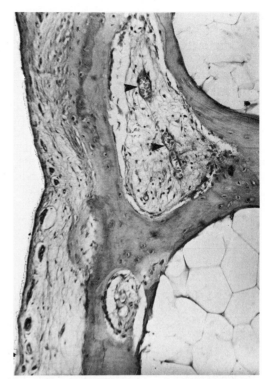

Figure 47–11. Microradiograph of pedunculated body of osteochondromatosis. Notice the presence of a vascular supply (arrows), and mature bone nidus. (From Henderson, M. S., and Jones, H. T.: Loose bodies in joints and bursae due to synovial osteochondromatosis. J. Bone Joint Surg. 5:400, 1923.)

changes.[13] Primary degenerative arthritis of the elbow is not common and has been discussed above. Bullock and Goodfellow have studied primary degenerative changes of the radiohumeral joint; this process could certainly give rise to the formation of a nidus and the subsequent development of a loose body.[7] Bell reviewed 52 instances of loose bodies occurring in the elbow and concluded that most were related to primary or secondary osteoarthritis.[3] This investigator pointed out that most occurred in the anterior aspect of the joint (Fig. 47–10). Small osteophytes may be observed at the tips of both the olecranon and the coronoid process with degenerative disease, either of which could give rise to the eventual development of a joint loose body (Fig. 47–6D).

Synovial Chondromatosis

Since the initial description of the entity in 1558[18] much has been written about synovial chondromatosis or osteochondromatosis, and the topic is discussed further in Chapter 46. Henderson reviewed the literature and reported the Mayo Clinic experience of 25 cases in 1923.[9] He concluded that this entity was

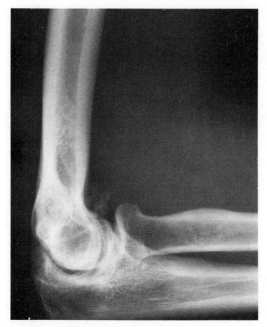

Figure 47–10. Anterior loose bodies of the elbow joint with no history of a single event of trauma.

separate from traumatic or degenerative loose body formation and that the nidus originated from the synovial tissue (Fig. 47–11). More specifically, the condition is felt to represent a proliferative disorder of the subsynovial soft tissue.[6] Milgram has identified three phases of the process.[14] In the active initial phase, no free or loose bodies are present. In the transitional phase, osteochondral nodules form in the synovial membrane, and nonossified free bodies are found in the joint (Fig. 47–12). In the final phase, free osteochondral bodies apparently herald the quiescent phase of the disease (Fig. 47-13).

In the second phase, the cartilaginous component becomes symptomatic before it ossifies, producing symptoms of elbow pain and loss of motion even in the presence of a relatively normal radiograph (Fig. 47-12). Enchondral bone formation replaces the cartilaginous component, and this gives rise to the obvious radiographic demonstration of multiple loose bodies (Fig. 47–13). Hence, the condition may present with multiple (up to 100) radiolucent (cartilaginous, Fig. 47–12) or radiopaque (ossified, Fig. 47–13) loose bodies. When the bodies are ossified, a possible cartilaginous neoplasm might be considered, but, as discussed in Chapter 46, the occurrence of cartilaginous sarcomas about the elbow is extremely rare. This disease is a self-limiting process that runs a rather predictable course.[14] Treatment consists of removal of symptomatic loose bodies. Synovectomy is not routinely

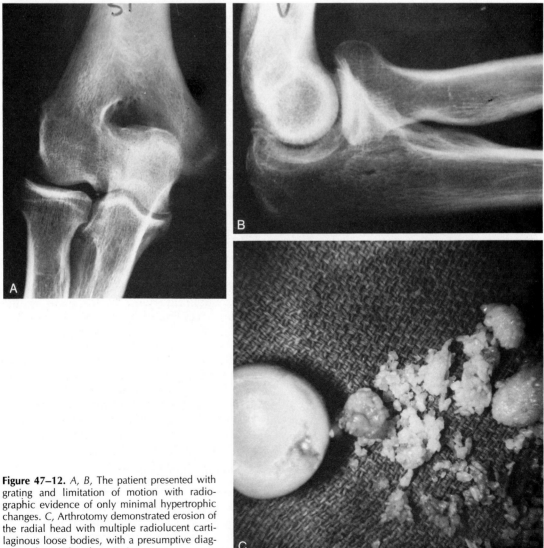

Figure 47–12. *A, B,* The patient presented with grating and limitation of motion with radiographic evidence of only minimal hypertrophic changes. *C,* Arthrotomy demonstrated erosion of the radial head with multiple radiolucent cartilaginous loose bodies, with a presumptive diagnosis of osteochondromatosis.

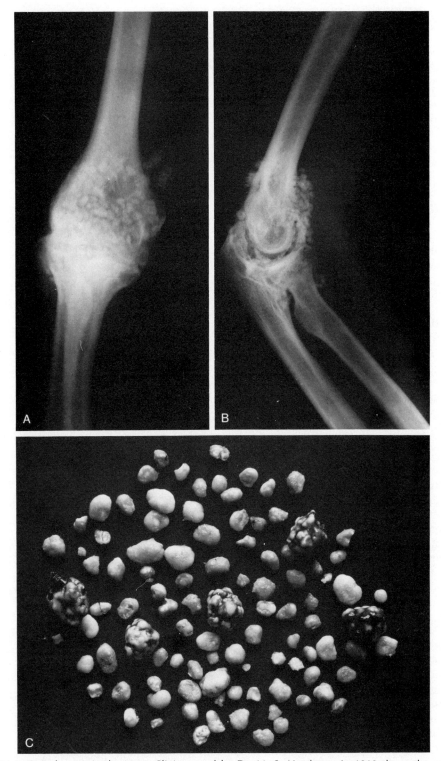

Figure 47–13. *A, B,* Early case in the Mayo Clinic treated by Dr. M. S. Henderson in 1918 shows the ossified form of osteochondromatosis. *C,* Arthrotomy resulted in multiple (over 100) loose bodies.

necessary, and recurrence of loose bodies may occur after surgery.

SIGNS AND SYMPTOMS

The occurrence of loose bodies is more frequent in males regardless of etiology: traumatic, degenerative, or from proliferative synovium.[9] Among Bell's 52 cases, most presented with loss of motion, usually extension.[3] Symptoms are often of a catching nature but rarely are disabling. Pain is variably present and usually occurs with a sensation of locking or grating. The patient may be able to localize the origin or location of the posterior or anterior ossicles, but with multiple site involvement the discomfort is generalized. The radiograph is helpful for large lesions but can be deceptively negative if the loose bodies have not calcified, if small ossicles are present in the ulnohumeral joint (Fig. 47-4**B**), if the location is obscured by the surrounding anatomy, or if the traumatic lesion contains little osseous tissue. These difficulties in diagnosis can be overcome by multiple views including oblique views or tomograms. Arthroscopy may also be helpful in some instances to identify these lesions (see Chapter 7).

TREATMENT

Simple removal is the treatment of choice for symptomatic loose bodies. Replacement of a large fragment of the capitellum in osteochondritis dissecans has been discussed in Chapter 30. We have no experience with this. The treatment of fractures of the medial epicondyle has been discussed in Chapter 13 and fractures of the capitellum in Chapter 18. We see little value in abrasion or drilling of the site of origin unless the diagnosis is made in the very acute stage. Such a procedure only adds to the surgical trauma and may result in an irritative hemarthrosis with secondary soft tissue contracture. Removal of loose bodies with the aid of the arthroscope should enhance the diagnosis, localization, and removal of these structures (Chapter 7).

The surgical approach for arthrotomy depends on the precise localization of the ossicle. Usually, the loose bodies may be removed through a limited incision directly over their anatomic location. In fact, removal of the loose body is probably the only indication for a posterior or medial approach to the joint (see Chapter 8).

References

1. Atsatt, S.: Loose Bodies of the Elbow Joint: An Unusual Location and Form. J. Bone Joint Surg. **15**:1008, 1933.
2. Bassett, L. W., Mirra, J. M., Forrester, D. M., Gold, R. H., Bernstein, M. L., and Rollins, J. S.: Post-Traumatic Osteochondral "Loose Body" of the Olecranon Fossa. Radiology **141**:635, 1981.
3. Bell, M. S.: Loose Bodies in the Elbow. Br. J. Surg. **62**:921, 1975.
4. Birsner, J. W., and DeSmet, D. H.: Patella Cubiti With Fracture. Ann. West Med. Surg. **4**:744, 1950.
5. Burman, M. S.: Unusual Locking of the Elbow Joint by the Sesamum Cubiti and a Free Joint Body. Am. J. Radiol. **45**:731, 1941.
6. Fisher, A. G. T.: A Study of Loose Bodies Composed of Cartilage or of Cartilage and Bone Occurring in Joints. Br. J. Surg. **8**:493, 1931.
7. Bullock, P. G., and Goodfellow, J. W.: Pattern of Aging of the Articular Cartilage of the Elbow Joint. J. Bone Joint Surg. **49B**:175, 1967.
8. Habbe, J. E.: Patella Cubiti, A Report of Four Cases. Am. J. Roentgenol. **48**:513, 1942.
9. Henderson, M. S., and Jones, H. T.: Loose Bodies in Joints and Bursae Due to Synovial Osteochondromatosis. J. Bone Joint Surg. **5**:400, 1923.
10. Keates, T. E.: An Atlas of Normal Roentgen Variants That May Simulate Disease. Chicago, Year Book Medical Publishers, 1979, pp. 251-252.
11. Kienbock, R.: Desenfans. G. über Anomalien am Ellbogengelenk Patella Cubiti. Beitr. Klin. Chir. **165**:524, 1937.
11a. Kohler, A., and Zimmer, E. A.: Borderlands of the Normal and Early Pathologic in Skeletal Anatomy, 3rd ed. Translated by S. P. Wilk. New York, Grune & Stratton, 1968.
12. Milgram, J. W.: The Classification of Loose Bodies in Human Joints. Clin. Orthop. **124**:282, 1977.
13. Milgram, J. W.: The Development of Loose Bodies in Human Joints. Clin. Orthop. **124**:292, 1977.
14. Milgram, J. W.: Synovial Osteochondromatosis. J. Bone Joint Surg. **59B**:492, 1977.
15. Morgan, P. W.: Osteochondritis Dissecans of the Supratrochlear Septum. Radiology **60**:241, 1953.
16. Morton, H. S., and Crysler, W. E.: Osteochondritis Dissecans of the Supratrochlear Septum. J. Bone Joint Surg. **27**:12, 1945.
17. Obermann, W. R., and Loose, H. W. C.: The Os Supratrochlear Dorsale: A Normal Variant That May Cause Symptoms. Am. J. Roentgenol. **141**:123, 1963.
18. Paré, A.: As quoted by Henderson, M. S., and Jones, H. T.: J. Bone Joint Surg. **5**:400, 1923.
19. Phemister, D. B.: The Causes and Changes in Loose Bodies Arising From the Articular Surface of the Joint. J. Bone Joint Surg. **6**:278, 1924.
20. Sachs, J.: Degenskein G. Patellar Cubiti. Arch. Surg. **57**:675, 1948.
21. Tullos, H. S., and King, J. W.: Lesions of the Pitching Arm in Adolescents. J.A.M.A. **220**:264, 1972.
22. Zietlin, A.: The Traumatic Origin of Accessory Bones at the Elbow. J. Bone Joint Surg. **17**:933, 1935.

CHAPTER 48

Bursitis

B. F. MORREY

"Ensuring the smooth and frictionless working of the body corporate, usually uncomplaining, inconspicuous, hard-working, and very modest in their requirements, the bursae have been so neglected that, even when one of them misbehaves, this is usually misattributed to be some more important structure." It is unlikely that the following discussion will do a great deal to dispel this rather menial position attributed to the bursae. With the exception of the olecranon bursa, bursal afflictions seem to be relatively uncommon about the elbow.

ANATOMY

In 1788 Monro described several deep bursae about the elbow (Fig. 48-1). Through the years, additional bursae have been described and may be divided into deep or superficial types (Fig. 48–2). Anatomically, the deep bursae are situated between muscle and muscle or between muscle and bone, thus making anatomic recognition somewhat difficult and clinical involvement almost impossible to diagnose. The superficial bursae consist only of those over the epicondyles and that overlying

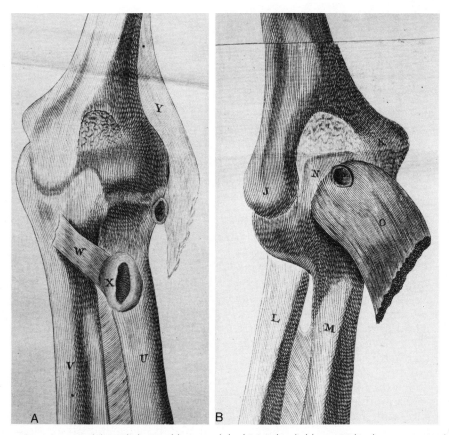

Figure 48–1. *A,* The existence of the radiohumeral bursa and the bicipital radial bursa (X) has been recognized for over 200 years, as demonstrated by this original 1788 illustration from Monro. *B,* Similarly, the subtendinous olecranon bursa has been well illustrated in this monograph.

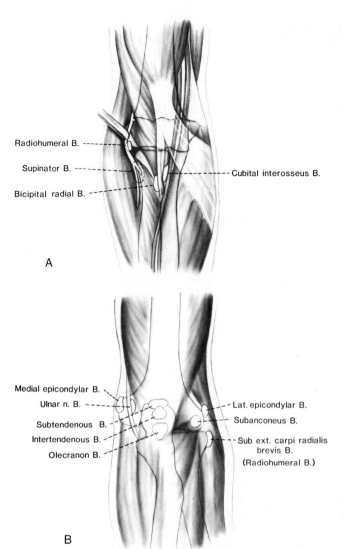

Radiohumeral B.

Supinator B.

Bicipital radial B.

Cubital interosseus B.

A

Medial epicondylar B.
Ulnar n. B.
Subtendenous B.
Intertendenous B.
Olecranon B.

Lat. epicondylar B.
Subanconeus B.
Sub ext. carpi radialis brevis B.
(Radiohumeral B.)

B

Figure 48–2. *A,* Many deep bursae have been reported to exist in the region of the elbow, usually interposed between muscle and muscle or tendon and bone. *B,* The exception is the subcutaneous bursae of the olecranon, which, with the bursae of the medial and lateral epicondyles, are the most commonly recognized and clinically important of these bursae.

the olecranon, which is by far the most important.

CLINICAL SIGNIFICANCE

The diagnosis of pathologic involvement of any of the deep bursal structures is rather uncommon. This fact, coupled with the difficulty of defining some of these structures by anatomic dissection, brings into question the very reality of some. The existence of the bicipital radial bursa is well established (Fig. 48–1 and 48–2), and we have observed inflammation of this structure at surgery in a patient with partial rupture of the insertion of the bicipital tendon at the tuberosity. Usually the diagnosis is presumptive, and the treatment is symptomatic—rest, ice or heat, and anti-inflammatory agents.

Tennis elbow and irritation of the radial nerve have been reported to result from an inflamed radiohumeral bursa that lies under the extensor carpi radialis brevis.[4, 17, 20] Thought to be a common cause of tennis elbow in the past, this association seems to be uncommon according to our present understanding of lateral epicondylitis. Yet this structure does exist and has been demonstrated in anatomic dissections,[16, 17] and it continues to be discussed as a possible etiology of this clinical condition in relatively recent texts.[9, 10, 19] In our opinion, the radiohumeral bursa must be an uncommon primary cause of tennis elbow.

The deep bursae associated with the triceps tendon are discussed below. The remainder of the deep bursae are of academic interest only at this time. The presence of these structures is variable and is probably developmental because not all of these bursae are present at birth.[22] In fact, the anatomic reality of some may be questioned, and we have not

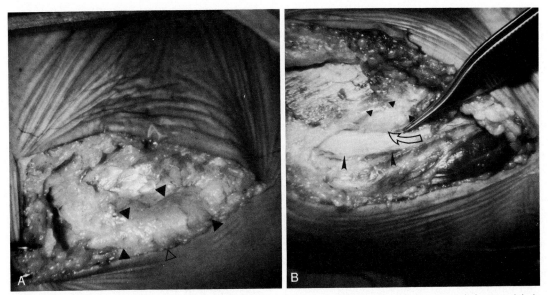

Figure 48–3. *A*, A refractory medial epicondylitis was shown to be due to or the cause of a chronic medial epicondyle bursa (arrows). *B*, With flexion, the nerve subluxed over the epicondyle, causing irritation of the bursa.

been able to find any clinical syndromes or a detailed anatomic discussion of many of these structures.

SUPERFICIAL BURSAE

The olecranon and the medial and lateral epicondylar bursae are the only superficial bursae about the elbow. We have observed one instance of an inflamed medial epicondylar bursa associated with chronic subluxation of the ulnar nerve (Fig. 48–3). This is probably rather uncommon and is treated by attending to the primary pathology, the ulnar nerve. Bursae in the olecranon region have been reported to exist in three locations: (1) the subcutaneous bursa so commonly seen clinically, (2) an intratendinous bursa in the substance of the triceps tendon near its insertion; and (3) a subtendinous bursa between the tendon and the capsule (Fig. 48–4). The significance of the two deep bursae is probably speculative because no recognizable clinical presentation has been documented with these structures. It is quite possible that inflammation of either the intratendinous or subtendinous bursae could be mistaken for tendinitis, synovitis, or capsulitis. In fact, spontaneous rupture of the triceps tendon (see Chapter 25) may be related to degeneration of the bicipital tendon, as has been documented with disruptions of the insertion of the bicipital tendon.[5]

Idiopathic calcific involvement of the subtendinous bursae has been described.[21] Yet calcification of bursae around the elbow is distinctly unusual in contrast to calcific tendonitis in the region of the shoulder. Calcium appears to form owing to anoxia, causing a cellular response with giant cell reaction, and the presentation is one of an inflamed "hot"-looking joint.

Olecranon Bursitis

Inflammation of the superficial olecranon bursae may result from either direct trauma or repetitive stress, the so-called miner's elbow or student's elbow. Larson and Osternig have also shown that olecranon bursitis is a common football injury, especially when associated with artificial turf.[11]

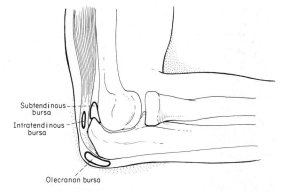

Subtendinous bursa

Intratendinous bursa

Olecranon bursa

Figure 48–4. Lateral illustration of the elbow demonstrating the superficial subcutaneous olecranon bursa, the intratendinous bursa found in the substance of the tendon, and the subtendinous bursa lying between the tip of the olecranon and the triceps tendon.

Involvement with systemic inflammatory processes such as rheumatoid arthritis, gout, chondrocalcinosis,[7] or hydroxy apatite crystal deposition[15] has been reported. Diffuse pigmented villonodular synovitis has also been shown to give rise to olecranon synovitis, and xanthoma has been reported to involve this region.[19] In instances due to a chronic overuse syndrome, for example, "coalminer's bursitis," synovial cells that are least subject to mechanical stress have been shown to be those elaborating the synovial fluid.[13]

The distinction and differentiation between a septic and a nonseptic inflammatory bursitis has been the subject of a detailed study by Ho and Tice[8] and is discussed in Chapter 42. Clinical presentation of fever, tenderness, and parabursal cellulitis is common with the septic etiology. The correct diagnosis is suggested when aspiration of the bursa demonstrates a high leukocyte count and a positive Gram stain. Thus a presumptive diagnosis can usually be made before the culture results have been obtained to confirm or exclude sepsis as the cause of the inflammation. Concern that a septic olecranon bursitis may lead to a contiguous spread causing osteomyelitis of the olecranon has been considered possible, although it probably rarely occurs. Excision of the olecranon has been recommended to avoid this possibility.[12]

Clinical Presentation

A distended olecranon bursa is usually painless unless the occurrence is associated with a septic or crystalline inflammatory process. Even traumatic bursitis is surprisingly painless after the initial event. When symptomatic, flexion of the elbow of more than 90 degrees causes most symptoms. In fact, positions between 60 and 90 degrees have been shown in the laboratory to produce a considerably greater pressure within the bursa compared with the extended elbow.[3] Canoso noted no pain with flexion even when the bursa is distended and speculated that discomfort probably is caused by nerve endings in the osseous tendinous attachment rather than by those in the roof of the bursa.

Canoso has also characterized the clinical features of 30 patients with noninflammatory olecranon bursitis.[2] Repetitive trauma was present in 14 instances and discrete, single-event trauma in 7, leaving 9 cases that might be considered idiopathic. An olecranon spur was present in 10 of 30 (Fig. 48–5). If symptoms were present more than 2 weeks, the bursa appeared discretely swollen; if less than 2 weeks, parabursal edema was observed in the arm and forearm in half of the patients (Fig. 48–6).

Aspiration showed evidence of hemorrhage in cases with a post-traumatic etiology. The synovial fluid was further characterized by a low white blood cell count averaging only 878 cells per high-power field with 84 per cent monocytes. This is in contrast to the high leukocyte count with a predominance of polymorphonuclear cells that is present in a septic bursa.

Treatment

If the olecranon bursitis is associated with a systemic inflammatory process, control of the underlying disease is the obvious first step in treatment. Communication with the joint is sometimes present in rheumatoid arthritis and is generally considered a secondary process.[9] If the bursa is not painful, local measures to prevent injury are all that is required. The

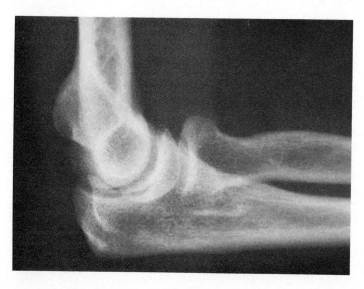

Figure 48–5. Lateral radiograph of the elbow in a patient with long-standing recurrent olecranon bursitis. The typical spur is demonstrated at the tip of the olecranon.

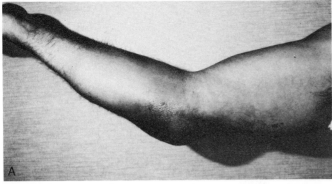

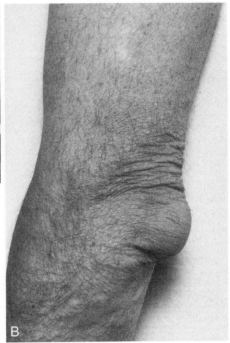

Figure 48–6. *A,* In acute olecranon bursitis, rather diffuse swelling is noted about the distal brachium and proximal forearm. There is variable inflammation depending on the cause. *B,* In more chronic conditions, however, the swelling is more discrete and is localized to the bursa itself, with no suggestion of inflammation.

use of a resting splint and compression may be necessary, and this is the usual treatment in the early stages. Acute traumatic or idiopathic bursitis is also treated symptomatically. If the traumatic impact is predictable, pads are useful (Fig. 48–7).

If the bursa is painful and prevents daily or occupational activity, aspiration is indicated. However, the swelling usually recurs, especially when joint communication is present.

If the process does not show rapid resolution, if pain persists and if parabursal swelling or erythema is present and is not resolving, septic bursitis is suspected, and the bursa must be aspirated. If this has already been done and the initial aspirate revealed no bacteria, repeat aspiration is indicated; a positive culture is occasionally found.

Treatment for Chronic Bursitis. Chronic recurrent or painful olecranon bursitis may require more definitive measures. A 16-gauge angiograph inserted with a compressive dressing for about 3 days has been used and is recommended as effective in lessening the

Figure 48–7. Traumatic olecranon bursitis from artificial turf treated by protection with an elbow pad. The ideal pad should be relieved somewhat over the olecranon. (From Larson, R. L., and Osternig, L. R.: Traumatic bursitis and artificial turf. J. Sports Med. 2(4):183, 1974.)

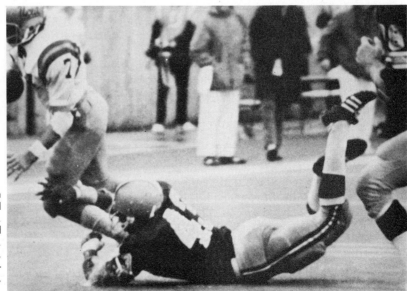

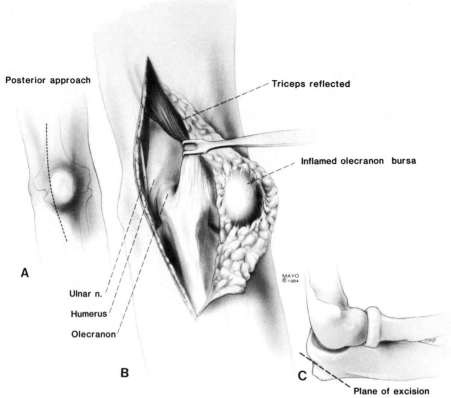

Figure 48–8. Surgical treatment for chronic olecranon bursitis recommended by Quayle and Robinson. *A*, A straight medial incision is preferred. The skin flap that includes the bursa is reflected laterally. *B*, The triceps is reflected laterally, revealing the tip of the olecranon. *C*, A generous osteotomy is recommended.

tendency for recurrence of bursal swelling.[6] Surgery is not commonly indicated; however, when the process is recalcitrant to nonoperative measures and is interfering with occupational or daily activities, operative intervention should be considered.

Operative Intervention. A longitudinal incision medial to the midline[10] or a transverse incision has been recommended.[19] All bursal tissue is removed, and the joint is immobilized in flexion or extreme flexion[10] for approximately 2 weeks. Freeing the bursa from the skin can devitalize the skin over the olecranon process or cause problems with healing; hence, we recommend a compressive dressing in about 45 degrees of flexion. To avoid this, a rather unusual approach to the problem has been reported by Quayle and Robinson (Fig. 48–8).[18] The concern about wound healing attendant to the subdermal dissection of the bursa is avoided by reflecting the skin with the bursal tissue from the tip of the olecranon from a lateral to medial or a medial to lateral direction. At this point the tip of the olecranon is obliquely osteotomized, leaving the bursal tissue intact. The triceps mechanism is then reflected back over the

olecranon, and the wound is closed with a drain. Eleven patients have been treated by this technique without recurrence.[18]

Complications. Wound healing is the most common recognized complication of excision of the olecranon bursa. No data have been found to allow an estimate of the frequency or management of this complication. Although we have had no personal experience with wound problems after excision of the olecranon bursa, similar problems following some total elbow procedures are encountered. Muscle flap transfers, either free or local, have been used in this instance with success. The indiscriminate removal of the olecranon bursa must be seriously questioned in light of the possibility and magnitude of this complication.

References

1. Bywaters, E. G.: The Bursae of the Body. Ann. Rheum. Dis. **24**:215, 1965.
2. Canoso, J. J.: Idiopathic or Traumatic Olecranon Bursitis. Clinical Features and Bursal Fluid Analysis. Arth. Rheum. **20**:1213, 1977.
3. Canoso, J. J.: Intrabursal Pressures in the Olecranon and Prepatellar Bursae. J. Rheum. **7(4)**:570, 1980.
4. Carp, L.: Tennis Elbow. Arch. Surg. **24**:905, 1932.

5. Davis, W. M., and Yassine, Z.: An Etiologic Factor in Tear of the Distal Tendon of the Biceps Brachii. J. Bone Joint Surg. **38A**:1365, 1956.

6. Fisher, R. H.: Conservative Treatment of Disturbed Patellae and Olecranon Bursae. Clin. Orthop. **123**:98, 1977.

7. Gerster, J. C., Lagier, R., and Boivin, G.: Olecranon Bursitis Related to Calcium Pyrophosphate Dihydrate Crystal Deposition Disease. Arth. Rheum. **25**:989, 1982.

8. Ho, G., and Tice, A. D.: Comparison of Nonseptic and Septic Bursitis. Arch. Int. Med. **139**:1269, 1979.

9. Hollinshead, W. H.: Anatomy for Surgeons, 2nd ed. Vol. 3, The Back and Limbs. New York, Hoeber, 1969.

10. Justis, E. J.: Affection of Fascia and Bursae. In Crenshaw, A. H. (ed.): Campbell's Operative Orthopedics, Vol. 2. St. Louis, C. V. Mosby, 1971.

11. Larson, R. L., and Osternig, L. R.: Traumatic Bursitis and Artificial Turf. J. Sports Med. **2(4)**:183, 1974.

12. Lasher, W. W., and Mathewson, L. M.: Olecranon Bursitis. J.A.M.A. **90**:1030, 1928.

13. Letizia, G., Piccione, F., Ridola, C., and Zummo, G.: Ultrastructural Comparisons of Human Synovial Membrane in Joints Exposed to Varying Stresses. Ital. J. Orthop. Traumatol. **6(2)**:279, 1980.

14. Mathews, R. E., Gould, J. S., and Kashlan, M. B.: Diffuse Pigmented Villonodular Tenosynovitis of the Ulnar Bursa—A Case Report. J. Hand Surg. **6**:64, 1981.

15. McCarty, D. J., Gatter, R. A.: Recurrent Acute Inflammation Associated with Focal Apatite Crystal Deposition. Arth Rheum. **9**:84, 1966.

16. Monro, A.: A Description of All the Bursae Mucose of the Human Body. Edinburgh, Elliot, 1788.

17. Osgood, R. B.: Radiohumeral Bursitis, Epicondylitis, Epicondylalgia (Tennis Elbow). Arch. Surg. **4**:420, 1922.

18. Quayle, J. B., and Robinson, M. P.: A Useful Procedure in the Treatment of Chronic Olecranon Bursitis. Injury, **9**:299, 1976.

19. Smith, F. M.: Surgery of the Elbow, 2nd ed. Philadelphia, W. B. Saunders Co., 1972.

20. Spinner, M.: Injuries to the Major Branches of Peripheral Nerves of the Forearm, 2nd ed. Philadelphia, W. B. Saunders Co., 1978.

21. Vizkelety, T., and Aszodi, K.: Bilateral Calcareous Bursitis at the Elbow. J. Bone Joint Surg. **50B**:644, 1968.

22. Whittaker, C. R.: The Arrangement of the Bursae in the Superior Extremities of the Fullterm Fetus. J. Anat. Physiol. **44**:133, 1910.

CHAPTER 49

The Elbow in Metabolic Disease

B. F. MORREY

With the possible exception of tumoral calcinosis, unlike the situation at other anatomic sites, there are no metabolic diseases with a special predilection for or a characteristic presentation at or about the elbow joint.[3, 12] Rather limited information, therefore, is available concerning the effect of metabolic disease at the elbow. In fact, the roentgenographic bone survey routinely taken to assess the extent of involvement of these diseases at the Mayo Clinic does not include the elbow region. No attempt will be made here to mention all the conditions that may incidentally involve the elbow. There are, however, several conditions that are regularly manifested at this joint: gout, pseudogout, and inborn errors of metabolism causing congenital abnormalities (Chapters 11 and 41). Paget's disease may, of course, involve any part of the body including the elbow (see Chapter 46).

It seems appropriate to discuss the appearance of and the effect of several of the more common or characteristic metabolic disorders involving the elbow region.

RICKETS

Vitamin D deficiency of the immature skeleton classically causes widening of the physis and cupping of the metaphysis, which is well represented at the wrist. Interestingly, although it has not been emphasized in the literature, a rather dramatic widening of the radiohumeral joint is typical of this disease (Fig. 49–1). The deficiency will obviously be better demonstrated in the more rapidly growing bones, and the physes of the distal humerus and proximal forearm are relatively slow growing.[3] Thus the manifestation of rickets in the region of the elbow is usually not dramatic.

OSTEOMALACIA

Vitamin D deficiency of the mature skeleton results in the production of uncalcified osteoid due to one of several mechanisms—nutritional intake deficiencies, absorption abnormalities, and utilization abnormalities.[8, 9] Radiographically, a marked loss of bone density is usually observed along with a coarsening of the trabecular pattern. There are no characteristic features at the elbow (Fig.

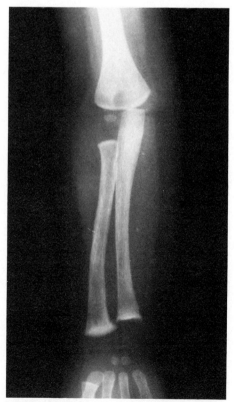

Figure 49–1. Six-month-old infant was slow to roll over or attempt sitting. The diagnosis of rickets was made. This radiograph demonstrates the marked widening of the radiohumeral growth region.

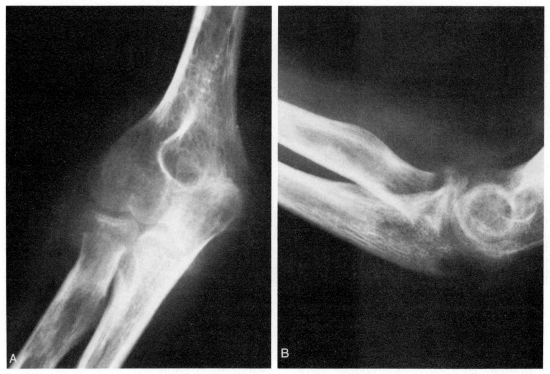

Figure 49–2. *A, B,* Blurred trabecular pattern and mottled decrease in bone density typical of osteomalacia without distinguishing features at the elbow joint. Primary disease was renal tubular dysfunction.

49–2). The lack of structural integrity causes bowing deformities of the weight-bearing extremities, but this is uncommon in the upper limb.

TUMORAL CALCINOSIS

Extensive para-articular calcification, so-called tumoral calcinosis, does have a certain predilection for the elbow region, although it is more commonly seen at the hip and shoulder.[4] First described by Inclan et al. in 1943,[5] the association with hyperphosphatemia has suggested a metabolic etiology for this disease.[2, 7] The exact cause of the condition is obscure, but deposition of calcium salts occurs in the posterior or anterior extraarticular regions of the elbow. The calcium salt is usually calcium phosphate or carbonate. A recent report, however, has demonstrated a similar radiographic appearance due to the deposition of hydroxyapatite crystals.[4] The intra-articular nature of this deposition serves to distinguish this presentation from true tumoral calcinoses (Fig. 49–3). Treatment is excision if the condition is symptomatic. However, the process may be extensive involving the substance of the triceps tendon, thus making excision difficult and recurrence common.[2]

HYPERPARATHYROIDISM

Primary hyperparathyroidism may be due to an adenoma, hyperplasia, carcinoma, or aberrant tumor secreting the parathyroid

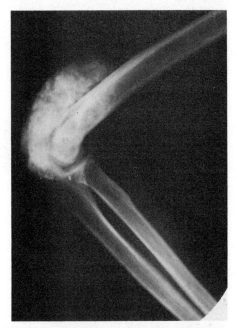

Figure 49–3. Extensive periarticular calcification in the region of the posterior aspect of the elbow was diagnosed as tumoral calcinosis. A metabolic etiology of this condition is likely.

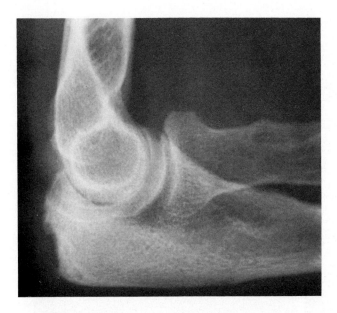

Figure 49–4. Hyperparathyroidism from renal failure is manifest in the region of the elbow by resorption and osteoporosis of the anterior proximal ulna, the so-called brown tumor. Subperiosteal resorption of the tip of the olecranon is also demonstrated.

hormone[15] as well as to type II multiple endocrine neoplasia. Secondary hyperparathyroidism occurs due to a chronic hypocalcemic state, which stimulates the production of parathyroid hormone. The classic radiographic appearance of hyperparathyroidism is subperiosteal resorption especially along the radial margin of the middle phalanges of the hand. More advanced but less common changes involve resorption of large amounts of bone, resulting in the radiographic appearance of the so-called brown tumor. Hyperparathyroidism rarely demonstrates any features in the region of the elbow but occasionally periosteal resorption or a brown tumor may be observed (Fig. 49–4).

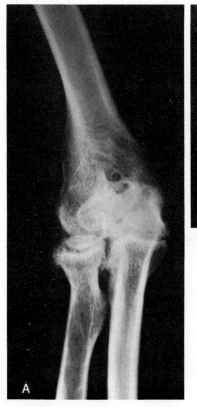
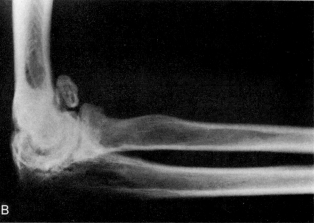

Figure 49–5. Wilson's disease involving the elbow with the classic appearance of fragmentation and periarticular calcification. A, Anteroposterior view. B, Lateral view.

WILSON'S DISEASE (HEPATOLENTICULAR DEGENERATION)

Caused by an inborn error of copper metabolism, this disease is best known for renal, hepatic, and neurologic symptoms. However, its effect on the bones and joints has been well recognized.[11, 14, 15] Osteoporosis occurs in about 75 per cent of patients,[11] and the appearance of osteomalacia is also common.[14] Joint involvement includes degenerative changes, sclerosis, fragmentation, and periarticular calcification (Fig. 49–5).

The roentgenographic appearance often correlates poorly with the clinical findings. The treatment of this disease is to decrease copper accumulation in the body by treatment with penicillamine. On occasion, the severity of the joint involvement requires surgical intervention. We have replaced the knee joint in patients with this condition but have not surgically treated the elbow joint.

HYPERLIPOPROTEINEMIA TYPE II (FAMILIAL ESSENTIAL HYPERCHOLESTEROLEMIA)

Periosteal xanthomatosis and tendon xanthomas result from an increased serum cholesterol level, which leads to the accumulation of cholesterol crystals. The olecranon bursa and the triceps tendon are commonly susceptible to this disorder.[16] If the process is symptomatic in the olecranon bursa, excision may be indicated. Care should be taken, however, before excising these deposits in the triceps tendon because this can weaken the extensor mechanism. The usual treatment is of the underlying disease state, as with diet and atromid.

OSTEOPOROSIS

Osteoporosis may be defined in the broadest sense as a decrease of bone substance that becomes a pathologic entity with the appearance of spontaneous fractures.[6] These usually occur in the spine, distal radius, and hip; recently, proximal humeral[13] and pelvic fractures[10] with minimal trauma have been associated with osteoporosis. The effects at the elbow are most commonly manifest with type III radial head fractures or comminuted olecranon fractures occurring in the older person with relatively little trauma. Unlike the spine and hip, there are no particular radiographic features characteristic of osteoporosis in the elbow region.

References

1. Aegerter, E., and Kirkpatrick, J. A.: Orthopedic Diseases, 4th ed. Philadelphia, W. B. Saunders Co., 1975.
2. Baldursson, H., Evans, E. B., Dodge, W. F., and Jackson, W. T.: Tumoral Calcinosis With Hyperphosphatemia. J. Bone Joint Surg. **51A**:913, 1969.
3. Greenfield, G. B.: Radiology of Bone Diseases, 2nd ed. Philadelphia, J. B. Lippincott Co., 1975.
4. Hensley, D. C., and Lin, J. J.: Massive Intra-Synovial Deposition of Calcium Pyrophosphate in the Elbow. J. Bone Joint Surg. **66A**:133, 1984.
5. Inclan, A., Leon, P., and Gomez, C. M.: Tumoral Calcinosis. J.A.M.A. **121**:490, 1943.
6. Jowsey, J.: Metabolic Diseases of Bone. Philadelphia, W. B. Saunders Co., 1977.
7. Lafferty, F. W., Reynolds, E. S., and Pearson, O. H.: Tumoral Calcinosis: A Metabolic Disease of Obscure Etiology. Am. J. Med. **38**:105, 1965.
8. Mankin, H. J.: Rickets, Osteomalasia, and Renal Osteodystrophy, Part I (review article). J. Bone Joint Surg. **56A**:101, 1974.
9. Mankin, H. J.: Rickets, Osteomalacia, and Renal Osteodystrophy, Part II (review article). J. Bone Joint Surg. **56A**:352, 1974.
10. Melton, L. J., Sampson, J. M., Morrey, B. F., and Ilstrup, D. M.: Epidemiologic Features of Pelvic Fractures. Clin. Orthop. **155**:43, 1981.
11. Mindelzun, R., Elkin, M., Scheinberg, I. H., and Sternlieb, I.: Skeletal Changes in Wilson's Disease. A Radiological Study. Radiology **94**:127, 1970.
12. Pugh, D. G.: Radiographic Diagnosis of Diseases of the Bone. New York, Thomas Nelson, 1951.
13. Rose, S. H., Melton, L. J., Morrey, B. F., Ilstrup, D. M., and Riggs, B. L.: Epidemiologic Features of Humeral Fractures. Clin. Orthop. **168**:24, 1982.
14. Rosenoer, V. M., and Mitchell, R. C.: Skeletal Changes in Wilson's Disease. (Hepatolenticular Degeneration). B. J. Radiol. **32**:805, 1959.
15. Salassa, R. M., Jowsey, J., and Arnaud, C. D.: Hypophosphatemic Osteomalacia Associated With "Non-Endocrine Tumors." N. Engl. J. Med. **283**:65, 1970.
16. Smith, F. M.: Surgery of the Elbow, 2nd ed., Philadelphia, W. B. Saunders, 1972.

Index

Note: Page numbers in *italics* indicate illustrations; numbers followed by (t) indicate tables.